WILLARD & SPACKMAN'S

Occupational Therapy

WILLARD & SPACKMAN'S

Occupational Therapy

Ninth Edition

Maureen E. Neistadt
ScD, OTR/L, FAOTA

Associate Professor
University of New Hampshire
School of Health and Human Services
Occupational Therapy Department
Durham, New Hampshire

Elizabeth Blesedell Crepeau
PhD, OTR/L, FAOTA

Associate Professor
University of New Hampshire
School of Health and Human Services
Occupational Therapy Department
Durham, New Hampshire

81 Contributors

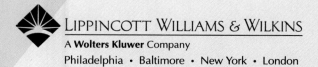
LIPPINCOTT WILLIAMS & WILKINS
A **Wolters Kluwer** Company
Philadelphia · Baltimore · New York · London
Buenos Aires · Hong Kong · Sydney · Tokyo

Executive Editor: Margaret Biblis
Assistant Editor: Patricia Moore
Project Editor: Sandra Cherrey Scheinin
Production Manager: Helen Ewan
Production Coordinator: Patricia McCloskey
Design Coordinator: Doug Smock

9th Edition

9   8   7   6   5   4

Library of Congress Cataloging-in-Publication Data
Occupation therapy.
    Willard and Spackman's occupational therapy. — 9th ed. / [edited
by] Maureen E. Neistadt, Elizabeth Blesedell Crepeau.
        p.   cm.
    Includes bibliographical references and index.
    ISBN 0-397-55192-4
    1. Occupational therapy.   I. Willard, Helen S.   II. Spackman,
Clare S.   III. Neistadt, Maureen E.   IV. Crepeau, Elizabeth
Blesedell.   V. Title.
RM735.029 1998
615.8′9515—dc21   97-15395
                                                   CIP

It is neither wealth nor splendor
but tranquility and occupation
which give happiness

THOMAS JEFFERSON

CONTRIBUTORS

Claudia Kay Allen, MA, OTR/L, FAOTA
Chief of Occupational Therapy,
  Psychiatry
Harbor-University of Southern
  California Medical Center
Torrance, California

Judith A. Atkins, BS, OTR
Clinical Specialist/Occupational Therapy
  Riley Hospital for Children
Indiana University Medical Center
Clarian Health Partners
Indianapolis, Indiana

Diana M. Bailey, EDD, OTR, FAOTA
Associate Professor
Boston School of Occupational Therapy
Tufts University
Medford, Massachusetts

Beverly K. Bain, EDD, OTR, FAOTA
Associate Adjunct Professor
Coordinator, Assistive Technology
  Project
Department of Occupational Therapy
New York University
New York, New York

Olga Baloueff, SCD, PT, OTR/L, BCP
Associate Professor
Boston School of Occupational Therapy
Tufts University
Medford, Massachusetts

Laura J. Barrett, MS, OTR/L
Occupational Therapy Program
  Coordinator
Department of Human Services
Chicago-Read Mental Health Center
Chicago, Illinois

Gary Bedell, MA, OTR
Adjunct Associate Professor
Coordinator, Post-Professional Program
  in Pediatric/ Developmental
  Disabilities
Department of Occupational Therapy
New York University
New York, New York

David W. Beer, MA, PHD (CAND)
Assistant Professor
Department of Occupational Therapy
College of Associated Health Professions
University of Illinois at Chicago
Chicago, Illinois

**Rosemarie Bigsby, SCD, BCP, OTR/L,
FAOTA**
Clinical Assistant Professor of Pediatrics
Brown University School of Medicine
Infant Development Center
Women and Infants Hospital
Providence, Rhode Island

Catana Brown, MA, OTR
Assistant Professor
Department of Occupational Therapy
  Education
School of Allied Health
University of Kansas Medical Center
Kansas City, Kansas

Ann Burkhardt, MA, OTR/L, BCN
Assistant Director, Occupational Therapy
Columbia-Presbyterian Medical Center
Clinical Instructor, Programs in
  Occupational Therapy
Columbia University
New York, New York

Florence A. Clark, PHD, OTR, FAOTA
Professor and Chair
Department of Occupational Science
  and Occupational Therapy
University of Southern California
Los Angeles, California

Ellen S. Cohn, EDM, OTR/L, FAOTA
Lecturer
Boston School of Occupational Therapy
Tufts University
Medford, Massachusetts

Kathleen Hilko Culler, MS, OTR/L
Clinical Educator
Center for Clinical Excellence
Rehabilitation Institute of Chicago
Chicago, Illinois

Debora A. Davidson, MS, OTR
Instructor
Program in Occupational Therapy
Washington University Medical School
St. Louis, Missouri

Jean Crosetto Deitz, PHD, OTR/L, FAOTA
Professor
Department of Rehabilitation Medicine
University of Washington
Seattle, Washington

Winnie Dunn, PHD, OTR, FAOTA
Professor and Chair
Department of Occupational Therapy
  Education
School of Allied Health
University Kansas Medical Center
Kansas City, Kansas

Rebecca Dutton, MS, OTR/L
Assistant Professor
Occupational Therapy Department
Kean College
Union, New Jersey

Joyce M. Engel, PHD, OTR/L, FAOTA
Associate Professor
Division of Occupational Therapy
Department of Rehabilitation Medicine
University of Washington
Seattle, Washington

Rhoda P. Erhardt, MS, OTR, FAOTA
Consultant in Pediatric Occupational
  Therapy
Private Practice
Maplewood, Minnesota

Sherlyn L. Fenton, MS, OTR, CWCE
Director of Rehabilitation
Saint Camillus Health Center
Whitinsville, Massachusetts

Regina Ferraro, MS, OTR/L
Coordinator, Inpatient/Acute Care
  Services
Occupational Therapy Department
Massachusetts General Hospital
Boston, Massachusetts

Elaine Ewing Fess, MS, OTR, FAOTA, CHT
Private Practice
Hand Research
Zionsville, Indiana

Linda L. Florey, MA, OTR, FAOTA, PHD
Chief of Rehabilitation Services
University of Southern California at Los Angeles
Neuropsychiatric Institute and Hospital
Los Angeles, California

Maureen Freda, MS, OTR/L
Director of MEDBridge Operations
Manor Care Health Services
Wheaton, Maryland

Patricia A. Gagnon, OTR/L, CWCE
Program Manager, The Therapy Center of Peabody
Work Venture Industrial Rehabilitation Program
The Arthritis Center
Shaugnessy Kaplan Rehabilitation Hospital
Peabody, Massachusetts

Gordon Muir Giles, MA, DIPCOT, OTR
Assistant Professor
Department of Occupational Therapy
Samuel Merritt College
Clinical Director
Neurobehavioral Program
Highview Hospital
Oakland, California

Clare Giuffrida, PHD, OTR/L, FAOTA
Assistant Professor
Department of Occupational Therapy
Duquesne University
Pittsburgh, Pennsylvania

Kathleen Golisz, MA, OTR/L
Associate Director of Clinical Education
Occupational Therapy Graduate Program
Mercy College
Dobbs Ferry, New York

Lou Ann Sooy Griswold, PHD, OTR
Associate Professor
Occupational Therapy Department
School of Health and Human Services
University of New Hampshire
Durham, New Hampshire

Ruth Ann Hansen, PHD, FAOTA
Professor
Associated Health Professions
Eastern Michigan University
Ypsilanti, Michigan

Betty R. Hasselkus, PHD, OTR, FAOTA
Associate Professor
Occupational Therapy Program
University of Wisconsin-Madison
Madison, Wisconsin

Alexis D. Henry, SCD, OTR/L, FAOTA
Research Assistant Professor
Department of Psychiatry
Center for Psychosocial and Forensic Services Research
University of Massachusetts Medical Center
Worcester, Massachusetts

James Hinojosa, PHD, OTR, FAOTA
Associate Professor
Director of Post Professional Programs
Department of Occupational Therapy
New York University
New York, New York

Margo B. Holm, PHD, OTR/L, FAOTA
Professor, Department of Occupational Therapy
College Misericordia
Dallas, Pennsylvania
Adjunct Assistant Professor of Psychiatry
School of Medicine
University of Pittsburgh
Pittsburgh, Pennsylvania

Anne B. James, MS, OTR/L
Assistant Professor
Occupational Therapy Program
College of Education, Nursing and Health Professions
University of Hartford
West Hartford, Connecticut

Cheryl Leman Jordan, MA, OTR/L, FAOTA
Burn Rehabilitation Research Coordinator
Burn Division
Washington Hospital Center
Washington, District of Columbia

Margaret Kaplan, MA, OTR
Clinical Assistant Professor
Occupational Therapy Program
State University of New York
Health Science Center at Brooklyn
Brooklyn, New York

Judith Hunt Kiel, MS, OTR
Clinical Associate Professor
Occupational Therapy Program
School of Allied Health Sciences
Indiana University School of Medicine
Indianapolis, Indiana

Gary Kielhofner, DRPH, OTR, FAOTA
Professor and Department Head
Department of Occupational Therapy
University of Illinois at Chicago
Chicago, Illinois

Susan H. Knox, PHD, OTR, FAOTA
Clinic Director
Hyland Clinic
Van Nuys, California

Kirsten M. Kohlmeyer, MS, OTR/L
Clinical Specialist
Rehabilitation Institute of Chicago
Chicago, Illinois

Wendy Kraft, OTR
Senior Clinical Supervisor
New England Rehabilitation Hospital
Woburn, Massachusetts

Penny L. Kyler, MA, OTR/L, FAOTA
Ethics Program Manager
American Occupational Therapy Association
Bethesda, Maryland

Elizabeth A. Larson, PHD, OTR
Pediatric Private Practice
South Pasadena, California

Mary Lawlor, SCD, OTR/L, FAOTA
Associate Professor
Department of Occupational Science and Occupational Therapy
University of Southern California
Los Angeles, California

Cheryl Mattingly, PHD
Associate Professor
Department of Occupational Science and Occupational Therapy
University of Southern California
Los Angeles, California

Linda McClain, PHD, OTR/L, FAOTA
Associate Professor
Occupational Therapy Program
University of New Mexico
Albuquerque, New Mexico

Juli H. McGruder, PHD (CAND)
Professor
School of Occupational Therapy and Physical Therapy
University of Puget Sound
Tacoma, Washington

Susan Cook Merrill, MA, OTR/L
Academic Fieldwork Coordinator
Assistant Professor
Occupational Therapy Department
School of Health and Human Services
University of New Hampshire
Durham, New Hampshire

Elizabeth Newman, OTR/L
Clinical Supervisor, Occupational
Therapy
National Rehabilitation Hospital
Occupational Therapy Department
Washington, District of Columbia

Kenneth J. Ottenbacher, PHD, OTR
Professor and Vice Dean
School of Allied Health Sciences
University of Texas Medical Branch
Galveston, Texas

Suzanne M. Peloquin, PHD, OTR, FAOTA
Professor
Department of Occupational Therapy
School of Allied Health Sciences
University of Texas Medical Branch
Galveston, Texas

Judith M. Perinchief, MS, OTR/L
Chair and Assistant Professor
College of Allied Health Professions
Temple University
Philadelphia, Pennsylvania

Debbie Pinet, MA, OTR/L
Occupational Therapist
Optima Health-Catholic Medical
Center
Manchester, New Hampshire

Michael Pizzi, MS, OTR/L, CHES, FAOTA
Executive Director
National Center for Wellness and Health
Promotion
Chief Executive Officer
Positive Images and Wellness, Inc.
Silver Spring, Maryland

Janice Miller Polgar, PHD, OT
Assistant Professor
Department of Occupational Therapy
Elborn College
University of Western Ontario
London, Ontario, Canada

Karen Halliday Pulaski, MS, OTR/L
Supervisor, Brain and Spinal Cord Injury
Rehabilitation
Moses Cone Health Systems
Rehabilitation Center
Greensboro, North Carolina

Kathlyn L. Reed, PHD, OTR, FAOTA
Adjunct Professor
School of Occupational Therapy
Texas Woman's University
Houston, Texas

Elizabeth A. Rivers, OTR, RN
Burn Rehabilitation Specialist
Health Partners St. Paul/Ramsey
Medical Center
St. Paul, Minnesota

Susan Robertson, MS, OTR/L, FAOTA
Mental Health Specialist
Rehabilitation Medicine Department
National Institutes of Health
Bethesda, Maryland

Joan C. Rogers, PHD, OTR/L, FAOTA
Professor of Occupational Therapy
School of Health and Rehabilitation
Sciences
Assistant Professor of Psychiatry
School of Medicine
University of Pittsburgh
Pittsburgh, Pennsylvania

Mary Sands, MSED, OTR, FAOTA
Chair, Occupational Therapy Assistant
Department
Orange Country Community College
Middletown, New York
Partner, Occupational Therapy Plus
Goshen, New York

Barbara A. Schell, PHD, OTR, FAOTA
Associate Professor and Program
Director
Occupational Therapy
Brenau University
Gainesville, Georgia

Janette K. Schkade, PHD, OTR
Professor and Dean
School of Occupational Therapy
Texas Woman's University
Denton, Texas

Sally Schultz, PHD, OTR
Associate Professor
Coordinator of Graduate Programs
School of Occupational Therapy
Texas Woman's University
Denton, Texas

Kathleen Barker Schwartz, EDD, OTR, FAOTA
Professor
Department of Occupational Therapy
San Jose State University
San Jose, California

Sharan L. Schwartzberg, EDD, OTR, FAOTA
Professor and Chair
Boston School of Occupational Therapy
Tufts University
Medford, Massachusetts
Associate Staff
Departments of Psychiatry and
Occupational Therapy
Mount Auburn Hospital
Cambridge, Massachusetts

Alice C. Seidel, EDD, OTR/L
Associate Professor
Occupational Therapy Department
School of Health and Human Services
University of New Hampshire
Durham, New Hampshire

Susanne Garred Seymour, OTR/L
Occupational Therapist
Sundance Rehabilitation Corporation
Clipper House of Rochester
Rochester, New Hampshire

Elinor Anne Spencer, MA, OTR/L, FAOTA
Director of Occupational Therapy
Services
Blue Hill Memorial Hospital
Blue Hill, Maine
Consultant in Occupational Therapy
Calais Regional Hospital
Calais, Maine

Jean Cole Spencer, PHD, OTR
Professor and Doctoral Program
Coordinator
School of Occupational Therapy
Texas Woman's University
Houston, Texas

Ronald G. Stone, MS
Professor
School of Occupational Therapy and
Physical Therapy
University of Puget Sound
Tacoma, Washington

Barbara B. Sussenberger, MS, OTR
Associate Professor
Occupational Therapy Department
School of Health and Human Services
University of New Hampshire
Durham, New Hampshire

Joan Pascale Toglia, MA, OTR/L
Program Director
Occupational Therapy Graduate
Program
Mercy College
Dobbs Ferry, New York

Judith D. Ward, PHD, OTR/L
Associate Professor
Occupational Therapy Department
School of Health and Human Services
University of New Hampshire
Durham, New Hampshire

Janet Waylett-Rendall, OTR, CHT
Chief Executive Officer
Rehabilitation Technology Works
San Bernardino, California

Mary Feldhaus Weber
Head Injury Survivor

Wendy Wood, PHD, OTR/L
Assistant Professor
Division of Occupational Therapy
Department of Medical Allied Health
    Professions
University of North Carolina at Chapel
    Hill
Chapel Hill, North Carolina

Elizabeth J. Yerxa, EDD, LHD (hon),
OTR, FAOTA
Distinguished Professor Emerita
University of Southern California
Los Angeles, California

Mary Jane Youngstrom, MS, OTR
Teaching Associate
University of Kansas Medical Center
Kansas City, Kansas

FOREWORD

In 1947, although the profession was 30 years old, there had been no books published that were written by occupational therapists. All of the books that had been published for this relatively new profession of occupational therapy had been written by physicians or nurses who discussed the value of occupation for intervention in the care of physical and mental conditions. The first book in this vein was written in 1910 by Susan E. Tracy, a nurse. *Studies in Invalid Occupations—A Manual For Nurses and Attendants* was primarily a craft book that explained the rationale for use of specific activities for many patient diagnoses in different types of settings. In 1915, William Rush Dunton Jr., a psychiatrist, wrote a complete textbook on occupational therapy, *Occupational Therapy—A Manual for Nurses.* Following this, other physicians wrote textbooks on occupational therapy, but none were written by occupational therapists.

In addition, except for Eleanor Clarke Slagle, all of the presidents of the American Occupational Therapy Association (AOTA) were physicians until 1947, when Winifred Kahmann was elected president. By this time standards for education had been established, schools of occupational therapy were evaluated in order to be qualified, and only those persons who met qualifications were listed in a registry that allowed them to practice as occupational therapists.

In the Preface of the book published in 1947, entitled *Principles of Occupational Therapy* and edited by Helen S. Willard and Clare S. Spackman—both leaders in occupational therapy—the editors noted: "There has been a woeful lack of adequate literature on occupational therapy. With the increased number of training schools, the greater demand for occupational therapists, and the wider use of this treatment, there is a greater need for education in the principles of the profession." There were twenty contributors to this book, of whom five were physicians, and the remaining fifteen were occupational therapists.

Published by J.B. Lippincott of Philadelphia, *Principles of Occupational Therapy* was the first edition of the textbook that has been used by occupational therapy students and practitioners in the United States and abroad. Helen S. Willard and Clare S. Spackman edited four editions of the textbook in 1947, 1954, 1963 and 1971. When both Helen Willard and Clare Spackman retired, they sought new editors for the book. In 1976 when we were approached to take over the editorship, we agreed to take on the task. Because of the importance of these two pioneers and leaders, we decided to call the textbook *Willard and Spackman's Occupational Therapy.*

In the Foreword to the fifth edition of the book, Miss Willard and Miss Spackman wrote, "When thirty-two years ago we agreed to edit what was then called *Principles of Occupational Therapy* it never occurred to us that in 1976 we should at last be passing on the editorship of *Occupational Therapy.* It is with pleasure that we give this task to two of our coworkers and friends—Helen L. Hopkins and Helen D. Smith—who have accepted the responsibility of editing the fifth edition while we become editors emeriti. . . . The third and fourth editions were translated into Japanese and the fourth into Spanish. . . . Forty-two authors contributed to the first four editions. . . . During this time our field has changed and grown immeasurably. The present edition reflects recent changes and will add much to the knowledge and understanding of occupational therapy today."

We were the editors of the fifth (1978), sixth (1983), seventh (1988), and eighth (1993) editions of *Willard and Spackman's Occupational Therapy.* The growth in knowledge in occupational therapy over the years was obvious by the size and length of each successive edition. The complexity of the profession can also be judged by the number of contributors to the editions, which increased from twenty-eight authors in 1978 to sixty-five in 1993. The fifth and sixth editions were translated into Japanese.

We thank all the authors for their contributions to the four editions that we have edited. It is now time to pass the responsibility for future editions on to two of our colleagues and friends, Maureen Neistadt and Elizabeth Crepeau. They are aware of the increase of knowledge in our profession and the need to prepare occupational therapists for the many changes occurring in our society and profession. The ninth edition will reflect these changes and the status of our profession in our ever changing world.

Helen L. Hopkins, EDD, OTR/L, FAOTA
Professor Emeritus
Temple University
College of Allied Health Professions
Department of Occupational Therapy
Philadelphia, Pennsylvania

Helen D. Smith, MOT, OTR/L, FAOTA
Associate Professor
Tufts University-Boston School of Occupational Therapy
Medford, Massachusetts

PREFACE

This edition marks the 50th anniversary of the first edition of *Principles of Occupational Therapy,* now called *Willard and Spackman's Occupational Therapy.* The transformation of this book over the past 50 years reflects the development and growth of the profession. In fact, some people have used the size of the successive volumes to demonstrate the growth of knowledge in the field. As we planned this edition we were mindful of the tradition of this text in the socialization of several generations of occupational therapy students and our responsibility to continue this tradition.

Today, unlike 1947, there are many specialized texts in occupational therapy. *Willard and Spackman's Occupational Therapy* no longer reflects the entire knowledge base of the field, nor does it serve as the only text for occupational therapy students. Still, many consider it to be the text that most comprehensively addresses the major practice and professional issues in occupational therapy. Consequently, our challenge in planning this book was to be comprehensive, yet stay within the page limits established in our contract.

We organized the book to answer student-oriented questions. Students want to know about occupational therapy and the people who will be seeking occupational therapy. Unit I defines the scope of the field and the emerging academic discipline of occupational science. Unit II is concerned with the people who seek and receive our services—who they are as individuals embedded in cultural, socioeconomic, and family systems. Students want to learn about their occupational therapy colleagues and what they will be doing together. Unit III begins to answer that question with a discussion of the roles of occupational therapists and occupational therapy assistants and the clinical reasoning process. Units IV and V address the therapeutic relationship and activity analysis, both precursors to occupational therapy intervention. Subsequent units further articulate aspects of the clinical role of occupational therapy practitioners. Units VI and VII delineate the evaluation and treatment principles of the field. Unit VIII follows with a review of the theories that support practice. Units IX and X address the specific diagnoses or problems that bring people to occupational therapy. Finally, Units XI and XII discuss issues related to working in the health care system, ethics, research, our historical heritage, and challenges for the future.

There are several things that are unique about this edition. First, is the reliance on first person narratives and stories. Unit II begins with a first person narrative that demonstrates the power of the human spirit to transcend disability and to create a new and fulfilling life. Many other chapters include narrative components that enable the reader to understand the meaning of illness and disability from the perspective of the individual, the family, or the occupational therapy practitioner. Second, is the emphasis on the broad values and principles upon which occupational therapy practice is based. Two units are devoted to understanding the perspective of the people seeking our care and fostering the development of a collaborative relationship. The evaluation and treatment units are very comprehensive, providing the basis for knowing how to approach the evaluation and treatment process for anyone seeking occupational therapy services. The diagnostic chapters, in contrast, are briefer, providing information about how to begin thinking about a particular problem and its impact on the life of the individual. We expect that students will use the more specialized texts available in the field for greater detail and depth on these topics. Third, theory is introduced after the evaluation and treatment units. In our experience, when theory is presented first, students have a hard time seeing how it relates to the day-to-day realities of practice. Students seem anxious to know what they will be doing. Once they know what they will be doing, they can see and appreciate the relationship between theory and practice. Fourth, are the history, ethics, and research notes throughout the text. These provide periodic opportunities to reflect on our past, the ethical dilemmas confronted by occupational therapy practitioners today, and the research challenges for our profession.

Because we are aware of the power of language to influence the way we think, we have attempted to be as inclusive as possible in the descriptors of individuals. Consequently, to the extent possible we used the term occupational therapy practitioner to represent the certified occupational therapist and certified occupational therapy assistant. We have tried to avoid language that reflects bias and labels people with disabilities. We have used nonmedical model language to the extent that this was appropriate. And we have struggled with terminology that refers to the individual who seeks occupational therapy—be that a patient, client, consumer, student, and so on.

We appreciate the faith that Helen Hopkins and Helen Smith placed in us when they approached us to edit the ninth edition of *Willard and Spackman's Occupational Therapy.* We hope this 50th anniversary edition reflects the collective efforts of all the previous editors and authors, as well as those in the current edition.

Maureen E. Neistadt, SCD, OTR/L, FAOTA
Elizabeth Blesedell Crepeau, PHD, OTR/L, FAOTA

ACKNOWLEDGMENTS

This book, as most others, reflects the collective efforts of many individuals. As we began planning its organization in 1994, we reviewed our preliminary ideas with our colleagues at the University of New Hampshire. Based on these discussions in July 1994, we shared our outline with several focus groups at the AOTA Annual Conference in Boston. The participants were Janice Posatery Burke, Florence Clark, Jean Deitz, Betty Hasselkus, Suzanne Peloquin, Jan Polgar, Susan Robertson, and Mary Sands. Using the outline derived from these meetings, we surveyed all occupational therapy and occupational therapy assistant programs. We are grateful for the detailed and thoughtful feedback from these educators. Based on feedback from this survey and ongoing discussions as the book evolved, we continued to revise the outline that is reflected in the table of contents.

A book of this size involves attention to detail and a lot of xeroxing, typing, and reference checking—the type of work that takes endless time and never seems to be finished. A cohort of students and recent graduates of the University of New Hampshire assisted us with these very pesky details. For over 6 months Susanne Seymour worked several hours each week, using her skills at the library to track down incomplete references or to verify others. She also helped consolidate the information that was scattered on numerous disks and papers for the unit opening pages. Kathleen Grundy read many chapters over the summer to "test" them from a student perspective and to check the in-text citations against the reference list. Her attention to detail on this latter task was of considerable assistance to us, and her "consumer" perspective helped us to verify that the material was at the appropriate level for students. PatSue Spear volunteered to help with filing early on; however, her primary contribution was her assistance in the development of the Glossary. Linda Fairbanks assisted with the compilation of several of the long multisection chapters, also a task that requires close attention to detail and judgment. Finally, we are grateful to Judith Churchill, who found the Thomas Jefferson quotation that opens the book. We cannot overstate our appreciation to all of these individuals for their willingness to assist us so readily and cheerfully. They are our colleagues in the best sense of the word.

Textbooks require pictures. It is as simple as that, though finding the right pictures is not an easy proposition. William Sturtevandt, Nancy Lang, Karen Pettigrew, and Diane Murphy of Rockingham County Home assisted in obtaining permissions for pictures taken over 12 years ago. Jennifer Manning orchestrated an efficient and very effective photo shoot of the occupational therapy staff and clients at Dover Rehabilitation and Living Center. Lou Ann Griswold assisted in locating photographs of children. Many of the pictures in this book were taken by the talented photographers at the University of New Hampshire—John Adam (now retired), Gary Samson, and Ron Bergeron. Mary Binderman at the Wilma L. West Library and AOTA Archives helped find the historical photographs. We are grateful to the collective contribution of all of these individuals.

Editing a book of this size requires a lot of solitary time reading chapters, editing, and reflecting on the relationship of each chapter to the unit and entire book. We appreciate the willing ears of many of our colleagues who helped us problem solve when we needed feedback. In particular, we would like to thank our colleagues at the University of New Hampshire, as well as Ellen S. Cohn, Ruth Ann Hansen, Betty Risteen Hasselkus, Suzanne Peloquin, Kathlyn Reed, Barbara A. Boyt Schell, and Elinor Anne Spencer. Several individuals assisted in a more formal review of chapters and units of the book. In particular we would like to thank Margaret Kaplan, Charlotte Brasic Royeen, and Susan Cook Merrill. Germaine Nadeau and Alice Vosburg, occupational therapy department secretaries, facilitated several large mailings and helped manage the faxes, mail, and the many computer glitches we encountered. Andrew Allen, former editor at Lippincott-Raven, helped keep us on track and offered many valuable suggestions and words of encouragement along the way. Patricia Moore, also at Lippincott-Raven, facilitated the process of obtaining contracts and permissions and shepherding the many details inherent in producing a book of this size and complexity. Sandy Cherrey Scheinin remained unflappable through multiple sets of page proofs.

Finally, our families. Our husbands, Jerry and Rod, provided the necessary ballast to keep us on course. They helped with the practical day-to-day aspects of living, with some of the mundane tasks of editing, and provided a willing ear when we needed to think out loud. Betty's children, now grown and living away from home, were a cheering section for yet another of their mother's projects. And our cats, Anthony (Maureen's), Scamper, George, and Fluffy (Betty's), did what only cats can do. They assisted with the typing by walking on our keyboards and with phone conversations by "butting heads." Most important, each day they demonstrated that rest and play are an essential aspect of living—for cats, as well as for human beings.

Collaboration is an essential aspect of occupational therapy practice. This book reflects the collaboration of many people, as these acknowledgements and the list of contributors demonstrates. Our work as editors, was to reflect and distill this work. We hope that in doing so, we have sustained, enhanced, and honored the 50 years contribution *Willard and Spackman's Occupational Therapy* has made to the field.

CONTENTS

SUMMARY OF RECURRING DISPLAYS

Penny Kyler and Ruth A. Hansen are the authors of Ethics Notes.
Kenneth J. Ottenbacher is the author of Research Notes.
Suzanne M. Peloquin is the author of Historical Notes.

WILLARD & SPACKMAN'S

Occupational Therapy

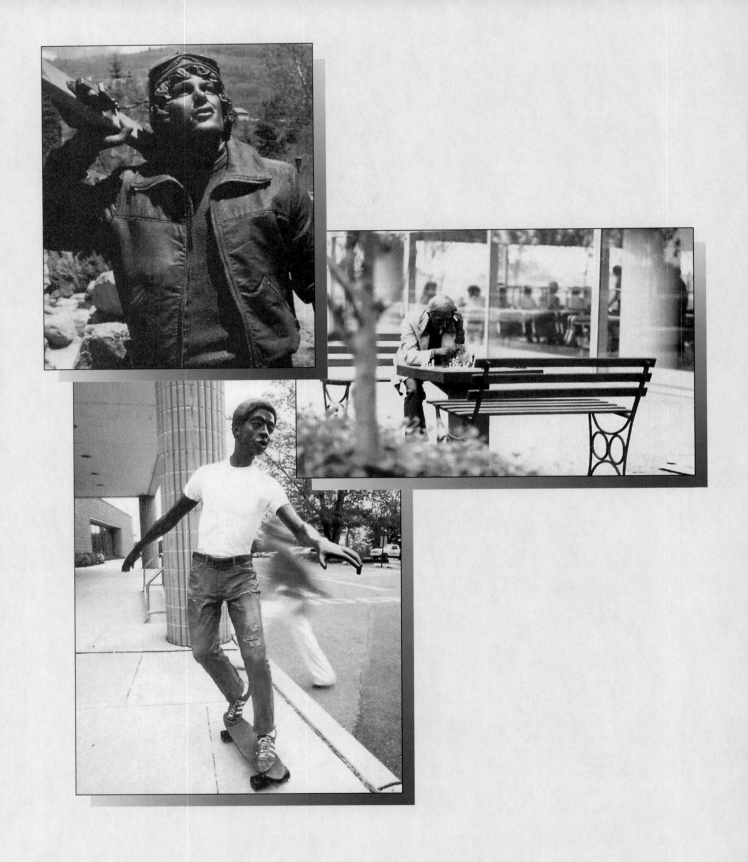

J. Seward Johnson's sculptures represent various contemporary occupations.
(Photos courtesy of Sculpture Placement, Ltd., Washington, DC.)

Unit I

Occupational Therapy and Occupational Science

LEARNING OBJECTIVES

After completing this unit, readers will be able to:

▶ Define occupational therapy and its scope of practice.

▶ Explain how the practice of occupational therapy gave direction to the domain of scientific concern embraced by occupational science.

▶ Delineate beliefs that have persevered throughout the profession's history concerning the relation of occupation to adaptation.

▶ Explain the value of developing an academic discipline based upon a science of occupation.

▶ Define the form, the function, and the meaning of occupation and give examples of research that address these aspects.

These opening chapters address the scope of practice of occupational therapy and the emerging discipline of occupational science. Occupational science provides us with an understanding of the relations between our daily round of activities, the meaning in our lives, and our state of health or well-being. This understanding in turn, has the potential to influence occupational therapy intervention and shape the future of the profession. It is through the multiple and interdependent roles of practitioner, manager, consultant, educator, and researcher that the profession has grown in strength and vitality. This unit introduces the reader to these roles, forming the foundation for the chapters that follow. (*Note:* Words in **bold** type are defined in the Glossary.)

Chapter 1

Introduction to Occupational Therapy

Maureen E. Neistadt and Elizabeth Blesedell Crepeau

- Peter is a 60-year-old divorced tugboat captain with two grown sons. He is currently in a rehabilitation unit in a hospital because he had a stroke.
- Linda is a 35-year-old single carpenter who accidently cut the tendons across the back of her right, dominant hand at work.
- Paul is a 7-year-old second grader. His teacher has asked for an occupational therapy consultation because he is clumsy in school and avoids the playground. His printing is larger than would be expected for someone his age, and he draws his letters very slowly.
- Jennifer is a 16-year-old single young woman in a psychiatric day program for treatment of alcohol abuse and other behaviors.

These four people have one thing in common. They are experiencing problems that impair their ability to carry out their daily activities. Consequently, they are unable to meet their life goals, fulfill their social roles, and participate fully in living. All could benefit from occupational therapy services. Occupational therapy practitioners provide not just direct treatment, but they also serve as managers, consultants, educators, and researchers. These roles, though less readily apparent, influence the interventions provided to Peter, Linda, Paul, and Jennifer. This chapter provides an overview of the range of occupational therapy roles—from clinician to consultant, manager, educator, and researcher. It addresses how each role contributes to the intervention received by these individuals and describes the interdependence among these roles.

▼ OCCUPATIONAL THERAPY

Occupational therapy is the art and science of helping people do the day-to-day activities that are important to them despite impairment, disability, or handicap. "Occupation" in occupational therapy does not simply refer to jobs or job training; occupation in occupational therapy refers to all of the activities that occupy people's time and give meaning to their lives. In occupational therapy terminology, these activities are called occupational performance areas. These occupational performance areas can be divided into Activities of Daily Living, Work and Productive Activities, and Play and Leisure Activities (AOTA, 1994) (Box 1-1).

The terms, impairment, disability, and handicap come from the World Health Organization (WHO, 1980). Impairment refers to a loss or abnormality of physical or psychological structures or functions. For example, a person who has fractured his or her left hip in a fall has an impairment of the left leg, or lower extremity. When an impairment is severe enough to limit a person's ability to perform the activities of daily living, work and productive activities, or play and leisure activities, the individual has a disability. The person with the fractured hip and impaired left lower extremity will be unable to bend and reach the left foot and so will need help to put on pants, or a sock and shoe on the left foot; therefore, he or she has a disability. When an impairment or disability interferes with a person's ability to complete activities that fulfill the essential responsibilities and duties of a social role, he or she is handicapped (WHO, 1980). The person with the fractured hip cannot take grandchildren to the park if he or she cannot get dressed. Handi-

Occupational Performance Areas as Defined by The American Occupational Therapy Association's Uniform Terminology (1994)

Activities of Daily Living: grooming, oral hygiene, bathing or showering, toilet hygiene, personal device care, dressing, feeding and eating, medication routine, health maintenance, socialization, functional communication, functional mobility, community mobility, emergency response, and sexual expression.

Work and Productive Activities: home management (clothing care, cleaning, meal preparation or cleanup, shopping, money management, household maintenance, safety procedures), care of others, educational activities, and vocational activities (vocational exploration, job acquisition, work or job performance, retirement planning, volunteer participation).

Play or Leisure Activities: play or leisure exploration and play or leisure performance

caps are often the result of inadequate access to health care or inaccessible environments. For example, the person with the fractured hip would be able to dress independently using a long-handled reacher; this adaptation is not possible for someone who cannot afford a long-handled reacher.

To help people "do the day-to-day activities that are important to them despite impairment, disability, or handicap," occupational therapy practitioners deliver a wide range of services, as illustrated in the case studies on this page and on pages 7 and 8.

All of these case studies have several things in common:

1. *The occupational therapy practitioners in all of these case studies focused on helping clients assume or return to valued day-to-day activities.* In some cases, as with Linda and Jennifer, the occupational therapy practitioner and client worked at the impairment level on prerequisite skills for occupational performance activities—movement in Linda's case, social skills in Jennifer's case. The **American Occupational Therapy Association's (AOTA) Uniform Terminology** terms these skills "component skills" (see Appendix F). In other cases, as with Peter, the occupational therapy program involved working at the level of disability, practicing occupational performance activities such as dressing and homemaking. Often, practitioners also work at the level of handicap, trying to eliminate physical and social barriers in their clients' communities. In Peter's case, this meant recommending (1) a wheelchair ramp to make his home accessible and (2) home health aide services to help Peter with some of his activities of daily living. In Linda's case, this meant talking to her employer to help negotiate altered job responsibilities for Linda during her recovery. For Paul, it meant recommending activity adaptations so that he could participate in his classes more fully. For Jennifer, it meant suggesting participation in community groups, such as AA, to help her maintain sobriety after discharge.

2. *The occupational therapy practitioners in all of these case studies collaborated with the client and the client's family or friends in setting up treatment goals that were important to the client and his or her social support network.* This type of collaboration is a central tenet of occupational therapy practice and distinguishes occupational therapy from helping professions that emphasize a helper as an expert model of client—professional interaction. In a expert or authoritarian model, the professional sets the treatment goals for the client without client input (Peloquin, 1990); in this model, clients are expected to be relatively passive recipients of services. In occupational therapy, clients are expected to be active participants and partners in treatment (Mattingly & Fleming, 1994). Clients who are active part-

CASE STUDY

PETER

Peter is a 60-year-old divorced tugboat captain with two grown sons. He is currently in the rehabilitation unit of a hospital because he had a stroke that paralyzed his left arm and leg. Given the severity of his stroke, Peter is not likely to recover enough movement in the left side of his body to walk or go back to work. Before his stroke, Peter lived alone in his own single-family house. His sons have expressed concern about Peter returning to that living situation, but Peter values his independence and has said he wants to return to his own home. Consequently, Peter and his occupational therapist have agreed to *practice activities of daily living and home-making from a wheelchair, using one-handed techniques,* so that Peter can become as independent as possible at home. The therapist has talked to the rest of Peter's treatment team and discovered that Peter will be eligible for only a few hours a day of home health aide services after discharge from the hospital. His sons are willing to help Peter return to his own home by building the wheelchair ramp recommended by the occupational therapy practitioner, if he can become independent and safe with the activities he would do when the home health aide was not around.

CASE STUDY

LINDA

Linda is a 35-year-old single carpenter who accidently cut the tendons across the back of her right, dominant hand at work. Linda has had surgery to repair the cut tendons, but this repair is not permanent—it only holds the tendon ends together until Linda's body can lay down new tissue at the injury site. Consequently, Linda will not be able to straighten her fingers and use her right hand until her recovery is complete. She has been referred to occupational therapy in an outpatient hand rehabilitation center. Linda lives in an apartment near the center with her female partner. The occupational therapist working with Linda has talked with her surgeon to determine the most appropriate schedule for gradually increasing Linda's right hand movement. Linda is concerned about being able to return to work. The occupational therapy program Linda's therapist recommends in-

cludes *(1) education about the exact nature of Linda's injury and the process of healing, (2) splinting, first to restrict movement in Linda's hand and later to provide limited mobility, (3) exercises to help control the swelling in Linda's hand, (4) exercises and activities, when appropriate, to help Linda strengthen her affected tendons and muscles, and (5) contact with Linda's employer to explain the time frame and extent of Linda's limitation and talk about what jobs Linda might do at her employer's business during her recovery.* Linda has agreed to this treatment program; she would like her sessions scheduled around her partner's work hours so her partner can also learn about Linda's home program. Linda's occupational therapist schedules treatment sessions that are convenient for both Linda and her partner and explains Linda's home program to both women.

ners in shaping their treatment goals have better treatment outcomes than clients who have goals imposed on them by health care providers (Czar, 1987; Neistadt, 1987; Neistadt & Marques, 1984; Shendell-Falik, 1990). Clients who feel their priorities are being respected in treatment are more likely to work harder in therapy than those who feel their priorities are being ignored (Hasselkus, 1989; Spencer, Young, Ritala, & Bates, 1995). Linda, for example, is much more likely to follow through with her

splinting and exercise program than she would be if her therapist ignored her concerns about work.

3. *The occupational therapy practitioners in all of these case studies collaborated with other professionals in each of the settings where treatment took place.* The ability to communicate and work effectively with other professionals is essential to quality service delivery. Clients benefit from the perspective and services of multiple professions. Paul's occupational therapy practitioners, for instance, cannot be the sole providers

CASE STUDY

PAUL

Paul is a 7-year-old second grader who lives with his parents and two older siblings—a 10-year-old brother, and a 13-year-old sister. Paul's teacher has asked for an occupational therapy consultation for Paul because he is clumsy in school and avoids the playground. His printing is larger than would be expected for someone his age, and he draws his letters very slowly. Paul's physical education (PE) teacher reports that in PE class Paul sits silently huddled up against the wall of the gym, refusing to participate. The occupational therapist observed Paul in his classroom and on the playground and gave Paul some standardized tests of gross and fine motor coordination and perception. These assessments suggested that Paul has difficulty with fine and gross motor coordination. The

occupational therapy program Paul's therapist recommends includes *(1) collaboration with the PE teacher to develop group gross motor activities that will not be too hard for Paul, (2) consultation with Paul's family to develop games that Paul could play with his siblings to improve his fine and gross motor coordination, and (3) consultation with Paul's classroom teacher to suggest strategies to help Paul with his handwriting (eg, use of commercially available paper with raised lines to give Paul physical cues about staying within the lines as he writes).* The certified occupational therapy assistant working at the school will assist the PE teacher and classroom teacher with these interventions each day. She will meet weekly with the therapist to review Paul's progress. Paul seems pleased with the idea of being able to participate more in school.

CASE STUDY

JENNIFER

Jennifer is a 16-year-old, single, young woman in a psychiatric day program for treatment of alcohol abuse and other behaviors. She lives with her father and stepmother. Over the past 6 months, Jennifer has been repeatedly truant from school and has been arrested several times for shoplifting. She also habitually sneaks out of her parents house after curfew, and stays out drinking with her friends until the early morning. With Jennifer's approval, her occupational therapy practitioners are providing her with the following services: *(1) stress management groups, (2) social skill groups, (3) encouragement to attend an Alcoholics Anonymous (AA) group for young people, (4)* *a vocational exploration group, (5) individual work related to study habits and strategies.* The groups on the unit are colead by team members. The certified occupational therapy assistant and occupational therapist on the unit colead the stress management and vocational exploration group. Jennifer spends part of each day with a tutor provided by her school; her occupational therapy practitioners are careful to schedule treatment around this tutoring time so Jennifer will not fall behind in her school work while she is in the day-treatment program. The occupational therapy practitioners also work closely with other members of Jennifer's treatment team and with her family.

of his education. He will be helped by the practitioners' knowledge of strategies to improve his handwriting, but he also needs instruction from his teachers.

These case studies may well trigger other questions about your future role as an occupational therapy practitioner. Questions such as, "Who am I going to work with?" "What will I be doing?" "Where will I be doing it?" and "When am I likely to work?" The following sections will address these questions.

▼ CLINICAL ROLE

The clinical role includes evaluation and treatment, professional communication, meetings, documentation, and the maintenance of professional credentials. It is in this role that practitioners typically enter the field. Practitioners working in clinical settings sometimes develop advanced competencies in their area of practice, such as certification as a hand or pediatric therapist.

Who

CLIENTS

Occupational therapy practitioners work with people of all ages, from infancy through old age. These individuals come from a variety of socioeconomic and cultural groups, and experience a variety of health problems. Some persons seeking occupational therapy services have physical diagnoses such as heart disease or burns. Others are experiencing psychological problems such as depression or eating disorders. Some will have problems related to atypical development, such as developmental delay. Units II and IV provide information about understanding the range of perspectives a client may bring to therapy and how these perspectives may influence the communication process; Units

IX and X provide more detail about the various diagnoses occupational therapy clients might have and about how these diagnoses affect occupational therapy services.

FAMILIES AND OTHER SUPPORT NETWORKS

Impairments, disabilities, or handicaps affect not only the individuals living with clients, but also their families and friends. Occupational therapy treatment is generally a relatively brief chapter in a person's life. When treatment is over, the client must rely on families and friends to maintain the gains achieved in therapy. Therefore, it is important for occupational therapy practitioners to include significant people in a client's life in the treatment process. Practitioners need to be prepared to deal with a wide range of social support networks with varied group dynamics and values relative to independence and interdependence (see Unit II).

OTHER PROFESSIONALS

Occupational therapy practitioners typically work as members of treatment teams, not as solo practitioners. The members of the treatment team will vary depending on the setting in which a practitioner works. In a school system, for instance, teachers would be important members of a treatment team; teachers would not be part of a treatment team in a nursing home. Chapter 44 provides more detail about working with other professionals. Chapter 8 addresses the collaborative relationships between **certified occupational therapists** and **certified occupational therapy assistants**.

What

EVALUATION AND TREATMENT

Occupational therapy services include **evaluation** and **treatment**. Evaluation in occupational therapy is the process of determining how a client's physical or psychological problems are interfering with competence in occupational **performance areas**. Occupational therapy evaluation would also yield a picture of the **performance components** affected by a client's medical or psychiatric diagnosis. Occupational therapists use a variety of methods and instruments during evaluation. Unit VI describes these.

Occupational therapy treatment ultimately aims to improve clients' abilities to perform the occupational performance activities that are important to them. As these case studies demonstrate, practitioners might do a wide range of things in treatment, from designing and making a splint to running a stress management group. Unit VII provides more detail about the many different interventions occupational therapy practitioners use.

PROFESSIONAL COMMUNICATION

A significant chunk of any practitioner's day is spent communicating with other professionals and insurance companies. Some of that communication takes place in meetings and telephone conversations, and some of it is done in writing. Chapter 44 address aspects of the communication process.

Meetings

In meetings with other professionals, occupational therapy practitioners typically are expected to report on (1) the types of services they are providing and (2) clients' responses to those services. It is often necessary for occupational therapy practitioners to advocate for a particular team treatment approach or discharge plan for a given client. Therefore, occupational therapy practitioners need to be assertive and confident when making oral reports or contributing to meetings.

Documentation

All occupational therapy practitioners keep written records of evaluation and treatment. These records serve as (1) feedback to the client about progress; (2) communication with other staff, especially those whose work schedules preclude attendance at team meetings; (3) legal evidence that services were delivered; and (4) support for billing of insurance companies, health plans, or private individuals.

Occupational therapy **documentation** should focus on function and answer two major questions:

1. How does the client's diagnoses affect his or her ability to perform occupational activities?
2. How will occupational therapy affect the client's ability to perform occupational activities?

Occupational therapy treatment goals should always be measurable (Box 1-2). Without measurable goals, practitioners have no way to demonstrate their interventions were effective. Insurance companies, health plans, or private individuals will not pay for services that are not effective in producing changes in clients' functional abilities. Chapter 43 provides additional information about documentation.

PROFESSIONAL CREDENTIALS

Members of all professions must meet certain education and competency requirements to practice in their professions. Professional credentials are proof of meeting those requirements. Credentials protect clients from being harmed by unqualified practitioners. In the United States, occupational therapy practitioners must have the following credentials:

1. Proof of graduation from an occupational therapy program accredited by the **Accreditation Council of Occupational Therapy Education of the AOTA**.
2. Proof of a passing grade on the examinations adminis-

▼ **BOX 1-2**

Measurable Documentation: Writing Behavioral Objectives

Occupational therapy treatment goals should be written as measurable behavioral objectives. All behavioral objectives should have the following elements:

Behavior: An expected behavioral outcome that can be seen or heard (eg, dressing or speaking)
Criteria: Expected level of performance (eg, "with minimal assistance" or "independently")
Conditions: How the client will perform the behavior (eg, seated or standing, using adapted equipment)
Time frame: Length of time it will take the client to achieve the target behavior
Example: Within 1 week, client will put her pants on independently using a long-handled reacher while seated.

    Behavior: = Put her pants on
    Criteria: = Independently
    Conditions: = Using a long-handled reacher while seated
    Time frame: = Within 1 week

tered by the **National Board of Certification in Occupational Therapy (NBCOT)**. These are competency examinations taken by occupational therapy and occupational therapy assistant students after the completion of their course work and fieldwork.

3. Proof of a **license** obtained from the state government in those states that require licenses.

In addition to these minimum requirements, some settings may also require specialty certifications (ie, proof of additional training in a particular area of practice). Other countries have their own credentialing processes.

RESOURCES: PROFESSIONAL ORGANIZATIONS

Local, national, and worldwide occupational therapy professional organizations are an important information resource for practitioners. The AOTA is the national professional organization. This organization establishes professional and educational standards, supports the development of occupational therapy practitioners through publications and continuing education programs, supports research through the **American Occupational Therapy Foundation (AOTF)**, and promotes the profession through public relations and legislative efforts. AOTA and other professional organizations publish newsletters, journals, and other resource materials to keep practitioners informed. They also organize conferences to disseminate professional information. Membership fees fund these services.

Where

Occupational therapy practitioners work in a variety of facility-based and community-based settings. Facility-based settings include general hospitals, outpatient clinics, rehabilitation hospitals, subacute or long-term rehabilitation centers, or nursing homes. Community-based settings include school systems, day-treatment programs, group homes, or clients' own homes. Some practitioners work in one place all the time; others, such as school or home health practitioners, travel from place to place during the workday. Some practitioners work for traveling companies that assign them to given facilities for a few weeks or months at a time, and then reassign them to other facilities. The logistics of the workday will vary depending on the type of setting. Unit XI provides more detail about different environments for practice.

When

Occupational therapy practitioner work schedules will also vary from setting to setting. Occupational therapy is generally not a 9 AM to 5 PM, Monday through Friday job. Those in facility-based practice will find that most facilities offer therapy services on weekends. Consequently, practitioners can expect to work a certain number of weekend days per year. Some outpatient settings have early-morning and

evening hours so clients do not have to miss work to attend therapy sessions. School system practitioners may work only during school hours and have all school holidays and vacations off.

▼ MANAGEMENT ROLE

Occupational therapy managers perform the administrative functions necessary for an occupational therapy department to survive and thrive. This is especially true in today's rapidly changing health care environment. For example, Peter's occupational therapy practitioner is skilled in discharge planning and collaboration with community agencies. She acquired these skills because the director of the occupational therapy department recognized their importance and developed a series of in-service programs. The director also implemented a quality assurance program that has improved documentation of services. Because of this, Peter's occupational therapy practitioner's documentation is excellent, and when it was reviewed, the department received full reimbursement for the services provided to Peter. Chapter 43 addresses the role of the manager in greater detail.

▼ CONSULTANT ROLE

Occupational therapy consultants provide indirect service to clients, agencies, and groups. Beyond knowledge of the practice setting, consultation requires excellent communication and collaboration skills. For example, an occupational therapy practitioner may work with a nursing home activity coordinator to help the coordinator plan programs that meet the needs of the residents of the nursing home. To be successful in this role, the occupational therapist must have an understanding of (1) the federal and state rules and regulations regarding activity programs in nursing homes, (2) the needs of the residents in this nursing home, (3) knowledge about the skills and knowledge of the activity coordinator, (4) understanding of this particular nursing home environment, and (5) knowledge of a variety of approaches to planning and implementing activities programs in nursing homes.

Paul's occupational therapist recommended limited direct intervention after her initial evaluation because in her judgment, direct service was not the most effective way to help Paul. Rather, she worked with the teachers in the school, helping them to modify Paul's learning environment so that he could function optimally. She asked the certified occupational therapy assistant to support the teachers in implementing this program. This approach keeps Paul with his classmates and integrates occupational therapy intervention with his educational program. As a consultant, Paul's occupational therapist must have an excellent understanding about what is possible and practical to suggest to teachers in a school setting, as well as excellent communication and collaboration skills. In this role, she will meet weekly with the certified occupational therapy assistant, observe Paul periodically to gauge his progress, and meet with the teachers to provide them with additional assistance if this is needed.

Linda's occupational therapist will most likely do an additional work site consultation toward the end of Linda's recovery. This consultation will address any residual disability Linda may have relative to her job as a carpenter and work site modifications that will be necessary to assure Linda's safety and minimize her functional limitations.

▼ EDUCATOR ROLE

Occupational therapy educators contribute to the development and socialization of the next generation of occupational therapy practitioners. They work in colleges and universities as faculty members in occupational therapy educational programs and in practice settings as fieldwork educators. Both of Jennifer's occupational therapy practitioners have been fieldwork educators since their second year of practice. Each began by having occupational therapy and occupational therapy assistant students observe in her groups for level I fieldwork experiences. The occupational therapist also initiated a level II fieldwork program with a local community college that has an occupational therapy assistant program and a local university that has an occupational therapy program. Level II fieldwork students from both programs are scheduled regularly on the unit, often together. By scheduling occupational therapy and occupational therapy assistant students at the same time, these practitioners are able to model the collaborative relationship so necessary for today's practice environment.

Both give guest lectures about the role of task groups in mental health practice settings. Because of their involvement in the education of future occupational therapy practitioners, Jennifer's occupational therapy practitioners learn from the students and are able to extend their services to more clients because the fieldwork students can assist and eventually lead some of the groups.

Involvement in fieldwork and guest lecturing may provide the catalyst for a practitioner to consider the role of academician. Many full-time faculty members enter academia through fieldwork education, guest lectures, and part-time teaching. The role of an occupational therapy faculty member involves teaching, research, and community service. Typically, occupational therapy faculty have a master's or doctoral degree in occupational therapy or a related field.

▼ RESEARCHER ROLE

Research provides the knowledge base for occupational therapy practice. It is through research that the assumptions and beliefs of the profession are tested and the efficacy of occupational therapy intervention is verified. Through clinically based research we are able to discover which evaluation and intervention methods are most effective; that is, which ones enable our clients to be able to meet their goals and carry out their daily round of activities with as much autonomy as possible. Research is typically conducted by individuals with a master's or doctoral degree. Practitioners with less formal education may be involved in research by assisting in data collection and analysis. Research is an exciting opportunity for professional growth for it enables practitioners to explore questions emanating from their work

RESEARCH NOTE
THE KNOWLEDGE BASE OF OCCUPATIONAL SCIENCE AND OCCUPATIONAL THERAPY

Kenneth J. Ottenbacher

The practice of occupational therapy is a synthesis of scholarly knowledge and technical skills. The challenge of research is not only to produce more and better scientific investigations, but also to transform research findings into useful knowledge and skills. An important question regarding this challenge is: Are professional educational curriculums skill-based or knowledge-based? Skill-based curriculums are focused on the present. Skill-based curriculums emphasize teaching the technologies of treatment. Skill-based curriculums provide *How to* information. Research is not an essential component of skill-based curriculums because the knowledge underpinning the skills is often generated by members of other disciplines.

Knowledge-based curriculums are proactive. Knowledge-based curriculums focus on imparting the critical reasoning skills needed to meet the challenges of a diversified

and changing practice. Knowledge-based curriculums focus on asking *Why* questions associated with clinical practice. Research is an integral component of knowledge-based curriculums. A knowledge-based curriculum cannot exist without research.

Developing a knowledge-based curriculum does not mean that professional skills are ignored. The question is not whether students should be taught skills. They must have skills to be competent practitioners. The question is, where do the technical skills come from and where will they lead professional practice? In a true profession, the skills come from a clearly defined and well-developed knowledge base generated by members of the discipline. The knowledge base provides the core of occupational science and generates the skills that constitute the practice of occupational therapy. ■

with clients. For more information about research in occupational therapy see Chapter 48.

Clinically based research is needed to identify the most effective ways to restore clients to independent function. For example, Jennifer's practitioners would benefit from research studies that showed the relative effectiveness of different groups on function after discharge. Because of their close relationship to several occupational therapy programs, they may have the opportunity to participate in collaborative research with one of the faculty members. They may also pursue additional education to develop their competencies. For example, Jennifer's therapist might pursue a master's degree and use this opportunity to develop a thesis topic on the clinical effectiveness of groups.

▶ CONCLUSION

Occupational therapy is an extremely varied and exciting field. Entry-level practitioners looking for work can choose from a wide range of settings and client populations. With experience and perhaps additional education, occupational therapy practitioners may expand from their clinical roles to those of consultant, manager, educator, researcher or a combination thereof. No matter where or with whom they choose to work, occupational therapy practitioners have a lifelong opportunity to make a significant difference in the lives of the people they serve, and to learn about themselves in the process. We hope you will embrace the many opportunities for caring and growing in your newly chosen profession.

REFERENCES

American Occupational Therapy Association (1994). Uniform terminology for occupational therapy—third edition. *American Journal of Occupational Therapy, 48,* 1047–1054.

Czar, M. (1987). Two methods of goal setting in middle-aged adults facing critical life changes. *Clinical Nurse Specialist, 1,* 171–177.

Hasselkus, B.R. (1989). Occupational and physical therapy in geriatric rehabilitation. *Physical & Occupational Therapy in Geriatrics, 73* (3), 3–19.

Mattingly, C. & Fleming, M. H. (1994). *Clinical reasoning: Forms of inquiry in a therapeutic practice.* Philadelphia: F. A. Davis Company.

Neistadt, M. E. (1987). An occupational therapy program for adults with developmental disabilities. *American Journal Occupational Therapy, 41,* 433–438.

Neistadt, M. E. & Marques, K. (1984). An independent living skills training program. *American Journal Occupational Therapy, 38,* 671–676.

Peloquin, S. M. (1990). The patient–therapist relationship in occupational therapy: Understanding visions and images. *American Journal of Occupational Therapy, 44,* 13–22.

Shendell-Falik, N. (1990). Creating self-care units in the acute care setting: A case study. *Patient Education and Counseling, 15,* 39–45.

Spencer, J., Young, M. E., Rintala, D., Bates, S. (1995). Socialization to the culture of a rehabilitation hospital: An ethnographic study. *American Journal of Occupational Therapy, 49,* 53–62.

World Health Organization. (1980). *International classification of impairments, disabilities and handicaps* (ICIDH). Geneva, Switzerland: Author.

Chapter 2

Occupational Science: Occupational Therapy's Legacy for the 21st Century

Florence Clark, Wendy Wood, and Elizabeth A. Larson

Occupational science emerged out of the early 20th century values and beliefs of occupational therapy practitioners and has promised in the upcoming century to nurture the profession of occupational therapy (University of Southern California, 1989). Although both occupational science and occupational therapy focus on occupation they differ in that occupational therapy is a profession, and occupational science is an academic discipline. A profession is a form of paid employment distinguished from other kinds by its service to the public through schooled application of a specialized knowledge base and skill (Freidson, 1994). In contrast, an academic discipline is a "branch of knowledge or learning recognized by the university community as legitimate for scholarly investigation" (University of Southern California, 1989, p. 143).

As an academic discipline, occupational science is focused on the study of the form, function, and meaning of human occupation. Founded by Elizabeth June Yerxa, it has also been described as the study of the human as an occupational being, centering on how human beings realize their sense of meaning through occupation (Yerxa et al., 1990; Clark et al., 1991). It addresses what anthropologists call the activity spectrum or stream, that is, the range of activities that fill the day for a given species (White, 1991). In occupational science, **occupations** are defined as the daily activities that can be named in the lexicon of the culture and that fill the stream of time (Yerxa et al., 1990; Clark et al., 1991). Occupational science is not a single theory, model, or frame of reference; rather, it is a social science similar in form to academic disciplines such as anthropology, sociology, or psychology (Yerxa et al., 1990). It is classified as falling within the sciences (rather than the humanities) because its methods of data collection are systematic, disciplined, and subject to public scrutiny (Carlson & Clark, 1991). Carlson and Clark (1991) define science "as a systematic (rule-bound) and empirically based form of human inquiry undertaken by a community of scholars" (p. 236). Occupational science is considered to be more closely aligned to the social sciences than the physical sciences because its subject matter deals with human behavior (Homans, 1967).

Occupational science can be expected to generate numerous theories about occupation that are likely to be applied to practice by occupational therapy practitioners in concert with other theories, models, or frames of reference that practitioners find particularly useful. Its unique and primary contribution to occupational therapy will be, however, that of providing a corpus of knowledge sharply focused on the concept of occupation. This contribution can build professional unity by giving practitioners a more explicit and expansive sense of the complexity and power of human occupation employed to serve the public good.

This chapter begins by bringing into sharp focus core beliefs about occupations and their underlying values that gave rise to occupational therapy in the early 20th century. These beliefs have subsequently persevered to provide a humanitarian and conceptual foundation to occupational science. The science of occupation is then further described as an academic discipline concerned with the form, function, and meaning of occupation. Subsequent sections address how occupational scientists go about studying each of these aspects.

13

▼ THE ROOTS OF OCCUPATIONAL SCIENCE IN OCCUPATIONAL THERAPY

Harold Bell Wright wrote that "Occupation is the very life of life" (cited in Dunton, 1915, p. 6). Nearly 100 years later, in 1995, Robert Bing stated the following: "[Historians] realize that there is something curiously special about the last decade of each century, an unusual surge of energy to clear the old century's agenda and make ready for the new century. The syndrome of the '90s focuses on both the past and the future" (p. 4).

That "occupation is the very life of life" is a notion as old as the millennia. That an unusual surge of energy has allowed occupational science to take root and begin to flourish in the 1990s represents a serious grappling with a philosophical view of occupation embraced by many of occupational therapy's most influential leaders in the early 20th century. Thus, although formally founded at the University of Southern California in 1989, occupational science is rooted in the same humanitarian and philosophical ground that gave rise to the profession of occupational therapy some 90 years ago. The emergence of occupational science constitutes a vital step in modernizing knowledge about occupation that will be of profound relevance to issues of health and daily living in the 21st century. In essence, therefore, the rise of occupational science, and its beginning yield, are both timely and timeless.

Convergence of Progressive Social Movements in the Early 1900s

Occupational therapy was preceded in the 1800s by the moral treatment movement which recognized the health-promoting benefits of engagement in a broad spectrum of what we today call occupations (see Chap. 49). Yet the precedence of moral treatment alone cannot account for why occupational therapy emerged when it did. Rather, the profession's rise is attributable to a confluence of diverse social movements near the turn of the 20th century that were congruent with the humanitarian principles of moral treatment (Quiroga, 1995). One of the most pivotal of these movements was known as the settlement movement.

Eleanor Clarke Slagle, an influential early leader of occupational therapy, studied under Jane Addams, the leader of the settlement movement, at a dynamic center of reform activities by women in America: the Hull House Settlement in Chicago, Illinois (Quiroga, 1995). The settlement movement embraced progressive social activism, largely carried out by women, to ameliorate the debilitating effects of poverty, industrialization, and cultural alienation on disenfranchised persons, particularly immigrants. Its proponents believed in the power of creative activity, such as art, music, drama, writing, or craft work, to address problems of an individual, societal, as well as cultural (Addams, 1961).

Yet the settlement movement's influence on occupational therapy is attributable not only to its use of occupation, but also to its success in bringing together proponents of other social movements, most notably those of the mental hygiene movement, the philosophy of pragmatism, and the arts and crafts movement. The work of Slagle as well as that of Adolph Meyer, a psychiatrist and a pioneer in occupational therapy, illustrate this contribution of the settlement movement to occupational therapy. While living at the Hull House, Slagle studied under Julia Lathrop in a course on "curative occupations and recreations" at the Chicago School of Civics and Philanthropy (Quiroga, 1995). Lathrop was a leader of the mental hygiene movement which sought to reform the treatment of persons with mental illness. Meyer also had direct connections to Hull House and its progressive intellectual community associated with the University of Chicago (Breines, 1986). Moreover, similar to Lathrop, Meyer (1922) was an advocate of the mental hygiene movement. When he wrote that psychiatric diseases were "largely problems of **adaptation**" (p. 639) that could be addressed through occupation and the restitution of a healthful temporal rhythm of work, play, rest, and sleep, Meyer's thinking reflected the views of mental hygienists (1922). Meyer was also influenced by the philosophy of pragmatism then being advanced by John Dewey, the educator, and George Herbert Meade, the sociologist. As stated by Breines (1986), "With the pragmatists, Meyer professes that doing, action and experience are being. . . [and] demonstrate a mind/body synthesis" (p. 46). As both a pragmatist and a mental hygienist, Meyer advocated on behalf of persons with mental illness insisting that occupation could be used as a powerful organizer of time and medium to develop vital living skills.

Houses of the settlement movement additionally provided laboratories for applying the humanitarian values associated with the arts and crafts movement (Reed, 1986). The arts and crafts movement originated in England and later spread to the United States out of reaction against the culturally alienating and demoralizing effects of industrialization (Levine, 1986). As well as railing against industrialization, arts and crafts proponents viewed idleness as a potentially devastating state of being. As expressed by John Ruskin, the founder of the movement, "God intends no man to live in this world without working; but it seems to me no less evident that He intends every man to be happy in his work" (cited by Levine, 1986, p. 262). The belief that creative manual work could help reconstruct one's sense of self and purpose was strongly endorsed by three founding physicians of occupational therapy—Adolph Meyer, Herbert Hall, and William Dunton (Levine, 1986). These men sought to integrate the humanistic values of the arts and crafts movement with medicine's increasingly scientific world view. Indeed, the rise of occupational therapy corresponded with a fall from prominence of the previously popular rest cure that had pursued "complete bed rest and a bland diet. . . [as] the only hope of restoring the exhausted

HISTORICAL NOTE
WILLIAM DUNTON'S CREED: THE CENTRAL ROLE OF OCCUPATION

Suzanne M. Peloquin

William Rush Dunton, Jr. (1919) shared a creed that introduced his book on wartime therapy:

> That occupation is as necessary to life as food and drink. That every human being should have both physical and mental occupation. . . . That sick minds, sick bodies, sick souls, may be healed through occupation (p. 17).

The creed asks therapists to see occupation as a life-giving staple and to engage persons toward the actions that help them build their lives.

Dunton (1955) also cited others who had used occupation as part of moral treatment in the 19th century, men such as the physician Brush:

Occupation is undoubtedly of very great importance in the treatment of the insane, but the idea of occupation which is satisfied by putting a row of twenty dements to picking hair or making fiber matts is far short of the true aim of occupation. (p. 17)

Comments such as these are cogent reminders that occupation occupies the body, mind, and spirit. Meaningful occupation must drive our inquiry and distinguish our practice. When our therapies fail to engage body, mind, and spirit, our credibility as occupational therapists is at stake. ■

Dunton, W. R. (1919). *Reconstruction therapy.* Philadelphia: W. B. Saunders.
Dunton, W. R. (1955). Today's principles reflected in early literature. *American Journal of Occupational Therapy, 9,* 17–18.

---

patient to health" (Quiroga, 1995, p. 74). In direct contrast to proponents of the rest cure, early occupational therapists considered boredom and idleness as deleterious to health and worked hard so that patients would enjoy a rich and productive menu of daily activities.

In addition to its influence by the settlement movement, the mental hygiene movement, pragmatism, and the arts and crafts movement, the rise of occupational therapy occurred in concert with a movement toward improved treatment of persons with tuberculosis as well as contemporary beliefs of a connection between the medical and spiritual dimensions of healing. At the turn of the century, tuberculosis was a highly dreaded contagious disease. Progressive treatment of tuberculous patients occurred in sanitariums offering a well-regulated balance of rest, with graduated involvement in a variety of occupations such as light household tasks, outdoor work, leisure activities, or craft work (Brown, 1922; Kidner, 1922). Because daily patterns of rest and activity per se, and not imposed medical treatments, were believed to constitute the essential curative dynamic, patients were responsible for monitoring their activities. In short, human agency, or the active participation of the individual in his or her own recovery, was thought to play a central role in regaining health. Beyond the tuberculous movement, human agency was also thought to provide a critical link between the physical and spiritual sides of healing. For example, Herbert Hall endorsed many beliefs associated with a theologically based self-help movement known as Emmanualism that believed in the inextricable interdependence of body, mind, and spirit. Hall viewed human agency as part of a "divine plan" for curing and preventing disease and, thereby, as manifesting the role of spirituality in healing (Quiroga, 1995, p. 106).

Finally, the rise of occupational therapy must be understood in the context of a wave of women's reform and professional activities that occurred near the turn of the 20th century (Quiroga, 1995). These activities transformed the traditional volunteerism of women into a new era of paid professionalism, thereby paving the way for predominantly female professions, such as occupational therapy, to arise and be supported by the larger American society. Early pioneers such as Eleanor Clarke Slagle, Susan Tracy, Susan Cox Johnson, or Elizabeth Greene Upham represented a transitional generation of women who enacted a delicate balance between the socially proscribed altruism and subservience expected of women and their personal efforts to advance occupational therapy as a legitimate profession. To preserve this balance, women of this transitional generation built occupational therapy from the inside, relying heavily on connections with women's reform networks; they also were the "doers" of the field who worked directly with patients. In contrast, the founding generation of men such as William Dunton, Adolph Meyer, Herbert Hall, George Barton, or Thomas Kidner convinced outsiders (often male physicians) of the value of occupational therapy. They also engaged in theorizing that sought to put occupational therapy on a scientific basis (Quiroga, 1995). In sum, prevailing beliefs about gender were simultaneously observed, stretched, and resisted (albeit unobtrusively) so that the profession of occupational therapy could take hold.

Occupational Therapy's Legacy to Occupational Science

Although it is true that occupation is as old as the millennia, it is also true that our understanding of occupation is now in the process of being vigorously modernized to meet the challenges of the 21st century. Clearly, a confluence of progressive social movements in the late 1800s and early 1900s generated a cross-pollination of ideas about occupation from such diverse fields as nursing, medicine, psychiatry, social work, sociology, education, philosophy, architecture, the arts, and theology (Quiroga, 1995). The legacy of this cross-pollination was a remarkable moral philosophy that the emerging profession of occupational therapy would soon endorse. Most fundamentally, that philosophy recognized the central role of occupation in daily living and health; it did not relegate occupation to one of many different types of treatment modalities to be inserted here or there in the day to achieve discrete therapeutic goals (Clark & Larson, 1993). In that the richness of this legacy has yet to be mined by any academic discipline, the concept of occupation constitutes the central focus of inquiry in occupational science today. Furthermore, because occupational science seeks to integrate interdisciplinary knowledge to elucidate the form, function, and meaning of occupation as "the very life of life," the science's range of inquiry includes, yet goes well beyond, therapeutic uses of occupation within medical contexts. By generating and organizing knowledge about occupation as a core phenomenon of daily living, occupational science will help meet the demands of an inevitably far more complex, as well as greatly expanded, practice in the 21st century. It will also help clarify to the general public the centrality of occupation to health, a critical first step if occupational therapy is to be appropriately and sufficiently valued.

In addition to recognizing the centrality of occupation, the moral philosophy that occupational therapy adopted recognized the inherent value of each human being, no matter how poor, socially devalued, or disabled. Early practitioners applied this philosophy when they respected the dignity and potential of their patients and, given that respect, helped their patients participate in personally meaningful and socially valued rounds of activity. Occupational science today consequently places great emphasis on subjective experiences of occupation as well as the function of occupation in society and culture. Occupational science also represents a coming of age, whereby the diverse activities necessary to maintain a discipline are no longer consigned by gender. Thus, the legacy of a schism between male "thinking" activities and female "doing" activities has been transcended. Should occupational science flourish in the 21st century, it is reasonable to anticipate that the traditionally subservient place of occupational therapy relative to predominantly male professions such as medicine shall be a thing of the past. The success of occupational science will also mean that occupational therapy can at last claim to have its own academic discipline, as opposed to being based mostly on knowledge borrowed from other disciplines, much of which has not been synthesized into a cogent understanding of occupation.

▼ CONTEMPORARY RESEARCH OF THE FORM, FUNCTION, AND MEANING OF OCCUPATION

The Form of Occupation

When occupational scientists study the form of occupation they focus on those aspects of occupation that are directly observable. We believe that what Nelson (1988) has chosen to call occupational form and occupational performance are, in actuality, both aspects of occupational form, because both can be readily observed, although we acknowledge that Nelson's distinction is useful for certain purposes. In Nelson's typology the environmental context as well as the demands of the task are classified as aspects of occupational form, whereas the act of doing as occupation is labeled performance. However, both are directly observable and, therefore, fall within our singular category of occupational form. One has no trouble recognizing the occupation of skiing, which entails certain task demands and recognizable patterns of movement. However, if instead of a snowsuit, the performer is wearing a bathing suit and the occupation is happening on a lake, rather than on a snow covered mountain, simply through observation one discerns that this is an instance of water rather than Alpine skiing. Studies that address what people do, the circumstances under which they do it, and how they do it in relation to time, space, and performance, are studies of occupational form. Traditional studies that have used time diaries, time logs, and observations of performance during engagement in occupation are examples of investigations of occupational form. However, recently, innovative qualitative research methodologies have been used by occupational scientists and other social scientists to uncover complex issues related to the form of occupation and the inextricable links between the acting individual and the context in generating occupational form (Fig. 2-1).

For example, Pierce (1996a) used qualitative interview techniques to provide an in-depth description of how scholars manage to stay productive. After interviewing ten full professors who taught at the University of Southern California, she found that the scholars structured their daily routines and activities in accord with their physiological needs. For example, they would use such activities as swimming or taking walks to adjust their physiological state for days of major writing. The scholars also reported needing to use preferred tools, including specific kinds of writing implements or computers, and they seemed dependent on being situated in customized office spaces. They also executed their scholarly activities in accord with specific temporal rhythms. Although this study additionally addressed certain emotional and psychological dimensions that influenced productivity, much of the study focused on occupational form as we have defined it; that is, on those aspects that are directly observable (Fig. 2-2).

1

FORM

Directly observable aspects of occupation

2

FUNCTION

Ways in which occupation serves adaptation

3

MEANING

The significance of occupation within the context of real lives and in the culture

▲

Figure 2-1. Occupational science: Three major research orientations.

Pierce (1996b) again studied occupational form in her longitudinal work on infant object play. The research methods were highly innovative, combining videotaping that adapted methods used by ethologists in naturalistic settings, maternal interviews in the home context, and computer-assisted qualitative analysis. Instead of replicating conventional methods in which infants of different ages are given standardized objects with which to interact in laboratory settings, Pierce videotaped the infants from birth through 18 months interacting with objects that were naturally available in their home settings. This technique allowed her to document how infants begin to structure their own play when given the spaces and objects readily available and accessible in the home, the constraints imposed and freedoms appropriated by the mothers, the child's developmental readiness at the time of videotaping, and other characteristics of the

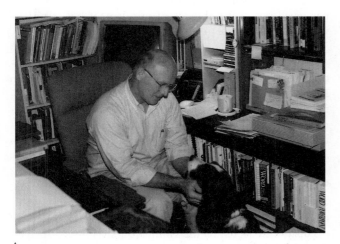

▲

Figure 2-2. Scholars appear to be dependent on highly customized spaces to execute their occupation. They also need to pace their work in accord with temporal rhythms. Here a scholar is "taking a break" from a long day of writing in his customized work space equipped with his preferred tools. (Photo courtesy of John Wolcott.)

child and home. Although, at each age during which the infants were videotaped, certain kinds of play seemed typical, this method enabled Pierce to detect the ways in which the play becomes customized in each setting and for each infant (Pierce, 1996b). One of the key findings of Pierce's work was the extent to which the particular "form" the play took was context-dependent.

Pierce's findings show certain similarities to those reported by Lave (1988) on the occupation of supermarket shopping. Lave found that even an activity that is seemingly as routinized as supermarket shopping actually involved a complex dialectical relation between the person acting (shopper) and the arena (the supermarket). Each shopper would customize his or her approach to shopping based on certain structural features of the market (displays, sequencing of goods on aisles, physical spaces) and his or her own priorities, shopping lists, values, and computational skills. Lave synthesized her findings into a theory of practice that suggests that how persons actually perform occupations is a function of a complex intersection of the person acting and the settings. She goes on to question the concept of goal-directed activity purporting that activity is "not compatible with a linear view of action as directed towards established goals" (Lave, 1988, p. 183). Instead, she sees experience in the lived-in world as constructed on the basis of expectations. She maintains people "act inventively in terms of expectations about what has happened, is happening, and may happen" (Lave, 1988, p. 185). Thus, Lave's work calls into question notions of occupation as solely goal-directed activity.

Studies of occupational orchestration are also studies of occupational form as we have defined it. Conventionally, orchestration means to compose or arrange (music) for an orchestra. However, in occupational science, the term occupational orchestration is used to refer "to ideation, composition, execution, ordering and other qualitative aspects of occupations" (University of Southern California, 1989, p. 148). It includes timing, rhythm, and tone. Recently, Larson

(1996) used qualitative research methods to describe the processes by which Mexican-American mothers, living in poverty and parenting a child with severe disability, orchestrated their daily occupations. The presence of the child imposed an enormous burden of care, one for which it was likely there would be only minimal relief over time. Larson's (1996) dissertation catalogues the many strategies these mothers employed so that they could plan, organize, and balance their daily occupations to successfully meet these challenges.

Occupations are historically and culturally situated. As a consequence, what constituted typical occupations in classical Greece only partially resembles what people spend their time doing today. Chariot riding on some level resembles driving a car, yet the two are probably more different than similar. Similarly, Martha Ballard, a woman who lived in New England from 1755 to 1812, spent much of her day overseeing and engaging in weaving and other aspects of textile production, necessary work if her family was to have clothing (Ulrich, 1991). However, by the time occupational therapy was founded, weaving was seen as a discretionary craft and was not routinely performed as part of the "work" of households. Today, we are witnessing another revolution in how people are occupying their time because of the advent of computer technology. When occupational scientists study historical changes in how people spend their time, they are investigating historical and cultural occupational forms. Turn of the 19th century Americans would, no doubt, be puzzled by the time their contemporary counterparts invest in surfing the Internet, driving on freeways, and watching television.

The Function of Occupation

When occupational scientists address the function of occupation they are particularly concerned with the ways in which occupation serves adaptation (Wilcock, 1993). Just as particular occupations may promote health and well-being in individuals, so may the patterns of occupation that characterize particular **cultures** affect the health of towns, nations, cities, neighborhoods, and communities. Whereas some occupations and patterns of occupation are health promoting, others may be health compromising. For example, *The Los Angeles Times* (Nazario, June 23, 1996) recently reported that in Palmdale, California, a newly developed Los Angeles suburb, where 36.9% of the residents spend two hours or more commuting to work, the incidence of wife beating, child abuse, divorce, and teenage truancy and delinquency far exceed national averages. Furthermore, among all police stations in Los Angeles County, more domestic violence felony arrests are made in this area and the rate of child abuse is greater than most other California communities and twice as high as other areas in Los Angeles County. Although the article implies that the daily commute is causing these deleterious effects, no formal research that established causality is reported in the article. A study on the effect of daily commuting on child delinquency, child abuse, and wife beating, would constitute a study on the potentially negative effects of a particular occupational pattern on individuals. Recently, Primeau (1996), an occupational scientist, published a review paper on travel as an occupation. As occupational scientists generate knowledge about the effects of travel patterns on health, occupational therapy practitioners may be inspired to carefully consider the demands travel makes on the well-being and functional performances of their clients.

Questions such as those addressing the relation of occupation to health, subjective well-being, daily functioning, stress management, the development of mastery and competence, and the quality of life, all are related to the function of occupation—what occupations do—how do they influence people and communities? Occupations also influence culture, for it is partially through occupations that cultures are constituted and transformed. For example, anthropologist Victor Turner (1987) proposes that certain occupations, in the form of rituals and social dramas, challenge prevailing cultural norms and are crucial to bring about cultural change.

Occupational scientist, Ann Wilcock (1993) has proposed a convincing theoretical argument to support the notion that humans have a biological need for occupations. She maintains that occupations have the following three functions: "(1) to provide for immediate bodily needs of sustenance, self-care, shelter, and safety; (2) develop skills, social structures and technology aimed at superiority over predators and the environment; (3) exercise and develop personal capacities enabling the organism to be maintained and flourish" (p. 20). Without engagement in occupations that achieve these ends, Wilcock is concerned that human beings cannot stay healthy and flourish. Wilcock's perspective is consistent with Yerxa's view, influenced by the Finnish philosopher Pörn (1993), that "health will ultimately be perceived not as the absence of impairment but as possession of a repertoire of skills to achieve one's purposes" (Yerxa, 1994, p. 589).

Recently, Wood (1995) investigated the effect of occupation on health using a definition of health derived from Pörn's (1993) work. The research approach integrated qualitative and quantitative methods to study how the environment influenced occupations, adaptation, and health of captive chimpanzees. Wood (1995) reasoned that both humans and chimpanzees, in so far as they share 97.6% of their genetic makeup, may both require occupation to stay healthy. She found that environmental opportunities for occupation, or the lack thereof, influenced frequencies of various occupations as well as the overall complexities of the rounds of occupations enacted by the chimpanzees. Moreover, behavioral flexibility and innovation was observed to vary in important primate occupations, especially playing and object-using, as a function of the chimpanzees acting, in effect, to force their living environment to support their biological need for challenging occupations. Wood's research has particular applicability to persons living within institutional settings that control the daily rounds of occupations made available to residents.

Various studies have demonstrated that engagement in occupations, including hobbies, clubs, and religious activities, is correlated with older adult health, cognitive functioning, and subjective well-being. As an example, Clarkson-Smith and Hartley (1990) found that older adults who participated in bridge clubs, in contrast with those who did not, scored higher on measures of working memory and cognitive processing. Similarly, research on successful aging suggests that both paid and unpaid productive activity correlates with both physical and psychological well-being of older adults (Herzog, House, & Morgan, 1991; Adelmann, 1994; Glass, Seeman, Herzog, Kahn, & Berkamn, 1995). More studies of this kind, as well as studies that more clearly specify causality to document the health-promoting and health-compromising effects of particular patterns and choices of occupation in all age groups and across the life span are needed. Findings from these studies will be particularly useful to occupational therapy practitioners whose responsibility it is to help their patients prevent and cope with disability and illness; they can also be used to guide interventions in community mental health, delinquency prevention, substance abuse and violence prevention. Just as dietitians make recommendations about balanced meals, occupational therapists will have data available through which they can recommend occupations to promote health and well-being. This research focus clearly echoes the issues already discussed that were of concern to the founders of the profession.

The Meaning of Occupation

People see occupations as important when they are meaningful within the context of their lives (Trombly, 1995). As Trombly (1995) has pointed out, "only meaningful occupation remains in a person's life repertoire" (p. 963). Therefore, it is crucial that occupational scientists study how occupations and their meaning influence performance, or what people choose to actually do in their customary rounds of daily activities. Occupational scientists must also study how occupations are symbolically constituted in the culture. As individuals attempt to make sense of their occupations, the personal interpretations they give are inevitably infused with the cultural meanings they absorb (Bruner, 1990). White (1996) in his analysis of Miles Davis's biography provides an understanding of how a life trajectory unfolds when it is guided by total investment in a single occupation: jazz playing. However, he also illustrates how prevailing cultural narratives about the African American population influenced the way Davis approached and dealt with audiences, music, critics, and record companies. In other words, Davis, in part, assigned meaning to his experiences based on overarching cultural myths and narratives.

Occupations, it seems, are one of the most potent vehicles through which cultural values are sanctioned and should not be underestimated in terms of their power. Although they often appear light and festive, occupations may, in fact, be subtly reinforcing normative practices through their symbolic meaning. Consider, for example, the occupation of going to a baby shower. Baby showers are typically understood as a chance to celebrate the anticipated birth of a baby. It is a time to symbolically and concretely give support to a woman who is in the last month of pregnancy. A time of celebration, it may serve to boost the spirits of the mother just a few weeks before delivery, an impending event of which the mother may be fearful. Thus, symbolically, the event serves the culture by "priming" the mother for a successful birthing. However, on another level, baby showers may be interpreted as subtly sanctioning heterosexuality and, in turn, as symbolically marginalizing those who are not heterosexual. Occupational scientist Jeanne Jackson's study of the occupations of lesbian occupational therapists and lesbian women with disabilities revealed that these respondents often interpreted the meaning of occupations, which are taken for granted in the culture, as powerful vehicles for privileging heterosexuals (Jackson, 1995). As another example of how occupations reinforce social structures, DeVault (1991) has shown how the practice of feeding the family is crucial to constituting families as interacting and bonding units. Finally, in her book, *Age of Innocence*, Edith Wharton (1920/1968) provides a picture of how an elegant dinner party becomes the arena in which 19th century New York society conspires to pressure a countess suspected of adultery to return to Europe. These examples illustrate that although occupations may appear light and innocuous, in fact, when we scratch beneath the surface they may be embedded with meaning that contributes to the preservation of cultural norms, and also they may serve to constitute social structures such as the family.

Occupations are meaningful to individuals in part because they become projects through which people can express emotion. The anthropologist, Renato Rosaldo, quoted John Lennon as saying "Life is what happens while you're making other plans" (Rosaldo, 1993, p. 91). Rosaldo suggests this means that often passion, rather than cognition, impels us to act. Rosaldo, during his field work in Manilla asked an Illongot why he head hunted. The Illongot replied, "It is rage, born of grief" (Rosaldo, p. 1). Only after Rosaldo's wife suddenly died during fieldwork, did Rosaldo feel compelled to write the book *Culture and Truth*. That book was also motivated by grief, and for Rosaldo, the experience demonstrated that emotion often inspires everyday action. Grieving is not limited to the formal cultural ritual of the funeral, but rather, it may continue in its expression through daily occupations. As occupational scientists continue to study the meaning of occupation, they hope to create an understanding of the connection between occupation and emotion. In turn, when occupational therapy practitioners draw from this knowledge, they may be more effective in inspiring patients to invest in occupation, because they are better able to tap the passions that drive it.

Finally, in studying the meaning of occupation, occupational scientists are interested in how one's sense of self emerges out of daily experiences and how those experiences become linked in a meaningful life story. Within the context of occupations, one begins to build an identity. The sculptor J. Seward Johnson, who has immortalized people doing occupations in life-size ultrarealistic bronze sculptures, has stated the following: "In occupational science and its therapeutic application, we know what we do, describes in great part, who we are" (Johnson, 1996, p. 25)(Fig. 2-3). For example, if a teenager spent an abundance of time playing tennis at a country club, she might develop a sense of herself as athletic, hardworking, aggressive, and well-to-do. Beyond this, one wonders how this occupation would eventually fit into her overall life narrative. Did she become an Olympic tennis player, hurt herself on the court and need rehabilitation, or simply give the game up out of disenchantment? When one begins to make sense of one's occupations in relation to an unfolding story, one is involved in the process of narrative configuration. Polkinghorne (1988) suggests:

We achieve our personal identities and self-concept through the use of narrative configuration, and make our existence into a whole by understanding it as an expression of a single unfolding and developing story. We are in the middle of our stories and cannot be sure how they will end; we are constantly having to revise the plot as new events are added to our lives (p. 150).

Clark (1993) and Price-Lackey and Cashman (1996) have published life histories that indicate how the recursive relation between engagement in occupation and meaningful interpretation of it in relation to an unfolding life story became therapeutic for two survivors of catastrophic accidents. These two life histories demonstrate the emergence of the occupational self through childhood, the reemergence of a newly constructed self following traumatic disability, and the centrality of meaningful occupations in the therapeutic process and recovery.

►CONCLUSION

Influenced by the arts and crafts movement, feminism, the mental hygiene movement, pragmatism, and the settlement movement, the founders of occupational therapy possessed a strong belief that engagement in occupation was health promoting. Today, occupational scientists are conducting systematic studies on the form, function, and meaning of occupation. Occupational science promises to nurture occupational therapy by providing a substantive knowledge base that can be applied to treatment. In these days of managed care, professions must demonstrate that their practitioners possess specialized knowledge and skills. Occupational science promises to provide a scientifically validated foundation that will better enable practitioners to serve the public good. As Eliot Friedson (1994) has eloquently stated: "Professionalism entails commitment to a particular body of knowledge and skill. . ., that is to say, commitment to preserve, refine, and elaborate that knowledge. . . [in order] to do good works" (p. 210). We envision that to be effective practitioners, occupational therapists and occupational therapy assistants, in the future, will increasingly draw from knowledge generated in occupational science.

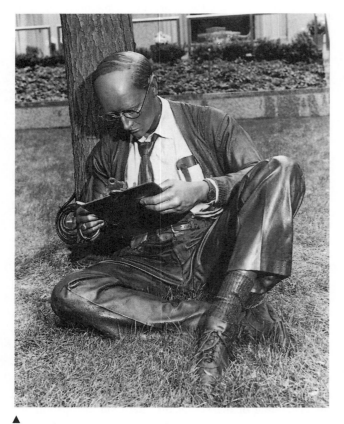

▲
Figure 2-3. Sculptor J. Seward Johnson believes what we do describes, in part, who we are. In this sculpture entitled "Creating" a man is absorbed in a task of obvious significance to him. (Photo courtesy of Sculpture Placement, Ltd., Washington, DC.)

REFERENCES

Addams, J. (1961). *Twenty years at Hull-House: With autobiographical notes.* New York: Signet.

Adelmann, P. K. (1994). Multiple roles and psychological well-being in a national sample of older adults. *Journal of Gerontology: Social Sciences, 49,* 277–288.

Bing, R. K. (1995). Foreword. In M. Quiroga, *Occupational Therapy: The First 30 Years 1900 to 1930* (pp. 1–10). Bethesda, MD: American Occupational Therapy Association.

Breines, E. (1986). *Origins and adaptations: A philosophy of practice.* Lebanon, NJ: Geri-Rehab, Inc.

Brown, P. K. (1922). The problem of our physically handicapped. *Archives of Occupational Therapy, 2,* 171–178.

Bruner, J. (1990). *Acts of meaning.* Cambridge, MA: Harvard University Press.

Carlson, M., & Clark, F. (1991). The search for useful methodologies in occupational science. *American Journal of Occupational Therapy, 45,* 235–241.

Clark, F. (1993). Occupation embedded in a real life: Interweaving occupational science and occupational therapy. *American Journal of Occupational Therapy, 47,* 1067–1078.

Clark, F., & Larson, E. A. (1993). Developing an academic discipline: The science of occupation. In H. Hopkins & H. D. Smith (Eds.), *Willard and Spackman's Occupational Therapy* (8th ed., pp. 44–57). Philadelphia: J. B. Lippincott.

Clark, F., Parham, D., Carlson, M., Frank, G., Jackson, J., Pierce, D., Wolfe, R. J., & Zemke, R. (1991). Occupational science: Academic innovation in the service of occupational therapy's future. *American Journal of Occupational Therapy, 45,* 300–310.

Clarkson-Smith, L., & Hartley, A. A. (1990). The game of bridge as an exercise in working memory and reasoning. *Journal of Gerontology, 45,* 233–238.

DeVault, M. L. (1991). *Feeding the family.* Chicago: University of Chicago Press.

Dunton W. R. (1915). *Occupational therapy: A manual for nurses.* Philadelphia: W. B. Saunders.

Freidson, E. (1994). *Professionalism reborn: Theory, prophecy, and policy.* Chicago: The University of Chicago Press.

Glass, T. A., Seeman, T. E., Herzog, A. R., Kahn, R., & Berkamn, L. F. (1995). *Journal of Gerontology: Social Sciences, 50B,* 65–76.

Herzog, A. R., House, J. S., & Morgan, J. N. (1991). Relation of work and retirement to health and well-being in old age. *Psychology and Aging, 6,* 202–211.

Homans, G. (1967). *The nature of science.* New York: Harbinger.

Jackson, J. M. (1995). *Lesbian identities, daily occupations, and health care experiences.* Unpublished doctoral dissertation, University of Southern California, Los Angeles.

Johnson, J. S. (1996). Realistic expressions: Statements of being. In R. Zemke and F. Clark (Eds.), *Occupational science: The evolving discipline* (pp. 23–25). Philadelphia: F. A. Davis.

Kidner, T. (1922). Work for the tuberculous during and after the cure. *Archives of Occupational Therapy, 1,* 363–377.

Larson, E. A. (1996). *Embracing paradox: The daily experience and subjective well-being of Mexican-origin mothers parenting children with disabilities.* Unpublished doctoral dissertation, University of Southern California, Los Angeles.

Lave, J. (1988). *Cognition in practice.* Cambridge, UK: Cambridge University Press.

Levine, R. (1986). Historical research: Ordering the past to chart our future. *Occupational Therapy Journal of Research, 6* (5), 32–42.

Meyer, A. (1922). Philosophy of occupation therapy. *Archives of Occupational Therapy, 1,* 1–10. (Reprinted in *American Journal of Occupational Therapy, 31,* 639–642, 1977.)

Nazario, S. (1996, June 23). Suburban dreams hit roadblock. *Los Angeles Times,* A1, A26, A27.

Nelson, D. L. (1988). Occupation: Form and performance. *American Journal of Occupational Therapy, 42,* 633-641.

Pierce, D. (1996a). The work on scholars. In R. Zemke and F. Clark (Eds.), *Occupational science: The evolving discipline* (pp. 125–142). Philadelphia: F. A. Davis.

Pierce, D. (1996b). *Conceptualizing infant object play: Development of temporal and spatial negotiation from 1 to 18 months.* Unpublished doctoral dissertation, University of Southern California, Los Angeles.

Polkinghorne, D. (1988). *Narrative knowing and the human sciences.* Albany, NY: SUNY Press.

Pörn, I. (1993). Health and adaptedness. *Theoretical Medicine, 14,* 295-303.

Price-Lackey, P. & Cashman, J. (1996). Jenny's story: Reinventing oneself through occupation and narrative configuration. *American Journal of Occupational Therapy, 50,* 306–313.

Primeau, L. A. (1996). Human daily travel: Personal choices and external constraints. In R. Zemke and F. Clark (Eds.), *Occupational Science: The Evolving Discipline* (pp. 115–124). Philadelphia: F. A. Davis.

Quiroga, V. (1995). *Occupational therapy: The first 30 years 1900 to 1930.* Bethesda, MD: The American Occupational Therapy Association.

Reed, K. L. (1986). Eleanor Clarke Slagle Lecture. Tools of practice: Heritage or baggage? *American Journal of Occupational Therapy, 40,* 597–605.

Rosaldo, R. (1993). *Culture and truth: The remaking of social analyses.* Boston: Beacon Press.

Trombly, C. A. (1995). Occupation: Purposefulness and meaningfulness as therapeutic mechanisms: 1995 Eleanor Clarke Slagle Lecture. *American Journal of Occupational Therapy, 49,* 960–972.

Turner, V. (1987). *The anthropology of performance.* New York: PAJ Publications.

Ulrich, L. T. (1991). *A midwife's tale.* New York: Vintage Books.

University of Southern California, Department of Occupational Therapy. (1989). *Proposal for a doctoral program in occupational science.* Unpublished manuscript.

Wharton, E. (1968). *The age of innocence.* New York: Charles Scribner's & Sons. (Original work published 1920).

White, D. (1991). *Human activity systems and the theory of cultural evolution.* Presented at the annual meeting of the Society for Applied Anthropology, Charleston, SC, March, 1991.

White, J. A. (1996). Miles Davis: Occupations in the extreme. In R. Zemke and F. Clark (Eds.), *Occupational science: The evolving discipline* (pp. 259–273). Philadelphia: F. A. Davis.

Wilcock, A. (1993). A theory of the human need for occupation. *Occupational Science: Australia, 1,* 17–24.

Wood, W. H. (1995). *Environmental influences upon the relationship of engagement in occupation to adaptation among captive chimpanzees.* Unpublished doctoral dissertation, University of Southern California, Los Angeles.

Yerxa, E. J. (1994). Dreams, dilemmas, and decisions for occupational therapy practice in a new millennium: An American perspective. *American Journal of Occupational Therapy, 48,* 586–589.

Yerxa, E., Clark, F., Frank, G., Jackson, J., Parham, D., Pierce, D., Stein, C., & Zemke, R. (1990). An introduction to occupational science: A foundation for occupational therapy in the 21st century. *Occupational Therapy in Health Care, 6,* 1–17.

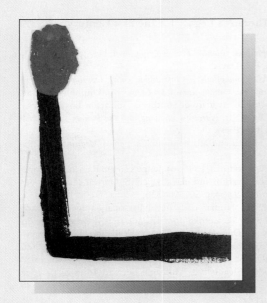

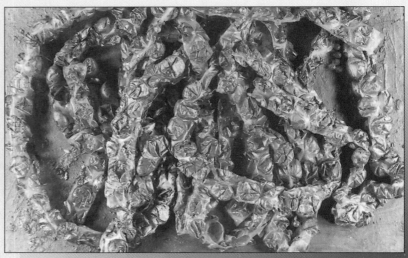

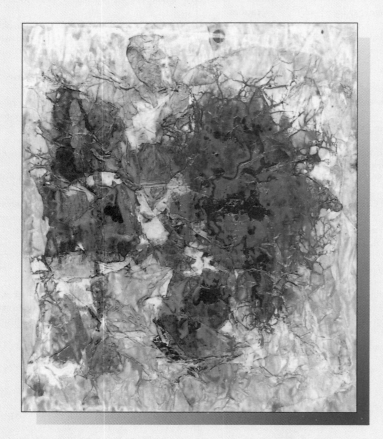

(top) Intersection: *For a long time after the accident I played and replayed the car crash. I painted it—there was the intersection and there was the car I was in—and here was the collision, the smashing of the car and of me.*

(middle) Dimensional brain: *I tried to create the pathways in the brain, what the brain would look like if it was reduced to the pathways.*

(bottom) Red seizure: *I imagined this is what my brain might look or feel like when I had a seizure—that the parts of the brain would dissolve, cease to exist. (Photos courtesy of Mary Feldhaus-Weber.)*

Unit II

Persons Seeking Occupational Therapy

LEARNING OBJECTIVES

After completing this unit, readers will be able to:

▶ Begin to explore the experience of brain injury from the perspective of one person.

▶ Explain the effect of illness or disability on the family.

▶ Explain the effect of illness or disability on occupation.

▶ Define culture and its influence on occupation and occupational therapy intervention.

▶ Define socioeconomic status and the influence of social inequities on occupation and occupational therapy intervention.

▶ Identify themes related to illness experience, culture, and socioeconomic status in Mary Feldhaus Weber's story.

People seek occupational therapy intervention typically because they are unable to carry out tasks and activities that are important to them in their day-to-day lives. The priorities they set in therapy reflect their particular life experiences and circumstances. For example, their family situation, work, socioeconomic, and cultural status, may constrain or facilitate their response to illness and disability. This unit opens with a first-person account of Mary Feldhaus Weber's experience following a **traumatic brain injury**. The chapters that follow address disability experience from the individual and family perspectives as well as the influence of cultural and socioeconomic issues on illness, disability, and occupational performance. These chapters provide the information to assist occupational therapy practitioners in being sensitive to the individuality of each person seen in occupational therapy and to use each person's particular strengths to foster his or her recovery. (*Note*: Words in **bold** type are defined in the Glossary.)

Chapter 3

An Excerpt from *The Book of Sorrows, Book of Dreams: A First Person Narrative*

Mary Feldhaus Weber

▼ EDITORS' PROLOGUE

At the age of 37, Mary Feldhaus Weber was a successful poet, playwright, film maker, and television producer. She had written, directed, or produced many programs for national public television. Her plays had been produced off off Broadway and published. She had just finished making *Joan Robinson: One Woman's Story*, an award-winning documentary film about her friend's 3-year struggle with and death from ovarian cancer. In December 1979, 3 weeks before this film was to be telecast on national public television, Mary was the passenger in a car that was struck on the passenger side by a drunk driver. Mary was taken from the demolished car and rushed to a hospital emergency room. Even though her head had smashed the car window during the accident, she was released from the hospital that very night. Three days later Mary began to have seizures. Months later she was diagnosed as having epilepsy—a seizure disorder—caused by traumatic brain injury. Her brain had been injured when she hit her head during the car accident. She was never hospitalized for this traumatic injury. Her seizures have never been well controlled with medication, and she has not been able to return to work.

What follows is the story of Mary's struggle to live with the effects of her brain injury and seizure disorder—in her own words. This excerpt was taken from her book in progress, *The Book of Sorrows, Book of Dreams*. The first part of the story covers the years 1979 to 1981. Mary dictated this part of her story to friends and occupational therapy students who were working with her. She says this writing would not have occurred without the help of her friends and the occupational therapy students because she was not

able to write at that time. The Epilogue is set in 1996. Mary was able to write this part of her story by herself.

▼ 1979 TO 1981

The Accident

A friend and I were driving home at 3 am after working on the "Joan Robinson" film, getting it ready for its national air date. A large American car, going at a high rate of speed, hit the small foreign car I was in, on the passenger side (I was the passenger). The car I was in was hit with such intensity that both cars were demolished, totaled. My head went through the passenger window sideways. The side of my head above the temple totally shattered the glass, hit with such impact that every piece of glass had been knocked out. People in the emergency room were astonished that I had no facial cuts. I told them my hard Scandinavian head was harder than glass—like stone or a diamond, I said at the time.

I can remember the car lights coming at us. I can remember the sense that we could not get out of the way. I can remember shouting to my friend, "watch out," and then the impact of the car. But strangely, when the car hit, I had the sense that it had not really hit me or the car I was in, that there had been a buffer that was made of time and space, was eternal, and does not break, a shield.

I was also sure that the driver of my car, my beloved friend Sally Schreiber-Cohn, had reached out way around at the moment of impact and shielded me with her own body. I was absolutely sure this had happened. When I asked her at the hospital, she said, "Oh no, I kept both hands on the wheel, of course." I told her I experienced some kind of shielding protection at impact. If the other car had hit a few inches further back, I probably would have been decapitated. But, it hit where it hit. All the damage has been inside my brain.

One doctor described it as if someone were to have taken jello, the consistency of the brain, and thrown it at a wall as hard as one could. That's how hard the brain hit one side of the skull, and then ricocheted back and hit the other side of the skull, leaving me with right and left side brain injuries. Even though only one side of my head hit the window, both sides of my brain are damaged.

Six Months After the Accident

Six months after the accident when I started to have more and more seizures, it became clear that I could no longer live alone and so I had to ask my mother to come from South Dakota to stay with me. I did this with great reluctance because she was 78 and my father wanted her there, taking care of him. When she got here, the thing I remember her saying was that she hadn't realized it had been so bad. Why hadn't I called her sooner? This was the time before the seizures were under any kind of control at all, which is to say, I was very sick.

I sat in the corner day after day, noticing that it was light or dark, noticing that my mother was busy, or sleeping, or crying, noticing that sometimes the phone rang, or that it was the day to see the doctor, noticing that sometimes I had pain in my head. My mother said, "I wonder if a cold wet towel on your head would help?" I think we both remembered that if a horse sprains its leg, you wrap its leg in towels. And so mother would get wet towels from the bathroom and wrap them around my head, my brain becoming like a sprained leg, a muscle that wasn't working. Cramped and tense. Convulsing. Filled with fear.

And then because things change and time moves on, the pain would stop, and I would become briefly aware that the couch cover was blue, or that the dog had been rolling in the dust, or that mother wanted to fix soup for lunch.

And we discovered that after I had a seizure, or as one doctor called them "spells," I didn't have the coordination, or was too confused, to drink soup or hold a spoon. Because mother liked soup so much, we seemed to try this many times, larger spoons, smaller spoons, bigger cups, smaller cups. It was decided that tomato soup was the easiest. Why, I'm not sure. Finally, I told mother I did not like soup and had not for years. Therefore could we try something else?

At this time, I was having constant seizures. There was no time that I was not either having one, getting ready to have one, feeling "spacey," with a strong metallic taste in my mouth, or feeling confused and disoriented after having had one. I felt like the seizures were a powerful force outside of me that suddenly grabbed my brain, me, the essence of me, and with the kind of fury of winds, blizzards, and driving

rain, held me under ice. While the me that was present could breathe the water under the ice, I knew I was caught, forced to be there. I knew if I struggled even slightly, the pain, the terror, became worse. And for the time the active seizure was roaring on inside me, I had to concentrate on total stillness until the fury dissipated and I was released.

All of the drive, the tenacity, the ambition, the creativity, all of the things that had made me who I was did not help in this place. I was terrified, and I was alone. I no longer knew the words to ask or tell anyone what I was living through. I could just sense what hurt, and it hurt less to be absolutely still until the force chose to release me. I had no control of when it seized me or when it chose to release me.

My friend, Sally, tells me now that looking at me was like watching a candle about to go out. It seemed to her that only 3 percent of me was left.

I felt that I was being annihilated. The me that I had become, lived with, was ceasing to be over and over and over again. It occurred to me that this was what it felt like to die and, for whatever reason, I was dying again and again.

One Year After the Accident

My mother had to return to South Dakota, so I was living alone. One day at the doctor's office, a year after the accident and when I was still in a fog, I noticed the doctor's tie. It was a bright, clear yellow Marimeco tie. I stared at the color yellow, and it was the first thing to make sense to me since the accident. I understood what I was seeing. The color yellow. The fog lifted for a minute. I understood something, and I had not had to struggle to understand it. I can remember thinking, I am going to be all right.

When I got home that day someone got me a set of poster paints and I painted a small, bright, vivid, yellow daisy (Fig. 3-1). And I started painting.

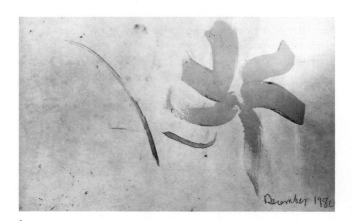

▲

Figure 3-1. Daisy: One year after the accident I painted this modest yellow daisy. I had never studied painting, but I knew I had to fight to work or I would be lost. The color of the daisy was the color of my neurologist's tie (Photo courtesy of Mary Feldhaus-Weber.)

When I began painting I was surprised to find that it didn't turn out so badly; the people who came and went who saw the paintings, were very kind, even effusive about them. I wasn't sure I believed what they were saying. I had an idea that they were just trying to be nice. Or, worse yet, felt sorry for me and were trying to be kind.

Painting was, however, one thing I could do all by myself, whether anyone was there or not. It didn't matter if I was spacey or sick. I could just lay down the piece of paper I was working on and continue again after the spell had come and gone.

Some days I did as many as ten paintings working with acrylic paint, wet tissue paper, and poster paints. Because I was interested in the color and shapes of things and had no training in drawing, it was all abstraction-representational. I was interested, however, in drawing brains and in trying to paint the experience of seizures, which I did over and over again (Fig. 3-2).

In a strange kind of way it was like having an artist's model for myself, not a model I could see, but a model which was myself, an internal experience that I then tried to translate into color. The painting gave me something to do and something to talk about other than myself. Something to talk about when people came to the house. It was a relief to have something to show someone, to have them look at pieces of paper, not to look at me. It also gave me a way to try to talk about what I was living through.

It was hard work to concentrate on what I was doing. Part of me hoped that the paintings weren't pitiful, because of all the things I did not want to be, to be pitied seemed the very worst. I was also aware that I had to start from scratch with painting, that I had developed such expertise in film making, that I had literally been able to make film do anything I wanted to.

I had reached a place in my career where I had control over my art, and now I had to struggle to squeeze the paint tubes. I was at the very beginning and grateful to be there.

Two Years After the Accident

I had no real picture of what happened to my brain, to me. I spent a great deal of time thinking about it. Trying to think about it.

I had listened to explanations from doctors, nurses, social workers, and none of them had made sense. All I knew was that I was unable to do the simplest thing, make a bed, tell time, count. Add or subtract. Recognize faces. Tell right from left. Read. Understand what people said to me. Remember things. And perhaps worst of all I did not feel like myself, like "me." I felt like someone, but not like any one I knew. I was a stranger to myself. **I** was lost (Fig. 3-3).

On days that I had constant seizures I had to ask my friend Sally to come and stay with me. It was at these times we were aware that I was not getting better, in fact I was barely hanging on.

The everyday litany was long and grim: I fell all the time, I was covered with black and blue marks everywhere. I would come to from a seizure to find that I had bitten the inside of my mouth and was bleeding and had a shard of my broken front tooth sticking out of my bottom lip. Some-

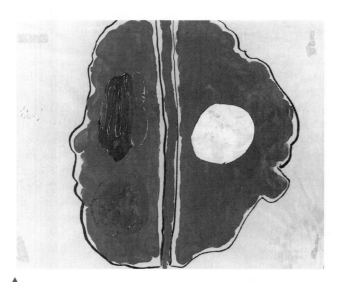

Figure 3-2. Damaged brain: I tried to explain to myself what my damaged brain looked like—where the damage was. In this painting, done when I was still very sick, I painted a brain that had damage on both sides. Several years later when I had MRIs (brain scans) done, indeed my brain was damaged on both sides (Photo courtesy of Mary Feldhaus-Weber.)

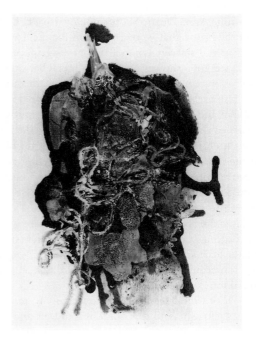

Figure 3-3. Self-portrait: The tiny knob on the top was my head. I felt I had ceased to have intelligence, a head. I was just a confused body (Photo courtesy of Mary Feldhaus-Weber.)

times I would put my finger in my eyes during a seizure, and the eye would be red and swollen for days. I hit my head. I broke my elbow. It did not seem safe for me to live alone.

I had lost my income when my film company closed after the accident and I had lost my health insurance with it. Because of these factors my only option would have been to go on welfare and go into a nursing home. My neurologist felt that if I did that I would likely never come out. I think he had seen too many people become institutionalized. In other words, they had become helpless and had given up.

I still had some small fight left in me; I had been a functional, successful adult. The 3 percent of me that was left was 3 percent of a fighter. We were all counting on the fact that I would keep fighting and I would get better. That somehow I would manage. I also knew I desperately needed someone to help me help myself.

Finally, more than 2 years after the accident, we found someone to help me. Sally had called a therapist friend who said she did know someone who was a gifted occupational therapist and liked dogs. And who was kind. When Sally called the occupational therapist—Anna Deane Scott—she said that she knew very little about head injury. She was a professor at Boston University and the coauthor of a famous occupational therapy textbook and, yes, she did like dogs. She agreed to come to my house to meet me.

When she first met me Anna Deane told me later that I was sitting in the dark on a couch, crying. We talked; she admired my dogs and told me about her own dog. After she left I called her to ask what she thought of the meeting. I was afraid that she might have felt I was beyond help. I asked her how she felt about meeting me. Anna Deane said "I felt sad." I knew I could trust her.

Every time Anna Deane Scott came over we talked about things in the house that were a problem for me. I was afraid of falling in the shower when I was getting spacey from a seizure, so we got a shower chair and a metal bar on the wall and rubber rugs inside the tub and outside the tub. Each one of these areas we worked on took months to identify the problem and with trial and error find the solutions. But in the case of the shower, finally I was able to take a shower and I was no longer afraid. I was also afraid of burning myself on the flames of my gas stove if I was feeling confused, so we got a large electric hot plate and I could heat something up without being afraid of lighting myself or my clothes on fire.

I had lost the ability to do things; I knew there were steps to take to do any task, but I had no idea which step came first. I later learned that I had lost the ability to sequence, a loss that sometimes occurs when you have had an injury to the frontal lobe of the brain.

Anna Deane and I set out to discover how to teach me to do things again. She said that there was always another way to do something. First we had to find out how I was still able to learn. You will notice when I speak of Anna Deane and myself I always say WE did this, WE decided that. Unlike other health professionals, Anna Deane felt her role was not to tell me what to do, but to work with me, to empower me. She asked me constantly what was important to me. What did I think of something. What did I want to do. And she LISTENED to me. Extraordinary!

One problem in my life was how to unlock my front door. My house has two doors, an outside door and an inner door, and therefore I have two different keys. If someone would bring me home from the doctor's office, one of the few places that I went, I would often try to get the key in the lock and not be able to. I would try to unlock the door for what felt like hours, over and over again. Desperately trying to get into my own house.

I asked whoever dropped me off to see that I got into the house before they drove off. Often they would have to open the door for me. I felt stupid, unable to do the simplest thing.

Anna Deane watched me try to get into the house and said she understood what the problem was. She said when I couldn't get in the outside door with one key, that I should *try the other key*. It had not occurred to me to try the other key. I would stand endlessly with the wrong key doing it over and over again, but when I had this new strategy, it freed me to get into my own house, and each time I opened the door myself it was such a victory. And I began to feel hope for myself.

Anna Deane and I discovered that while it was impossible for me to just follow or understand verbal directions, if I could also watch someone do a task, listen to the directions, even place my hands on the things at the same time, I could after a number of tries, do it again myself.

Anna Deane said we could not be sure which parts of my brain were still working, but we had the best chance for success if we used as many senses as possible, hoping we could tap into the areas in my brain that still functioned. When Anna Deane first said this it sounded like the most primitive kind of investigation into unknown territories, all of which were inside me. We were searching for the me that was still there. But she was right. With Anna Deane's help I have learned to do everything [day-to-day self-maintenance activities] over again. Absolutely everything. It is not too strong to say that she gave me my life back.

Another thing that Anna Deane and I worked on was a chart that monitored my daily activities. One of the problems was that I had lost any sense of time. With epilepsy it is important that you take a certain amount of pills, at a certain time every day. It's very simple—if you don't, the seizures come back. You also have to eat and rest regularly in relationship to taking the pills, and before I met Anna Deane, I could not remember if I'd taken a pill, had lunch, let the dogs out; I couldn't tell if it were afternoon or morning, or what day it was.

Gradually, over a period of months and many failures, we worked out a chart on a magnetic blackboard that we divided into morning, afternoon, and evening. We used different colored magnets for different parts of the day, as we discovered that I could understand colors better than words.

For every victory, such as the discovery that I still remembered colors, there were dozens of defeats.

Anna Deane said over and over that there was always another way to do something. We just had to find the other way. And every time we failed she learned that much more about my brain, what still worked and how it was working. She said there was no such thing as a "failure." She learned something each time we tried something new.

I, on the other hand, felt the failures very keenly. Because I had been quick and life had come easily to me, I was not used to trying and failing at something simple again and again and again. The things we were trying to do, like a system to get me to remember to take my pills, were both very simple and very important. I was impatient with myself and judged myself by who I had been. For each failure I shed many tears.

I tried not to cry in front of Anna Deane. My dogs, Desmond and Todd, listened to my crying. I would go to pet them and their fur would be wet. I would be puzzled at first and then remembered I had been crying. And they had been sitting beside me on the couch, wet with my tears.

Anna Deane said that I was doing what I needed to do, grieving over my losses. I had lost a great deal. And that if one didn't grieve and let the past go, it was harder to do new things. That grief could stand in the way of progress. But on the other hand I also needed to look to the balance of things. I needed to find things that still made me happy, gave me pleasure. It became my job each day to do one thing that gave me pleasure. This sometimes was as hard to do as the task of grieving. It became obvious to me that the two were connected.

So we refined the magnetic board system further: colored magnets for each time of day, further divided into "take pill;" "have lunch;" "feed dogs;" etc. When the activity had been completed I moved the magnet from the *not-done* category to the *done* category. The chart is large and colorful and I can look at it from across the room and tell what I've done and what I haven't done yet, and how I'm doing. . . and so, eventually, time and memory seemed somewhat under my control again.

Anna Deane came to my house every week for an hour and we talked on the phone a number of times between the visits. In the year that I worked with her I could see small changes in my life and as I got greater control over the details of my life again, the person who I had been started to reemerge. I wasn't making films, but I could change the sheets on my bed. I wasn't writing poetry, but I could dress myself. These may seem like small things, but with each skill I regained I could feel life flowing back into me again.

Another triumph that stands out was the ability to get in and out of buildings. There are many buildings in Boston where you have to buzz the company or office that you are going to, and then they buzz you back and the door opens. I was no more able to decipher this than the Rosetta Stone. It was impossibly complex for me and therefore overwhelming, and therefore tear-producing, and therefore one more thing that I couldn't do.

Anna Deane and I talked about every possible kind of solution and came up with one that worked. The solution was: To stand and watch until someone else came along and pushed a button and got in the door; watch how they did it; and either go in with them or do the same thing they did. And it worked.

In large buildings it's still a problem finding the correct office if I haven't been there before because in the elevator I am not able to understand if 5 is the same as 7 is the same as 9 when the elevator opens. So, I have been lost in the best hospitals in Boston. The people that have taken me went to park their car and against their better judgment let me out, me telling them not to worry about it, that I would meet them at the office. And then, 45 minutes later when I did not show up at the office, and it became clear that there was

---

HISTORICAL NOTE

THE POWER OF PATIENTS IN SHAPING THERAPY: THE STORY OF CLIFFORD BEERS

Suzanne M. Peloquin

Clifford Beers, a patient admitted for depression to three mental institutions between 1900 and 1905, framed an articulate plea for reform. In his book, *A Mind That Found Itself*, Beers (1917) used his own experiences to promote change: "For one year no further attention was paid to me than to see that I had three meals a day, the requisite number of baths, and a sufficient amount of exercise" (p. 68). He described his struggle to get simple materials, such as a book or paper and pencil, items with which he might occupy himself. After he finally procured these, Beers felt that his reading, writing, and drawing led to his cure. He argued that occupation held healing potential for others. He started the National Committee for Mental Hygiene, and through this group, advocated many hospital changes, including the use of occupation and recreation.

This story shows us the power of occupation, but also shows that persons can shape their destinies and the therapies of their culture. If we stay mindful of the experience of Beers, we might more readily see the strength that dwells in the persons who seek our therapy. ■

Beers, C. W. (1917). *A mind that found itself.* New York: Longmans, Green.

a problem, various people would be sent to find me. For my part, I would be asking people if this was the fourth floor, etc., etc.

Among the least helpful people to give this kind of simple directions are doctors, nurses, or anyone else from "The Allied Health Professions." Among the most helpful, of course, are the other patients, and all the cleaning and maintenance people. However, Anna Deane and I have not figured a way around this problem. A way to make me independent, to do it all on my own. It is still, sadly, something that makes me cry.

With Anna Deane's help I listened to talking books for reading, used a calculator to add and subtract, told time with a digital clock, asked people to take me places and not just give me directions, used the brightly colored arrows that told me which way to turn the thermostat to heat my house, and turned on the water faucets in the shower. In other words, many victories. And more to come.

Sometimes people ask me what kind of fee Anna Deane charged me for this amount of work, of devotion. The answer is—not one cent. She told me she did not know enough about head injury to charge for her services, it was a learning experience for her too. And, she did not say it, but I knew she knew I did not have a cent to my name.

▼ EPILOGUE: MAY 1996, SIXTEEN YEARS AFTER THE CAR ACCIDENT

How am I now? I was told that if a function did not come back after a year it would not come back. They were wrong about this in some cases. I have continued to regain things over a period of 12 years. I can discriminate between right and left again, I am much better at recognizing faces—not perfect, but better. I can understand poetry and most abstractions again. I regained my sense of smell. I can read a bit if the print is big. I can write again.

I still can't count. I still can't do multiplication tables, or months of the year. I still see double out of one eye. I still have to sit and think a long time about what steps go into a task like putting the laundry in the washing machine and what order those steps should take. I still have balance problems. I still have a lot of seizures—several a day most of the time. I have learned to live with these things—the things that are lost to me and the things that have come back but are different.

I had a battery of [neuropsychological] tests done on me recently and I still do badly on a number of them. You are reading the writing of someone who now has an IQ still considerably under 100.

I was surprised how many strong feelings I had when I started to answer the simple sounding question—how are you? First of all, it is not until I started to get better that I realized how much I had lost. Before that I was too sick or too overwhelmed to notice, to understand the breadth of the loss.

In broad strokes, I lost 10 years of my life where I almost ceased to exist. And I still grieve over that loss; some days it feels like a very big loss, other days it doesn't.

So how am I now? I am doing better without having gotten better. In other words, I learned to do a lot of things in new ways just as Anna Deane Scott, the occupational therapist who worked with me, said I would—tell time with a digital clock, read with talking books, write with a large screen, large print computer.

I feel like myself again. I am happy most of the time. . . in fact I seem to be one of the more happy and contented people I know. I have become grateful for things large and small. I am more appreciative of other people. In fact, I think we should all gets stars and blue birds for getting up in the morning.

The head injury has forced me to look at myself. Look at all the sad, angry parts of me that I did not consider when I was a hotshot television producer. I was too busy working 18-hour days. Being very busy in a high visibility job can be seductive. What you are doing seems so important that you can easily push everything else into a corner. But when you are sitting home, day after day, when the phone isn't ringing off the hook, it is less possible to ignore things.

Being head injured has given me time to look at who I was, how I got there, and to ask myself what I want to do about it. Counseling also helped me to survive the many assaults to the spirit that can occur when you are forced to endlessly deal with health care providers. Being a patient can be a grueling life.

I know this will seem strange, it seems strange to me even as I write it down. There is a belief that if you have some sense like sight taken away your hearing becomes more acute to compensate. In order to understand my own suffering, I have come to better understand the suffering of others.

I also laugh more, am made happy more easily. I am much more at ease with myself. I feel quite literally that I walked and walked and walked through the valley of the shadow of death, stumbling, crying, falling, breaking bones, and finally came out on the other side. When asked about the head injury, I tell people I would not wish it on my worst enemy. Yet strangely, I am also grateful for the journey.

▼ POSTSCRIPT: THOUGHTS FOR OCCUPATIONAL THERAPY PRACTITIONERS

One more thought I want to share with you. I have spent a lot of time thinking about what "helps" in the kind of situation I have been in with my head injury. Why could some people get through to me and not others? Why did some people comfort and heal me and other seemingly well-meaning people shame or humiliate me? In other words, what works, what heals? What helps?

I discovered that power is at the heart of living with an injury, and power is at the heart of getting better. Many of us, particularly women, don't think of ourselves as having power. It is just a word, not something we own or think much about. Yet power is the ability to make things happen.

When I was at my most diminished it felt like everyone was more powerful than I was. From the secretary in the doctor's office who had to take the time to push the right elevator button for me to the cab driver I had to trust to count the money I gave him and give me back the correct change because I could not count. The people who had to show me to the rest room when I was not capable of finding it. The doctors who filled out the insurance forms documenting my disability so I would get disability payments to live on. It was a very long list and I was at the bottom. I had to depend on everyone.

Because of the power issues (who has it, who wants it, who needs it, who can share it), I think it is important to check why you are going into the healing professions. Ask yourself tough questions and keep asking them. Questions like, "What do I get out of this work?" "How does this situation make me feel about myself?" "Do I need to have things in black and white or can I bear the uncertainty of all the shades of gray that illness and sorrow present us with?" "Can I trust people, however damaged, to know what is best for themselves?"

So the question I am asking you is this—can you give over power to another person? Can you honor their own wishes, dreams, abilities? Can you be as interested in their abilities as you are in their disabilities? Can you give them the tools to get their own lives back on track?

And do you listen to people? Do you HEAR what they are telling you? I believe that we are far wiser than we give ourselves or each other credit for.

So I am telling you that the two most important things you can do as occupational therapy practitioners are to listen and to empower. The people who helped me the most did both of those things. I continue to bless them and to use what they have taught me every day.

You have chosen a profession that helps, restores, teaches, and gives comfort. Some of the finest human beings I have ever met are occupational therapy practitioners.

You speak for us, the people you serve. You are in our corner.

▶ EDITORS' COMMENT

Mary's story eloquently illustrates concepts we need to think about for all of our clients' stories—the illness experience and the influences of illness, cultural systems, socioeconomic systems, and nonhuman environments on occupation. Think about Mary's story as you read the following chapters about these concepts.

Chapter 4

The Illness and Disability Experience from an Individual Perspective

David W. Beer

In this chapter I consider the perspectives of occupational therapy practitioner and client as healer and sufferer, respectively. I am interested to draw out some of the dimensions of this difference, because as occupational therapy practitioners our understanding of the sufferer's point of view has significant implications for our capacity to engage him or her in meaningful activities. Yet there are characteristics of the roles and experience of practitioners and clients that tend to separate their perspectives. A practitioner has a professional understanding of the body and the person that is based on training which the client, generally, does not have. How many clients, for instance, have actually seen and handled the muscles, tendons, and ligaments of the human arm? Also, many practitioners work in settings that encourage them to restrict their view of clients, reducing them to characteristics directly linked to their afflictions or deficits as exemplars of a disease or syndrome. These settings, and the payment systems that support them, measure client progress (and practitioner effectiveness) against changes in such decontextualized characteristics.

Illness experience, however, is particular to the afflicted person and the world(s) in which he or she lives. An **illness** initially interferes with, and later becomes intertwined with, a particular life, complicating particular relationships, interfering with particular pleasures and activities, requiring particular adaptations and, ultimately, coming to have original significance for a particular person. The generalizing and reducing tendencies of what Arthur Frank calls "disease talk" (Frank 1991, pp. 12–15) run counter to development of relationships and understandings out of which can develop a partnership centered on activities that are meaningful to the client. In approaching this topic I shall explore the perspectives of occupational therapy practitioner and client through use of constructs that have gained acceptance in anthropological and sociological studies of practitioner and patient or client experiences, including illness and **disease**, sickness, deviance, **liminality**, and **explanatory models**.

▼ ILLNESS AND DISEASE

Over the past quarter century, medical sociology and anthropology have suggested a conceptual distinction between **illness** and **disease**, intended to describe the contrast between the perspectives of patients and healing professionals, and to place those differing perspectives in their appropriate social and cultural contexts (eg, Kleinman, Eisenberg, & Good, 1978; Frankenberg, 1980). This contrast is a useful one, although potentially problematic (see Hahn, 1984). It reminds us that the perceptions and understandings of this aspect of human experience are positioned—that is, they partly depend on the social and cultural location of the perceiver.

Among other things, this implies that the perceptions of neither client nor healer are completely consistent with reality, meaning with bias- and prejudice-free understandings of the world. Both are influenced by who holds them, why they hold them, what they plan to do with the information, and other concerns. The following conversation, recounted by Arthur Kleinman, is useful in illustrating this point. Mrs. Lawler, who has had psoriasis for some time, has come to consult with Dr. Jones, who is reported to be an expert in administering a new treatment for psoriasis:

Dr. Jones: How long have you had psoriasis?
Mrs. Lawler: Oh, about 15 years.
Dr. Jones: Where did it begin?
Mrs. Lawler: I was in college, under lots of pressure from ex-

ams, and there is a family history of skin problems. It was winter and I was wearing heavy woolen sweaters that seemed to bother my skin. My diet was. . .

Dr. Jones: No, No! I meant where on your skin did you first notice plaques?

Mrs. Lawler: My shoulders and knees. But I had a problem for some time with my scalp that I never...

Dr. Jones: How has it progressed the past few years?

Mrs. Lawler: These have been difficult years. I mean I have been under great stress at work and in my personal life. I...

Dr. Jones: I meant, how has your skin problem progressed? (Kleinman, 1988, pp. 128–129)

As shown in their conversation, Mrs. Lawler and Dr. Jones take substantially different views of psoriasis. Mrs. Lawler thinks of psoriasis as she experiences it—as integrated into her ongoing life experience. She locates its beginnings in life events and situations—college, examinations, a family history of skin troubles, winter and scratchy sweaters, diet. She remembers that it was preceded by a scalp problem. She describes its progress in terms of its effect on her life, adding to already significant stress at work and in her personal life.

Dr. Jones thinks of psoriasis as a skin condition that afflicts many people. Psoriasis can be subdivided into different types, each of which has certain causes, follows a certain course, and shares certain characteristics. He wants to know when the first plaques appeared, how far and how rapidly the psoriasis has spread. All of this will help Dr. Jones know what variety of psoriasis Mrs. Lawler has contracted and whether the new treatment will help.

Mrs. Lawler's understanding of psoriasis is personal. Psoriatic plaques, peeling, itching, and skin disfiguration have become a painful part of the last 15 years of Mrs. Lawler's life, causing her both physical and social suffering. Thinking about psoriasis without thinking about the events and experiences of her life with which it is associated would be impossible. Dr. Jones, on the other hand, must determine whether the psoriasis experienced by Mrs. Lawler is amenable to the new treatment. He must compare certain nonexperiential characteristics of her sickness (eg, length of time she has suffered, which parts of the body are affected) with those of other patients to know which category of psoriasis this is. Because he is acting as a dermatologist, Dr. Jones ignores much of the personal detail of Mrs. Lawler's story. It is not that he does not care about her, it is that he has a different job to do. He is to attack psoriasis itself, located in the body of Mrs. Lawler. Whereas Mrs. Lawler may not easily be able to separate her body, her self, and her life, Dr. Jones does so as a matter of course. For Dr. Jones, Mrs. Lawler's body is not an inseparable part of who she is and how she travels through her world, it is simply the battleground on which he will fight the war against psoriasis.

We construe the terms disease and illness to refer to the perspectives of the professional healer (in this example, the physician) and the patient, respectively. Which perspective is correct? Should we believe Mrs. Lawler or Dr. Jones? Both accounts can be correct. Mrs. Lawler might very well accept Dr. Jones's entire explanation, and likely would approve of the way Dr. Jones uses his account of psoriasis in determining whether and how to treat her. But Mrs. Lawler would never state that Dr. Jones's account explained her experience of psoriasis.

It is important to emphasize just what it is that the patient and professional perspectives are about. Some accounts suggest that the physician perspective is about reality and the client perspective is about perception, equating the former with hard science and the latter with emotion. A perspective which seems sounder is that outlined by Hahn (1984), in which some form of suffering or disorder is the common denominator in all therapeutic exchanges, and different parties to the suffering or disorder draw upon different sets of ideas and interests, or ideologies, to generate an appropriate explanation for and response to the suffering. In Hahn's conceptualization, illness and disease correspond to the patient and physician views about suffering or disorder.

Occupational therapy practitioners, who often find themselves acting as brokers between physicians and clients, will find in Hahn's conceptualization room for a third point of view concerning the challenges confronted by a given client. Joan Rogers (1982) suggested that much of the difference in viewpoint between medicine and occupational therapy stems from their differential understandings of order and disorder. Medicine uses the presence or absence of disease and functional deficit as the basis for perceiving the presence of order or disorder. Occupational therapy, on the other hand, bases its understanding of order and disorder on the occupational performance of the person in question. Occupational performance may be affected by active pathologies, or it may be diminished by capacity changes that are part of normal development. Performance occurs in normal life **contexts**, not just in clinical settings isolated from regular activity. Performance problems often can only be detected in natural settings; they can seldom be well understood without reference to such settings. A person may have a disease or functional deficit without experiencing disruptions in occupational performance. Likewise, a person may experience a disruption in occupational performance without any disease or functional deficit (Rogers, 1982).

Rogers' (1982) distinction between and among types of order and disorder provides a way to distinguish the practice paradigm of occupational therapy from that of medicine. By itself, however, it does not guarantee that the occupational therapy practitioner will adopt a stance in treatment that includes the client perspective. Occupational therapy practitioners, similar to other therapeutic professionals, are prone to fail to take the client's perspective seriously. This tendency is related to society's view that occupational performance-related disorders are forms of social deviance, and occupational therapy intervention is part of society's effort to control such disorder.

▼ SICKNESS, RECOVERY, LIMINALITY, AND EXPERIENCE

Deviance became an explicit part of formal sociological thought about disease and illness with the work of Talcott Parsons (eg, Parsons, 1951). Parsons noted that persons experiencing illness do not perform their assigned roles in a normal fashion, and that, under certain circumstances, there seems to be social acceptance for this deviation from the norm. Parsons termed this situation or condition sickness. When people contract disease, they are exempted, temporarily, from their normal social roles. They may stay home from work, miss class, or in other ways avoid normal role behaviors. They are not, however, role-free. Instead, sick persons take the sick role, meaning that they are expected to conduct themselves in a way such that they alleviate the conditions that exempt them from normal activity. If one breaks a bone, he or she must have it set and wear a cast. If someone suffers from exhaustion, he or she must rest. In many cases people must seek the advice of physicians and other health care professionals, and they must follow that advice. The sick role is temporary; it obtains under the presumption that the condition that has forced the person out of his or her normal roles will last only a short time. That condition is itself a kind of deviation from the norm (health), and the person is bound by social convention to do whatever is required to alleviate it. In fact, it is the correction of this deviance (sickness) that leads society to permit taking on the sick role, a deviation from the normal performance of social roles. Once the condition has been alleviated, the person, it is assumed, will resume his or her normal roles and activities.

It will be clear to the reader, on reflection, that in our society, the notions of sickness and sick role are related to the notion of disease. I am entitled to take sick leave, and receive sick pay covered by sick days, provided either I have something wrong with me that is rooted in a disease, or I am pursuing medical advice about a complaint that may, ultimately, turn out to be rooted in a disease. Under some rules, I am permitted to take sick leave to assist with the care of a family member who is suffering from the aforementioned conditions. Nearly always, when there is a dispute, it is the word of a physician that is considered to be the ultimate authority on whether taking sick days is a legitimate response to what ails *me*.

Our need to regulate sickness, to prescribe a role for those who become ill, and to regulate who can and cannot enter into that role, suggests a further assumption embedded in the sick role: that sickness is a form of deviance. In this view, participation in activities socially assigned to a particular period of life—school for children, work for adults—constitutes normal activity. Sickness, which excuses one from such activities, is a form of social deviance; hence, it must be carefully regulated. Disease, which causes the condition of sickness, is itself a deviation from health. Fighting or working to alleviate disease is the major justification for the sick role.

Occupational therapy practitioners, however, treat many clients who are not going to get better. Because these clients will not, ultimately, be "cured," the sick role and its associated model of social deviance, do not really apply. They may experience release from social roles to attend to their rehabilitation, but the resumption of these roles, especially for someone with severe disability or chronic illness, may remain a question. Whether and if so, how and when, they will resume these roles becomes the object of their rehabilitative process—and the focus of much of occupational therapy intervention. This is also the experience of clients recovering from such unpredictable diseases as cancer. Arthur Frank describes his permanent membership in what he calls the "remission society," a category of people joined by the common knowledge that one telephone call can return them instantly to the tunnel of treatment and uncertainty that the reappearance of cancer cells occasions (Frank, 1991). One cannot, he suggests, go back to the way things were before one developed cancer. One's life has been permanently changed. What is normal for such a person has been transformed.

These considerations suggest that we need to rethink the nature of the experience of disablement. Robert Murphy suggests that his experience of being physically disabled, "neither sick nor well, neither dead nor fully alive, neither out of society nor wholly in it" is more like a state of permanent liminality than a temporary state of sickness (Murphy, 1990, p. 131).

The notion of liminality is drawn from the writings of anthropologists who study rites of passage, rituals that mark the movement of persons from one status to another (eg, from child to adult). Such rituals mark not only changes in status, but also are considered to be transformative. The Christian ritual of baptism, for instance, not only symbolizes acceptance of certain beliefs, but is also felt to cleanse the soul of the baptized person. The anthropologist Victor Turner observed that such rituals first separate participants from their roles in social life. While participants are separated from their former roles, they undergo transformation through instruction, endowment, surgery, pronouncement, covenant, or magic. Following their transformation, they emerge from their separation and are reintegrated into society, as persons with a new status (Turner, 1967).

For instance, the bride and groom, before their wedding, separate from the rest of the world by changing clothes, by preparing in isolation from one another, by occupying certain spaces. Then, when it is time for the ceremony, they stand together before a ritual officiant who is vested with the capacity to make their covenant to live together legally recognized, who evokes promises and intentions from them and pronounces them "man and wife." Once this transformation from being unmarried to being married, from being unrelated to being legally bound has occurred, the man and woman become a legally recognized family, meaning, among other things, that their future offspring will be considered the legal heirs of both members of this couple. The new husband and wife emerge from the sacred edifice, home, or courthouse into the world, often to a celebration during which they eat, drink, dance, and engage in other forms of social intercourse with family and friends. Then, finally they retire together to their home, enacting for the first time, their new status in society as married partners.

During the time when persons are undergoing change in status, they belong neither to their former nor their future status. They are liminal because they are betwixt and between social roles. During this time they are, in many rituals, considered dangerous to normal persons because of their liminality. But the promise exists that they will be, when all is said and done, reintegrated into society, occupying or enacting a new role, holding a new status, carrying on social life as before. With many disabled persons, such reintegration never occurs. They seem dangerous to those nonafflicted persons Goffman (1963) called "normals," precisely because they are physically or psychosocially anomalous. They are not sick, not well, neither dead, nor fully alive. They embody disorder. They are never recovered, can never return to the way things used to be.

> The disabled person fits into the mold of liminality far better than into the model of social deviance followed by sociologists. Writing about ritual process in primitive societies, Victor Turner says, ". . . liminality is frequently likened to death, to being in the womb, to invisibility, to darkness, to bisexuality, to the wilderness, and to an eclipse of the sun or the moon." How well this fits everything we have discussed: the occasional rumor of my death, the social invisibility of the disabled, the attribution of asexuality in the popular mind, the unisex hospital room, and the blurring of roles within the community of the handicapped. The disabled are more than deviants. They are the antiphony of everyday life.
>
> Just as the bodies of the disabled are permanently impaired, so also is their standing as members of society. The lasting indeterminacy of their state of being produces a similar lack of definition of their social roles, which are in any event superseded and obscured by submersion of their identities. Their persons are regarded as contaminated; eyes are averted and people take care not to approach wheelchairs too closely. (Murphy, 1990, p. 135)

In addition to painting a more realistic description of the social standing of disabled persons, Murphy's use of the notion of liminality augments the deviance model of disability and illness in another way. Absent from Parson's account of sickness is any careful attention to the variegated and compelling experience of the sick person. The notion of liminality neatly summarizes one vector of the experience of disabled persons living in the contemporary United States, the feeling that one is not quite human, not quite ill, yet not quite well. This is the feeling to which Murphy, John Hockenberry, and other wheelchair users refer when they describe brief encounters with so-called normals. Persons who do not use wheelchairs act as though the mere presence of a wheelchair gives a normal permission to ignore the person using it, step on him, or treat him as an insentient obstacle (Hockenberry, 1995, pp. 308–316). When such persons do speak, although the disability is often at the forefront of the

minds of both parties to the interaction, both conscientiously avoid mentioning the subject (Murphy 1990, pp. 121–124). Such behaviors mark the stigma that attaches to both physical and psychosocial disablement in the contemporary United States. The experience of shame that this stigma engenders in the person with disability is a critical part of the state of being a disabled member of our society.

But the problem with the deviance model goes deeper. Arthur Frank (1991) wrote, "Being ill is just another way of living . . ."; it is "nothing special" (p. 3). Suffering illness or injury is a part of normal human life; few of us live out our lives without suffering from some form of affliction. As Frank points out, by focusing on recovery to the exclusion of the experience of illness, we risk missing completely that part of life (p. 2). This is even more true for those who suffer from disability or chronic illness. To continue to speak of such conditions in terms of deviance is to deny the degree to which they become integrated with or define the lived world of the afflicted person. John Hockenberry, radio and television correspondent, piano student, trainer of developmentally disabled adults, world traveler, never ceases being a "crip." Although he vigorously resists limitations that normal society attempts to impose on him because of his paraplegia, he does have to deal daily with the personal and social consequences of not having any sensation below the nipples. But for Hockenberry, this is a permanent state; in such circumstances it makes little sense, and no difference, whether suffering from paraplegia is "normal" or not. In this case, being "abnormal" has become Hockenberry's "normality" (Hockenberry, 1995). There is nothing special to be served by knowing whether Hockenberry's body is normal or not. There is nothing special about knowing the physical details of what is now part of his everyday life, the pathologies, impairments, and functional limitations he suffers, which make him diagnostically similar to some paraplegics, but different from others. What *is* something special is how he lives, experiences, and describes his life.

▼ EXPLANATORY MODELS AND NARRATIVES

Liminality is only one aspect of the experience of disablement. Others we may glean from accounts written by persons experiencing disablement: frustration, anger, loss, isolation, guilt, helplessness, personal worthlessness, depression, and pain. All of these feelings are important parts of the experience of disablement. In addition, there are positive feelings: joy, excitement, pride, accomplishment, power, intelligence, fulfillment, triumph. Such feelings have meaning, ultimately, in the context of a person's life. But how might we best learn of such feelings and the associated events and perspectives that accompany them?

Experience suggests that if we desire to understand our clients, we must invite them to talk about their disabilities or illnesses and listen carefully. Two different (but not mutually exclusive) approaches to conceptualizing this process are explanatory models and illness–disability narratives (IDNs). Explanatory models are personal, often implicit, accounts of illness, held by both practitioners and professionals that describe the nature and origins of the problem and what can be done about it (Kleinman 1987). IDNs are developing chronicles of key events, situations, personalities, and factors that tell the story of illness. IDNs may also be elicited from both professionals and lay persons (Mattingly, 1994).

Explanatory Models

Kleinman suggests that explanatory models answer five major questions concerning illness: (1) what is the etiology of the affliction, (2) when and how did it begin, (3) what is its pathophysiology or nature, (4) what has been or will be the course of sickness (including degree of severity and type of sick role—acute, chronic, impaired, or other), and (5) what are or should be the available courses of treatment? The notion of explanatory model reminds practitioners that they are not alone in actively seeking to comprehend and give meaning to the problems confronted by their clients. Practitioner explanations of the problem do not encounter a vacuum. The client, the client's family, and other close associates of the client are likely to actively attempt to make sense of the disruption and discomfort caused by the problem at hand as well. These "theorists" may apply a much wider range of causes and remedies to the problems at hand than practitioners.

An example will help clarify the meaning and importance of explanatory models. Donald was born with apparent neurological sequelae from his mother's heroin abuse during the first trimester of her pregnancy and his gestation. Within a week of birth Donald had had a seizure. He showed the signs of problematic neurologic state regulation, alternating between tension and tightness on the one hand, and floppiness on the other. Early in life it was hard to get Donald aroused to full wakefulness. The occupational therapist who worked with Donald treated him both while he was a patient in the neonatal intensive care unit (NICU) and as an outpatient following his discharge from the hospital. The excerpts in the following case story are taken from interviews with Donald's therapist and his mother, conducted by an occupational therapy graduate student during the period when Donald was receiving occupational therapy as an outpatient (Beer, Lawlor, & Mattingly, 1994).

The occupational therapist and the mother have different understandings of Donald's condition and talk about their understandings in very different ways. Thinking of their statements as representing underlying explanatory models, even if we must think of those models as partly formed, is quite useful. Kleinman's (1988) construct gives us a way to organize the comments of each person into a more coherent point of view, as well as providing us with some points of contrast.

For instance, we see that the therapist and the mother have defined Donald's problem in different ways, that they use different information to describe the problem, and that their definitions are works in progress, at different stages of completion. The therapist does not give a name to Donald's condition, but instead tells us through use of a variety of specific physiological details that Donald is suffering from as yet undetermined–unspecified aftereffects of his mother's heroin abuse. She mentions edema of the temporal lobe, symptoms of withdrawal, a seizure, poor state regulation, poor coordination of the suck–swallow mechanism, not achieving full alertness, alternating floppiness and tightness when she sees Donald in the NICU. When she sees Donald as an outpatient, she observes some relaxation of tightness, independent movement of fingers, back arching, more alertness, and improvements in visual tracking. Overall her statements suggest she sees improvement. In contrast, Donald's mother defines his problem more narrowly as a seizure disorder; she notes that there has only been one seizure thus far and that seizures are being controlled by medication.

That Donald's occupational therapist and his mother understand his problem differently is not trivial. Each organizes her description of Donald and of her activities to assist him around her understanding of Donald's problems. His therapist focuses on activities intended to assess and encourage Donald's neurological development. His mother focuses on personal and family efforts intended to prevent a recurrence of the seizure.

Donald's therapist identifies the mother's heroin abuse as one of the potential causes of his problems, indicating that he did exhibit signs of withdrawal in the NICU. This is consistent with the focus of her description of Donald on signs related to or indicative of neurologic functioning. Donald's mother mentions her drug use, but does not link it directly to Donald's seizure disorder. In fact, she states her understanding of the problem in a way that supports the family efforts being made to avoid another seizure: "We don't know what caused it an' I don't know when one could be triggered." In related interviews Donald's mother tells us that she received conflicting information about the role of her heroin use in causing Donald's problems. She does, ultimately, identify the use of heroin as a contributor to Donald's problems. At that point, the explanatory models of therapist and mother come to overlap.

Looking toward the future, there is complementarity, but not agreement, between the explanatory models of Donald's therapist and his mother. Donald's therapist did not know what the future would bring for Donald, partly because of her understanding of the workings of the body. It would be hard to tell the extent and permanence of any neurological damage to Donald's body until it developed further. The seizure, a week after birth, the lack of alertness, the variation between floppiness and tightness, and the inconsistent sucking all suggested to Donald's therapist that something neurological might be wrong. On the other hand, such effects can be (in whole or in part) transient. Donald's increased

DONALD, ACCORDING TO THE OCCUPATIONAL THERAPIST AND MOTHER

[Donald's occupational therapist speaks:] I met this baby first . . . when he was in the neonatal intensive care unit. I'll give you a little bit of statistics [picks up chart to read information from]. He was born full term . . . um . . . on May 29, 1992, and um . . . he was born because of a ruptured membrane. So labor was induced and so it wasn't a . . . a normal birth . . . He was initially floppy, and they had to give him a bit of oxygen and he had, um, a seizure about a week later. Um . . . his mother was also on methadone. She had been doing heroin and then found out she was pregnant, pretty early on in the pregnancy . . . I'm not sure exactly when, but um . . . went to a methadone program right away as soon as she found out. And he did show, . . . his name is Donald Peterson . . . he did show some signs of withdrawal . . . After, um . . . while being in the nursery. Let's see . . . what else can I tell you about him? Um, he had a little bit of edema—that was shown on the CAT scan, so, so . . . I'm not sure where it was in his brain, but he had some edema somewhere in his brain um . . . I think it was in the temporal area . . . So we were called in to evaluate him, um, when he was in the intensive care unit. He was reported to be a poor feeder and they were worried about some tightness in his lower extremities too. So I, I saw him . . . once. And um, he was very hard to wake up and to get to an alert stage, even though he was full-term, and he was about a month old when I saw him. And he was tight. His shoulders were tight, his hands were tight, he was irritable . . . and I never did really get him to that full awake stage. So I saw him one other time and tried to feed him, and um, he, he was a very in— inconsistent sucker. He couldn't coordinate the suck–swallow mechanism. He was just having a hard time. And again, just wasn't alert and just didn't look very good. Um, he was a good-sized baby, he was a big baby, so he wasn't little or frail, um, just had a lot of trouble with state regulation and being tight and just, um, not a calm baby. Um, and when he left I did meet his mother, an-an, mother and his father and his little brother—her name is Paula—and set up an appointment for her to come as an outpatient. I explained to her what we had seen—that he was a little bit tight, he was irritable and having trouble with feedings—and told her that um, we would like to monitor that to make sure he won't have problems when he gets older. And, um, she was—she seemed to understand and was very agreeable and, um—we

scheduled an appointment, and, um, so I've seen him—oh, I think four or five times since then. So, um, and they, she comes consistently and will call if she can't come, and, um, Donald is now going to be 3 months old, I believe, so . . . he's still tiny. Um, and he's gotten al—his picture has changed since he's— since I've been seeing him. He's now, um, an alert baby. He now tracks visually, which he wasn't doing before. Um, he doesn't cry as much. He can, he calms easier with, um, a pacifier or holding—um, he's still got some, he's got some arching and some tightness in his shoulders and in his back. He tends to keep his hands fisted though that's—the last time I saw him, he looked better with that, with, um, showing some more isolated finger movements and, um, exploring things a little bit with his fingers, fingers on his body or fingers on your hand, um, and I've also worked with the mother a lot, trying to tell her, explain to her what I'm looking at, um, what I'd like to see, what I'd like to see go away, um, like the arching and the tightness, um, and how we can facilitate him in different positions to get him to move and explore optimally without that tightness interfering . . . And, um, she comes back and she—"Well, I tried putting something behind his head, but—now watch—but he'll lean back anyway and it doesn't really seem to . . ." So we'll try to work together um . . . to problem solve around that.

[Donald's mother speaks:] Donald is a star. Donald is my pride and joy. Donald is my little star . . . Well (takes deep breath) . . . As as you already know, that Donald has a seizure disorder. Where it's, it's controllable now. When I first had him, he had a real trauma seizure . . . and they put him on medication. You know? And he's supposed to be on his medication until he either grows out of it or 3 years old. But I believe he's gonna go further than that. Cause you can't estimate on a newborn, what's gonna happen in the future. You know? Like we can't see the future. We don't know how Donald's gonna be when he gets older. We don't know if when he make one he might have more seizures, cause he only really had one. So far his medications been controlling it. Everybody in my house been real careful with him, you know? So, it's been controllable. It's alright now but we don't know how he might look in the future. You know, we don't know tomorrow until tomorrow gets here. But . . . like

(continued)

(Continued)

I said, um . . . it's still considered a disorder because he's taking medication. Dependin' on medication everyday. Takin' phenobarbital everyday . . .So . . . he's spoiled. He want you ta hold him. He's a sweet baby. Don't get me wrong. But I knew from the day that he went to intensive care. Like my mother says, she knew from that day that I told her that Donald was going to be pinpointed as a special child—special attention—because he had that seizure. So you know everybody really was like watchin' him real close? Now we gettin' a little bit more confidence. Everybody watchin'. Don't get me wrong. They still watchin'. They don't let him cry. He go through like seven arms in my house. He'll be cryin' and somebody pickin' him up. You know? So . . . he, you know? He . . . he be attached to that now. If he whine, he know you gonna pick him up [both laugh]. That's all I have ta do is whhhaaa. `Then somebody will come and pick me up!' So . . . it's not no problem though. Because, like I said, I'm not workin' now so I . . . I don't have nothin' else ta do but enjoy my baby's childhood life. An, you know? Watch 'em grow up. It's kind of scary because I don't know what the future look like for me as far as him havin' that seizure. We don't know what caused it an' I don't know when one could be triggered. You know? Like when I take him to the doctor to get his um . . . baby shot? They tell me that a a fever can trigger a seizure. An' I be so scared when I get him home that he might have a fever, you know, might catch a fever. But so far, since Donald's been takin' his baby shots? I've been lucky. He hasn't had no temperature. He haven't been real irritable. Been sweet ta be honest with ya. I ain't really had no problems. Not as far as gettin' him a shot. Like I said, when you got God behind you. I know I did some real devious things, but I been an angel too—don't get me wrong. I think the worst thing in my life that I have done is when I got wrapped up into drugs. You know? But God forgave me. And it's like, he be behind me so . . . I'm okay. An' I got Him . . . you know, He watchin' over Donald. I have so many. I have a lot of people prayin' for him. You know, my grandmother inta church, my uncle inta church. I got an uncle that's a preacher. You know, I have a lot with the church, by me goin' to the church, I have a lot . . . I have a lot of people prayin' for Donald. An' when you have people behind you like that, you know, it makes it better. But that's basically all about Donald.

alertness, his visual tracking, and the reduction of tightness in some parts of his body all suggested that he might grow out of some of the difficulties. The therapist based her estimations on her observations of and interactions with the child, on the knowledge of neurological and motor development she obtained from formal education and experience, and on the comments and observations of others whom she consulted about Donald's condition. Her response to her evolving understanding of Donald's condition was threefold. She continued trying to assess his developing capacities and deficiencies. She addressed specific problems, such as fisting of the hands or arching of the back, with specific postures, movements, and activities. And she used activities to support Donald's development—to increase his flexibility and strength, to stimulate his perception, and to help him master developmentally appropriate activities and skills.

Donald's mother also did not know what the future would bring for Donald, but her response to not knowing was different than that of Donald's occupational therapist. Donald's mother expressed her immediate concern that Donald would have another seizure. She, with other family members, responded to this concern by making sure Donald took his phenobarbital and by exercising care and watchfulness. Donald's mother credited both strategies with helping avoid further seizures. Embedded in the family's watchfulness were theories about the kinds of events that might bring on another seizure—fevers induced by inoculations, agitation, or long periods of crying. Family members would not let Donald cry much, and Donald's mother was very careful with inoculations. This line of defense had been successful thus far, as a result of which Donald's family was beginning to feel confident that there might be no more seizures. If Donald reaches the age of 3 years without incident, he likely will have grown out of seizures and the need to take medication. Donald's mother attributed the fact that Donald has not had another seizure at least partly to having God supporting her. Although she has done some "devious things," the worst of which was her drug abuse, Donald's mother has been "an angel" since that time and feels that God has forgiven her. In addition to her own reformation, Donald's mother points to the number of people who are praying for Donald, including a grandmother and an uncle who are "inta church," and an uncle who is a preacher.

Donald's therapist and mother draw on different sets of resources in responding to Donald's condition. Donald's therapist relies primarily on her interactions with Donald, viewing the problem primarily as a developmental–neurological problem which, while located in Donald's body, can be affected by the appropriate kinds of interaction between Donald and his environment. She extends this idea to Donald's mother and his family when she describes ways to adjust the home environment to support Donald in more appropriate postures. Donald's mother draws on substantial social and religious resources in her efforts to prevent future seizures. Family efforts are organized around seeing to it that Donald takes his medication and avoids circumstances that might bring on a seizure. Extended family efforts add the power of God to the efforts of the family, as if to counter the uncertainties of Donald's future well-being.

Explanatory models can be, then, a powerful approach to transforming statements and descriptions into perspectives. Practitioners can elicit material that can be interpreted using the construct of explanatory models through directed, open-ended interview questions such as the following: "Tell me about your problem." "How did it begin?" "What seems to cause it?" "What can you do about it?" "If you did nothing about it, what would happen?" Statements and ideas that allow the construction of such models can also be collected one statement at a time. Remembering that both clients and practitioners have such models can help practitioners to recognize the efforts of clients to understand, interpret, and respond to their ailments, as well as provide practitioners one means of understanding the bases of client behaviors that do not seem logical (Beer, Lawlor, & Mattingly, 1994).

Illness and Disability Narratives

Illness and disability narratives (IDNs) are developing chronicles of key events, situations, personalities, and factors that tell the story of illness or disability. IDNs share a number of elements with other forms of narrative—actors, setting, plot, desire, dramatic tension, and resolution. IDNs, similar to explanatory models, may be elicited from professionals and lay persons, or they may be constructed from their accounts. They are different from explanatory models, however, in their degree of temporal particularity—their connection to specific events occurring at specific times in particular contexts, as well as to specific actors acting at certain times in certain contexts with specific motives. They also differ in the role of temporal ordering and unfolding. In explanatory models, temporality appears, primarily, in the service of causal explanations. In IDNs, temporality is a central structure for organizing plot and tracing the development and resolution of dramatic tension (Mattingly, 1994).

There is a common confusion between chronological accounts of events and stories, as the term is used here. Any account that includes actors, provides some sort of setting, and moves in a time-ordered fashion may be considered a chronological account, but a story is different. The actors in a story have concerns, interests, and desires that are either in conflict with one another or with events or circumstances that seem to be out of their control. It is not known if the actors will receive fulfillment of their desires. This question, embedded in the telling of the story, creates an experience of uncertainty for the listener or reader, which may be termed narrative or dramatic tension. This tension is what

gives a story its life. It animates its plot, its temporal structure of events, and keeps the listener listening or the reader turning the pages. The listener or reader listens for and looks forward to a resolution, some determination as to whether, and if so, how, the dramatic tension will be resolved. Often there is a moral or point embedded in the story, which points to how the story is to be made sense of in the context of its telling, and which is key to interpreting the story outside the context of its telling.

The term *story* is used here in full knowledge of its common connection to falsehoods and fictions. In fact, stories *are* constructions, often telescoping years of living and experience into a few hours of talking, or even a few paragraphs of transcribed text. But they are not simply made up. Stories about illness or disability are efforts to describe real events and experiences from the perspective of one observer or actor. Although they may not provide us accounts that are objectively accurate when mapped onto constant chronological time, stories do give us insight into the lives and perspectives of story tellers. They indicate (by their presence or absence in the story) which events are significant enough to be recounted. They give meaning to those events, shedding further light on the perspective of the story teller. And they communicate something of the teller's experience of them, as we experience the ebb and flow of dramatic tension and draw analogies to our own experience. Whether a story accurately reflects its teller's original experience at the historical time of the recounted events is a significant issue, but for a practitioner listening to a client, what is important is the client's experience of those events at the time the events are recounted.

In some of our most moving accounts of illness and disability (eg, Robert Murphy's *The Body Silent*, John Hockenberry's *Moving Violations*), we know the general outcome before we begin reading. Robert Murphy died in 1990 of respiratory failure, a consequence of increasing pressure from the tumor growing inside his spinal cavity. John Hockenberry has become a successful correspondent for NBC news, his third major correspondent position in radio and television reporting. There is, in reading their stories, little tension related to events themselves. These accounts are worth reading for other reasons. Murphy's description of his steadily increasing impairments and functional limitations and of his increasing social isolation, anger, loss, and sense of guilt over the burden he is to his wife Yolanda, provide an opportunity for him to turn his anthropological gaze on the meaning and experience of disablement in the contemporary United States. As Murphy reflects on his progressing disability, he draws on his knowledge of Mundurucu society, on his Irish Catholic upbringing, and on his experience of alcoholism. He draws on sociologist Erving Goffman's writings about stigma and social interaction, on Oliver Sacks' account of Christina, the "disembodied lady," and on the reactions of his friends, colleagues, and neighbors to his increasing disablement. He weaves these and other materials into his own feelings about his increasing disembodiment and its effect on himself and his family. The resulting IDN is, essentially, a semantic map of Murphy's world.

Hockenberry's account is different. Hockenberry's disablement stems from a single accident, an irruption into his biography, and his story is about living in and adjusting to a body that has changed. But it is also about learning what it means to use a wheelchair, and figuring out what sorts of uses (eg, mobility, political activism, social panhandling, personal advantage) for which wheelchairs are appropriate, moral, or healthy. His book makes an interesting contrast with Murphy's. Murphy, an anthropologist, turns his cross-cultural eye inward onto his own life world, defining for his reader the meaning and experience of disability. Hockenberry, with his wheelchair, travels all over the world, demonstrating in societies from New York to Somalia that it is he, not social or cultural attitudes toward disablement, who will define the limits of his world. His account highlights the practices and attitudes that variously circumscribe and expand the world of the disabled.

Long narrative works, such as *The Body Silent* and *Moving Violations*, not only show us how actors attribute meaning to disablement and its interface with their lived worlds, they show us these meanings unfolding across time. One of the critical features of the disablement experience, which the structure of therapy obscures, is its temporal length. Disablement, whether temporary or permanent, is constant and pervasive, and the experience of living it is always more comprehensive than the staccato sequence of therapy appointments. Reading lengthy disablement stories, seeing the meaning of disability unfold in the life of the teller, gives the reader a sense of the temporal extent of the experience of disability. This is important, because the interest of the disabled client nearly always has more temporal breadth than the interest of the practitioner.

In the accounts of Donald, given in the foregoing, the temporal period that is the focus of Donald's mother is nearly 3 years long, and implied in her discussion of that period is a concern about the future beyond that initial 3 years. One tension in her account pivots on the question of whether Donald will have another seizure before his third birthday, as well as on whether avoiding a seizure will assure that Donald will grow into a relatively normal, independent adult. Another tension, not entirely clear in this excerpt, has to do with the extent to which her drug abuse is to blame for Donald's condition. The therapist, in contrast, has a shorter-term interest. For her there are at least two tensions—how will Donald respond to her efforts to reduce the tightness in his fists and the arching of his back, and will she be able to help Donald explore the world in a way that will facilitate the rest of his development, in spite of whatever tightness is present? The temporal span of the narrative tension in the therapist's account is relatively narrow compared with the temporal period that is of interest to the mother.

The purposeful elicitation of stories is an art for experienced interviewers, but the human propensity for story telling means that almost anyone will tell an illness or disability narrative, given enough time and a willing listener. Therapeutic settings often provide the rhythm and predictability necessary for a client to feel willing to tell a story, and therapeutic activities may instigate the telling. In addition, a narrative orientation can be used as a frame for combining and interpreting statements made by clients on different occasions over a time period. Either way, a sense of narrative, that actors attribute meaning to their illness or disability by acting and seeing its significance unfold as they live it, makes it possible for practitioners to appreciate the disability experience of the actors. Likewise, the notion that

RESEARCH NOTE
RESEARCH IN OCCUPATIONAL THERAPY INVOLVES PEOPLE

Kenneth J. Ottenbacher

Research in occupational therapy involves people. Often the participants in occupational therapy investigations are persons with some level of impairment, disability, or handicap. These persons function in a complex social ecology where they are engaged in multiple roles. The presence of tangled contextual factors means that research conducted in occupational therapy is often functionally and philosophically different from that conducted in other medical and health disciplines. In many traditional medical specialties, the unit of analysis is an organ, body system, or particular type of pathology. In fact, much of traditional medicine is organized around the treatment of specific organs and systems, for example, cardiology, neurology, and orthopedics are all disciplines with an organ or system focus. Within these disciplines the goal of intervention is cure, and research methods are developed and used accordingly.

In occupational therapy, the unit of analysis is the person and the person's relation to his or her achievement. The ultimate goal is not cure, but enhanced function; that is, the ability to function as independently as possible in the most natural and least restrictive environment. Research approaches and outcome measures used in occupational therapy must reflect this complexity and diversity. Persons who are involved in occupational therapy studies often become active participants in the planning, implementation, and interpretation of research activities. In person-centered research, the opportunity exists for the individual consumer of occupational therapy research to also be directly involved in its production. ∎

persons suffering disability or illness are actively trying to make sense out of what is happening in their lives with explanatory models, by determining what caused the problem, what can be done about it, and what effect doing that will have, suggests to the practitioner that apparently irrational or meaningless statements or actions by clients may, in fact, make perfect sense, from the client perspective. These approaches to understanding the statements of clients constitute a powerful set of tools for understanding the client perspective.

►CONCLUSION: DISABLEMENT, LIMINALITY, AND LIVING

Robert Murphy (1990) has suggested that the state of being disabled is a kind of permanent liminality. He suggests that, once separated from normal social intercourse, persons with disabilities are never fully reintegrated. They are left on the margins of social life, partly integrated and partly not, anomalous for the remainder of their lives. As a conclusion to this reflection on the experience of illness and disablement, I would like to suggest an alternative interpretation of what happens to the person who suffers a disorder that results in disablement.

Were disabled people to be permanently consigned to separation from the rest of society, they would be institutionalized in isolated facilities, never having social interaction with so-called normal persons. Because this is true for only a few such people, to say that they are permanently liminal is to wrest the meaning of liminality. Turner (1967) uses the term liminal to describe the state of those ritually separated from day-to-day social intercourse because they are undergoing social and personal transformation. While they are undergoing this process, they are considered to be dangerous, shifting, anomalous, and even dead. But people who become disabled are more and more often reintegrated into the world. Murphy taught at Columbia. Hockenberry continues to report for television. Donald lives at home with his family. All have left the hospital, graduated from the rehabilitation clinic, and reside in normal settings. All interact regularly (or are at least available for interaction) with normals who are not wheelchair users, who are not slowly losing control of more and more of their body, who are not in danger of seizure at any moment. It seems that all have been reintegrated into society, but not as normals.

Being not-normal or other-than-normal has its dangers in this society. For years we have sent anthropologists and other observers off to strange societies to chronicle how "other peoples" are different from "us," as part of a cultural project of comparative self-definition (Fabian, 1983; Wolf, 1982). Part of this process of self-definition is the assumption that "others" are inferior to "us," that "otherness" is, in fact, prima facie evidence of inferiority. Similar processes of collective self-definition have af-

fected our understanding of the mentally ill, whom we have used to define our sanity and our civility (Foucault, 1972). The construction of "minorities," groups of persons racially or ethnically or linguistically different from "us" (in this case, the white middle-class mainstream of American society), has been a way of justifying unequal distributions of resources and opportunities in our supposedly democratic society.

Now we confront another construction of "other"—the disabled. In our society, people with disabilities culturally define the boundaries of "ableness," through existing just across those arbitrary boundaries from able, or normal persons. Their existence as outliers, as others, is critical to maintaining the physical and psychosocial aspects of normalcy. Normals look through them, step on them, bump around them, and obstruct them, because they are positioned just beyond the physical or psychosocial horizon of humanity. When people with disabilities are reintegrated into society they are reintegrated as markers, as personifications of the margins, as not-quite-human beings. But they are fully integrated in the sense that the meaning of their existence—in opposition to normalcy—is critical to the maintenance of the notion of normalcy itself. In other words, the transformation that happens in the treatment and rehabilitation process is partly a transformation from normal to abnormal, from able to disabled, from disorder to disordered. Along with this transformation come indications that what has occurred is irreversible and permanent, that there is no road back to what society has defined as normal. However, as Hockenberry demonstrates, the definition of what is normal is also a personal one. Hockenberry incorporates his disability so completely into his daily routine, that it is an aspect of himself that he would not change—for to change it would be to deny much of his adult life. This is just the point that people without disabilities miss, that the discomfort they may experience around people with disabilities emanates from themselves and their lack of understanding of the experience of disability.

Fortunately, this is not the end of the story. Persons with disabilities know that one disability differs from another, that the effect of disability differs from one life to another, and that individual persons differ in their capacity to recognize the person who is disabled as more than the disability. Similar to illness, disability is a normal part of life, suffered to some degree by most of us during some part of our lives. Each of us responds to our disability differently. And like illness narratives, disability stories are stories about humanity, about meaning and significance, about challenge and triumph and defeat. Occupational therapy practitioners have opportunities to interact with people with disabilities on a regular basis, and with this comes the opportunity to ask and to listen as such persons talk about their experience. Understanding the perspective of people struggling with disabling conditions helps creative practitioners devise treatment that is meaningful to their clients. Knowing how disability affects a person's life, how the person thinks about it, what personal resources a person has to cope, all help practitioners understand the way a person responds to treatment. All of this increases the likelihood that treatment will be meaningful.

Moreover, listening to and understanding the perspective of a person with a disability confirms the right of such a person to have a perspective and places a value on it. As participants in the rehabilitation process, practitioners cannot change the response of the world outside rehabilitation to the person with a disability. But they can give these people a sense of their importance; of their humanity; of the legitimacy of their struggles and losses, grief and pain, defeats and triumphs; as well as of their interest to other human beings. Practitioners can counter the tendency in rehabilitation to define people in terms of their disorder, by paying attention to them as whole people, with abilities and disabilities. Practitioners can avoid premature conclusions about their limitations, instead helping them to learn to assess and extend their abilities. Practitioners can help clients learn to respond to their social and physical environment creatively, especially in those cases where the environment does not give adequate support. Finally, practitioners can help clients understand that, whatever limitations they may experience, their biography has not yet been written. Ultimately, as Murphy and Hockenberry demonstrate, living is the antidote for the experience of disability.

REFERENCES

Beer, D. W., Lawlor, M., Mattingly, C. (1994). *Collaboration, coercion, and compliance in therapeutic relationships.* Paper presented at American Occupational Therapy Association Annual Conference, Boston, MA.

Fabian, J. (1983). *Time and the other: How anthropology makes its objects.* New York: Columbia University Press.

Foucault, M. (1972). *Madness and civilization* (A. M. Sheridan Smith, Trans.). New York: Vintage Press.

Frank, A. (1991). *At the will of the body: Reflections on illness.* Boston: Houghton Mifflin Company.

Frankenberg, R. (1980). Medical anthropology and development: A theoretical perspective. *Social Science and Medicine, 14B,* 197–207.

Goffman, E. (1963). *Stigma: Notes on the management of spoiled identity.* Englewood Cliffs, NJ: Prentice Hall .

Hahn, R. A. (1984). Rethinking "illness" and "disease." In E. V. Daniel & J. F. Pugh (Eds.), *South Asian systems of healing: Contributions to Asian studies,* Vol. 18 (pp. 1–23). Leiden: E. J. Brill.

Hockenberry, J. (1995). *Moving violations: War zones, wheelchairs, and declarations of independence.* New York: Hyperion.

Kleinman, A. (1988). *The illness narratives: Suffering, healing, and the human condition.* New York: Basic Books.

Kleinman, A., Eisenberg, L., and Good, B. (1978). Culture, illness, and care. *Annals of Internal Medicine, 88,* 251–258.

Mattingly, C. (1994). Therapeutic emplotment. *Social Science and Medicine, 36,* 811–822.

Murphy, R. (1990). *The body silent.* New York: W. W. Norton.

Parsons, T. (1951). *The social system.* New York: The Free Press.

Rogers, J. (1982). Order and disorder in medicine and occupational therapy. *American Journal of Occupational Therapy, 36,* 29-35.

Turner, V. (1967). *The forest of symbols: Aspects of Ndembu ritual.* Ithaca, NY: Cornell University Press.

Wolf, E. (1982). *Europe and the people without history.* Berkeley: University of California Press.

Chapter 5

Disability Experience from a Family Perspective

Cheryl F. Mattingly and Mary C. Lawlor

Common sense tells us that most people who come to occupational therapy practitioners live in families of some kind. Even when clients live apart from their families, if they need consistent care, it is very likely that some family members will be instrumental in this care-giving. And even in those instances where no family member is actively involved in care, it is likely that someone from a client's family will be concerned with this care, including the services of the occupational therapy practitioner. Furthermore, the way disability is experienced by clients, and how it affects their functioning in the world, is often heavily dependent on their relationships with family members. This is most obvious in pediatric care when the client is a very young child, and in geriatric care when spouses and children become involved; but for most people, no matter what the age, ethnicity, socioeconomic status, or geographical location, at times of severe illness or disability, families tend to matter.

Not only do families matter, families shift in response to the issues raised by having a family member with an illness or disability. Roles change. Power relations change. Activities change. The way meals are eaten, vacations are taken, arguments are had, beds are made, money is earned, houses are organized, and a myriad other aspects of family life are likely to be affected.

Even though there is nothing startling about any of these statements, families are systematically underconsidered in health care. Professional training, institutional structures, reimbursement procedures, and reward systems, all tend to contribute to the marginalization of families. When occupational therapy practitioners do try to consider the needs of their clients and of family caregivers, they can find themselves addressing a range of issues and facing a number of

dilemmas for which they were not prepared. This chapter addresses the place of the family in occupational therapy care and the need to attend to family perspectives in providing services to people with chronic illnesses or disabilities. It highlights some of the interesting problems and opportunities that emerge when practitioners look to involve families actively in the therapeutic process. We begin by arguing the need to bring families into the picture and by discussing the recent movement (largely in pediatrics) toward "**family-centered care**," raising some questions about what this term might mean in practice. We then look at why families have been so peripheral in the way most health care professions have defined their practice. The heart of the chapter moves from these more general considerations to an analysis of case stories in which practitioners and family members describe their efforts to collaborate in the therapeutic process. In the context of these cases, we highlight some of the intricacies, dilemmas, surprises, and richness of therapeutic work where families play a central role.

▼ WHY ARE FAMILIES IMPORTANT IN HEALTH CARE?

Public policy efforts related to promoting the health and development of children have been traced to the turn of the century (Hanft, 1991). The implementation of federal initiatives related to providing services for children with special health care needs and their families has been documented as early as 1912, with the establishment of the Children's Bureau in Maternal and Child Health (Hanft, 1991) and expanded with the implementation of Title V legislation in

1935 (Colman, 1988). The implementation of **PL 94-142, Part B**, amendment to the Education for the Handicapped Act (EHA) in 1975, and **PL 99-457, Part H**, amendment to the EHA in 1986; have prompted dramatic changes in the nature of service delivery to children in educational and early childhood settings (Hanft, 1991; Lawlor, 1991). Implementation of these services placed new demands on practitioners to reframe traditional medical models of practice to accommodate to the needs of families as well as the child who was referred for services.

Although the initiative for developing services centered around the needs and values of families began in early childhood programs, many of the principles apply to services for people of all ages. As human service systems moved into the community and people began providing home care, practitioners developed a deeper appreciation of the centrality of families in healing, recovery, and adaptation. Practitioners also recognized that family members often had different perspectives about the needs, priorities, and strengths than the professionals. A shift is occurring from perceiving the family members as people who will carry out the doctor's and practitioners' orders to perceiving family members as people who are most knowledgeable about the client and who are partners in decision making. Family members' perspectives about how the client is doing, what the client needs, what the family needs, and what is most important and meaningful become part of the clinical dialogue.

The challenge for the occupational therapy practitioner is to collaborate with clients, their families and other team members in designing a program that builds on a family's strengths and addresses its needs. When done successfully, intervention services are individualized to each family and reflect their unique cultural world. We have defined family centered-care as an experience that happens when practitioners effectively and compassionately listen to the concerns, address the needs, and support the hopes of people and their families (Lawlor & Cada, 1993). Sometimes, practitioners can best involve clients and families in the decision-making process by offering multiple options for interventions (Rosen & Granger, 1992). This type of engagement is often described as a means of enabling and empowering families (Deal, Dunst, & Trivette, 1989).

Family-centered care is enacted through the collaborative efforts of family members and practitioners (Edelman, Greenland, & Mills, 1993) and typically provided through multidisciplinary and interdisciplinary team structures. Partnerships are created based on the establishment of trust and rapport, as well as respect for family values, beliefs, and routines (Hanft, 1989). Additional elements of successful collaboration include clarity and honesty in communication, mutual agreements on goals, effective information sharing, accessibility, and absence of blame (McGonigel, Kaufmann, & Johnson, 1991). Collaboration is successful when practitioners and family members form relationships that foster a shared understanding of the needs, hopes, expectations, and contributions of all partners (Lawlor & Cada, 1993). Collaboration is much more than being "nice." It involves complex interpretive acts in which the practitioner must understand the meanings of interventions, the meanings of illness or disability in a person and family's life, and the feelings that accompany these experiences.

▼ WHY HAVE FAMILIES BEEN SO MARGINAL AND MISUNDERSTOOD IN HEALTH CARE?

The easiest way to understand why families have not traditionally been better included in decisions about health care is to remember that health care professionals, including occupational therapy practitioners, are members of professional cultures and work in settings that have institutional cultures. All health care professions have been powerfully influenced by what anthropologists sometimes call the "culture of Western **biomedicine**" (Hahn & Gaines, 1985; Locke & Gordon, 1988). It is a bit deceptive to speak of one monolithic culture of biomedicine, as though this were some single, homogeneous entity. Occupational therapy practitioners, for example, may find they only partly live in the same professional culture as, say, neurosurgeons. And practitioners working within one setting may find that this institutional culture is quite different from another setting where they have practiced. This can hold true even if both organizations appear outwardly similar—two different rehabilitation hospitals, for instance. But even keeping all these differences and nuances in mind, there are a number of powerful assumptions shared at some level by nearly all health professionals working across a wide variety of settings.

Not only do professionals such as occupational therapy practitioners learn professional skills when they enter the field, they also assimilate a set of values and beliefs that make them members of a professional culture. The culture of biomedicine has developed over the past 250 years (For a detailed reading of this history as a cultural phenomena, see, for example, Foucault, 1973; 1979). In its development, this culture has provided a powerful view of what it means to be ill, what is expected of the client, the health care professional and the client's family or key caregivers. There are some deeply held beliefs about what constitutes an appropriate relationship among professional, client, and family caregivers. These assumptions about the professional–client–caregiver relationship are influenced, in turn, by other basic assumptions about the nature of illness and how it is best treated. Some of these assumptions are especially problematic for rehabilitation professionals such as occupational therapy practitioners who treat clients with chronic illnesses and disabling conditions.

▼ TROUBLESOME ASSUMPTIONS ABOUT DISABILITY, THE "ILLNESS EXPERIENCE," AND FAMILIES

Several key assumptions that are particularly potent and particularly "tenacious" (Gordon, 1988) in the culture of biomedicine, and in occupational therapy, have significantly influenced the way families are drawn into the therapeutic process. We will present some case examples written by therapists that illustrate how these assumptions play out in concrete cases. Case examples are particularly useful as a way to look at a professional's assumptions and beliefs, for these are often held so unconsciously that the therapist is not even aware he or she holds them until, in some specific situation, they are violated. These cases tend to concern surprises as the therapists come to learn something about a client's family that turns out to be extremely important in influencing the meaning and value of therapy and helps the therapist redirect therapeutic interventions in a more efficacious way.

The Disability Belongs to the Individual

One of the most pervasive assumptions in biomedicine is that the professional's task is to treat the individual who has the illness. Sometimes this is very narrowly interpreted among health professionals as "treating the pathology," but occupational therapy practitioners are usually very sensitive in trying to remember that they are also treating a person who has a disabling condition. The hand therapist is not only treating a hand injury, for example, but also an out of work auto mechanic with a wife and three children whose hand was injured on the job and who is fearful about his ability to regain his role as family breadwinner.

Put differently, practitioners try to treat what anthropologists speak of as the "illness experience," rather than simply the disease (Good, 1993; Good & Good, 1994; Kleinman, 1988). In the context of occupational therapy, a more accurate term is probably the "disability experience," for it is certainly possible to have a disability, even one that requires therapy, without being ill. Practitioners try to attend both to the disability as a physiological condition and to the meaning this particular condition carries for the person who has the disability (Mattingly, 1991; Mattingly & Fleming, 1994). If a practitioner knows a client wants to relearn how to drive, dress independently, eat out at restaurants, or continue to work as an auto mechanic, the practitioner may be able to organize therapeutic tasks that aid the client in carrying out these activities.

However, some goals are far less tangible. This is especially true for goals that concern the social world of the client and the connection between functional skills and social relationships. It is artificial to treat only narrowly defined functional skills as though these were unrelated to a client's social world, for a key aspect of the meaning of a condition is how it affects an individual's personal relationships; this is one of the trickier aspects of therapeutic work. By contrast with such goals as learning how to dress oneself, or learning wheelchair motility, goals and concerns connected to family relations are much more difficult to define, and they are certainly likely to be hard to measure. Helping a client reclaim his identity as a good father to his 5-year-old daughter even though he has a spinal cord injury, for example, is harder to translate into discrete, skill-based goals than learning how to increase upper body strength or learning how to feed oneself. Family-oriented goals are likely to be tied to outcomes that are diffuse, complex, subtle, and difficult to measure, even when they are deeply significant to the client and family. When a client's goals and concerns are tied to shifting family relationships, these may seem out of professional bounds for the occupational therapy practitioner.

Despite the many difficulties in trying to understand a disabling condition as it pertains to a client's role in the family, ignoring this aspect often means being blind to the most significant aspects of the illness (or disability) experience. Ignoring family-oriented goals or the meaning of a disability as it ties to family concerns and family relationships may mean ignoring the person altogether.

The following case provided by Mary Black illustrates the very different identity a client assumes once her family relationships are known. This client, a woman in her 70s with significant health problems, is almost invisible to the professional staff, except in the psychiatric unit where she resides as an inconvenient collection of medical difficulties. During the course of treatment, the occupational therapist listens to stories she tells about her long marriage and family life. Through these stories, the client is transformed for the therapist into a mother and wife, and her deeper identity, her personhood one might say, is revealed. An abbreviated version of this case, written by the treating occupational therapist, follows on p. 46.

Mary Black's case also suggests the difficulty family members may have as they try to interact with health care professionals in making decisions about the care of their family member. In Mary's example, the staff perceived Lily as a burden because she "misfit" the kinds of psychiatric patients they were accustomed to treating. Her psychiatric diagnosis was vague (and, in Mary's view, probably inappropriate), but her medical problems required intense attention. The burden felt by the staff spilled into their relations with the family so that family members, such that two of Lily's sons also came to be perceived and treated as a "burden," needlessly inconveniencing the staff by coming for a visit at the wrong hours. Although it is easy to understand the staff members' frustration in trying to care for Lily, this case vividly illustrates how family members might feel when they are trying to deal with a very difficult family transition

LILY AND HER FAMILY

Mary Black

This story is about a woman I worked with for a short time; no longer than 1 or 2 weeks. I met her about 3 years ago when I was working on a contractual basis on an inpatient psychiatric unit for older adults. I cannot even remember her name, or why exactly she was on the psychiatric unit, but I can picture her clearly and remember stories she told me about herself. What I do recall is that her declining health and loss of independence resulted in major transitions for herself and her family. Her future plans for her living arrangements were decided by her family during her stay in the hospital.

Lily was admitted to the psychiatric unit from the medical floor under confusing circumstances. The feeling conveyed in the morning rounds was that she required more medical management than the psychiatric unit staff could provide, and it was unclear whether she was depressed or disoriented.

Lily had diabetes for many years, and came to the unit in a very weakened state and needed maximum assistance with self-care and transfers. She had intravenous tubes in her arm and took frequent rests during the day. Most of the time I saw Lily individually at her bedside, but on a couple of occasions she was able, once in a geri-chair, to attend an afternoon group.

When I first met Lily she did not strike me as confused or depressed, but rather sturdying herself for the inevitable upcoming changes through taking account of her life. Lily was a black woman in her 70s. She told me she was married at 16 to the only man she ever loved. They were married where they grew up, in Mississippi. She wore a "tomato red" dress, and had the loan of a car to drive them from the church to the house where they had a party. At the party, the roof or the floor broke (I can't remember which) but she told me, "It was some party." Lily and her husband had 13 children, all now grown. She was very proud that most of them were college educated. This was the first time she had been separated from her husband for so many weeks. She told me they both shared one long pillow. She and her husband, who was also ill, were both going to move into a nursing home together, but it was not yet determined where.

This may sound nostalgic. It was! But through her reminiscing she was able to paint—vividly—highlights and everyday aspects of her life. She had spent her whole life at home, and her family was everything to her. What jolted me then was the re-ception her children received. Because of the extra care the nursing staff had to provide, they were understandably frustrated. The resentment seemed to be deflected to the family though. Two of Lily's sons came to see her in the morning, and were chastised for not being here during visiting hours. They were questioned "Your brothers and sisters knew, why didn't you?" The family, in turn, did not understand why their mother was on a psychiatric unit, and were not given any reasonable answers, because the communication channels between medicine and psychiatry were so ambiguous. They had the feeling their mother was "dumped" here. There were efforts by staff to have her transferred off the floor, but it was unclear as to where. Luckily, the social worker was able to see beyond the internal politics and work with the family on their immediate concern—easing the transition into a nursing home and finding one that would provide care for both their mother and father.

Together the social worker and I met with seven or eight of Lily's children to work on this transition. I felt like I was able to confirm to them some of her strengths through my work with her, including interests in working with her hands, efforts in self-care, and brightness of spirit despite her failing health, as well as her quite normal reactions to the losses she felt, of her home, independence, and concern about her husband. Lily had ultimate trust that her family would provide the best they could for her. The social worker was able to provide information and contacts at nursing homes he felt reputable. We were both able to suggest questions and issues to address when investigating a home. What I remember as well, from the meeting, and individually, was just being able to listen to how hard this was for them. It was impossible for anyone of them to care for both of their parents, and they were very ambivalent about a nursing home. The consolation was that their parents would be together. The family found a home they thought suitable and near enough for most to visit, and Lily was then transferred. I do not know anymore about her after that.

What I found remarkable was the family's closeness, but conversely many of the staff's judgments to the contrary. A "they cannot get it together" and "we want her out of here" attitude prevailed among the staff. I also recognized, coming from a big family myself, that I was easily defensive about these

(continued)

(Continued)

judgments. What I think often happens, as did here, is that "territorial issues" took precedence over the patient and family concerns. Because of Lily's lovely personality and her family's keen interest and perse-

verance, the image of her as a "burden" diminished by her departure, but it was unfortunate her family was not included earlier and that the staff was not more supportive.

and are not supported by many of the professionals. This case also reveals how internal staff issues and other organizational difficulties can cloud the health professionals' recognition of the strengths a family offers and families, too, can appear as just one more irritation (rather than a resource) in providing services to a client.

The Professional Is the Expert

Traditionally, Western biomedicine has been concerned with curing people. The notion of the professional as healer is important here. The healer is an expert who can both ascertain what is wrong (assess and diagnose) and identify the correct intervention to cure the ailment (treat). The patient's role is a submissive one, offering information as requested, submitting to physical examination, and following the expert's directives for treatment. In this view, health care professionals make people healthy by curing disease. The concern of the professional is largely with the disease, rather than the person who has the disease (the oncologist "fighting" the cancer cells with radiation, for instance). The patient's personal history, family situation, and work history are usually of only peripheral importance in the healer's task of diagnosing and treating the pathological condition that is causing the illness.

Sometimes, this model works. But this is almost never true with the clients occupational therapists treat. Occupational therapy practitioners are well aware that their clients have medical conditions that, by and large, mean living with disabilities. Whereas the hope of medicine has been "curing" or "healing," which implies the ability of the health professional to bring a person from a state of illness to some state of "normalcy" or "premorbidity," occupational therapy practitioners are rarely in a position to cure anyone. The people they treat may have rich, full lives, but they are usually living these lives with an impairment that cannot be "fixed."

Practices steeped in medical traditions frequently adopt professional–client relationships based on hierarchical models or expert-driven models. The expert model remains prevalent within early childhood practices despite increasing recognition that elements of this model create barriers to developing collaborative partnerships and understanding family life. The expert model tends to promote dependence within recipients of services, limit opportunities for families to contribute insights and have their specific concerns and

needs addressed, burden the professional with the unrealistic expectation of always having the expertise to respond to all issues (Cunningham & Davis, 1985), and organize services in ways that are self-serving to the expert (Howard & Strauss, 1975).

Not surprisingly, reliance on expert models fosters relationships between practitioners and family members that incorporate compliance and coercion strategies. Practitioners and family members are often engaged in relationships in which there is considerable confusion about whether the "story" is one of collaboration, coercion, or compliance (Beer, Lawlor & Mattingly, 1994). The issue is not merely a semantics problem. Each approach to working relationships creates distinctly different experiences for all parties. Practitioner judgments that a person is "noncompliant," or in the terms used by family members—"bad parent," "bad daughter," and the like—diverts energies away from more reflective analysis or direct attempts to understand alternative perspectives (Trostle, 1988).

The Client Is the Recipient of Care

Another interrelated assumption quite pervasive in biomedicine is that health professionals deliver treatment "to" the person with the disease; they treat a passive patient whose primary task is to receive the cure (eg, take the medications, undergo the surgery, and the like). Although occupational therapy practitioners are well aware that they need "active clients," rather than passive ones, and that clients must learn to "do for themselves," the recipient role reasserts itself in another guise.

Practitioners know that therapy will be successful only if their clients (and often the key family caregivers as well) become motivated to work hard at it. But even as active participants, the clients and family members are often assigned a role as recipients of the instructions offered by occupational therapy practitioners and other rehabilitation experts. While these "active recipients" are sometimes offered a range of choices of goals or preferred activities, and practitioners often try to accommodate therapeutic goals into the life of the client or family, practitioners still tend to equate "good patients" and "good families" with compliant ones. Thus, a quite typical scenario is for the practitioner to assign "homework" for the client to do between therapy sessions. When family members are involved in therapy, they too are assigned roles as facilitators of the home therapy program.

The client and family's primary task is to do their homework faithfully. This family role is regularly underscored by the usual practice of devoting a few minutes of any session to a discussion about how the homework went.

Even though there is nothing necessarily wrong with this kind of collaborative relationship between practitioner and family, it carries some dangers, especially when practitioners are unaware of their power to shift family dynamics and family relationships by pressing family caregivers to become responsible for therapeutic gains. One critical danger is that both practitioners and family members may unconsciously begin to presume that the family's primary role is as a kind of adjunct practitioner. This danger is well illustrated by the following case.

CASE STORY

MY THERAPIST'S TALE

Beth Korby Elenko

I recently began treatment of a little boy named Sam. Sam was born with a hemangioma and multiple congenital anomalies. Sam's family includes a mom, a dad, and a 2-year-old sister, Dawn. This family was unusual to me because they came from suburban Chicago, had insurance and regularly attended treatment, which is very unique to my work environment. Sam was a child who needed to attend numerous specialists in addition to physical and occupational therapies. His mom never went without her appointment book and never missed an appointment unless she called to reschedule it.

Sam began ocupational therapy at 8 months of age after being involved in physical therapy (PT) since 3 months of age. It was the physical therapist who impressed on both mom and the physician the importance of occupational therapy intervention. My first visit with Sam was a cotreatment transition with PT. During this visit, I spoke to mom about providing Sam with more "normal" experiences of sensory-stimulating activities. This mom amazed me; she repeated back everything I told her with those, "So, you're saying, I should . . ." phrases.

On the next appointment, Sam's mom told me all about the new experiences they had had and how she tried everything I told her. I was amazed and excited that this mom would carryover all my treatment goals—this was a therapist's ideal situation.

From then on, Sam's mom would come to therapy reiterating what she had done the previous week and asking what she should work on for the next time. She told me that she set aside an hour each day of "therapy time," during which she carried out the physical therapist's and my instructions. It was always during the evenings so that her husband could occupy Dawn's time. Her husband would also work with Sam an additional hour, and then on weekends when Dawn could spend time at her grandma's house, they would work with Sam together. She told me how difficult it was to live each day running from doctor to doctor to therapists for Sam while trying to maintain a normal family life for Dawn and her husband. If she only knew how much work having a disabled child could be, she would have had Sam first and not had another child.

All of a sudden, I realized that in my excitement of having a mom who would carry out my treatment goals, I forgot to empower this family with just being a family. I then gave Sam's mom "permission" to take a break. A break, which I told her meant time for Sam to be just a baby, just a brother, just a son; a time for Dawn to be just a sister, just a daughter; a time for mom to be just a mom, just a wife; a time for dad to be just a dad, just a husband, and for all to be just a family, with all the things a family includes. Once I gave that signal that it was okay to be just Sam's mom, I saw the biggest weight lifted off her shoulders, but she looked as if she didn't believe me. I gave her no "assignment" for the following week saying that they had lots to work on just learning to be a family. When Sam and his mom returned the following week; the first thing she said was:

> Thank you, Beth. I never realized how much we had forgotten how to just be anything but Sam's everything since he was born. I also thought that if I didn't do his therapy time religiously everyday that I would be a bad mom and Sam would never develop and catch up. Now I can see that I really need time to enjoy being Sam's as well as Dawn's mom and that Sam needs time just being a baby. We all need a vacation once in awhile. Thank you for reminding me that we're all only human, I really appreciated that.

This case reveals how powerful a therapist can be in family life, even when she is not present. Practitioners, as we can see, play a role in a family system whether they are aware of it or not. The stronger the partnership between practitioner, client, and family members, the more likely that the practitioner will influence the family outside therapy time in ways he or she had not thought about. In this example, where clearly Beth and the mother develop an effective partnership, Beth enters the family world as a kind of absent voice in which she unintentionally reinforces the guilt and sense of inadequacy so prevalent among family caregivers who struggle to care for their family member with a disability.

Ironically, in her attempts to involve this very cooperative and willing family in therapy and to create a partnership with the mother, Beth may have added pressure to a family already overloaded with responsibility. When the mother begins to voice her weariness at her task, Beth suddenly recognizes what has happened. Her clever intervention was to suggest that the family take a vacation from therapeutic "homework." In her eloquent appeal to the mother to carry out these new instructions, she offers the mother reasons to return family members to being members of a family rather, than helpers in a complicated therapeutic home team. The importance of this, and the power of the practitioner to influence family dynamics, is captured in the mother's thank you the following week. The mother's grateful response also shows how often practitioners may unwittingly be giving family members messages about whether they are "good" or not based on how faithfully they carry out therapeutic activities. As this mother tells Beth, she thought if she "didn't do his therapy time religiously everyday" she would be a "bad Mom."

Illness and Disability Generate Only Negative Experiences

There has been, and continues to be, an assumption that all the effects of illness and disability on a family are negative. This belief also leads to the erroneous conclusion that family reactions to illness and disability are both predictable and shared. In other words, the practitioner might presume to know about the effect of an illness or disability on the family, without fully understanding a particular family. These notions get dismissed once one listens to families talk about their experiences. We have been struck by the incredible richness of their stories and the difficulty people have reducing their complex reactions to a few discrete categories such as stress, grief, or acceptance. Some theorists have also attempted to develop theories based on stages of reactions, but the fixedness of these stages has been criticized (Moses, 1983).

Much of the research that has been conducted related to the response of family members to illness or disability has been conducted with parents of children with special health care needs. Recently, parents and other family members have offered critiques of this body of research (eg, Lipsky, 1985) citing the failure of researchers to recognize positive outcomes from these experiences. Researchers have tended to measure such predetermined variables as maternal depression and stress. Critics report that personal reports of other effects, including positive changes in family life, have been discounted. Advocates of the family-centered care movement note the failure of many researchers and practitioners to understand the unique features of family adaptation and coping and assert the need for further research that is grounded in the perspectives of family members. Although it is beyond the scope of this chapter to summarize this body of literature, the assumption that effects of disability are unilateral and negative must be challenged as both simplistic and inadequate.

Practitioners need to seek understanding of the effects and affects of illness and disability on the families of the people who come to them for assistance. These effects will likely change over time, and the perceptions of the relative stress of families will be shaped by other events in the family and the availability of resources. The presumption that the entirety of a family's experience can be summarized as stressful often leads to misunderstandings and lost opportunities to promote any positive effects. For example, parents who were interviewed in focus groups concerning their experiences with therapists (Lawlor & Cada, 1993), commented on their disappointment that therapists did not tend to celebrate successes with them.

There is One Family Perspective per Family

Although much of the literature on family-centered care presumes that practitioners come to know all members of the family, we have found that often one member of the family, typically a mother or spouse, serves as the primary contact for the practitioner. It is this individual's perspective that practitioners understand; however, this may be only one of several perspectives held by family members. The case story on p. 50 illustrates how misunderstandings about the family can occur.

In many ways, Elizabeth had an extremely difficult job as she tried to negotiate the expectations of the professionals and the views of Jorge held by her husband and his extended family. She was acting as a type of "cultural broker" (Lawlor & Mattingly, 1994) trying to represent the clinical world to the family and the family world to the clinical staff. The team presumed that Elizabeth's view and the view of her husband and family were highly consistent. Once the team recognized the flaws in their assumptions, they were able to focus on understanding how to ease the burden of being the broker between these two different views, how to promote better communication, and how to better collabo-

THE WHOLE FAMILY

This is a story about Jorge and his family and our attempts as an interdisciplinary team to meet their requests for help in promoting Jorge's development. I was working as an occupational therapist at a regional diagnostic center as a member of a highly cohesive interdisciplinary team. We devoted considerable time toward developing strategies to help families feel more comfortable with the process and prided ourselves in how responsive we were to families. "Morning Team" (a title based purely on scheduling) was considered to be the "best team."

We received a referral on a child who was about 18 months old, who was reportedly not progressing well developmentally. His parents were both highly educated and had recently immigrated to the United States from Mexico while the husband, Raul, was completing his doctoral work at a prestigious university. Elizabeth was trained as a teacher, but had not gone to work since coming to the United States so that she could devote more time to Jorge and getting the family situated.

When we first met the family, we were surprised with the parents' fluency in English and only detected a slight accent in Raul's speech. The family assured us that they used English primarily, although they continued to speak some Spanish in the home, and would prefer our communication to be in English. They were a striking couple, and I recall our initial conversations and meetings to be unusually comfortable, and there was a sense of immediate rapport that I and several colleagues noted. Jorge was a very "syndromey"-looking child. A term which sounds offensive, but reflected our clinical jargon. His somewhat dysmorphic features were particularly apparent because both parents were so striking in their physical attributes. We found Jorge to be developmentally delayed, and I recall my concern that most of his developmental milestones were between 2 and 6 months of age. Jorge was able to propel himself forward on his feet in a manner that simulated walking, but his balance was very poor and he would inevitably crash (into walls, furniture, or the floor) because he was unable to control the forward momentum that he would generate. I remember this sense of how active, out of control, and socially disconnected this child appeared and can still visualize him, even though it has been at least 7 years since I last saw the family.

As a group, we were disappointed in our evaluation findings and were somewhat overwhelmed by the "sadness" of the story as we found little to be optimistic about for Jorge's future development. We felt that the family was the primary strength, but expressed concern that Elizabeth might easily become overburdened with the full-time care of this infant, who seemed to give so little back in terms of social responsiveness. In addition, we decided to focus on safety concerns and identify some other means of mobility while we worked on promoting more age-appropriate development. We continued to see the family for a period of several weeks while we made arrangements for early intervention services in their community.

One morning I was scheduled for a follow-up visit with Jorge and Elizabeth and the speech and physical therapists. We had not seen them for several weeks because they had canceled an appointment. When they came in, I was shocked to see wounds around Jorge's mouth. Elizabeth was also quite anxious about this and told us that Jorge had bitten into a live electrical wire. She saw this as a violation of her commitment to us to work and keep Jorge safe and clearly was horrified that the accident had happened. We at first assumed that her distress was primarily due to guilt, but sensed that there was a lot more she had to tell us. We were all standing awkwardly at the entrance of the clinic when she proceeded to tell us what a "living hell" her life was. Her efforts to follow our direction by keeping Jorge safe and providing more meaningful developmental experiences were viewed by her husband as poor mothering, giving up on his first-born son, and failing to provide the appropriate home environment. In addition, Raul's extended family called from Mexico regularly to remind her that their first-born son would carry the family name and needed to be encouraged to his full potential. For example, using the helmet, trying to facilitate more mature walking patterns, and adapting the home to make it safer were viewed as "signs" of her inadequacies. Our view that we were family-oriented and working collaboratively with the family was clearly out of focus.

rate with the family in identifying intervention priorities and more effective strategies.

▼ THE OCCUPATIONAL THERAPY PRACTITIONER AS THE AGENT OF FAMILY-CENTERED CARE

One of the greatest challenges for practitioners is understanding how their own lived experience shapes their interactions with family members in the course of providing services for patients and clients. Conceptual models of practice, theory regarding family systems and human development, ethics, and public and institutional policies, all contribute to our framework for family-centered interventions. However, practitioners, as the instruments for intervention, bring their selves and their cultural views of families into clinical interactions.

Occupational therapy practitioners come to their profession with life experiences of being a member of a family. This lived experience of growing up in a family significantly shapes who we are as practitioners, particularly in situations in which practitioners are getting to know a family and seeking to understand their needs, priorities, values, hopes, and resources. These assumptions about family life tend to be quite tacit, and we are often not aware of their influence unless we actively reflect on our actions. Guided reflection through mentorship and supervision, as well as discussions with other team members concerning beliefs about specific families, are essential components of intervention planning and implementation with clients and their families.

The following story was shared by one of the chapter authors to illustrate how these multiple perspectives on families intersect in the course of clinical interactions.

CASE STORY

MY FATHER

My father was terminally ill and in a coronary intensive care unit. I caught a flight, as I had done many times over the spring, and joined my gathering siblings. I went directly from the airport to the hospital and met a brother. A friendly and sympathetic nurse approached us and talked about her approach to care. When she described herself as "family-centered," I felt both relieved and jarred by her comments, because family-centered care had been the focus of my research and teaching. When I have thought about this encounter, which I have many times, I conjure up the theme from Twilight Zone as a kind of background music.

Shortly after we entered his room, the nurse returned and asked us to leave because she had some procedures to do. My sister questioned her a little bit about this because she had been with my father during the day and evening shifts and had been allowed to stay.

We were troubled about leaving the room because we had made a promise to my father that he would not die alone. My professional self knew that this was quite presumptuous, given the nature of hospital life and the fact that many hospitals require that you follow visiting hours, particularly in intensive care units. However, as a member of a family that loved this man deeply we just knew that we would need to be there. We left the room and waited in the unit day room. After over 20 minutes had gone by, my brother and I returned to check. The nurse was doing an invasive procedure that we

had understood would not be done. When we spoke to the nurse, she talked about the fact that she was the one with the nurse's license and we should not be challenging her. She indicated that she did not agree with our decision not to continue procedures. We tried to find out why she did not agree, because we obviously wanted to do the right thing, and I was still very much hoping that someone would come up with something that would turn things for the better. However, our efforts to understand where she was coming from seemed to generate more defensive reactions. I am sure we were also not the easiest people to talk with at the time because of our stress and distress. Needless to say, a difficult and disturbing series of discussions followed.

The next day another nurse came on duty who cared for my father. At one point she came into the room and asked how my sister and I were doing. She then started crying and apologizing profusely for her tears which she feared were very "unprofessional." As she tried to explain why she was so upset, she began talking about why she had grown so fond of our father. Many of the characteristics she spoke about were aspects that were also very endearing to the family. I was struck by how much this nurse, who was providing the care, cared. She also shared that watching us with our father made her think about her own father and that "She couldn't do it" (presumably referring to our kind of deathbed vigil).

The first nurse spoke eloquently about the principles of family-centered care, but our experience with her was quite contradictory to her espoused beliefs. The second nurse, who we found to be truly a partner in this ordeal, perceived her caring actions as unprofessional. As family members, we felt much more supported by the second nurse and also felt that we were active participants in making decisions for my father. The first nurse seemed to understand the principles of providing family-centered care, but our experiences left us confused, upset, and chastised for interfering with the work of the nurse.

Why did these two experiences feel so different? These two nurses were colleagues and worked under the prevailing philosophy of the unit that included being responsive to the needs of families and developing effective partnerships with family members. Perhaps the difference can be partially explained by the fact that the first nurse seemed to perceive the involvement of family members as interfering with her role as the nurse. The second nurse also had confusion about her perceptions of how a nurse behaved and her personal response to the situation. She seemed to fear that sharing emotions and getting "personally involved" diminished her professionalism. In implementing family-centered care, practitioners must move beyond the rhetoric and develop roles as practitioners that integrate the need for supportive relationships within the context of the "work" of providing care.

►CONCLUSION

In the foregoing sections, we have highlighted many of the challenges involved in attempting to respond to the needs of clients and their families. Challenges are coupled with opportunities. As practitioners discover ways of getting to know families and understanding their perspectives, opportunities emerge for practitioners to construct richer, more meaningful experiences. The more meaningful the experience the more likely treatment will be efficacious.

We have found that discussions of opportunities must be tempered with specific cautions. Approaches to getting to know families must be noninvasive, sensitive, nonjudgmental, and respectful of the parameters for privacy and disclosure that individuals indicate. Understanding a perspective does not presume that as an occupational therapy practitioner you are responsible for intervening around every dimension of that perspective. Family-centered care is implemented most effectively in situations in which interdisciplinary efforts are well coordinated and effectively communicated. In situations in which practitioners are working in relative isolation, caution must be exercised to ensure that they are practicing within the bounds of their expertise and appropriately facilitating access to other resources as needed.

We intuitively recognize that such things as our ethnicity, nationality, geographical home, perhaps even our religion, provide us powerful cultural worlds. These aspects of our background help make us who we are, culturally speaking. We are often less aware that our profession and our family also offer cultural worlds that shape some of our deepest assumptions, beliefs, and values. This chapter concerns a kind of cultural intersection between the practitioner (acting as a member of a professional culture) and a client (acting as a member of a family culture). Practitioners, of course, have families, and clients often have professions. However, when practitioners and clients meet in a treatment situation, the practitioner's professional and institutional cultures are particularly significant in shaping how the practitioner defines good treatment and a good professional–client relationship.

REFERENCES

Beer, D., Lawlor, M., & Mattingly, C. (1994). Collaboration, coercion, or compliance? (Paper presented at American Occupational Therapy Annual Conference).

Colman, W. (1988). The evolution of occupational therapy in the public schools: The laws mandating practice. *American Journal of Occupational Therapy, 42,* 701–705.

Cunningham, C., & Davis, H. (1985). *Working with parents: Frameworks for collaboration.* Philadelphia: Open University Press.

Deal, A., Dunst, C., & Trivette, C. (1989). A flexible and functional approach to developing individualized family support plans. *Infants and Young Children, 1*(4), 32–43.

Edelman, L., Greenland, B., & Mills, B. (1993). *Building parent professional collaboration: Facilitator's guide.* St. Paul: Pathfinder Resources.

Foucault, M. (1973). *The birth of the clinic: An archaeology of medical perception.* New York: Vintage Books.

Foucault, M. (1979). *Discipline and punish: The birth of the prison.* New York: Vintage Books.

Good, B. (1993). *Medicine, rationality, and experience.* Cambridge: Cambridge University Press.

Good, B., & Good, M.D. (1994). In the subjunctive mode: Epilepsy narratives in Turkey. *Social Science in Medicine, 38,* 835–842.

Gordon, D. (1988). Clinical science and clinical experience: Changing boundaries between art and science in medicine. In M. Locke & D. Gordon (Eds.), *Biomedicine examined* (pp. 257–295). Dordrecht: Kluwer Academic.

Hahn, R. A., & Gaines, A. D. (Eds.). (1985). *Physicians of Western medicine.* Norwell, MA: D. Reidel Publishing Company.

Hanft, B. (1989). *Family-centered care: An early intervention resource manual.* Rockville, MD: American Occupational Therapy Association.

Hanft, B. E. (1991). Impact of public policy on pediatric health and education programs. In W. Dunn (Ed.), *Pediatric occupational therapy: Facilitating effective service provision* (pp. 273–284). Thoroughfare, NJ: Slack.

Howard, J., & Strauss, A. (1975). *Humanizing health care.* New York: John Wiley & Sons.

Kleinman, A. (1988). *The illness narratives: Suffering, healing, and the human condition.* New York: Basic Books.

Lawlor, M. C. (1991). Historical and societal influences on school system practice. In A. Bundy (Ed.), *Making a difference: OTs and PTs in public schools* (pp. 1–15). Chicago: The University of Illinois.

Lawlor, M. C., & Cada, E. (1993). Partnerships between therapists, parents, and children. *OSERS News in Print, V*(4), 27–30.

Lawlor, M. C., & Mattingly, C. (1994). *Understanding family-centered care.* (Concept paper).

Lipsky, D. K. (1985). A parental perspective in stress and coping. *American Journal of Orthopsychiatry, 55*, 614–617.

Locke, M., & Gordon, D. (Eds.). (1988). *Biomedicine examined.* Dordrecht: Kluwer Academic.

Mattingly, C. (1991). What is clinical reasoning? *American Journal of Occupational Therapy, 45*, 979–998.

Mattingly, C. & Fleming, M. (1994). *Clinical reasoning: Forms of inquiry in a therapeutic practice.* Philadelphia: F. A. Davis.

McGonigel, M. J., Kaufmann, R. K., & Johnson, B. H. (Eds.). (1991). *Guidelines and recommended practices for the individualized family service plan.* Bethesda: Association for the Care of Children's Health.

Moses, K. L. (1983). The impact of initial diagnosis: Mobilizing family resources. In J. Mulick & S. Pueschel (Eds.), *Parent-professional partnerships in developmental disability services* (pp. 11–34). Cambridge, MA: Academic Guild.

Rosen, S. & Granger, M. (1992). Early intervention and school programs. In A. Crocker, H. Cohen, & T. Kastner (Eds.), *HIV infection and developmental disabilities: A resource for service providers* (pp. 75–84). Baltimore: Paul Brookes.

Trostle, J. A. (1988). Medical compliance as an ideology. *Social Sciences in Medicine, 27*, 1299–1308.

Chapter 6

Culture and Other Forms of Human Diversity in Occupational Therapy

Juli McGruder

C ulture can be defined in many ways. In occupational therapy, culture has been defined as learned, shared experience that provides "the individual and the group with effective mechanisms for interacting both with others and with the surrounding environment." (Krefting & Krefting, 1991, p. 102). "To belong to a culture is to have become socialized into a whole series of life worlds" (Mattingly & Beer, 1993, p. 156).

The concept of culture can be misused in occupational therapy. Isabel Dyck wrote:

. . . a reliance on culture as distinct beliefs, values, and customary practices to explain nonadherence and difficulties in the therapeutic process is misguided. The everyday social and work conditions that shape health experiences and behaviors must also be recognized. These, in turn, are forged within a socio-economic and political environment (1992, p. 696)

This specific criticism of the use of the concept of culture in occupational therapy is informed by three more general criticisms of conceptualizations of culture; that is, the concept, misused, has a tendency to essentialize, reify, and mystify human difference.

To essentialize is to take complex multifaceted phenomena, such as the lifeways, ideas, and all that a group of humans has acquired by learning, and reduce them to a few basic "essences" that explain this group in totality. To reify is to "thing-ify," to take an abstract and to treat it as a concrete tangible thing with definable boundaries. "Culture is not a thing," wrote Mattingly and Beer (1993, p. 157). Treating culture as a thing may have some usefulness, they argued, but it also promotes stereotyping. To mystify is to obscure important causes, contributing factors, results, or other relevancies

of a phenomenon. Any attempt to define or discuss culture must avoid reproducing these errors and fallacies. With that precaution in mind, let us examine a list of defining attributes of culture on which most students of culture can agree.

▼ WHAT CULTURE IS: AN AGREED UPON LIST

Culture is real, learned, shared, malleable and dynamic, and invisible. Although not concrete and tangible, culture is real. When someone falls ill because of a curse, the illness is real. When someone resolves a conflict of opinion with reference to axioms about individuality, personal rights, or individual uniqueness—everyone is entitled to his or her own opinion—he or she enacts a cultural reality that revolves around this conception of personhood. We cannot see or touch culture, but its effects surround us, rendering it a very real force.

Culture is not inherited, it is learned. Beliefs and values are taught to us both explicitly and tacitly in our families and communities and by mass media. Most readers of this chapter will not have learned much about spirits, curses, or propitiation rituals, but will have been taught in more than a thousand ways that they are each unique individuals with unalienable rights. The idea that we are individuals with a free will and a "natural" right to our own opinions seems a given to 20th century Americans, but is quite foreign to others. It is a cultural idea.

Culture is not idiosyncratic, but is shared in human society. Even though it may be carried in the minds of individuals, as some have argued, culture's manifestations are social.

How do you greet your grandfather? With a kiss on the cheek? A hug? A "hello?" A kiss on the back of his hand? Or do you shake his hand and then kiss your own and place it over your heart, as a respectful child in Zanzibar would? Scholars of culture may dispute whether it is the greeting behavior itself or the shared understanding that underlies it that is the locus of culture, but all would agree that culture is shared socially. As such, it is most easily perceived in interactions between and among people.

Although culture is real and has incredible staying power, it is not static, fixed, or immutable. Values, attitudes, lifeways, arts, morals, customs, laws, and the many other things that are included in culture can change in response to the forces of history, politics, and economics. Culture is malleable and dynamic. Even a cursory glance at the advertising media of the United States in the late 20th century would reveal that we think light brown or beige skin, narrow muscular buttocks, large chests, and full lips are aesthetically pleasing in either gender. Was it always so? No. For example, before the industrial revolution, when peasants labored outdoors, suntanned skin was not considered aesthetically pleasing, but a mark of low class. The leisured classes of the preindustrial years in North America and Europe took great pains to protect the whiteness of their skin, even while enjoying outdoor activities. It was not until workers went indoors to sunless factories that suntanning became a mark of expendable income and leisure time and, thus, became culturally valued.

Cultures change as human groups come in contact with each other. A 10-year-old child who is a family friend and a recent immigrant from the Philippines made us chuckle when she asked if we knew the Filipino dish, "spaghetti." But spaghetti is Italian, right? Unless you remember that Marco Polo brought pasta to Italy from Asia.

Culture is invisible, especially to the one who carries it and participates in it. It is taken for granted. When we come in contact with cultural ways that are different from our own we perceive the "otherness," the strangeness of the other groups' ways. But it takes repeated experiences with entering other cultural spaces, coupled with introspection, just to make our own cultural assumptions visible to us. In Western culture people accept without question the unitariness and continuity of personhood as a given, as natural. But the "nature" of human nature is a culturally constructed entity, invisible to us, because we are immersed in it.

▼ WHAT CULTURE IS NOT: RACIAL AND ETHNIC DIVERSITY

Although the terms are often used interchangeably, culture is not the same as race or ethnicity. Culture is not a polite synonym for race, although it is sometimes employed as such by people who are uncomfortable with discussing race and ethnicity. Racial and ethnic groups are often too large

to share much overlap in cultural beliefs, attitudes, and practices.

Ethnicity is commonly defined as membership, conveyed by birth, in a racial, religious, national, or linguistic group. But it is important to distinguish between ethnic or racial identity that is self-selected versus imposed on a group from outside. Race and ethnicity are socially constructed categories, concepts agreed on in public and private discourse, which can only be understood in the context of the history of their employment in a particular place.

Moreover, race, although an operative concept in American social life, politics, economics, and entertainment marketing, is biologically a nonentity. Biologists have proved many times that there is more variation within than between the so-called races of humans, thereby invalidating the categorization on a statistical basis. To say that race is a bogus concept biologically or that it is socially constructed, however, does not mean that race is not psychologically or socially real. Dealing with race relations is a very real part of life for many humans. Humans are killed, denied or given rights and privileges on the basis of race. Even though race and ethnicity are not the same as culture, the historical experience of oppression or, for that matter, of privilege, based on racial or ethnic group membership can shape culture.

▼ LANGUAGE GROUP DIVERSITY

Because occupational therapy practitioners rely on interviews for gathering data relevant to treatment planning at the level of typical activities, role performance, and environmental constraints and demands, perhaps the diversity that most complicates the treatment process is language diversity.

Some practitioners are naive relative to issues surrounding language diversity and communication (Wardin, 1996). For example, some occupational therapists who were interviewed by Wardin indicated that, when family members or professional translators were not available, gestural communication could be relied on. Yet, gestures are not universal, and without an understanding of what gestures mean in different cultural contexts, occupational therapy practitioners run the risk of insulting their clients. In North America when people gesture for someone to come close they flex the index finger and, the more pleading and apologetic they are, the more likely they are to minimize the range and the size of this beckoning gesture. In East Africa, a polite "come here" must be beckoned with the whole hand and forearm and to use a digit or minimize the size of the gesture is a serious insult. Even a smile can be misinterpreted. Foreign visitors to North America have commented on how embarrassed they have felt by North Americans' persistent smiling at them. Cross-cultural communication literature has described how smiles may be misinterpreted, for example, as sly indications of the smiler's superiority and as an indication that the one smiled at is appearing foolish. One foreign student told of how he felt he must return to his room to check his clothing and make certain his trouser fly was closed and his attire neat as he could think of no other reason that the other students would persist in grinning at him so. Clearly, nonverbal communication is an inadequate basis on which to form a therapeutic relationship across cultures.

More reliable than gestural communication, but not without difficulties, is the use of translators. Instead of having professional translation services, many respondents apparently worked in systems that led them to rely on family members for translation (Wardin, 1996). Problems that occurred in the use of family members as translators, most frequently related to family members giving too much help or suggesting responses on evaluations (Wardin). Furthermore, practitioners should be sensitive to the role strain caused when junior members are required to ask personal questions of, or assertively give directions to, more senior members.

This recounting of some practitioners' lack of knowledge on language diversity and cross-cultural communication is not meant to criticize or indict occupational therapy practitioners as a group. Any lack of sophistication apparent in the respondents to Wardin's (1996) survey simply mirrors that seen in the United States population generally. Compared to citizens of other nations, those of the United States are more monolingual and less aware of cross-cultural communication conventions than most. The more positive findings of Wardin's study, on the other hand, showed that therapists treated significantly more clients with limited English than monolingual therapists did; undertook more assessments in these clients' first languages; reported understanding their clients' needs more; and appeared more knowledgeable about how to get translator services.

In any language there are individual variations, called idiolects, and group variations, called dialects. Dialects have systematic variations from one another, at the phonological (sound), grammatical (rules for combining), and lexical (vocabulary) levels, but are mutually intelligible; that is, speakers of different dialects of the same language can understand each other. Variations that are merely phonological are called accents.

Although all languages are made up of dialects, many people think that there is one right way, well-defined and fixed, that forms the standard version of a language. However, no dialect or language is considered deficient, bad, or inadequate. A multiculturally competent practitioner must remember that clients have a right to express themselves in the language and dialect that they choose.

Within a language, there are also specialized vocabularies specific to some function or profession. These are called jargon or argot. Consider the impenetrability of some common occupational therapy jargon, from a new client's perspective. If a practitioner approached me saying she was there to retrain me in activities of daily living, I might well mistake her for a reading teacher, for reading is an activity I perform daily and value highly. I would be disappointed when I learned we were to work on hair combing or tooth brushing. To a Buddhist monk, self-care might mean med-

itation. As with all words, the meanings of these phrases are not inherent in their shapes or sounds, but are assigned arbitrarily and then agreed on through their use. Practitioners become adept at changing their style of communication from speaking "medical" or "therapy" jargon to speaking common English more understandable to their clients.

Remember that communication is not a simple or straightforward process. When analyzed closely, it can be seen as fraught with so many complications that one is amazed we understand each other at all. Practitioners acknowledge the need for active listening that checks to see that the meaning received is the one intended, and that attends to both verbal and nonverbal aspects of communication.

▼ MYTHS, STEREOTYPES, XENOPHOBIA, AND GENERALIZATIONS

In multicultural awareness, a myth is defined as an unfounded or poorly founded belief that is given uncritical acceptance by members of a group. Myths operate in support of existing or traditional practices and institutions. Stereotypes are mental pictures based on myths that lead people to associate a characteristic or set of characteristics with particular groups of people. An experienced cultural awareness trainer provided the following short list of the most frequent stereotypes that he has elicited from mixed groups of social service workers over the years (M. McGruder, personal communication, 1996). Given permission and encouragement to share myths they had heard or stereotypes they had formed, learners most frequently admitted to the following associations: homosexuals with **acquired immunodeficiency syndrome (AIDS)**, Native Americans with **alcoholism**, African Americans with low intelligence and a lack of education, European Americans with arrogance, Asian Americans with good math skills, Mexican Americans with laziness, Jewish Americans with stinginess and property ownership, men with sexual aggression, and women with weakness and emotionality. This same cultural awareness trainer also noted, however, that education has a profound influence on stereotypes. He has watched, over the years, a weakening of the association between homosexuality and AIDS.

Xenophobia is defined as an unreasonable fear or hatred of those different from ourselves. Is xenophobia just part of human nature, as some have argued, or is it taught and learned, handed down from adults to children, as part and parcel of a social group's culture? The fact that xenophobia can be unlearned and that some humans are consistently attracted to those who are different from themselves seems to argue against a view of humans as naturally suspicious of other humans not of their own group.

The tendency to generalize, however, and to cluster perceptions in memory, does appear to be an inherent part of the human mental apparatus. Piaget (1969) wrote about the development of children's thinking in terms of forming and refining schemata to group objects and creatures in the natural world around them. Thinking about such cognitive clustering can provide some insights into how myths and stereotypes about groups of "others" are formed. It is a way to begin to undo some of the myths and stereotypes we may have incorporated into our own thinking about human diversity.

Let us say that at some point in your youth you heard the phrase "woman driver." Circumstances under which you heard this bit of language employed allowed you to rather quickly understand that this was a phrase meant to disparage the abilities of women to operate motor vehicles safely and efficiently. Having heard the phrase used once or twice, you internalized this concept, even if just on a trial basis. With this concept embedded in your mental apparatus, however, you were readily able to incorporate and file away in this conceptual category any and all instances you may have noted personally or heard about in which a woman indeed did operate a motor vehicle in an ineffective or unsafe manner. Conversely, there was no handy cognitive schema in which you might mentally record, in a ready-made category, all incidents or reports of men driving poorly. Challenged to recall instances of or anecdotes about bad driving by women and by men, you would much more readily retrieve from memory all those precoded instances of bad driving by women. A concept is introduced and, as with a self-fulfilling prophecy, evidence begins to be amassed through experience—experience filtered through previously learned cognitive categories. You might well conclude that women are worse drivers than men. Then you would be confronted with a different reality. Insurance actuarial tables show that, in fact, women are better drivers than men and insurance companies, large and small, honor that truth in the way they structure differential rates for coverage by gender.

Humans cannot turn off the grouping, generalizing, and schemata-building aspects of their minds. They can, however, rigorously examine the **generalizations** they make about other humans and the conclusions they draw. To practice competently and ethically in working with a diversity of individuals and groups, occupational therapy practitioners and other health care professionals accept the responsibility of examining their generalizations.

Generalizations about cultural or racial groups need not be as negative or destructive as were most of the stereotypes listed in the first paragraph of this section. Health professionals have found it useful to generalize from published lists of characterizations of particular ethnic, cultural, or language groups. One such list contrasts beliefs, values, and practices of American Indians with those of Anglo-European Americans, so all statements included are considered as relative comparisons. In contrast to European Americans, American Indians are characterized as: more group than individual oriented, having respect for elders and experts,

viewing time and place as permanent and settled, being introverted and avoiding ridicule or criticism of others, being pragmatic and accepting of "what is," emphasizing responsibility for family and self more than authority over or responsibility for larger social groups, attending to how others behave more so than to what they say they think or feel, and seeking harmony (Joe & Malch, 1992). This may be very useful information to have as a starting point for observations of and conversations with a particular Native American client or family, but it is important to remain open to the possibility that the individual or various family members may espouse and enact all, some, or none of these beliefs and values. If, for example, the hypothetical client were an urban American Indian Movement activist leader, it would be unlikely that he would concern himself only with self and family or pragmatically accept the status quo. The more information that you have about social history and context of an individual or family group, the better able you will be to discern whether published descriptions of these cultural "others" will apply.

Attempts to generalize from knowledge of another's religion present particular difficulties. While North Americans and Europeans may tend to select a religious tradition and give it complete allegiance, excluding the possibility of participating in religious practices springing from other traditions, this is not the rule worldwide. Moslems in North, West, and East Africa, for example, do not experience rituals aimed at recognizing or propitiating capricious and problematic spirits as contradictory to or disrespectful of their Islamic faith. Similarly, spirit possession and animal sacrifice practices by Brazilians practicing candomblé or Cubans practicing santeria, both of which blend elements of Christianity with worship of West African deities, do not see these as interfering with their practice of Roman Catholicism. Conservative orthodox leaders of Sunni Islam or of Roman Catholicism may frown on such practices, but their disapproval is somewhat moot from the perspective of the practitioner-client relationship and attempts at cross-cultural understanding. Medical anthropologists have long observed that, faced with adversity, humans will generally try any and all remedies they perceive as useful, even if these remedies do not fit into one systematic world view or set of beliefs in the supernatural.

Another caution in applying generalizations is to consider the forces of assimilation. As previously mentioned, mass media and interactions with other social group members provide a powerful impetus for cultural or racial minorities to adopt dominant group values, beliefs, and practices. This is seen most readily in generations born to immigrant citizens. A client's personal ethos (world view and approach to life) may well be a creative blend of cultural elements from the previous society, or older generation's culture, and the new society and culture he or she has entered. For example, Yasuda (1994) studied Issei (first-generation Japanese American immigrants) and Nisei (second-generation) adults who lived in a long-term care facility that

TABLE 6-1. Review of Occupational Therapy Literature on Culturally Sensitive Assessment

Author	Year	Description of Work	Conclusions About Effects of Diversity on Test Scores
Bowman & Wallace	1990	Quasi-experimental study, N = 22 white preschoolers of low SES compared with 22 higher SES preschoolers (matched for age, race, sex, hand dominance, height, and weight) on a battery of 12 assessments.	Lower SES subjects scored as functioning at significantly lower developmental levels in hand strength, visuomotor integration, and praxis development. Therapist should consider the effects of social class when interpreting results of tests of hand strength, of the Beery Test of Visual-Motor Integration and the Praxis on Verbal Command subtest of the SIPT. Vestibular functioning and other SIPT measures of praxis did not differ significantly between the two groups.
Janelle	1992	Quasi-experimental study, N = 13 nondisabled and 8 congenitally physically disabled adolescents (matched for IQ, age, race, and SES) compared for locus of control, as measured by the Nowicki–Strickland Locus of Control Scale	Unanticipated finding that disability status did not correlate with locus of control. Rather, race was the only variable correlated significantly with locus of control scores, with African American subjects in both groups scoring more external than European American subjects. Given small number of African American subjects, author viewed this result with caution, considered that SES might have been a hidden factor in difference by race and recommended further research. See also Elliot (1995) in Table 6-2.
Myers	1992	Description and discussion based on clinical observation of Hmong children and their families in an early-intervention program.	No standardized test of development, motor functioning, or sensory integration has included the Hmong population in norming. Approach to interpretation of standardized testing should be one of item analysis, description of patterns of behavior, and augmentation of test results through extended or multiple observations in child's home environment. Some often-tested skills may be absent or delayed secondary, not due to developmental delay, but to lack of family expectation, exposure, and practice.
Miller	1992	Description and discussion of observations based on experience of trying to administer standardized tests, such as the Peabody Test of Motor Development to orphans in Cambodia.	Children had such limited experience with toys and with one-on-one mental play stimulation with an adult that therapist had to quickly abandon this assessment strategy. Devising an observation checklist, therapist used her knowledge of development and neurodevelopmental treatment to make judgments about children's areas of competence.
Fudge	1992	Description and discussion of observations based on the experience of administering the Peabody to children with kwashiorkor and other types of malnutrition in Guatemala.	Therapist concluded that children's limited exposure to test materials made it impossible to interpret test results as indicators of motor function. Rather, as children responded to novel play tasks, Peabody format allowed observations about early cognitive functioning and imitative learning.
Packir	1994	Quasi-experimental study, comparison of 15 Sri Lankan mother–child dyads to U.S.-established norms for the Nursing Child Assessment Satellite Training scales (NCAST)	Sri Lankan subject dyads scored significantly below norms on cognitive and social emotional growth-fostering subscales. Norms are unlikely to apply to this population, as cultural differences in parenting, differential valuing of various temperaments of infants and children and different social norms of parent–child interaction (eg, frequency of sustained direct eye contact) limit application of this instrument across cultures.
Cermack et al.	1995	Quasi-experimental study, N = 25 North Americans N = 56 Israelis all post CVA, compared on the Loewstein Occupational Therapy Cognitive Assessment	Only one subtest, the Orientation to Time test, revealed significant difference between American and Israeli groups for subjects with either L or R CVA. Researchers unsure whether age differences between the two groups or cultural differences underlay better performance by Israeli group with lower mean age. Paper also deals with differences between performance of subjects with L vs. R CVA, not summarized here.
Colonius	1995	Quasi-experimental study, N = 27 Alaskan Native (Tlingit and Haida) children, N = 7 non-Native children from same preschools, compared with norms for the FirstSTEP, developmental screening test.	Native Alaskan children scored significantly higher than norms in the motor domain and significantly lower than norms in the cognitive and language domains. Non-Native peers of a similar SES (based on their inclusion in Head Start preschool) scored at or above normative means. Given norms and performance of small sample of non-Native children, differences in performance across groups seem related to culture more than to SES. Researcher recommended caution in application of FirstSTEP norms to Alaskan Native children.

(SES = socioeconomic status; SIPT = Sensory Integration and Praxis Test; CVA = cerebrovascular accident; L or R = left or right) catered specifically to Japanese Americans. Meals, many activities and opportunities for Buddhist religious participation at this facility reflected Japanese culture. The two groups were compared for morale and time spent in activity participation. The Issei group spent significantly more time in religious activity, and expressed overall more subjective well-being, more positive attitudes, less agitation, and less loneliness. Yasuda surmised that the Nisei elders were more assimilated into North American mainstream culture and thus, perhaps, their needs were less well met by the culture-specific program of the nursing home.

Finally, it is also very important to realize that the process of generalizing about culturally different others is multidirectional. As you interact with those different from you, and test hypotheses based on your learned generalizations, others will be doing the same for you. Myths and stereotypes about all cultural and racial groups, including European Americans, abound. The reader is directed to books such as Henry Louis Gates' *Colored People*, and Anna Deavere Smith's *Twilight, Los Angeles, 1992* or *Fires in the Mirror* for priceless insights into cultural and racial myth-making and stereotyping in America.

▼ CULTURE AND OTHER FORMS OF DIVERSITY IN OCCUPATIONAL THERAPY PROCESSES

Mattingly and Beer (1993) offered two straightforward reasons for occupational therapy practitioners to strive for an accurate understanding of their clients' cultural backgrounds: (1) to allow for collaboration in goal setting and treatment planning and (2) to individualize therapy. To these I would add two others: (1) to ensure accurate assessment and (2) to increase the likelihood of equitable intervention. Underlying all of these goals of culturally sensitive intervention is the practitioner's need to establish accurate empathy for the client.

More than 90% of occupational therapy practitioners are European Americans (AOTA, 1991). Only 76% of the U. S. population is European American. African Americans, Hispanic and Latino Americans, and Native Americans are underrepresented in our profession. Even if race and ethnicity are not the same as culture, they are attributes that, similar to culture, are marked as differences in North American society. As such, they can represent challenges to interpersonal understanding between individuals coming from different groups, just as class and culture do. The American Occupational Therapy Association (AOTA) does not keep statistics on the class backgrounds of practitioners, but it seems safe to hypothesize that occupational therapy practitioners come from a narrower range of class backgrounds than those of their clients. Furthermore, all practitioners share the socializing influence of higher education. A recent study showed strong agreement among occupational therapy practitioners of different races on a list of beliefs and values, whereas these same practitioners ascribed different sets of values to racial or ethnic groups other than their own (Pineda, 1996).

An occupational therapist interviewing to discover the activity goals of a client and the meaning that activities hold for a client is sometimes likely to elicit stories that make no sense to him or her. The ethical practitioners' challenge is to push themselves outside the comfortable but invisible confines of their culture and class to attempt an accurate understanding of their clients' world view and life situation. Doing so is a necessary step in collaborative goal setting and treatment planning, accurate assessment, individualizing therapy, and ensuring equitable intervention.

Cultural differences enter into the process of evaluation not only at the level of achieving understanding and empathy for the client, but also at the level of choosing assessment instruments and strategies and interpreting results. By their very nature, standardized norm-referenced assessment tools make assumptions about normalcy that may be culturally bound. Most testing instruments assume characteristics of modal individuals often based on middle-class European or European American lifeways and experiences. For example, Law (1993) asserted that current activities of daily living (ADL) and **instrumental activities of daily living (IADL)** instruments reflected North American dominant cultural values concerning independence and individual rights. Investigations by occupational practitioners examining cultural differences have often revealed a conflict over how much independence and how much interdependence with family members is ideal (Skawski, 1987; Pineda, 1996; Wardin, 1996). Table 6-1 summarizes other occupational therapy literature that supports the need to tailor assessment strategies with care, given cultural, racial, ethnic, and class diversity.

In the United States, racial minorities, particularly African Americans, have less access to health care than do European Americans, and suffer higher mortality and morbidity rates from a host of common disease processes (AMA, 1990; Evans, 1992a). Limited access to health care services seems especially evident for high-technology interventions, costly surgical procedures, and lengthy rehabilitation services. Once an accurate understanding of the client is achieved and valid assessment strategies selected, the practitioner's role is as an advocate for the client to receive needed services. Evans (1992a) recommended that European Americans carefully reexamine their assumptions any time they perceive a client of color as unlikely to benefit from rehabilitation services to be certain that myths, stereotypes, or generalizations do not cloud their vision.

▼ CULTURE AND OTHER FORMS OF DIVERSITY IN OCCUPATIONAL THERAPY THEORY

Humphry (1995) described how chronic poverty, an experience unequally shared across cultural and racial groups in the United States, depersonalizes and erodes the sense of

TABLE 6-2. Criticism of the Model of Human Occupation (MOHO) Based on Research in Various Cultures

Author	Year	Description of Work	Conclusions and Criticism of MOHO
Wieringa & McColl	1987	Description and theoretical discussion, observational data, Native Canadians: Cree and Ojibway	MOHO definitions of temporal adaptation and dysfunction and emphasis on productivity and individualism belie cultural bias that potentially limits the model's applicability to intervention with this population. Some concepts of the model (open system, person–environment interaction) resonate well with Native Canadian ethos, however. Model is flexible and can be adapted for use with Canadian Native populations.
Evans	1992b	Description and theoretical discussion, observation and interview with persons with schizophrenia and their families in two cultures	Concepts of personal causation, temporal adaptation, valued goals, and personal interests are shaped by North American-dominant culture. These concepts limit application of the model in Swahili culture and to some North American groups as well.
Evans & Salim	1992	Validity study. Hospital sample, $N = 50$ persons with schizophrenia, $N = 10$ nondysfunctional subjects. Correlation between and among psychosocial assessment measures and measures of illness.	A test of sensory integration distinguished between normals and schizophrenic patients in an African psychiatric setting better than did an interview score based on assumptions of the model of human occupation. The sensory integration assessment correlated more highly with a culture-specific test of functional skills than did the MOHO interview assessment. The MOHO-inspired interview measure did not correlate with seriousness of illness measures. MOHO was criticized for prematurely attempting to quantify assumptions about relationships among temporal adaptation, agency, control, and normalcy without sufficient regard for cultural variation.
Spadone	1992	Quasi-experimental study. Purposive sample $N = 88$; 29 Thai and 31 Khmer Buddhists and 28 white Methodists; all nondysfunctional. Compared on Rotter Internal–External Locus of Control Scale and Time Reference Inventory (TRI).	No significant differences between groups on locus of control, but all groups scored more external than Rotter's original norms and nearer to a sample of psychiatric inpatients reported by Oakley et al. (1985). On TRI Thai selected more past-oriented statements, white Americans more present-oriented ones. White Americans projected farther into the future than did Thai or Khmer subjects, but *all* three groups had a greater past than future extensions. Calls into question MOHO assumptions that nondysfunctional persons have an internal locus of control and a strong future time orientation.
Wood	1992	Pilot study. Convenience sample, $N = 16$, 7 gay men, 9 lesbian women. Effectiveness of Role Checklist in identifying meaningful time use and occupational roles of gays and lesbians explored.	Sexual orientation relates to a variety of occupational roles, but current MOHO instruments are not designed to capture the existence or meaning of this connection. Sociologic role theory, which undergirds the Role Checklist and informs occupational therapy practice, assumes conformity to societal role expectations that invalidates its use with gay or lesbian people in a homophobic-dominant culture. Values that support occupation science incompatible with those of sociologic role theory.
Jackson	1995a, b	Description and theoretical discussion (1992); $N = 20$, 10 lesbian occupational therapists, 10 lesbian women with disabilities. Feminist and qualitative narrative analysis (1995).	Lesbian sexual orientation and identity organized and gave meaning to occupations and narratives about occupations for all subjects to varying degrees. Symbolic meaning of occupation in lesbian narratives showed dissonance between lesbian identity and heterosexist social surround. Keilhofner has argued that sexual, social, survival, and spiritual activities are outside the purview of occupational therapy, but sexual orientation shapes more than just occupations related to intimacy. Thus, ignoring sexual orientation renders some important symbolic aspects of occupation invisible.
Elliot	1995	Quasi-experimental study. Purposive sample, $N = 43$; 19 African Americans, 24 European Americans. Compared using Rotter Internal–External Locus of Control and Reid–Ware Three-Factor Internal–External scale	African Americans more external than norms on Rotter and on Reid–Ware fatalism factor. With age differences neutralized by analysis of covariance (ANCOVA), scores on Rotter and Reid–Ware fatalism factor varied by race, with African Americans scoring significantly more external than European Americans. Fatalism on Reid–Ware scale is related to degree of control over life events and societal rewards, and is probably sensitive to the effects of external forces such as racism. Use of internal locus of control as characteristic of normalcy in MOHO is questioned.

NEGOTIATING ACROSS MULTIPLE LAYERS OF DIVERSITY

Material for this case study is based in part on interview transcripts from a study conducted by Crenshaw (1996). Some names and circumstances have been altered to protect informant anonymity and provide closure on the case study.

John is a 41-year-old African American father of nine children, the youngest of whom, Tyler, has multiple disabilities and medical conditions related to a chromosomal anomaly. Joanne, John's wife, works full time as a secretary and has health care benefits through a health maintenance organization (HMO). John chooses to work part time so that the family will not be disqualified for Medicaid assistance. The family's income at the poverty level places them among our country's many "working poor." John and Joanne agree that the specialty children's hospital, to which they have access through their Medicaid coverage, provides better, more complete and more sophisticated therapy services than does the HMO. John, Joanne, and the other eight children in the family are able-bodied and generally healthy. John is very involved in the care of his son, Tyler, who is now 3 years old and functions at approximately the 6-month level. On days when John does not work, he is Tyler's primary caregiver. John attends all parent–professional case conferences related to Tyler's ongoing early intervention program.

John has attended parent support group meetings and within the last 2 years has joined a state-level policy-planning council for early intervention services, as a parent member. Through these experiences John has become very knowledgeable about the services available in the state, but very frustrated with state level agencies' perceived slowness and lack of responsiveness to the needs of families with disabled children.

Currently, John and Rita, a 26-year-old European American who is Tyler's occupational therapist, are involved in a conflict about the elements of programming on Tyler's care plan. The occupational therapist has recommended play therapy and is standing firm behind that suggestion. John is seeking expensive exercise equipment and a power wheelchair for Tyler and is refusing play therapy for him. The therapist does not agree that Tyler needs the exercise equipment or is ready for power mobility. She has the power to block John's request for these items by not providing the state with the necessary therapeutic rationale for their procurement. She reports that she sees John as unrealistic and in denial. John is angry about the therapist's interference with his obtaining for his child what he believes the child truly needs.

A second occupational therapist, an African American, intervened by meeting with John and giving him an uninterrupted time to talk about his son, his perceptions of therapy, and his feelings.

During the interview John revealed the following:

- His perception that the range of services available is not communicated to the African American community, asking "Why would they have these services and then hide the fact that they provide these services?"

- His perception that as an African American man he is often disrespected and challenged by European American care providers to prove that he is not "trying to get something for nothing." African American parents, said John, often see the health care system as adversarial and exclusive. He related this to the dominant cultural myth that many African Americans are welfare frauds.

- His perception that the family had received services that were "human and sincere" from some European American care providers; that is, that the problem was not inherent in racial differences. He related several stories about a very caring woman European American pediatrician who had left the area.

- His spiritual beliefs and the deep intangible connection he shares with his nonverbal child. John commented that "the spirituality that is in African American culture is not one that is understood in the European American culture." John related how from the first instant that he saw an early ultrasound image of his son, before any problems were even diagnosed, he had a spiritual connection to the child: "The spirit spoke out to me and I cried . . . I sat on the edge of the bed, picked up the picture and cried. I knew immediately something was wrong." He went on to say that he and Joanne never considered abortion as an option, but decided to let their son's spirit determine his fate. John sees his son as having a very strong spirit and will to live.

- His idea that play therapy would be frivolous and that Tyler needs to work hard, with the most intense therapy possible during the early intervention period because this will determine his course later on. "We don't have time to waste with play, we need to work."

The following elements of cross-cultural conflict are apparent in the case study:

1. A **class** and race conflict based on the historical denial and continuing barriers to equal access to health care for African Americans that makes it

(continued)

difficult for John to trust that the therapist has his or Tyler's best interests at heart. This is intensified by the current struggle over health care reform, and John's fear that he will lose access to the children's hospital.

2. A cultural conflict involving values related to work. John may be misperceived as having a weak work ethic because of his rational choice to limit his income earning so that he does not lose **Medicaid** benefits and because of myths and stereotypes that exist in the dominant culture about both African Americans and welfare recipients.

3. A potential cultural conflict between John and the therapist over the relative values of spirituality and science–technology, given John's assertion that European Americans don't understand his spirituality and occupational therapy's position as an allied medical service in the children's hospital.

4. A potential gender-based cultural conflict with John favoring strength, exercise, technology, and motor skills (male ideal) while the occupational therapist values (or is perceived as valuing) social–emotional, cognitive, and interaction skills (female ideal) to be developed through play.

At the same time, carefully listening to John reveals many bases for agreement and keys to cooperation.

1. John and Joanne have enjoyed very good relations with specific European American care providers in the past, so the trust barrier can be overcome. They have a history of very good relations with a European American woman who was perceived as "human and sincere."

2. John's remarks about work being more necessary and more serious than play actually reveal a strong valuing of work, a work ethic perhaps stronger than the therapist's.

3. John's desire for high-technology exercise equipment and power mobility devices belies a faith in science and technology that is typically considered a mainstream, dominant culture value. He likely does not experience his spiritual beliefs as being in conflict with this faith in technology as an aid to human progress.

4. John's belief in the existence and strength of Tyler's spirit opens a door to an understanding of play as a developer of that spirit.

5. John has clearly internalized the importance of early intervention and has learned to be an advocate for his child within a complex system.

Here is a list of things that Rita can do to rebuild a cooperative working relationship with John so that Tyler can benefit from both of their good intentions. As a professional service provider, it is Rita's responsibility to begin the process of resolving the conflict.

1. Accord John respect. Use his surname in addressing him. He is her senior and in accordance with norms of African American culture should be addressed formally until he explicitly gives permission for her to call him "John" (Evans, 1992a; Willis, 1992).

2. Assume that John earnestly seeks what is best for his child. Convey this assumption to him and, for that matter, to all parents (Crenshaw, 1996). Convey that Tyler has a right to the best combination of services possible and work diligently toward that end. Elicit and respect John and Joanne's opinions on Tyler's care.

3. Rigorously avoid conversing with coworkers about personal matters while providing care to Tyler, or indulging in idle chitchat during sessions. These kinds of behavior are read as a lack of concern and not having one's mind on one's work. Adopt a serious, but warm attitude (Willis, 1992).

4. Rigorously avoid conveying agreement with any stereotypes of African Americans or welfare recipients as somehow not worthy of the best services available. Similarly, if Rita disagrees with or disproves of the family's decisions about the pregnancy, the size of their family, or work schedules she must keep these entirely out of the conversation. Her role is to help the family, not to judge it. Poverty is not, in and of itself, a dysfunction (Willis, 1992; Humphry, 1995).

5. Open a discussion with John about his spiritual connection with Tyler and seek to understand and appreciate it. It is an asset to Tyler's development.

6. Elicit from John his aims and goals for the desired exercise equipment and power mobility devices. Remain open and use active listening.

7. Once these views of John's are understood, build from them, negotiating a view of the problem and its treatment that both practitioner and client's parents can agree on (Kleinman, 1988). For example, present the occupational therapy belief that play is the antecedent of work. Present play therapy as a way to exercise Tyler's spirit through awakening his understanding of cause and effect and the way that the physical world works. Given John's interest in high technology and Tyler's limited motor control, plan to incorporate in play therapy some work with microswitches or computer keyboards to activate toys or games. Explain the skills of understanding cause and effect and operating switches as prerequisites to learning to use power mobility equipment and augmentative communication devices. Offer hope that Tyler will one day be able to profit from these high-technology assistive devices.

self, alters children's developmental progression, and causes potential conflicts between practitioners and clients or their caregivers around the five universal problems of time orientation, activity, human relationships, human nature, and control of natural forces. These value-conflicts have implications, not only for testing that purports to measure locus of control and human motivation, but also for how we represent humans and human occupation in occupational therapy theory. Occupational therapy theoreticians continually build and refine models for practice. The profession values this scholarly activity. Refinement takes place as scholars open their work for criticism and debate among their peers. Rigorously examining the culture-based assumptions of a practice model is one way to test it.

The **model of human occupation**, one of the more encompassing frames of reference in occupational therapy, incorporates multiple levels of data gathering about humans' skill, habits and roles, and their interests and motivations embedded in a social and cultural environment. Because the model of human occupation emphasizes temporal adaptation, is concerned with volition as a regulator of playful and productive output, and includes locus of control as an element in the volitional subsystem, it incorporates concepts the configurations of which vary widely across cultures. Although the model is valued for its attempts to attend to issues of culture and social environment, descriptions of the aforementioned elements of the model, especially in its earlier articulations, showed a distinct North American dominant culture bias (Kielhofner & Henry, 1988; Kielhofner, 1985; Neville, Kreisberg & Kielhofner, 1985; Oakley, Kielhofner & Barris, 1985). Table 6-2 summarizes studies that tested the model of human occupation in a variety of cultures and suggested ways to improve the applicability of the model across cultures. A more recent focus among model of human occupation theoreticians has been assessment of the model's volitional subsystem components through narrative analysis, rather than formal quantification-oriented assessment (Helfrich & Kielhofner, 1994; Helfrich, Kielhofner & Mattingly, 1994; Mallinson & Kielhofner, 1995). This work strengthens the model and answers some of the criticisms of the studies in Table 6-2.

Occupational science, the more recently developed academic discipline underlying occupational therapy, from its inception has embraced narrative, or story making, as the best means to understand clients' experiences of their illness or disability (Clark, 1993). The emphasis in occupational science on emic (insider's) perspectives gives it the potential to cross cultural barriers. Moreover, concern with the client's own account of his or her life is part of the occupational therapy tradition (Frank, 1996). In the application of narrative methods of assessment across cultures, however, it is important to recognize that what is a satisfying narrative to Western minds has a particular linear structure. That structure has been discussed (and prescribed) in Western culture since Aristotle's time. Proponents of narrative methods of evaluation admit that the "story" arrived at by the client (and family) and therapist is the result of a negotiation between the client's telling and the therapist's reconstruction of the story (Frank). Recognizing, and being able to accept and incorporate, culturally distinct narrative structures will be a challenge in employment of narrative analysis as a technique in occupational therapy.

▼ ACHIEVING MULTICULTURAL COMPETENCE AS AN OCCUPATIONAL THERAPY PRACTITIONER

Approaches to **multicultural competence** education are sometimes dichotomized as "culture-specific" and "culture-universal" or "culture-general" models (Bandy, 1994; Bennet, 1986; Freeman, 1993). Culture-specific models endeavor to inform learners about expected differences between groups, usually in a didactic way. "Others" are described by way of lists of traits, beliefs, or customary practices. These models are aimed at increasing "cultural sensitivity," defined as an openness to the cultural values of others (Dillard, Andonian, Flores, MacRae, & Shakir, 1992). In contrast, culture-general or culture-universal models emphasize that all humans have culture and thereby attempt to avoid reifying differences between self and others. The approach to understanding others is through self-awareness. The assumption is made that those who understand themselves better will understand their own culture better and, thus, be enabled to understand that of others. This component of multicultural competence training has been called "cultural awareness" (Dillard et al, 1992). Bandy after reviewing multicultural competence education literature concluded that both activities and experiences aimed at increasing cultural awareness and cultural sensitivity are important and that, used together, they have the potential to offset deficiencies inherent in using only one or the other.

Programs aimed at increasing awareness of one's own culture often begin with examination of the dominant North American cultural values, so that dominant cultural values become less invisible to those who have assimilated them. Table 6-3 lists some areas for which the values orientation of the dominant culture and those of the occupational therapy profession come together to create a strong bias that we must be aware of, and be willing to give up, in working with others whose values may be different (Humphry, 1995; Pineda, 1996; Sanchez, 1964).

For European American practitioners, learning to establish accurate empathy begins with acknowledgement of the privileges and advantages inherent in membership in the dominant group (Evans, 1992a; Matala, 1993). This is not an

TABLE 6-3. Values Orientations of Dominant European American Culture Shared by Occupational Therapy Practitioners on Which Many Clients Will Differ

Dominant European American Culture and OT Profession	As Evidenced by, for Example:
Value the future over the present, value long-range planning, and delaying gratification	Writing plans with long-term goals, undergoing discomfort now with the idea that a better result will occur later (burn garments), emphasizing saving (the grasshopper and ant morality tale)
Value individuality, and will place the good of one individual over that of the rest of the social group	Feeling parents should orient the family's emotional or financial resources toward the developmental needs of a child with a disability
See the locus of identity as the individual and define the social unit primarily as the nuclear family	Expecting patients to have individual goals for their well-being without consultation with socially significant others, or if others are involved in goal setting, often select one (spouse, parent, or offspring)
Value independence over interdependence and group members doing for themselves over being served by others	Assuming that one will want to perform own hygiene, grooming, toileting, and other ADLs and that independence in these activities is far better than reliance on another. Assuming that it is unfair if others are expected to care for patient. Having concept such as "caregiver burden."
Desire and value control and do not readily acquiesce to situations others may see as fate	Assuming everything has a cause. Relentlessly seeking a natural cause to explain the incidence of disease. Having a book on the best seller list that tries to solve the conundrum "Why Bad Things Happen to Good People." Seeing a belief in personal causation and an internal locus of control as marks of normalcy.
See science and technology as a source of control over the natural world, including humans	Elaboration of technological assistive devices, weather prediction and measurement equipment, nuclear weapons, genetic engineering. "The Lord helps those who help themselves."
Value physicality and doing over introspection and being	Expenditures on sporting and gaming equipment overwhelm expenditures on books. Images of activity far outnumber depictions of thinking, conversing, reading, or other less active pursuits in mass media.
Believe that humans are nearly perfectible, value discipline and learning as a means toward that end	The proliferation of self-help books, infant learning protocols, and flash cards. "Spare the rod and spoil the child."

(Summarized from Humphrey, 1995; Pineda, 1996; Sanchez, 1964)

easy step, but it is a necessary one. Dominant cultural group members may have been raised with the myth that one may "pull himself up by his boot straps," and that hard work pays off. Moreover, they may have worked very hard. Thus, they come to see their status as a just reward and wonder why others have not achieved similarly. The privileges, small and large, that accompany dominant group status may be invisible to them. Box 6-1, shows a sampling of such privileges, taken from a longer list by McIntosh (1988).

Cultural sensitivity follows when the learner is aware of her or his own values' orientation and is ready to explore that of others nonjudgmentally. Contact with empowered people whose cultural, racial, ethnic, class, gender, or sexual orientation is different from one's own is the most highly valued sort of activity for increasing cultural sensitivity (Bandy, 1994). The learner must be willing to leave his or her own comfort zone and enter environments in which he or she will have the experience of being the numerical minority. While face-to-face contact and immersion in culturally distinct environments is extremely useful, much can also be learned from reading autobiographies and novels written by those different from oneself. Sometimes a well written novel does more to pull the reader into the protagonist's perspective and helps her or him develop empathy than hours of lecture on the same cultural group could accomplish. Didactic works that take a positive approach in employing cross-cultural generalizations with caution include: Wells' *Developing Multicultural Competency: An Educational and Resource Manual for Educators and Practitioners* (1993) and Lynch and Hanson's *Developing Cross Cultural Competence* (1992), the former written specifically for occupational therapy practitioners.

▼ BOX 6-1

Acknowledging Privilege Inherent in Dominant Group Membership

- I can if I wish arrange to be in the company of people of my race most of the time.
- I can avoid spending time with people who I was trained to mistrust and who have learned to mistrust my kind or me.
- If I should need to move, I can be pretty sure of renting or purchasing housing in an area that I can afford and in which I would want to live.
- I can be pretty sure that my neighbors in such a location will be neutral or pleasant to me.
- I can go shopping alone most of the time, pretty well assured that I will not be followed or harassed.
- I can turn on the television or open to the front page of the paper and see people of my race widely represented.
- When I am told about our national heritage or about "civilization," I am shown that people of my color made it what it is.
- I can be sure that my children will be given curricular materials that testify to the existence of their race. . . .
- Whether I use checks, credit cards, or cash, I can count on my skin color not to work against the appearance of financial reliability.

- I can arrange to protect my children most of the time from people who might not like them.
- I do not have to educate my children to be aware of systemic racism for their own daily physical protection.
- I can be pretty sure that my children's teachers and employers will tolerate them if they fit school and workplace norms; my chief worries about them do not concern others' attitudes toward their race. . . .
- I am never asked to speak for all the people of my racial group.
- I can remain oblivious of the language and customs of persons of color who constitute the world's majority without feeling in my culture any penalty for such oblivion.
- I can criticize our government and talk about how much I fear its policies and behavior without being seen as a cultural outsider.
- I can be pretty sure that if I ask to talk to "the person in charge," I will be facing a person of my race. . . .
- I can expect figurative language and imagery in all of the arts to testify to experiences of my life.

[McIntosh, P. (1988). White privilege and male privilege: A personal account of coming to see correspondences through women's studies. Working Paper No. 189, Wellesley College Center for Research on Women.]

▶ CONCLUSION

Developing multicultural competence is a challenge, but the learning that occurs along the way can be a joy. Nothing is more interesting than the varieties of ways humans use to solve the problems of daily living. Looking for culture through careful observation of and interaction with others, coupled with introspection of self, enables the establishment of accurate empathy between practitioner and client. Cultural difference then becomes a basis for understanding and working together and not a barrier to therapeutic gains.

REFERENCES

American Medical Association (AMA) Council on Ethical and Judicial Affairs. (1990). Black-white disparities in health care. *Journal of the American Medical Association, 263,* 2344-2346.

American Occupational Therapy Association (AOTA). (1991). 1990 Member data survey.

Bennet, J. (1986). Modes of cross-cultural training: Conceptualizing cross-cultural training as education. *International Journal of Cultural Relations, 10,* 179-196.

Bandy, N. (1994). *Educating occupational therapists for multicultural competence.* Unpublished master's thesis: University of Puget Sound, Tacoma, WA.

Bowman, O. J. & Wallace, B. A. (1990). The effects of socioeconomic status on hand size and strength, vestibular function, visuomotor integration and praxis in preschool children. *American Journal of Occupational Therapy, 44,* 610-622.

Cermack, S. A., Katz, N., McGuire, E., Greenbaum, S., Peralta, C., & Maser-Flanagan, V. (1995). Performance of Americans and Israelis with cerebrovascular accident on the Loewenstein Occupational Therapy Cognitive Assessment (LOTCA). *American Journal of Occupational Therapy, 49,* 500-506.

Clark, F. (1993). Occupation embedded in a real life: Interweaving occupational science and occupational therapy. *American Journal of Occupational Therapy, 47,* 1067-1078.

Colonius, G. (1995). *Measurement accuracy of the FirstSTEP: A comparison between Alaska Native children and the FirstSTEP norms.* Unpublished master's thesis: University of Puget Sound, Tacoma, WA.

Crenshaw, B. (1996). *Parent satisfaction with family-centered services in African American families: A pilot study.* Unpublished master's thesis: University of Puget Sound, Tacoma, WA.

Dillard, M., Andonian, L., Flores, O., MacRae, A., & Shakir, M. (1992) Culturally competent occupational therapy in a diversely populated mental health setting. *American Journal of Occupational Therapy, 46,* 721-726.

Dyck, I. (1992). Managing chronic illness: An immigrant woman's acquisition and use of health care knowledge. *American Journal of Occupational Therapy, 46,* 696-705

Elliot, S. (1995). Locus of control differences between African and European Americans. Paper presented at the Annual Conference of the American Occupational Therapy Association, Denver, CO, April 1995.

Evans, J. (1992a). Nationally speaking—what occupational therapists can do to eliminate racial barriers to health care access. *American Journal of Occupational Therapy, 46,* 679-683.

Evans, J. (1992b) Schizophrenia: Living with madness here and in Zanzibar. *Occupational Therapy in Health Care, 8*, 53–71.

Evans, J. & Salim, A.A. (1992). A cross-cultural test of the validity of occupational therapy assessments with patients with schizophrenia. *American Journal of Occupational Therapy, 46*, 685-695.

Frank, G. (1996). Life histories in occupational therapy clinical practice. *American Journal of Occupational Therapy, 50*, 251-264.

Freeman, S. (1993). Client-centered therapy: The universal within the specific. *Journal of Multicultural Counseling and Development, 18*, 173-179.

Fudge, S. (1992). A perspective on consulting in Guatemala. *Occupational Therapy in Health Care, 8*, 15-37.

Helfrich, C. & Kielhofner, G. (1994). Volitional narratives and the meaning of therapy. *American Journal of Occupational Therapy, 48*, 319-326.

Helfrich, C., Kielhofner, G., & Mattingly, C. (1994). Volition as narrative: Understanding motivation in chronic illness. *American Journal of Occupational Therapy, 48*, 311-317.

Humphry, R. (1995). Families who live in chronic poverty: Meeting the challenge of family-centered services. *American Journal of Occupational Therapy, 49*, 687-693.

Jackson, J.M. (1995a). *Lesbian identities, daily occupations, and health care experience.* Unpublished doctoral dissertation, University of Southern California, Los Angeles.

Jackson, J. M. (1995b). Sexual orientation: Its relevance to occupational science and the practice of occupational therapy. *American Journal of Occupational Therapy, 49*, 669-679.

Janelle, S. (1992). Locus of control in nondisabled versus congenitally physically disabled adolescents. *American Journal of Occupational Therapy, 46*, 334-342.

Joe, J. R. & Malach, R. S. (1992). Families with Native American roots. In Lynch, E. W. & Hanson, M. J. (Eds.), *Developing cross-cultural competence: A guide for working with young children and their families.* Baltimore: Paul H. Brooks.

Kielhofner, G. (Ed.). (1985). *A model of human occupation.* Baltimore: Williams & Wilkins.

Kielhofner, G. & Henry, A. (1988). Development and investigation of the occupational performance history interview. *American Journal of Occupational Therapy, 42*, 489-498.

Kleinman, A. (1988). *The illness narratives: Suffering, healing and the human condition.* New York: Basic Books.

Krefting, L. & Krefting, D. (1991). Cultural influences on performance. In C. Christiansen and C. M. Baum (Eds.), *Occupational therapy: Overcoming human performance deficits.* Thorofare, NJ: Slack.

Kroeber, A. L. & Kluckholn, C. (1963). *Culture: A critical review.* New York: Vintage Books.

Law, M. (1993). Evaluating activities of daily living: Directions for the future. *American Journal of Occupational Therapy, 47*, 233-237.

Lynch, E. W. & Hanson, M. J. (Eds.). (1992). *Developing cross-cultural competence: A guide for working with young children and their families.* Baltimore: Paul H. Brooks.

Mallinson, T. & Kielhofner, G. (1995). Like being stuck in flypaper: Understanding volition through metaphor. Paper presented at the Annual Conference of the American Occupational Therapy Association, Denver, CO, April 1995. Tape A6 a & b, Palm Dessert, CA: Convention Cassettes Unlimited.

Matala, M. R. (1993). Race relations at work: A challenge to occupational therapy. *British Journal of Occupational Therapy, 56*, 434–436.

Mattingly, C. & Beer, D. (1993). Interpreting culture in a therapeutic context. In H. L. Hopkins & H. D. Smith (Eds.), *Willard and Spackman's occupational therapy* (8th ed., pp. 154-161). Philadelphia: J. B. Lippincott.

McIntosh, P. (1988). White privilege and male privilege: A personal account of coming to see correspondences through work in women's studies. Working Paper No. 189, Wellesley College Center for Research on Women.

Miller, L. (1992). Evaluating the developmental skills of Cambodian orphans. *Occupational Therapy in Health Care, 8*, 73-87.

Myers, C. (1992). Hmong children and their families: Consideration of cultural influences in assessment. *American Journal of Occupational Therapy, 46*, 737-744.

Neville, A., Kreisberg A., & Kielhofner, G. (1985). Temporal dysfunction in schizophrenia. *Occupational Therapy in Mental Health, 5*, 1-19.

Oakley, F., Kielhofner, G., & Barris, R. (1985). An occupational therapy approach to assessing psychiatric patients' adaptive functioning. *American Journal of Occupational Therapy, 39*, 147-154.

Packir, R. (1994). *Comparison of Sri Lankan and American mother-child dyads on the NCAST.* Unpublished master's thesis: University of Puget Sound, Tacoma, WA.

Piaget, J. (1969). *Science of education and the psychology of the child.* Translated by D. Coltman. New York: Viking Press.

Pineda, L. (1996). *Occupational therapists' multicultural competence and attitudes toward ethnically and culturally different clients.* Unpublished master's thesis: University of Puget Sound, Tacoma, WA.

Sanchez, V. (1964). Relevance of cultural values for occupational therapy programs. *American Journal of Occupational Therapy, 18*, 1–5.

Skawski, K. (1987). Ethnic/racial considerations in occupational therapy: A survey of attitudes. *Occupational Therapy in Health Care, 4*, 37-48.

Spadone, R. (1992). Internal-external control and temporal orientation among Southeast Asians and white Americans. *American Journal of Occupational Therapy, 46*, 713-719.

Wardin, K. (1996). A comparison of verbal assessment of clients with limited English proficiency and English speaking clients in physical rehabilitation settings. *American Journal of Occupational Therapy.*

Wells, S. (1993). *Development of multicultural competence: An education and resource manual for educators and practitioners.* AOTA, Rockville, MD.

Wieringa, N. & McColl, M. (1987). Implications of the model of human occupation for intervention with native Canadians. *Occupational Therapy in Health Care, 4*, 73-91.

Willis, W. (1992). Families with African American roots. In Lynch, E. W. & Hanson, M. J. (Eds.). *Developing cross-cultural competence: A guide for working with young children and their families.* Baltimore: Paul H. Brooks.

Wood, W. (1992). Temporal adaptation and self-identification as lesbian or gay. Paper presented at the Annual Conference of the American Occupational Therapy Association, Houston, TX, March 1992.

Yasuda, E. K. (1994). *Well-being and activity participation in Japanese-American older adults.* Unpublished master's thesis: University of Puget Sound, Tacoma, WA.

Chapter 7

Socioeconomic Factors and Their Influence on Occupational Performance

Barbara Biggs Sussenberger

The focus of this chapter is to discuss the influence of socioeconomic factors on people seeking occupational therapy. How do social and economic factors influence individual occupation in health and illness? Why and how do we need to take this into account as occupational therapy practitioners? Essentially we are talking about the importance of recognizing that there are supports for and constraints on the options available to individuals in their occupational performance; this means that the kinds of choices and chances people have open to them in their education, jobs, leisure interests, living arrangements, self-care, and well-being are significantly affected by socioeconomic factors. Each of us occupies a "social position" that is individually and socially defined and constructed by the differences and inequities between people or groups of people "that are consequential for the lives they lead, most particularly for the rights or opportunities they exercise and the rewards or privileges they enjoy" (Grabb, 1997, pp. 1–2). Social and material inequities refer to such resources as education, jobs, housing, or health care. At the individual level our social position shapes our values, beliefs, and view of the world. As you can imagine, all of these have a direct relation to our interactions with a client and the effectiveness of any of our occupational therapy interventions and outcomes. The values, beliefs, and material resources of our clients have a high degree of variation and may be quite different from our own. We have to ensure that our services are directed to clients' needs and values and that client-practitioner communications are mutually understood. This means that the occupational therapy practitioner has to develop the ability to look at the world in the way the individual client sees it. Issues such as these need discussion and study in the educational preparation and day-to-day practice of occupational therapy practitioners.

The human-biological science courses required in occupational therapy education enable us to have a knowledge base of the structure and function of the human body and its systems, but we must take that knowledge and put it into the social context of each individual with whom we work. Occupational performance has to be recognized as being profoundly social, which means that occupational therapy practitioners must acquire knowledge of social institutions and constructs with the same care as we attend to the inner constructs and functions of the human body.

This chapter examines some of the ways in which socioeconomic factors influence individual choice and opportunity, and how and why occupational therapy practitioners can increase their knowledge of these factors in the occupational therapy process. We will discuss linkages between education, work, leisure, health and well-being, and **socioeconomic status** (SES). We will examine some of the assumptions underlying occupational therapy services in relation to socioeconomic factors and ethical considerations of equity in our practice settings. When working at its best, occupational therapy services can assist clients to maximize and expand their choices and resources.

▼ DEFINING AND CONTEXTUALIZING SOCIOECONOMIC FACTORS

First, we should come to an understanding of how the term *socioeconomic factors* is used in this chapter. On the surface, it may seem as if the meaning is self-evident, but there are several terms that are used to indicate a recognition of social inequalities and each has a slightly different meaning. *SES* is often used in the social sciences to indicate social and economic differences. Gilbert and Kahl (1993) use the definition of SES as "...The inequalities among individuals in occupational prestige, income, and education" (p. 165).

You may be more familiar with the term class to indicate differences. We often hear such differences through use of the terms lower-class, working-class, middle-class, or upper-class. Class is often used interchangeably with SES, and the two are closely interrelated (Bee, 1996, p. 41). However, whereas SES refers to differences among individuals, class is used as a way to indicate differences between groups (Gilbert & Kahl, 1993, p. 16). To varying degrees all societies are stratified by classes or class divisions; in some societies classes are rigid and legally defined, whereas others (such as the United States) have "open" class systems, meaning that the differences are not legally enforced and that there is room for potential mobility between classes. The term stratification is used by sociologists to refer to "studies of structured social inequality" (Marshall, 1994, p. 512). The United States, which is an industrialized, free-market society is stratified largely according to economic rewards, and as Scase (1992) observes, such a social system is divided into "patterns of opportunity" (p. 42). Social inequality is used to refer to the unequal rewards and opportunities for different individuals or groups within a group or groups within a society (Marshall, 1994, p. 246).

Changing one's social or economic position in the social system, even if it is an open system, such as in the United States, is not a straightforward matter of individual desire or ambition. Inequality is a persistent social problem and at the same time, there is the "American Dream" of achievement. Generational mobility can be observed at the individual SES level when a member of the younger generation has achieved more years of education, followed by employment in a prestigious profession, compared with the background of her or his parents. Upward mobility can be observed during the course of an individual's life span often through what we sometimes call "career ladders" (Gilbert & Kahl, 1993, p. 17). It is also possible for a person to experience downward mobility through such life events as illness, job loss, or unanticipated family difficulties. In our work settings, occupational therapy practitioners are often in a posi-

tion to see people at a time in their personal history when they are struggling with losing their social, economic, and physical well-being. Illness or many other difficult life events can easily destabilize and shift the life course of a person. These are some of the factors we have to consider when we approach a new client.

In this chapter, socioeconomic factors is used to focus and stress the need to recognize that there are inequities of material resources and opportunities between and among individuals and groups of people in our society, all of which have multiple implications for the many facets of a person's occupational performance. A large share of our clients and their families are poor. They are struggling, not only with the health-related issues that brought them into contact with occupational therapy, but also with meeting their personal and financial responsibilities day-by-day or week-to-week. In addition, as health care professionals, we have to remember that there are many people who do not even have access to health care because of their economic status. One of the roles of occupational therapy practitioners is a concern for the health and well-being of all members of our society. The individual practitioner may act on this level of social concern through social or political advocacy activities in our state and national associations.

▼ THE INTERSECTIONS OF CLASS, GENDER, RACE, ETHNICITY, AGE, AND DISABILITY

The notion of status, class differences, or inequalities in the United States is not an appealing one (Fig. 7-1). The idea that we all have equal chances and equal opportunities is one that we want to believe is true; to go to the schools of our choice, to enter any occupation we desire, and to be free to participate in any leisure activity that appeals to us is the idealized version of our social system. On the other hand, we know from our individual experiences that this ideal is not so easily realized. Most of us have had to change or modify our plans or hopes and desires because we did not have the necessary resources to obtain what we wanted. The word resources is used broadly to include both material and social factors. The ability to meet our needs or achieve what we want out of life depends on a variety of factors, quite often it is financial, but not entirely. Our individual support system may help us get through a difficult period more successfully than having substantial financial assets, yet so much in society is dependent on having material resources. There are multiple socioeconomic barriers confronting individuals and groups of people as they attempt to actively achieve their hopes and ambitions.

Inequalities are socially and materially enacted through the dynamic and changing interrelationships of such variables as class, gender, race, ethnicity, age, or disability. There are "moments" when these variables may intersect and we

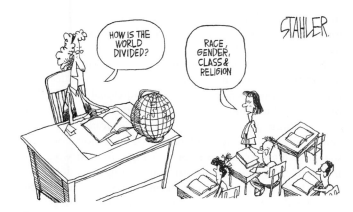

Figure 7-1. Divisions in our society are frequently unstated; however, they are implicitly understood through personal observations and experiences. (Jeff Stahler, reprinted by permission of Newspaper Association, Inc.)

discover that one may take primacy over another. An example might be membership in a country club. Membership fees at an "exclusive" country club in your home town may be very expensive, costing thousands of dollars. But there may also be unstated criteria about membership that prevents the entry of a person, it may be race, ethnicity, marital status, or occupation; the person may have the financial resources for the membership fee, but another dynamic of our stratified social system intersects and acts as a barrier to joining the club.

Having the necessary financial resources or educational preparation is not all that affects entry into certain occupations. The road to one's ambitions can be blocked by other forms of social inequities. Women have found it particularly difficult to enter certain professions or jobs, or to participate in certain activities because of gender bias. Although opportunities have been rapidly changing and expanding, there continue to be fields that are hostile terrain for women. And there continue to be roles that are predominately perceived to be "women's work" (Apter, 1993).

Race and ethnicity are two significant variables that affect the chances and choices of individuals. Educational opportunities and career paths are not equally open or accessible, and levels of health status are affected. Some examples from the literature illustrate the problems: The Children's Defense Fund reports, "In 1993, 46% of all African-American children and 41% of all Latino children lived in families with incomes below the poverty level" (as cited in Albelda, Folbre, & The Centre for Popular Economics, 1996, p. 27). And Bee (1996) discusses that health studies consistently show that "African Americans have shorter life expectancies, more chronic illnesses and disabilities, and are more likely than whites to suffer from certain specific diseases, such as many forms of cancer" (p. 139). Many of the health-related issues of minority groups refer to inadequate or unavailable medical care for poor people. However, people who are poor do not form a homogeneous group, and we

cannot equate race or ethnicity with being poor, but we do need to recognize that members of minority groups are at a greater risk of living in poverty because of racism. Some of the discussions of economic inequality that follow in this chapter refer to the experiences of members of minority groups, because the issues of racism and poverty are so closely interrelated.

Age is another variable recognized as a factor that shapes opportunity. Bee (1996) refers to Riley's term "age strata" to describe how all societies have some sorts of shared expectations and demands of its members based on age (p. 6). Ageism is used to identify and describe discrimination based on age, but not all cultures perceive aging in a negative way (Bee, 1996, p. 6). Aging generally does not receive positive attributions in the United States. Despite substantial research to the contrary about the ability to maintain high cognitive levels of functional abilities, people in the age category we might call "middle adulthood," are often seen as "over the hill" and too old to perform certain educational or vocational tasks (Bee, p. 264). One ex-Wall Street executive is quoted as reporting that "Employers think that over forty you can't think anymore. Over fifty and you're burned out" (Newman, 1988, p. 65). Although it is against the law to discriminate when hiring people for jobs, the 50-year-old man or woman who wants to (or needs to) make a career change does not find many open doors, regardless of their experience, skills, or educational background. Perhaps we will see a real decrease in ageism in this country because of the aging of the population as a whole. There may be more social changes demanded by members of the older generation in the United States as they forge new models of aging and force all of us to develop new ways of looking at role performance in the later years of life.

People with disabilities have found educational, employment, and leisure opportunities blocked, regardless of their individual skills and abilities or financial resources. Accessible recreational resources are only recently being expanded or developed for people with disabilities. Medical and technological advances have enabled people to be independent in the community, but that independence cannot be fully realized without access to education, jobs, or recreational resources. The social and political actions at the basis of the **Americans with Disabilities Act**, and earlier legislation aimed at equal opportunities for people with disabilities, reflect the efforts and outcomes to influence the inequities of the legal and social structures. It is as important to alter the popular misperceptions of disability as it is to pass legislation, and occupational therapy practitioners are in a unique position to help to make these changes (Barlow, 1992).

Despite the legislation intended to eliminate or reduce the social and economic inequalities that exist, and regardless of our professed beliefs in equal opportunity, life's choices and chances are not equal. This means that the occupational performance of an individual is mediated by many social and economic variables. The foregoing discussion is intended to point out variables that dynamically intersect. Sometimes the constraint on the individual is primarily because of economic disadvantages, but other times it might be gender, or race–ethnicity, or age, or disability that intervenes and blocks the person's choices. The intersections of race, ethnicity, gender, age, disability, and sometimes geographic region are dynamic and specific, they change with the situation, and they change across time. This chapter is broadly focused on structured inequality and the effect on individual occupational performance, but we need to recognize the multiple complexities of the social system.

▼ HOW IS POVERTY DEFINED?

Issues of poverty are long-standing in the United States, but the roots of our current understanding of how poverty is defined and measured can be traced to the 1960s. Of particular importance is a book written by Michael Harrington in 1962, titled, *The Other America: Poverty in the United States.* Harrington's book conveyed human dimensions to what before was an abstract concept of poverty used for policy deliberations. America's poor were everywhere, urban and rural, African American and white, young and old, unemployed, and poorly employed, and yet they were "hidden" from the public understanding until Harrington's account of the situation brought it into the spotlight and onto the public agenda (Gilbert & Kahl, 1993, pp. 270-277; Trattner, 1994, pp. 316–318).

Poverty refers to the lack of material resources that are necessary for subsistence. To help people acquire the necessary material resources and to determine who qualifies for assistance, poverty has to be defined in a way that it can be measured, this is what is called the poverty line. In the United States, the first definition of the poverty line at the federal level was developed in 1963 by taking "the cost of a minimum nutritious diet for a typical family of four and the proportion of income (approximately one-third) that the average family spent on food. Multiplying the price of the food budget by three to allow for non-food costs . . . an income 'poverty line' [is calculated]" (Gilbert & Kahl, 1993, p. 274). The poverty line has to be regularly adjusted for inflation because costs rise, and it also has to be adjusted for the size of the family, and region. "In 1995, the poverty line for a single person was $7,470 and for a family of three it was $12,590" (Albelda et al., 1996, p. 12).

This kind of definition lends itself to a great deal of debate, for it does not account for relative standards of living or the quality of life. Some adjustments for minimum standards have been made at local levels over time, based on such assumptions as considering that a minimum standard of living includes having electricity or a full bath. However, at the federal level, the basis for establishing the poverty line in relation to food costs remains the same (Albelda et al., 1996, pp. 12-13; Gilbert & Kahl, 1993, pp. 275–276). Another of the difficulties with the fundamental formula for the poverty line is that food costs have come to represent a smaller proportion of a family's overall expenses since the formula was originally conceived, while other kinds of costs have risen (Sidel, 1996, p. 73).

Sidel (1996) cites Schwarz and Vogel's description of living on the poverty line that has a series of implications for the occupational performance of an individual or members of a family. The kind of budget required to stay within the financial limits at, or near, the poverty line would impose severe constraints on the smallest kind of recreational outings, such as ball games, concerts, or movies; eating out would be impossible, baby sitters, or summer camp would be too costly; books, or tapes, or toys, or music lessons could not be considered; gifts or parties, or special kinds of food for birthdays and holidays would have to be planned and saved for across the whole year, and even then they would have to be kept at a minimum (Sidel, 1996, p.74).

There are misconceptions and debates about how many people are poor, who are the poor, and who is at risk of being poor. Most researchers and human service agencies begin to examine those questions by using statistics collected by the U. S. Census Bureau, with the poverty line as a measure. Here are some of the answers:

1. In 1991, 13.5% of the population (33.6 million people) were identified as being at, or below the poverty line (Gilbert & Kahl, 1993, pp. 279–280).
2. In 1993, 15.1% of the population (39,265,000 million people) were designated as being in poverty (Sidel, 1996, p. xiii).
3. In 1995, the percentage of those in poverty dropped to 13.8% (Holmes, *The New York Times*, September 27, 1996).

From just these few "official" numbers, we can see that although there are shifts in the numbers, the problem persists. While there have been gains in trying to reduce poverty in some categories, the numbers have been growing since the 1980s.

▼ WHO IS POOR? WHO IS AT RISK OF BEING POOR?

Risk means that certain categories of people are more vulnerable than others to being in poverty. Risk, or incidence of poverty refers to "the percentage of the people in a specific group that fall below the poverty line" (Gilbert & Kahl, 1993, p. 280).

Sidel (1996, p. 70) points out some of those who are at risk from 1993 figures:

1. The number of children in poverty has always represented the largest category. In 1993, 15.7 million children (younger than 18) were designated as being in poverty.
2. In the same year, 1993, 14.7 million women (older than 18) were designated as being in poverty.
3. African Americans and Hispanics represented poverty rates three times higher than whites in 1993.

4. The 1993 rate of poverty for families headed by women was five times greater than that of two-parent families.

These figures give us some idea about the extent of poverty and of categories of the population who are most vulnerable to the problem, those who are at the greatest risk are women and children. But statistics can be, and often are, used in ways that mislead us into constructing stereotypes of who the poor are. In many ways, the distribution of poverty continues to be the way Harrington discussed it in the 1960s: poverty is everywhere. Much of the stigma about poverty is directed toward those who are at risk, and this tends to hide the issues. The tendency in our social system is to look at individuals or groups as "the problem." rather than looking at the social structural constraints that produce the problems (Scase, 1992, p. 65).

Gilbert and Kahl's (1993, p. 281) analysis of the distribution of poverty in 1990 demonstrates some of the contradictions between the myths and the facts.

1. Poverty is not primarily in central cities, it is spread out among suburbs, small towns, and rural areas.
2. In 1990, more whites than African Americans or Hispanics were in poverty: 22.3 million white people were reported as being in poverty compared with 9.8 million African Americans or 6 million Hispanics.
3. In 1990, more people in the age category 18 to 64 (16.5 million) were reported as being in poverty than those who were younger than 18 (13.4 million).

The foregoing figures represent complexities embedded in our social system, the composition of the census categories shift and change with time as the political economy and the demographics change. The terms "working poor" and the "new poor" are used to identify what some of those complexities are, and how some of those changes happen to individuals.

The working poor refers to a growing number of people who are working full time, but whose wages do not raise them or their families above the poverty line. A full-time worker in a job that paid the minimum wage rate in 1994 ($4.25/hour) would not have been able to make an adequate salary (Albelda et al., 1996). The new poor is used to describe "a group of people who did not grow up in poverty, some of whom grew up working class, middle class, or even upper middle class but, because of events in their lives—divorce, death, illness, unemployment, an untimely birth, or other precipitating events— have fallen into poverty" (Sidel, 1996, pp. 59–60).

One of the changes that has been happening since the 1980s is what is called the "shrinking middle class" and the growing polarization between the rich and poor. We are seeing a rising tendency for a group of working poor and a downward slide for many who were once in the middle income bracket. As Sidel (1996) observes, "By 1993, the top 20 percent of U.S. households received nearly half of all household income (48.2 percent). . . while the bottom 20 percent received 3.6 percent of all income" (p. xiv).

▼ THE EFFECTS OF SOCIOECONOMIC FACTORS ON OCCUPATIONAL PERFORMANCE

Much of the social science research indicates that there are degrees of stratification both internally and externally imposed. There is a "strong tendency for people to associate with class equals in friendships, marriages, organizational memberships and residential choices" (Gilbert & Kahl, 1993, p.131). It is easy to see how this happens at the individual level, we develop our view of the world through the world in which we live. We want to join clubs and live in neighborhoods where we know people and where we feel comfortable. It also refers to the observation about the tendency of the stratified social system to reproduce itself. But Gilbert and Kahl (1993) remind us that the changes in society are continuous and that they transform lives and expectations and possibilities. Shifts in the economy change job opportunities, technological developments cause some fields to become obsolete while creating entirely new occupations, and mass media shows us varieties of life styles that influence our ideas (pp. 137-138). There is a constant tension between change and continuity in the social system, and the individual experience is a part of that dichotomy (Fig. 7-2).

Now we return to the leading question in this section: What are some of the ways in which socioeconomic factors influence education, work, leisure, and self-care? The discussion that follows examines some of the research in poverty as it applies to domains of concern in occupational therapy.

Education

The extent and quality of education is a critical factor in the life course of an individual. Bee (1996) notes that "In our culture . . . variation in the years of education is the mecha-

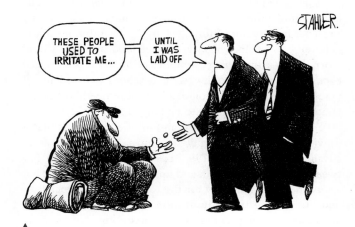

▲
Figure 7-2. Our ability to empathize with people is often limited by the view from our own "social position." (Jeff Stahler, reprinted by permission of Newspaper Enterprise Association, Inc.)

nism that tends to perpetuate existing class differences. But education is also the vehicle for change in status" (p. 46).

There are social and economic advantages associated with more education, such as better mental and physical health, higher satisfaction with jobs and relationships, and a greater involvement in social and political activities (Bee, 1996). Access to public education is a fundamental part of realizing the American Dream of being able to advance. The institution of the public school system played a "major role in establishing the democratic values of the nation" (Peterson, 1994, p. 234). But neither educational opportunities nor the quality of educational experiences are equitably distributed in our social system (Sennet & Cobb, 1972, p. 187).

Studies show that there is a positive correlation between school quality and the rate of future earnings (Albelda et al., 1996, p. 83). Schools in neighborhoods where the poverty rates are high tend to be overcrowded, understaffed, and undersupplied; their maintenance and repair is neglected, the nonhuman environment unsafe, and the human environment is often violent (Kozol, 1991, 1995). It is not hard to imagine that given school environments such as these, students "get the message" that they are not considered as valuable resources for the future of society. A 15-year-old girl described her perceptions to Kozol (1995), "It's more like being 'hidden.' It's as if you have been put in a garage where, if they don't have room for something but aren't sure if they should throw it out, they put it where they don't need to think of it again" (pp. 37–38). It is also easy to understand that the views of the world that children develop in settings such as these can differ substantially from those of children in well-financed school systems.

Levinson's theory of development includes the concept of "the dream" and its importance in young adulthood (Bee, 1996, pp. 65–66). The ability to see oneself in a future role can actually help in the achievement of one's dream. You begin to see yourself as capable and competent through envisioning yourself in the future, this is really the foundation of life goals. But what vision of the future can you have if you feel society has hidden you away? Kozol (1995) relates an illustration of a dream limited by opportunity told to him by a teacher in the South Bronx, "Many of the ambitions of the children . . . are locked in at a level suburban kids would scorn. It's as if the very possibilities of life have been scaled back. Boys who are doing well in school will tell me, 'I would like to be a sanitation man'. . . in this neighborhood, a sanitation job is something to be longed for" (p. 125).

One of the roles of the expansion of education is that it provides more "opportunity structures" for individuals to advance in jobs (Scase, 1992, p. 43). The connection between education and work and upward mobility is clear, but again, there is a tendency for the reproduction of social inequalities. Educational institutions in some high-poverty areas may provide programs to fill certain kinds of job markets that are low in status, low in salary, and offer no security or advancement possibilities (Gilbert & Kahl, 1993, p. 182).

Students are channeled into those jobs without having other kinds of options available (Kozol 1995, p. 203).

Economic and social science research shows a growing disparity in the 1990s between those who can attend college and those who find the economic barriers too great for them or their children. Reasons for this are identified as being largely due to increased tuition rates combined with decreased availability of tuition assistance. This means that families in the higher-income brackets can more readily ensure that their children can have "the college education that makes possible entry into higher paying jobs in management and the professions" (Peterson, 1994, p. 65). Because education is such a critical element in one's ability to lessen the risk of being in poverty or to achieve upward mobility, the effect of the gaps in who can and who cannot attend college has enormous consequences for the future of the children who are now in poverty.

Work

In the occupational therapy process, as we collaborate with clients to develop their long-term goals and objectives, education and paid work are often central concerns. Our direct services focus on the client's abilities and functional skills in relation to their short-term and long-term goals, but we do not always consider the goals in the context of the trends and issues of the economy. When a client is ready to return to work, it can be an indicator of success of our interventions, but can we describe the labor market to the client to assist in developing alternative strategies as certain kinds of jobs become scarce or as their skills become less marketable?

The upward mobility of an individual, or the reduction of risk of falling into poverty depends on the availability of educational opportunities and access to particular forms of work. Mobility is also inspired by the dream to enter a particular profession or a job. From the examples cited earlier, we know that dreams have to be nurtured; in the absence of support and material resources aspirations are reduced or "scaled back." Research consistently shows that parents' occupations influence children's choices of work (Bee, 1996, p. 259). Children growing up in areas with high unemployment and poor jobs will have fewer chances and choices about work, and they will perceive their choices as limited. Children will have fewer models of worker roles if their parents or other family members are unemployed or underemployed; the environment and its limitations promote the tendency to the reproduction of stratification.

Entry into work is the active process of matching available opportunities with a person's skills and interests. Skill development depends on the person's innate abilities and also on the quality of his or her educational preparation. We see the combined problem of poor education, poor job skills, and limited jobs for people with minimum skills. Not surprisingly, the unemployment rate is higher in areas where the poverty rate is high, especially for young African Americans and Hispanics in poor urban neighborhoods. There are fewer job possibilities in these neighborhoods, and the quality of the schools is generally poor. This means that young people with poor educational backgrounds have less competitive job market skills. The kinds of jobs that are available in neighborhoods with high poverty rates often offer few benefits, such as health care, nor do they open up chances for security or advancement (Albelda et al., 1996, p. 78).

In addition to problems of unemployment, there are the working poor, defined earlier as those who are working, but with wages so low they are unable to avoid living in poverty. We often think of minimum wage earners as teenagers in summer jobs, but estimates of up to 43% of the minimum wage earners were working full time in 1994, and 64% of them were women (Albelda, 1996, p. 81). Work for many people at the lower end of the occupational scale is not the success story that we would envision for our clients when we discontinue our services with the client ready to enter the job market. Satisfaction with work declines as you move down the occupational ladder (Schor, 1992, p. 71).

Handler (1995) asks the question: "If the problem is poverty, and the vast majority of the poor are working and not on welfare, then what is the problem with work?" (p. 39). Trends in the labor market have implications for our future and for our clients who need to return to work. Over the years there has been an overall decline in real wages, the better jobs have increasingly higher education and skill requirements, a decrease in the availability of jobs in the manufacturing sector, an increase in part time work, and an increase in jobs without benefits (Handler, p. 44). The loss of manufacturing jobs in the United States since the 1980s to shifts in the global economy is significant, because these typically offered opportunities for people with low educational backgrounds and minimum skills (Peterson, 1994, p. 190).

Another problem with work is the increase in downward mobility that has been growing since the 1980s with corporate downsizing and mergers. Newman (1988) tells about a well-to-do corporate executive who was given 9 months notice that the company was closing out the division that he headed. During the 9 months, he searched, but could find no equivalent job. He and his family moved from their comfortable suburban home into a modest apartment. The social life of the entire family changed because they no longer had the same financial resources; as they lost contact with their old friends, tensions built up in the family, which heightened the feelings of instability and anxiety (pp. 64-67). This story is not about the experience of living at the poverty line, but instead, it tells us that downward mobility can happen at any income level and that it reverberates through every activity of the whole family system.

People who have fewer skills and less education run a higher risk of falling into poverty. Sidel (1996, p. 59) tells about a woman who, after 23 years of marriage, was divorced by her husband who left the state and provided no financial support for her or the children. In a few months, she found that her income went from $70,000 to $7,000/ year. Her job as a home health aide was not enough to keep her out of poverty. Although she and the children went without heating oil for a winter and sold household appliances, such as the dishwasher, she was unable to keep up payments on their home. The bank foreclosed on the mortgage, and she and her children found themselves homeless. Although she was able to find work, she had a relatively limited educational background and no prior work experience to enable her to compete in the job market for work that would pay her an adequate salary.

In general, women's work and career patterns have differed from men's, largely because they have taken time out for child rearing or other caretaker roles. This interrupted pattern of employment increases women's economic vulnerability because career achievement and economic success are associated with working continuously.

Work interrelates with many socioeconomic factors, for the individual it is family background, parental occupations, location, and the quality and extent of educational preparation that influence perceptions and decisions about work. At the level of the social system, the dynamics of the local, national, and international political economies affect the kinds of jobs that are available in each neighborhood.

Play and Leisure

Kelly and Godbey (1992) describe the importance of leisure in individual development and in the context of the broader social system as being "a realm of openness in which individuals take action that has consequences for who they are and what they are becoming. Children learn and develop in play. In fact, most critical early socialization occurs in play" (pp. 25-26). The neighborhoods described by Kozol (1991, 1995) are in areas wracked by poverty, crime, neglect, and abuse, in the form of polluting industries and incinerators. These are the environments where children play and learn who they are becoming. In some instances, parents are afraid to let their children play outdoors because of the high rate of crime and violence in the neighborhood. As we noted earlier, the budgets required for living at the poverty line provide little room for toys, games, or such luxuries as music or sports lessons.

"Leisure, like work is stratified" (Kelly & Godbey, 1992, p. 120). You can see socioeconomic gradations in travel advertisements in your Sunday papers directed at specialized groups for "luxury class" or "budget" accommodations. You can observe parents who opt to take their children to a fast food outlet because it would be too costly to go to a gourmet restaurant with three children. Some of the leisure research indicates that there are class differences, not just with the economic differences of recreational choices, but also with the type of activities in which people participate. Many of these patterns are linked to family and educational backgrounds that tend to be repeated by the children as they grow into adulthood (Gilbert & Kahl, 1992, p. 131-138).

There is a concern that there is a growing loss of leisure time for people in the United States (Schor, 1992). The reasons given for this trend are generally related to problems about trends in the job market. As companies cut back on the number of employees, the people who are kept on are afraid to lose their jobs; they feel they cannot refuse when asked to work overtime. For some people, they invest more and more hours in their work to stay competitive in the job market in case their company merges or downsizes. And other people are simply working at more than one job, as many hours as they can to avoid or escape poverty. In situations such as these, leisure becomes even more important to a person's health and well-being, but time for leisure is problematic. Schor (1992) tells us that "people report their leisure time has declined by as much as one third since the 1970s. Predictably, they are spending less time on the basics, like sleeping and eating. Parents are devoting less time to their children. Stress is on the rise, partly owing to the 'balancing act' of reconciling the demands of work and family life" (p. 5). And the juggling act of time and work for women is typically complicated by their additional hours of responsibilities in nonwaged household chores. Bee (1996, p. 278) cites studies that compare the number of hours invested in household chores by men and women that show that women consistently spend more hours on housework than their spouses. Hochschild (1989) found that even when the division of household labor was more equitable, it was women who performed two-thirds of the daily jobs at home, such as cooking and cleaning.

Health and Illness

Studies of socioeconomic differences in health and illness consistently illustrate patterns of relationships. The increase in chronic health conditions and limitations in daily activities is "earlier and steeper for the poor and the working class" (Bee, 1996, p. 137). One of the explanations for this relation is that for people in lower levels of income there is reduced access to medical care. Another explanation is the connection between poverty or low income and poor housing and the quality of the environment.

The higher poverty rates associated with race and ethnic groups are also reflected in studies of their health status. Native Americans have the shortest life expectancy of any group and suffer more from specific diseases, such as diabetes, than other groups. African Americans also have shorter life expectancies than whites, and have higher rates of specific diseases, including certain forms of cancer (Bee,1996, pp. 138-139; Berger, 1994, pp. 9-10).

Some of the large-scale, longitudinal research undertaken to examine the relations between class and health status have shown that even if specific causes of death are eliminated, there are still class differences in health status (Marmot, et al., 1994). This means the focus of the solution cannot be disease-specific; what seems to be the explanation are the characteristically low birth weights of infants at the lower end of the economic scale. Low birth weight places the individual at risk for many forms of health related problems and diseases throughout adulthood (Rice, 1994). These findings point up the importance for the availability of resources for mothers and infants.

The health of an individual is not largely determined by the health system, rather it has more to do with "our environment, our relations with friends and enemies, the quality of our education, our status in the community and how we think about ourselves" (Kelly & Godbey, 1992, p. 503). Everyday activities and routines can make the difference in our health status, but given the descriptions of the everyday problems people encounter, a healthy life style is not that simple to establish or sustain. Some of the differences in social class related health habits are in smoking, diet, and exercise; poorer health habits are associated with lower education and lower income (Bee, 1996, p. 140–141; Rice, 1994). There is a strong connection between good health habits and a sense of personal control (Bee, 1996, pp.144-145). But personal control, or autonomy is what a lot of people feel they are losing; more people are experiencing stress and a loss of security in their jobs, more are working harder to escape poverty. Furthermore, maintaining a nutritious diet at the poverty level is a challenge for even the most informed consumer and creative cook.

▼ THE POLITICAL ECONOMY OF THE HEALTH CARE SYSTEM

The health care system of the United States is a highly dynamic, complex, and stratified system of competition, regulation, and reimbursement (Fig. 7-3). As Brennan and Berwick (1996) acknowledge, "it goes without saying that the uninsured do not receive the same standard of care as that received by the insured" (p. 391). Reports indicate higher death rates for the uninsured (Albelda et al, 1996, p. 37). The system is described as being the least responsive to the most needy and least powerful members of the social system; "reserving its greatest hardships for the following groups: the poor and near poor, workers, the unemployed, the disabled, displaced, homemakers, the elderly, and children" (Friedman, 1994, p. 303). Kozol (1991) tells of reports about the quality of health care in New York hospitals intended to serve the poor where there is "no working microscope to study sputum samples, no gauze or syringes" and where they were "running out of sutures in the operating room" (p.116). Many times people choose not to seek health care in places such as this because they know the system itself is dangerous to their health.

Health care is not accessible to a significant and increasing number of people, up to 40 million people are estimated to have no private health insurance. And although Medicaid

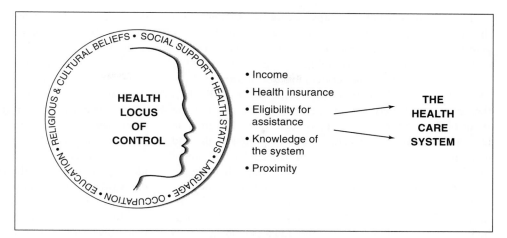

▶

Figure 7-3. Individual decisions to seek and use services in the health care system are based on the influence and interaction of many internal and external factors.

was intended to assist the poor who have no health coverage, many are not covered because of eligibility requirements. Despite the recognition that millions of people in the United States are uninsured or underinsured for their health needs, the arguments around reforming the system show little tendency to coming to agreement about how to "fix" it. The shifts in the economy since the 1980s and the mix of jobs and industries in it have added to the numbers of uninsured because so much of our health care coverage is linked to jobs. Another factor that compounds the problem is that many of the new jobs that have been created recently are part-time and offer no health benefits (Lee, Soffel, & Luft, 1994, p. 207).

Illness can create a series of events that place a family in poverty. One story reported by Allen (*The New York Times,* December 31, 1995) illustrates how this can happen. A 46-year-old woman, single parent of two boys, who had worked for 26 years in a billing department of a hospital became seriously ill and was hospitalized for 2 weeks. Her illness caused her to lose more time at work and eventually she used up all her vacation and sick time and began to lose her income because of lost work time. As the bills accumulated, her older son's tuition at school had to be put on hold; she turned off her telephone and stopped the cable television services. She eliminated all the expenses she could, but still faced eviction and homelessness because she was behind in rent.

▼ OCCUPATIONAL THERAPY SERVICES: ARE THEY EQUITABLE? WHOM DO WE SERVE?

The preceding discussion on socioeconomic factors focused on domains of concern for occupational therapy practitioners: education, work, play and leisure, and health and illness. We have examined and discussed issues of social and economic inequities of a stratified social system. The ways in

which health care is organized and delivered is a reflection of the larger system. Peloquin (1993) notes that one of the constructs that compromises the caring expressions of health practitioners is the "health care provision system that is driven by business, efficiency, and profit" (p. 936). We need to recognize that occupational therapy is a part of the health care system and that our patterns of practice may also reflect aspects of the inequities we have discussed.

One of the "occupational hazards" of a health care professional is a tendency to begin to think of our clients in categories; patients, clients, consumers, or students. We have a "case load" or a "really interesting **TBI** [traumatic brain injury]," and we have required numbers of treatment units per day. All of these terms are abstractions of what we really intend to offer in the occupational therapy process. As occupational therapy practitioners, we like to argue that one of the strengths of the profession is that we gear our approach to the "whole person," but do we? or how do we? That phrase does not simply mean that we address the physical and psychosocial domains in our outcome goals for a consumer with carpal tunnel syndrome. It means we have to learn about the consumer as "Ms. Smith" in the terms of her world, her perceptions, her experiences, and her realities of it. We have to develop "multicultural competencies" (Pope-Davis, 1993) and understand the cultural complexities we encounter in our practice through the kind of active—reflective process discussed in the preceding chapter. And we have to learn and understand the socioeconomic supports and constraints of Ms. Smith's world and integrate that knowledge into our work with her. We have to do this to be effective in our services to each person (client) with whom we work. Without this, the follow-through or carryover of our services is unlikely. This is becoming harder to do in today's health care system where we may only see Ms. Smith for two to five times, and those limited times are highly structured around specific outcome goals. For our interventions to be truly effective, they have to be geared to the contextual realities of the individual client. We have to consciously incorporate it in our everyday ethical practice.

The **Occupational Therapy Code of Ethics** states that we are responsible for providing services without regard to "race, creed, national origin, sex, age, handicap, disease entity, social status, or religious affiliation" (AOTA, 1994); but sometimes our services are discriminatory. Purtilo and Haddad (1996) point out some of the difficulties that may emerge between a practitioner and a client as the result of (SES) differences. They observe that "The income level and accompanying status of health professionals tend to create barriers to interacting with patients" (p. 56). These differences can influence how we feel and what we do about our therapeutic interventions with clients in such dimensions as our capacity to empathize or our ability to understand daily routines and priorities that differ from our own (p. 56). In addition to our individual personalities and experiences that affect our relationships with clients, all the attributes that make the practitioner a "professional" may be factors that contribute to a "distancing" between the client and the practitioner.

Many of our assessment tools contain categories of occupational performance skills and habits. Because we have to objectify our documentation, the content implied by the categories of occupational performance become abstract, and we tend to lose sight of the complexities. This problem is clearly illustrated in the preceding chapter. Although the effect of economic factors on occupational performance are not directly addressed, Dunn, Brown, and McGuigan (1994) refer to the need for us to consider the effect of "context" and questions if "standardized functional assessments are valid for capturing what is actually known about the person's performance in the natural context" (p. 605). On-site home and job visits are examples of where the practitioner can come in direct contact and observation of the client in her or his own environment. Knowledge and understanding of the client's home and work environments greatly increase the effectiveness of our interventions. However, the context of these visits may also bring the practitioner into conflict with values, priorities, and resources available for self-care, diet, or other occupational performance components. Practitioners find themselves overwhelmed and intimidated at times by the social and economic barriers that challenge their clients. Home or job-site visits are not always possible to undertake, but we can become more familiar with the neighborhoods in which our clients live and work as a matter of our own orientation to our work settings.

As occupational therapy practitioners, we often feel compromised by what services we can offer our clients compared with what we want to offer. Our services are constrained by the particulars of reimbursement, and the system of reimbursement in health care does take such things as the social–economic status of our clients into account through the inequities of the private or public health insurance programs. So how do you give the maximum to all and each of your clients and stay within the constraints of the system? We want to keep our focus on the ideals of what services we could offer. One occupational therapist made a decision to always include a note or a list of occupational therapy services recommended as the "ideal" for her clients with the documentation for services that were "allowed" for reimbursement. This kind of daily practice habit of the therapist's documentation keeps the gaps between the ideal and the real in the forefront. It helps us keep a focus on ethical practice and it communicates the gaps to third-party payers. There are active and proactive approaches the practitioner can take individually or through organizations to promote and support change in the system, but our focus on ethical ideals of occupational therapy have to become a part of our day-to-day work, otherwise we become a part of the problem, not a part of the solution.

Most health and human service professionals would say that they learned their most important lessons from their clients. These stories are usually about how the professional lacked an understanding of the situation and the client "set them straight" about "how things really were." This means we have to listen, and in order to listen we have to ask the right questions and give the time and space for the answers. Studies have shown that on average, physicians interrupt their patients after 18 seconds of their attempts to describe or explain their symptoms or problems (Frishman, 1996). We do not know how long occupational therapy practitioners wait and listen to clients' responses before trying to categorize them or attempting to resolve a problem based on personal ideas and assumptions about what would be best. Fortunately, there are some very instructive lessons in the occupational therapy literature in the form of qualitative research contributions that show us the benefits of asking and listening (Peloquin, 1993, 1995; Wood, 1996).

Clark and colleagues (1996) identify, what they call "adaptive strategies" of a group of low-income, older, well, adults as a way to describe how and what they did to successfully maintain their engagement in activities that were of personal and individual significance. They recognized that the environment required particular kinds of adaptation, such issues as safety in the neighborhood had to be taken into account, as did financial resources available for recreation or activities of daily living. This study places "personal importance" as a first consideration and puts it in the context of the older adults' living environment and financial constraints. The authors have enabled us to see the potential for preventive services that are informed by the values and beliefs of individuals as well as socioeconomic constraints.

Fidler's (1996) Life-style Performance Model also offers a construct that would "listen" to clients and take the environmental context into account. She says that the model "stresses an initial focus on individual interests, capacities, and customary patterns of daily living as the basis for defining and prioritizing any intervention" (p. 141). Whatever assessment tools we choose to use, we need to put the emphasis on the individual's priorities, resources, and constraints. This means that we have to integrate knowledge and consideration of socioeconomic factors. A large part of the occupational therapy process is enabling our clients' problem solving; we need to know how to assist in realizing goals, which means we have to know how clients can obtain necessary resources. If we can do this, we can help people break through some of the barriers to their goals.

▼ INCORPORATING KNOWLEDGE OF SOCIOECONOMIC FACTORS INTO OUR PRACTICE

At the beginning of the chapter, occupational therapy services are described as most effective when they assist clients to expand to maximize the choices and resources that are available to them. To accomplish this promise of occupational therapy requires knowledge of the communities in which we work; the networks of social, medical, educational, voluntary public, and private organizations that make up potential resources. It requires knowledge of the policy definitions of eligibility for various forms of assistance. And it involves experience in the community, knowing its politics and its economy, and asking questions. Where are the jobs? What is the unemployment rate? What are the schools like? What are the characteristics of the population in the communities served by your agency? A lot of this kind of knowledge and experience we learn first hand, and we learn from others, professionals, volunteers, and our clients. Very often, the issues themselves can shape the focus of group sessions with some of our clients in which all members contribute to each others' knowledge base; for example job readiness groups, money management groups, or cooking (on a poverty line budget) groups, all are excellent vehicles for learning new strategies and resources, but they have to draw on the experience and knowledge of the clients' environments.

▼ LESSONS FROM CLIENTS

The following vignettes describe four lessons learned from clients to illustrate some of the points discussed throughout the chapter about the effect of socioeconomic factors on occupational performance.

Work

I once observed an occupational therapy group at a day-treatment center. The group was intended to enable its members to build job readiness skills in eight sessions. Two sessions of this group were devoted to "how to write resumes." However, when you took into account the membership of the group and the jobs clients were hoping to get, writing resumes was not a necessary skill. The kinds of jobs people were looking for included waitress, hardware store clerk, janitor, and counter help in a fast food chain; jobs such as these do not require a resume, they require be-

ing able to fill out forms, and most importantly, being able to effectively interact and communicate in a short-term interview. The notion of a resume being such an important tool in the clients' job searches came from the occupational therapist's own experience as a health care professional. The two sessions of the group that were devoted to resume writing were valuable lost time that could have been spent role playing the kind of interviews the clients might encounter, instead, other forms of skill building were used doing activities that were not meaningful or transferrable for the clients' needs.

Play and Leisure

A client at a mental health center gave me an effective lesson in choices. I asked the client to complete an interest inventory of leisure activities, a commonly used tool in assessment. He was asked to check those activities that he enjoyed doing and those he did not enjoy. A third column asked him to check any of the activities that he would like to learn to do. His response was to check the third column for the entire list. When I asked him to discuss his responses, he explained that he had never had the opportunity to learn to do any of the activities on the list. His background information confirmed his explanation; his childhood was spent moving from one foster home to another, and he had few memories of play or toys. Some of the activities on the list required special equipment or instruction, in other words, they required resources that were unavailable to him. Later, he was able to make up his own list of leisure interests based on his experiences that were not on the original "occupational therapy list" he was given to complete.

One Monday morning a client told me about taking her children "on a trip" over the weekend. As she described the "trip," it became clear that her experiences and mine were very different. She finally got up the courage to take the public bus to a city park where she and her children had a picnic lunch and a paddle boat tour around the pond in the center of the park. The bus trip was less than 5 miles, but she and her children had never been in that section of the city before because, as she explained, she had never thought about being able to leave the housing project or the neighborhood where she lived. Furthermore, neither she nor her two school-aged children had ever been on a picnic. Her weekend activity with her children was an adventure that took a lot of courage to try out some new skills and ideas that were inspired by the encouragement and coaching of other group members in the program.

Self Care

An occupational therapy colleague once told me about a client she worked with on transfer skills for bathing and toileting. More by chance than design, the therapist did a follow-up home visit a few weeks after discharge. To the therapist's surprise, the client's home had no indoor plumbing.

The occasional showers that were accessible to the former client were at the home of a friend a few miles away. The client had been too self-conscious to tell the therapist at the rehabilitation center that the resources that were available at home for personal hygiene were different from the therapist's assumptions. Needless to say, the skills the client needed at home were not the same as those that were worked on during the therapy sessions at the rehabilitation center, but they could have been if the therapist had known more about the client.

►CONCLUSION

The foregoing examples all indicate that despite the very best intentions, it is quite possible for an occupational therapy practitioner to implement an intervention strategy without adequate or accurate client information. Within the client-practitioner relationship there is a power dynamic that is often intimidating for clients because of the professional-client roles. Even when we feel as if our planning with a client is a collaborative effort, we may have imposed our ideas and values in such a way that the client feels compelled to comply. This may be especially true for clients who have less education than the health professionals. The socioeconomic factors discussed throughout this chapter come into play in our own relationships with clients and their families. While the importance of listening and learning from individual clients is paramount to effective occupational therapy interventions, we also have to remember that this approach individualizes the underlying problems of the social structural constraints. The social system has a tendency to produce and reproduce problems of stratification (Scase, 1992, p. 65). On the one hand, we have to work with and understand each client individually with knowledge of the particulars of their resources, but this can obscure the larger issues resulting from the kind of social and material inequities we have discussed. We have to be able to work at both levels, the individual and the social system–social policy level to offer occupational therapy services that are ethical, effective, and equitable.

Acknowledgments

I would like to express my thanks to Hilary Lyle who worked with me during her senior year in the Occupational Therapy Department at the University of New Hampshire. Her assistance, resourcefulness, and interest in this project are greatly appreciated. And to Helen Gilmour, graphic designer at the University of New Hampshire, my sincere appreciation for her expertise and help.

REFERENCES

Albelda, R., Folbre, N., & The Centre for Popular Economics (1996). *The war on the poor: A defense manual.* New York: The New Press.

Allen, L. (1995, December 31). Family's careful balance collapses during illness. *The New York Times,* p. 27.

American Occupational Therapy Association (AOTA). (1994). Occupational therapy code of ethics. *American Journal of Occupational Therapy, 48,* 1034.

Apter, T. (1993). *Working women don't have wives: Professional success in the 1990s.* New York: St. Martin's Press.

Barlow, O. J. (1992). Special issue on the Americans with Disabilities Act. *American Journal of Occupational Therapy, 46* (5).

Bee, H. L. (1996). *The journey of adulthood* (3rd ed.). Upper Saddle River, NJ: Prentice-Hall.

Berger, K. S. (1994). *The developing person through the life span.* New York: Worth Publishers.

Brennan, T. & Berwick D. (1996). *New rules: Regulation, markets, and the quality of American health care.* San Francisco: Jossey-Bass.

Clark, F., Carlson, M., Zemke, R., Frank, G., Patterson, K., Ennevor, B. L., Rankin-Martinez, A., Hobson, L., Crandall, J., Mandel, D., & Lipson, L. (1996). Life domains and adaptive strategies of a group of low-income, well older adults. *American Journal of Occupational Therapy, 50,* 99-108.

Dunn, W., Brown, C., & McGuigan, A. (1994). The ecology of human performance: A framework for considering the effect of context. *The American Journal of Occupational Therapy, 48,* 595-607.

Fidler, G. (1996). Life-style performance: From profile to conceptual model. *The American Journal of Occupational Therapy, 50,* 139-147.

Friedman, E. (1994). The uninsured: From dilemma to crisis. In P. Lee & C. Estes (Eds.), *The nation's health* (4th ed., pp. 302–308). Boston: Jones and Bartlett Publishers.

Frishman, R. (1996, August). Quality of care: Don't be a wimp in the doctor's office. *Harvard Health Letter, 21,* 1-2.

Gilbert, D. & Kahl, J. (1993). *The American class structure: A new synthesis* (4th ed.). Belmont, CA: Wadsworth Publishing.

Grabb, E. G. (1997). *Theories of social inequality: Classical and contemporary perspectives* (3rd ed.). New York: Harcourt Brace.

Handler, J. H. (1995). *The poverty of welfare reform.* New Haven, CT: Yale University Press.

Hochschild, A. (1989). *The second shift.* New York: Avon Books.

Holmes, S. (1996, September 27). U. S. census finds first income rise in past six years. *The New York Times,* pp. A1, A23.

Kelly, J. & Godbey, G. (1992). *The sociology of leisure.* State College, PA: Venture Publishing.

Kozol, J. (1995). *Amazing grace.* New York. Crown Publishers.

Kozol, J. (1991). *Savage inequalities: Children in America's schools.* New York: Harper Collins.

Lee, P., Soffel, D., & Luft, H. (1994). Costs and coverage: Pressures toward health care reform. In P. Lee & C. Estes (Eds.), *The nation's health* (4th ed., pp. 204–213). Boston: Jones and Bartlett Publishers.

Marmot, M. G., Smith, G. D., Stansfeld, S., Patel, C., North, F., Head, J., White, I., Brunner, E., & Feeney, A. (1994). Health inequalities and social class. In P. Lee & C. Estes (Eds.), *The nation's health* (4th ed., pp. 34–40). Boston: Jones and Bartlett Publishers.

Marshall, G. (Ed.). (1994). *The concise Oxford dictionary of sociology.* Oxford: Oxford University Press.

Newman, K. S. (1988). *Falling from grace: The experience of downward mobility in the American middle class.* New York: Vintage Books.

Peterson, W. C. (1994). *Silent depression: The fate of the American dream.* New York: W. W. Norton.

Peloquin, S. M. (1995). The fullness of empathy: Reflections and illustrations. *The American Journal of Occupational Therapy, 1,* 24-31.

Peloquin, S. M. (1993). The patient-therapist relationship: Beliefs that shape care. *The American Journal of Occupational Therapy, 10,* 935-942.

Pope-Davis, D.B., (1993). Exploring multicultural competencies of occupational therapists: Implications for education and training. *The American Journal of Occupational Therapy, 9,* 838-844.

Purtilo, R. & Haddad, A. (1996). *Health professional and patient interaction* (5th ed.). Philadelphia: W. B. Saunders.

Rice, D. P. (1994). Health status and national health priorities. In P. Lee & C. Estes (Eds.) *The nation's health* (4th ed., pp. 45–58). Boston: Jones and Bartlett Publishers.

Scase, R. (1992). *Class.* Minneapolis: University of Minnesota Press.

Schor, J. (1992). *The overworked American: The unexpected decline of leisure.* New York: Basic Books.

Sidel, R. (1996). *Keeping women and children last: America's war on the poor.* New York: Penguin Books.

Trattner, W. (1994). *From poor law to welfare state: A history of social welfare in America* (5th ed.). New York: The Free Press.

Wood, W. (1996). Delivering occupational therapy's fullest promise: Clinical interpretations of "life domains and adaptive strategies of a group of low-income, well older adults." *American Journal of Occupational Therapy, 50,* 109-112.

UNIT II
Narrative Analysis

Elizabeth Blesedell Crepeau

Mary Feldhaus Weber's powerful story never fails to move me, although I have read it numerous times in preparing this book. What can we learn from her story, about living, about adapting, and about helping others with their recovery from devastating illness or disability? I would like to pose a few questions for you to consider, both in thinking about Mary's story and in thinking about the stories of all the people who you will treat in the future. All of the people who seek occupational therapy have personal histories which are largely hidden from us—seldom do they write stories such as this one to facilitate our understanding. So, similar to Anna Deane, we must learn about them through ongoing conversations with them and with their families. Anna Deane Scott's success with Mary was based on her ability to listen empathically to Mary and her concerns. As she listened, she talked with Mary about their mutual love of dogs. She focused on Mary's concerns of maintaining her safety and her ability to live independently. She avoided the formal evaluations that served only to reinforce Mary's sense of loss. She was honest with Mary, acknowledging her feelings when Mary asked her about their first meeting by saying, "I felt sad" (see Chap. 3, p. 28). Mary concluded, "I knew I could trust her" (see Chap. 3, p. 28). As you will read repeatedly in this book, listening is the essence of occupational therapy practice, for it is through achieving an understanding of the experience of the person before you that you will be able to form trusting partnerships with them, much as Mary and Anna Deane did.

Mary was a very successful movie producer before her accident. She had a network of friends and a life that was full and satisfying. What strengths can you discern from the story directly? What strengths can you infer? How did she use her dogs and art to help herself? What were the roles of her friends and family in this process? Despite her efforts to help herself after 2 years she said,

I was unable to do the simplest thing, make a bed, tell time, count . . . I felt like someone, but not like anyone I knew. I was a stranger to myself. **I** was lost . . . I still had some fight left in me; I had been a functional, successful adult. The three percent of me that was left was three percent of a fighter. We were all counting on the fact that I would keep fighting and I would get better. That somehow I would manage. I also knew I desperately needed someone to help me help myself (see Chap. 3, pp. 27–28).

Through her friend Sally she found Anna Deane Scott. Together, Anna Deane and Mary began reconstructing Mary's life. This reconstruction, based on the foundation of Mary's goals and needs and enacted through mutual problem solving, is the essence of occupational therapy practice. The chapters in this unit provide you with a way to begin to understand the values, beliefs, and assumptions we and the people we serve bring to the therapeutic encounter. By making these aspects more explicit we can improve our ability to serve others with the empathy and compassion demonstrated by Anna Deane Scott. In doing so we can achieve Mary's challenge to us:

So I am telling you that the two most important things you can do as an occupational therapy practitioner are to listen and to empower. The people who helped me most did both of those things. I continue to bless them and to use what they have taught me every day (see Chap. 3, p. 31).

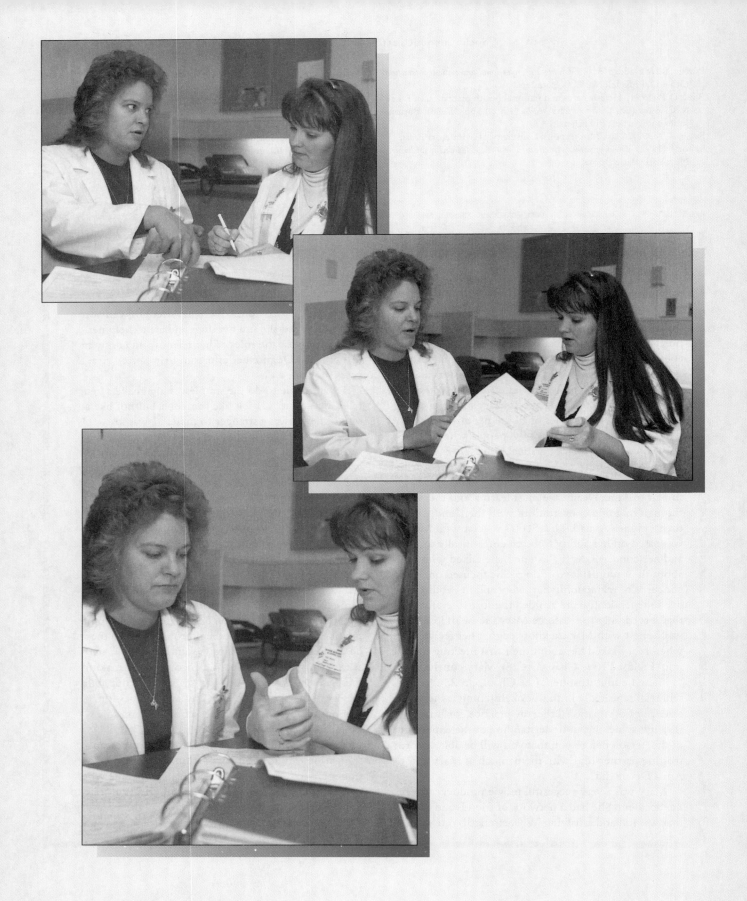

An occupational therapist (OTR) and certified occupational therapy assistant (COTA) work together reviewing the progress of one of their clients. (Photos by Gary Samson, Instructional Services, Dimond Library, University of New Hampshire.)

UNIT III

Occupational Therapy Practitioners: The Occupational Therapist and the Occupational Therapy Assistant

LEARNING OBJECTIVES

After completing this unit, readers will be able to:

▶ Define the role of the occupational therapist (OTR) and the role of the certified occupational therapy assistant (COTA) when collaborating to provide quality occupational therapy services.

▶ Define clinical reasoning and describe four important facets of the clinical reasoning process.

▶ Identify the different facets of clinical reasoning when observing others in practice or when presented with case materials.

Occupational therapy practitioners, working together in partnership, are the focus of the first chapter in this unit. Mary Sands demonstrates the interdependence that is essential for two individuals to work together to achieve common goals. She accomplishes this by linking conversations with OTR/COTA teams with the professional standards that guide practice. Our primary work is to help people do the things that are important to them so they can achieve their goals. We accomplish this through clinical reasoning. In the second chapter, Barbara Schell describes this multifaceted process and the interrelation among its scientific, narrative, pragmatic, and ethical components. (*Note*: Words in **bold** type are defined in the Glossary.)

Chapter 8

Practitioners' Perspectives on the Occupational Therapist and Occupational Therapy Assistant Partnership

Mary Sands

In many practice settings, occupational therapy (OT) services are delivered by a team consisting of an occupational therapist, registered (OTR) and a certified occupational therapy assistant (COTA). The roles of these two practitioners, and the relationship in which these roles flourish, are explored through first-person narratives. Practitioners who work as occupational therapist—occupational therapy assistant teams in different practice settings discuss their partnerships in stories and conversations about their work together.

The key to team work is collaboration. Meaningful collaboration results when each team member has mastered two requirements: (1) a clear understanding of each role; and (2) respect for the differences and similarities of each role. Roles are defined by more than a list of duties and responsibilities. Roles reflect values, customs, culture, and commitments. The roles of OTRs and COTAs at entry level have changed over time. Documents delineating entry level roles have served as guidelines for practice and education. The current guideline, *Occupational Therapy Roles* (AOTA, 1993), provides a framework from which an occupational therapy team can test and validate their individual model of practice. The Occupational Therapy Roles document provides definitions of professional roles. The stories and conversations that follow reveal the values, customs, culture, and commitments that shape and reinforce these roles.

▼ CLARIFYING EACH OTHER'S ROLE

The ability to act, based on an understanding of the roles of the two practitioners, is primary to the success of the occupational therapy team. Kathleen (Katie) Wilson, OTR and Celeste McAteer, COTA work in a public school practice setting. They have worked together for over 10 years as subcontractors in a private practice agency. The following conversation with this treatment team demonstrates the dynamics, subtlety, and value of their understanding.

Katie, OTR:

When we first started to work together, I included Celeste in the evaluation process. We started by doing evaluations together, then she did some parts and I watched, then she would do certain parts independently, and we would discuss what she did. I always evaluate the students, but I'm comfortable that Celeste, with her experience, can use the results I get to select correct treatment interventions. She can look at the evaluation, read the goals, and figure out what needs to be done. She has excellent ideas on projects, and I tend to be more technical. Celeste is good at finding projects that fit the treatment focus.

Celeste, COTA:

I bring all information about treatment to Katie (eg, a request for an evaluation, a teacher wanting a child's schedule changed, every-

HISTORICAL NOTE

THE SCRUBWOMEN OF WORLD WAR I: THE CHALLENGES OF PRACTICE

Suzanne M. Peloquin

Many see World War I reconstruction aides as the forebears of occupational therapy practitioners. Most are less familiar with the circumstances of the aides' recruitment. Dr. Frankwood Williams hoped to have occupational workers on his staff for Base Hospital 117. Although he had gathered several women who wanted to serve, he could not get Washington officials to appoint them. He read about openings for civilian aides: scrubwomen with no official connection to the army. Williams suggested that he get his recruits overseas by calling them scrubwomen, and they agreed (Myers, 1948).

These early "scrubwomen" were Mrs. Clyde Myers, a graduate of Columbia University; Eleanor Johnson, a psy-

chologist; Amy Drevenstedt, a history teacher at Hunter College; Corrine Dezeller, another Columbia graduate; and Laura LaForce, a graduate nurse. They were "divided into squads to clean the quarters assigned" on Ellis Island and moved on from there to reconstruction work overseas (Myers, p. 209).

If we choose to see these women as individuals whose passion for a cause carried them past the hurdles that blocked their way to practice, we might muster a similar passion in the face of circumstances that challenge us today. ■

Meyers, C. M. (1948). Pioneer occupational therapists in World War I. *American Journal of Occupational Therapy, 2,* 208–215.

---

thing). I do make treatment decisions independently, but I always let Katie know what I have done.

A slightly different approach to establishing a comfort level of understanding is discussed by another OTR and COTA team who collaborate on providing home-based treatment to children younger than the age of 4. Katherine Ferrara, OTR and Patricia (Pat) Schneider, COTA have worked together in clinical and nonclinical settings for 5 years. Both bring considerable past practice experience to the partnership.

Katherine, OTR:

I have to feel comfortable with the child before I will consider using a COTA. I need to have clearly defined goals and objectives; I have to feel confident that the occupational therapy assistant will be comfortable working with the child. As an OTR, if I don't feel comfortable treating a child with a certain type of problem, I seek supervision. If a COTA is uncomfortable in a treatment situation, [he or she] should receive adequate supervision and support. There has to be increased communication; the COTA must be able to say I'm really not comfortable with this, I'm going to need more supervision. There may need to be more opportunities for cotreating, more working together.

Pat, COTA:

Normally, I come in after the evaluation is completed and the type of treatment needed has been determined. Katherine has done the evaluation; we go over the evaluation and discuss the child before we actually begin treatment. You need a good support system, someone you can speak to at any time. In some places where I have worked, you have a set ½ hour of time per week for supervision. This is your supervision time whether you have anything to discuss at that point or not. I find it works better if you are able to ask questions as they come up, or even at the end of the day.

Katherine, OTR:

Or being able to ask, will you see this child with me? Can you take a minute to come over and feel this or see that?

▼ RESPECTING DIFFERENCES AND SIMILARITIES

The individuals in these treatment teams base their working relationships on a clear and mutual understanding of each other's roles. To develop an understanding of roles, one needs to develop respect for the differences and similarities in the roles that each person plays. According to Holmes (1993), "When the terms partner and collaboration are used to describe the relationship between the occupational therapist and the certified occupational therapy assistant, these words imply such elements as regard and respect for and knowledge of one's coworker" (p. 3). Swedberg (1993), in her discussion on supervising the COTA in a private practice setting, stressed the importance of (1) effective communication, (2) clear role delineation, (3) understanding of mutual expectations, and (4) mutual agreement on who is responsible for which aspects of the treatment process.

Occupational Therapy Roles (AOTA, 1993) identifies the major functions of OTR and COTA practitioners. The major function of the OTR is to, "Provide quality occupational therapy services, including assessment, intervention, program planning and implementation, discharge planning-related documentation and communication" (p. 1088). The major function of the COTA is to, "Provide quality occupational therapy services to assigned individuals under the supervision of a certified occupational therapist" (p. 1089).

With these definitions of function as a guide, it follows that a major difference in roles is responsibility for development and implementation of an occupational therapy treatment program. The OTR has this responsibility. The therapist may (1) select appropriate assessment and intervention techniques and carry them out unassisted, (2) assign procedures to the COTA based on previously established service competencies, or (3) assign cases to the COTA as the primary service provider by matching the client's needs with the skill and knowledge levels the COTA has achieved. In using any one of these options, the OTR and the COTA will need to rely heavily on effective supervision and communication.

The establishment of service competency plays a vital role in shaping the type of collaborative relationship an OTR–COTA team will have. Service competency is defined as "the ability to use the identified intervention in a safe and effective manner" (AOTA, 1993, p. 1090). The concept of service competency implies that the OTR delegates a specific task or tasks to the COTA based on the level of professional competence demonstrated by the assistant in performing the task or tasks in other situations. Stated more simply, the OTR must be confident that the COTA will achieve the same results or outcomes as the OTR would, even if the techniques used are slightly different. Because the OTR is responsible for all aspects of occupational therapy service delivery, service competency is critical to the collaborative process. Service competency sets the framework for effective supervision. *The Guide for Supervision of Occupational Therapy Personnel* (AOTA, 1994) describes quality supervision as "a mutual undertaking between the supervisor and the supervisee that fosters growth and development; assures appropriate use of training and potential; encourages creativity and innovation; and provides guidance, support, encouragement, and respect, while working toward a goal" (p. 1045).

Communication facilitates effective supervision. "Mutual trust and respect are necessary for communication to take place" (Swedberg, 1993, p. 4). When mutual trust and respect exists, the COTA can comfortably report what is going on in the treatment process, ask for assistance or support when needed, and make and share an honest assessment of his or her skill and knowledge levels. The OTR can assign tasks for the treatment process based on informed decisions that reflect a clear understanding of the contributions that each member of the occupational therapy team will make.

The following conversations demonstrate how trust and respect provide a basis on which the practitioners build their collaborative experiences through supervision and communication.

Katie, OTR:

I feel comfortable handing Celeste an evaluation because I know she can interpret the technical language and understand what it means relative to what needs be done. I wouldn't feel comfortable doing this if I didn't know her skills. I trust that if Celeste has to make a decision about treatment, it will be a good decision, it will work out, and it won't be a problem. I also know that she's aware of when a decision has to be made by me. An example is a recent

Committee on Special Education meeting that Celeste attended in my absence. There were requests made for major changes in a child's treatment program and Celeste informed the people at the meeting that the requested changes would have to be considered and approved by the OTR.

Being together on a weekly basis really helps. Telephone calls are good, but you also need to see what's going on. You have to make sure you meet once a week as a minimum. I definitely have to feel comfortable with my COTA partner because I don't know the children as well as I would if I were treating them by myself.

Celeste, COTA:

Speaking from past experiences, when I worked at a different setting as a new graduate, I didn't always have a supervisor. I didn't know if that was okay or what to do about it. I think as a COTA you need supervision, you need a resource, someone to go to. You need to know that there are some responsibilities that should not fall on you. You shouldn't be afraid to speak out; you should know that there are ways to correct uncomfortable situations. I finally had to go to my administrator and say, I should be supervised.

I gained my confidence through observing Katie; being trusted with certain responsibilities in the treatment process; and being allowed to share in decision making. Working together, we take up each other's slack. There is a lot of trust; we can rely on each other. I know that Katie's evaluation is a true representation of a child's abilities and deficits. When I am treating and I have a question, I know I can go to Katie and get the answer. Even on days when I am treating alone, I'm comfortable knowing she is only a phone call away.

Katie, OTR:

As an OTR supervisor, I feel I have to be flexible. If a COTA doesn't feel comfortable doing certain treatment activities, that's okay because people have different comfort levels. On the other hand, if a COTA demonstrates that he or she can do more and wants to do more, [he or she] should be given the opportunity to do more. I try to remember that COTAs, similar to OTRs, function at different skill levels. The key to working well together is being able to get along. You can't be rigid or have the attitude that this is what an OTR does; don't do my job. Or, I'm not an OTR; don't expect me to do that. I think the team approach can work in any situation. If you work with someone that you know has the necessary skills and you feel comfortable that the person will come to you when there is something he or she doesn't understand, you have the makings of a great collaborative team.

Katie and Celeste have developed their own unique and successful way of communicating with each other. In the following conversation they tell us how it facilitates their collaborative process.

Katie, OTR:

We have a running list, each of us writes down information that we want to share with each other. We are in the school district 2 days a week. Celeste sees one group of children on Monday and I see another group. The next week we switch groups. This way, we both see everybody. We each see something different, and we leave notes for each other about our observations. This is helpful not only as a stimulus for our weekly meetings, but also the list is always there as a reminder. For example, I can look back at the notes Celeste wrote about a particular child when she worked with him the week before and be reminded that certain things she tried didn't appear to work, or that the child has a more pronounced problem in a particular area than I originally thought. It helps me adapt my approach with the child.

In the next narratives, the practitioners discuss one way of establishing service competency that fosters communication, develops skills, and ultimately, leads to better supervision.

Pat, COTA:

Being able to cotreat is helpful. As a COTA, I am constantly learning by observing my supervisor. When we cotreat, I observe the different things she does with the child and I pick up on it and use it later on. Sometimes when I'm treating alone, I will use a technique that I am comfortable in applying, but I'm not sure why it works. When I observe Katherine do the same technique, I can actually see the end results. After discussing it, I gain a better understanding for why I do it.

Katherine, OTR:

With cotreatments, I get to have a hands on approach in treatment implementation. I look at the progress the person has made, and I see how the short-term and long-term goals are being reached. I develop a feeling for what is being done when I'm not there; what is working or not working. Pat will start an activity with the child while I sit and observe, and then I introduce a different activity and she observes. Afterward, we talk about what we did and the results we obtained. We share ideas and problem solve together. Mutual respect is a key element in the OTR/COTA partnership. Each person must use professional interpersonal skills at all times.

▼ IMPLEMENTING THE COLLABORATIVE PROCESS

When a referral or prescription for occupational therapy services is received, the occupational therapy team begins the process of defining and addressing problems that interfere with function. Screening, evaluation, treatment planning, and goal setting lead to treatment intervention strategies selected to address the unique and specific problems of the person receiving treatment. The team must identify problems to be addressed and methods to address them. The OTR has the primary responsibility for problem identification and the COTA may contribute to the collection of data that will facilitate framing problems for therapeutic intervention. The application of theory in problem setting is uniquely the responsibility of the OTR. The therapist may use one or more theoretical frames of reference in setting clinical problems. Parham (1986), in discussing the importance of applying theory to practice, states that "problem setting is as important as problem solving. Problem setting refers to identifying the appropriate problem to solve" (p. 120). She describes it as a conceptual process in which the therapist names what will be attended to in practice, and frames the context for intervention. "Once the problem has been set, the problem solving process can begin. Here technical procedures are applied" (Parham, p. 120). The application of technical

procedures, under the supervision of the OTR, is the primary role of the COTA. "Problem solving . . . may be done by the occupational therapist or by the occupational therapy assistant working under the supervision of, and in collaboration with, the occupational therapist" (Sands, 1986, p. 125).

The components of collaboration are varied and personal. Each team will need to define the parameters of their collaborative efforts:

Katie, OTR:

When we receive a referral, the first thing we do is gather information on the child's general background. We speak to the classroom teacher and we may speak to the psychologist or the gym teacher. I like to obtain this information before I do the evaluation so that I have a general picture of the child; it helps to know what to zero in on. When the referral comes in, regardless of who's providing services that day, we start to collect information. Celeste may leave me a note that she spoke with the teacher and what was said. Because I will be doing the evaluation, I usually try to talk to the major people. If Celeste has spoken with someone, we discuss what she found out. I also read reports from other services that may be treating the child.

After I complete the evaluation, I go back to the teacher and share what I saw in doing the evaluation and what my feelings are; and I ask if this fits what is being seen in the classroom. The next step is to document the evaluation results and my recommendations in a report to the Committee on Special Education. Once the committee approves the recommendations, the parents are notified, a referral is obtained, and either Celeste or I contact the teacher to setup a schedule to see the child. Most children are seen twice a week. Celeste will see the child one day and I will see the child alone or with her on the second day. We communicate with each other on each child in weekly face-to-face meetings and in writing, using our running list of comments, questions, and suggestions that we both contribute to regularly. We write treatment notes after each treatment session. The notes are for us, we use them to keep a record of treatment and as a way to communicate with each other—highlighting the things you want the other person to be aware of.

Celeste, COTA:

Once a year we do an **Individual Education Plan (IEP)** for each child. Katie reevaluates the child and checks goals. Together we decide whether to change goals, increase or decrease treatment sessions, change the treatment format (group versus individual), or to discontinue the child.

Katie, OTR:

We go back and forth with comments such as: I think we should increase the time, I think we should keep it the same, I think the child should be grouped. For example, Celeste may make a point that the child is not consistently demonstrating a certain skill and we discuss it and agree that we should continue to see the child for individual sessions, or we should increase our focus on a particular desired outcome.

Celeste, COTA:

Based on our individual experiences with a child, we each give input on the plans for the next school year. We share the task of writing the IEPs, and we read each others and sometimes add things. Katie will usually add evaluation data, and I may do a summary of treatment activities. If our decision is to discontinue a child, Katie will write the discharge summary.

The occupational therapy team working in home care describes their collaboration as fairly traditional. The OTR receives the referral for service, performs the evaluation, and designs the treatment plan. The COTA implements the treatment plan under the supervision of the OTR. The assistant provides direct service to the client on a predetermined schedule. The therapist sees the client with the assistant once a week or once a month, depending on the frequency of treatment and the status of the client's condition. When working with a child in the home, the COTA explains the importance of communication in preparing the OTR for changes in the child's behavior:

Pat, COTA:

When working with young children, you can never predict how they will respond on any given day. What worked on Monday may

not work on Friday. One child started biting when she became upset. I saw the child on Monday and Katherine was going to see her on Friday. I was really concerned that she might get bitten; so I called to let her know about this new behavior and we talked about why this was happening and how we could address it. I discuss any changes I see with Katherine, whether the child is making terrific gains or no gains.

Katherine, OTR:

I'm aware before I go in to see a child of what has been working and what hasn't. Without constant communication I'm not able to facilitate treatment or provide the necessary supervision appropriately.

Each occupational therapy team should develop their own model for collaboration, and it should reflect the personal and professional uniqueness of the team members. Guidelines exist to assist practitioners in selecting and delineating responsibilities. Guidelines, such as *Occupational Therapy Roles* (AOTA, 1993), can be especially helpful to new practitioners (see Appendix C for this document). Table 8-1 summarizes some of the key performance areas identified in

TABLE 8-1. OTR/COTA Collaboration at Entry Level*

Responsibilities	OTR	COTA
Responds to request for services in accordance with service agency's policies and procedures	x	x
Initiates referrals when appropriate	x	
Screens to determine need for intervention	x	
Evaluates to obtain and interpret data necessary for treatment planning and intervention	x	
Assists with data collection and evaluation		x With supervision
Interprets evaluation findings	x	
Develops and coordinates intervention plan	x	
Develops treatment goals	x	x With supervision
Implements intervention plan (provides direct service)	x	x With supervision
Adapts environment according to needs of the individual	x	x With supervision
Monitors individual's response to intervention and modifies plan if needed	x	
Communicates and collaborates with other team members, family and caregivers	x	x In collaboration with OTR
Maintains records and documentation required by practice setting	x	x With supervision
Terminates services when maximum benefit is received	x	
Maintains treatment area, equipment, and supply inventory	x	x
Follows policy and procedures required in the setting	x	x
Performs continuous quality improvement activities	x	x In collaboration with OTR
Identifies and pursues own professional growth and development	x	x
Schedules and prioritizes own workload	x	
Participates in professional and community activities	x	x
Monitors own performance and identifies supervisory needs	x	
Functions according to the AOTA *Code of Ethics and Standards of Practice* (AOTA, 1994) of the profession	x	x

*(Note: The performance areas in the first column are from Occupational Therapy Roles, American Occupational Therapy Association (1993). American Journal of Occupational Therapy, 47, 1088–1090. Copyright 1993 by American Occupational Therapy Association, Inc. Adapted with permission.)

the roles document for OTR and COTA practitioners, and delineates responsibilities for these areas.

It is expected that as OTRs and COTAs gain experience, develop new skills, and improve and refine old ones, they will enhance their professional development and function at progressively more advanced levels. As knowledge and skill levels change, so will the conditions of collaboration. Because supervision provides a foundation for collaboration, changes in the focus and substance of supervision should match changes in performance of the practitioners involved. The document, *Roles of Occupational Therapists and Occupational Therapy Assistants in Schools* (AOTA, 1987), outlines a well-defined model for supervision and collaboration between the OTR and the COTA. It suggest that both members of the team have a responsibility for facilitating and strengthening the collaborative process, and that "methods of professional supervision should be . . . periodically reevaluated for effectiveness" (p. 799).

The OTR and COTA teams we spoke with are experienced practitioners, and they identified their awareness of changes in their levels of performance in the following ways:

Pat, COTA:

You develop skills each time you work with an individual, and you draw on them each time you work with a new person. You don't group people (ie, this is a person with a stroke so you do A and B). As you treat, you draw on past experiences, embellish what you know, and learn new things.

Katie, OTR:

I assess my skills by considering the questions teachers in the schools ask and how prepared I feel to answer them. A teacher may ask about a specific evaluation technique that I don't know, and this will spark an initiative; as will a student with a diagnosis or problem that I have never worked with. The skills that you need to sharpen will depend on where you are working. In schools, I spend a good amount of time working with children on fine motor skills, so I concentrate on handwriting, and this has been a focus for my continuing education activities.

▼ ASSESSING THE VALUE OF THE OTR/COTA PARTNERSHIP

Increases in levels of service productivity, increased access to occupational therapy services, reduced intervention time frames, and increases in the severity and longevity of treatable disorders have all influenced service delivery models in occupational therapy, and will continue to do so. According to Gilfoyle (1993), roles for OTRs and COTAs will change significantly as we prepare to enter the 21st century. Social, economic, political, and technologic changes will influence on what they do and how they do it. Gilfoyle (1993) predicts an increased need for services to the elderly, prompted by the growing number of persons older than 75. She sug-

gests that COTAs will be increasingly more responsible for direct service delivery to this population, and OTRs will have increased responsibility for research, education, consultation, and supervision (p. 316). In anticipation of these and other changes, the promotion of effective OTR/COTA teams should be a primary focus within the profession.

The quality of occupational therapy services is embedded in a commitment to holistic intervention. Changing models of practice should embrace this tradition; therefore, the partnership between the therapist and the assistant should be viewed in the holistic nature of occupational therapy intervention. The OTR and the COTA who have a partnership in a public school setting share their feelings and humanistic professional beliefs about practice:

Katie, OTR:

I have an eclectic approach to treatment. Every child will respond to more than one approach. I always rely on development, what's missing and how can we get what is needed from a particular treatment approach. We try to address everything because the child is a whole person. You can address the whole child by incorporating tasks that are school related with tasks that address other areas of need (eg, an obstacle course for gross motor coordination can be integrated with doing a puzzle to address fine motor skills). Sometimes we use more traditional occupational therapy projects in place of neurodevelopmental and sensory integration techniques to increase a child's self-esteem: something that is familiar, is of interest to the child, and incorporates fine motor skills.

Working with the total child is important in the school setting. If a child is having trouble academically, it doesn't always mean it's because the child can't do 2 + 2. It's because of a whole multitude of problems that often are ignored. We try to address these other needs and make suggestions to teachers to help them address them also. Teachers appreciate the input because it works, it focuses on the child's self-image and self-confidence.

Celeste, COTA:

We give teachers information on home programs and relate them to the types of things the teacher can do in the classroom and pass on to parents. Over the years, we have earned the respect of the teachers by being consistent in what we say and by talking with them when miscommunication has occurred. That has been an important part of our relationship with them. The child's environment and culture play a big part in the results we get. It's difficult when there is no carryover at home. We write notes to parents or call them, but even then things are not always carried through. Some parents will bring problems to our attention, such as trouble tying shoes, and this is a good indication that the parent will follow through on our suggestions.

Katie, OTR:

Being consistent is important. We will discuss and debate the pros and cons of taking a particular stance about a child's treatment program. We come to a conclusion, and if we really feel strongly about it, we go with it, even though others may challenge our position. We may ask for input on legal issues and then consider what we feel is right. Our recommendations may not be accepted by the

Committee on Special Education, but we stick with what we believe. The decision may be to do the opposite of what we recommend, and we say that's fine, this is our report and this is how we stand on this issue.

Adopting a holistic approach to service intervention involves promoting and facilitating productive interactions between the person and the environment. The practitioners delivering home care services discuss the influence occupational therapy had on a family member–caregiver in a home-based treatment setting.

Katherine, OTR:

I think the real difference with home-based treatment is the direct contact with the caregiver. The communication is constant and you are a role model for the caregiver. They see what you do with the family member and you ask them to follow through with the things you do. When doing home-based treatment, you really get a feel for family dynamics and what the person does 24 hours a day. You don't get that with a 1-hour, twice a week, in the clinic arrangement. You get a view of their performance that you would never get seeing the person in the clinic.

Pat, COTA:

An example is the 3-year-old twins we recently started seeing in the home. When they were coming to the clinic, we asked the mother if the girls were eating normally and she said they were. They looked healthy, and we had no way of knowing that they were still on baby food until we went to the home and saw the baby food jars lined up on the kitchen counter. Mom had never mentioned that they were still on baby food, a status that neither we or the speech therapist wanted to encourage. By being in the home, we can find out things like this, and we have the opportunity to suggest and facilitate more appropriate options.

I can see a change in the mother with the twins. She is able to play with them more comfortably. She didn't know how to play with them, nor how to discipline them. She sees us say no to the girls and not give in to their temper tantrums. The mom is learning from watching how we handle the children.

I find that I draw on my own experiences as a parent, and I try to stress the positive. I also make a point to show the parents the positive, because they already know the negative. The mom doesn't need me to tell her what they are unable to do, she is aware of that. At the end of each treatment session, I make a point to share the things the girls were able to do. You treat the whole family, because the disability affects the whole family.

CONCLUSION

Prerequisites for successful collaboration are an understanding and respect for the similarities and the differences in roles, trust, communication, and the ability to effectively participate in the supervisory process. The OTR is responsible for supervising the COTA whenever the assistant is performing service intervention. The degree of supervision will depend on the assistant's level of experience and expertise and the level of service competency established for a given intervention technique. Service competency is the ability to use an intervention in a safe and effective manner (AOTA, 1993).

Collaboration is accomplished when each member of the partnership understands and respects the contribution of the other. Collaboration implies a full commitment to working together by listening to, accepting, and valuing each other's input. Collaboration between occupational therapy practitioners is important to providers of service, receivers of service, and to the viability of the profession.

Acknowledgments
The author wishes to thank Kathleen Wilson, OTR, Celeste McAteer, COTA, Katherine Ferrara, OTR, and Patricia Schneider, COTA for their candid and enthusiastic participation in conversations about their partnerships.

▼ REFERENCES

American Occupational Therapy Association (AOTA). (1987). Roles of occupational therapists and occupational therapy assistants in schools. *American Journal of Occupational Therapy, 41,* 798–803.

American Occupational Therapy Association. (1993). Occupational therapy roles. *American Journal of Occupational Therapy, 47,* 1087–1099.

American Occupational Therapy Association. (1994). Guide for supervision of occupational therapy personnel. *American Journal of Occupational Therapy, 48,* 1045–1046.

Gilfoyle, E. M. (1993). The future of occupational therapy. In S. E. Ryan (Ed.), *Practice issues in occupational therapy intraprofessional team building* (pp. 315–329). Thorofare, NJ: Slack.

Holmes, C. (1993, September). Challenging old paradigms. *Administration & Management Special Interest Section Newsletter, 9,* 3–4.

Parham, L. D. (1986). Applying theory to practice. In *Occupational Therapy Education: Target 2000* (pp. 119–122). Rockville, MD: American Occupational Therapy Association.

Sands, M. (1986). Applying theory to practice: A response from technical education. In *Occupational Therapy Education: Target 2000* (pp. 125–126). Rockville, MD: American Occupational Therapy Association.

Swedberg, L. (1993, September). Supervising the advanced certified occupational therapy assistant in a private practice setting. *Administration & Management Special Interest Section Newsletter, 9,* 4–5.

Chapter 9

Clinical Reasoning: The Basis of Practice

Barbara Boyt Schell

Clinical reasoning is the process used by practitioners to plan, direct, perform, and reflect on client care. It is a complex and multifaceted process. To consider clinical reasoning requires engaging in a metacognitive analysis. In simple terms, that means we are thinking about thinking. This is important, because newcomers to the field may incorrectly understand clinical reasoning as something that one "chooses to do" or as a form of occupational therapy treatment theory. It is neither of those things. Whenever you are engaged in planning, doing, or thinking about occupational therapy for an identified individual or group, you are engaged in clinical reasoning. It is not a question of whether you are doing it, only a question of how well. Furthermore, there are many evaluation and treatment theories that are discussed throughout this text that may become part of your clinical reasoning process. However, the theories about clinical reasoning discussed in this chapter are theories about occupational therapy practitioners and their reasoning processes, not about clients. Keep in mind these important distinctions as you become mindful of your own clinical reasoning processes.

In this chapter, clinical reasoning is examined from several perspectives. First, it is discussed as a multisensory process that involves the whole body. Second, the practical nature of clinical reasoning is described, along with the relation between formal theory and clinical reasoning. Next is a discussion of some current understandings of the many facets of clinical reasoning. This leads to the final section about the development of clinical reasoning and strategies to improve clinical reasoning throughout your career.

To make this discussion more reality-based for you, a description of a typical clinical situation is first presented that illustrates many of the issues discussed. The case study on the facing page is adapted from an actual observation by the author during the course of a research study on clinical reasoning. Read the case study before continuing with the text. Pay special attention to the different kinds of issues and problems that the therapist has to address. In particular, look for how the therapist views issues related to (1) the client's occupational performance, medical prognosis, and financial issues; (2) coordination with team members; and (3) ethical dilemmas.

▼ CLINICAL REASONING: A WHOLE BODY PRACTICE

With this case study in mind, the following discussion will explore the nature of clinical reasoning. Perhaps one of the first things to note is that clinical reasoning is a whole-body process. This is one reason that it is a different experience to read about a case study, such as the one just described, and to actually be the practitioner in the situation. Some aspects of clinical reasoning seem to involve some straightforward thinking processes that an occupational therapy practitioner can easily describe. Examples include evaluating and treating occupational performance areas, such as self-care or work. Practitioners use their observations and theoretical knowledge to identify relevant performance components that may be contributing to performance problems. Practitioners also attend to the contextual factors affecting perfor-

CAN SHE GO HOME?

Terry, an occupational therapist, goes to a client's room in the neurology unit of a regional medical center. Along the way, she shares her thoughts with Barb, a researcher who is observing her practice. Terry fills Barb in on the client they are about to see. The client, Mrs. Munro (a pseudonym), is a widow who lives alone in a house in town. A couple of days ago, she suffered a stroke [right **cerebrovascular accident (CVA)**] and was brought by a neighbor to the hospital. Mrs. Munro has made a rapid recovery, and is demonstrating good return of her motor skills. She still has some left-sided weakness and incoordination, along with some cognitive problems. She is a delightfully pleasant older woman, and is anxious to return home. Terry, the occupational therapist, is seeing this client for the third time, and her primary concern is to evaluate whether Mrs. Munro has any residual cognitive deficits from her stroke that would put her at serious risk if she returns home alone. Terry plans to do some more in-depth activities of daily living (ADL) with her, to see how well Mrs. Munro demonstrates safety awareness. Terry thinks she will probably have Mrs. Munro get out of bed, obtain her clothing and hygiene supplies, perform her morning hygiene routines at the sink, and then get dressed. Terry wants to see the degree to which Mrs. Munro is able to spontaneously manage these tasks, as well as how good her judgment appears to be. Terry's thought is that if she can engage Mrs. Munro in several multistep activities that also require her to perform in different positions, Terry should be able to detect any cognitive and motor problems that pose a serious safety threat.

When Terry arrives at the room, she greets Mrs. Munro who says: "I am so excited. The doctor says I can go home tomorrow." Terry turns to Barb and raises her eyebrows, as if to say "I told you so." On the way to the room, Terry had told Barb that she was worried that the physician managing Mrs. Munro's case tended to think that as soon as clients can get up, they can go home. Terry went on to defend the physician by saying that in today's cost-conscious environment, the doctors were under a lot of pressure not to keep clients in the hospital.

As Terry talks with Mrs. Munro about generalities, she notices that Mrs. Munro is already dressed in her housecoat. When she talks to Mrs. Munro about doing some self-care activities, it becomes apparent that Mrs. Munro has already completed her bathing and dressing routines, with help from nursing. When Terry suggests that they perhaps brush her teeth and comb her hair, Mrs. Munro is happy to get up out of bed, but notes that her neighbor never did bring in her dentures. Mrs. Munro sits on the edge of the bed, and after a reminder from Terry, puts on her slippers. She then stands and walks to the nearby sink, finds her comb and combs her hair. While she is doing this Terry looks around for some other ideas about what to do, because Mrs. Munro has already completed the self-care tasks Terry had planned to do with her. Terry's eyes light on some flowers by the bed that are wilted. She suggests to Mrs. Munro that she might want to dispose of the flowers, and clean the vase. Then the vase will be ready to pack when it comes time to go home. Mrs. Munro agrees, and proceeds to walk somewhat unsteadily over to the vase. Picking it up, she carries it to the sink, where she pulls out the dead flowers. Terry follows her, staying slightly behind and within reach of Mrs. Munro. When Mrs. Munro stops after removing the flowers, Terry suggests she rinse out the vase, which she does. She then dries it and returns the vase to the bedside table. Terry reminds her to throw out the dead flowers. While Mrs. Munro does this, they begin to talk some more about her plans to return home.

Mrs. Munro tells Terry that she has lived in her home for 40 years, and even though her husband died over 10 years ago, she still feels his presence there. He used to love her cooking, and she still cooks herself three meals a day. She starts to cry when they talk about cooking, but then cheers up. Terry tells her that it might be safer if she had someone around the house for a few weeks, until she gets a little more recovered from her stroke. Mrs. Munro thinks she can get some help from her neighbor. Terry says she is also going to suggest some home care therapy, just to make sure she is safe in the kitchen, bathroom, and so on, noting that "We sure don't want to see you have a bad fall just when you are doing so well after your stroke." After reviewing some coordination exercises for her left hand, Terry says good-bye. Terry and Barb leave the room. Terry stops at the nurses station to note in the chart that Mrs. Munro demonstrated good safety awareness in familiar tasks at bedside, but did require cuing to complete multistep tasks. Terry also notes some motor instability in task performance during ambulation. Terry recommends a referral to

(continued)

(Continued)

a home health occupational therapist "to assess safety and equipment needs during bathroom activities, meal preparation, and routine homemaking tasks." Terry comments to Barb, as they walk off the unit, that she thinks Mrs. Munro did pretty well, but Terry remains concerned about the risks once she goes home, and particularly when she is tired. Terry is also concerned that someone monitor Mrs. Munro in a familiar setting to see if she handles her daily routines adequately. Terry would really like to see Mrs. Munro go to a rehabilitation center, but she has no insurance funding to support that. Terry notes that at least she might be able to get some home care, for there are a few programs around that provide some services to indigent elderly. Staying in her own home seems to be Mrs. Munro's major goal, and Terry is going to do what she can to try to help her attain that goal. She'll catch up with the social worker later to discuss the need for Mrs. Munro to have good support from any neighbors, friends, or relatives.

mance. For instance, Terry was able to describe her concerns about Mrs. Munro's safety in returning home. In particular, Terry was addressing self-care and homemaking activities. She had analyzed relevant contextual factors about the home setting, and Mrs. Munro's social and financial situation. Terry had identified the performance component areas of cognition and motor control as impaired areas that were affecting occupational performance. This was all information that Terry could readily share with Barb. However, there were many more kinds of information in the therapy session that represented knowledge that Terry used, but either did not or could not put into words.

Some of the knowledge that Terry did not put into words involved information gained from other senses. Part of Terry's clinical reasoning involved body-based knowledge. For instance, Terry used her sense of touch to feel the muscle tension (or lack of tension) in Mrs. Munro's affected arm when she was doing an activity or home exercise program. During her evaluation, Terry did some quick stretches to Mrs. Munro's elbow and wrist to see if she could feel evidence of spasticity, an abnormal reflex response commonly found in individuals recovering from a stroke. When Mrs. Munro stood up, Terry carefully gauged the distance she stood from Mrs. Munro, because Mrs. Munro was at some risk of falling. Terry was careful not to stand too close so that she did not crowd or overprotect Mrs. Munro, but close enough to protect her should she lose her balance. While close to Mrs. Munro, Terry could smell her, gaining a quick sense of possible hygiene or continence problems. Terry used her voice quality to display encouragement and support. She watched and listened carefully for clues about the nature of Mrs. Munro's emotional state. In particular she watched facial expressions and listened for evidence of fear or insecurity during Mrs. Munro's performance of activities.

Even beyond the clinical knowledge that is based in the senses we can describe, there are many aspects of the process for which we do not have clear words. Fleming describes this as "knowing more than we can tell" (1994a, p. 24). She goes on to explain that much of the profession's knowledge is practical knowledge, which is "seldom discussed and rarely described" (p. 25). This tacit (unspoken) knowledge, combined with the rich sensory aspects of actual practice, helps explain why reading about therapy and doing therapy are such different experiences. With this understanding of clinical reasoning as a whole-body practice, we turn next to a discussion about the role of theory in practice, and how theoretical knowledge and clinical reasoning are related.

▼ THEORY AND PRACTICE

There has been a long-standing discussion in many professions about the role of theory in professional practice (Casteless & Korthagen, 1996). In occupational therapy, these discussions have most often concerned the problems students experience in moving from the classroom into clinical practice (Cohn, 1989). Although many leaders (Parham, 1987; Rogers 1983, 1986) argue the benefits of theory-based practice, Cohn (1989) notes that the problems of practice rarely present themselves in the straightforward manner described in textbook theories. Building on Schon's (1983) work, a consensus seems to be evolving that advocates a reflective stance toward the therapeutic process. Reflective practice involves the use of theories and research-based knowledge to consciously examine daily practices to identify ways to improve both the theories and individual practice routines. This is where theory and practice meet in the clinical-reasoning process.

A theory is a set of interconnected propositions about a subject area. It consists of concepts and the relations among these concepts, sometimes called principles (Miller, 1993). As Mosey described it, "the theoretical foundation of a profession consists of selected theories and empirical [observable] data that serve as the scientific basis for practice" (1992, p. 63). Because theory is, by nature, an abstraction of the real world, theory is always too general to fully guide practice (Argyris & Schon, 1974). On the other hand, practitioners need some way of making sound clinical choices and predicting outcomes associated with those choices. That is where theory and clinical reasoning come together. Clinical reasoning involves the naming and framing of problems based on a personal understanding of the client's situation (Schon, 1983). In problem identification and problem solution, clinicians use a blend of theories. Because clinical reasoning is a practical process, directed toward action, practitioners routinely make decisions in the absence of clear data. However, theoretical knowledge aids the clinician to (1) avoid unjustified assumptions or the use of ineffective clinical techniques, and (2) reflect on how the clinical experience is similar or different from theoretical understandings. This issue is revisited at the end of this chapter in relation to advancing practitioner expertise. For the moment, let us turn our attention to the different facets of clinical reasoning.

▼ FACETS OF CLINICAL REASONING

When early researchers of clinical reasoning in occupational therapy first began to examine the nature of occupational therapists thinking, they thought in terms of a single clinical-reasoning process (Fleming 1991; Rogers & Masagatani, 1982). Fleming was the first within occupational therapy to describe how therapists used different modes of thinking, depending on the nature of the clinical problem they were addressing. She referred to this process as the "therapist with the three-track mind" (Fleming, 1991, p. 1007). Since that time, others have examined the different aspects of therapists clinical reasoning. These will be summarized in the following under the headings of scientific, narrative, pragmatic, and ethical reasoning.

Scientific Reasoning

Scientific reasoning is used to understand the condition that is affecting an individual, and to decide on treatment interventions that are in the best interest of the client. It is a logical process, which parallels scientific inquiry. Two forms of scientific reasoning identified in occupational therapy are diagnostic reasoning (Rogers & Holm, 1991) and procedural reasoning (Fleming, 1994b). Scientific reasoning may also be referred to as occupational therapy "treatment planning" (Pelland, 1987, p. 353), in which the therapist uses selected theories both to identify problems and to guide clinical decision making. Much like the experimental approaches used in science, data about clients' problems are systematically gathered and treatment approaches are based on hypotheses about the causes of the client's condition. Treatment procedures are selected based on scientifically researched knowledge, and treatment effectiveness is carefully monitored through reevaluation. Much of the information contained in this text reflects current scientific reasoning in occupational therapy.

Two forms of scientific reasoning are diagnostic reasoning and procedural reasoning. Diagnostic reasoning is concerned with clinical problem sensing and problem definition. The process starts in advance of seeing a client. For instance, occupational therapy practitioners already have a mindset about the kinds of problems they are looking for: occupational performance problems. Additionally, the nature of the problems they expect to find are influenced by the information in the request for services. The person's age, the nature and severity of the medical condition, and the reason for referral, all influence the therapist's expectations. Finally, the therapist will likely reflect on similar cases that he or she has seen. All of this occurs before the therapist even sees the client. In the case study described earlier, some of these issues can be seen. For example, Terry knew, from her understanding of brain functioning and pathology, that most individuals who have a stroke experience both motor and cognitive problems. Terry also knew that older women often live alone, and have outlived their spouses. Therefore, to some degree she knew the kinds of discharge planning issues that were likely to arise.

From the initial encounter, the occupational therapy practitioner begins to collect cues, and uses systematic strategies to understand the client's condition. Fleming described this as procedural reasoning in which therapists were "thinking about the disease or disability and deciding which treatment activities (procedures) they might employ to remediate the people functional performance problems" (1991, p. 1008). This may involve an interview, an observation of the person engaged in a task, or formal evaluations using standardized tools. In the case study, Terry used a combination of interview and observation, both of which were guided by her working hypothesis that Mrs. Munro may have a cognitive problem that could affect her safe performance at home. As intervention begins, more data is collected, and the occupational therapy practitioner gains a sharper clinical image. This clinical image represents an interplay between what the practitioner expects to see (such as the usual course of the disease or disability) and the actual performance of the client. In our case study, there was congruence between Mrs. Munro's abilities and problems in performing activities of daily living and Terry's expectations of someone making a good recovery from a stroke.

Mattingly has made the point that occupational therapists have a "two-body practice" (1994a, p. 37). By that she means that occupational therapists view a person in two ways: the body as a machine, in which parts may be broken; and the person as a life filled with personal meanings and hopes. Much of the scientific reasoning in occupational therapy addresses issues related to the "body as machine." The next form of clinical reasoning, narrative reasoning, provides the practitioner with a vehicle for understanding a person's illness experience.

Narrative Reasoning

Understanding the meaning that a disease, illness, or disability has to an individual is a task that goes beyond the scientific understanding of disease processes and organ systems. Rather, it requires that clinicians find a way to understand the meaning of this experience from the client's perspective. Mattingly (1994b) has suggested that practitioners do this through a form of reasoning she called narrative reasoning. Narrative reasoning is so named because it involves thinking in story form. It is not uncommon for one practitioner who is getting ready to substitute for another with a client to ask "So what is her story?" Kielhofner suggests that narrative thinking "is oriented to making sense of human experience in terms of understanding motives" (1992, p. 260).

In the case study, part of Terry's clinical reasoning was directed at making decisions in light of what was important to Mrs. Munro. Clark, Ennevor, and Richardson (1996) have described this process of collaboration and empathy as one of "building a communal horizon of understanding" (p. 376). Terry gains understanding by listening attentively to Mrs. Munro's stories about her husband and how he loved her cooking. It is apparent from this session that Mrs. Munro's home is more than just a house. It is the place in which she lived with her husband, where he died, and where she still felt his presence. Part of Mrs. Munro's story is that going home is going back to her husband. Should this stroke prevent that, Mrs. Munro would lose more than her independence; she would lose symbolic connections to her husband. Although a logical case might be made that Mrs. Munro should start considering a more supportive-living environment, Terry understands that for Mrs. Munro this would not be an acceptable ending. Consequently, Terry works hard to obtain the support systems that will be necessary for Mrs. Munro to function in her chosen environment, where she will continue her life story.

Often, occupational therapy practitioners work with individuals whose life stories are so severely disrupted that they cannot imagine what their lives will look like. Mattingly (1994b) believes that in these situations, skillful practitioners help their clients invent new life stories. To some degree, these stories become visible as the practitioner and the client develop goals together. The use of life stories are also apparent when activities are selected for both their healing potential and their particular significance to the person. To do this, one must first solicit occupational stories from the individual (Clark et al., 1996), such as the stories Mrs. Munro told Terry of how much her husband liked her cooking. With an understanding of clients' past occupational stories, practitioners can help individuals create new stories and new futures for themselves. If Mrs. Munro were more significantly disabled, and in a more extended therapy process, Terry might explore her interest in cooking as an activity that Mrs. Munro liked and that offers many therapeutic opportunities. Furthermore, Mrs. Munro might find that she could express her pleasure in cooking for others by making special treats, first for other clients, and then perhaps for neighbors in exchange for the help they had given her. By engaging in meaningful occupation, Mrs. Munro would not only be regaining coordination and dexterity, she would

also be regaining her sense of self as a productive person. This view of clinical reasoning as a narrative process seems to provide a link between the founding values of the profession and current scientifically oriented practice demands (Clark, 1993; Clark et al, 1996; Katzman, 1993; Peloquin, 1993).

Pragmatic Reasoning

Pragmatic reasoning is yet another strand of clinical reasoning that goes beyond the practitioner-client relationship and addresses the world in which therapy occurs (Schell & Cervero, 1993). This world is considered from two perspectives: the practice context, and the personal context. Because clinical reasoning is a practical activity, there are several everyday issues that have been identified over the years that affect the therapy process. These include treatment resources, organizational culture, power relations among team members, reimbursement issues, and practice trends in the profession (Barris, 1987; Howard, 1991; Neuhaus, 1988; Rogers & Holm, 1991). Recent studies examining clinical reasoning are confirming that practitioners both actively consider and are influenced by the situations that occur in their occupational therapy practice (Creighton, Dijkers, Bennett, & Brown, 1995; Schell, 1994; Strong, Gilbert, Cassidy, & Bennett, 1995). An example of pragmatic reasoning in the case study was Terry's use of immediate resources (the flower vase) in the client's room as a therapy tool. Although Terry had thought of appropriate activities related to self-care, she had to quickly identify practical alternatives when it turned out that Mrs. Munro was already dressed. Practical constraints for Terry included (1) the time it would take to move Mrs. Munro to the clinic where there might be more resources, (2) the need to get the required information on that day, because Mrs. Munro was going home, and (3) the physical constraints of what was available to work within the room. Terry's invention of a feasible alternative was a product of both her therapeutic imagination and the cues provided within her practice setting.

Terry's attention to the influence of team members demonstrates pragmatic reasoning directed to interpersonal and group issues. She knew the physician had the power to make discharge decisions. She was aware of the pressures on the physician by the payers to discharge clients as quickly as possible. Furthermore, Terry planned to enlist the social worker to mobilize necessary caregiver support for Mrs. Munro's return home. Much of occupational therapy practice requires that practitioners reason about how to negotiate their clients' interests within the practice culture.

Similar to the practice context, the practitioner's personal situation is also part of the pragmatic reasoning process. A person's clinical competencies, preferences, commitment to the profession, and life role demands outside of work influence his or her clinical reasoning. For instance, if a practitioner does not feel safe in helping a client stand or transfer to a bed, he or she is more likely to use table-top based activities that can be done from a wheelchair. Alternatively, another practitioner may feel uncomfortable in dealing with depressed individuals, and avoid treating them, suggesting that such individuals are not motivated for therapy. Furthermore, if a practitioner has a young family to go home to, he or she may opt not to schedule clients later in the day, so that he or she can return home as soon as possible. These simple personal issues become clinical decisions that affect the scope and timing of therapy services. Underlying these aspects of pragmatic reasoning are the values that shape each practitioner's choices. This leads us to a discussion of the last form of clinical reasoning, ethical reasoning.

Ethical Reasoning

All of the forms of reasoning described so far help the practitioner respond to the questions: "What is this person's current occupational situation?" and "What can be done to enhance the person's situation?" Ethical reasoning goes one step farther, and asks the question "What should be done?" Joan Rogers framed these three questions (here paraphrased) in her Eleanor Clark Slagle lecture, and went on to state that "The clinical reasoning process terminates in an ethical decision, rather than a scientific one, and the ethical nature of the goal of clinical reasoning projects itself over the entire sequence" (1983, p. 602). In the case study, Terry's ethical dilemma is to understand Mrs. Munro's personal wishes and to honor these in the development of a therapy plan that realistically addresses her limitations. This can be particularly challenging when the pressures of financial realities (such as Mrs. Munro's lack of insurance) affect available options. Various occupational therapy authors have addressed the ethical aspect of clinical reasoning (Fondiller, Rosage, & Neuhaus; 1990; Howard, 1991; Neuhaus, 1988; Peloquin, 1993). Because of the importance of this aspect of clinical reasoning, there is an entire chapter addressing the ethics of the profession later in this text (see Chap. 47). The purpose here is to introduce ethical reasoning as yet another of the components of clinical reasoning in occupational therapy.

▼ CLINICAL REASONING: A PROCESS OF SYNTHESIS

The different aspects of clinical reasoning were analyzed separately in the last section to help you understand the different parts of the process. However, it is a disservice if you are left thinking of these as separate or parallel processes, when the opposite appears to be true. Figure 9-1 summarizes the different aspects of clinical reasoning, along with examples of typical problems addressed by each facet. Virtually all the research about clinical reasoning suggests that these different forms interact with each other. How this occurs is discussed next.

Interactive Process

Scientific, narrative, pragmatic, and ethical reasoning processes are intertwined throughout therapy. Indeed, each perspective informs the other. In the case study, Terry's understanding of medical science helped her know what might be potential impairments or disabilities, but her narrative reasoning helped her understand the importance for Mrs. Munro of returning home. Put together, these two forms of reasoning helped Terry arrive at an unsaid understanding that there would be a high risk for depression (which could worsen Mrs. Munro's medical condition) if she were not returned to her home that meant so much to her. Furthermore, the practical constraints associated with the setting and Mrs. Munro's reimbursement prompted Terry to reason about the ethics of referring Mrs. Munro to a rehabilitation center (which she could not afford), to home alone (where she might not be safe), and finally to home with the support of home health care and neighbors.

Underlying the view of clinical reasoning as an interactive process is the communicative nature of occupational therapy practice. This is because occupational therapy involves "doing with" as opposed to "doing to" clients (Mattingly & Fleming, 1994b, p. 178). Practitioners must gain the trust of their clients and of those people important in their

---

ETHICS NOTE
WHAT ARE ROBERT'S THERAPIST'S ETHICAL OBLIGATIONS TO HIM?
Penny Kyler & Ruth Ann Hansen

Robert is a 25-year-old with sickle cell anemia. Medicaid provides coverage for his health care. He has been in the hospital 11 times in the past year with severe abdominal pain and joint pain. During each hospitalization, he receives occupational therapy instruction in energy conservation and joint protection. Today, the occupational therapist walks into the clinic and sees Robert waiting. She turns and walks out mumbling to herself, "It's a waste of my time to treat 'him.' He doesn't follow through on any of my suggestions."

1. What are some of the possible reasons that the OTR is reluctant to treat Robert? Can you justify any of them either ethically or legally?
2. Are Robert's goals important? Should his priorities make a difference in setting treatment goals?
3. What are possible reasons for Robert's lack of compliance? ■

Primary Clinical Reasoning Concerns

What are the person's occupational performance concerns?

What is the person's occupational performance status and potential?

What will be done to improve occupational performance?

How effective are interventions?

When and how should interventions stop?

Scientific Used to understand nature of condition	Narrative Used to understand meaning of condition to person	Pragmatic Used to understand practical issues affecting clinical action	Ethical Used to choose morally defensible action, given competing interests
What is the nature of the illness, injury or development problem? What are common disabilities resulting from this condition? What are the typical performance components affected by this condition? What are typical contextual factors that affect performance? What theories and research are available to guide assessment and intervention? What intervention protocols are applicable to this person's condition?	What is this person's life story? What is the nature of this person as an occupational being? How has the health condition affected the person's life story or ability to continue his or her life story? What occupational activities are most important to this person? What occupational activities are both meaningful to this person and useful to meet therapy goals?	Who referred this person and why? Who is paying for services, and what are their expectations? What family or caregiver resources are there to support intervention? What are the expectations of my supervisor and workplace? How much time is there to see this person? What therapy space and equipment is available? What are my clinical competencies?	What are the benefits and risks to the person related to service provision and do the benefits warrant the risks? In the face of limited time and resources, what is the fairest way to prioritize care? How can I balance the goals of the person receiving services with those of the caregiver, when they don't agree? To what degree should I customize documentation of services to improve reimbursement? What should I do when other members of the treatment team are operating in ways that I feel conflict with the goals of the person receiving services?

▲

Figure 9-1. Aspects and examples of clinical reasoning process.

world. They do this by entering the life-world of the person (Crepeau, 1991). Once they are in that life-world, practitioners can better understand how to help the individual resolve performance problems.

Conditional Process

Not only must occupational therapy practitioners blend different aspects of clinical reasoning to interact effectively with their clients, they must also be highly flexible in their ability to modify treatment in response to changing conditions. In the case study, this was demonstrated by Terry's flexibility in finding alternate activities when the one she had planned did not work out. Creighton and her colleagues (1995) noticed that therapists preplanned treatments in a hierarchical manner. They described how therapists typ-

ically brought several sets of supplies to a treatment session. One set would be directed to the expected level of performance, and the others to a stage higher and lower than expected performance. As an example, one therapist, in preparation for a writing activity with a person with spinal cord injury, brought a short writing splint and unlined paper. This therapist also brought a longer splint providing wrist support (in case the client's hand control was worse than expected) and lined paper requiring more precision (in case his hand control was better than expected). This shows how this therapist not only blended scientific and pragmatic concerns, but also did so in a way such as to anticipate several possible conditions that might occur.

On a larger scale, Fleming described the ability of skilled therapists to "form an image of future life possibilities for the person" (1994c, p. 234). The ability to form these images seems to require a blend of all the forms of clinical reasoning, along with sufficient clinical experiences to have seen a variety of different outcomes with former clients. These images helped practitioners select therapeutic activities on a day-to-day basis. For instance, the writing activity for the young man with spinal cord injury is not only a good activity to increase coordination, it also presages regaining control of life through writing his own checks, signing his name on legal documents, and using various forms of technology for work and play. If this young man had been an accountant, these might be powerful images. Conversely, if the young man had been a professional athlete, the therapists might have to create different activities that would allow him to bridge the vision of himself as a possible future coach or teacher. The daily treatment activities used in occupational therapy, when selected in light of possible future images, serve not only to meet specific short-term goals, but also to set expectations of these possible futures. It is in this way that occupational therapy practitioners help individuals reinvent themselves through the use of meaningful occupations.

▼ DEVELOPING EXPERT CLINICAL-REASONING SKILLS

An understanding of the development of clinical-reasoning skills and related implications for teaching these skills have been a challenge to educators and supervisors throughout the profession's history. Dreyfus and Dreyfus (1986) have a framework of professional expertise that has been applied to occupational therapy (Slater & Cohn, 1991). This model, summarized in Table 9-1, identifies characteristics associated with different stages of expertise.

There is actually relatively little research that has directly examined the development from one stage to the next, particularly beyond entry level into the profession. However, the increasingly richer understanding of clinical reasoning, when combined with an understanding of the stages of expertise, does lead to some logical implications that are supported by research in occupational therapy and in other health professions (Benner, 1984; Gambrill, 1990; Slater & Cohn, 1991).

TABLE 9-1. Developmental Stages and Characteristics of Clinical Reasoning in Occupational Therapy Practice

Stage	Years of Reflective Practice	Characteristics
Novice	0	No experience, and therefore dependent on theory to guide practice. Uses rule-based procedural reasoning to guide actions, but doesn't recognize contextual cues, and therefore not skillful in adapting rules to fit situation. Narrative reasoning used to establish social relationships, but does not significantly inform practice. Pragmatic reasoning stressed in terms of job survival skills. Recognizes overt ethical issues.
Advanced beginner	<1	Begins to incorporate contextual information into rule-based thinking. Recognizes differences between theoretic expectations and presenting problems. Limited experience impedes recognition of patterns, consequently doesn't prioritize well. Gaining skill in pragmatic and narrative reasoning. Begins to recognize more subtle ethical issues.
Competent	3	Automatically performs more therapeutic skills and attends to more issues. Able to develop communal horizon with persons receiving service. Sorts relevant data and able to prioritize treatment in light of discharge goals. Planning is deliberate, efficient, and responsive to contextual issues. Uses conditional reasoning to shift treatment during sessions and to anticipate discharge needs, but lacks flexibility of more advanced practitioners. Recognizes ethical dilemmas posed by practice setting, but may be less sensitive to justifiably different ethnical responses.
Proficient	5	Perceives situations as wholes. Brings deeper store of experiences, which permits more targeted evaluation, more flexibility in treatment. Creatively combines different diagnostic and procedural approaches. More attentive to occupational stories and relevance for treatment. More skillful in negotiating resources to meet patient/client needs. Increased sophistication in recognizing situational nature of ethical reasoning.
Expert	10	Clinical reasoning becomes a quick intuitive process which is deeply internalized and imbedded in an extensive store of case experiences. This permits practice with less routine analysis, except when confronted with situations where approach is not working. Highly skillful use of occupational story making during intervention to promote long term occupational performance satisfaction.

(Based on Dreyfus & Dreyfus, 1986 and modified in light of Benner, 1984; Clark, 1996; Creighton et al, 1995; Mattingly & Fleming, 1994a; Slater & Cohn, 1991; and Strong et al, 1995.)

Clinical Experience

Experience in occupational therapy practice is required to develop and advance clinical reasoning skills. To some degree, this is an issue of attention. Because therapy is a complex process, newcomers to the field have difficulty concentrating on everything at once. It is not until some skills become more automatic that practitioners can free up their minds to concentrate on other parts of the process. Furthermore, it is a matter of shifting from theoretical knowledge to practical knowledge. Practical, first-hand knowledge takes into account many of the details of the practice context that cannot be addressed in more abstract formal theory.

In addition to the development of more automatic skills, experience also allows the practitioner to gain first-hand knowledge of the usual course of events associated with client care. This knowledge is stored in mental files or case stories, which serve to inform practice over time. The understanding of possible futures, along with ease in performing a variety of technical skills, permits the use of conditional reasoning to guide treatment.

An important aspect of experience is that it may not reliably generalize to situations different from the one in which one has gained some expertise. This observation has led Benner (1984) to suggest that expert professionals are only expert relative to particular situations. This same person in an unfamiliar situation may not be expert at all. It is this sort of observation that has led to suggestions that sustained experience in a particular practice situation may be more effective in developing clinical reasoning than a variety of more superficial experiences in many situations.

Personal Experience

Personal experiences can serve to enrich clinical reasoning by serving as the basis for empathetic understanding. This, in turn, helps the practitioner enter the life-world of another, supporting narrative reasoning. For instance, a clinician who is also a parent may well be more realistic about what sort of home program is feasible for a disabled infant's mother to accomplish. Conversely, powerful personal experiences may also impede the clinical reasoning process, particularly when one assumes another's experience will be just like one's own. In spite of these risks, practitioners do find that skillful therapeutic use of self requires a reservoir of personal stories useful in gaining empathy with the client.

Reflection on Experiences

There is virtually unanimous agreement that experience alone, although it may be necessary, is not sufficient to ensure advancement in clinical reasoning skills. Schon (1983) coined the term "reflective practitioner" to describe how experts typically think critically about their own experience. This happens in two ways. First, practitioners "reflect-in-action" (p. 49). This involves thinking about what you are doing at the same time that you are doing it, and changing the game plan as needed. "Reflection-on-action" (p. 61) is the term Schon used for critical thinking that occurs after the fact. Reflection about practice, identifying what worked and what did not, and being open to alternative conceptions are necessary to support the learning associated with advancing expertise. As discussed earlier, formal theories, along

---

RESEARCH NOTE
INTEGRATION OF RESEARCH IN OCCUPATIONAL THERAPY PRACTICE

Kenneth J. Ottenbacher

A primary characteristic of a profession is that the body of knowledge that defines and guides practice is produced by members of the discipline. In contrast, technologists have a high degree of skill in the application of specific procedures, but they are usually not responsible for generating the knowledge base that underlies the technical skills they apply. True professionals are responsible for developing, refining, and controlling the body of knowledge on which their practice is based. To develop a body of knowledge requires professionals who conduct and disseminate research, and practitioners who not only are consumers of the professional literature, but also understand how to integrate research findings into clinical practice. There are three strategies for integration of research in occupational therapy practice.

- *Methodological integration* Occurs when the technology used in research, for example, a method of systematic collection of client performance, is adopted for use in a clinical setting.
- *Empirical integration* Occurs when findings from a specific study are directly applied to a clinical problem. For instance, a splint described in an article using subjects with arthritis is applied to a client with arthritis being treated in a specific clinic.
- *Theoretical integration* Occurs when a theory that has been supported by previous research investigations is used to develop an intervention program for a client.

All occupational therapy practitioners must become experts in clinical reasoning and research integration if practice is to evolve based on evidence instead of anecdote. ■

with systematic data collection can be invaluable aids to the reflection process (Gambrill, 1990; Parham, 1987).

Education

The need for ongoing education to continue development and refinement of clinical reasoning skills is well accepted in most professions, including occupational therapy. The value of education is twofold: it provides an arena for the development of new skills, and it supports systematic reflection about past and current practices. This education can take the form of self-directed inquiry, continuing education, and formal education. Self-directed inquiry includes reading or viewing relevant educational resources, as well as networking with others through meetings, study groups, and electronic means. Continuing education involves the completion of short courses of study, such as inservices, workshops, and seminars. Formal education requires enrollment in programs at degree-granting institutions. Each form of education can support the development of clinical reasoning. Critical to effective education is the learner's willingness to engage in a dialogue, whether imaginative (as when reading an article) or real (as in a workshop), which challenges his or her current views and opens new perspectives to the clinical-reasoning process.

▶ CONCLUSION

Clinical reasoning is the process used by practitioners to plan, direct, perform, and reflect on client care. It is a whole-body and multisensory process. It is multifaceted, because occupational therapy requires an understanding of client issues from multiple perspectives. Practitioners use the logical processes associated with scientific reasoning to (1) understand an individual's impairments, disabilities, and performance contexts; and (2) predict the effect these have on occupational performance. Narrative reasoning helps practitioners personalize treatment, by helping them understand the meaning that occupational performance limitations have for an individual. Practitioners use pragmatic reasoning when they address the practical realities associated with service delivery. All of these forms of reasoning lead to an ethical reasoning process in which practitioners must select the best therapeutic intervention to respond to the person's occupational performance needs. Clinical reasoning is an interactive and conditional process in which all aspects of clinical reasoning are integrated to resolve both current and future occupational performance issues. The development of clinical reasoning occurs as a function of experience and the reflection on that experience. This development is aided through lifelong learning strategies of self-directed, continuing, and formal education.

▶ REFERENCES

Argyris, C., & Schon, D. A. (1974). *Theory in practice: Increasing professional effectiveness.* San Francisco, CA: Jossey-Bass.

Barris, R. (1987). Clinical reasoning in psychosocial occupational therapy: The evaluation process. *Occupational Therapy Journal of Research, 7,* 147–162.

Benner, P. (1984). *From novice to expert.* Menlo Park, CA Addison-Wesley.

Casteless, J. P. A. M., & Korthagen, F. A. (1996). The relationship between theory and practice: Back to the classics. *Educational Researcher, 25* (32), 17–22.

Clark, F. (1993). Occupation embedded in real life: Interweaving occupational science and occupational therapy. *American Journal of Occupational Therapy, 47,* 1067–1078.

Clark, F., Ennevor, B. L., & Richardson, P. L. (1996). A grounded theory of techniques for occupational storytelling and occupational story making. In R. Zemke & F. Clark (Eds.), *Occupational science: The evolving discipline* (pp. 373–392). Philadelphia, PA: F. A. Davis.

Cohn, E. S. (1989). Fieldwork education: Shaping a foundation for clinical reasoning. *American Journal of Occupational Therapy, 43,* 240–244.

Creighton, C., Dijkers, M., Bennett, N., & Brown, K. (1995). Reasoning and the art of therapy for spinal cord injury. *American Journal of Occupational Therapy, 49,* 311–317.

Crepeau, E. B. (1991). Achieving intersubjective understanding: Examples from an occupational therapy treatment session. *American Journal of Occupational Therapy, 44 ,* 1016–1024.

Dreyfus, H. L., & Dreyfus, S. E. (1986). *Mind over machine: The power of human intuition and expertise in the era of the computer.* New York: Free Press.

Fondiller, E. D., Rosage, L. J., & Neuhaus, B. E. (1990). Values influencing clinical reasoning in occupational therapy: An exploratory study. *Occupational Therapy Journal of Research, 10,* 41–55.

Fleming, M. H. (1991). The therapist with the three track mind. *American Journal of Occupational Therapy, 45,* 1007–1015.

Fleming, M. H. (1994a). The search for tacit knowledge. In C. Mattingly & M. H. Fleming (Eds.), *Clinical reasoning: Forms of inquiry in a therapeutic practice* (pp. 22–33). Philadelphia: F. A. Davis.

Fleming, M. H. (1994b). Procedural reasoning: Addressing functional limitations. In C. Mattingly & M. H. Fleming (Eds.), *Clinical reasoning: Forms of inquiry in a therapeutic practice.* (pp. 137–177). Philadelphia: F. A. Davis.

Fleming, M. H. (1994c). Conditional reasoning: Creating meaningful experiences. In C. Mattingly & M. H. Fleming (Eds.), *Clinical reasoning: Forms of inquiry in a therapeutic practice.* (pp. 197–235). Philadelphia: F. A. Davis.

Gambrill, E. (1990). *Critical thinking in clinical practice: Improving the accuracy of judgments and decisions about clients.* San Francisco: Jossey–Bass.

Howard, B. S. (1991). How high do we jump? The effect of reimbursement on occupational therapy. *American Journal of Occupational Therapy, 45,* 875–881.

Katzman, L. N. (1993). Linking patient and family stories to caregivers' use of clinical reasoning. *American Journal of Occupational Therapy, 47,* 169–173.

Kielhofner, G. (1992). *Conceptual foundations of occupational therapy.* Philadelphia: F. A. Davis.

Mattingly, C. (1994a). Occupational therapy as a two body practice: Body as machine. In C. Mattingly & M. H. Fleming (Eds.), *Clinical reasoning: Forms of inquiry in a therapeutic practice* (pp. 37–63). Philadelphia: F. A. Davis.

Mattingly, C. (1994b). The narrative nature of clinical reasoning. In C. Mattingly & M. H. Fleming (Eds.), *Clinical reasoning: Forms of inquiry in a therapeutic practice* (pp. 239–269). Philadelphia: F. A. Davis.

Mattingly, C. & Fleming, M. H. (1994a). *Clinical reasoning: Forms of inquiry in a therapeutic practice.* Philadelphia: F. A. Davis.

Mattingly, C., & Fleming, M. H. (1994b). Interactive reasoning: Collaborating with the person. In C. Mattingly & M. H. Fleming (Eds.), *Clinical reasoning: Forms of inquiry in a therapeutic practice* (pp. 137–177). Philadelphia: F. A. Davis.

Miller, R. J. (1993). What is theory and why does it matter?. In R.J. Miller & K. F. Walker (Eds.), *Perspectives on theory for the practice of occupational therapy* (pp. 1–16). Gaithersburg, MD: Aspen.

Mosey, A. C. (1992). *Applied scientific inquiry in the health professions: An epistemological orientation.* Rockville, MD: American Occupational Therapy Association.

Neuhaus, B. E. (1988). Ethical considerations in clinical reasoning: The impact of technology and cost containment. *American Journal of Occupational Therapy, 42,* 288–294.

Parham, D. (1987). Nationally speaking—toward professionalism: The reflective therapist. *American Journal of Occupational Therapy, 41,* 555–561.

Pelland, M. J. (1987). A conceptual model for the instruction and supervision of treatment planning. *American Journal of Occupational Therapy, 41,* 351–359.

Peloquin, S. M. (1993). The depersonalization of patients: A profile gleaned from narratives. *American Journal of Occupational Therapy, 49,* 830–837.

Rogers, J. C. (1983). Clinical reasoning: The ethics, science, and art. *American Journal of Occupational Therapy, 37,* 601–616.

Rogers, J. C. (1986). Clinical judgment: The bridge between theory and practice. In *Target 2000: Occupational therapy education* (pp. 123–130). Rockville, MD: American Occupational Therapy Association.

Rogers, J. C., & Holm, M. B. (1991). Occupational therapy diagnostic reasoning: A component of clinical reasoning. *American Journal of Occupational Therapy, 45,* 1045–1053.

Rogers, J. C., & Masagatani, G. (1982). Clinical reasoning of occupational therapists during initial assessment of physically disabled patients. *Occupational Therapy Journal of Research, 2,* 195–219.

Schell, B. A. B. (1994). *The effect of practice context on occupational therapist's clinical reasoning* (Doctoral dissertation, University of Georgia, 1994).

Schell, B. A., & Cervero, R. M. (1993). Clinical reasoning in occupational therapy: An integrative review. *The American Journal of Occupational Therapy, 47,* 605–610.

Schon, D. A. (1983). *The reflective practitioner: How professionals think in action.* New York: Basic Books.

Slater, D. Y., & Cohn, E. S. (1991). Staff development through analysis of practice. *American Journal of Occupational Therapy, 45,* 1038–1044.

Strong, J., Gilbert, J., Cassidy, S., & Bennett, S. (1995). Expert clinicians and student view on clinical reasoning in occupational therapy. *British Journal of Occupational Therapy, 58,* 119–123.

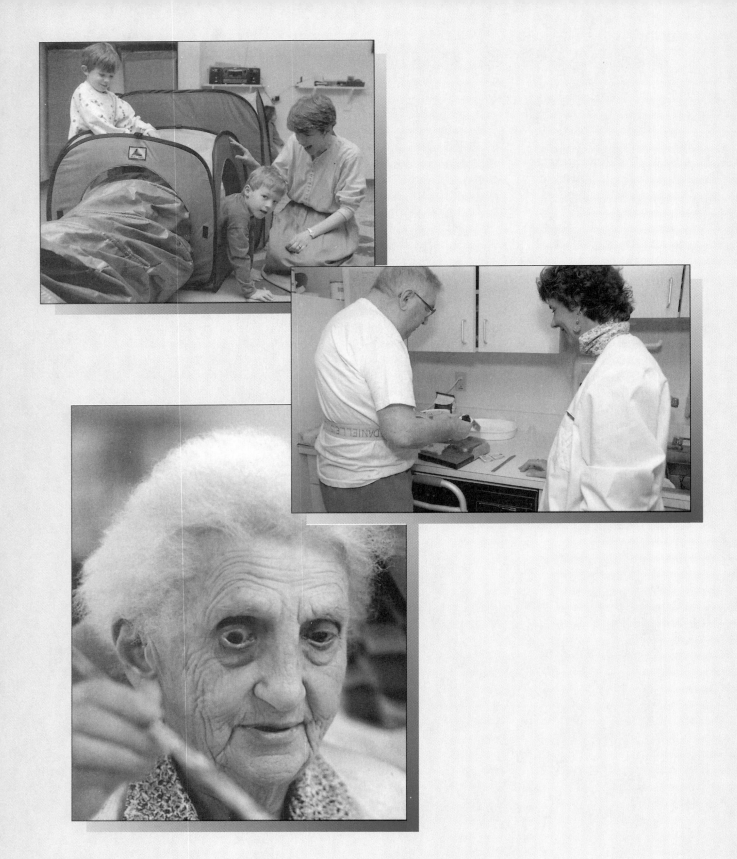

These occupational therapy practitioners have designed interventions that meet the interests and goals of the persons seeking their care, an essential aspect of the therapeutic alliance. (Photos: (top) by Ron Bergeron, Instructional Services, Dimond Library, University of New Hampshire; (middle) by Gary Samson, Instructional Services, Dimond Library, University of New Hampshire; (bottom) by John Adams, Instructional Services, Dimond Library, University of New Hampshire)

UNIT IV

Establishing the Therapeutic Alliance

LEARNING OBJECTIVES

After completing this unit, readers will be able to:

▶ Describe the manner in which occupational therapy practitioners form alliances that honor dignity and convey caring.

▶ Describe the history and present role, types, purposes, and models of group work in occupational therapy.

The challenge of occupational therapy practice is to mobilize people to work toward their own recovery. Although it might seem obvious that they would be motivated to do so, this is not always true. Discouragement, depression, and other factors may interfere with full involvement. By establishing a therapeutic alliance with those who seek our care, we, as occupational therapy practitioners, provide the catalyst to help them engage fully in the process of occupational therapy and achieve their goals. The chapters in this unit provide insights into this process, from the perspectives of the person–practitioner dyad and the therapeutic use of groups. (*Note*: Words in **bold** type are defined in the Glossary.)

Chapter 10

The Therapeutic Relationship

Suzanne M. Peloquin

▼ THE CHARACTER OF THE RELATIONSHIP

The Art of Practice

Occupational therapy practice is "the art and science of directing man's [sic] participation in selected tasks . . . " (AOTA, 1972, p. 204). There is an artistry to most practices, even those seen as scientific, and especially those known as therapy. In her discussion of the art of practice, Mosey (1981) first defined it negatively, stating that the art is not (1) a desire to help others, (2) the skilled application of scientific knowledge, or (3) simply being a systematic or sympathetic listener. She wrote, "The capacity to establish rapport, to empathize, and to guide others to know and make use of their potential as participants in a community of others illustrates the art of occupational therapy" (p. 4). The art of practice, as is most art, is a process of making connections and finding meaning. Without its art, Mosey (1981) claimed, occupational therapy would be an application of knowledge in a sterile vacuum.

According to Mosey (1981), one who masters the art of practice perceives the individual as a whole, indivisible into parts or subsystems. Although practitioners must often reduce the complexity of human organisms to more clearly understand, those who use artistry, Mosey said, reintegrate those parts to clearly see the person. Seeing the person lets the practitioner empathize with the feelings and values that make life meaningful.

In her reflections about the art of practice, Devereaux (1984) wrote, "Occupational therapists are specialists in making care happen" (p. 794). She characterized the caring of occupational therapists as singular: helping persons to connect with those occupations that are meaningful.

A CORE VALUE: PERSONAL DIGNITY

The American Occupational Therapy Association (AOTA) in 1993 identified seven core values that characterize the profession and clarify expectations for the therapeutic relationship: altruism, equality, freedom, justice, dignity, truth, and prudence. These values derive from the documents that guide practice. For practitioners who work among divergent populations and in varied settings, with distinct frames of reference, this affirmation of values shapes the character of alliances and sparks the commitment to care.

Within the AOTA's identification of core values, personal dignity seems primary; a sound grasp of dignity will catalyze the other values. A practitioner who honors dignity, the core document reads, has an "attitude of empathy" (AOTA, 1993, p. 1086). The phrase is familiar, but its meaning must be made clear. What does empathy *look* like? More pointedly, what does it mean to be empathic in a practice that holds occupation at its center?

THE REQUISITE DISPOSITION: EMPATHY

Some individuals want to dismiss a discussion of **empathy**, thinking, "Oh, another rehash of how to decode body language and paraphrase what the patient says." Any such dismissal would be hasty, because empathy is much more. Katz (1963) articulated the challenge: "To be a man [sic] means to be a fellow man. The human personality becomes human through its association with others" (p. 189). Those who aim for therapeutic alliances must see them as forms of fellowship and chances to hone their humanity.

How can practitioners establish fellowship with those who seek therapy? Thomas (1983) explained that fellowship rests first on a willingness to *be* there. The disposition to be there is central to Buber's (1965) concept of dialogue, in which one person turns toward the other, "of course with the body, but also in requisite measure with the soul" (p. 10). The turning in dialogue is an empathic action that transcends procedures; it asks more of who one is than of what one does. Likening it to love, Hackney (1978) saw empathy as a qualitative response to people, a potential possessed by most.

Adler (1931) believed that if practitioners did attend to others, they would see this potential: "to connect ourselves in a common meaning with other people, to be controlled by the common sense of all mankind [sic]" (p. 254). Empathy is the common sense of people. It spins connections through which helpers see their likeness to others, in eyes that widen, brows that furrow, hands that clench. But empathy also quickens a respect for differences. At its deepest level, Egan (1986) explained, empathy is a way of seeing with the eyes of others to appreciate their views of the world. To be present to others empathically is to take a stand from which one shares in their experiences. Such a stance is aptly named an understanding.

Perhaps the description of empathy that is most cited is that of Rogers (1975):

It means entering the private world of the other and becoming thoroughly at home in it. In involves being sensitive, moment to moment, to the changing felt meanings which flow in this other person, to the fear or rage or tenderness or confusion or whatever, that he/she is experiencing. It means temporarily living in his/her life, moving about in it delicately without making judgments . . . as you look with fresh and unfrightened eyes at elements of which the individual is fearful. . . . In some sense it means that you lay aside your self and this can only be done by a person who is secure enough in himself that he knows he will not get lost in what may turn out to be the strange and bizarre world of the other. (p. 3)

In his early writings, Rogers (1957) underscored the as–if cognition of empathy; one thinks and feels and moves *as if* one were in the other's world. This imaginative presence lets caregivers distinguish their patients' experiences from their own. If practitioners aim to help, Reiser and Schroder (1980) explained that they must know how to be there, fiercely caring, while standing as themselves. This is the hallmark of empathy: "In order to help people who are sick, we must know what it is like to be in their shoes but, at the same time, also know very well that we are not in their shoes" (Reiser and Schroder, p. 46).

Practitioners sometimes seem ambivalent about the intimacy of empathy. They worry that "they may not be able to extricate themselves from the net of feeling" (Katz, 1963, p. 25). When they stand overwhelmed with feelings, it is not empathy that they enact, but sympathy. Olinick found sympathy "an immature, imperfect empathy" (1984, p. 139). Sympathetic helpers never quite get out of themselves; they touch the other's feelings but duck back into their own worlds, nursing the pain from that touch. The true empathizer, said Katz, "tends to abandon his self-conscious-

ness" in the encounter (p. 9). And even when a helper engages in a profound act of empathy, "the power to recover" remains (Katz, p. 42).

Empathy does not exact a fusion, but a connection. It implies an experience not only of the pain of another, but also of integrity and courage alongside the pain. Empathy, in health care practice, is the enactment of the conviction that, empowered by someone's willingness to understand, a person will gather the requisite courage. The empathic way of being conveys a fierce faith in personal dignity. It is the art of therapy.

Empathy: Reaching for Hands and Heart

Because the manner of *being with* in occupational therapy is a unique enactment of *doing with*, portrayals of that enactment are important to the profession's vision. A vibrant image emerges within the book *The Healing Heart*. This story of Ora Ruggles, reconstruction aide, chronicles some early history of occupational therapy from World War I through the 1950s. Because it deals openly with the values that Ruggles held and the relationships that she formed, the story serves well as a lesson in empathy.

The title of the book derives from a comment made twice by Ruggles, once at the start of the book and again at the end. On the first occasion, Ruggles went into the barracks at Fort McPherson and was strangely quiet. When pressed to share her thoughts, Ruggles said: "It is not enough to give a patient something to do with his hands. It's the heart that really does the healing" (Carlova & Ruggles, 1946, p. 69). On the occasion of her retirement from Children's Hospital, when asked about the most important part of her work, she echoed her discovery: a patient's heart must be reached.

In *The Healing Heart* Ruggles exemplifies an empathic disposition and caring actions. At Fort McPherson, she worked among soldiers with amputations because of war injuries. Her two enormous wards were the scenes of much horseplay among those who could hobble, much stone-faced staring from those who could not. A tall and attractive redhead, Ruggles drew much attention on the day she first walked the wards. One patient named Hap, who had no legs and one arm, made Ruggles laugh with his flirtatious comments and impish grin. When she said that she would keep the men occupied with basket weaving, Hap quipped that he'd rather keep *her* occupied. Another patient, Kilgore, called Hap a legless clown, not man enough to keep anyone occupied. The men grew silent. Ruggles moved to Hap's side and put her hand on his shoulder, saying, "Don't mind him, Hap! Man is far more than an arm or leg" (p. 57). Her words went deep. Within minutes, more than 20 men clamored into her class.

Because of his disability, Hap could only pass reeds to the other men; Ruggles felt his silence as his incapacity grew clear. She spent much time thinking about what Hap could do. She went to the artificial limb shop where limb-making was still rather crude. She described and sketched what she wanted: a leather device from which metal braces and a clamp would protrude. Later she approached Hap, cautioning him against too much hope as she slipped the breeching over his stump and secured a brush in the clamp. As Hap painted tentative lines of color onto the rim of a basket, he whooped with joy. He practiced secretly for days before showing his skill. The men responded with delight; even Kilgore was impressed. Overwhelmed with feeling, Ruggles began a practice that she kept for years. She slipped away into a closet and let the tears flow. That closet was the first of Ruggles' many "crying corners" (p. 63).

Kilgore worried Ruggles. During one class a soldier said that Kilgore did not try basket weaving because he knew he would fail. Challenged, Kilgore sat for an hour weaving furiously. When one soldier judged the result "not bad," Kilgore drove his fist down to destroy the basket. Ruggles asked the physician about Kilgore's behavior. The physician told her that the man had been a cowboy and he now felt revulsion over the acts of war. Ruggles consulted the foreman of the blacksmith shop and then looked for Kilgore. When she found him and he told her he would not make more baskets, Ruggles showed him a design for spurs and asked if he would help her start a metalwork class. Within the hour he was in the shop, where he mastered the work quickly. His drinking, gambling, and outbursts stopped, and after discharge he started an ironwork plant that grew to be the largest in the Southwest. Kilgore wrote Ruggles, years later:

I've been doing a lot of thinking lately, Ruggie. It started out last week when some of the boys around town asked me to run for mayor. It makes me realize, again, Ruggie, how much I owe you. I wonder what the boys who asked me to run for mayor would think if they knew an army doctor once scribbled on my medical record, "This man is a menace to society." (p. 91)

Ruggles's treatment of Hap and Kilgore depicts a person whose *doing with* others reflects the best of clinical reasoning alongside fellowship. Ruggles reached for the heart as well as the hands. She made care happen, and she practiced with artistry.

THE ENACTMENT OF EMPATHY: POIGNANT ILLUSTRATIONS

Scenes within *The Healing Heart* show other aspects of empathy. Beyond its communication of fellowship, empathy has been said to consist of (1) a turning of the soul, (2) a recognition of likeness and uniqueness in the other, (3) an entry into the other's experience, (4) a connection with the other's feelings, (5) a power to recover from that connection, and (6) a personal enrichment that derives from these actions.

Each of these aspects of empathy assumes a unique character in occupational therapy, an encounter within which a practitioner brings not just the self, but the trappings of occupation: objects, tools, and activities.

A Turning of the Soul

Empathy requires a turning to another that is a *turning of the soul*. One example of Ruggles' turning, not just to solve a problem but to capture its deeper meaning, was her treatment of a child named Ruby. When Ruggles first met Ruby, she saw a most unattractive 12-year-old who retaliated against the taunts of other children by ruining their work. Hoping to learn the child's interests, Ruggles asked Ruby if she might like sewing. The child responded, "Why? So I can grow up and be an old maid and sit at home with my sewing? Is that what you do?" (Carlova & Ruggles, p. 215) Although Ruggles' initial urge was to "wallop" Ruby, she checked her temper and thought, "This girl dislikes people because she can see they dislike her. I must alter my attitude. I must change my hate to love. I must show Ruby that I love her" (Carlova & Ruggles, p. 215). This turn of soul prompted Ruggles to ask what Ruby aimed to be when she grew up. In a tiny voice, Ruby said she hoped to work in a beauty parlor. Ruggles softened as she saw this child in light of her yearning for beauty. She taught Ruby how to shampoo and set her hair, and she arranged for her to spend time in a beauty shop. Over time, Ruggles noticed a change; as Ruby connected with others, her beauty emerged. Ruggles' turning of the soul prompted a similar turning in Ruby.

A Recognition of Likeness

Another aspect of empathy is a *recognition of likeness* in another, a grasp of the commonality of personal problems. Ruggles' work with an 11-year-old boy named Ramon exemplifies her capacity to see his need for belonging and to structure occupations to meet that need. Ramon was thought to be incapacitated. He had little muscular control, and he twitched and jerked constantly. Painfully shy, he hid himself in dark corners so he would not be noticed. One day, when the rest of Ruggles' charges complained that their clay was so lumpy that they were wasting time pressing it through a screen, Ruggles thought of Ramon. She walked him from a corner into the workroom. As soon as he saw the others making clay figures, he reproached Ruggles for suggesting that he join this group. Ruggles countered by showing him how to press clay through the screen. His uncontrolled shaking worked to his advantage, and the other children patted him on the back and thanked him for producing clay with such fine texture. Ramon felt useful and appreciated and after a short period was no longer shy. The task gave Ramon a chance to connect with others in a venture that highlighted fellowship more than differences.

A Recognition of Uniqueness

Empathy also requires a recognition of uniqueness in the other, and Ruggles' practice in a "mental ward" at Fort McPherson introduced her to some dramatic examples of the unique behaviors of schizophrenia during an era before psychotropic medications. One day a patient announced that he was General Pershing and that Ruggles ought to salute. She did. Another patient whispered as they were working that he was a German spy. He and Ruggles agreed on a set of signals to use. Ruggles knew another patient to be a bird lover. He stood for hours by the barred windows. One day while hallucinating, he asked what the birds were doing in Ruggles' hair. Without pausing, Ruggles said, "Oh those. Their nest was blown away and I'm sort of helping them out until I find another one" (Carlova & Ruggles, 1946, p. 100). Calmed, he commended the quality of her nest. She learned to salute, pass secret signals, and live with the birds as she worked with the men. Her matter-of-fact acceptance of their uniqueness permitted their engagement with her and with the work that calmed them.

An Entering into the Experience of the Other

Central to empathy is the act of entering into the experience of another to understand what it must be like. Ruggles' interaction with a man named Leo shows her sensitive participation in the lives of her patients. Poverty troubled many of the patients at the Olive View sanatorium, especially those with families. Ruggles ran a shop in the hospital where patients sold crafts to defray expenses. After Leo arrived he was sent to bed with a high fever. He was restless and troubled; he had a wife and four children to support, and his small farm was mortgaged. His family needed $15.25 a month to keep the farm. The physician thought Leo's temperature too high and work with Ruggles too risky. Although Ruggles accepted that decision at first, as Leo's condition worsened she reopened the question. Ruggles thought that his deterioration was more mental than physical. She proposed to work with Leo at bedside but to stop if his temperature rose. The physician agreed.

Ruggles told Leo that he could make $20 a month selling leather work. Although his first efforts were crude, before long he was producing fine items. His first earnings amounted to $22.65 and the physician's pronouncement that he was well enough to work outside the ward. Leo became Ruggles' assistant, helping other patients as soon as he secured his $15.25. Ruggles' work was credited with saving Leo's farm, his pride, and his life. Her willingness to enter into his situation had engaged him.

A Connection with Feelings

Ruggles' work among people with so much pain offered many occasions to connect with their feelings. Ruggles helped patients turn to their courage even when her own feelings were at risk. While Ruggles was on the ward one day, a young soldier shot with shrapnel in 65 places caught her eye as he frantically scanned the room. Kilgore warned her that the young man was about to explode his feelings, and that she'd better go. "They pour it all out at once, then they never talk about it again," Kilgore said (p. 87). Ruggles told Kilgore that she would stay. The soldier spoke of screams in a trench where he sank into the flesh of his buddies. Suddenly an artillery blast blew him free, and he woke

to find parts of bodies, naked, torn, and bloody, scattered all over. "I was the only man alive," he said, "and I wished I was dead" (p. 88). Ruggles sat near the boy for a long time feeling sick and weak. Kilgore whispered that now she too had been through the war, but that she would know better the next time. "No," Ruggles said, "if I can help, I'll stay" (p. 88). Ruggles' patients often needed to speak their anguish and share their pain. Her staying power in the face of their feelings confirmed her empathy.

Her many connections with others led Ruggles to crying corners where she faced the depth of her feelings:

The many patients who reached out for her help pained her with the ever increasing pressure of their demands and needs. She stared into the darkness and, assailed by a crushing feeling of futility and helplessness, turned her face to the pillow and wept. (p. 84)

A Power to Recover from the Connection

But Ruggles' power to recover from connecting, another of the actions that earmarks empathy, stayed strong. She turned to friends who would listen. She changed jobs to work with different populations. She applied to herself the principles of her therapy, finding strength in occupations. And always, Ruggles saw her practice as one from which she drew the personal enrichment that is the promise of empathy. She saw the results of her efforts; through occupational therapy, patients found their courage. And Ruggles knew that in "helping others, she helped herself" (p. 191). As the years passed and she felt the growing presence of a supreme spirit, she "felt more than rich" (p. 192).

Empathy assumes a unique character in occupational therapy, a practice to which people bring the trappings of occupation. The story of Ora Ruggles portrays a caring alliance: a doing-with that showed others their inner strength—a reaching for hearts as well as hands.

Visions of the Relationship

The AOTA's (1993) articulation of the core values that shape the therapeutic alliance might be called the vision of the 1990s. In the absence of a formal document on core values, practitioners previously turned to other sources—such as the story of Ora Ruggles—for clarity about how they should be in practice. Perhaps no source better illustrates the evolution of the profession's vision of the therapeutic relationship than *Willard and Spackman's Occupational Therapy*. From the first edition to the present, this text has offered contributions from individuals working in a variety of practice arenas. It has been a primary tool in educating students and has often introduced the vision of the relationship.

The vision presented in *Willard and Spackman's Occupational Therapy* has changed over the years. Earlier contributors proposed skill-oriented and professional (impersonal) relationships; their emphasis was on competence. Later contributors focused on the personal character of the relationship, with an emphasis on caring.

THE VISION OF THE 1940s

In the 1947 edition of *Willard and Spackman's Occupational Therapy*, Wade described the requisite approach to those with mental illness:

The development of a good psychiatric approach does not occur spontaneously, nor is it a natural gift but, like many other accomplishments, it is acquired through diligent effort, study and experience. (p. 83)

Wade viewed a good relationship as one in which a skilled therapist would "command respect, admiration, hope and confidence" (p. 83). She named "courage, patience, tolerance and friendliness" as traits for achieving a "good approach" (p. 83). Wade saw the successful therapist as one who had mastered two skills that "supported patient equilibrium." First was the skill of "tact," in which "adjustment is always made to the patient by the worker" (p. 84). Wade explained her rationale: "These patients are hypersensitive to implications expressed in words, by tone of voice, mannerism or facial expression" (p. 84). The second skill was "complete self-control in order to prevent untimely expression of a spontaneous emotional reaction" (p. 84). A therapist's self-control supported patient equanimity; spontaneity and personal expression were suspect.

Reaching out was thought important, but it was always done with objectivity. The therapist had to identify with the patient's situation but still keep an objective attitude: "The technic [*sic*] of doing this is similar to that used by the adult in correlating his thoughts with those of a child" (Wade, 1947, p. 84). The therapeutic goal was primary; good communication led to that goal. If the therapist had to be a good listener, it was because "it is frequently necessary to play this role" (Wade, p. 84). The "good approach" needed to be "within normal limits" and "restricted to matters of impersonal interests" (Wade, p. 85). The bottom line was that one be "impersonal in relationships" (Wade, p. 84).

This press for impersonality was not limited to mental health practice. Fay and March (1947) discussed the therapeutic relationship in general and special hospitals, enumerating several directives, a few of which follow:

Do's

3. Stand or sit where you can be seen easily.
4. Be encouraging and hopeful and foster a desire in the patient to get well.
5. Be understandingly sympathetic.
6. Be friendly and sincere.
7. Be courteous, not flippant or bold.
11. Be patient and resourceful.
12. Be impersonally personal.

Don't's [*sic*]

3. Don't show alarm, horror or sorrow.
5. Don't be physically objectionable by body odor, the use of strong perfume or by having the clothes permeated with cigarette smoke.
7. Don't argue. Be a good listener.
8. Don't talk of depressing or distressing subjects.
9. Don't make promises that cannot be kept.
10. Don't hit or jar the bed.
12. Don't show racial, religious or political prejudices. (pp. 125-126).

The vision of the patient-therapist relationship in this 1947 edition reflects a conscious striving for skills that would objectify and professionalize the encounter. Warm traits and spontaneous expressions warranted vigilance. Perhaps the closest any contributor in the 1947 edition came to the idea of caring was Gleave in her chapter on pediatric services:

The occupational therapist should be an understanding, friendly and rather cheerful person. . . . Ability to talk with children rather than to or at them is an asset. Every effort should be made to bring out the child's ideas, to get him [*sic*] to express himself freely and naturally. In all contacts with the patient, the therapist should strive to keep the tone of her voice pleasant and well modulated. She must make the child feel that she is his friend while holding his respect and maintaining discipline when problems arise. (p. 148)

Gleave alone alluded to friendship. Her position seemed acceptable within the context of working with children, for whom, perhaps, the need for impersonality seemed less crucial.

THE VISION OF THE 1980s

By the 1983 edition of *Willard and Spackman's Occupational Therapy*, the term therapeutic relationship had taken hold, and a therapist's caring attitude assumed more significance. The knowledge of self was deemed "most important," and Frank's (1958) work on the therapeutic use of self (the use of one's personal strengths as a tool in therapy), was cited. As if in recognition of prior emphasis on professionalism, Hopkins and Tiffany (1983) cited a new image: Purtilo's characterization of "the personal-professional self" (p. 95). Purtilo (1978), a physical therapist, had proposed a blend of characteristics. She tried to minimize conflicts for those who struggled with a personal-professional tension in their relationships:

[The personal-professional self] incorporates actions that communicate caring into the patient health professional interaction; he [*sic*] recognizes efficiency as a trait which can express caring when it does not impose rigid limits on the interaction. He is interested in the patient as a person with values, needs, and beliefs, but does not encourage a relationship that will lead to over-dependence (detrimental dependence). (p. 148)

This view conveyed a sense of helping. Hopkins and Tiffany (1983) thought that individuals needed to feel that they could be helped; they argued that "the therapist in a treatment setting is by definition a helper" (p. 94). The helping process required a trust that built on confidence and respect.

Without the establishment of trust between the client and therapist, it is unlikely that a truly collaborative effort will be possible. . . . The therapist's own self-confidence, the therapist's ability to be honest and open in the relationship, and the extent to which the therapist is able to communicate "unconditional positive regard" and empathy for the client will affect the client's ability to invest in the relationship. (pp. 94–95)

Tiffany (1983) underscored the therapist's role: "Occupational therapy is attuned to the principle of facilitating the client's own personal search for purpose, meaning, and self-actualization" (p. 291). Open and personal communication seemed vital to understanding aims and values.

It was the relationship that might well "determine the success or failure of the treatment plan" (Hopkins & Tiffany, 1983, p. 94), and within that relationship, "activities are used as facilitators for transactions between people" (Hopkins & Tiffany, p. 95). This distinction ought not be forgotten; occupational therapy's vision has always been one of doing with.

The therapeutic relationship envisaged in occupational therapy has presented variable features. Practitioners have interacted in a number of ways, depending in part on their grasp of the occupational therapy vision. When one pieces together ideas about the therapeutic alliance from 1947 and 1983, the ensuing vision may lend itself to individual interpretation. One practitioner may feel that directives to be impersonally personal should yield to more warmth; another may favor a relationship marked by objectivity. If practitioners enact the alliance differently in contemporary practice, this difference is consistent with their having been exposed to a changing vision of the relationship over the years.

Collaboration: A Fundamental Action

A practitioner who collaborates in treatment does so because the vision of the alliance is that of a partnership. Assumptions that support a collaborative approach are well represented in the occupational therapy literature of 50 years ago, even when the relationship was kept impersonal. These assumptions can be summarized: The patient is rational. The patient is free to choose or reject therapeutic services. The therapist is a teacher and a motivator in the therapeutic process.

Excerpts taken once again from *Willard and Spackman's Occupational Therapy* highlight these assumptions. McNary (1947) wrote: "An activity entered into without a purpose is not occupational therapy" (p. 10). If an individual enters into the activity, he or she must understand its purpose. It then becomes the practitioner's task to state the purpose. Edgerton (1947) said that "the ability to relate an activity to the need of the individual is one of the characteristics that distinguishes the occupational therapist from . . . crafts instructor" (p. 42). Here is clear support for sharing the meaning of any plan. Occupational therapy practitioners who resent having their role minimized must determine whether they present their work as therapy.

Wade (1947) said that "if the patient is unable to participate actively in the plan, its existence should be kept in his [*sic*] consciousness as a justification for the task" (p. 90). When collaboration is not possible, she suggested the therapist must explain. If the person who seeks therapy is old or young or cognitively impaired, although it may seem easy to abandon explanations, Wade (1947) advised that therapists explain at whatever level of understanding is possible. The information could be brief and simple but still "placed in the patient's consciousness." When in doubt, one communicates.

Later literature about collaboration supports these examples from the 1940s. Reed and Sanderson (1983), in describing the assumptions that drive the occupational therapy process, emphasized points made more subtly 50 years ago. They asked practitioners to see a "valuable, worthwhile person, even if the client does not respond readily to the program" (p. 153). Any right to challenge services offered, they said, shaped a responsibility to give helpful information "in a manner that is comprehensive and at a rate that can be absorbed by the client" (p. 154).

Reed and Sanderson (1983) listed patient's rights to include:

1. A person has the right to decide whether to seek and accept health care services within legal limitations.
3. A person has the right to be consulted regarding the objectives, goals and methods to be used in individual health care plans. (p. 71)

These rights should prevail; the habitual gift of information and choice will let them.

Within the context of the patient's right to choose, motivation becomes a shared task, meaningfulness a shared perspective. Reed and Sanderson (1983) thus saw the last step of the occupational therapy process as being "to facilitate and influence client participation and investment" (p. 81). This step is a directive to evoke investment by stating the relevance and rationale of therapy. The occupational therapy literature turns consistently to the idea that practitioners must work with those who seek their help. This colaboring is collaboration.

The Other Side: Images of Practitioners

The stories patients tell about their experiences with occupational therapists share their views of the alliance more colorfully than do structured responses to surveys. The following fictional story says much about one relationship:

Brunhilde, the misplaced Viking Lady, comes tapping on my door every afternoon in an effort to intimidate me into going to Occupational Therapy. She marches around the seventh floor telling all the patients that their doctor has "ordered" Occupational Therapy, and they must come IMMEDIATELY. She herds them out in the hall and they mill around until she lines them up in two columns and goosesteps them out the door. (Rebeta-Burditt, 1977, p. 114)

A fuller reading of the story shows that this patient, Cassie, felt concern from other professionals. Her satirical barbs targeted only those whose demands for control threatened her autonomy. Because Brunhilde seems uncaring, this image is disturbing.

Clinically, patients derive images of their therapists from their interactions with them. Image-forming includes an exchange; the therapist brings to each exchange some understanding, or vision, of what a therapeutic relationship (and perhaps what a "good patient") should be, and the patient brings needs, memories of past experiences, and expectations of how a helpful caregiver should behave. The exchange of need, vision, and expectation helps shape the image that each person will hold of the other. In the story of Brunhilde, Cassie was frustrated by an occupational therapist who did not show the caring—either fellowship or collaboration—that she wanted and expected. She saw a paternalistic therapist, an intimidating Viking Lady.

Not all images of occupational therapists convey the fullness of empathy shown by Ruggles. Some stories present therapists who seem bossy—such as Brunhilde—or preoccupied. One wonders how to characterize these images, how to begin to name them, to better understand and evaluate them.

THE PRACTITIONER SEEN AS TECHNICIAN, PARENT, OR COVENANTER

It may help to turn to the writings of May (1983), a physician who thought about relationships in terms of images. May (1983) found images helpful, both in clarifying the functions of individuals and in setting standards for their performance. He argued that "the image tells a kind of compressed story" (p. 17) in that it describes not only the basic actor (in this case the physician), but also the person with whom the actor relates. The image characterizes the alliance. If one thinks of a physician as a priest, for example, one sees in that image a mystical power and the awe that it will evoke.

May (1983) discussed various images that characterize physicians. Three of the images—technician, parent, and covenanter—seem relevant to this discussion because they also emerge from stories about occupational therapists. Technical practitioners are concerned with technique, parental practitioners treat people as dependents, and covenanting practitioners see partners pursuing shared goals. Each of these images reflects a markedly different enactment of a practitioner's competence and caring.

The Practitioner as Technician

The occupational therapy practitioner who functions as a technician commits to competence in procedures (May, 1983), honing technical skills above all else. Although the image may seem cold, the basic aim is humanitarian, because the technical practitioner sees caring in superior performances and best procedures. An individual whose primary focus is on methodology, return of function, or task at hand is seen as a technician.

In *No Laughing Matter* (Heller & Vogel, 1986), Heller described his ordeal with Guillain-Barre syndrome and his time with an occupational therapist who "possibly will be surprised or contrite to find out now of the very considerable anguish I experienced so often in my sessions with her" (p. 166). Methodology and gain were overly important:

But in occupational therapy, as soon as I could sand a block of wood (with a need to rest both arms, it was written, after seven repetitions), a change was made to a coarser grade of sandpaper, increasing the amount of force required, and it was just as punishing and demoralizing for me to have to execute them as it had been in the beginning. (pp. 166–167)

Heller's impression was that "what they intended was to keep me always at a standstill" (p. 166). His personal need seems clear—to make and then savor some gain. The therapist, oblivious to his need, used a strategy to treat a condition. Treatment goals were hers and did not come from collaboration.

Seabrook (1935) told of his time in an institution for his dependence on alcohol. Although his experience was generally positive, Seabrook saw his occupational therapy worker as "conscientious and probably having a kind heart, but nobody like[s] him" (p. 62). This practitioner valued technique over relationship. Any collaborative function that could be linked with occupational therapy rested with Paschal, the psychiatrist. Paschal pressed for different crafts and a more personalized approach. The occupational therapist gave competence, the psychiatrist caring.

The next story, in verse, also portrays a technician. The opening lines introduce the dilemma: "Preserve me from the occupational therapist, God. She means well, but I'm too busy to make baskets" (McClay, 1977, p. 106). This therapist pushed activity for its own sake. She made no attempt to hear the patient or discuss meaningful occupations; the exchange mocked the idea of relationship:

Oh, here she comes, the therapist, with
scissors and paste,
Would I like to try decoupage?
"No," I say, "I haven't got time."
"Nonsense," she says, "You're going to
live a long, long time."
That's not what I mean,
I mean that all my life I've been
doing things
for people, with people. I have to
catch up
on my thinking and feeling. . . . (p. 107)

The concept of occupational therapy as a process that uses meaningful occupation rests on some mutual pursuit of meaning. This therapist matched technique to problem; she used age, diagnosis, and disability to determine the choice of activity, without regard for the patient's perception or need. Activities chosen because either protocol or provider consider them significant may be purposeful, but they are questionable therapy when they lack meaning. An overzealous commitment to competence, even for the sake of others, leaves them wondering if practitioners care.

The Practitioner as Parent

The image of parent is no doubt more personal to most than that of a crisp technician. But the parental image, typically associated with order and nurturance, can be either positive or negative, depending on the manner in which the order or nurturing is given (May, 1983). An excess of either can squelch the relationship and make it seem uncaring; when helpers become paternalistic, patients rebel against the order or overly depend on the nurturing. The best parental figure, superior in knowledge and skill, bridges the gap through compassion (May). The practitioner who supports another, while trying to meet some need, conveys the image of a good parent. Conversely, the negative parental helper threatens individual autonomy by enforcing rules or preempting decisions.

Brunhilde, the fictional therapist named Viking Lady, was an authoritative figure wielding power for the patient's own good. Rule-bound Brunhilde eschewed her patients' autonomy; caring, for her, was parenting gone awry. By contrast, Hanlan (1979) praised the parental therapists who treated her husband:

I was . . . impressed with the equanimity of occupational and physical therapists as they worked all day with severely handicapped people, some with terminal illnesses. . . . If helping personnel—social workers, physicians, or whoever—conceived of their function with the terminally ill as helping with discrete, day-to-day problems, I believe they would have less trouble just "hanging in there," which is really the most essential ingredient. (p. 28)

The steadfastness of practitioners who help with simple activities creates a benign parental image.

The fictional story about an activities therapist named Meg shows a parental therapist's vigilance against overnurture and overorder (Gibson, 1979). Meg had patients in a private psychiatric hospital design and make living room drapery. She manipulated them into seeing the idea as their own, and they were enthusiastic about "their" project. The psychiatrist later commended her skilled handling of the situation. She acknowledged that it was a "handling" and questioned the appropriateness of the act. Her psychiatrist friend answered:

I don't think you did any—violence to their being; the idea was in them or you couldn't have wooed it out. And dealing with patients always takes some handling, the question is only is it for their benefit or yours. (Gibson, 1979, p. 51)

The psychiatrist's rationale for this intervention is common; paternalism is justified if for the person's own good. The parental practitioner assumes greater wisdom, always, and the balance of power tips toward practitioner competence.

The Practitioner as Covenanter

May's (1983) image of the physician as covenanter yields a sense of friendship. A covenanter acknowledges the gift in any relationship. For one who covenants with another, reciprocity grounds the exchange. Steeped in a spirit of covenant the professional sees skills as gifts to be shared. Services rendered occur within the context of a trusted relationship, and both parties take as well as give. The stronger partner uses personal strengths and professional skills to build strength in the weaker (May). Above all, the covenanted person supports the other's actualization.

Petersen (1976) described a way of infusing occupation into self-actualization:

There is a shouting spirit deep inside me:
Take clay, it cries,
Take pen and ink,
Take flour and water,
Take a scrub brush,
Take a yellow crayon
Take another's hand
And with all these
Say you,
Say loving.

The voice of the poem, the shouting spirit deep inside, seems much like the voice of a friend.

Other stories portray practitioners as friends who share the goals of those they would help. Benziger (1969), for example, described her hospitalization for depression, remembering the occupational therapist as her "new friend" (p. 48). She shared her first impression of the therapist:

A few days later the first person I had met there who made any real sense came into my room. She was the occupational therapist—a term I've always hated. She was kind, interested, enthusiastic, full of ideas, and intelligent. (p. 47)

The therapist trusted Benziger, followed through on promises, and supported a will to get well. Crafts served as catalysts for their discussions of life. The following exchange shows how the therapist befriended Benziger and valued her strengths:

"You know, you go at your work too hard, too fast, too desperately—and too frenetically."

"I guess I do, but that's the way I feel. Time stands still for me now, it is endless, and yet if I have something to do, I get the sense that there will not be time enough to finish it, or that someone will stop me . . ."

She said, "You are an intelligent person, and you will help yourself to get well quickly."

"You know," I answered, "you're the first person who has mentioned intelligence versus non intelligence, instead of sanity. You make me feel like a human being. . . ." I was grateful. I should not forget her. (p. 49)

A third image of practitioner as friend appeared in Donaldson's (1976) account of his unwarranted 15-year confinement in mental institutions. That Donaldson could perceive any staff as friendly is surprising. Nonetheless, Donaldson saw in "Baldylocks" a friend:

While I waited, I found OT fun. Young, overweight Baldylocks had about five of us. He was a zealous worker in his church, and did not swear, drink, or smoke. He translated his religion to his work by showing compassion and understanding to all of us. He let me spend afternoons learning the touch system of typing. . . . Baldylocks started taking the OT men and a half dozen from upstairs for a two-hour walk on the grounds each Wednesday. Under the umbrella of all this warmth, I began watching the news on TV again. (pp. 245–246)

Donaldson exercised, cooked, and learned lathe work—all satisfying activities he helped choose. He saw and valued his therapist's commitment to caring, trust, and respect.

Collectively, patients' stories suggest that occupational therapy practitioners can project an image of technician, parent, or covenanter. Images from such stories shed light on the manner in which patients can experience rather varied displays of competence and care.

VARIABLE EMPHASES ON COMPETENCE AND CARING

Patients' positive images of occupational therapists reflect the actions of therapists who use competence and caring to match a patient's needs. Each of May's three images—technician, parent, and covenanter—emphasizes competence and caring in a slightly different way. The challenge for practitioners is to consider what each person needs; ideally, individual need will give cues about how to respond. Although some individuals will want practitioners to function as technicians or parents, most will ask for a way of being that equalizes competence and caring and creates an image of partner or friend.

Growing distress over impersonal care has resulted in measures that acknowledge personal rights: quality assurance requirements, the Patient's Bill of Rights, and informed consent laws. These measures defend against systems that demand technical competence, but not caring; laws counter that imbalance with prompts that honor rights. Although a commitment to caring cannot be legislated, it can be inspired by a vision that keeps caring central.

▼ THE CONTEXT OF THE RELATIONSHIP

Visions of the therapeutic relationship in occupational therapy are shaped by contexts that are temporal, social, or physical. Any alliance can be seen as embedded within some context. The therapeutic alliance of the 1940s, for example, differed from that of the 1980s, showing responsivity to the times. Social and physical environments also shape the features of the relationship. It would be an oversimplification to see any therapeutic connection only in terms of the dynamics between the person who gives therapy and the person who seeks it. Individuals who partner in any venture will find opportunity and constraint from the locale, group, or culture within which their alliance occurs. And so it is with therapy.

Societal Beliefs that Shape Care

Prevalent beliefs shape societal forces into trends for practice. Such forces have shaped occupational therapy since its inception, when as Yerxa (1980) said, "it began in a climate of caring" (p. 532). One notable change in the latter part of this century is the growing complaint from those who seek care that the climate of practice is changing. Patients say that their experiences with practitioners are difficult, describing their grasp of the problem with the words dehumanizing or depersonalizing. These abstractions have become the shorthand expression for a dismay that people are often treated carelessly.

Woven through a large number of patients' stories is a profile of impersonal attitudes and behaviors that patients say discourage them when they most need courage. Patients say that helpers depersonalize practice by failing to see the personal consequences of illness and disability. They deny the feelings of those whom they treat; they dismiss patients and their concerns. They fail to show, in even small ways, that they are people who feel, who participate in their patients' pain. Instead, they engage in distancing behaviors and harmful withholdings; they are silent, aloof, and brusque. They misuse their power. The personal hurts in such narratives call for serious reflection.

If practitioners can give both competence and caring, what societal beliefs cause them to act impersonally? Three constructs surface as shaping forces that compromise caring: (1) an emphasis on the rational fixing of problems; (2) an overreliance on methods and protocols; and (3) delivery systems that are driven by business, efficiency, and profit. These forces can prompt caregivers to act in ways that cause them to be seen as controlling parents or cold technicians, rather than as partners who cherish dignity.

THE EMPHASIS ON RATIONAL FIXING

One societal force that compromises caring actions is the belief that health problems should be solved rationally. When Hodgins wrote in 1964 after his stroke, it was about a form of disregard. He described the patient and the caregiver perceiving illness differently.

In stroke two basic sets of assumptions could govern treatment. One set proceeds from what the patient perceives or thinks he perceives; the other comes from what the doctor knows or thinks he knows. The two are very different sets of things. (p. 842)

Many health care narratives show helpers rendering some aspects of care while withholding others that patients value. Sir Dominic Corrigan, a physician, argued as long as a century ago that the trouble with doctors is "not that they don't know enough, but that they don't see enough" (cited in Taylor, 1972, p. 6).

Van Eys (1988), also a physician, regretted the hemisected worldview in which "diseases become problems, and patients become dissected into such problems" (p. 21). Patients resent this narrowness of view because it feels uncaring. They complain that caregivers see their disease, the physiology and the mechanism of their bodies, but not their experience of illness and unease, not its meaning, and surely not their feelings.

Disregard for parts of people disturbed Murphy (1987), an anthropologist who wrote of his disabling illness: "The full subjective states of the patient are of little concern in the medical model of disability, which holds that the problem arises wholly from some atomic or physiological disorder and is correctable by standard modes of therapy—drugs, surgery, radiation, or whatever" (p. 88). Sarton (1988) remembered that after a stroke she was made to feel like "so many pounds of meat, filled with potentially interesting mechanical parts and neurochemical combinations" (p. 106). Leder (1984) argued that a person is never so many pounds of meat, that the human body is "not a mere extrinsic machine but our living center" (p. 34).

The question for practitioners becomes: What is the problem with treating bodies when they need fixing? Most narratives answer that "when a patient appears as a physiological mechanism, the doctor may neglect personal communication in favor of the immediate scientific task at hand" (Leder, 1984, p. 36). The preference for fixing makes it easier for a helper to neglect feelings and easier to justify being silent, curt, or aloof. The resulting problem is impersonal care.

Any caregiver can fall short of seeing the person and focus narrowly on a fixing function. Gebolys (1990) remembered this incident:

A male therapist came in whistling and cheerfully setting up his equipment. He stuck the breathing tube into my mouth and told me to "breathe" which I did while he walked around the room admiring my flowers, gazing out the window and remarking what a lovely day it was. (p. 13)

The consequence of a too-strong commitment to rational fixing—of the disease, the body, or the dysfunction—is a disregard that feels careless. And although practitioners mean well, physician-educator Moore (1978) grasped the problem: "Professions tend to be right in what they affirm and wrong in what they ignore" (p. 3).

Are occupational therapy practitioners among those who commit to rational fixing? Mattingly (1991) gave most pause when she said that "therapists can come to reduce their practice to a manipulation of the physical body, forgetting how much their interventions are directed to a person's life" (p. 986). Schultz and Schkade (1992) shared a similar concern: "The current demand for therapists to base occupational therapy on acquisition of functional skills . . . may actually limit the contribution of occupational therapy" (p. 918). When practitioners focus on functional skills with scant attention to feelings or meaning, their fixing preempts

fellowship. There is no art to alliances that lack feeling or meaning.

THE RELIANCE ON METHODS AND PROTOCOL

A second societal force that compromises caring is an over-reliance on the techniques, procedures, and modalities that solve the problem. When they are ill, patients seek concern as well as solutions, and they grieve when they find something else. Hodgins (1964) loathed the discovery:

For the physician, of course, it must have been wonderful, indeed, when true specifics began to arrive on the scene to supplant beef, iron, and wine or syrup of hypophosphates. . . . As so-called science more and more enters medicine, the heedless or routine physician will be accordingly tempted to withdraw his humanity and wait for specifics. (p. 843)

Hodgins considered the specifics needed for cure and the humanity needed for care as different but inseparable parts of care. Flagg (1923), a physician who practiced at the turn of the century, agreed; he regretted "the unwise employment of laboratory methods to the exclusion of personal attention" (p. 5).

When a drug or a procedure suffices, a practitioner may think less about the need to make personal connections. Sacks (1983) rejected the argument that helpers must use only treatments or protocols. When facing surgery, he wondered,

What sort of man would Swan be? I know he was a good surgeon, but it was not the surgeon but the person that I would stand in relation to, or, rather, the man in whom, I hoped, the surgeon and the person would be wholly fused. (p. 92)

Cassell (1985), another physician, shared this belief: "Doctors who lack developed personal powers are inadequately trained. . . . Doctors are themselves instruments of patient care" (p. 1).

When they are effective, however, methods and protocols can take the upper hand. Helpers side with what works, so that a challenge to the procedure also threatens them. Martha Lear (1980) remembered the upshot of such an identification when her husband Hal, a urologist, requested a milder painkiller: "The resident got angry. He said, 'There is a medication ordered for pain for you. If you want it, you can have it. If not, you'll get nothing.' And he walked out" (p. 41). But patients, wrote the physician Pellegrino (1979), do not want practitioners to fuse with their skills: "Physicians have a medical education, an M.D. degree, a set of skills, knowledge, prestige, titles. They possess many things by which they mistakenly identify themselves" (p. 228).

Helpers wrap themselves in their procedural authority, binding themselves so tightly in their concern for the right method and latest technique, that it is no wonder they seem constrained. Helpers can never be seen as personal if they offer knowledge or skills instead of themselves. Murphy (1987) resented the trade: "What I needed was not a new instrument, but an old-fashioned clinician with plenty of intuition" (p. 14). Patients argue that their helpers dismiss their feelings, that they have bought the argument in favor of impersonality.

Hodgins (1964) argued that encounters felt as personal are often what patients need most: "[The patient] will draw courage as he perceives human understanding underlying the professional techniques of those into whose care he has been given" (p. 841). Unhappily, concern for personal issues seems to matter little in this formulaic belief: correct procedures produce superior results.

Occupational therapy practitioners admit that techniques can preempt caring. Yerxa (1980) argued that "technique, once employed in the service of human needs, is rapidly moving us toward a society of total technology in which our ways of thinking and being themselves become so technical that we lose sight of other ways of thinking and being" (p. 530). Parham (1987) discussed the case of Longmore, a former faculty member at the University of Southern California Program in Disability and Society:

He was subjected to long hours of occupational therapy training for self-care skills although he had no intention of performing these time-consuming tasks independently at home. He planned to hire an attendant who would expedite the process, freeing him to use his time and energy to pursue more stimulating and productive activities. (p. 556)

Situations such as this one no doubt led King (1980) to conclude that "therapists have ignored their instinct for caring." (p. 525)

DELIVERY SYSTEMS DRIVEN BY BUSINESS, EFFICIENCY, AND PROFIT

Francis Peabody (1930) stated the problem well when he argued that "hospitals, like other institutions, founded with the highest human ideals, are apt to deteriorate into dehumanized machines" (p. 33). Many narratives suggest that this dehumanization plagues systems that build on business, efficiency, and profit.

The Business

Any business that aims to offer individual service to large numbers of people—whether a hospital, prison, or school—may suffer from its clients' criticisms about being ignored. Sarton's (1988) is one such complaint:

A small incident at the hairdresser's has given me something to try to understand. . . . While Donna was securing my hair into curlers, an old lady who was waiting to be picked up came and stood beside us and talked cheerfully about herself and her daughters and Donna responded. It was as though I did not exist, was an animal being groomed. (p. 255)

The sheer number of individuals who seek treatment can compromise the attention that is felt as caring. As Sarason (1985) wrote, "The clinician becomes a rationer of time, and that obviously sets drastic limits on the degree to which the ever-present client need for caring and compassion can be met" (p. 170). The result of that rationing is the feeling expressed by a young man with acquired immunodeficiency syndrome (AIDS) visiting a busy clinic: "I just feel like they don't care" (Peabody, 1986, p. 172). Additional complications associate with the business of hospitals because of their lifesaving function. Hodgins (1964) discussed the estrangement that occurs with life-threatening illness:

The stroke victim is most likely to encounter, as his first medical ministrant, a physician to whom he is a total stranger. Since speedy hospitalization is usually a first goal in stroke, treatment by strangers is likely to continue. (p. 839)

Peabody (1930) explained one consequence to the patient of a lifesaving business among strangers:

He loses his personal identity. He is generally referred to, not as Henry Jones, but as "that case of mitral stenosis in the second bed on the left". . . . It leads, more or less directly, to the patient being treated as a case of mitral stenosis, and not a sick man. (p. 31)

The problem is a matter of focus; the institutional eye sees the relevance of saving Henry's life but does not capture the wider clinical picture—that although "Henry happens to have heart disease, he is not disturbed so much by dyspnea as he is by anxiety for the future" (Peabody, 1930, p. 34).

The Efficiency

Murphy (1987) spoke to the kind of ordering in institutions, renaming the hospital an island invaded by a rationalized system of schedules and shifts: "The hospital has all the features of a bureaucracy, and, like bureaucracies everywhere, it both breeds and feeds on impersonality" (p. 21). The impersonality is well illustrated in Saxton's (1987) account:

The scariest part of the hospitalization for me was not the surgery but the doctor rounds. On the mornings when these rituals were scheduled, the nurses and aides awakened us much earlier that usual. Meals and wash-ups were rushed. . . . Then they would come, the surgeons, the residents, the interns. . . . They entered our ward, about fifteen adults. . . . Strange long words were uttered; bandages were opened and quickly closed. (p. 53)

Gebolys (1990) recalled that only on the fourth day of her hospital stay did a nurse's aide wash her hair, bloody and dirty from an automobile accident. The aide did so after her shift was over because the highly regulated day precluded this helping task. Sacks (1983) concluded that "the hospital, in short, is a singular mixture, where freedom and bondage, warmth and coldness, human and mechanical, life and death, are locked together in perpetual combat" (p. 24).

The battle sometimes seems insane, Murphy (1987) said, because like most bureaucracies, the hospital has turned "capricious, arbitrary, and irresponsible as Wonderland's Red Queen" (p. 44). One feels this capriciousness in Beisser's (1989) experience with heartless caretakers:

In one hospital, the first hour of the nurses' shift was spent in a detailed discussion of who would take coffee breaks when. Medications, patient needs, all other things paled in comparison. Sometimes people would literally leave you in midair in a lift to go on a coffee break, or leave you in some other awkward position, and just say, "It's my break time." (p. 35)

Brice (1987) recalled a nurse in the recovery room whom she asked for a blanket. The nurse, seeming much like the Red Queen, "barked 'I just brought you one; I'm not going to bring you another' and disappeared" (p. 31). People are a care system's conveyors of feeling; there can be no fellowship if helpers are capricious. Sarton (1988) wearied of her experience that was "bland at best, cold and inhuman at worst" (p. 103).

The Profit of Service Provision

Hodgins (1964) thought that helpers produce mostly problems with the profit-driven system of care:

We have heard much sentimental lamentation over the disappearance of the old "family physician"—dear, lovable old Dr. Peatmoss, who delivered all the babies, saw them through diphtheria, whooping cough and scarlet fever, sat at deathbeds of the elderly, and never sent anyone a bill. This last lovable quality is, I suppose, why he disappeared. I felt no sense of personal loss at his passing because I never knew him. I should have liked to. The physicians in my life all had very efficient accounting systems—if not actual departments. (p. 840)

Longcope (1962) had argued even earlier that a business orientation causes "the quantification, mechanization and standardization which are said to characterize this country" (p. 547). Within a business view of service, knowledge takes coin value, cure is a high-priced commodity, and ill people become buyers. Success and solvency turn into treatment goals and efficiency the means to achieve them. In this scheme, more accrues from procedures that cure than manners that care. Rabin (1982), a physician with amyotrophic lateral sclerosis, remembered that his physician gave him a pamphlet outlining the course of a disease that he already knew too well. He regretted that this physician gave him no suggestions about "how to muster the emotional strength to cope with a progressive degenerative disease" (p. 307).

Practitioners face a major quandary when the need for time and compassion competes with the agency's need to prosper. When high regard falls to those who accumulate the most billable units of time, moments spend noticing, listening, or communicating are harder to justify. Sarason (1985) explained: "Whose agent I was became a pressing, daily, moral problem. I know what it is to have divided loyalties, to want to give up the fight, to rationalize away the internalized conflict" (pp. 170–171). And although few helpers buy the idea that patients are mere customers, many budget their caring actions. Individuals feel the cuts as hurtful. Lear (1980) wrote of her husband's regret that he had not attended to his patients' experiences. He thought: "Damn it, doctors should know. They should care. Say how're they treating you? How's the food? Accommoda-

tions comfortable? Staff courteous? . . . . He himself would never even have thought to ask. Didn't that make him negligent too? Ah. Bingo!" (p. 43).

Occupational therapy practitioners speak openly about their frustrations. Growing caseloads are a concern because "productivity and efficiency are becoming high-priority goals" (Howard, 1991, p. 878). Howard argued that technological approaches are thus "valued more than the holistic use of a variety of methods" (p. 880). The climate often seems one of "cost containment," rather than caring (Howard, p. 878). Burke and Cassidy (1991) named it a "disparity between reimbursement driven practice and the humanistic values of occupational therapy" (p. 173). The enormity of the challenge pressed Grady (1992) to ask: "Is there still enjoyment in occupational therapy, or have we become so controlled with the realities of productivity, reimbursement, and modalities that we are failing to see the process as part of the outcome (p. 1063)? And, of course, blindness to the process can mean disregard for the person.

The Profession's Affirmation of a Climate of Caring

At about the same time that a number of individuals were recording their depersonalizing experiences within various delivery systems, several leaders in the profession endorsed a climate of caring at the 60th Annual Conference of the AOTA. Together they shared a vision of practice as a caring relationship. They spoke of a climate of caring because they saw dangers fomenting in delivery systems "not oriented to the human being" (Baum, 1980, p. 514).

In an effort to sharpen the profession's view of caring, Baum (1980) said, "We are nothing more than a bystander in the life of [the patient] until a relationship is formed" (p. 514). She clarified her meaning: "Occupational therapy harnesses will and gives the individual control through activity. That is human, that is care" (p. 515). Technical skills, these leaders argued, work well if they "promote movement and flexibility within our therapeutic relationships" (Gilfoyle, 1980, p. 520).

Caring, they said, needs to be rooted in commitment to a person who seeks therapy. Gilfoyle (1980) wrote:

The caring therapist directly knows a client as a unique individual, as someone in his or her own right, not as an average, a generality, or number on the Gaussian curve. . . . Implicit knowledge is the art of "being with the person"; it is something you feel. (p. 520)

"The caring," said Gilfoyle, "is not the taking-care-of the person, but helping the person learn to take care of himself/herself" (1980, p. 519). The same principle, stated differently, is this: "Through our professional relationships we reach out and with empathy show that we care, hoping that from this caring . . . the person will find his or her own strength" (Baum, 1980, p. 515).

Yerxa (1980) saw deliberations on caring as calibrations of the profession's success. She said, "Our practice in the future should be evaluated not only on the basis of measurable scientific outcomes, but also by what it contributes to individual human dignity, a sense of mastery and self-respect" (p. 534). She identified the challenge of the future as that of preserving and embracing a climate of caring "in the face of a society increasingly dominated by technique and objectivism" (p. 532). The challenge seems clear.

Preserving the Relationship
SUSTAINING THE ART OF PRACTICE

Reflections about the art of occupational therapy are less widespread in the professional literature than reflections about its science. This reality is a matter of concern because practice needs both. Without caring in the relationship, occupational therapy is sterile technique. Many delivery systems within which practitioners work fail to nurture the art of practice, but the art needs validation if it is to flourish.

Therapy as an art is an old theme; literature as a nurturer of the soul is an older theme still. Practitioners committed to the artistry of practice can sustain themselves by reflecting about images of caring in the phenomenological literature. The story of Ruggles, for example, exemplifies the enactment of empathy: a doing-with that leads people to their inner strengths. The therapeutic alliance in *The Healing Heart* (Carlova and Ruggles, 1946) consists of one person reaching for the hands and heart of another; it portrays respect for human dignity.

Engaging with the arts can also yield sustaining images—of relationships, of qualities that make relationships meaningful, and of the meaning of occupation in a life. Responsivity to these images can renew the energy for caring. If the arts hold unsavory images, such as Brunhilde the Viking Lady (Rebeta-Burditt, 1977), they also show real care.

CONCLUSION: INSPIRING CARE

The therapeutic relationship that has characterized occupational therapy over the years will survive only if it is encouraged. Practitioners will need to determine to which resources they must turn for the requisite courage. Some may turn to the reflections of those who have written about the art of practice or the therapeutic encounter. Others may find support in professional documents that clarify core values. Others may draw and create support from informal exchanges or from formal presentations about caring.

In his reflections about education, Davies (1991) said much that may help this discussion. From his position on a state governing board, he saw that the essential function of board members was to inspire education. A question that he thought they must ask is this: "Are we helping to create an environment in which teaching and learning are honored and can flourish?" (p. 58). He said that the making of that environment is a call to (1) engender a restlessness throughout the system, (2) disturb complacency, and (3) insist that rules be broken when there is good and sufficient reason.

Many human services invite a like response. Occupational therapy practitioners must see their business and technical functions—one mark of their competence—as a background to good practice. But they must also ask if they are making an environment in which care can flourish. They might then name and frame an essential function—inspire care. As he spoke to a group of graduating students, one of the founders of the Society for the Promotion of Occupational Therapy named the inspiration that nourishes care:

> May you realize in increasing measure the value of certain spiritual things which are the real making of life, but

---

ETHICS NOTE
HOW CAN A PRACTITIONER BALANCE CONFLICTING ETHICAL OBLIGATIONS?
Penny Kyler and Ruth A. Hansen

Jamie, a 14-year-old, has an attention deficit disorder and juvenile-onset diabetes. Some of the kids in his neighborhood know that Jamie has needles for insulin injections. They have forced him to give them some of the needles. Then they sell them to substance abusers. Jamie has confided to his occupational therapy practitioner that he is afraid to tell his parents about this and is afraid of what the kids will do to him if he does tell.

1. The occupational therapy practitioner has obligations and duties to several individuals and groups. Identify

them. Which group or individual should receive the highest priority?
2. What conflicts are present between the role of being a caring professional and that of preventing harm?
3. Discuss the concepts of personal autonomy, the right to privacy, the right to confidentiality, and the obligations to do good and avoid doing harm as they relate to this situation. ■

which we call by many common names. Kindness, humanity, decency, honor, good faith—to give these up under any circumstances whatever would be a loss greater than any defeat, or even death itself. (Kidner, 1929, p. 385)

The message from our forebears has meaning today; we can touch hearts as well as hands—if we choose to reach for them. We can make care happen—if we choose to be there. We can practice our art—if we choose to make meaningful connections. The challenge is real, and it can be framed with this question: "As I engage others in occupation, am I making a climate in which caring is honored and fellowship grows?"

Acknowledgment

The American Occupational Therapy Association granted permission to revise the author's original works from the *American Journal of Occupational Therapy*: Linking purpose to procedure during interactions with patients, *42* (12), 775–781; Sustaining the art of practice, *43* (4), 219–226; The patient–therapist relationship in occupational therapy: Understanding visions and images, *44* (1), 13–21; The depersonalization of patients: A profile gleaned from narratives, *47* (9), 830–837; The patient–therapist relationship: Beliefs that shape care, *47* (10), 935–942; The fullness of empathy: Reflections and illustrations, *49* (1), 24–31.

▶ REFERENCES

Adler, A. (1931). *What life should mean to you.* Boston: Little, Brown.

American Occupational Therapy Association Council on Standards. (1972). Occupational therapy: Its definition and functions. *American Journal of Occupational Therapy, 26*, 204–205.

American Occupational Therapy Association (AOTA). (1993). Core values and attitudes of occupational therapy practice. *American Journal of Occupational Therapy, 47*, 1085–1086.

Baum, C. M. (1980). Eleanor Clarke Slagle lecture—Occupational therapists put care in the health system. *American Journal of Occupational Therapy, 34*, 505–516.

Beisser, A. (1989). *Flying without wings: Personal reflections on becoming disabled.* New York: Doubleday.

Benziger, B. (1969). *The prison of my mind.* New York: Walker.

Brice, J. (1987). Empathy lost. *Harvard Medical Letter, 60*, 28–32.

Buber, M. (1965). *Between man and man.* New York: Macmillan.

Burke, J. P., & Cassidy, J. C. (1991). Disparity between reimbursement–driven practice and humanistic values of occupational therapy. *American Journal of Occupational Therapy, 45*, 173–176.

Carlova, J., & Ruggles, O. (1946). *The healing heart.* New York: Julian Messner.

Cassell, E. J. (1985). *Talking with patients: Volume 1.* The theory of doctor–patient communication. Cambridge: MIT Press.

Davies, G. K. (1991). Teaching and learning: What are the questions? *Teaching Education, 4*, 57–61.

Devereaux, E. B. (1984). Occupational therapy's challenge: The caring relationship. *American Journal of Occupational Therapy, 38*, 791–798.

Donaldson, K. (1976). *Insanity inside out.* New York: Crown.

Edgerton, W. B. (1947). Activities in occupational therapy. In H. Willard & C. Spackman (Eds.), *Principles of occupational therapy* (pp. 40–59). Philadelphia: J. B. Lippincott.

Egan, G. (1986). *The skilled helper: A systematic approach to effective helping.* Monterey: Brooks/Cole.

Fay, E. V., & March, I. (1983). Occupational therapy in general and special hospitals. In H. S. Willard & C. S. Spackman (Eds), *Principles of occupational therapy* 6th ed., (pp. 118–137). Philadelphia: J. B. Lippincott.

Flagg, P. (1923). *The patient's viewpoint.* Milwaukee: Bruce Publishing.

Frank, J. (1958). The therapeutic use of self. *American Journal of Occupational Therapy, 12*, 215.

Gebolys, E. (1990). Inadequacies, inequities and inanities in modern medicine—a personal experience. *Occupational Therapy Forum, 12*, 6–7, 13–18.

Gibson, W. (1979). *The cobweb.* New York: Atheneum Press.

Gilfoyle, E. (1980). Caring: A philosophy of practice. *American Journal of Occupational Therapy, 34*, 517–521.

Gleave, G. M. (1947). Occupational therapy in children's hospitals and pediatric services. In H. S. Willard & C. S. Spackman (Eds.), *Principles of occupational therapy* (pp. 141–174). Philadelphia: J. B. Lippincott.

Grady, A. P. (1992). Nationally speaking—occupation as vision. *American Journal of Occupational Therapy, 46*, 1062–1065.

Hackney, H. (1978). The evolution of empathy. *Personnel and Guidance Journal, 56*, 35–38.

Hanlan, M. (1979, November). Living with a dying husband. *Pennsylvania Gazette*, pp. 25–28.

Heller, J., & Vogel, S. (1986). *No laughing matter.* New York: Avon.

Hodgins, E. (1964). Whatever became of the healing art? *Annals of the New York Academy of Sciences, 164*, 838–846.

Hopkins, H. L. & Smith, H. D. (Eds.). (1983). *Willard and Spackman's occupational therapy* (6th ed.). Philadelphia: J. B. Lippincott.

Hopkins, H. L., & Tiffany, E. G. (1983). Occupational therapy: A problem solving process. In H. L. Hopkins & H. D. Smith (Eds.). *Willard & Spackman's occupational therapy* (6th ed., pp. 89–100). Philadelphia: J. B. Lippincott.

Howard, B. S. (1991). How high do we jump? The effect of reimbursement on occupational therapy. *American Journal of Occupational Therapy, 45*, 875–881.

Katz, R. L. (1963). *Empathy: Its nature and uses.* London: Free Press of Glencoe.

Kidner, T. B. (1929). Address to graduates. *Occupational Therapy and Rehabilitation, 8*, 379–385.

King, L. J. (1980). Creative caring. *American Journal of Occupational Therapy, 34*, 522–528.

Lear, M. (1980). *Heartsounds.* New York: Simon & Schuster.

Leder, D. (1984). Medicine and paradigms of embodiment. *Journal of Medicine and Philosophy, 9* (1), 29–43.

Longcope, W. (1962). Methods and medicine. In W. H. Davenport (Ed.), *The good physician: A treasury of medicine* (pp. 546–559). New York: Macmillan.

Mattingly, C. (1991). The narrative nature of clinical reasoning. *American Journal of Occupational Therapy, 45*, 998–1005.

May, W. (1983). *The physician's covenant: Images of the healer in medical ethics.* Philadelphia: Westminster Press.

McClay, E. (1977). *Green winter: Celebrations of old age.* New York: Reader's Digest Press.

McNary, H. (1947). The scope of occupational therapy. In H. Willard & C. Spackman (Eds.), *Principles of occupational therapy* (pp. 10–22). Philadelphia: J. B. Lippincott.

Moore, A. R. (1978). *The missing medical text: Humane patient care.* Melbourne, Australia: Melbourne University Press.

Mosey, A. C. (1981). *Occupational therapy: Configuration of a profession.* New York: Raven Press.

Murphy, R. F. (1987). *The body silent.* New York: Henry Holt.

Olinick, S. L. (1984). Empathy and sympathy. In J. Lichtenberg, M. Bornstein & D. Silver (Eds.), *Empathy I* (pp. 25–166). New York: Analytic.

Parham, D. (1987). Nationally speaking—toward professionalism: The reflective therapist. *American Journal of Occupational Therapy, 41*, 555–561.

Peabody, B. (1986). *The screaming room: A mother's journal of her son's struggle with AIDS.* New York: Avon.

Peabody, F. W. (1930). *Doctor and patient papers on the relationship of the physician to men and institutions.* New York: Macmillan.

Pellegrino, E. (1979). *Humanism and the physician.* Knoxville: University of Tennessee Press.

Petersen, J. (1976). *A book of yes.* Illinois: Argus Communications

Purtilo, R. (1978). *Health professional/patient interaction.* Philadelphia: W. B. Saunders.

Rabin, D., Rabin, P., & Rabin, R. (1982). Compounding the ordeal of ALS. *New England Journal of Medicine, 307*, 506–509.

Rebeta–Burditt, J. (1977). *The cracker factory.* New York: Macmillan.

Reed, K. L., & Sanderson, S. R. (1983). *Concepts of occupational therapy.* Baltimore: Williams & Wilkins.

Reiser, D., & Schroder, A. K. (1980). *Patient interviewing: The human dimension.* Baltimore: Williams & Wilkins.

Rogers, C. R. (1975). The necessary and sufficient conditions of therapeutic personality change. *Journal of Consulting Psychology, 21*, 95–103.

Rogers, C. R. (1975). Empathic: An unappreciated way of being. *Counseling Psychologist, 5* (2), 2–10.

Sacks, O. (1983). *Awakenings.* New York: Dutton.

Sarason, S. B. (1985). *Caring and compassion in clinical practice.* San Francisco: Jossey–Bass.

Sarton, M. (1988). *After the stroke: A journal.* New York: Norton.

Saxton, M. (1987). In M. Saxton & F. Howe (Eds.), *With wings: An anthology of literature by and about women with disabilities* (pp. 51–57). New York: Feminist Press.

Schultz, S., & Schkade, J. K. (1992). Occupational adaptation: Toward a holistic approach for contemporary practice, Part 2. *American Journal of Occupational Therapy, 46*, 917–925.

Seabrook, W. (1935). *Asylum.* New York: Harcourt, Brace.

Taylor, R. (1972). *The practical art of medicine.* New York: Harper & Row.

Thomas, L. (1983). *The youngest science: Notes of a medicine–watcher.* New York: Viking.

Tiffany, E. G. (1983). Psychiatry and mental health. In H. L. Hopkins & H. D. Smith (Eds.), *Willard and Spackman's occupational therapy* (6th ed., pp. 267–229). Philadelphia: J. B. Lippincott.

Van Eys, J. & McGovern, J. P., (Eds.). (1988). *The doctor as a person.* Illinois: Charles C. Thomas.

Wade, B. D. (1947). Occupational therapy for patients with mental disease. In H. Willard & C. Spackman (Eds.) *Principles of occupational therapy* (pp. 81–117). Philadelphia: Lippincott.

Willard, H. S., & Spackman, C. S. (Eds.). (1947). *Principles of occupational therapy.* Philadelphia: J. B. Lippincott.

Yerxa, E. J. (1980). Occupational therapy's role in creating a future climate of caring. *American Journal of Occupational Therapy, 34*, 529–534.

Chapter 11

Group Process

Sharan L. Schwartzberg

G roup process skills are essential to therapeutic alliances in occupational therapy. This chapter explains the theory, history, and uses of group process and applies therapeutic reasoning and procedural guidelines to situations in practice.

Occupational therapy practitioners work within large group systems, such as schools and hospitals, and in small task groups designed for therapeutic aims, peer support, organizational goals, and evaluation purposes. In a hospital setting, occupational therapy practitioners may lead adaptive equipment groups for clients with hip fractures. In the community, occupational therapy practitioners may facilitate peer support groups for people who have sustained a head injury or who are coping with chronic mental illness. Therapists may use group process skills during consultation with community organizations concerning accessibility of facilities or when assisting families or other caretakers to learn feeding techniques for a child with difficulty swallowing.

▼ GROUP THEORY RELATED TO LARGE GROUP SYSTEMS AND SMALL TASK GROUPS

Ecological Systems Analysis

To fully appreciate group process, an integrative perspective of the individual, interpersonal relationships, and the environment is helpful. The ecological systems model in occupa-

tional therapy (Howe & Briggs, 1982) draws upon Bronfenbrenner's (1979) work in human development and on general systems theory. This model presents behavior as a result of interactions between (1) an individual with an inherent biopsychosocial makeup and (2) a given environmental system.

Large Groups

The ecological notion of relationship between person and environment is central to an integrative perspective on large groups. The community or institutional setting provides the context for individual and interpersonal relationships. Human behavior and performance cannot be understood outside of context (ie, physical, temporal, social, and cultural features) (Dunn, Brown, & McGuigan, 1994).

COMMUNITY

Understanding the community as a large group can tell practitioners about the various sociocultural perspectives of individuals and subgroups. An analysis may look at the range of options in a community for factors such as racial and ethnic backgrounds, religious affiliations, educational backgrounds, occupational roles, sexual orientation, as well as community resources for vocational, cultural, leisure, and educational pursuits. Of equal importance, but not as easy to identify, are the various values, beliefs, and attitudes of a community.

INSTITUTIONAL SETTINGS

Traditional institutions, such as hospitals, clinics, and schools, are standard working environments for occupational therapy practitioners. Each setting has its own mission and philosophy, values, and hierarchy, all of which influence individuals in that institution—be they client, staff, or administrative personnel. As in the community setting, institutional norms may be covert. When norms are covert they may be an unidentified source of conflict; hence, they should be made explicit. With rapid change in health service delivery systems one can expect frustration as a result of clashes in values. For example, practitioners and consumers accustomed to unlimited care may question the ethics of managed care. When angry and disillusioned, they may appear resistant in group meetings.

Small Task Groups

There are many types of small **task groups** in occupational therapy. They can be broadly classified by purpose: (1) therapeutic, (2) peer support, (3) focus or study, and (4) consultation and supervision.

THERAPEUTIC GROUPS

Most task groups in this category are aimed primarily at facilitating change in individual group members and have individual change as a primary aim. The therapeutic tasks are designed for restoration or development of function in components skills and areas of occupational performance; these tasks prevent further problems and support existing strengths. Group membership is usually small, ordinarily from six to ten clients.

PEER SUPPORT GROUPS

These groups are designed to provide support for individuals, families, caretakers, and partners, who have a medically related problem, diagnosis, or disability in common. The degree to which professionals are involved varies a great deal, from active involvement as teacher and leader to a more consultative role as facilitator. These task groups can be quite large or small, depending on the format. If the material is instructional, rather than process-oriented, a larger group can be accommodated.

FOCUS GROUPS

These task groups are designed to generate research hypotheses about a specific theme, or to organize discussion of material on a given topic. Meetings are structured around a specific question or set of semistructured questions. The group facilitator uses the questions to engage the group in discussion of common concerns. We can expect focus groups to gain popularity in occupational therapy with the need for more qualitative research related to function. Practitioners working in an institutional setting, for example, may wish to have a focus group or interdisciplinary group to address quality of care issues relative to length of stay.

The focus group is also useful as a time-limited therapy format and is increasingly prevalent in practice because of pressures to contain costs. The structure is well suited for specific populations and chronic illnesses, in which clients have common problems and experiences related to difficulties in functioning.

CONSULTATION AND SUPERVISION GROUPS

As therapists work more independently there will be an increased need for peer support, **supervision**, and **consulta-**

RESEARCH NOTE
CLINICAL RESEARCH REQUIRES SOCIAL AND SCIENTIFIC SKILLS

Kenneth J. Ottenbacher

The therapeutic process demands sharing and cooperation, and that is why therapeutic intervention is planned, implemented, and evaluated by teams. Contemporary versions of therapeutic teams are often labeled as transdisciplinary and include the client as a contributing member. Transdisciplinary teams require role sharing, role reversal, and a high degree of interaction and cooperation among team members. The planning, implementation, and dissemination of clinical research is also enhanced by transdisciplinary teams. Clinical research is a collaborative process involving social as well as scientific skills. In describing the cooperative nature of the research process, Lewis Thomas (1974) makes the following observation:

It [research] sometimes looks like a lonely activity, but it is as much the opposite of lonely as human behavior can be. There is nothing so social, so communal, so interdependent. An active field of science is like an immense intellectual anthill; the individual almost vanishes into the mass of minds tumbling over each other, carrying information from place to place, passing it around at the speed of light. (p. 101)

Establishing a body of knowledge requires building therapeutic alliances and research teams at multiple levels. These teams will contribute to the "*immense intellectual anthill*" of occupational science. ■

Thomas, L. (1974). *The lives of a cell: Notes of a biology watcher.* New York: Viking Press.

tion. Group supervision of professional practice, both disciplinary and interdisciplinary, is a viable option to meet this need, one that is more cost-effective than one-to-one supervision. One can expect a trend in this direction as departments are pressured to spend less time in nonrevenue-generating activities such as supervision and consultation. The health care trend toward increased utilization of less costly staff will also require more occupational therapy supervision of aides and other caretakers. Provision of this consultation or supervision in a group format should meet this need both educationally and economically.

▼ PAST AND PRESENT TRENDS IN THERAPEUTIC GROUPS

Occupational therapy group treatment is the combination of structured, group process and adapted tasks or activities aimed at fostering change and adaptation in persons with acute or chronic illness, impairments, or disabilities. The use of group process requires knowledge of theories of group process and dynamics, understanding of conceptual models that describe group principles and parallel therapeutic techniques, and knowledge of empirical research on variables related to the small, task-oriented group, both nonclinical and therapeutic. Group leaders must be able to use this information, along with their knowledge of pathology, wellness, and the use of purposeful activity, to reason about the individual client in the group context.

Historical Overview

A contemporary occupational therapy group consists of more than simply two or three persons doing solitary activities in the same room. Nevertheless, it was not uncommon to find such parallel interaction constituting group treatment in the profession's early years (Howe & Schwartzberg, 1986).

Today, it is incongruous to have occupational therapy conducted in groups without practitioner consideration of the unique properties of the group format. Occupational therapy groups place different emphasis on group properties than verbal psychotherapy and peer support groups (see Table 11-1). Group properties refer to the structure and interactions of a given group. A comparison of the relative importance of the group properties for the three aforementioned group types is given in Table 11-1. Separate historical periods have been identified in occupational therapy group work (Howe & Schwartzberg, 1986, 1995) (Table 11-2).

Current Occupational Therapy Group Approaches Across Practice Settings

The use of group treatment in occupational therapy is often mistakenly perceived as primarily restricted to practice in mental health or to the treatment of children or the elderly. Duncombe and Howe (1985) established that "60% of occupational therapists in all areas of practice lead groups in treatment" (p. 163). Ten years later they found a slight decrease to 52% (Duncombe & Howe, 1995). This negligible difference, they surmise, is due to a decrease in occupational practitioners working in large hospitals and psychiatric hospitals. Shifts toward community and school-based practice and cost-containment measures, including managed care, will probably increase the use of group treatment in the future. The role of a group leader as educator and consultant should grow as occupational therapy practitioners form partnerships with consumers in peer support groups and family care, as well as with other care-extenders and health professionals in group practice plans.

Reports also specifically document the value of group occupational therapy for clients with physical problems, such as **Parkinson disease** (Gauthier, Dalziel, & Gauthier, 1987), head injuries (Lundgren & Persechino, 1986), and rheumatoid arthritis (Van Deusen & Harlowe, 1987). Individual treatment is fast becoming viewed as a luxury as practitioners move toward interdisciplinary group treatment models that are more cost-efficient and capitalize on the therapeutic properties of groups (Marmer, 1995; Morris, Andreassi, & Lichtenberg, 1994). Projects similar to Trahey's (1991) study of services to individuals with total hip replacements demonstrate not only the therapeutic value, but

Group Properties	Occupational Therapy	Verbal Psychotherapy	Peer Support
Leader involvement	Very central	Not central	Not central
Purposeful activity	Very central	Not central	Not central
Structure and format	Very central	Not central	Somewhat central
Practice	Very central	Somewhat central	Not central
Teaching and learning	Very central	Somewhat central	Very central
Socialization and outside action	Somewhat central	Not central	Very central
There-and-then	Not central	Very central	Somewhat central
Here-and-now	Very central	Very central	Very central

TABLE 11-1. Comparison of Therapeutic Uses of Group Properties

TABLE 11-2. Eras of Group Work in Occupational Therapy	
Era	**Focus of Group Involvement**
Project Era, 1922–1936	Project completion
Socialization Era, 1937–1953	Social activity
Group Dynamics-Process Era, 1954–1961	Interpersonal dynamics
Ego-Building–Psychodynamic Era, 1962–1969	Ego reconstitution
Adaptation Era, 1970–1990s	Social adaptation

Historical analysis is from Howe, M. C., & Schwartzberg, S. L. (1995). A functional approach to group work in occupational therapy (2nd ed.). Philadelphia: J. B. Lippincott.

also the cost-effectiveness of occupational therapy group treatment, when compared with individual treatment, as the primary format for care in physical disabilities practice.

Definitions and Types of Occupational Therapy Groups

Duncombe and Howe (1985) identified ten types of groups commonly used in occupational therapy: (1) exercise, (2) cooking, (3) tasks, (4) activities of daily living, (5) arts and crafts, (6) self-expression, (7) feelings-oriented discussion, (8) reality-oriented discussion, (9) sensorimotor or sensory integration, and (10) educational. Occupational therapy groups, for the most part, remain small-sized activity groups (fewer than ten members; usually about six) that are focused on therapeutic goals such as task skills, communication and socialization skills, and physical abilities (Duncombe & Howe, 1995).

At least 12 group variables describe an occupational therapy group; these are listed in Box 11-1. Each needs to be considered in the formation and design of a therapeutic group. One of the most important of these variables, the group setting (inpatient or outpatient) influences the group

▼ **BOX 11-1**

Occupational Therapy Group Variables

Setting
Therapeutic factors
Goals: Short-term and long-term
Duration of group
Composition of group
Time frame and format
Population
Group size
Frame of reference
Open versus time-limited, closed membership
Member selection and preparation
Contraindications

goals and techniques used. The relationship between group orientation or format and therapeutic focus in different settings is shown in Table 11-3.

Models in Occupational Therapy: Roles of Leader, Group Member, and Activity

Several different group approaches are used in occupational therapy and, to varying degrees, each has its own articulated theoretical perspective. Selected occupational therapy group approaches are identified in Box 11-2. The roles of the leader, group member, and activity vary among the models. Each deserves attention when the models are applied to practice. The reader is referred to the original works for details about each approach.

The Functional Group Model (Howe & Schwartzberg, 1986, 1988, 1995; Kielhofner, 1992) is considered a generic group model in occupational therapy. It incorporates four key concepts: "purposeful activity," "self-initiated action," "spontaneous action," and "group-centered action." Howe and Schwartzberg (1988) explain how to enhance group process through group structure:

To accomplish this result within the functional group model, the following factors should be considered in planning, running, and reviewing the group: (1) maximum involvement through group-centered action, (2) a maximum sense of individual and group identity, (3) a "flow" experience, (4) spontaneous involvement of members, and (5) member support and feedback. These five major categories should be reviewed individually in terms of the parameters to be considered by the leader or co-leaders. (p. 3)

Leader techniques and procedures for conducting a group are described later in this section.

Comparison with Group Formats of Other Professions

As was depicted in Table 11-1, the occupational therapy group format is significantly different from verbal psychotherapy groups conducted by other professionals, such as psychiatrists, psychologists, nurses, and social workers. In verbal group psychotherapy, for example, the emphasis is

TABLE 11-3. Occupational Therapy Group Settings, Goals, and Techniques		
Group Orientation or Format*	Inpatient Goals and Techniques	Outpatient Goals and Techniques
Interpersonal and dynamic	Support, containment	Social change, insight
Behavioral and educational	New skills and attitudes, structure, here-and-now experiences	Same as inpatient
Support	Acceptance	Legitimization, information, decreased isolation
Maintenance and rehabilitation	Safety, reevaluation, discharge planning	Adaptation, resources; minimize stress

*These categories were adapted for this purpose from Vinogradov and Yalom's (1989) classification of outpatient groups.

often on talking, insight, and understanding. In a psychodynamic or interpersonal model of group treatment, the *there-and-then experience*, or past experience, which is often familial, is used as a means to understand present-day conflicts. The *here-and-now experience*, or immediate experience, in the group is examined as a projection of the client's past and provides members with an opportunity to test new and more adaptive interpersonal styles. These groups require members to have a fair degree of abstract capability and self-control over their behavior.

In contrast, as a general rule, occupational therapy groups focus as much as possible on shared "doing" and adjusted experience within the here-and-now experience. Groups are structured and graded so that members with modest to more advanced social and cognitive skills may participate. Mosey's (1973a) classification of group interaction skills is often used to designate the type and level of interaction required in an activity group. These levels are designated as (1) "parallel group," (2) "project group," (3) "egocentric-coop-

erative group," (4) "cooperative group," and (5) "mature group." They range from the parallel level, with maximal leader support and structure and little expectation for interaction around a task, to the mature level, with minimal leader intervention and a high degree of interaction required for task completion and social-emotional satisfaction.

A nonprogressing but multilevel scheme is the hierarchical task analysis developed by Allen (1985). This task analysis is used to group clients according to their cognitive capabilities; these capabilities are designated by cognitive levels numbered 1 through 6. Group tasks of varying complexity are chosen accordingly. Activities are gauged to the client's level and adjusted as acute symptoms remit. At the lowest level for which group treatment is possible (level 2 groups), movement activities with demonstrated directions are indicated. At the higher levels (level 5 and 6 groups) more complex tasks are suggested, such as craft or cooking activities, that have several steps demonstrated at one time; planning may be involved as the practitioner continues to monitor the group for safety and ability to follow directions (Cole, 1993).

▼ BOX 11-2

Selected Occupational Therapy Group Approaches

Task-Oriented Group (Fidler, 1969)
Functional Group Model (Howe & Schwartzberg, 1986; 1995)
Directive Group Therapy (Kaplan, 1988)
Activity Group (Borg & Bruce, 1991; Mosey, 1973a, 1973b)
Developmental Group (Mosey, 1970)
Psychoeducational Group (Lillie & Armstrong, 1982)
Integrative Group Therapy Structured Five-Stage Approach (Ross, 1991)
Peer Support Group (Schwartzberg, 1994)

▼ GROUP PROCESS AND SMALL TASK GROUPS

The practice of group work in occupational therapy involves observation and interaction as well as the procedures of evaluation, designing, planning, analyzing, responding, and documenting.

Observation

The leader looks for information about the group's process in several areas. All aspects of the group are dynamic and constantly changing, which makes observation difficult and challenging. Leaders observe the following aspects of groups.

GROUP AS SYSTEM: GROUP PROCESS AND DYNAMICS

Groups progress through stages of development when the therapeutic conditions of clear, mutual goals and trust have been achieved. Group phases indicating the stages of group development in terms of leader, group member, and activity roles are identified in Table 11-4. In observing the group's development, leaders look at the group's phase in relation to (1) decision-making patterns, (2) membership and leadership roles, and (3) the level and type of participation patterns, such as who initiates communication, who talks to whom, and the tone of voice members and leaders use.

INDIVIDUAL MEMBER IN SYSTEM

In addition to the group as a whole, the leader observes individual group members in relation to other members, the leader, and the group task. These observations of group dynamics may be informal, or be structured around a task designed to demonstrate certain skills and behaviors such as cooperativeness, mobility, attention span, memory, concentration, and assertiveness. The observation task may also include functional activities, such as collaborative work, cooking, or other activities of daily living. Depending on the setting and length of treatment, when possible, the practitioner may also conduct pregroup interviews as a means to observe, establish **rapport** with, and gain information about a potential group member.

LEADER AND COLEADER SELF-AWARENESS

An equally important area of observation is the leader's own behavior and internal reactions. It is good practice for group leaders to write group process notes after each group meeting. In these notes, practitioners describe their personal reactions, thoughts, and the critical events in the group. It is beneficial to share observations of the group and of each other with a coleader. These observations are helpful in clinical supervision and in analysis of countertransference.

GROUP, MEMBER, AND LEADER INTERACTIONS

The observation of group process (interactions within the group) is conducted at levels of (1) the group, (2) the individual members in relation to the group, (3) the individual members and the group in relation to the leader or coleaders, and (4) all in relation to a task or activity. In addition, for the purposes of feedback, the practitioner may look for opportunities to observe the group member in functional contexts outside the group (eg, community, school, work, and family environments).

Establishing a Therapeutic Alliance Through Group Process

Therapeutic factors unique to occupational therapy groups have been isolated in preliminary studies. They include creativity and self-esteem, relaxation and diversion, enjoyment, increased skills, and concentration (Finn, 1989; Webster, 1988; Webster & Schwartzberg, 1992). Given the extensive research on therapeutic factors in verbal psychotherapy groups, those factors found in common with occupational therapy groups deserve emphasis. The therapeutic factors identified by Yalom (1985) found in both occupational therapy and psychotherapy groups are group cohesiveness, interpersonal learning-output, and instillation of hope (Falk-Kessler, Momich, & Perel, 1991; Finn, 1989; Howe & Schwartzberg, 1986; Webster & Schwartzberg, 1992). Leadership strategies should be chosen to promote these factors for group members.

LEADER TO MEMBER INTERACTIONS

An important aspect of group therapy practice as well as individual therapy practice is the practitioner's use of self in the group. Leaders serve particular roles and use techniques that they are continually attempting to perfect to achieve therapeutic goals. The primary roles of the leader include observer, group designer, role model, and climate setter (supporting and substituting actions as needed in the group). A skilled leader is continually weighing individual and group needs and chooses the strategies and techniques she or he will use by considering past responses and immediate as well as long-term therapeutic goals.

The leadership strategies commonly used include genuineness and empathy, modeling behavior, reality testing, communicating, and planning the group activity through activity analysis and adaptation (Howe & Schwartzberg, 1986, 1995). Particular use of these strategies and related techniques is dependent upon the group's goals and conceptual framework, the group's phase of development, and the practitioner's relationship with the clients.

TABLE 11-4. Sample Roles and Phases of Group Development			
Roles	**Formation**	**Development**	**Termination**
Leader	Set climate, provide structure, offer support	Grade actions, facilitate	Aid separation, reinforce gains
Member	Identify purpose	Collaborate, initiate	Evaluate, express reactions
Activity	Form goals, establish trust	Purposeful action	Review

GROUP MEMBER TO GROUP MEMBER INTERACTIONS

The practitioner and members of a group have work to accomplish in a group. Nevertheless, some problems commonly surface in group work, including: (1) difficulty establishing trust with the leader and other group members; (2) dependency on the leader; (3) difficulty setting goals; (4) misdirected anger, competition among group members, subgrouping, and withdrawal from the group or task; (5) lack of skill; (6) absenteeism, members leaving the group meeting, and premature termination from the group; (7) external conflicts and pressure (eg, from family); and (8) interference from outside the group (eg, interruptions from other services such as the laboratory). When one of these problems arises, it must be examined separately and interpreted differently depending on the clinician's theoretical framework.

COLEADER INTERACTIONS

In working together, coleaders assist in the physical and emotional management of the group. This is particularly important when the group is large or when members require considerable individual attention because of cognitive, physical, or social-emotional limitations. In addition, coleaders are model participants in the group, demonstrating healthy interaction and ways of resolving conflict with others.

It is useful to have supervision with both leaders present. These sessions help the leaders work out differences of opinion, conflicts, and rivalry that inevitably exist when coleading a group. Where possible, a more experienced practitioner coleads with a beginning practitioner. The experienced practitioner serves as a model and can also provide supervision. Often the coleaders' relationship draws attention from the group. For example, members may be competitive with a novice practitioner in fear of losing the more senior leader's attention. Through an accepting relationship with both leaders, members can alter their perceptions. They may react differently when expected to share in the future. As model participants in groups, the coleaders provide members an opportunity to observe a working, productive, teaching-learning relationship.

Interactive and Procedural Reasoning

Group leadership in occupational therapy requires time to design the overall group plan and individual session plans. The leader also evaluates individual sessions and members' progress and the overall group's progress. These professional tasks require both interactive reasoning that focuses on the client's disability experience and procedural reasoning that focuses on the client's disability and its affect on functioning.

EVALUATING INDIVIDUAL MEMBERS AND THE GROUP

Evaluation is an ongoing process that usually begins with meeting the client before the first session. The therapist may have a formal referral or see a group member as part of a larger program. Groups may also be used for the sole purpose of evaluation. This is common in inpatient settings, when clients are discharged rapidly and the main goal of hospitalization is evaluation and discharge planning.

Through "interactive reasoning" the leader comes to (1) know how members experience their disability (Fleming, 1991) and (2) understand how the disability affects their function. Interactive reasoning enables the practitioner to be truly empathic. This empathy forms the basis for trust to develop within the group. In coming to know the members, the leader conveys and models warmth, support, and acceptance. In the group setting, interactive reasoning occurs not only between the practitioner and the client, but also between other group members and within the group as a whole. The relative success of this interactive reasoning influences the degree to which therapeutic factors of cohesiveness, interpersonal learning, and instillation of hope are achieved.

In some settings the registered occupational therapist evaluates clients and develops a plan and the certified occupational therapy assistant actually conducts the group. The registered therapist provides supervision for the occupational therapy assistant as well. Service delivery arrangements and use of staff resources vary from setting to setting.

DESIGNING

The group's design has several components. The design is usually written in the form of a group protocol that includes (1) group, and if possible, individual member short-term and long-term goals; (2) selection criteria for membership; (3) group size and composition; (4) group methods, techniques, and activity modalities; (5) time and location of the group meeting and group leaders' names; and (6) referral procedures. Protocols aid practitioners in communicating with other professionals and prospective group members.

PLANNING AND EVALUATING

Evaluation is continuous throughout the group's existence and when possible involves the group members. After evaluating each session, the leaders create detailed individual group session plans with categories similar to the overall, more generalized plan. When there is a major shift in client population, the leader may also modify the general group plan. In time-limited groups (MacKenzie, 1995) sessions are highly focused, and circumscribed goals are made explicit to members. The practitioner must be highly active in promoting a therapeutic climate conducive to goal achievement.

ANALYZING AND RESPONDING

Each group situation is analyzed separately and continuously if the group is ongoing. To respond, the leader uses the group's history as well as individual members' histories of strategies that were successful or unsuccessful. In an open group with changing membership, the leader's experience with similar situations becomes particularly useful. In a closed or time-limited group, the membership remains consistent from session to session. In these situations, the leader can use prior experience for analyzing and responding, and the group can become its own control.

▼ THERAPEUTIC FACTOR CASE STUDIES

To illustrate the reasoning involved in analyzing and responding to group process, the three previously mentioned therapeutic factors will be used as a focus for the case studies: group cohesiveness, interpersonal learning, and instillation of hope. Although presented separately, multiple goals are the norm, and a leadership strategy often promotes more than one factor and outcome. The strategies detailed here are those commonly applicable to occupational therapy (Andrews, 1995; Howe & Schwartzberg, 1995; Mattingly & Fleming, 1994). However, this is not an exhaustive list.

Group Cohesiveness

Cohesiveness refers to the attraction that members have for their group and for the other members. The members of a cohesive group are accepting of one another, supportive, and inclined to form meaningful relationships in the group. Cohesiveness seems to be a significant factor in successful group therapy outcome (Yalom, 1985, p. 69).

Leadership Strategies

1. Design activities that have "maximal involvement of members through group-centered action" (Howe & Schwartzberg, 1995).
2. Maintain "maximal sense of individual and group identity" (Howe & Schwartzberg, 1995).
3. Provide and invite member support.
4. Demonstrate genuineness and empathy.
5. Self-disclose own feelings and reactions in an authentic and prudent fashion.
6. Be active in listening and responding.
7. Consider judiciously "doing for patients" (Mattingly & Fleming, 1994).
8. Look for ways to encourage joint problem solving.
9. Demonstrate acceptance and affirmation.
10. Contemplate reframing problems in a more positive manner (Andrews, 1995).

CASE STUDY

Mrs. Clark was looking forward to a vacation in Florida, although somewhat apprehensive about her husband's upcoming retirement. He had worked hard as a loyal employee of a men's clothing store; however, he had no other interests or involvement in his home. The latter was "wife business." The store was about to go into bankruptcy and now at age 68 Mr. Clark was forced to retire. Despite trepidations about these events, Mrs. Clark was pleased with an opportunity to go to her niece's wedding, and put on her best new high-heeled shoes for an evening of dancing. Hours later Mrs. Clark slipped while dancing and broke her hip and several bones in the wrist of her dominant hand. She was rushed to a local emergency room and four days later a rehabilitation hospital. The recovery seemed to go well until she got home. Mr. Clark was of no help. Beyond his lack of involvement in managing their home, he had become depressed and agitated since his retirement. Mrs. Clark felt angry, unsupported, and frustrated with her limited mobility and loss of homemaker role. The occupational practitioner providing services in the Clarks' home tried to intervene with the family dynamics without success. Once the visiting nurses association stopped home services, Mrs. Clark went for outpatient occupational therapy at the rehabilitation center.

In attending one of the occupational therapy groups for clients with hip replacements, Mrs. Clark found relief. Many of the other clients were older than Mrs. Clark, and she had an opportunity to help them and, at the same time, be nurtured. Many stories were told about husbands retiring and acting "helpless," children not visiting, and so on. This support had been unavailable to her when she was being treated at home.

Summary: From the perspective of group cohesiveness, which calls attention to member support, acceptance, and individual identity, we would be alert to the following questions:

1. How can the leader structure range of motion and functional activities to promote maximal sharing and joint problem solving?
2. What role can the leader play in helping the members reframe their problems in a more positive way?

Interpersonal Learning—Output

Interpersonal learning is the group therapy equivalent of such individual therapy factors as self-understanding or insight, working through the transference, and the corrective emotional experience. Interpersonal learning involves the identification, the elucidation, and the modification of maladaptive interpersonal relationships. . . . three basic assumptions upon [which] it rests: 1.interpersonal theory 2. the group as a social microcosm and 3. the here-and-now (Yalom, 1983, p. 45).

Interpersonal learning output involves "improving . . . skills in getting along with people."(Yalom, 1985, Table 4.1).

Leadership Strategies

1. Invite spontaneous involvement.
2. Invite member feedback.
3. Model desired behaviors.
4. Clarify, explain, understand, and interpret what is happening in the group as a framework for change.
5. Reality test.
6. Encourage feedback and consensual validation.
7. Be concrete and bridge group experiences to situations outside of the group.
8. Invite gentle confrontation.
9. Look for ways to create choices (Mattingly & Fleming, 1994).
10. Encourage members to compare experiences and impressions.
11. Encourage members to identify problems in group that are familiar and similar to difficulties in outside functioning.

CASE STUDY

The head injury support group is assembling for the usual weekly meeting. The group has been meeting at the founding member's home (Facilitator A) for its second year. An occupational therapist is present as cofacilitator (Facilitator B).

Facilitator B: I would like to have the older members introduce themselves and tell their stories and have other people have a chance to tell their story. (This is a group ritual for starting meetings.)

Member A: I'm not going first.

Facilitator A: Should we get labels?

Facilitator B: Yes, that helps.

Facilitator A: I will go and get labels for everybody because that helps a lot.

Member A: I really don't like that.

Facilitator B: Why is that?

Member A: Because it really bothers me.

Facilitator B: What bothers you?

Member A: Labels.

Facilitator B: You mean name tags? Why?

Member B: Because it's distracting?

Member A: Because it's insulting.

Member B: Why?

Member C: For brain injured people?

Member D: For anyone.

Member C: My ability before my brain injury was to remember everything about a person. Now I forget their names. But I remember everything about them. I guess. . .

Member B: Member A was saying that she objected, Facilitator A, to name tags.

Facilitator A: But why?

Facilitator B: I think that we just starting out talking. . .

Member A: That was a very noncompassionate thing for me to say because I strengthen my memory by not having things like name tags so I can really work on remembering names. I have to be compassionate that there are people who have strength in other things that I have more trouble with, and that name tags are necessary.

Member D: Since we're not together every day. If we were, we might remember.

Member B: So Member A said she didn't want to be the first one to tell her story.

Facilitator B: Facilitator A?

Facilitator A: I had a car accident 4´ years ago. . .

Summary: From the perspective of interpersonal learning, which calls attention to understanding and interpreting what is happening within the group, concreteness, and comparing experiences, we would be mindful of the following questions:

1. In what ways can the facilitator use the group process so that Member A feels accepted and understood, rather than encouraged to further castigate herself for lacking "compassion," and at the same time get feedback from other members about their impressions?
2. How might the facilitator create new choices by relating this exchange to outside experiences? Typically individuals with a head injury may be unaware or attempt to conceal problems in functioning to avoid be viewed as disabled and, in doing so, may sabotage assistance offered.

CASE STUDY

Maria, a teenage mother, entered the hospital after slashing her wrists and threatening to throw her baby out the window. John, a teenage young man, entered the hospital after repeated attempts to beat his father. He was smoking pot at school, truant most of the time, and, when at home, spent most of his days locked in his room not eating or sleeping.

Terry, an anorexic adolescent, entered the hospital after she returned from a college semester abroad. Her parents found that she had not eaten in a week. The event was apparently precipitated by receiving a B average grade on her report card.

The group was making holiday greeting cards using stencils, stamps, and silk screens. Options ranged from placing stickers on a preworded card to creating designs for silk screening. While doing the activity members talked about their family disappointments, hopes, and accomplishments, and losses of confidence. The practitioner structured the activity so that everyone succeeded in making an attractive product.

Summary: From the perspective of instillation of hope, which calls attention to structuring success experiences, exchange of personal stories, and supporting positive themes in the group, we would be alert to the following questions:

1. How can the activity be graded from simple to fairly complex so that members' decrease in perceptual, cognitive, and social functioning is not apparent and the developmental needs of adolescents and the 3- to 5-day hospital length of stay is taken into consideration?
2. Parallel task groups intrinsically create conditions that promote interaction between clients (Schwartzberg, Howe, & McDermott, 1982). How can the leader gently invite members to share feelings of hope, being sensitive to members' feelings of disappointment, and at the same time not contaminate the natural flow of communication?

Instillation of Hope

Group members are at different points along a collapse–coping continuum and can gain hope from observing others, especially others with similar problems, who have profited from therapy. (Yalom, 1983, p. 41)

Leadership Strategies

1. Design the group so that there is a "flow experience" (Csikszentmihalyi cited in Howe & Schwartzberg, 1995).
2. Structure success into activities and process.
3. Encourage exchange of "personal stories" (Mattingly & Fleming, 1994).

HISTORICAL NOTE

THE STORY OF THE HEALING HEART: DOING WITH PERSONS AS A UNIQUE ALLIANCE

Suzanne M. Peloquin

The biography of Ora Ruggles chronicled the kind of service that reconstruction aides rendered during World War I. A schoolteacher who had graduated from San Diego Normal School and taken courses in the manual arts, Ruggles quickly engaged each of her patients. Her competence, warmth, and concern inspired awe and gratitude in many of them.

The title of her biography, *The Healing Heart* (1946), derives from a comment Ruggles made to her peers. As she walked into the army barracks at Fort McPherson one evening, her friends asked about her unusual silence. Rug-

gles explained that she had made a great discovery, simple yet so effective. When pressed to share, she offered this fine keepsake: "It is not enough to give a patient something to do with his hands. You must reach for the heart as well as the hands. It's the heart that really does the healing" (Carlova and Ruggles, 1946, p. 69). The comment has meaning five decades later. Ruggles described an interactive form of doing with others that transforms the use of occupation into an alliance named occupational therapy. Within a health care system that presses so many to do things to their clients, this alliance is remarkable. ■

Carlova, J. and Ruggles, O. (1946). *The healing heart.* New York: Julian Messner.

4. Comment on member successes as they happen (Andrews, 1995).
5. Highlight positive themes in the group (Andrews, 1995).

▼ DOCUMENTATION

Clinicians must consult their individual facilities, third-party payers, and state requirements for specific information concerning appropriate documentation and billing for group evaluation and treatment. Practitioners usually document each client's progress separately after group sessions. Ideally, they would also keep records of the group's progress as a whole for the purposes of analysis and supervision. As mentioned earlier, group protocols, session plans, and process notes are other forms of documentation commonly used in group practice.

►RESEARCH AND CONCLUSIONS
PROBLEMS AND STRENGTHS

Much remains to be understood about the use of group process in occupational therapy and about the best methods for teaching students and practitioners how to use this important tool. Group approaches have two strengths. First, groups enable members to achieve their goals in ways that individual therapy cannot match. Second, group approaches are cost-effective—an increasingly important characteristic in a climate that emphasizes cost containment.

The practice of documenting group process and content is diminishing as practitioners are under increasing pressures to be efficient and cost-effective. Duncombe and Howe (1995) recently found that 55% of 75 therapists in their study reported no difference in the rate charged for individual versus group treatment. Furthermore, they reported that 94% of the 219 respondents kept individual documentation, rather than for the group as a whole, or both. Even though invaluable, it takes time to write and analyze group process notes. There is a danger that economic incentives will undermine this process. Practitioners mistakenly may not take time or be permitted adequate time for this task. The practice of documenting and examining the relationship between the individual and the group as a whole must be safeguarded, for it is inherent to the therapeutic value of group treatment.

Current Research

Recent studies strongly suggest differences in outcomes when activity groups are compared with psychotherapy groups (DeCarlo & Mann, 1985; Klyczek & Mann, 1986; McDermott, 1988; Mumford, 1974; Schwartzberg et al., 1982). In contrast, although differences have been noted (Finn, 1989; Webster, 1988), similarities have also been found between members' percep-

tions of the therapeutic value of occupational therapy groups and the perspectives of members of psychotherapy groups (Falk-Kessler et al, 1991; Webster & Schwartzberg, 1992). In addition, there appear to exist unique roles and helping factors when peer-led groups are compared with professional-led groups in occupational therapy (Sacenti, 1988; Schwartzberg, 1994). Furthermore, Howe and Schwartzberg (1995) "demonstrate that group format has an effect on the quality and quantity of interaction, meaning assigned to the group action, and members' functional status" (p. 221).

Future research in all settings where occupational therapy practitioners use group treatment should address both outcomes related to function and client perceptions of group treatment. Regardless of group format, it would be of interest to know, for example, if client perceptions of therapeutic factors are related to functional outcomes, or vice versa. Further studies in activity group analysis and the meaning of restricted variables would also support the endeavor to explain the therapeutic use of group process in occupational therapy (Adelstein & Nelson, 1985; Henry, Nelson, & Duncombe, 1984; Kremer, Nelson, & Duncombe, 1984; Nelson, Peterson, Smith, Boughton, & Whalen, 1988; Steffan & Nelson, 1987; Steffan, 1990). Finally, in this era of managed and rationed care, it would be of interest to study (1) individual and group treatment outcomes in relation to the amount of treatment time required and staff resources; (2) treatment time required with various occupational therapy group modalities and strategies in relation to diagnosis, functional problems, resources, and severity of illness; and (3) therapeutic factors in occupational therapy groups in comparison with verbally oriented, interdisciplinary, and peer formats.

► REFERENCES

Adelstein, L. A., & Nelson, D. L. (1985). Effects of sharing versus non-sharing on affective meaning in collage activities. *Occupational Therapy in Mental Health: A Journal of Psychosocial Practice and Research, 5* (2), 29–45.

Allen, C. K. (1985). *Occupational therapy for psychiatric diseases: Measurement and management of cognitive disabilities.* Boston: Little, Brown & Company.

Andrews, H. B. (1995). *Group design and leadership: Strategies for creating successful common theme groups.* Boston: Allyn and Bacon.

Borg, B., & Bruce, M. A. (1991). *The group system: The therapeutic activity group in occupational therapy.* Thorofare, NJ: Slack.

Bronfenbrenner, U. (1979). *The ecology of human development: Experiments by nature and design.* Cambridge: Harvard University Press.

Cole, M. B. (1993). *Group dynamics in occupational therapy: The theoretical basis and practice application of group treatment.* Thorofare, NJ: Slack.

DeCarlo, J. J., & Mann, W. C. (1985). The effectiveness of verbal versus activity groups in improving self-perceptions of interpersonal communication skills. *American Journal of Occupational Therapy, 39,* 20–27.

Duncombe, L. W., & Howe, M. C. (1985). Group work in occupational therapy: A survey of practice. *American Journal of Occupational Therapy, 39,* 163–170.

Duncombe, L. W., & Howe, M. C. (1995). Group treatment: Goals, tasks, and economic implications. *American Journal of Occupational Therapy, 49*, 199–205.

Dunn, W., Brown, C., & McGuigan, A. (1994). The ecology of human performance: A framework for considering the effect of context. *American Journal of Occupational Therapy, 48*, 595–607.

Falk-Kessler, J., Momich, C., & Perel, S. (1991). Therapeutic factors in occupational therapy groups. *American Journal of Occupational Therapy, 45*, 59–66.

Fidler, G. S. (1969). The task-oriented group as a context for treatment. *American Journal of Occupational Therapy, 23*, 43–48.

Finn, M. (1989). *Patients' perceptions of occupational therapy groups: Interview generated factors.* Unpublished master's thesis, Tufts University-Boston School of Occupational Therapy, Medford, MA.

Fleming, M. H. (1991). The therapist with the three-track mind. *American Journal of Occupational Therapy, 45*, 1007–1014.

Gauthier, L., Dalziel, S., & Gauthier, S. (1987). The benefits of group occupational therapy for patients with Parkinson's disease. *American Journal of Occupational Therapy, 41*, 360–365.

Henry, A. D., Nelson, D. L., & Duncombe, L. W. (1984). Choice making in group and individual activity. *American Journal of Occupational Therapy, 38*, 245–251.

Howe, M. C., & Briggs, A. K. (1982). Ecological systems model for occupational therapy. *American Journal of Occupational Therapy, 36*, 322–327.

Howe, M. C., & Schwartzberg, S. L. (1986). *A functional approach to group work in occupational therapy.* Philadelphia: J.B. Lippincott.

Howe, M. C., & Schwartzberg, S. L. (1988). Structure and process in designing a functional group. *Occupational Therapy in Mental Health: A Journal of Psychosocial Practice and Research, 8* (3), 1–8.

Howe, M. C., & Schwartzberg, S. L. (1995). *A functional approach to group work in occupational therapy* (2nd ed.). Philadelphia: J.B. Lippincott.

Kaplan, K. L. (1988). *Directive group therapy: Innovative mental health treatment.* Thorofare, NJ: Slack.

Kielhofner, G. (1992). *Conceptual foundations in occupational therapy.* Philadelphia: F. A. Davis.

Klyczek, J. P., & Mann, W. C. (1986). Therapeutic modality comparisons in day treatment. *American Journal of Occupational Therapy, 40*, 606–611.

Kremer, E. R. H., Nelson, D. L., & Duncombe, L. W. (1984). Effects of selected activities on affective meaning in psychiatric patients. *American Journal of Occupational Therapy, 38*, 522–528.

Lillie, M., & Armstrong, H. (1982). Contributions to the development of psychoeducational approaches to mental health service. *American Journal of Occupational Therapy, 36*, 438–443.

Lundgren, C. C., & Persechino, E. L. (1986). Cognitive group: A treatment program for head injured adults. *American Journal of Occupational Therapy, 40*, 397–401.

MacKenzie, K. R. (1995). Rationale for group psychotherapy in managed care. In K. R. MacKenzie (Ed.), *Effective use of group therapy in managed care* (pp. 1–25). Washington, DC: American Psychiatric Press.

Marmer, L. (1995, October 2). Group treatment works well in stroke recovery. *Advance for Occupational Therapists*, 13.

Mattingly, C., & Fleming, M. H. (1994). Interactive reasoning: Collaborating with the person. In C. Mattingly & M. H. Fleming, *Clinical reasoning: Forms of inquiry in a therapeutic practice* (pp. 178–196). Philadelphia: F. A. Davis.

McDermott, A. A. (1988). The effect of three group formats on group interaction patterns. *Occupational Therapy in Mental Health: A Journal of Psychosocial Practice and Research, 8* (3), 69–89.

Morris, P. A., Andreassi, E., & Lichtenberg, P. (1994, August 25). Preparing for community living. *OT Week*, 20–21.

Mosey, A. C. (1970). The concept and use of developmental groups. *American Journal of Occupational Therapy, 24*, 272–275.

Mosey, A. C. (1973a). *Activities therapy.* New York: Raven Press.

Mosey, A. C. (1973b). Meeting health needs. *American Journal of Occupational Therapy, 27*, 14–17.

Mumford, M. S. (1974). A comparison of interpersonal skills in verbal and activity groups. *American Journal of Occupational Therapy, 28*, 281–283.

Nelson, D. L., Peterson, C., Smith, D. A., Boughton, J. A., & Whalen, G. M. (1988). Effects of project versus parallel groups on social interaction and affective responses in senior citizens. *American Journal of Occupational Therapy, 42*, 23–29.

Ross, M. (1991). *Integrative group therapy: The structured five-stage approach* (2nd ed.). Thorofare, NJ: Slack.

Sacenti, L. (1988). *Mastery and levels of participation in members of two groups for chronic pain: Self-help and professionally led.* Unpublished master's thesis, Tufts University-Boston School of Occupational Therapy, Medford, MA.

Schwartzberg, S. L. (1994). Helping factors in a peer-developed support group for persons with head injury, Part 1: Participant observer perspective. *American Journal of Occupational Therapy, 48*, 297–304.

Schwartzberg, S. L., Howe, M. C., & McDermott, A. (1982). A comparison of three treatment group formats for facilitating social interaction. *Occupational Therapy in Mental Health: A Journal of Psychosocial Practice and Research, 2* (4), 1–16.

Steffan, J. A. (1990). Productive occupation in small task groups of adults: Synthesis and annotations of the social psychology literature. In A. C. Bundy, N. D. Prendergast, J. A. Steffan, & D. Thorn (Eds.), *Review of selected literature on occupation and health* (pp. 175–281). Rockville, MD: American Occupational Therapy Association.

Steffan, J. A., & Nelson, D. L. (1987). The effects of tool scarcity on group climate and affective meaning within the context of a stenciling activity. *American Journal of Occupational Therapy, 41*, 449–453.

Trahey, P. J. (1991). A comparison of the cost-effectiveness of two types of occupational therapy services. *American Journal of Occupational Therapy, 45*, 397–400.

Van Deusen, J., & Harlowe, D. (1987). The efficacy of the ROM dance program for adults with rheumatoid arthritis. *American Journal of Occupational Therapy, 41*, 90–95.

Vinogradov, S., & Yalom, I. D. (1989). *A concise guide to group psychotherapy.* Washington, DC: American Psychiatric Press.

Webster, D. (1988). *Patients' perceptions of therapeutic factors in occupational therapy groups.* Unpublished master's thesis, Tufts University-Boston School of Occupational Therapy, Medford, MA.

Webster, D., & Schwartzberg, S. L. (1992). Patients' perception of curative factors in occupational therapy groups. *Occupational Therapy in Mental Health: A Journal of Psychosocial Practice and Research, 12* (1), 3–24.

Yalom, I. D. (1983). *Inpatient group psychotherapy.* New York: Basic Books.

Yalom, I. D. (1985). *The theory and practice of group psychotherapy* (3rd ed.). New York: Basic Books.

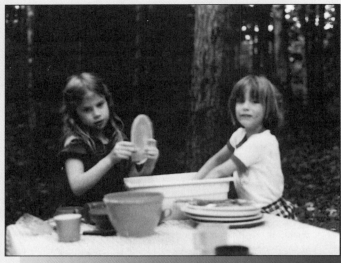

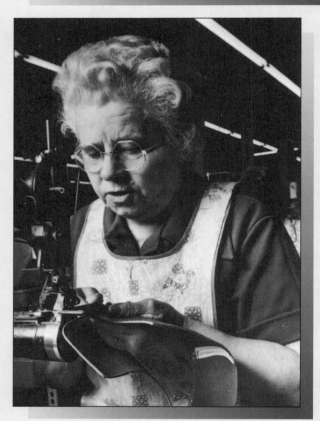

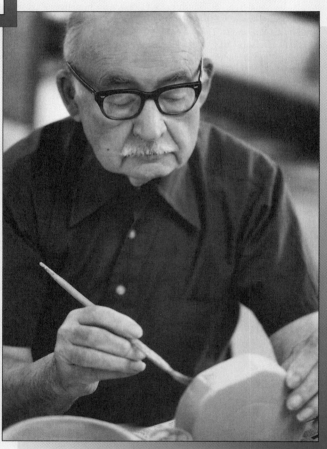

(top left) Dishwashing takes on a different character when children are camping. (Photo courtesy of Elizabeth Crepeau.)

(bottom left) The context and meaning of sewing differs if one is sewing shoes versus making clothing for the family. (Photo courtesy of Dennis Abbott.)

(bottom right) New leisure pursuits are offered to this man in an adult day program. (Photo courtesy of John Adams, Instructional Services, Dimond Library, University of New Hampshire.)

UNIT V

Activity Analysis

LEARNING OBJECTIVES

After completing this unit, readers will be able to:

▶ Analyze activities for occupational performance components.

▶ Define and explain activity analysis and its relation to occupational therapy practice.

Activity analysis is a way of thinking used by occupational therapy practitioners to develop an understanding of activities, their component parts, their meaning to clients, and their therapeutic potential. Activities are at the center of occupational therapy intervention; consequently, the ability to analyze activity and use activity therapeutically is at the core of occupational therapy practice. This unit describes activity analysis and links it to the clinical reasoning process and occupational therapy interventions. (*Note*: Words in **bold** type are defined in the Glossary.)

Chapter 12

Activity Analysis: A Way of Thinking About Occupational Performance

Elizabeth Blesedell Crepeau

This chapter describes activity analysis, a way of thinking used by occupational therapy practitioners to understand activities, the performance components required to do them, and the cultural meanings typically ascribed to them. This analysis contributes to the clinical reasoning of occupational therapy practitioners and is the basis for the selection, adaptation, and grading of the activities used in occupational therapy intervention. When occupational therapy practitioners analyze activities, they typically focus on the task or activity level. Activities are goal-directed tasks that require skills and resources to meet personal and social needs. Thus activities can range from simple, such as tying our shoes or brushing our teeth, to complex, such as preparing a meal. Tasks and activities cluster together to support occupational roles. For example, a variety of activities, such as peeling potatoes, making salad, and cooking chicken, are involved in the activity of meal preparation that is part of the occupational role of family member. Although some have attempted to make a distinction between the terms tasks and activities (Trombly, 1995), there is no consensus in the field concerning this distinction (American Occupational Therapy Association [AOTA], 1995). Therefore, for the purpose of this chapter the terms tasks and activities will be used interchangeably.

Occupational therapy practitioners draw on their education, knowledge of activities, and clinical experience when analyzing activities (Neistadt, McCauley, Zecha, and Shannon, 1993). Their analysis is also based on access to particular activities and the degree to which they are willing to engage in trial and error or experimentation to understand activities more fully. Activity analysis is an aspect of clinical practice that is so automatic that it is often ignored or unappreciated. The vignette about Terry and Mrs. Munro in Chapter 9 demonstrates Terry's ability to quickly identify an appropriate activity when she discovered that Mrs. Munro was already bathed and dressed, activities she had planned to use to evaluate Mrs. Munro's safety and cognitive function. Because Mrs. Munro was being discharged, Terry needed to do this evaluation that day. So she scanned the room for substitute activities. Terry decided to use grooming, taking care of flowers, and washing a vase, as appropriate activities for Mrs. Munro's interests and Terry's evaluation goals. Terry's knowledge of the skills she wanted to evaluate and Mrs. Munro's interests, as well as her ability to quickly analyze the available activities, enabled her to conduct this evaluation despite the initial mix-up. Terry's account of this interaction treats the change in activities as an expected and usual part of her day as an occupational therapy practitioner. This shows how embedded activity analysis is in the clinical reasoning process.

Although there has been a call to make activity analysis an objective process, studies that have attempted to achieve this goal have demonstrated that the number of variables are so great that the goal of objectivity would be exceedingly difficult to achieve (Llorens, 1986; Neistadt et al., 1993; and Trombly, 1995). If the outcome of activity analysis is understanding the potential demands of an activity in relation to a particular person's performance problems, then objectivity is not so important. Rather, the understanding of the interaction between the person, the person's occupational performance problems, and the **performance context** is primary because it is through this understanding that the analysis becomes meaningful for that particular individual and occupational therapy intervention.

Activity analysis occurs at three levels: task-focused, theory-focused, and individual-focused. Task-focused activity analysis addresses (1) the typical methods and context of activity performance, (2) the range of skills involved in this performance, and (3) the various cultural meanings that might be ascribed to the activity. Students initially learn to analyze activity in this way. Occupational therapy practitioners may also think about activities from this perspective, sizing up new games, cooking gadgets, and other objects or activities for their therapeutic potential. Task-focused activity analysis pertains to the task itself, the skills required to do it, its cultural meaning, and therapeutic potential. Theory-focused activity analysis has a different perspective. Rather than examining the properties of an activity to understand its demands in general, theory-focused activity analysis examines these properties from a theoretical perspective. By using the principles of a particular **practice theory**, occupational therapy practitioners analyze activities as they think about performance problems addressed by this theory. The potential therapeutic intervention should be consistent with the theory and will likely entail grading and adapting activity. These two ways of analyzing activity can occur without a client, for they involve exploring and understanding the activity itself in relation to occupational therapy intervention.

In contrast, individual-focused activity analysis places the client in the foreground. It takes into account the particular person's interests, goals, abilities, and functional limitations, as well as his or her temporal and environmental performance contexts. These considerations shape the practitioner's efforts to help the client reach his or her goals through carefully designed intervention. The selection and design of the particular therapeutic activities are derived from the practitioner's understanding of the client, the task demands of the activities important to this client, and the relation between these activities and occupational therapy theories. This is a highly specific and contextualized way of thinking. Consequently, activity analysis, at least as it is typically learned by occupational therapy students, proceeds

from the more general task-focused and theory-focused perspectives, to the highly specific and contextualized individual-focused perspective. Figure 12-1 demonstrates the relation between these three perspectives with individual-focused activity analysis incorporating the previous two perspectives.

▼ TASK-FOCUSED ACTIVITY ANALYSIS

The goal of task-focused activity analysis is to understand as much as possible, about an activity including the particular skills required to do it competently and its relation to participation in the world at large (Cynkin, 1995). When you analyze activities from this perspective you will ask questions such as these. "What are the skills people generally use who do this activity in a typical way?" "What is the cultural meaning of this activity?" "How could this activity be used therapeutically?" By analyzing a wide range of activities, you will develop an appreciation of the skills required to participate in self-care, work, and play or leisure. You will also gain an appreciation of the relations between these activities and everyday life. It is this aspect of your knowledge of activities, their properties, and cultural meanings that you will draw on to suggest particular activities to clients.

Task-focused activity analysis is also a way of thinking about activities. It is that aspect of clinical reasoning that enables practitioners to identify quickly the demands of activities and to use them when working with clients. Terry used task-focused activity analysis when she scanned the room for possible activities for Mrs. Munro. Imagine her standing there, looking around Mrs. Munro's room and asking herself, "What is in this room that requires similar physical and cognitive skills as bathing and dressing."

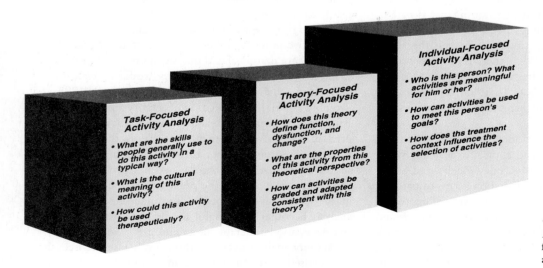

Figure 12-1. Task-focused, theory-focused, and individual-focused activity analysis

HISTORICAL NOTE
THE LONGSTANDING NEED FOR ACTIVITY ANALYSIS: GEORGE BARTON'S BELIEFS

Suzanne M. Peloquin

George Edward Barton, originator of the idea of founding a society to promote occupation as therapy, grasped the concept of activity analysis. He often used medical analogies to explain the therapeutic effects of occupation. He suggested that when Adam was cast from the Garden of Eden, he was given this divine prescription: "Work by the sweat of the brow" (Barton, 1915a).

More specifically, Barton thought that any medicine listed as a therapeutic agent in the *Materia Medica* had an occupational parallel. He explained that if a doctor might pre-scribe the leukotoxin benzol to a patient with leukemia, the occupational therapist could lead that same person to work in a canning factory where the fumes of hot benzine would have a similar effect (Barton, 1915b).

The specifics of Barton's analysis now seem quaint. The fact remains, however, that if an occupation is to be deemed therapeutic, it must withstand a rigorous analysis of its possible benefits. If the specifics are outdated, the concept endures. ■

Barton, G. E. (1915a). Occupational nursing. *Trained Nurse and Hospital Review, 54,* 138–140.
Barton, G. E. (1915b). Occupational therapy. *Trained Nurse and Hospital Review, 54,* 335–338.

Task-Focused Activity Analysis Format

The task-focused activity analysis format (Fig. 12-2) follows the organization of the third edition of the Uniform Terminology for Occupational Therapy (AOTA, 1994). The uniform terminology is designed to provide a common language for the profession and is divided into three interrelated parts: performance areas, performance components, and performance contexts. Task-focused activity analysis addresses the performance components and the environmental aspect of performance contexts of the uniform terminology. Performance components fall into three broad categories: (1) sensorimotor, (2) cognitive integrative and cognitive, and (3) psychosocial skills and psychological. Performance components are the skills we use to engage in the performance areas of activities of daily living (ADL), work and productive activities, and play or leisure activities (AOTA, 1994). When we bathe, dress, use a computer, or play tennis, we draw on the performance component skills needed to do each particular activity. The environmental aspects of performance contexts relate to the physical, social, and cultural world in which the individual lives. The following sections provide instructions for using this format.

Task Description

Task-focused activity analysis begins with task description. This description takes into account all aspects of doing the activity from the initial planning to cleaning up. Use steps 1 through 6 of Figure 12-2, to begin this descriptive process. By completing these steps, you are beginning to engage in the exploration of this activity, including its meaning, its performance context, and the steps used to complete the activity.

STEP 1: DESCRIBE THE ACTIVITY
Describe this activity in one or two sentences.

STEP 2: DESCRIBE THE TYPICAL AGE RANGE OF PEOPLE WHO ENGAGE IN THIS ACTIVITY
Many activities have developmental components that are related to the skills required to do the activity as well as the social and cultural meaning of the activity. For example, Go Fish and Concentration are very elementary card games for children, whereas Bridge requires the higher levels of cognitive and psychosocial abilities typical of adults. The social and cultural meanings of the activity also influence the typical age range. Go Fish has a childish connotation, and it is unlikely that adults would choose to play this game except when playing with children. In contrast, Yatzee is also a game appropriate for children, but is more age-neutral and may be played by age-segregated or intergenerational groups. A knowledge of the typical age range for a particular activity enables you to make some initial judgments about its appropriateness for your clients.

STEP 3: DESCRIBE THE ENVIRONMENTAL ASPECTS OF THE PERFORMANCE CONTEXT
a. *Physical:* Describe the physical context in which this activity will be analyzed. Be specific. Describe the arrangement of furniture, the placement of equipment, the lighting, the level of noise, and other distractions that will be present.
b. *Social:* Describe the other persons who will be present. Describe the social roles of the persons present in relation to the activity. Describe the behavioral expectations for this context. For example, normative behavior in a classroom is very different from behavior at a basketball game.

1. Briefly (one or two sentences) describe the activity. . . . .
. . . .
. . . .
. . . .
. . . .

2. Describe the typical age range of people who engage in this
activity
. . . .

3. Describe the environmental aspects of the performance context in which the activity is being
analyzed.
   a. physical. . . . .

   b. social. . . . .
      . . . .
   c. cultural . . . .
      . . . .
4. List the supplies and equipment needed to carry out the activity . . . .
. . . .
. . . .
. . . .

5. Describe the safety hazards inherent in this activity . . . .
. . . .
. . . .
. . . .

6. List the sequential steps of the activity. Depending upon the activity there may be 10 to 20
steps. Each step should not take more than two sentences to explain. . . . .
. . . .
. . . .
. . . .

7. Summary of activity analysis of performance components. Review the summaries of the performance components.
   a. Write a paragraph identifying and describing the major performance components needed
      for this activity.
   b. Write a paragraph identifying and describing the performance components least needed
      for this activity.
8. Describe how to grade and adapt this activity.
   a. List and describe approximately 6 to 10 performance components that could be devel-
      oped using this activity. . . . .
      . . . .
   b. Select two performance components from this list. For each performance component, de-
      scribe how this activity could be graded to increase function. *Note:* You will have a sepa-
      rate description for each performance component. . . . .
      . . . .
   c. Select two additional performance components. For each performance component, de-
      scribe how this activity could be graded to enable someone to continue to perform this ac-
      tivity despite declining function. . . . .
      . . . .
   d. Select two additional performance components. For each performance component, de-
      scribe how this activity could be adapted for someone with a stable disability. . . . .
      . . . .

◄

Figure 12-2. Task-focused activity analysis format.

c. *Cultural:* Any activity can have a wide range of meanings. For example, cooking in our culture may be viewed from a nutritional–utilitarian perspective, as an opportunity to be creative, or as an opportunity to care for others. The context contributes to these different interpretations. At a symbolic level, cooking may represent nurturance and love. You should describe as many of the potential meanings of the activity you are analyzing as possible, recognizing that it is virtually impossible to identify all of the meanings different persons may attribute to a single activity. As you work with clients, your appreciation for the variety of meanings possible for a particular activity will grow.

STEP 4: LIST SUPPLIES AND EQUIPMENT NEEDED TO CARRY OUT THE ACTIVITY

Ingredients for a recipe, or the paper, paint, and glue for a collage, are supplies. Small tools such as scissors, knitting needles, and measuring cups are also considered supplies because they may need to be replaced periodically. In other words, supplies are relatively inexpensive items that may be either consumed, worn out, broken, or lost during the activity. In contrast, equipment includes items that are replaced infrequently because they are so expensive. Stoves, sewing machines, games, and compact disc (CD) players are examples of equipment.

STEP 5: DESCRIBE THE SAFETY HAZARDS INHERENT IN THIS ACTIVITY

Describe the safety hazards for persons without impaired function. Consider developmental issues, such as the use of scissors or toxic substances, with small children. Describe potential safety hazards that might be present for persons with such disabilities as impaired sensation, movement, cognition, or judgment. Are there special considerations you would need to take with clients who are deemed to be suicide risks or dangerous to others?

STEP 6: LIST THE SEQUENTIAL STEPS OF THE ACTIVITY

Outline these steps, including all of the important components of the activity. The number of steps should be limited to 10 to 20 for most activities. Be sure to include the steps required for preparation and clean up. For example, cooking involves assembling the ingredients, utensils, and recipe, through the final steps of cleaning up the kitchen. This list should describe how the activity will be accomplished in the performance context in which it is being analyzed.

Activity Analysis of Performance Components

In Steps 1 through 6 you described the activity and the environmental aspect of the performance context. In Step 7, you will identify the most essential and least essential performance components needed for this activity. To do so you should review the steps of the activity in relation to the performance components listed in the following. Identify the performance components necessary for each step of the activity. When you are finished, summarize your findings by responding to the questions listed in step 7 of Figure 12-2.

The following text defines each performance component and poses analysis questions for each. Please note, all italicized material is directly quoted from the Uniform Terminology (AOTA, 1994, pp. 1047–1054) (Copyright 1994 by the American Occupational Therapy Association, Inc. Reprinted with permission.)

SENSORIMOTOR: THE ABILITY TO RECEIVE INPUT, PROCESS INFORMATION, AND PRODUCE OUTPUT (AOTA, 1994, P. 1052).

In this definition of sensorimotor, "receive input" refers to information from the senses; "process information" refers to the analysis of sensory information; "produce output" refers to muscle contractions that result in movement, speech, or nonverbal communication. The sensorimotor component has three subcomponents: sensory, neuromusculoskeletal, and motor.

Sensory

The sensory component of this process includes sensory awareness and sensory processing. The perceptual component involves recognition and interpretation of sensory stimuli.

Sensory Awareness: Receiving and differentiating sensory stimuli. At the awareness level the basic requirement is intact sensory receptors. Sensory awareness involves being able to see, hear, taste, and smell. It also involves less obvious senses such as the sense of touch, balance, and joint movement.

▶ **Think about** the activity you are analyzing. What senses are necessary for engagement in this activity? For example, what parts of the activity require vision, hearing, or other?

Sensory Processing: Interpreting sensory stimuli. Sensory processing involves the ability to interpret or make meaning from the incoming sensory stimuli so that they can be responded to in an appropriate way. This processing includes the interpretation of a variety of sensory stimuli including tactile, proprioceptive, visual, auditory, or other.

Tactile: Interpreting light touch, pressure, temperature, pain, and vibration through skin contact/receptors. The tactile sense is especially important during infancy, for it is through tactile exploration that children learn about the world around them (Parham & Mallioux, 1996). It continues to be important throughout the life span for the individual to receive feedback from the environment.

Proprioceptive: Interpreting stimuli originating in muscles, joints, and other internal tissues that give information about the position of one body part in relation to another. Proprioception enables us to understand the position of our body parts when we are sitting in a chair reading or standing at the sink washing dishes. Proprioception or awareness of position is closely connected to kinesthesia which is the awareness and interpretation of joint motion.

Vestibular: Interpreting stimuli from the inner ear receptors regarding head position and movement. The vestibular system is critical for the maintenance of balance and position sense (Anderson, 1994). It contributes to our ability to move in and through our world by giving us feedback about our position in space (Snow, 1996).

Visual: Interpreting stimuli through the eyes, including peripheral vision and acuity, and awareness of color and pattern. Vision enables us to interpret the world around us, most especially the relations between ourselves and objects in our environment (Snow, 1996).

Auditory: Interpreting and localizing sounds, and discriminating background sounds. The auditory system enables us to tell the difference between various sounds and to understand the meaning of sounds (Snow, 1996). It is through our ability to localize sound that we know where to go if someone is calling us from another room in the house and to determine which family member is calling.

Gustatory: Interpreting tastes. Taste is a multisensory process that takes place through receptors on the tongue, soft palate, and upper part of the throat (Corsini, 1994). Our sense of taste lends pleasure to our lives as we eat the foods we enjoy.

Olfactory: Interpreting odors. The ability to smell is dependent on receptors in the nose and contributes to our sense of taste. It makes an important contribution to personal safety, for example, the ability to smell smoke or food that has spoiled.

▶ **Think about** the activity you are analyzing. What sensory processing components are necessary for engagement in this activity? For example, what parts of the activity require proprioception, olfaction, and so on?

Perceptual Processing: Organizing sensory input into meaningful patterns. Perception serves as the basis for understanding the world around us and for learning. It involves recognition and interpretation of sensory stimuli (Anderson, 1994).

Stereognosis: Identifying objects through proprioception, cognition, and the sense of touch. Stereognosis is that perceptual process that enables us to reach into our coat pockets to pull out our car keys. This entails being able to discriminate between the car keys and any other small objects that might be in our pockets.

Kinesthesia: Identifying the excursion and direction of joint movement. This ability to interpret joint motion is closely linked to proprioceptive (interpretation of position) and vestibular (balance) processes which combine with kinesthesia to enable us to move effectively and efficiently (Pedretti, 1996).

Pain Response: Interpreting noxious stimuli. Pain is a subjective process that varies from individual to individual (Anderson, 1994).

Body Scheme: Acquiring an internal awareness of the body and the relations of body parts to each other. During the first 2 years of life children learn to differentiate between themselves and the world around them (Anderson, 1994). This perception of the body and the relation of body parts to each other is necessary before we can understand the relation between ourselves and the objects in the world around us. The ability to dress is dependent in part on an intact body scheme.

Right–Left Discrimination: Differentiating one side from the other. This perceptual skill entails understanding right from left in relation to ourselves and to our external world. Right–left discrimination is necessary for following directions and, again, contributes to our ability to dress ourselves (Quintana, 1995).

Form Constancy: Recognizing forms and objects as the same in various environments, positions, and sizes. This ability enables us to recognize a mug as a mug, regardless of its shape, size, and color. Form constancy is important in reading because it enables us to read a particular letter as that letter, regardless of how it is printed or written. Consequently, form constancy enables us to understand that an "*A*," "a," and "A" are all "A's" (Schneck, 1996).

Position in Space: Determining the spatial relation of figures and objects to self or other forms and objects. This perceptual skill entails understanding such concepts as up and down, over and under, and so forth, and being able to interpret them in relation to ourselves and between objects (Quintana, 1995). This ability enables us to understand that a ball has rolled under the table. It also contributes to our ability to interpret a group of letters as a word, and words as a sentence (Schneck, 1996), as well as to dress and to navigate through a crowded space (Quintana, 1995).

Visual-Closure: Identifying forms or objects from incomplete presentations. This enables us to understand that a book is a book, even if we only see its spine on the shelf.

Figure Ground: Differentiating between foreground and background from objects. No matter what we do we need to be able to focus on the most pertinent aspects of the external environment. This entails focusing on the figure, or the object or objects that are essential for what we are doing and attending less to other aspects of the environment that we put in the background. This is a fluid process, in that we can shift our attention and, consequently, shift what has been a "figure" to the background and visa versa (Schneck, 1996). Figure ground abilities enable us to focus on the road when we are driving and to ignore other aspects of the environment that are not essential for our safety. This ability may also be applied to hearing and enables us to listen to a particular conversation in a room filled with other people speaking.

Depth Perception: Determining the relative difference between objects, figures, or landmarks and the observer. This is the perceptual ability we use to go up and down stairs and, when we drive, to determine how far oncoming cars are from us before we turn across traffic. Consequently, this ability contributes to our ability to move through space effectively and safely (Schneck, 1996).

Spatial Relations: Determining the position of objects relative to each other. This ability involves understanding the relation between objects in the environment and ourselves. It is closely related to the abilities described in position in space and contributes to activities such as moving through space and dressing. Because transferring requires judging the distance between objects (ie, the distance between a wheelchair and toilet), it is a necessary perceptual skill for safe transfers (Quintana, 1995).

Topographical Orientation: Determining the location of objects and setting and the route to the location. To find our way from one place to another we need to construct a cognitive map of the environment (Schneck, 1996). This entails being able to envision the relations between places in the environment and how to get from one place to another. This perceptual ability is called into play when we move from one room to another in our homes, find a store in the mall, or travel to a different part of our town or city.

▶ **Think about** the activity you are analyzing. What perceptual components are necessary for engagement in this activity? For example, what parts of the activity require form constancy, spatial relations, and such?

Neuromusculoskeletal

The neuromusculoskeletal component pertains to biomechanical aspects of movement.

Reflex: Eliciting an involuntary muscle response by sensory input. Reflexes occur immediately after the stimulus, without any voluntary action on the part of the individual (Anderson, 1994).

Range of Motion: Moving body parts through an arc. This entails the maximum movement through all the planes of movement possible for any given joint.

Muscle Tone: Demonstrating a degree of tension or resistance in a muscle at rest and in response to stretch. Muscle tone is the state of balanced tension that exists in intact muscles, so that when the muscle is stretched it offers some resistance, but not enough to impede movement. Muscle tone provides stability for joints that are needed to maintain position and perform smooth, controlled movement (Undzis, Zoltan, & Pedretti, 1996).

Strength: Demonstrating a degree of muscle power when movement is resisted, as with objects or gravity. Muscle strength is required to produce and control movement, as well as to maintain posture (Zemke, 1995).

Endurance: Sustaining cardiac, pulmonary, and musculoskeletal exertion over time. Endurance enables us to perform activities for an extended time. It is related to strength in that weak muscles also tend to have lower levels of endurance (Anderson, 1994).

Postural Control: Using righting and equilibrium adjustments to maintain balance during functional movements. This is a dynamic process that provides a stable posture from which skilled movement can occur. For example, bending over to pick something from the floor requires a stable base of support, which shifts as we bend over and straighten up. Being able to do this without falling is a characteristic of postural control.

Postural Alignment: Maintaining biomechanical integrity among body parts. The alignment of joints is necessary to maintain good posture and body mechanics. Poor postural alignment may occur in work settings that require persons to work in awkward positions. These awkward working positions may lead to repetitive trauma injuries such as back strain.

Soft Tissue Integrity: Maintaining anatomical and physiological condition of interstitial tissue and skin. Skin breakdown or decubitus ulcers, resulting from prolonged pressure on the skin, may occur in persons who cannot move well enough to change positions frequently.

▶ **Think about** the activity you are analyzing. What neuromusculoskeletal components are necessary for engagement in this activity? For example, what parts of the activity require strength, postural control, and such?

Motor

The motor component concerns the quality of movement.

Gross Coordination: Using large muscle groups for controlled, goal directed movements. Coordinated movement is smooth, accurate, and seemingly effortless. Gross coordination involves large muscle groups, typically walking, running, and many sports and activities of daily living involve gross coordination.

Crossing the Midline: Moving limbs and eyes across the midsagittal plane of the body. The ability to cross the midline is necessary to engage in many activities requiring skilled movement on the opposite side of the body. For example, it is necessary to cross the midline to put on a jacket or shirt, to button the cuffs of long sleeves, and so forth.

Laterality: Using a preferred unilateral body part for activities requiring a high level of skill. Laterality refers to the preference most people have for using either the right or left hand for highly skilled activities, such as writing and eating.

Bilateral Integration: Coordinating both body sides during activity. Bilateral integration is important for any activity that typically requires the use of both hands or feet (eg, rowing a boat or walking).

Motor Control: Using the body in functional and versatile movement patterns. Motor control is dynamic, goal-directed movement that reflects the individual's preferred patterns of movement (Mathiowetz & Haugen, 1995).

Praxis: Conceiving and planning a new motor act in response to an environmental demand. Praxis entails the mental activities of planning actions. In other words, it is the ability to know that to comb our hair we have to hold a comb with the teeth in position to move through our hair, raise an arm repeatedly, and move the comb through our hair until it is styled in a way that is satisfactory (Quintana, 1995).

Fine Coordination and Dexterity: Using small muscle groups for controlled movements, particularly object manipulation. Fine coordination involves skilled hand use, most especially isolated use of the fingers (Mathiowetz & Haugen, 1995). Sewing, woodworking, playing the piano, buttoning buttons, and many kitchen activities require a high level of dexterity.

Oral–Motor Control: Coordinating oropharyngeal musculature for controlled movements. Oral motor control is needed for eating and speaking.

▶ **Think about** the activity you are analyzing. What motor skills are necessary for engagement in this activity? For example, what parts of the activity require motor control, fine coordination, or other like activities?

Summary of the Sensorimotor Components

List the five most essential sensorimotor skills required by this activity. Explain what parts of the activity require each of these skills.

List the five least essential sensorimotor skills required by this activity. Explain what parts of the activity require each of these skills.

COGNITIVE INTEGRATION AND COGNITIVE COMPONENTS. THE ABILITY TO USE HIGHER BRAIN FUNCTIONS (AOTA, 1994, P. 1053).

Cognitive function pertains to the intellectual processes that enable people to attend to a task, reason, and problem solve.

Level of Arousal: Demonstrating alertness and responsiveness to environmental stimuli.

Responding to stimuli is necessary for engagement in any form of activity.

Orientation: Identifying person, place, time, and situation.

Being oriented enables us to function in our current environment or adapt to a new one (Anderson, 1994).

Recognition: Identifying familiar faces, objects, and other previously presented materials.

Recognition is necessary to interact with others, to find tools and equipment, and other such activities.

Attention Span: Focusing on a task over time.

This entails readiness to stay focused on a particular topic or activity. It is necessary for task completion and efficient performance.

Initiation of Activity: Starting a physical or mental activity.

We take starting an activity for granted; however, persons with frontal lobe or basal ganglia damage, or depression may not be able to start activities on their own. These persons will need practitioner cues to initiate activity.

Termination of Activity: Stopping a physical or mental activity.

This entails understanding when it is appropriate to stop an activity. Clients with frontal lobe damage may repeat activities or given steps of an activity over and over without stopping. For example, continuing to wipe a plate even when it is completely dry. This behavior is called perseveration. Clients who perseverate will need practitioner cues to stop one behavior and move on to another.

Memory: Recalling information after brief or long periods of time.

Memory involves the retrieval of information that is learned, as well as experiences and feelings. Some memory is very short-term such as remembering the seven digits of a phone number long enough to write it down. Other memories are very long-term such as the recollections of an 80-year-old woman about her childhood.

Sequencing: Placing information, concepts, and actions in order.

Sequencing is a necessary cognitive skill for many activities. For example, it is called into play for even the most basic of dressing skills, knowing that underwear goes on before outerwear, and socks before shoes.

Categorization: Identifying similarities of and differences among pieces of environmental information.

This skill is important for activities such as grocery shopping for which we need to see both how objects are similar (eg, two different brands of ketchup are still ketchup despite their different brand names) and how they are different (eg, price, amount of fat, sugar, or salt in the different brands).

Concept Formation: Organizing a variety of information to form thoughts and ideas.

For example, colors and shapes are concepts, as are our ideas about what is true, right, and good. Concepts aid in categorization, because they form a basis for clustering similar things together. For example, the concepts of color, car, and shape contribute to distinguishing cars from trucks, and then clustering cars in subgroups by color and shape (sedans, vans, convertibles).

Spatial Operations: Mentally manipulating the position of objects in various relationships.

This skill is important for activities, such as parking a car in a parking lot, for which you need to visualize how close your car will come to other vehicles throughout the parking process, before you begin to park. This skill requires good spatial relations abilities.

Problem Solving: Recognizing a problem, defining a problem, identifying alternative plans, selecting a plan, organizing steps in a plan, implementing a plan, and evaluating the outcome.

We use our problem-solving abilities any time we engage in a new activity, or encounter a difficulty in a familiar one. When we encounter a new situation, our ability to problem solve enables us to recognize possible solutions and try them out. Sometimes this is very organized, as the definition implies, at other times we may use a trial and error method to see which of a number of options is the most appropriate solution.

Learning: Acquiring new concepts and behaviors.

We learn by studying new concepts or ideas, through practice, and by direct experience. We know that someone has learned something when their behavior has changed, they can do something that they had not done before or explain something they previously had not understood. Learning can be demonstrated verbally, motorically, and through attitudes that are demonstrated behaviorally.

Generalization: Applying previously learned concepts and behaviors to a variety of new situations.

This is a form of categorization in which concepts or behaviors are clustered together into a general rule which then can be applied to a variety of different situations. If we stay at a concrete or specific level, what we learn in one situation cannot be used in a different situation. For example, knowing how to prune roses requires knowledge of how the plant grows and the best places on the stem to prune. Other plants and shrubs have similar pruning needs. If we were not able to generalize, we would fail to recognize the common elements between different shrubs and would need to approach pruning each as a new learning experience.

▶ **Think about** the activity you are analyzing. What cognitive integrative and cognitive are necessary for engagement in this activity? For example, what parts of the activity require memory, problem solving, and so forth?

Summary of the Cognitive Integrative and Cognitive Components

List the five most essential cognitive integrative and cognitive performance components required by this activity. Explain what parts of the activity require each of these skills.

List the five least essential cognitive integrative and cognitive performance components required by this activity. Explain what parts of the activity require each of these skills.

PSYCHOSOCIAL SKILLS AND PSYCHOLOGICAL COMPONENTS: THE ABILITY TO INTERACT IN SOCIETY AND TO PROCESS EMOTIONS (AOTA, 1994, P. 1054).

These components pertain to the interaction between individuals and the social environment in which they live. It focuses especially on attitudes and motivation and the resulting behavior. These performance components are highly individualistic and depend on the individual's culture, values, and beliefs. For the purpose of task-focused activity analysis it is useful to think about the possible meanings that could be attributed to this activity, even though they may not apply to everyone.

Psychological

Psychological components refer to the mental, motivational, and behavioral characteristics of an individual or a group.

Values: Identifying ideas or beliefs that are important to self and others. These ideas and beliefs are culturally determined and are shared by members of a group. For example the American culture values independence and autonomy, whereas other cultures value interdependence more highly (see Chap. 6). Values also influence our choice of activities because they reflect what we feel is important in our lives (Kielhofner, Borell, Burke, Helfrich, and Nygård, 1995).

Interests: Identifying mental or physical activities that create pleasure and maintain attention. We want to engage in activities that provide us with enjoyment and pleasure; that is, those activities in which we have an interest (Kielhofner, Borell, Burke, Helfrich, and Nygård, 1995).

Self-Concept: Developing the value of the physical, emotional, and sexual self. The self-concept entails our image of ourselves, one that we construct through our experience in the world. This is derived from our assessment of our actions as well as feedback from others.

▶ **Think about** the activity you are analyzing. What values and interests might be expressed through these activities? What opportunities for feedback about performance exists to influence the self-concept?

Social

The social performance component addresses skills that are required to live in a variety of groups such as families and organizations.

Role Performance: Identifying, maintaining, and balancing functions one assumes or acquires in society (eg, worker student, parent, friend, religious participant. Roles are normative behaviors that are expected of a group of individuals such as mothers, teachers, siblings, workers, and others. These roles are socially defined and tend to be relatively stable (Stephan and Stephan, 1985). As we enter new roles we must acquire the behavior expected of that role. This is often accomplished through play or practice (Mead, 1934).

Social Conduct: Interacting by using manners, personal space, eye contact, gestures, active listening, and self-expression appropriate to one's environment. Social conduct entails understanding the expectations of the social situation and modifying our way of interacting to be suitable for that situation. Being able to "read" subtle social situations enables us to avoid awkwardness and conflict. For example, knowing when to initiate a conversation with another person involves reading a number of verbal and nonverbal cues (Goffman, 1967).

Interpersonal Skills: Using verbal and nonverbal communication to interact in a variety of settings. Interpersonal skills involve knowing how to talk to other people and interact in different settings. In contrast, social conduct is the ability to choose the right behavior in a particular social situation (Goffman, 1967).

Self-Expression: Using a variety of styles and skills to express thoughts, feelings, and needs. Self-expression involves the flexibility to change the way we express ourselves to be consistent with the way we are thinking and feeling. In other words, to express anger when we are feeling it, to seek assistance when we need it.

▶ **Think about** the activity you are analyzing. What social skills are necessary for engagement in this activity? For example, what parts of the activity require interpersonal skills, self-expression, or others?

Self-Management

Self-management refers to those abilities that enable us to accomplish our goals, despite stress in our lives.

Coping Skills: Identifying and managing stress and related factors. When we are able to adapt and manage our daily lives, despite stressors such as illness, family, or financial problems, we are said to have the ability "to cope." Coping also refers to the actions we may take in an attempt to avoid or diminish the effect of stressors (Pearlin, 1989). For example, those who save and avoid excessive debt reduce the financial stress of unemployment or other unexpected financial losses. Although coping behavior is an individual characteristic, it is to some extent learned from others (Pearlin).

Time Management: Planning and participating in a balance of self-care, work, leisure, and rest activities to promote satisfaction and health. Time management involves knowing how to use our time to achieve our goals, to organize tasks so that they can be accomplished in a way that is satisfying to ourselves and meets our obligations to others. Occupational therapy practitioners are concerned with the balancing of these activities so that there is adequate time for both obligatory tasks, such as self-care and work, and for tasks and activities that are perceived to be related to leisure and play.

Self-Control: Modifying one's own behavior in response to environmental needs, demands, constraints, personal aspirations, and feedback from others. Self-control entails the management of our behavior so that it is appropriate to the social situation. It is called on most dramatically when we feel strong emotions that may not be appropriate to express with the full range of emotions that we are feeling. In other words, if we are very angry at someone, it is inappropriate to have the temper tantrum our 2-year-old selves would like to have.

▶ **Think about** the activity you are analyzing. What self-management skills are necessary for engagement in this activity? For example, what parts of the activity require time management, self-control, or other attributes?

Summary of the Psychosocial Skills and Psychological Components

List the five most essential psychosocial skills and psychological performance components required by this activity. Explain what parts of the activity require each of these skills.

List the five least essential psychosocial skills and psychological performance components required by this activity. Explain what parts of the activity require each of these skills.

Summary of Performance Components

Summarize your analysis in Step 7 of Figure 12-2 by identifying the most essential and least essential performance components needed for this activity. To do this, you should review your summaries of the performance components needed for the different steps of the activity. You have now completed an initial analysis of an activity. This first level of description addresses a single way of doing this activity. However, because we are all individuals, we perform even the simplest of tasks in slightly different ways. One way to discover this is to watch people put on their jackets, tie their shoes, or write. The variation in the ways of doing even these simple tasks is often very surprising. Consequently, task-focused activity analysis cannot begin to describe the full range of possibilities for either the methods or the meanings of the activity. However, you can begin to develop an idea of the task demands of an activity by analyzing it from one perspective and then exploring the potential variations later.

Grading and Adapting Activity

Step 8 of the Task-Focused Activity Analysis Format (see Fig. 12-2) asks you to think about grading and adapting the activity you are analyzing. Grading and adapting activity is an essential aspect of occupational therapy practice, for it is through grading and adapting activity that we bring about therapeutic change or support declining function. The grading of an activity involves sequentially increasing or decreasing the demands of the activity over time to stimulate improvement in the client's function or to respond to diminishing functional capacity. For example, by selectively increasing the resistance and repetitions for particular muscle groups using functional activities, occupational therapy practitioners increase muscle strength and endurance. Conversely, cooking can be graded to be less cognitively demanding by changing the type of food prepared to require fewer steps and less attention to detail. The activity of making pudding can be graded from a complicated recipe for custard, to packaged cooked pudding, to instant pudding, to premade pudding that only has to be opened.

Activity adaptation is the process of changing tasks and activities to promote independent function. That is, the activity is graded down to be easier physically, cognitive, or otherwise. Adaptation is especially appropriate for persons with performance problems that are not likely to improve any further (eg, a person with a spinal cord injury who is approaching discharge from occupational therapy or someone with a degenerative condition). Adaptation entails changing the task demands of the activity by making it simpler cognitively, reducing the amount of physical skill or the endurance required to do it. Adaptations may also involve adaptive equipment or changes in the environment to enable independent function, elimination of activities, the assistance of another person, or some combination thereof. In degenerative conditions, these adaptations may need to be made repeatedly. Conditions such as acquired immunodeficiency syndrome (AIDS) or cancer, and chronic illnesses, such as arthritis, may require grading on a daily basis to accommodate the fluctuating levels of function typical of these illnesses. (See Fig. 12-2 for the steps to follow for grading and adapting activity).

▼ THEORY-FOCUSED ACTIVITY ANALYSIS

Students also learn about occupational therapy theories and how to plan treatment from the perspective of particular practice theories (see Chap. 22). The particular practice theory or theories you select is influenced by the problems of the persons you are treating, your professional beliefs, and the philosophic perspective of your department or organization. In some instances you may combine several theories to provide a broader approach to your clients' problems.

Each theory shapes your view of function, dysfunction, and the use of activity to enable clients to improve their occupational performance. This understanding will direct you to the particular evaluation and intervention strategies of that theory. For example, motor performance is an important aspect of occupational therapy intervention. From a

---

RESEARCH NOTE
RESEARCH ABOUT ACTIVITY, ITS MEANINGS AND SKILLS—IS A PRIORITY FOR THE PROFESSION

Kenneth J. Ottenbacher

In a previous edition of this text, Simon (1993) wrote:

The scope and variety of activities in life allow for the idiosyncratic growth of a person and define who that person is by virtue of their choice of activities. Inherent in the pursuit of an activity is the concept of doing. Engaging in activity is not a passive act. One must make choices, use body parts, problem-solve, interact with others or the physical environment, and react to the outcome of success, failure, or perhaps frustration and anxiety (p. 282).

The day-to-day practice of occupational therapy reflects that our activities, behaviors, and the products of our occupations combine to give us a sense of who we are and help define us as social beings. Each of the activity-based functions identified by Hopkins and Smith (1983) represents important areas of research for occupational therapy. Research on activity begins with *activity analysis,* which was defined by Mosey (1981) as the process of determining the component parts of an activity and the skills necessary for completing the activity. The activity-based functions identified by Simon (1993) are essential components of occupational therapy practice and represent areas of high research priority. ■

Simon, C. J. (1993). Use of activity analysis. In H. L. Hopkins and H. D. Smith (Eds.), *Willard and Spackman's occupational therapy* (8th ed., pp. 281–291.). Philadelphia: J. B. Lippincott.
Mosey, A. C. (1981). *Configuration of a profession.* New York: Raven.

biomechanical theoretical perspective, motor performance is linked to strength and range of motion. Practitioners operating within this theoretical perspective bring about improvement by designing activities to improve strength through greater resistance to motion or increasing repetitions of the desired motion. Practitioners using the multi-context theoretical perspective for adults with brain injury are also concerned about movement; however, here, their concern is not with strength or range of motion, but with the complexity of the movement patterns. From this theoretical perspective activities would be graded from simple, overlearned, and repetitive movements to activities that required more complex movement patterns and greater motor planning (see Chap. 26, Section 4).

The theories you use will influence the way you grade or adapt activity. Grading and adaptation are processes designed to produce therapeutic change or promote function. Within a particular treatment session, grading and adaptation are called on by the need to constantly gauge the client's response to the intervention. Is the activity at the right level to create the appropriate challenge for the individual? Does it need to be graded to be easier or harder? For examples of theory-focused activity analysis, see Tables 20-5 through 20-8 in Chapter 20, Section 6.

Summary of Theory-Focused Activity Analysis

How does this theory define function, dysfunction, and change?

How does this theory define occupational performance components differently from the uniform terminology (AOTA, 1994)?

How can activities be graded and adapted consistent with this theory?

How do multiple frames of reference relate to each other? Are there areas of reinforcement or conflict that will influence the use of activity within a treatment session?

▼ INDIVIDUAL-FOCUSED ACTIVITY ANALYSIS

Individual-focused activity analysis integrates your knowledge of activities and their therapeutic properties to meet the goals of your client. Rather than being centered on the activity itself, analysis at this level focuses on the client. The client's goals, interests, strengths, needs, and performance context, all are central to this process. Consequently, task-focused and theory-focused activity analysis is embedded in the narrative, scientific, and pragmatic components of clinical reasoning.

The narrative component of the clinical reasoning process is based on developing an understanding of the client's goals, interests, occupational roles, and pattern of activities,

and how these have been influenced by his or her functional problems (Mattingly, 1994). This relates directly to the performance components this individual uses or needs to successfully perform valued activities to fulfill his or her life goals within home, work, and leisure environments. Task-focused activity analysis contributes to your understanding of the typical demands of many activities. This enables you to develop an initial image of this person as an occupational being.

Scientific reasoning influences the evaluation of the client's performance problems and the development of plans to ameliorate these problems. Scientific reasoning draws on your understanding of activities (task-focused activity analysis) and how to use activities to bring about therapeutic change (theory-focused activity analysis). Your understanding of the disease or disability and its functional implications combines with these activity analysis skills to assist you in developing ways of treating your clients.

Finally, pragmatic reasoning is influenced by the context of the treatment setting, such as the physical setting, anticipated number of treatment sessions allowed, and reimbursement issues. These pragmatic issues create the range of activities available for use in therapy. For example, a well-supplied clinic and unlimited money provide options that may not be available in other settings. Pragmatics will also come into play as you use your analytic skills to work with clients to design new ways of performing a valued activity within the anticipated environment. The particular characteristics of this environment will influence the options with which you and the client have to work. You and the client are likely to try the activity in a variety of ways until the best way to do the activity is found. For example, bathroom adaptations may be needed to enable a person to return home. Although many standard adaptations are known, their applicability to a particular client and context must be tried to be sure that they work in the particular situation. This involves detailed analysis of the problem and trying solutions until the most appropriate one is found.

All of these factors influenced Terry's selection of activities in the vignette described earlier in this chapter. Activity analysis was that process which enabled her to focus on Mrs. Munro's goal of returning home and to select activities from the hospital room that were appropriate for Mrs. Munro. The following questions, adapted from Chapter 9, are designed to address the individual-focused activity analysis as it is embedded in the clinical reasoning process.

Summary of Individual-Focused Activity Analysis

Narrative

What activities are most important to this person?

How have they been influenced by his or her functional problems?

Which of the activities listed in the foregoing could be used in occupational therapy intervention?

Scientific

What theory will be appropriate to evaluate and treat this problem?

How does this theory define function, dysfunction, change?

How does this theory categorize occupational performance components? What skills does the client have relative to these performance components? What deficits?

How can activities be graded or adapted within this theory?

For multiple theories, how do they relate to each other? Are there areas of conflict that would influence the use of activity within a treatment session?

Pragmatic

What resources are available in the treatment context?

What resources will the client have to draw on after discharge?

What constraints exist in the treatment context and the client's expected environment?

Summary

Based on this analysis what activities would be most appropriate to use for treatment with this individual. How might these activities be graded and adapted?

►CONCLUSION

This chapter has described activity analysis as a cognitive process that occupational therapy practitioners use every day. It involves a way of thinking about activities that entails (1) understanding their general properties, (2) understanding how to use them to bring about therapeutic change from the perspective of a variety of practice theories, and (3) understanding how to use activities to achieve client-centered goals. Learning how to analyze activity begins early in occupational therapy education at the task and theory-focused levels. Fieldwork and professional practice further develop and refine these skills as practitioners use them with their clients.

► REFERENCES

American Occupational Therapy Association (AOTA). (1994). Uniform terminology for occupational therapy. *American Journal of Occupational Therapy, 48*, 1047–1054.

American Occupational Therapy Association. (1995). Position Paper: Occupation. *American Journal of Occupational Therapy, 49*, 1015–1018.

Anderson, K. N. (Ed.). (1994). *Mosby's medical, nursing & allied health dictionary* (4th ed.). St. Louis: Mosby.

Corsini. R. J. (Ed.). (1994). *Encyclopedia of psychology* (2nd ed.). New York: John Wiley & Sons.

Cynkin, S. (1995). Activities. In C. B. Royeen (Ed.), *The practice of the future: Putting occupation back into therapy: AOTA self-study series* (Module 7). Rockville, MD: American Occupational Therapy Association.

Goffman, E. (1967). *Interaction ritual: Essays on face-to-face behavior.* New York: Pantheon.

Kielhofner, G., Borell, L., Burke, J., Helfrich, C., & Nygård, L. (1995). Volition subsystem. In G. Kielhofner (Ed.), *A model of human occupation: Theory and application* (2nd. ed., pp. 39–42). Baltimore: Williams & Wilkins.

Llorens, L. A. (1986). Activity analysis: Agreement among factors in a sensory processing model. *American Journal of Occupational Therapy, 40*, 103–110.

Mathiowetz, V., & Haugen, J. B. (1995). Evaluation of motor behavior: Traditional and contemporary views. In C. A. Trombly (Ed.), *Occupational therapy for physical dysfunction* (4th ed., pp. 157–185). Baltimore: William & Wilkins.

Mattingly, C. (1994). The narrative nature of clinical reasoning. In C. Mattingly and M. H. Fleming (Ed.), *Clinical reasoning: Forms of inquiry in a therapeutic practice* (pp. 239–269). Philadelphia: F. A. Davis.

Mead, G. H. (1934). *Mind, self and society: From the standpoint of a social behaviorist.* Chicago: University of Chicago Press.

Neistadt, M. E., McAuley, D., Zecha, D., & Shannon, R. (1993). An analysis of a board game as a treatment activity. *American Journal of Occupational Therapy, 47*, 154–160.

Parham, L. D., & Maillioux, Z. (1996). Sensory integration. In J. Case-Smith, A. S. Allen, & P. N. Pratt (Eds.), *Occupational therapy for children* (3rd ed., pp. 307–356). St. Louis: C.V. Mosby.

Pearlin, L. I. (1989). The sociological study of stress. *Journal of Health and Social Behavior, 30*, 241–256.

Pedretti, L. W. (1996). Evaluation of sensation and treatment of sensory dysfunction. In L. W. Pedretti (Ed.), *Occupational therapy: Practice skills for physical dysfunction.* (4th ed., pp. 213–230). St. Louis: C. V. Mosby.

Quintana, L. (1995). Evaluation of perception and cognition. In C. A. Trombly (Ed.), *Occupational therapy for physical dysfunction* (4th ed., pp. 201–223). Baltimore: William & Wilkins.

Schneck, C. M. (1996). Visual perception. In J. Case-Smith, A. S. Allen, & P. N. Pratt (Eds.), *Occupational therapy for children* (3rd ed., pp. 357–385). St. Louis: C.V. Mosby.

Snow, E. (1996). Services for children with visual or auditory impairment. In J. Case-Smith, A. S. Allen, & P. N. Pratt (Eds.), *Occupational therapy for children* (3rd ed., pp. 717–742). St. Louis: C.V. Mosby.

Stephan, C. W., & Stephan, W. G. (1985). *Two social psychologies: An integrative approach.* Homewood, IL: Dorsey Press.

Trombly, C. A. (1995). Occupation, purposefulness and meaningfulness as therapeutic mechanisms—1995 Eleanor Clarke Slagle lecture. *American Journal of Occupational Therapy, 49*, 960–972.

Undzis, M. F., Zoltan, B., & Pedretti, L. W. (1996). Evaluation of motor control. In L. W. Pedretti (Ed.), *Occupational therapy: Practice skills for physical dysfunction.* (4th ed., pp. 151–164). St. Louis: C.V. Mosby.

Zemke, R. (1995). Remediating biomechanical and physiological impairments in motor performance. In C. A. Trombly (Ed.). *Occupational therapy for physical dysfunction* (4th ed., pp. 405–422). Baltimore: William & Wilkins.

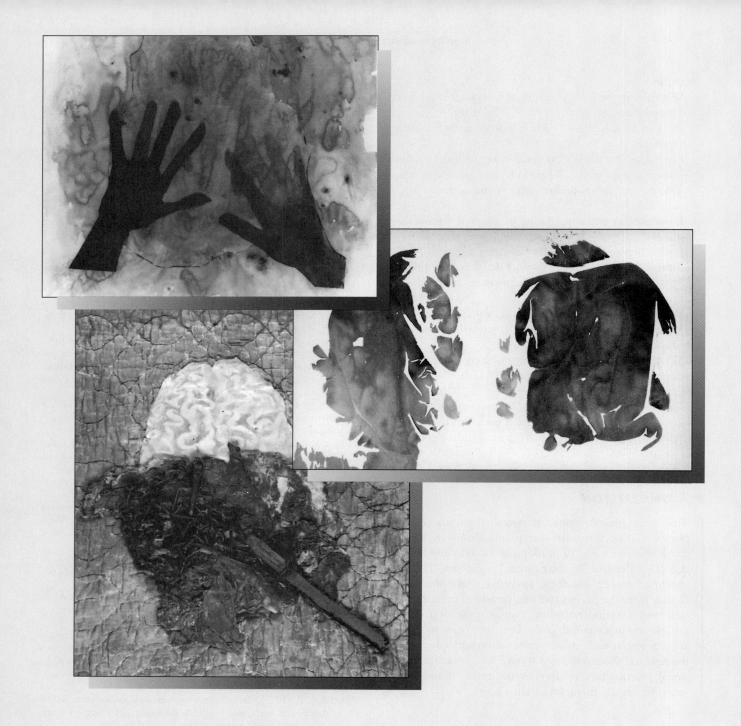

(top) Blue seizure: Before we discovered an epilepsy medication that worked I was having constant seizures. This is a picture of what it felt like—that a force outside myself (the hands) held my brain under ice. That it held me there helpless until it chose to release me. One of the fingers was red because I sometimes felt pain during the seizures.

(middle) Healing brain: This picture shows what I imagined the damaged brain and the healed brain would look like, side by side. (Photos courtesy of Mary Feldhaus-Weber.)

(bottom) Temporal lobe epilepsy: I used a brain picture painted gold and covered it with a rusted dog leash. There were many times I would forget I had epilepsy and be surprised, even afraid, of what was happening to me. The "leash" would snap me back again, control me. I could not get away from it.

UNIT VI

Occupational Therapy Evaluation

LEARNING OBJECTIVES

After completing this unit, readers will be able to:

▶ Describe a general sequence for an occupational therapy evaluation.

▶ Discuss the use of interviewing as an evaluation procedure in occupational therapy.

▶ List the purposes of evaluation in occupational therapy.

▶ Identify a framework or format for critiquing tests for both clinical practice and research purposes.

▶ List several formal assessments of activities of daily living (ADL).

▶ Describe methods for evaluating homemaking, budgeting, and health and safety awareness.

▶ Be familiar with a variety of assessment tools used to identify a worker's current level of functioning.

▶ Describe job site analysis.

▶ Define the components of a comprehensive driving evaluation.

▶ Describe a variety of play or leisure assessments and determine their usefulness for assessment and treatment planning.

▶ Describe several sensory, neuromuscular, and motor evaluation methods.

▶ Articulate a framework for prioritizing evaluations used in a clinic setting.

▶ Define specific cognitive and perceptual skills (orientation, attention, memory, visual processing, organization, problem solving, and executive functions) and identify methods and specific assessments for evaluating these skill areas.

▶ Describe several assessments of psychosocial skills.

▶ Describe alternative tools and approaches that can be used in clinical practice to assess temporal and environmental contexts of occupational therapy clients.

This unit deals with occupational therapy evaluation. Occupational therapy **evaluation** is the process of identifying clients' occupational **performance area**, **performance component**, and **performance context** problems. The results of this evaluation provide the basis for collaborative treatment and discharge planning with clients. The chapters in this unit are organized to give students a sequence and some methods for a general occupational therapy evaluation. The specific **assessments** (tests and measures) that would be used with any given client will vary depending on (1) the age and diagnosis of the client, (2) the reason the client was referred to occupational therapy, (3) the setting in which the evaluation will take place, and (4) the length of evaluation and treatment time approved by the client's insurance company or health plan. Later units on specific diagnostic conditions in children and adults will provide more detail about how therapists can tailor evaluations to particular client problems. (*Note*: Words in **bold** type are defined in the Glossary.)

Chapter 13

Introduction to Evaluation and Interviewing

Section 1: Overview of Evaluation

Section 2: The Interview Process in Occupational Therapy

Section I

Overview of Evaluation

Maureen E. Neistadt

Evaluation Overview
Initial Evaluation
    Review Preliminary Information
    Interview Client and Caregivers
    Observe Occupational Performance
    Evaluate Relevant Component Skills
    Synthesize and Summarize the Data
Interim Evaluations
Discharge Evaluations

This section describes the thought process occupational therapists use during evaluation, a thought process that can be used in any setting, with any client population. This thought process focuses on the client's occupational problems, because occupation is the central concern of occupational therapists. The occupational therapy evaluation process is grounded in an appreciation for the client as a person, and it requires therapists to engage in clinical reasoning, rapport building, and activity analysis.

▼ EVALUATION OVERVIEW

Evaluation is the information-gathering process health care professionals use to identify clients' health-related problems. Typically, evaluations are done at the beginning of treatment (initial evaluations), periodically during the treatment process (interim evaluations), and at the end of treatment (discharge evaluations). The initial evaluation is done to determine client problems, suggest treatments and goals for those problems, and document client performance before treatment begins. The interim evaluations are done to see if the client has progressed relative to the previous evaluations. The discharge evaluation is done to assess the overall effect of the treatment and to see what further treatment or follow-up care is necessary.

The type of evaluation any given professional might do depends on the types of client problems that a professional has been trained to treat. For example, a physician typically evaluates your physical status because he or she is interested primarily in treating your physical problems. Occupational therapy practitioners are concerned with clients' occupational functioning; that is, their abilities to successfully engage in their chosen day-to-day self-care, work, and leisure activities. Consequently, occupational therapists evaluate clients' occupational performance, performance components, and performance contexts.

Occupational performance areas can be categorized into **activities of daily living (ADL)**, **work and productive activities**, and play or **leisure activities** (see Table 1-1). Performance components include abilities such as strength, sensation, perception, and social skills. Performance contexts include the person's developmental stage and the physical and social environments in which activity performance occurs (American Occupational Therapy Association [AOTA], 1994). See Appendix F for a complete listing of occupational performance areas, performance components, and performance contexts.

Occupational performance areas are the day-to-day activities that help people fulfill the responsibilities of their **roles** (eg, student, spouse, parent, worker, or volunteer) and stay connected to other people. The particular occupations any given person chooses to do over time are a reflection of what that person considers important in life. Put together, our past, present, and planned activity choices make up our occupational narratives—the stories of our lives as told through our activity choices (Clarke, 1993). Occupational therapists are concerned with helping persons resume or reconstruct their occupational narratives (ie, with helping people to participate in the activities that are important to them), despite illness or disability. Therefore, occupational therapy evaluation should define the occupational problems of concern to the client. The general steps you need to follow to define those problems during initial, interim, and discharge occupational therapy evaluations are (1) review preliminary information (referral information, medical or educational records, record of occupational therapy treatment); (2) interview the client and his or her caregivers to determine what occupational performance areas are important to them; (3) observe the client's priority occupational performance areas; (4) evaluate component skill areas that looked problematic during occupational performance, and (5) synthesize and summarize the data you have collected during the entire evaluation process. In general, you need to be aware of how much evaluation time any given client's insurance carrier will allow; for shorter-time periods you may have to focus your evaluation quickly on a few occupational performance and component skill areas: the ones of most concern to the client.

▼ INITIAL EVALUATION

The initial evaluation sets up a contract between the professional and the recipient of services (the client) and between the professional and the party paying for the services (the client or a health insurance company). This contract is a promise for therapy services that will change the client's problems. Clients and their insurance carriers expect health care professionals to follow through with the interventions promised at the end of the initial evaluation; they will also expect those interventions to have some effect on the client's problems.

The purposes of an occupational therapy initial evaluation are to (1) establish the client's priorities for treatment; (2) briefly describe the client's potential post treatment situation; (3) establish an occupational therapy diagnosis—a list of occupational performance deficits and component skill deficits relevant to those performance deficits (Rogers & Holm, 1991); and (4) establish treatment goals that reflect the client's priorities and can be achieved within the time frame allotted for treatment by the client's insurance carrier. Occupational performance deficits are relevant only if those occupations are important to clients in their usual environments. For example, a wife and mother with a head injury, who does not have the judgment, memory, or sequencing skills to cook a meal, has an occupational performance deficit in meal preparation. However, if that wife and mother has typically hired someone to do the cooking in her home and still has the financial resources to do that, her meal preparation deficit is not a problem for her and should not be part of the occupational therapy diagnosis.

Treatment goals should always be measurable and tied to occupational performance. Insurance carriers are not interested and will generally not pay for changes in component skills, they are interested in how those changes affect function. A goal of "increase shoulder motion to 160 degrees," for example, is not as meaningful as "increase shoulder motion so that client can reach top of head to shampoo and groom hair independently." As a beginning therapist, you may have some difficulty predicting how much improvement any given client can make in occupational performance within a set amount of treatment time. With increased experience, you will be able to make good clinical judgements about clients' potential rates of improvement. Meanwhile, many facilities now have "critical paths" or lists of anticipated rates of progress for clients with particular sets of problems, given a certain frequency of treatment. These critical paths, which are established based on the history of client progress in that facility, may help you make accurate predictions of function even early in your practice. You need to go through the following steps to gather the data you will need to make predictions of clients' future functional abilities.

Review Preliminary Information

The occupational therapy diagnosis is a description of the functional effects of the client's medical or psychiatric diagnosis. This list of occupational performance and component skill deficits shows how the medical or psychiatric diagnosis has affected a client's ability to carry out his or her day-to-day activities. Medical and psychiatric diagnoses are associated with some predictable patterns of occupational performance and component skill deficits. For example, a person with **rheumatoid arthritis (RA)**, a connective tissue disease that can cause joint pain and deformity, could be expected to have deficits in the component skill of joint mobility and in a wide range of occupational performance areas, depending on the severity of the joint involvement. In contrast, a person recovering from a **myocardial infarction (MI)**, or heart attack, would be expected to have component skill deficits not in joint mobility but in endurance, secondary to a decrease in the heart's ability to pump blood throughout the body.

Knowing a client's diagnoses before you begin your evaluation can help you anticipate what types of occupational therapy problems the client may be experiencing and focus your thinking about what types of measures you may have to use during your evaluation. For example, you would want to be sure to have your goniometer, an instrument for measuring joint motion, with you before going to see the client with RA. Before going in to see the person with a diagnosis of MI, you would not be thinking of goniometers, but of observing the signs and symptoms of overexertion.

The diagnoses, and the client's medical or psychiatric history will also tell you what precautions you need to think about during evaluation and treatment with any given client. For the person with RA, for example, you would need to be aware of the client's pain and fatigue levels. For the person who is status post MI (just had an MI) you need to be aware of what activities might overtax the person's recovering heart.

You can obtain the client's diagnoses and medical history from the medical record, which you should review before going to see a client. You can find information about the client's current medical status, medications, or other treatments in the physician and nursing notes. The social service notes can give you information about the client's living situation and anticipated placement after discharge from your facility or agency. It is important for you to review the medical record before beginning your evaluation, but it is also important for you to remember that the medical record does not tell you who this client is as a person. You should not make decisions about someone's treatment potential based on only the medical record. Nor should you decide in advance what a client's personality will be, based on previous notes in the medical record. The medical record gives you preliminary information only—you must always stay open to meeting the person you will be evaluating.

Interview Client and Caregivers

In your initial meeting with your client, you need to first introduce yourself and explain the purpose of your visit. It is also important for you to ask the client or caregivers to tell you what brought them to your setting for treatment; the response to this question can tell you how a client and his or her caregivers understand and feel about this illness and the treatment they have received so far. Nearly all of your clients will be anxious about your evaluation, about the problems that have brought them into the health care system, and about the disruptions those problems have caused in their lives. It is your job to make clients feel comfortable and safe through respectful and empathetic interaction with them. This interaction starts during the interview. Section 2 of this chapter provides specific guidelines about how to conduct a good interview.

Observe Occupational Performance

After you have interviewed the client to learn about his or her occupational narrative, priorities for treatment, and posttreatment situation, you need to observe the client performing those ADL activities he or she has identified as routine, offering assistance as needed. (Because of time restraints, you will probably not be able to observe the client performing routine work or leisure activities for your initial evaluation.) During that observation, you need to note performance deficits and levels of assistance needed to complete ADL activities. You may use standardized assessments of ADL to do this part of your evaluation. Chapter 14 discusses the relative merits of formal versus informal evaluations and will help you select the types of assessments that are most appropriate for your evaluation needs. Chapter 15 offers detailed descriptions of various ADL, work, and play and leisure evaluations.

During your observations of the client's occupational performance, you also need to hypothesize or guess about what component skill deficits might be contributing to the performance problems. An occupational therapist generates these hypotheses or educated guesses about component skill deficits by using activity analysis.

As the activity analysis chapter (see Chap. 12) indicated, to be successful in occupational performance, you need to be proficient both in the skills that contribute to activity performance and in putting those skills together for any given activity. For example, to put on an over-the-head tee shirt, you need to have a certain amount of strength and joint flexibility in your arms. You need a certain amount of trunk balance so you do not fall over when you try to put on your shirt. You also need to be able to perceive the difference between the neck and armholes of the shirt, and know which body parts go into which holes. Once the shirt is over your head, you need to be able to feel the holes in the shirt to get the shirt on right. And you need the judgment to know if this particular tee shirt is an appropriate one to wear for your activities that day. So, to do something as simple as put on a tee shirt, you need motor, perceptual, sensory, and cognitive skills. And you need to be able to put all of those skills together for the task of putting on the tee shirt. You would need the same set of skills for putting on a sweatshirt, but you might put those skills together in a slightly different way to adjust to the differences in the garment.

A client who failed to put on a tee shirt independently has an occupational performance deficit in upper extremity dressing (occupational therapy jargon for difficulty in dressing the upper half of the body). The type of trouble the client had with this activity can suggest component skill deficits. For example, a client who could not put the tee shirt on because he or she is unable to raise one arm overhead might have component deficits in strength, joint flexibility, or sensation in that arm. In contrast, a client who can reach both arms overhead but looks confused and is not able to orient the shirt to his or her body could have component skill deficits in cognition or perception.

Evaluate Relevant Component Skills

Once you have established performance deficits and hypothesized component skill deficits, you need to test or check out your component skill hypotheses with specific component skill tests. In other words, you need to evaluate the component skills you suspect are problems to see which of your hypotheses or educated guesses are correct. For instance, for the client who could not put the tee shirt on because he or she was unable to raise one arm overhead, you would need to measure the joint flexibility and strength of the affected arm. If you can move the client's shoulder through its full range of motion while the client is relaxed and not trying to move the limb, then joint flexibility is not a component skill deficit. So you would have eliminated joint flexibility from your hypothesis list. Now you would need to check sensation and muscle strength to see if deficits in either of those component skills were contributing to the client's inability to move his or her arm overhead on his or her own. Chapter 16 contains detailed information about component skill evaluations.

Synthesize and Summarize the Data

Once you have completed your occupational therapy diagnosis, your list of occupational performance and component skill deficits, you need to revise it as needed to reflect the client's stated priorities and anticipated future living situation. Then you need to sit with the client and his or her caregivers to go over your occupational therapy diagnosis. You can also suggest some treatment goals and activities at that time. You need to be sure that your client and his or her caregivers agree with your occupational therapy diagnosis and accept your treatment goals and recommendations.

Occasionally, when you think a client's goals are unsafe, you may have to negotiate with a client about what the goals of treatment ought to be. For instance if an adolescent with **mental retardation**, who has poor judgement and very slow reaction times, wanted to learn how to drive, you could explain why you think that goal is unsafe by briefly describing how this client's slow reaction time could cause an automobile accident. You could then suggest working on learning how to use public transportation as an alternative way to meet this client's need and desire to get around his or her community independently.

In other cases, you may have to link what you consider to be priority treatment goals and activities to the client's goals. For example, if an elderly woman with a hip fracture who needed assistance to get out of bed and get dressed wanted to focus on dusting, you could suggest that getting dressed and out of bed are precursors to dusting, so it would be a good idea to work on dressing, bed mobility, and transfer skills first. You can also use clients' activity goals to work on multiple treatment goals. For instance, this woman with a hip fracture could work on dynamic standing balance and functional ambulation with a walker while doing her priority activity of dusting. You need to use your activity analysis skills to figure out how to accomplish as many treatment goals as possible with the activities clients see as priorities.

▼ INTERIM EVALUATIONS

Interim evaluations are done formally in some settings at set intervals determined by the policies of the setting and the requirements of insurance companies. In other settings interim evaluations are done informally, as part of treatment. The latter approach is not problematic because a good therapist measures and documents client progress in each treatment session, modifying treatment as appropriate. The steps of an interim evaluation would be the same as those for an initial evaluation, except that your preliminary information would include the record of the client's progress in occupational therapy treatment so far.

The purposes of an occupational therapy interim evaluation are to (1) reassess the client's priorities for treatment, (2) update the client's potential posttreatment situation, (3) revise the occupational therapy diagnosis, (4) assess the client's progress since the last evaluation, and (5) revise treatment goals to reflect the client's priorities given his or her change since the last evaluation.

For your interim evaluations, you may want to expand the occupational performance areas you observe to include work and play or leisure activities. The scope of occupational performance areas you evaluate will vary from setting to setting. In some settings, such as a work-hardening outpatient center, you will start with evaluations of work, because clients are referred to those settings specifically for evaluation and treatment of work issues. In most adult physical dysfunction settings, you will find that insurance companies will refuse to pay for evaluations of leisure activities.

RESEARCH NOTE
THE PRACTICE CLAIMS OF THE PROFESSION MUST BE VERIFIED BY RESEARCH

Kenneth J. Ottenbacher

The evaluation of clinical effectiveness should be an integral part of any intervention program carried out by occupational therapists. In the current economic and political climate, no health care professional can hope to defend his or her practice against skepticism and accusations of inefficiency or questionable ethical standards unless its treatment programs demonstrate improved therapeutic outcomes. More than a decade ago, Gillette noted that

the practice claims of the profession must be established in order to provide ample evidence of the value of occupational therapy to

consumers of the services and to other health care providers as well. In the absence of careful and thorough documentation, members of a profession such as occupational therapy will not receive appropriate recognition nor adequate reimbursement for their services (Gillette, 1982, p. 499).

In the present climate of managed care and health care reform these observations are as relevant now as they were in 1982. Only through carefully planned evaluation will we succeed in demonstrating the value of occupational therapy to our peers and consumers. ■

Gillette, N. (1982). Nationally speaking: A database for occupational therapy. *American Journal of Occupational Therapy, 36*, 499–501.

▼ DISCHARGE EVALUATIONS

Discharge evaluations are generally done formally shortly before a client is due to finish his or her course of occupational therapy treatment. When a client is being discharged to his or her home from a facility, the discharge evaluation often includes a home visit during which the occupational therapist assesses the safety and accessibility of the client's home. When the client is being discharged from a work-hardening program, the discharge evaluation often includes a therapist visit to the client's future place of employment to assess that work place's accessibility and design. Chapter 17 provides more detail about home, work, and other performance context evaluations. The steps of a discharge evaluation would be the same as those for an initial evaluation, except that your preliminary information would include the record of the client's progress in occupational therapy treatment.

The purposes of an occupational therapy discharge evaluation are to (1) assess client progress since the initial evaluation, (2) document the amount of assistance the client needs for occupational performance areas, (3) document the status of the client's identified component skill deficits, (4) document recommendations for adaptive equipment and modifications to the client's potential posttreatment situation, (5) document recommendations for continued or ongoing services for the client. When clients are being discharged to other facilities for continued rehabilitation or long-term care, the discharge evaluation can include recommendations for treatment or care of the client in that facility. When clients are being discharged to their homes, the occupational therapy discharge evaluation can include recommendations for homemaker services (someone to do housekeeping for a client), home health aides (someone to help a client with washing and dressing), outpatient or in-home therapy. The occupational therapy discharge evaluation needs to make recommendations for the services the client will need in the next part of the health care system he or she will be entering. See Unit XII for more detail about the continuum of health care services available in the United States.

Section 2

The Interview Process In Occupational Therapy

Alexis D. Henry

Interviewing is a valuable clinical strategy and one of the most common evaluation procedures used by occupational therapists. As a clinical strategy, interviewing involves both product and process—that is, interviews are usually done to obtain information (product), but also to further the development of a therapeutic alliance with the client (process).

▼ WHAT IS INTERVIEWING?

Interviewing has been defined as a shared verbal experience, jointly constructed by the interviewer and the interviewee, organized around the asking and answering of questions (Mishler, 1986). While your "job," as the interviewer, is primarily to ask the questions, and the client's "job," as the interviewee, is primarily to answer; effective interviewing does not proceed in a stilted, "stimulus-response" manner. Rather, you and the client are attempting to achieve some shared understanding of a particular reality. That reality is the client's story.

When a client newly enters your treatment setting, the piece of information that you are most likely to have is a label that identifies the client as having a particular type of problem. Most often this label takes the form of a diagnosis; for example, the client may have a diagnosis of **schizophrenia** or **arthritis** or a **learning disability**. And, this information is likely to lead you to make certain preliminary assumptions about the occupational performance problems this client might have, based on your past experience with other persons with that particular diagnosis. While information such as a client's diagnosis may have some usefulness in influencing the course of occupational therapy intervention (for example, knowing that a client has arthritis might mean that you would plan to teach the client **joint protection** techniques), by itself its usefulness is limited. To meaningfully plan for a client's treatment, you need to know the particulars of the client's situation, and you need to know them from the client's perspective. In other words, you need to hear the client's story.

When a therapist considers how the client's present situation fits into the larger life story that the client has been living, the therapist is thinking *narratively* about the client (Frank, 1996; Helfrich & Kielhofner, 1994; Mattingly, 1991; Mattingly & Fleming, 1994). A narrative or life story approach involves considering the particular set of circumstances that describe a client's life before he or she came into treatment, how the client views his or her life now, and where the client sees his or her life going after treatment is over. When thinking narratively about a client, the therapist strives to understand the client's **values** and motives to make the therapeutic experience meaningful.

Interviews are one important clinical strategy that can help you think about the client in narrative terms. The client's story is more important for determining the course of your intervention with the client than evaluations of motor skills, perceptual skills, or level of ADL independence. By having some understanding of the client's life before he or she came to therapy and where he or she hopes to go after therapy, you will be better able to make therapeutic experiences meaningful, because these experiences will relate to the values, goals, and concerns of the client. When there is a mismatch between your perception and the client's perception of what is needed in therapy, therapy is likely to become stalled (Mattingly, 1991). A shared perception of what is needed in therapy can really be achieved only through a dialogue between you and the client.

Interviews are generally structured strategies for engaging the client in a dialogue, although interviews perhaps function best when they proceed as normal conversation, rather than as a formal question-and-answer session. Usually, although not always, an interview takes place at the beginning of the therapy experience. At the beginning, one important goal of an interview is to gather specific information about the client. In this way, an interview is one of a battery of procedures that might be used in a comprehensive evaluation of a client. However, because it is an interaction between you and the client, an interview is also an intervention that can have therapeutic value in its own right. In the context of an interview, you and the client can together begin to construct a new life story for the client (Mattingly & Fleming, 1994).

▼ WHEN AND WHOM TO INTERVIEW

The Initial Interview: Interview as Evaluation

Because interviewing is an integral part of a comprehensive evaluation of a client's occupational functioning, it most frequently occurs at the beginning of a client's treatment. In my own practice in psychiatry, an interview was almost always my first significant interaction with a new client. Before administering any performance-based assessment, I would sit down with a client to talk. During that initial interaction, I would have two primary goals. The first would be to begin to understand the client's story. Who is this person? What brought him here? Where does he hope to go after he leaves? The answers to these questions would shape the suggestions that I might make for the work we could do together in the time we had. The second, but not unrelated, goal would be to begin to form a collaborative relationship with the client. These and other goals of interviewing will be discussed later in this section.

During the Course of Therapy: Interview as Intervention

Although interviewing is an important strategy to use at the beginning of the therapy experience, the beginning is not the only time an interview may be appropriate. An interview that occurs after therapy has begun can be both a form of re-evaluation and an intervention. An interview that takes place after therapy has been started is likely to be less structured than the data-gathering process used during the formal initial evaluation phase of a client's treatment. This more informal kind of interaction can involve you and the client reviewing what has happened in therapy, thus far, and anticipating and planning for the future. This kind of discussion can help the client construct an image of a future self who is able to do more than he or she can do now. Such images are important in making therapy something the client can commit to and invest in (Helfrich & Kielhofner, 1994; Polkinghorne, 1996). In addition, reviewing the therapy process together can be a useful strategy when you seem to be at a "stuck" point, when it seems that therapy is not progressing. Together, you and the client can ask "Why is this not working?" and "What can we do to make things better?" In these ways, interviewing is a collaborative tool that is used repeatedly throughout the therapy process.

Interviewing Older Adolescents and Adults

Most older adolescents and adults that occupational therapists encounter in clinical practice are appropriate candidates for interviewing. The techniques for interviewing and

HISTORICAL NOTE
RUGGLES' WORK WITH PERSON AS PART OF EVALUATION

Suzanne M. Peloquin

Ora Ruggles, reconstruction aide, helped many individuals through the use of occupation. One difficult patient at Fort McPherson initially worried her, so she consulted his doctor for more information. She learned that Kilgore was a cowboy whose wartime experience had fueled an anger he suppressed.

Ruggles approached the foreman of the blacksmith shop. She then found Kilgore, showed him a design for spurs, and asked him if he would help her start a metalwork class. Within the hour, Kilgore was busily working in the shop. Years later he wrote Ruggles (1946) about his personal reconstruction, made possible through her having correctly grasped his problems and strengths:

I've been doing a lot of thinking lately, Ruggie. It started out last week when some of the boys around town asked me to run for mayor. . . . It makes me realize again, Ruggie, how much I owe you. I wonder what the boys who asked me to run for mayor would think if they knew an army doctor once scribbled on my medical record, "This man is a menace to society." (p. 91)

Kilgore's gratitude is clear; it speaks to his having been seen not as the personification of a problem but as a person with real strengths. Such an evaluation can spark in many the courage that they need for change. ■

Carlova, J., & Ruggles, O. (1946). *The healing heart*. New York: Julian Messner.

---

the specific occupational therapy interviews that are discussed later in this section apply, for the most part, to interviewing persons of these ages. However, some persons are not appropriate candidates for interviews, or really, should be interviewed only in highly structured situations. For example, individuals with severe **depression** may have difficulty concentrating on and responding to interview questions; persons with mania may be too distracted by external stimuli to attend to an interview. Persons with psychosis may have such disorganized thinking that their answers to questions are difficult to understand. Persons with expressive or receptive language deficits (eg, **aphasia**) may either not comprehend questions or not be able to respond even if they understand. If an interview is approached as a conversation, a time when you and the client are going to "talk," rather than as a "formal evaluation" of the client, then either continuing or discontinuing the interview (if that seems necessary) can be done without making the client feel as if he or she has failed the evaluation.

Interviewing Children and Younger Adolescents

Although pediatrics is one of the largest specialty practice areas in occupational therapy, there have been virtually no interview procedures developed to gather data on children's occupational behavior directly from children (although some parent interviews relative to play have been developed), and there has been only one interview developed for use with adolescents (Black, 1976).

Children pose a unique challenge for the interviewer. The ability of children to describe their experiences and their feelings depends on their acquisition of the requisite cognitive, linguistic, and social skills (Stone & Lemanek, 1990). Before the age of 7 or 8, most children describe themselves only in terms of observable characteristics and behaviors, and make differentiations between themselves and others on the basis of these observable traits, rather than on internal states. For example, a young child may be able to describe herself in terms of the physical attributes (eg, "I have blue eyes."), or possessions (eg, "I have a cat."), or preferred activities (e.g. "I like to ride my bike."). However, these notions about the self are not integrated into a global self-concept (Stone & Lemanek, 1990). In addition, young children may have difficulty labeling or verbally communicating their subjective emotional state (LaGreca, 1990). Young children also have difficulty relating events in a temporal order, especially if the events happened in the (relatively) distant past.

At around age 8, children acquire a more global sense of the self. After this age, children are better able to report on their thoughts and feelings, and to provide more accurate information on diverse experiences and situations. During adolescence, the capacity for self-reflection increases further. Adolescents have the capacity to describe themselves in abstract psychological and interpersonal terms, rather than the concrete, physical terms used by younger children. In addition, adolescents begin to evaluate their own thoughts and behaviors critically, and to analyze others' reactions to their behavior (Stone & Lemanek, 1990). Thus, as self-awareness increases, older children and younger adolescents are able to respond to interview questions with increasing sophistication. However, the increased use of social comparisons and greater psychological awareness that come as children age may contribute to a tendency to respond to interview questions in a socially desirable manner (Stone & Lemanek, 1990).

Other factors may influence the way in which children and adolescents respond during interview situations. One of the most important to consider is the inherent power imbalance in the relationship between a child and an adult interviewer (Cohn, 1994). Adults, generally, have greater social power than children; children are, for the most part, socialized to respond to adults in ways they think adults want to hear. Because of the power imbalance, whether real or merely perceived, children may unintentionally fabricate answers to questions to please an adult interviewer (Cohn, 1994).

Establishing rapport and a sense of trust is critical to the successful interview. With children, engaging the child in a play activity or a discussion about a favorite book or movie before the interview can help establish rapport. With adolescents, honest communication about the reasons for the interview and the confidential nature of the interview can help instill trust. Age-appropriate communication is another key to a successful interview. With young children, the use of simple vocabulary, short sentences, and concrete, direct questions (eg, "What do you do during school?") are recommended (Cohn, 1994). Adolescents can usually answer more open-ended questions (eg, "Tell me about how school has been going for you.").

Finally, the process of gathering information concerning children's functioning should involve other people in the child's environment, including parents and teachers (LaGreca, 1990). Because children are under the social control of others, their behavior in one environment may not be the same as their behavior in another environment. Thus, it is important to gather information from the multiple contexts within which the child functions. Moreover, because children are usually referred for treatment by others, usually a parent, it is important to understand and respect the perspective of those who may be distressed by the child's behavior (LaGreca, 1990).

▼ WHY INTERVIEW

Understanding the Client's Story

The single most important reason to interview the client is so that you can better understand how the client sees things. As I have discussed previously, an interview is an opportunity for the client to tell you his or her story. Mattingly (1991) has noted, "a disability is something that interrupts and irreversibly changes a person's life story"; "therapy can be seen as a short story within the patient's longer life story" (p. 1000). During the course of the interview, you are trying to uncover the "plot" of the client's story. Before the initial interview, you might have some general information about the client. During the interview, you want to "fill in" the particulars of the story. So your main question should be, "What happened?" How did this person come to you? What

was her life like before she came to you? What was and is important to her? Where does she hope to go after she leaves you? The answers to these questions will guide and individualize your intervention with this particular client.

If therapy is a "short story" in an unfolding life story, then you are an actor in that story. Your primary role, as an actor in that story, is to offer advice and experiences that will help the client get to where he or she wants to go, and can realistically expect to go. In effect, you are a "life consultant." Therapy experiences can be made meaningful only when you see how therapy is an event that comes into a life in progress (Helfrich & Kielhofner, 1994). You can only fulfill the role of life consultant when you have some understanding of the life.

Building the Therapeutic Alliance

Because an interview is an interaction between two persons, a relationship begins to develop during the course of the interview. During the interview, you want to establish a relationship with the client that will facilitate the attainment of therapeutic goals. The manner in which you conduct the interview will either foster or inhibit the development of that relationship. As you are talking with a client, your ability to communicate a sense of concern and respect for the individual and the information being shared, and your ability to be real and genuine in the interaction will go a long way to establishing this relationship. The client has come to you for help. For the client to feel that you are someone who can be of help, a sense of safety, trust and, collaboration must develop between the two of you (Bruce & Borg, 1993). An interview can enhance a sense of collaboration between you and the client, because it gives you an opportunity to communicate that you care about what is important to the client. To the extent that you have a collaborative relationship with the client, you will be much more likely to achieve the goals of therapy (Tickle-Degnen, 1995; Neistadt, 1995).

Gathering Information

Obviously, one important reason to interview a client is to gather information. Occupational therapy interviews generally are used to gather information about the client's functioning in occupations. Most interviews consider the client's current or recent functioning; some also take a more historical perspective and seek to understand the client's functioning over time. Although the specific questions vary across different interviews, in general, interviews solicit information about the client's daily use of time, past and current productive role involvement (eg, worker, student, homemaker), social and play and leisure involvement, as well as his or her values, goals, and sense of competence relative to occupations. Some interviews also ask questions about the client's current environment (human and nonhuman), to evaluate whether the environment supports or constrains the person's functioning.

It is important to gather information about the client's functioning before he or she came to therapy, because past functioning is one of the best predictors of future functioning (Henry & Coster, 1996). The client's disability and the resulting functional impairments will predict his or her future functioning to some extent. But the successes that a person was able to achieve in the past, particularly the recent past, are often resources on which he or she can draw. Moreover, a person's goals and sense of competence are indicators of his or her desire and motivation to return to his or her prior life.

Observing Behavior

During the course of an interview, you have an opportunity to observe the person's behavior. The client's ability to participate in an interview can reveal much about his or her current functioning. You will be able to make observations about the client's energy level, stamina, **affect**, comprehension, **memory**, concentration, thought organization, physical appearance, and interpersonal behavior. Is the client able to actively engage with you through a 30 or 45 minute interview without fatiguing? Does he or she appear depressed, elated, or is the person's affect flat (an absence of emotion)? Does his or her memory seem intact? For example, is he or she able to remember the dates of his or her last five jobs, and relate them to you in chronological order? Does the person comprehend the questions being asked? Is he or she able to convey his or her history in a manner that you can understand and follow? Is the person's thinking organized and goal-directed, or is he or she tangential (ie, does he or she seem to get "off track")? Is the person appropriately dressed and groomed for the situation, or does he or she appear unkempt? Is the person being friendly and forthcoming with information, or does he or she seem angry, hostile, resistant to being interviewed? The extent to which the client engages with you during an interview may be some indication of the extent to which he or she will engage with you in therapy. Of course, if the client appears to be defensive or resistant during the interview, it is important to ask yourself if there is something that you are doing to make the client feel defensive.

In my own practice in mental health settings, I would make the kinds of behavioral observations described in the foregoing as I interviewed a client. In doing so, the initial interview served as a kind of "screening procedure" that would give indications of other, performance-based assessments that might be useful to administer to the client. For example, if a client's physical appearance was disheveled, I might administer an assessment such as the **Kohlman Evaluation of Living Skills** (Kohlman-Thompson, 1992) for a more in depth evaluation of the client's ADL skills.

Identifying Problems

As the interview progresses, and you begin to achieve a deeper understanding of the person's story and observe his or her behavior, you will begin to formulate, in your mind, an initial list of problems that might be addressed by occupational therapy interventions. (You might also recognize problems that would lead you to refer the client to someone else for intervention.) This problem list will begin to take shape from the things the client tells you and the things you observe. It is important to remember, however, that this initial idea about the problems is tentative, and subject to revision as you begin to know the client better through the treatment process. Moreover, your perspective of the problems the client faces may not be the same as the client's perspective. Occupational therapists often begin to see problems at the level of performance components, whereas clients often think of their problems at the level of roles. Obviously, you want to share your initial impression with the client, and to confirm the extent to which you are seeing things in the same way. This involves both restating what you have perceived as the client's major concerns, and also sharing your impressions and observations during the interview. By engaging in mutual problem-setting, you lay the ground work for a collaborative relationship. Toward the end of an interview, you might say to the client, "Well, from what you've told me, it sound like you are concerned about . . ., and it seems to me that you are also having some difficulty with. . . ." The goal is for the two of you to arrive at some agreement about the problems the client faces.

Clarifying Your Role in the Client's Treatment

You can also use the end of an interview to elaborate on and clarify your role in the client's treatment. Do not be surprised if the client does not know what occupational therapists do. At this point, you can explain what services occupational therapy offers in your facility, what activity choices might be available to the client, whether you might be cotreating the client with another professional (eg, physical therapy or nursing or social work), or whether you might refer the client to another clinician for a service not provided by occupational therapy. It is at this point that you can make initial recommendations about the client's treatment.

Establishing Priorities for Intervention

Once you and the client have agreed on the problems to be addressed, you have explained your role in the client's treatment and the services that occupational therapy can offer, and made some initial recommendations for treatment, then you and the client can work collaboratively to establish treatment priorities. Initially, your priorities may not be the client's, and vice versa. Although one hopes your priorities are influenced by the client's needs, it is important to recognize other factors that might influence the recommendations you make. For example, you might be influenced by the services most easily provided by your setting, your own interests and competencies, funding and reimbursement, among others. The client's goals and priorities must be central in determining the course of treatment; after all, the treatment plan belongs to the client. Engaging the client in active goal setting and goal prioritizing is a good way to finish up an interview.

▼ HOW TO INTERVIEW

It may seem that interviewing should be something that comes naturally; after all, you talk to people everyday. But, in fact, much of our day-to-day communication with other people is quite superficial. When you conduct an interview with a client, you are engaging in a dialogue with the express purpose of trying to understand that other person so that you can be helpful (Davis, 1994). Thus, "therapeutic communication" differs from day-to-day conversation in some fundamental ways. Developing communication skills needed to become an effective interviewer takes time and experience. The skills of effective interviewing and ways to structure a clinical interview are discussed below.

The Skills of Effective Interviewing

PREPARING
Preparing for the interview is an important first step. Before conducting an interview, you should prepare yourself, the client, and the environment.

In preparing yourself, you should obviously have some notion of the questions you want to ask the client. Several different occupational therapy interview procedures have been published in recent years, and these will be discussed later in this section. I strongly recommend using one of the existing interview procedures, rather than developing your own. (The efficacy of the field is enhanced when clinicians use standardized assessment procedures that have been subjected to examinations of reliability and validity.) If you are a novice interviewer, you will need to practice before interviewing your first client. Observing experienced interviewers, noting how they structure the interview, ask questions, and respond to information the client gives is a good way to begin to develop a sense of how an interview flows. You might also practice administering the interview to a colleague or clinical supervisor and have that person give you feedback. Videotaping and critiquing your practice interviews is another, very useful way of honing your interviewing skills.

Before conducting an interview with a client, you should read whatever preliminary information (eg, admission note, referral form) might be available on the client. This information may give you some initial ideas about areas that you might focus on during the interview. Also, information about the client's diagnosis or presenting problem will help you anticipate how actively the client can participate in the interview, whether he or she might tolerate only a short interview, or whether he or she might not be appropriate for an interview at this time. In addition, when I worked on an inpatient mental health unit, and was about to interview a new client or a client that I had not seen since the previous day, I would always ask someone on the nursing staff how the client was doing that day.

In addition to preparing yourself, you should prepare the client for the interview. Rarely, will I approach a person whom I have never met before and ask if I can interview him or her on the spot. Rather, I will approach a client, introduce myself and tell him or her briefly about my role in the setting. Then I will ask permission to do the interview, telling the client briefly about the content and purpose of the interview, and schedule an appointment. Scheduling an appointment (even if just for later that same day) gives the client a degree of control; the client has some choice about when he or she will see you. Some times of the day are better than others for many persons. For example, many persons with depression feel worse in the morning, and experience improvements in their mood and energy level as the day progresses. By allowing the client to have some degree of control in a situation where he or she is likely to feel out of control, you help set the tone for the collaborative relationship you want to have with the client.

Finally, you need to pay some attention to the environment in which you will conduct the interview. Obviously, a private space is the most desirable. Some of the questions you will be asking are highly personal, and a private space will make you both feel more comfortable. You should not make assumptions about what might and might not be personal questions for the client. I have often had the experience of a client having an emotional response to questions about a particular aspect of his or her prior functioning that I had not anticipated. Chairs should be an appropriate distance apart (3 or 4 feet). The room should be at a temperature that is comfortable for both of you and should be well-lighted. Have tissues and water available. If it is not possible to have a private space, then creating some sense of privacy in a more open space by arranging the chairs in a corner of the room would be suitable. If possible, I prefer not to interview a client when he or she is in bed.

QUESTIONING
Interviewing involves the asking of questions. The manner in which you pose questions to the client will influence the quality and amount of information you obtain, and thus, the level of understanding of the client's story you can achieve. How you ask questions will also influence how you are perceived by the client, and will influence the development of your relationship with the client.

In general, open-ended questions encourage the client to tell his or her story, and are more likely to yield meaningful information from a client than closed questions that require only a yes or no answer or a very brief response. For example, the question "Do (did) you like your job?', can be answered "yes" or "no." "Tell me what you liked about your job." is a question that will likely result in a more elaborated response by the client. In addition, the use of probes and follow-up questions (eg, "Tell me more about that.") encourage the client to relate his or her story. During the course of an interview, it is likely that you will ask two types of questions: those that are factual or descriptive in nature (eg, "What do you do for work?"), and those that are intended to elicit more narrative data. Narrative questions yield data on events in the client's life and the client's perceptions and motives concerning events (eg, "Tell me about a time when work was going very well for you."). Kielhofner and Mallinson (1995) suggest that effective interviewing involves a weaving of these two ways of questioning, and have provided some guidelines for narrative interviewing.

There may be certain clients for whom a more structured, factual approach to questioning is appropriate. For example, a client whose thinking is disorganized (eg, the client has psychotic symptoms) may have difficulty answering more open-ended or narrative questions in a coherent manner, but can respond to a more structured question such as "Where do you live?" It will usually be apparent when you need to use a more structured approach to the interview.

During the interview, you want to be conscious of whether the questions you are asking are making the client anxious or uncomfortable. Your intention should be to put the client at ease. To do this, it is best if your questions are open, clear, singular (ie, you ask only one question at a time), nonjudgmental, and encourage the client to tell his or her story. You want to avoid putting the client on the defensive. Sometimes, questions that begin with "why" (eg, "Why did you do that?") can have the unintended effect of making the client feel that he or she owes you an explanation about his or her feelings or behavior (Davis, 1994). Particularly during the initial interview, it is more useful to assume a neutral, nonjudgmental stance (Bradburn, 1992).

RESPONDING

For an interview to be a useful experience for both you and the client, the interview needs to be more than a series of questions on your part, interspersed with answers from the client. You will also frequently need to respond to the information that the client is sharing with you. There are many ways that you might respond. Often, because of a desire to help, our impulse is to respond with advice or suggestions. However, particularly during an initial interview, you want to resist this impulse, at least until you have come to the end of the interview. Before that, it is doubtful that you will have sufficient information on which to base advice. So, even though you want to resist giving advice until you have achieved some understanding of the client's story, you still need to respond. During the course of the interview, your

responses should primarily be attempts to paraphrase what the client has just said. Paraphrasing is more than just repeating what the client has just said. It involves trying to capture the essence of what the client has said and restating it in your own words to communicate your desire to understand (Denton, 1987). Paraphrasing helps you communicate to the client that you have listened to, heard, understood, and valued the information being shared with you. Paraphrasing also allows you to confirm that you have, in fact, clearly understood what the client has said.

There are two general types of responses that you can use during an interview: content responses and affective responses. Content responses are used when you want to clarify the facts or communicate that you have understood what the client means. A content response might begin "So, you're saying that. . . ." Content responses serve the purpose of clarifying information and meaning. Affective responses are used when you want to reflect the underlying affect or feeling tone that the client is communicating. An affective response might begin "It seems like you're feeling. . .," or "I might have felt very. . . in that situation." An affective response should be phrased somewhat tentatively until you have confirmed that the client feels this way. Affective responses serve the purpose of communicating that you are trying to understand and are concerned about how the client feels.

ATTENDING AND OBSERVING

Attending involves the use of both nonverbal and verbal behaviors that help communicate your interest in the client and can facilitate the development of therapeutic rapport. Nonverbal behaviors include positions and movements of the face and body, as well as qualities of the voice, such as tone, intensity, and speed (Tickle-Degnen, 1995). Having your chair and the client's chair either facing each other or slightly angled, about 3 feet apart, allows you to fully see the client and the client to see you. You can communicate your interest in the client by making frequent eye contact. Other nonverbal behaviors that communicate interest include head-nodding, smiling, and leaning forward. Verbal behaviors, such as saying "uh-huh," "humm," "yes," or "go on," let the client know that you are listening and encourage the client to continue with his or her story. Tickle-Degnen (1995) notes that tone of voice is an important attribute to attend to. A cheerful tone of voice is not always the most appropriate to use. Rather, a tone of voice that is genuine and conveys concern about the client may be more effective. Effective interviewers often accommodate their bodies, movements, and tone of voice to be "in sync" with the client's (Bradburn, 1992; Tickle-Degnen, 1995).

Attending also involves observing how the client seems to be feeling as the interview progresses. Does the client seem to be fatiguing? Does the interview content seem to be emotionally difficult for the client? If you sense that the client is finding the interview difficult, you should ask to verify this. For example, questions such as "How are you doing?" and "Are you getting tired?" communicate that you are concerned about the client. A common side effect of psychiatric medications is dry mouth; offering a class a water is another way of showing that you are attending. Observing also involves noting the client's behavior as the interview progresses.

LISTENING

Finally, although it seems obvious to say so, throughout the interview, you need to listen to the client. Listening effectively allows you to respond effectively. Paying close attention to both the content and the underlying feeling or affect takes energy. Listening is more difficult than it sound, because there are many distractions to effective listening. There can be external distractions, such as activity in the environment, or internal distractions, such as your thoughts about a meeting you just came from or your next client. Even when your attention is focused on the client, there can be distractions. Denton (1987) has identified certain blocks to effective listening to the client; she calls these *thinking about the person*, *thinking for the person*, and *thinking ahead of the person*.

Thinking about the person involves making judgments about the client's life style, morals, and motives; such judgments can create distance between you and the client and interfere with your being able to understand the client's perspective. When you think for the person, you prematurely think about solutions to the client's problems. Because one aim of the interview is to facilitate a collaborative problem-solving relationship with the client, prematurely offering solutions diminishes the client's role in the relationship and can reinforce the client's sense of helplessness. Thinking ahead of the person involves rushing the client through his or her story just to get the facts. This can happen when you feel you already know the story, when the client is relating too much or seemingly irrelevant details, or when you feel pressed for time (Denton, 1987). The reality is that you never already know the story; each person's story is unique. However, if the client is giving you more detail than you need at the moment and you begin to run out of time, you can respectfully redirect the client by saying, "I can hear that this topic is very important to you. Perhaps we should set another time to really talk about this. Right now, I need to ask you some questions about something else."

Finally, particularly if you are a novice interviewer, you can be distracted from listening because you are thinking about what you should say next. If you are thinking about what you should say next then you are not listening to the client. "Effective listening occurs only when you are paying attention to your patient instead of yourself" (Denton, 1987, p. 13). One way to improve your listening skills is to learn to use silence effectively. Most of us feel uncomfortable with silence and feel a need to fill a silent space as soon as it occurs. However, if you can feel comfortable taking a brief silent pause to think about what the client has just said

and about what you might say next, then you will not need to prepare your next question while the client is talking. You can even say to the client, "I'm just taking a moment to think about what you've said." Rarely, will you need more than 10 seconds to do this.

Structuring the Interview

Regardless of the type of interview you use, there are three phases to a clinical interview: the opening, the body of the interview, and closure (Davis, 1994; Denton, 1987).

OPENING

At the opening of the interview, you let the client know the purpose of the interview. Even though you probably did so when you made the appointment for the interview, you might want to reintroduce yourself to the client, to say again that you are an occupational therapist and to briefly describe your role in the client's treatment. You should then explain the purpose of the interview and the types of questions that you will be asking.

BODY

The body is the exploration and development phase of the interview; the time when you and the client are actively constructing the client's story. Although specific interview procedures often provide a recommended sequence of questions, it is good idea to enter into this phase of the interview with relatively general and neutral questions that allow you to begin to sketch the background of the story. Because I am interested in a client's occupations, I often begin by asking a client to tell me how he or she typically spent time before he or she came into treatment. Such a broad question tends to be nonthreatening, but allows me to begin to develop a picture of the client's roles. Subsequent questions serve to fill in the details. Some clients are very forthcoming and are able to relate their stories easily; others will need much support and structure. It is during this phase that you will be calling on your skills in listening, attending, responding, and questioning.

Closure

As the time that you have allotted for the interview comes to an end, you will need to put closure on the session. It is important not to end the interview abruptly. Make sure that you allow sufficient time to summarize information, identify important themes in the client's story, and address how you and the client will work together. This will often be the time that you and the client mutually begin to set goals for therapy. As the interview comes to an end, you should let the client know what the next step in the therapy process will be, and when he or she will see you again. You might set a time for your next appointment. You should also thank the client for sharing his or her story with you.

▼ OCCUPATIONAL THERAPY INTERVIEWS

Occupational therapists need to develop **standardized** data-gathering instruments and procedures for both clinical and research purposes (Bonder, 1993). Over the past two decades, there have been several attempts to develop interview procedures that allow the collection of clinically useful information and that demonstrate evidence of reliability and validity. Several interview procedures will be briefly reviewed next.

Adolescent Role Assessment

The **Adolescent Role Assessment (ARA)** (Black, 1976) is the only occupational therapy interview specifically targeted for adolescents. The ARA is a semistructured interview procedure that gathers information on the adolescent's occupational role involvement over time and across domains. The 21 questions of the ARA cover six areas: childhood play, socialization within the family, school functioning, socialization with peers, occupational choice, and anticipated adult work. The items are scored with a 3-point scale; (+) indicates appropriate behavior, (0) indicates marginal or borderline behavior, (−) indicates inappropriate behavior. Black (1982) reported a test-retest **reliability** coefficient of 0.91 for the rating scale in a pilot study with a small group of adolescents. In addition, the scores on the ARA were found to discriminate between psychiatrically hospitalized adolescents ($n = 12$) and nonhospitalized adolescents drawn from a high school ($n = 28$). The ARA appears to yield useful information on an adolescent's functioning in occupations. Given the paucity of interview procedures specifically targeted for children and adolescents, further development of the ARA and similar procedures should be a priority for the field.

The Occupational Case Analysis and Interview Rating Scale

The **Occupational Case Analysis Interview and Rating Scale (OCAIRS)** (Kaplan & Kielhofner, 1989) was the first interview procedure specifically designed to reflect the **model of human occupation (MOHO)** (Kielhofner, 1985, 1995) perspective. The OCAIRS was designed for use in short-term adult psychiatric settings. The OCAIRS is a semistructured interview of approximately 38 recommended questions that are designed to address MOHO components.

A 5-point rating scale, with 14 items, accompanies the interview. The items include personal causation, values and goals, interests, roles, **habits**, skills, output, physical environment, social environment, feedback, dynamic (gestalt functioning), historical (life history pattern), contextual (environmental influence), and system trajectory (occupational prognosis). The client's functioning relative to each item is rated from adaptive (5) to maladaptive (1). A detailed training manual on the administration and interpretation of the OCAIRS is available (Kaplan & Kielhofner, 1989). Several studies have established the interrater reliability and concurrent **validity** of the OCAIRS (Brollier, Watts, Bauer & Schmidt, 1988; Kaplan & Kielhofner, 1989; Watts, Brollier, Bauer & Schmidt, 1988a).

The Assessment of Occupational Functioning

The **Assessment of Occupational Functioning (AOF)** (Watts, Brollier, Bauer, & Schmidt 1988b) is also based on the MOHO. The AOF was initially developed as a screening tool for use with either physically or psychiatrically disabled clients in long-term care settings. However, the most recent version, published in *Occupational Therapy in Mental Health* (Watts et al., 1988b), has been revised to be appropriate for use in other settings.

The AOF is a semistructured interview with 23 questions that tap the client's current functioning consistent with MOHO constructs. The AOF rating scale consists of 20 items, with three to four items comprising each of six subscales: values, personal causation, interests, roles, habits, and skills. Each item poses a question (eg, "Does this person routinely pursue his/her interests?"), which is then rated from 5 (very highly) to 1 (very little). All 20 items may be summed for a total score (Watts et al., 1988b).

The original version of the AOF has both interrater and test-retest reliability (Watts et al., 1986). No reliability data on the most recent revised version of the AOF rating scale have been reported. Studies have shown both the original and revised versions of the AOF to have concurrent validity (Brollier et al., 1988; Watts et al., 1988). Moreover, the AOF was found to discriminate between healthy community subjects and subjects in institutions 94% of the time (Watts, Kielhofner, Bauer, Gregory, & Valentine, 1986).

The Occupational Performance History Interview

The **Occupational Performance History Interview (OPHI)** (Kielhofner, Henry, & Walens, 1989) is a semistructured interview designed to gather information about a client's occupational performance over time, and is intended for use with adolescent, adult, and geriatric clients with both physical and psychiatric diagnoses. Although consistent with the occupational behavior perspective, the OPHI was specifically designed to be compatible with more than one frame of reference.

The OPHI consists of 39 recommended questions covering five content areas: (1) organization of daily routines;

(2) life roles; (3) interests, values, and goals; (4) perception of ability and responsibility; and (5) environmental influences. In addition to the questions, separate sets of yield statements have been developed to guide the use of the interview from both an eclectic and a model of human occupation (MOHO) perspective. Information is gathered about the client's functioning in each of the five areas in both the past and the present. A critical event or time period that distinguishes past from present is decided on jointly by the interviewer and the client at the beginning of the interview, and is referred to throughout the interview (Kielhofner et al., 1989).

Accompanying the interview is a 5-point scale used to rate the client's adaptation in both the past and the present (5 = adaptation; 1 = maladaptation). Two items are rated for each content area; all ten items can be summed for a total score. In addition to the rating scale, the OPHI provides a format for reporting narrative data gathered during the interview called the Life History Narrative. A manual detailing the procedure for administering and scoring the OPHI is available from AOTA (Kielhofner et al., 1989).

Test-retest and interrater reliability of the first version of the OPHI was examined in a study involving 153 physically and psychiatrically disabled subjects, and 201 clinicians as data collectors. In both the test-retest and interrater reliability data analyses, past ratings were generally more stable than present ratings. The test-retest reliability coefficients for the past and present total scores were 0.73 and 0.53, respectively, whereas the interrater reliability coefficients for the past and present total scores were 0.63 and 0.48, respectively (Kielhofner & Henry, 1988).

Following revisions to the OPHI, a second interrater reliability study was conducted. Two groups of 20 subjects with psychiatric diagnoses were interviewed and rated by three formally trained raters from either an eclectic or MOHO perspective. The coefficients for the past and present total score were 0.73 and 0.72, respectively, for the eclectic raters, and 0.70 and 0.57, respectively, for the MOHO raters (Kielhofner, Henry, Walens, & Rogers, 1991). Overall, the revisions to the interview procedure and formally training the raters appeared to strengthen the interrater reliability of the OPHI. However, reliability of the present total score for the MOHO raters was somewhat lower than desirable.

Concurrent and predictive validity of the OPHI rating scale have been established in a study of 44 adolescents and young adults hospitalized for a first episode of psychosis (Henry, 1994). Validity of the OPHI has also been established in studies of individuals with physical disabilities (Mauras-Nelson & Oakley, 1996; Lynch & Bridle, 1993)

Role Activity Performance Scale

In somewhat of a departure from the instruments described in the foregoing, the **Role Activity Performance Scale (RAPS)** (Good-Ellis, Fine, Spencer, & DiVittis, 1987) is an interview procedure that focuses specifically on *role functioning*. Developed for use with adult psychiatric patients, the RAPS was designed to facilitate treatment planning and to be used as a research tool in treatment outcome studies (Good-Ellis et al., 1987).

The RAPS is a semistructured interview and rating procedure that assesses an individual's history of role performance over a period of up to 18 months. The RAPS covers role performance in 12 areas: work/work equivalent, education, home management, family relationships, mate relationships, parental role, social relationships, leisure activities, self-management, health care, hygiene and appearance, and health care role. The interviewer covers only those role areas that are relevant. Unlike the interviews described earlier, which rely only on client self-report, the RAPS allows data to be gathered from a variety of other sources, including family members, the medical record, and the treatment team. Before the interview, the interviewer asks the client to complete a self-report questionnaire, reviews the medical record for pertinent data, and contacts other sources to determine which role areas should be covered during the interview. A set of recommended question has been developed for each role area, and the format of the questions is similar across role areas (Good-Ellis et al., 1987).

Each relevant role area is rated using a 6-point scale, with a score of "1' denoting excellent or good role performance, and "6" indicating an inability to function in the role (Good-Ellis et al., 1987). In addition, because the RAPS is intended to evaluate role functioning over time, separate ratings in each role area are made retrospectively on a monthly basis up to 18 months before the interview. This retrospective rating allows for scores reflecting the person's performance within each role over time, as well as a total score reflecting the person's performance across roles over time (Good-Ellis et al., 1987). A manual detailing the administration and scoring of the RAPS is currently in production (Good-Ellis, personal communication, May 1996).

Several studies have shown the RAPS to have good interrater reliability (Good-Ellis et al., 1987), concurrent validity, (Good-Ellis et al., 1987) and criterion-related validity (Good-Ellis, Fine, Hass, Spencer, & Glick, 1986; Good-Ellis et al., 1987).

The Worker Role Interview

The **Worker Role Interview (WRI)** is a semistructured interview that gathers data on psychosocial and environmental factors related to work, and was designed to be used with injured workers (Velozo, Kielhofner, & Fisher, 1992). The WRI is comprised of a set of 28 recommended questions and an accompanying 17-item rating scale, and was developed to be compatible with the MOHO. The items form six subscales that reflect the worker's sense of personal causation, values, interests, roles and habits related to work, as well as the influence of the environment. Each of the 17 items is rated using a 4-point scale (4, strongly supports client returning to job; 1, strongly interferes with client returning to job).

Biernacki (1993) found good interrater and test–retest reliability for the WRI studies of adults with upper extremity injuries. Even though the WRI was originally developed for use with individuals with physical disabilities, it has recently been adapted for use with individuals with psychiatric disorders (Handelsman, 1994).

The Canadian Occupational Performance Measure

The **Canadian Occupational Performance Measure (COPM)** (Law et al, 1994) is a client-centered semistructured interview procedure designed to measure a client's perceptions of his or her occupational performance over time. During an initial evaluation, the therapist interviews the client about his or her functioning in the areas of **self-care**, productivity, and leisure. (A specific set of interview questions has not been developed for the COPM.) The client is asked to identify any activities that are difficult for him or her to do in each area, and to do indicate how important it is for him or her to be able to do those activities. Finally, the client is asked to identify his or her five most important problems, and to rate his or her performance and level of satisfaction in these activities. The importance of the activity to the client, the quality of the client's performance, and the client's level of satisfaction are all rated *by the client* using similar 10-point scales (1 = not important at all, not able to do it, and not satisfied at all; 10 = extremely important, able to do it extremely well, and extremely satisfied). The specific focus of the COPM on client-identified problems is intended to facilitate collaborative goal setting between the therapist and client. At a re-evaluation, the client is again asked to rate his or her performance and satisfaction relative to the problem areas identified in the initial evaluation. By doing this, changes in the client's perceptions over time can be detected (Law et al., 1994).

In a study of 27 older adults with a variety of physical disabilities, test–retest reliability coefficients were 0.63 and 0.84, respectively (Law et al., 1994). Studies have also suggested that the COPM ratings are a valid indicator of clients' perceptions of their occupational performance. The COPM is also sensitive to changes in clients' performance and satisfaction ratings following occupational therapy and other rehabilitative interventions (Law et al., 1994).

Discussion

Each of the interview procedures reviewed in the foregoing sections shows evidence of having acceptable reliability. The procedures appear to be roughly equivalent in terms of the time required to administer and rate the interview. Whereas some (OCAIRS, AOF, WRI) are grounded in a specific theoretical model (MOHO), all gather data on occupational functioning and, thus, address universal concerns of the field. The ARA, OCAIRS, AOF, and OPHI take fairly broad perspectives on occupational functioning, considering both role performance in multiple domains and the influence of routines, interests, goals, and self-esteem on role performance. The RAPS and WRI are somewhat more narrowly focused; the RAPS considers only role performance, and the WRI is concerned specifically with the worker role. The COPM is unique in it's client-centered focus on mutual problem identification and collaborative treatment goal setting. Collaborative goal setting is not specifically identified as a goal of any of the other interviews, although it could easily follow any of the procedures described. Interviews such as the ARA, OCAIRS, AOF, and OPHI are likely to generate more narrative data. In the clinical setting, it might be useful to use one of these interviews in conjunction with the COPM, to both understand the client's story and plan meaningfully for treatment.

▼ ADJUNCTS TO INTERVIEWS: SELF-REPORT MEASURES

In addition to interviewing, paper-and-pencil **self-report measures** can be a useful method of obtaining information from the client. Self-report measures include surveys, forms, and checklists that the client completes. Frequently, a client can complete the form or checklist on his or her own, making this a convenient way to obtain information. More often, however, you should be present when the client completes the self-report measure, to ensure that the client comprehends what is being asked by the measure and is responding appropriately. Just as with interviews, self-report measures may not be appropriate for all clients.

In the clinical setting, self-report measures should not be used to substitute for a face-to-face interview with the client. They can be a helpful adjunct, however, because they tend to gather detailed information on a specific topic, such as time use or interest patterns. They are most useful when used in conjunction with an interview. Once a client has completed a self-report measure, the client and therapist should review the form together. The self-report measure focuses the discussion around a particular topic or issue.

Interest Checklists

Among the most commonly used self-report measures are **interest checklists**. Interest checklists are generally used to tap a client's level of interest in a range of activities, most often (but not exclusively) leisure activities. One of the oldest and most widely used is the NPI interest checklist (Matsutsuyu, 1969). The NPI interest checklist contains 80 activity items, which can be grouped in five categories: activities of daily living, manual skills, cultural and educational activities, physical sports, and social and recreational activities. In completing the checklist, the client indicates strong, casual, or no interest in the activity (Rogers, 1988).

Test–retest reliability of the NPI interest checklist was examined by Weinstein (1979). Using a 5-point Likert-type scale, a reliability coefficient of 0.92 was obtained. Two studies have found scores on the interest checklist to discriminate between normal and psychosocially dysfunctional adolescents (Barris et al., 1986; Ebb, Coster, & Duncombe, 1989). Moreover, Henry (1994) found variables derived from the NPI interest checklist that reflect an interest in recreational activities to be predictive for functioning of adolescents and young adults with psychosis following hospitalization.

Other checklist-format measures of interest have been developed. Kielhofner and Neville (1983) modified the NPI interest checklist to include questions concerning changes in activity preferences over time, and the desire to participate in interests in the future. In 1983, Gregory described two self-report measures of activity involvement specifically designed for older adults. Total scores on both the Activity Index, which taps activity interest and participation, and on the Meaningfulness of Activity Scale, which taps feelings of enjoyment, autonomy, and competence relative to activities, demonstrated good test-retest reliability with small pilot samples (0.70 and 0.87, respectively). Scores on both measures were also correlated positively with a measure of life satisfaction.

Age-targeted measures of interest in activities are likely to yield more relevant data than a general measure, because leisure interests vary widely across the age span. Recently, Henry (1996), adapting the scales developed by Gregory (1983), developed a measure of leisure interest specifically targeted for adolescents. The Adolescent Leisure Interest Profile (ALIP), is an 86-item measure, designed to tap leisure interests, leisure participation, and feelings about leisure among adolescents. Preliminary studies with both normal adolescents and adolescents with disabilities indicate that the ALIP total scores demonstrate good test-retest reliability. Versions of the Leisure Interest Profile targeted for children, adults, and elders are currently being developed. Interest checklists are useful in identifying problems related to leisure and for identifying potential activities to use in treatment.

The Role Checklist

The Role Checklist (Oakley, Kielhofner, Barris, & Reichler, 1986) is a two-part, paper-and-pencil inventory of ten occupational roles, including worker, student, family member, homemaker, caregiver, volunteer, and hobbyist. The first part of the Role Checklist examines a client's past, present, and future intentions related to performance of each role. The second part examines the value assigned to each role by the client.

Studies have indicated that the Role Checklist has good test-retest reliability (Barris, Oakley, & Kielhofer, 1988) and

is valid (Barris, Dickie, & Baron, 1988; Ebb et al., 1989; Smyntek, Barris, & Kielhofer, 1985).

Self-Assessment of Occupational Functioning

The Self-Assessment of Occupational Functioning (SAOF) (Baron & Curtin, 1990) is a self-report measure designed to gather data on a person's perception of his or her strengths and weaknesses relative to occupational functioning. Moreover, the SAOF is a procedure designed to be used in collaborative problem identification and treatment goal setting between the client and the therapist, making it particularly useful to use in conjunction with an interview. The items of the SAOF reflect MOHO constructs; the areas of occupational functioning evaluated correspond directly to the volition, habituation, and performance subsystems, and the environment. Both adolescent–adult and child versions of the SAOF have been developed (Baron & Curtin, 1990). The adolescent–adult version of the SAOF includes 23 items, which are organized into four subscales; volition, habituation, performance, and environment. The child version includes 44 items, organized into the same four subscales. Preliminary examination of test-retest reliability of the adolescent–adult version of the SAOF with 37 normal female college students yielded test-retest reliability coefficients for the four subscales ranging from 0.68 to 0.75; the coefficient for the total scales was 0.87 (Mouradian et al, 1993). Henry (1994) found scores on the SAOF habituation subscale to predict functioning among adolescent and young adults with psychosis following hospitalization.

The Occupational Questionnaire

The **Occupational Questionnaire (OQ)** (Smith, Kielhofner, & Watts, 1986) is a paper-and-pencil measure that gathers data on time use patterns and feelings about time use. In completing the OQ, the person indicates his or her main activity during each half hour of a typical day, and classifies each activity as either school, work, activity of daily living (ADL), recreation, or rest. The person then rates each activity using a 5-point Likert-type scale, indicating how well he or she does the activity (competence), how important the activity is (value), and how enjoyable the activity is (enjoyment). Similar to the SAOF, the OQ is based on MOHO constructs.

In a test–retest reliability study of 20 elderly adults, 68% of a typical day's activities reported during the first administration were again reported during the same time period of the second administration. Agreement on activity categorization and feelings of competence, value, and enjoyment was also high. A study of concurrent validity using the Household Work Study Diary yielded high agreement in configuration of activities and in how subjects' classified activities (Smith et al, 1986).

► CONCLUSION

In addition to providing information about a client's functioning in specific occupations, interviews are among the useful strategies available to therapists to both better understand the client's perspective of his or her situation and to enhance the working relationship with the client. Each of the interviews and self-report measures discussed in this section has its unique characteristics. In clinical practice, therapists must choose the combination of interview and other assessments that best fits the needs of their clients and practice setting.

► REFERENCES

American Occupational Therapy Association (AOTA). (1994). Uniform terminology for occupational therapy—Third edition. *American Journal of Occupational Therapy, 48,* 1047–1054.

Baron K. B., & Curtin, C. (1990). *A manual for use with the self assessment of occupational functioning.* Department of Occupational Therapy, University of Illinois at Chicago.

Barris, R., Dickie, V., & Baron, K. B. (1988). A comparison of psychiatric patients and normal subjects based on the model of human occupation. *Occupational Therapy Journal of Research, 8,* 3–37.

Barris, R., Kielhofner, G., Burch, R. M., Gelinas, I., Klement, M., & Schultz, B. (1986). Occupational function and dysfunction in three groups of adolescents. *Occupational Therapy Journal of Research, 6, 301–317.*

Barris, R., Oakley, F., & Kielhofner, G. (1988). The role checklist. In B. Hemphill (Ed.), *Mental health assessment in occupational therapy. An integrative approach to the evaluation process* (pp. 73–91). Thorofare, NJ: Slack.

Biernacki, S. D. (1993). Reliability of the worker role interview. *American Journal of Occupational Therapy, 47,* 797–803.

Black, M. M. (1976). Adolescent role assessment. *American Journal of Occupational Therapy, 30,* 73–79.

Black, M. M. (1982). Adolescent role assessment. In B. Hemphill (Ed.), *The evaluative process in psychiatric occupational therapy.* (pp. 49–53). Thorofare, NJ: Slack.

Bonder, B. (1993). Issues in assessment of psychosocial components of function. *American Journal of Occupational Therapy, 47,* 211–216.

Bradburn, S. L. (1992). *Psychiatric occupational therapists' strategies for engaging patients in treatment during the initial interview.* Unpublished masters thesis, Tufts University.

Brollier, C., Watts, J. H., Bauer, D., & Schmidt. W. (1988). A concurrent validity study of two occupational therapy evaluation instruments. The AOF and OCAIRS. *Occupational Therapy in Mental Health, 8* (4), 49–60.

Bruce, B., & Borg, M. A. (1993). *Psychosocial occupational therapy frame of reference for intervention* (2nd ed.). Thorofare, NJ: Slack.

Clark, F. (1993). Eleanor Clarke Slagle Lectureship—1993; Occupation embedded in a real life: Interweaving occupational science and occupational therapy. *American Journal of Occupational Therapy, 47,* 1067–1078.

Cohn, E. (1994). *Interviewing children.* Unpublished manuscript, Boston University.

Davis, C. M. (1994). *Patient practitioner interaction. An experiential manual for developing the art of health care.* Thorofare, NJ: Slack.

Denton, P. L. (1987). *Psychiatric occupational therapy: A workbook of practical skills.* Boston: Little, Brown & Company.

Ebb, E. W., Coster, W., & Duncombe, L. (1989). Comparison of normal and psychosocially dysfunctional male adolescents. *Occupational Therapy in Mental Health, 9* (2), 53–74.

Frank, G. (1996). Life histories in occupational therapy clinical practice. *American Journal of Occupational Therapy, 50,* 251–264.

Good–Ellis, M. A., Fine S. B., Hass, G. L., Spencer, J. H., & Glick, I. D. (1986). Quantitative role and performance assessment: Implications and application to treatment of major affective disorders. In *Depression: Assessment and treatment update.* Proceedings from the AOTA Preconference Institute to the American Psychiatric Association's Institute on Hospital and Community Psychiatry. Rockville, MD: AOTA.

Good–Ellis, M. A., Fine, S. B., Spencer, J. H., & DiVittis, A. (1987). Developing a role activity performance scale. *American Journal of Occupational Therapy, 41,* 232–241.

Gregory, M. (1983). Occupational behavior and life satisfaction among retirees. *American Journal of Occupational Therapy, 37,* 548–552.

Handelsman, D. (1994). *The construct validity of the worker role interview for the chronic mentally ill.* Unpublished master's thesis, University of Illinois at Chicago.

Helfrich, C., & Kielhofner, G. (1994). Volitional narratives and the meaning of therapy. *American Journal of Occupational Therapy, 48,* 319–326.

Henry, A. D. (1994). *Predicting psychosocial functioning and symptomatic recovery of adolescents and young adults with a first psychotic episode: A six-month follow-up study.* Unpublished doctoral dissertation, Boston University.

Henry, A. (1996, April). *Development of a measure of adolescent leisure interests.* Poster presentation at the American Occupational Therapy Association Annual Conference, Chicago, IL.

Henry, A. D., & Coster, W. J. (1996). Predictors of functional outcome among adolescents and young adults with psychotic disorders. *American Journal of Occupational Therapy, 50,* 171–181.

Kaplan, K., & Kielhofner, G. (1989). *Occupational case analysis interview and rating scale.* Thorofare, NJ: Slack.

Kielhofner, G. (Ed.). (1985). *A model of human occupation. Theory and application.* Baltimore: Williams & Wilkins.

Kielhofner, G. (Ed.). (1995). *A model of human occupation. Theory and application.* (2nd ed.). Baltimore: Williams & Wilkins.

Kielhofner, G., & Henry, A. D. (1988). Development and investigation of the occupational performance history interview. *American Journal of Occupational Therapy, 42,* 489–498.

Kielhofner, G., Henry A. D., & Walens, D. (1989). *A user's guide to the occupational performance history interview.* Rockville, MD: American Occupational Therapy Association.

Kielhofner, G., Henry, A. D., Walens, D., & Rogers, E. S. (1991). A generalizability study of the occupational performance history interview. *Occupational Therapy Journal of Research, 11,* 292–306.

Kielhofner, G., & Mallinson, T. (1995). Gathering narrative data through interviews: Empirical observations and suggested guidelines. *Scandinavian Journal of Occupational Therapy, 2,* 63–68.

Kielhofner, G., & Neville, A. (1983). *The modified interest checklist.* Unpublished manuscript, University of Illinois at Chicago.

Kohlman-Thompson, L. (1992). *The Kohlman evaluation of living skills.* Rockville, MD: American Occupational Therapy Association.

LaGreca, A. M. (Ed.). (1990). *Through the eyes of the child. Obtaining self-reports from children and adolescents.* Boston: Allyn and Bacon.

Law, M., Baptiste, S., Carswell, A., McColl, M. A., Polatajko, H., & Pollock, N. (1994). *Canadian occupational performance measure.* (2nd ed.). Toronto: Canadian Association of Occupational Therapists.

Lynch, K. B., & Bridle, M. J. (1993). Construct validity of the occupational performance history interview. *Occupational Therapy Journal of Research, 13,* 231–240.

Matsutsuyu, J. (1969). The interest checklist. *American Journal of Occupational Therapy, 23,* 323–328.

Mattingly, C. (1991). The narrative nature of clinical reasoning. *American Journal of Occupational Therapy, 45,* 998–1005.

Mattingly, C., & Fleming, M. H. (1994). *Clinical reasoning. Forms of inquiry in a therapeutic practice.* Philadelphia: F. A. Davis Company.

Mauras-Nelson, E., & Oakley, F. (1996, April). *Bone marrow transplanta-*

tion: Implications on function. Poster presentation at the American Occupational Therapy Association Annual Conference, Chicago, IL.

Mishler, E. G. (1986). *Research interviewing: Context and narrative*. Cambridge, MA: Harvard University Press.

Mouradian, L., Anhalt, A., Aronowitz, L., Beauchamp, R., Benson, A., Burgos, L., Busker, D., Christopher, R., Dailey, J., Day, E., Mondschein, M., & Roelse, T. (1993, April). *Test-retest reliability of the self assessment of occupational functioning*. Poster presented at the Neurobehavioral Rehabilitation Research Center 1st Annual Research Colloquium, Boston University, Sargent College of Allied Health Professions.

Neistadt, M. E. (1995). Methods of assessing clients' priorities: A survey of adult physical dysfunction settings. *American Journal of Occupational Therapy, 49*, 428–436.

Oakley, F., Kielhofner, G., Barris, R., & Reichler, R. (1986). The role checklist: Development and empirical assessment of reliability. *Occupational Therapy Journal of Research, 6*, 157–170.

Polkinghorne, D. E. (1996). Transformative narratives: From victimic to agentic life plots. *American Journal of Occupational Therapy, 50*, 299–305.

Rogers, J. C. (1988). The NPI Interest Checklist. In B. J. Hemphill (Ed.), *Mental health assessment in occupational therapy. An integrative approach to the evaluation process*. Thorofare, NJ: Slack.

Rogers, J.C., & Holm, M.B. (1991). Occupational therapy diagnostic reasoning: A component of clinical reasoning. *American Journal of Occupational Therapy, 45*, 1045–1053.

Smith, N. R., Kielhofner, G., & Watts, J. H. (1986). The relationship be-

tween volition, activity pattern and life satisfaction in the elderly. *American Journal of Occupational Therapy, 40*, 278–283.

Smyntek, L., Barris, R., & Kielhofner, G. (1985). The model of human occupation applied to psychosocially functional and dysfunctional adolescents. *Occupational Therapy in Mental Health, 5* (1), 21–40.

Stone, W. L., & Lemanek, K. L. (1990). Developmental issues in children's self-reports. In A. M. LaGreca (Ed.), *Through the eyes of the child. Obtaining self-reports from children and adolescents.* (pp. 18–55). Boston: Allyn and Bacon.

Tickle-Degnen, L. (1995). Therapeutic rapport. In C. A. Trombly (Ed.), *Occupational therapy for physical dysfunction*. Fourth edition. (pp. 277–285). Baltimore: Williams & Wilkins.

Velozo, C., Kielhofner, G., & Fisher, G. (1992). *A user's guide to the worker role interview*. (Research version). Department of Occupational Therapy, University of Illinois at Chicago.

Watts, J. H., Brollier, C., Bauer, D., & Schmidt, W. (1988a). A comparison of two evaluation instruments used with psychiatric patients in occupational therapy. *Occupational Therapy in Mental Health, 8* (4), 7–27.

Watts, J. H., Brollier, C., Bauer, D., & Schmidt, W. (1988b). The assessment of occupational functioning: The second revision. *Occupational Therapy in Mental Health, 8* (4), 61–88.

Watts, J. H., Kielhofner, G., Bauer, D., Gregory, M., & Valentine, D. (1986). The assessment of occupational functioning: A screening tool for use in long-term care. *American Journal of Occupational Therapy, 40*, 231–240.

Weinstein, J. (1979). *The generation of profiles of adolescent interests*. Unpublished master's thesis, University of Southern California, Los Angeles.

Chapter 14

Critiquing Assessments

Janice Miller Polgar

O ccupational therapists evaluate all of their clients to understand their levels of function in **occupations**. Occasionally informal **assessments** are used, but on other occasions, standardized assessments are most appropriate. When a standardized assessment is used, it is crucial that the occupational therapist has critiqued the instrument to determine its ability to evaluate the areas under consideration. The occupational therapist must ensure that the method of test development, standardization, development of norms, and psychometric properties meet an acceptable standard when determining the test's clinical usefulness. This chapter will provide an understanding of why it is important to critically appraise these instruments and discuss each component of a thorough instrument critique.

The primary purpose of this chapter is to inform occupational therapists of the purposes of **evaluation** and the necessity of critiquing the assessments we use in our practice. A framework will be presented to organize the critique. Issues of test development and standardization, reliability and validity, and the influence of culture and disabilities on test use will also be presented. This chapter is meant to provide sufficient information to enable an adequate critique of instruments that are used in occupational therapy. It is not meant to provide the reader with a detailed discussion of the various statistical analyses involved in test development or establishment of psychometric properties. Sources for more detailed information will be identified at the end of the chapter. In the literature, various labels are used to identify a measurement tool, including "test," "instrument," "evaluation," "measurement," and "assessment." Either assessment, instrument, or test will be used as labels in this chapter.

▼ MEASUREMENT

Measurement is the process of assigning numbers to represent quantities of a trait, attribute, or characteristic, or to classify objects (Nunnally & Bernstein, 1995). It enables therapists to understand aspects of clients' function, abilities, or personal characteristics. An important distinction, here, is that measurement enables therapists to quantify aspects of persons, but not persons themselves (Nunnally & Bernstein, 1995). It provides a means to operationally define behaviors and, by quantifying these behaviors, to make comparisons between individuals, or to compare the same person at two different times (Law, 1987).

Some fundamental assumptions of measurement are critical to an understanding of the properties of psychometrically sound instruments (Barclay, 1991). The definition of measurement presented in the foregoing assumes that psychological, sociological, and biological functions are observable and thus, measurable. A second assumption is that what is observable and quantifiable corresponds to aspects of human behavior. For example, the Rotter I-E scale (Rotter, 1966) yields a numerical score that purports to measure the individual's level of personal causation; the pattern of responses on the test items is considered to represent the multifaceted construct of personal causation. Third, it is assumed that these measures have a normal distribution in the population; this concept will be discussed later. Finally, it is assumed that some traits are relatively stable across time. Measurements are used in different ways, depending on the purpose of a given evaluation.

▼ PURPOSES OF EVALUATION IN OCCUPATIONAL THERAPY

Three main purposes have been identified for evaluation (Kirshner & Guyatt, 1985). The first purpose is descriptive. When the occupational therapist's intent is to describe individuals within a group or to describe differences between members of a group, an instrument should be chosen that measures the desired attribute comprehensively (Law, 1987). For example, if an occupational therapist is interested in describing a child's ability to operate a powered wheelchair, the instrument should measure all components considered necessary for this task.

A second purpose is to predict either future function or function in a related area (Kirshner & Guyatt, 1985). The occupational therapist may be interested in understanding the relation between performance on a measure of motor skills in infancy and subsequent performance on a test of fine motor skills at the age of 5. Alternatively, the therapist may be interested in determining the relation between achievement of a certain score on a vocational test and function on the job site.

Finally, occupational therapists use measurement to evaluate outcomes of therapeutic intervention (Kirshner & Guyatt, 1985). In this instance, it is important to use an instrument that will detect change that has occurred (Gowland et al., 1991; Law, 1987). This last purpose is important to demonstrate the efficacy of our practice.

Whether an instrument is used to describe an individual or group, to predict function, or evaluate outcome, the results of testing are used to make decisions. From our testing, we determine the suitability of a person to return to work or to his or her community, whether a person is a suitable candidate for therapeutic intervention, or what types of intervention are likely to be most effective. We also make decisions about the efficacy of our practice. These decisions have important implications to our practice and to the lives of our clients. Because of the importance of our decisions, it is crucial that occupational therapists critique instruments relative to test construction, **reliability** and **validity,** and applicability to the client group under consideration.

▼ CRITIQUING ASSESSMENTS

An outline to guide the critique of an instrument can be seen in Box 14-1. Each of the major technical considerations will be discussed.

Test Construction

The test manual should explicate the manner in which the test has been constructed. It should give sufficient information for the individual evaluating the test to be able to determine that it was developed in a logical, systematic, and

▼ **BOX 14-1**

> ## A Format for Critiquing Assessments
>   ### I. GENERAL INFORMATION
>   Title
>   Author
>   Publisher
>   Time required to administer
>   Materials required
>   Cost
>   ### II. BRIEF DESCRIPTION OF PURPOSE OF TEST
>   Type/purpose of test (description, prediction, evaluation)
>   Target population
>   Item description (response format, content)
>   Traits or aptitudes evaluated (total score and subscales)
>   ### III. PRACTICAL ASSESSMENT
>   Ease of administration
>   Clarity of directions
>   Scoring procedures
>   Examiner qualifications and training
>   ### IV. TECHNICAL CONSIDERATIONS
>   #### A. NORMS
>   Type (percentiles, standard scores, etc.)
>   Standardization sample
>   Standardization procedures
>   #### B. RELIABILITY
>   Test–retest
>   Alternative form
>   Internal consistency
>   Split-half
>   Cronbach's alpha
>   Kuder–Richardson
>   #### C. VALIDITY
>   Construct
>   Criterion
>   Content
>   #### D. EVIDENCE OF TEST RESPONSIVENESS
>   ### V. EXTERNAL REVIEWERS COMMENTS
>   Include information from published evaluations of the test
>   ### VI. SUMMARY OF STRENGTHS AND WEAKNESSES OF THE TEST

stringent fashion. The following sections present information about how tests should be constructed and what should be considered when critiquing an unfamiliar test.

DEFINING THE CONSTRUCT

DePoy and Gitlin (1993) define a *construct* as something that is abstract and, therefore, cannot be directly measured. Constructs do not exist "as an observable dimension of behavior" (Nunnally & Bernstein, 1995). For example, self-efficacy is considered to be a construct because it is not a tangible entity that can be measured directly. Rather, hypotheses must be generated identifying which behaviors demonstrate high versus low levels of self-efficacy.

The first step in test construction is to define, explicitly, the construct or concept of interest and generate hypotheses about how this construct will manifest itself (Zeidner & Most, 1992). Definition of the construct requires that the test developers articulate their understanding of the construct and its content domain. The definition of the construct comes from a sound understanding of the relevant literature (Benson & Clark, 1982). From clinical experience and support from the literature, an operational definition of the construct is developed, and the significant factors contributing to it are identified and defined. An operational definition is one that states under which conditions behavior will be labeled as the desired construct (Pedhazur & Schmelkin, 1991). For example, the construct of arm coordination is operationally defined as the ability to bounce a ball, catch a beanbag and throw it through a target on the *McCarthy Scales of Children's Abilities* (McCarthy, 1972). The information concerning conceptualization and definition of the construct and related variables should be included in the test manual.

The potential users must go through a similar procedure to evaluate the suitability of the test. If the users are not familiar with the area, they too should review the pertinent literature (Zeidner & Most, 1992). The users must explicitly articulate their conceptualization of the construct and its dimensions to compare their understanding of the construct with that stated in the test manual. If this comparison yields a match between conceptualizations, support is gained for the clinical usefulness of the instrument.

ITEM DEVELOPMENT

Development of the test items is an involved process, detailed discussion of which is beyond the scope of this chapter. Relative to test critique, it is important to review test items for the following features:

1. Congruence of the items with the conceptualization of the construct found in the test manual or related literature
2. Representativeness of the dimensions of the construct
3. Clarity of items to avoid ambiguity
4. Possibility of bias for certain clients (Murphy & Davidshofer, 1991).

SCALES OF MEASUREMENT

It is important to determine the type of measurement scale that is used. There are four scales of measurement: nominal, ordinal, interval, and ratio (Pedhazur & Schmelkin, 1991; Salvia & Ysseldyke, 1985). The *nominal scale* involves mutually exclusive categories (eg, female versus male, or geographic location). Often these categories are given numbers (eg, male = 1 and female = 2), but these numbers are not meaningful in a quantitative way. This scale simply identifies differences with no attempt to quantify or order those differences.

A second level is the *ordinal scale*. This scale involves rank-ordering scores. The order indicates greater (or better) than, but no inference can be made about the magnitude of the difference between scores. *Interval scales* are a third level. This type of scale is the most common in measures found in occupational therapy. The intervals between scores are equal so

comparisons can be made between individuals (Pedhazur & Schmelkin, 1991). However, 0 is not an absolute point on these scales. Because 0 is arbitrary, ratio comparisons between scores cannot be made (Pedhazur & Schmelkin, 1991; Salvia & Ysseldyke, 1985). For example, if person A scores 20 on a test of self-esteem and person B scores 40 on the same test, it is not meaningful to say that person B has twice as much self-esteem as person A. To make this comparison meaningfully, 0 must be a fixed point.

On *ratio scales*, 0 does have a fixed point and ratio comparisons can be made (Pedhazur & Schmelkin, 1991). To use these scales, absence of the attribute being measured must be meaningful. When measuring volume, a score of 0 indicates the absence of liquid. In occupational therapy, range of motion can be understood as a ratio scale as there can be absence of measurable movement around a joint, and it is meaningful to indicate that a person has gained twice as much movement between measurements.

DEVELOPMENT OF NORMS

Many of the tests used by occupational therapists are norm-referenced (Anastasi, 1982; Murphy & Davidshofer, 1991). Norms are statistics that are generated from a well-defined group that has been evaluated using the test in a standardized manner (Wiersma & Jurs, 1990). Usually, but not necessarily, norms are measures of the average performance of this reference group. These statistics are used to make comparisons between the individual tested and this reference group (ie, the norms provide a point of reference for comparison of the individual's score).

It is crucial to understand that the norms provided in the manual are not *the* definitive norms (Murphy & Davidshofer, 1991). They represent the performance of those individuals who were tested for the development of the norms. The usefulness of the norms for making a meaningful interpretation of an individual's score is dependent on the information given about the characteristics of the sample used to create the norms, the method of recruiting the sample, and the degree to which the sample represents the test's target **population**.

At some point in the development of the test, a target population is identified (Murphy & Davidshofer, 1991; Wiersma & Jurs, 1990). The population defines the group for whom the test is intended. The test manual should clearly state the intended target population. Before using a test, the therapist must determine that it is intended to evaluate people with characteristics similar to those of the client.

Wiersma and Jurs (1990) list three criteria for evaluating the usefulness of the norms, related to the target population: They should be representative, relevant, and recent. The sample *represents* the target population when the distribution of characteristics of the population is reflected in the sample. A test that is targeted for national (or international) use must demonstrate that the norms were developed to represent the distribution of region, urban or rural living, gender, ethnicity, and any other relevant characteristics of the national or international population (Murphy & Davidshofer, 1991; Wiersma & Jurs, 1990). One that is intended to provide information about performance at different ages must use a sample including individuals of each age. For example, a test that provides norms for children at 6-month intervals should ensure that children at each of these ages were included in the norming sample.

The test manual should include clear information about the selection of the norming sample. Random-sampling procedures should be used. These involve selection based on the distribution of the characteristics of the population identified; not because of convenience (Wiersma & Jurs, 1990). The sample size should be sufficient to minimize measurement errors and to maximize the confidence the test user has in the norms provided. The procedures for administering the test to the sample and the time of administration should also be identified in the test manual (Wiersma & Jurs).

The norming sample should be *relevant* to the target population (Wiersma & Jurs, 1990). It should have characteristics similar to the population. Norms that have been developed from the motor performance of adults are of little use in providing a meaningful interpretation of the motor performance of preschoolers.

Finally, norms should be *recent* (Wiersma & Jurs, 1990). Test material can become dated. For example, tests developed before the mid-1970s that require knowledge of linear measurement will not reliably test this knowledge in Canadian children today. Before the mid-1970s measurement was expressed in Imperial units. At that time, the metric system was introduced and Canadian children no longer were taught Imperial units of measurement. Now, questions about Imperial units will not be meaningful to them. As well, over time, performance or attributes may change in the population.

STANDARDIZED SCORES

Raw scores are usually converted into another form to facilitate comparison and a meaningful interpretation. These forms include percentiles, stanines, standard scores, and age- or grade-equivalent scores (Murphy & Davidshofer, 1991; Wiersma & Jurs, 1990). These will be discussed presently but, first, some basic statistical concepts related to test scores will be briefly reviewed. There are three measures of central tendency: mean, median, and mode. The *mean* is the arithmetic average of the cumulative measures (Ferguson, 1981; Murphy & Davidshofer, 1991). The *median* is the point in the distribution of the scores that divides the scores in half (ie, 50% are above the median and 50% are below it). The *mode* is the most frequently occurring score. It is important to know which of these measures of central tendency is being reported.

For a given population, scores are considered to be distributed normally. In the *normal distribution*, the bulk of the scores are at the center of the range, with fewer scores found at the extremes of the range (Ferguson, 1981). The *range* of the distribution is the span between the lowest and highest score (Ferguson). The *variance* indicates the dispersion of the scores (Ferguson). *Standard deviation* (SD) is the square root of the variance and is the most common method of dividing the normal distribution. It represents the spread of the scores in the same units as the test score (Wiersma & Jurs, 1990). Approximately 68% of the scores fall within -1.0 and $+1.0$ SD, 95% fall within -2.0 and $+2.0$ SD, and 99% fall within -3.0 and $+3.0$ SD (Anastasi, 1982).

The *percentile rank* is expressed as a whole number between 1 and 99. The number represents the percentage of persons who scored at or below a given score (Anastasi, 1982; Wiersma & Jurs, 1990). An individual whose score is at the 75th percentile performed equal to or better than 75% of those tested. Percentile rank is an ordinal scale so the intervals between the ranks are not equal (Wiersma & Jurs, 1990). It is considered to have a normal distribution with the majority of the scores falling around the 50th percentile (Anastasi, 1982).

Stanine is an abbreviated form of standard-nine (Wiersma & Jurs, 1990). This method of standardizing scores divides the normal distribution into nine components, each comprising one-half of a standard deviation to provide equal units of measure. It minimizes a tendency to overinterpret small differences in scores, but it may not be sufficiently sensitive to detect small changes (Wiersma & Jurs).

Standard scores use the standard deviation to obtain a scale with equal intervals. These scores have been termed *z-scores* (Witt, Elliott, Gresham, & Kramer, 1988). The standard or z-scores express an individual's score in terms of standard deviation above or below the mean (Wiersma & Jurs, 1990) providing ease of interpretation.

Age- or grade-equivalent scores relate the individual's performance on the test to that of the typical individual of a particular age or grade (Murphy & Davidshofer, 1991). It is crucial that the sample used to create the norms has sufficient representation of the comparison grades or ages.

In summary, the norms of the test provide the comparison group needed to make a meaningful interpretation of the obtained score. The group used to create the norms should represent and be relevant to the test's target population and be current. The methods used for establishing the norms and the type of standardized score used should be clearly identified in the test manual.

TEST STANDARDIZATION

As stated earlier, tests are used to describe people, make comparisons, or evaluate performance. Because of the effect that decisions from test scores have on the lives of people, it is important that as many extraneous factors as possible are eliminated from the method of administering, scoring, and interpreting the scores (Murphy & Davidshofer, 1991). Test standardization procedures are used to ensure the maximum level of consistency in testing situations.

The test manual should clearly describe the arrangement of the testing environment, the presentation of materials, standardized instructions, and time limits (American Educational Research Association [AERA], 1985). When the test developers have made modifications to any of these areas to accommodate individuals with different abilities, these modifications should be clearly indicated so they can be replicated in appropriate situations. Moreover, the manual should indicate clear guidelines for scoring the test and interpreting the scores (AERA).

It is not possible to standardize all aspects of test administration. Aspects of the environment, such as noise, or the examinee's mood at the time of testing, are not controllable. Because of these uncontrollable factors, which can affect the reliability of the test, it is important to follow the standardized instructions of the test exactly. Failure to do so will affect the test's reliability (AERA, 1985). It is also important to ensure that the test user is adequately trained or prepared to administer the test. Some tests indicate the type of training necessary for administration. Indeed, some tests are not available except to those who hold the necessary qualifications.

Reliability

DEFINITION OF RELIABILITY

A standardized test used to evaluate the performance of an individual or to measure the existence of a specified trait yields a score. It is important to demonstrate that the score resulting from the use of a test is consistent and repeatable. Consistency and repeatability are aspects of *reliability*, defined as "the extent to which an experiment, test, or any measuring procedure yields the same results on repeated trials" (Carmines & Zeller, 1979, p. 11). All forms of reliability are based on the correlation coefficient and referred to as a reliability coefficient. The reliability coefficient can range from 0 to +1, with 0 indicating no consistency and +1 indicating perfect consistency. Reliability approaching +1 is desirable.

An instrument is considered to be reliable when a similar score is achieved on repeated administration. It is important to distinguish that a similar score, not an identical one, is the aim in reliability (Siegel, 1989). When an instrument is reliable, it is expected that on subsequent testing the individual will achieve scores that are consistent, but not identical with, previously achieved scores. To understand why identical scores are not expected, an explanation of some of the assumptions of reliability or classical test theory is important. A test score is considered to consist of three components:

1. The obtained score
2. The true score, considered to be a hypothetical, unobservable quantity of the specific attribute under consideration (Carmines & Zeller, 1979)
3. Measurement error

The relation between these components is expressed by:

Obtained score = true score + measurement error

In other words, every obtained score is made up of two components, a portion of the score that reflects the "true" quantity of an attribute and random errors that contribute to inconsistency in the measurement (Murphy & Davidshofer, 1991). It is assumed that no relation exists between true scores and the error component (1991). Reliability is high when the proportion of the obtained score owing to measurement error is low. The sources of measurement error will be discussed further.

FACTORS THAT CONTRIBUTE TO ERROR IN TESTING

There are several factors that contribute to error in testing. These factors can be classed as factors relating to the test itself, factors relating to the situation of testing, those related to the individual being tested, and factors related to the examiner. *Factors related to the test* include how stringently the test was constructed, the adequacy of the directions for administering and scoring the test, test length, homogeneity of test content, effect of bias, and the construction of the items (Isaac & Michael, 1971; Murphy & Davidshofer, 1991).

Various *environmental or situational factors* may contribute to error. The environment might be distracting, time limits may induce undue stress, or the length of the assessment may contribute to fatigue (Isaac & Michael, 1971).

Many *factors related to the individual* can contribute to variance in the obtained score. Some factors are relatively stable, such as level of ability, knowledge or skills, personality, or the level of comfort with a particular response mode (eg, multiple choice) (Murphy & Davidshofer, 1991). Other factors are more inconsistent, such as motivation, practice with test items, fatigue, anxiety, or other emotional states (1991). *Factors related to the examiner* include familiarity and training for the specific test and assessment process, adherence to standardized instructions, and the ability to establish an effective evaluation atmosphere (Isaac & Michael, 1971). These factors occur on a random basis and are not easily quantifiable. Therefore, we must estimate their potential influence on an individual's obtained test score.

TYPES OF RELIABILITY
Test–Retest Reliability
Test–retest reliability is a measure of the consistency of an assessment over time. It has also been termed "stability" (Jensen, 1980), for it estimates the stability of the measurement over time. This form of reliability is determined by administering an evaluation on two occasions, separated by a time interval. Nunnally and Bernstein (1995) suggest that a desirable separation is 2 weeks. With a shorter time period, the examinee may remember the test items; with a longer time period, actual changes might occur. Test–retest reliability is estimated by determining the correlation or associa-

tion between scores obtained on two testing occasions. A correlation approaching +1.0 suggests that a test is stable across time.

Test–retest reliability or stability is meaningful only when the trait being measured is expected to be stable over the testing interval (Carmines & Zeller, 1979). An evaluation of mood, for example, is not expected to yield consistent results over a period of weeks, for mood is considered to fluctuate. Alternatively, a trait such as height is stable and should yield little variability in the obtained scores over repeated measurements. Many attributes measured in occupational therapy are not as clearly consistent or inconsistent as the examples just given. In each case, individuals considering the test must compare their understanding of the construct or attribute being measured with that explicated in the test manual to assess whether that attribute is stable and, thus, whether an indication of stability is essential.

An estimate of the test's stability is necessary when the measurement is used as an outcome measure (Jensen, 1980). Test stability should not be affected by maturation unless such is accounted for in the scoring procedures (Murphy & Davidshofer, 1991).

Evaluation of a test's stability can be confounded by several factors. There may be changes in the individual on the trait being measured between the test administrations (Jensen, 1980). Sometimes, simple exposure to a test may cause the individual to reflect on the trait or attribute, resulting in a change in subsequent test performance. Carmines and Zeller (1979) have termed this phenomena "reactivity." A historical event may occur between administrations that could influence the score (Kerlinger, 1973). The individual may remember the test items or practice with the materials, which would result in inflation of the estimate of stability (Carmines & Zeller, 1979).

Alternative Form Reliability

The establishment of reliability using alternative forms has some similarities to test–retest reliability because it is estimated by testing the same group of people on two separate occasions (Carmines & Zeller, 1979). However, it differs from test–retest reliability estimation because of its use of two distinct, but parallel, forms of a test (1979). When estimating alternative forms reliability, the test administration should occur about 2 weeks apart to account for day-to-day fluctuations in performance (Nunnally & Bernstein, 1995).

Occasionally, in occupational therapy treatment, clients' performance in a specific area must be evaluated repeatedly. Repeated administrations of the same instrument causes problems because the persons may remember test items or practice them. Thus, repeated exposure to the same test may artificially inflate the obtained score. The use of parallel forms minimizes the influence that memory or practice can have on inflating the estimated reliability. These two forms should not differ in "any systematic way" (Carmines & Zeller, 1979, p. 40). Computation of the reliability coefficient between these forms establishes their equivalence.

Internal Consistency

Both the alternative form and test–retest reliabilities require two separate test administrations to determine reliability. As we have seen, this separation of administrations of the test may make it difficult to determine whether the difference between the scores is due to test unreliability or to other sources of error, such as the individual's memory, actual changes in the trait, or a historical event (Carmines & Zeller, 1979; Jensen, 1980; Kerlinger, 1973). One means of eliminating the influence of time separation is to estimate reliability from a single test administration. These methods determine the internal consistency of the test (Carmines & Zeller, 1979; Nunnally & Bernstein, 1995; Pedhazur & Schmelkin, 1991).

The simplest and crudest type of internal consistency is split-half reliability (Nunnally & Bernstein, 1995; Pedhazur & Schmelkin, 1991). Here, reliability is determined by dividing the test items in half and obtaining the correlation between these two halves. Commonly, performance is compared between even- and odd-numbered items or the first half of the items and the second half.

This method calculates the correlation between the two halves so, unless a correction is made, the resulting reliability coefficient will underestimate the reliability of the whole test (Carmines & Zeller, 1979). Use of the Spearman-Brown formula makes a statistical correction such that the estimated reliability reflects the total test and not the compared halves (Brown, 1910; Spearman, 1910 in Carmines & Zeller, 1979).

The limitation of the split-half method of estimating reliability is that the variety of ways of dividing the items can result in different reliability coefficients (Carmines & Zeller, 1979). More sophisticated methods of estimating internal consistency take into account the variety of ways of grouping the test items (Carmines & Zeller, 1979; Nunnally & Bernstein, 1995; Pedhazur & Schmelkin, 1991). These analyses give an indication of the consistency of the "responses across the various items of the test" (Zeidner & Most, 1992, p. 59). Internal consistency takes into account the correlation of each item with every other item as well as with the total score. These interitem and item-total correlations provide an estimate of how consistent the items are with each other.

High internal consistency suggests that the test items measure a homogeneous construct. When low internal consistency exists, the representation of a single construct in a test must be questioned. Those items that do not correlate highly with other items or with the total test may measure a different construct. A test that is intended to measure a narrowly defined construct should have high internal consistency (Zeidner & Most, 1992).

The most common ways to estimate the internal consistency are through the use of Cronbach's alpha (Cronbach, 1951) or the Kuder-Richardson formula (Kuder & Richardson, 1937). These methods provide the "theoretical average of all possible split-half correlations" (Green, 1991, p. 29). In other words, the formulas used to calculate internal consistency generate a matrix of the interitem correlations and the item-total correlations in the calculation of reliability. Cronbach's alpha is computed when the items are scored in a nondichotomous manner. When the scoring is dichotomous, the Kuder-Richardson formula (Kuder & Richardson, 1937) is used. For further information on the theory and calculations of internal consistency, refer to one of the books asterisked in the references at the end of this chapter.

STANDARD ERROR OF MEASUREMENT

Procedures used to establish reliability involve testing groups of individuals (Zeidner & Most, 1992). Reliability estimation gives the potential test user an indication of the test's consistency. In instances when the therapist would like to understand how close the obtained score is to the true score for an individual, the estimates from group data can be used to calculate the standard error of measurement (SEM). The standard error of measurement indicates how much variability in the test scores can be attributed to error (Murphy & Davidshofer, 1991). As can be seen from the following equation, as reliability increases, the standard error of measurement decreases:

$$\text{SEM} = \text{SD} \sqrt{1 - r_{xx}}$$

In this equation, SD refers to the standard deviation of the group from which the reliability is calculated. It can be seen that the SEM is always less than the standard deviation except in the unlikely occurrence that the reliability equals 0. In this extreme case, the SEM would equal the standard deviation.

Once the SEM has been calculated, a confidence interval can be constructed around the obtained score. A *confidence interval* is defined as the range in which it can be stated with a "known degree of confidence" that a specific score would fall (Ferguson, 1981, p. 158). The degree of confidence is determined from the properties of the normal distribution. Previously, the approximate distribution of scores within the normal distribution was identified for ease of understanding. To calculate a confidence interval, the precise SD that corresponds to 95% of the distribution, for example, must be used. Thus, from the normal distribution, 95% of the scores fall within −1.96 and +1.96 SD from the mean and 99% fall within −2.54 to +2.54 SD from the mean (Anastasi, 1982). To construct a 95% confidence interval, the SEM is multiplied by 1.96 (Murphy & Davidshofer, 1991). Thus, the true score is known, with 95% confidence, to fall between the [obtained score −1.96 (SEM)] and the [obtained score +1.96 (SEM)]. Similarly a 99% confidence interval is constructed by multiplying the SEM by 2.54.

Suppose a 5½-year-old child achieves a score of 55 on the *McCarthy Scales of Children's Abilities* (McCarthy, 1972). From the test manual, it is known that the standard deviation equals 7.3 and the reliability is 0.75. From the foregoing formula, the SEM is calculated at 3.65. To construct a 95% confidence interval, 3.65 (SEM) is multiplied by 1.96

(SD) resulting in 7.15, rounded to 7. The confidence interval is then 55, plus or minus 7, or 48 to 62. Thus, it can be said with a 95% level of confidence that the child's "true" score falls within the range of 48 to 62. It can be seen from this example how the standard error of measurement can be used to provide an estimate of the range in which the child's true score would fall, providing a more meaningful interpretation of performance.

HOW RELIABLE SHOULD A TEST BE?

The question "how reliable should a test be?" does not have a ready answer. The purpose of the test should be considered when deciding whether the reliability reported is acceptable (Salvia & Ysseldyke, 1985). Tests that are used to make decisions about a person, such as determining whether he or she is capable of returning to work, should have a higher level of reliability than those tests that are intended to serve as screening or descriptive instruments (King-Thomas & Hacker, 1987; Salvia & Ysseldyke, 1985; Murphy & Davidshofer, 1991). Similarly, those instruments that attempt to categorize persons, such as a test that is used to assign cognitive levels, should have a high degree of reliability (Murphy & Davidshofer, 1991).

The following minimal levels of reliability should be considered as guidelines. It is also useful to remember that the reliability coefficient estimates the proportion of the score comprising the true score. A reliability coefficient of 0.80 indicates that 80% of the variance in the score is true variance and 20% of the variance of the score is due to errors of measurement. Thus, when a reliability coefficient of 0.50 is reported, the amount of the score that can be attributed to the true score is equivalent to that attributed to error. Generally, a reliability coefficient of 0.90 is considered to be high, 0.80 moderate, 0.70 low, and 0.60 generally unacceptable for clinical use (Murphy & Davidshofer, 1991).

It is recommended that when a test score is to be used to make significant decisions about an individual, such as placement decisions, a minimum level of reliability of 0.90 should be reported (King-Thomas & Hacker, 1987; Nunnally & Bernstein, 1995; Salvia & Ysseldyke, 1985). When a test is to be used for screening, a minimum level of reliability of 0.80 is considered appropriate (King-Thomas & Hacker, 1987; Salvia & Ysseldyke, 1985). Wiersma and Jurs (1990) suggest that because attitudes are more difficult to quantify, reliability coefficients are likely to be lower, and that a minimum level of reliability of 0.70 is acceptable for attitude tests. If the test has been administered to a group and the data are reported for the group as a whole, a minimum level of 0.60 has been suggested (Salvia & Ysseldyke, 1985).

It is important to remember that the reliability reported reflects the specific situation and the sample used to collect the data. The method used to collect the data to establish reliability should be clearly stated in the test manual. The potential test users must ensure that they understand the type of reliability that has been reported, the appropriate means of establishing that specific reliability, and its applicability for the purpose of the test. Table 14-1 summarizes this information. With this information and the reported reliability coefficient, the potential test users can make an informed decision about the usefulness of the test for their purposes.

Validity

DEFINITION OF VALIDITY

When we question the extent to which an evaluation measures what it purports to measure, we are asking questions about validity. Validity is the most crucial psychometric property to consider when critiquing an assessment (Jensen, 1980). A test may be very reliable, achieving consistent results, but if it does not measure that which it is supposed to measure, the consistency is of no consequence. For example, consider an occupational therapist using a newly developed instrument reported to measure satisfaction with task performance. The instrument is used with a client on three occasions and a similar score is obtained each time. The therapist might interpret that the instrument provides a consistent measure of satisfaction with task performance. Subsequently, a research report of the criterion-related validity of the instrument indicates that it correlates highly with a measure of fine motor ability, but not with another measure of satisfaction with task performance. This information suggests that the initial instrument does not measure satisfaction with task performance, but rather measures fine motor ability. Therefore, although a consistent score is obtained, the test does not provide meaningful information about satisfaction with task performance. The test is reliable, but not valid for the stated purpose.

Messick (1995) defines *validity* as "an evaluative summary of both the evidence for and the actual—as well as potential—consequences of score interpretation and use" (p. 742).

The establishment of validity involves both empirical investigation and rational argument to support or refute inferences made from test scores. Cronbach (1990) suggests that validation is an ongoing process providing support for the internal structure and interpretation of a particular instrument. It is important to realize that validity is not a property of the test, but of the inferences made about the test results or score (Messick, 1995). Messick further suggests that these inferences carry both a theoretical and social consequence and that investigation into the validity of an instrument should consider both.

Traditionally, three classifications of validity have been identified: content, criterion-related, and construct (Anastasi, 1982; Carmines & Zeller, 1979; Nunnally & Bernstein, 1995). Recently, Messick (1995) has advocated validity as a unified concept concerned with establishing the "adequacy and appropriateness of interpretations and actions on the basis of test scores or other modes of assessment" (p. 741). He argues that all investigation into the meaning of test scores is informative about the construct. Content and criterion-related validity provide further support and information about the construct validity. In addition, he discusses the social consequences resulting from inferences made from the test scores. For clarity, the three traditional classifications of validity will be discussed individually, recognizing that content and criterion-related validity are now considered to be components of construct validity (Messick, 1995). A brief discussion of Messick's ideas concerning the social consequences of score use will follow.

Construct Validity

Recall that a construct is considered to be an abstract entity that cannot be measured directly (Depoy & Gitlin, 1993). Hypotheses must be generated about the nature of the construct, its relation to other variables, and the behaviors that

---

TABLE 14-1. Summary of Reliability Coefficients, Type of Reliability, and Sources of Variability

Reliability Coefficient	Type of Reliability	Sources of Variability
Test–retest	Stability	Length of time between testing, stability of trait measured, memory of test items, actual change in trait measured
Alternative form	Equivalence of parallel forms (equivalence and stability if forms are administered at two different times)	Ability to generate parallel forms
Split-half	Internal consistency	Method of splitting items, length of test, consistency of content of test
Cronbach's alpha Kuder-Richardson 20 Kuder-Richardson 21	Internal consistency	Consistency of content of test

provide evidence of this construct. The process of construct validation is thus the process of systematically researching the variable that is intended to be measured by the test and identifying the alternative factors that might account for performance on the test (Kerlinger, 1973).

Construct validation can be considered to be a process of hypothesis testing (Cronbach, 1990). Suppose it was hypothesized that a positive relation exists between internal locus of control and self-efficacy. An analysis to determine the correlation between measures of these two variables is completed and, indeed, yields a positive correlation between them. This analysis provides support for the existence of such a relation, but does not prove this existence. Further research is necessary to provide increasing evidence of the relation. It is obvious that construct validation is an ongoing process, with greater understanding gained about the construct with each successive analysis.

Jensen (1980) suggests that construct validation can be achieved in two ways. The first is as explained in the foregoing by hypothesis testing. In the presence of a theory related to the construct, various hypotheses about the nature of the construct can be generated. Empirical evaluation of these hypotheses adds evidence for the construct validity.

A second method is the use of factor analysis. Factor analysis involves the generation of correlations among items from a test to identify patterns in the correlations (Kerlinger, 1973; Nunnally & Bernstein, 1995). These patterns can then be interpreted as factors and labeled according to the common aspects among the items composing the patterns.

Because of the consequences of the decisions made based on the interpretation of test scores, the investigation of construct validity is critical. Evidence must be provided to support the meaning of test scores. We will now examine how content and criterion-related validity support the understanding of the construct.

Content Validity

Content validity refers to how well the test samples the domain or behaviors that are considered to represent a particular construct (Walsh & Betz, 1990). The initial steps in establishing content validity occur when the test content is defined during test development, as previously discussed. An instrument is judged to have acceptable content validity when it represents or samples the content domain adequately (Kerlinger, 1973).

There are no specific statistical procedures for establishing content validity. Usually experts in a given field are used to evaluate the ability of the test to sample the content domain. Kerlinger (1973) suggests that the determination of content validity is achieved through the examination of each individual item with subsequent evaluation of its relevance to the content domain. Ideally, the individual constructing the test, as well as experts in the field, are involved in making this determination.

For example, an instrument designed to measure performance in activities of daily living (ADL) must be shown to adequately sample those behaviors that constitute ADL. Most occupational therapists would be in agreement about what constitutes an activity of daily living and would even agree with the division of self-care, productivity, and leisure (Canadian Association of Occupational Therapists [CAOT], 1991). To establish content validity, occupational therapists, considered to be experts, must determine that the content domain of ADL and that the aspects of self-care, productivity, and leisure are adequately represented on this test.

Content validity, therefore, is the determination that the test's items adequately represent the content domain. Adequate representation of the domain is important for evaluation of performance (Anastasi, 1982). The relation to the construct is seen in the necessity for identification of the structure of the construct against which a comparison of the test's content is made. Expert support for this structure provides further evidence of the construct validity.

Criterion Validity

Criterion-related validity has also been termed predictive validity (Carmines & Zeller, 1979; Kerlinger, 1973). Jensen (1980) also presents the term concurrent criterion-related validity. Another label for this type of validity is congruent validity (Jensen, 1980) There is considerable diversity in the literature relative to the terminology for this form of validity. For the sake of clarity, the term criterion-related validity will be used throughout this discussion. Essentially, this type of validity is determined by correlating the scores from one instrument with those of another, external instrument, or criterion (Anastasi, 1982; Carmines & Zeller, 1979). It is essential that this external criterion has well-established psychometric properties, most importantly that it is readily identified to measure the construct under consideration (Messick, 1995).

When an instrument is compared with an external criterion that is established as a valid measure of the desired construct, concurrent criterion-related validity is investigated. If a positive relation is obtained between the two measures, it provides convergent information about the construct (Messick, 1995). Divergent information is provided when the expected relation is not found (Messick, 1995).

Concurrent criterion-related validity is difficult to establish in occupational therapy. Because we measure behavior considered indicative of a construct, the identification of an acceptable criterion with which to compare the instrument is difficult. For many constructs, no "gold standard" exists to make a comparison (Murphy & Davidshofer, 1991). Thus, limited potential exists for the establishment of concurrent criterion-related validity.

Criterion-related validity is more useful when the intent of the evaluation is to predict performance in the future or in a related area (Kerlinger, 1973; Jensen, 1980). For example, occupational therapists frequently use vocational tests to determine the client's readiness to return to a vocational situation. Criterion-related validity (or as some would term this instance, predictive validity) is established by demonstrating the relation between performance on the vocational test and that in the work situation. Another situation in which criterion validity is important is when a screening tool is used to predict future performance and thus suitability for involvement in treatment. Often an occupational therapist performs an initial assessment and, on the basis of that assessment, determines whether treatment is warranted or not. In these decision-making situations, it is important to demonstrate, empirically, that there is a strong relation between the test and the criterion.

It should be evident that criterion-related validity is not tied to any specific theoretical statement about the construct under consideration. Criterion-related validity is concerned only with the strength of the relation between the instrument and criterion (Carmines & Zeller, 1979). Theory may become important, however, for the selection of the criterion with which to compare the instrument.

In summary, a unified concept of validity has been proposed. Investigation of validity aims to understand the meaning of the construct and the effect of inferences made from obtained scores (Messick, 1995). Criterion-related and content validity contribute to an understanding of the construct. Table 14-2 summarizes these forms of validity.

SOCIAL CONSEQUENCES OF TEST SCORE INFERENCES

The decisions made based on the interpretation of test scores influence people's lives. The outcome may be positive as when an individual is accepted into graduate school based on their academic performance (Messick, 1995). Alternatively, the consequences may be negative if some aspect of the testing situation was biased, resulting in an unfair judgement about a person's performance (Messick, 1995).

The concern about social consequences, from a validity perspective, is that any negative consequences, resulting from testing, must not result from sources of test invalidity (Messick, 1995). Messick describes two sources contributing to construct invalidity: *Construct underrepresentation* refers to content, relevant to the construct, that is missing from the test. This bias occurs when test content is focused too narrowly. Inclusion of this content would result in improved performance of affected individuals. *Construct-irrelevant variance* occurs when unnecessary aspects of the test lower performance. An example of this type of variance is a test of arithmetic ability that requires reading comprehension to complete the problems satisfactorily.

This aspect of construct validity is not commonly discussed, nor is it likely to be available in test manuals. The lack of availability does not lessen its importance. When tests are used to make decisions affecting people's lives, it is imperative that the test user identifies information about the consequences of inferences made from test scores from the literature. As occupational therapists become increasingly accountable for the decisions based on test results, research investigating the social consequences of our decisions will become crucial.

Test Responsiveness

One aspect of validity that has received little attention in the literature is that of test responsiveness (Gowland et al, 1991; Guyatt, Walter, & Norman, 1987; Kirshner & Guyatt, 1985; Law, 1987). *Test responsiveness* is defined as "the capability of an instrument to detect clinically meaningful change in an attribute, characteristic, or function" (Guyatt et al., 1987, cited in Gowland et al., 1991, p. 7). This attribute is important when a test is being used for evaluative purposes (Gowland et al., 1991; Law, 1987). For example, suppose an occupational therapist wanted to determine whether the participants in a task group developed improved self-esteem as a result of involvement in the group. The therapist could measure the participants' self-esteem before they begin the group and, again, on its termination and determine if a significant difference existed between the two measures. To make a meaningful interpretation of the results, the therapist must be confident that the instrument was capable of detecting any change that had occurred.

TABLE 14-2. Summary of Types of Validity: Their Purpose and Method of Determination		
Type	**Purpose**	**Method of Determination**
Construct	Understand the nature of behavior, attribute measured by the test; identify related or constituent variables and their structure	Systematic, empirical investigation of hypotheses related to the structure and nature of the trait, and so on.
Content	To determine that the content adequately samples the domain of concern	Support for content is found in the literature and expert opinion
Criterion	Prediction of function in the future or in a related area; establish relation between test and gold standard of the construct	Correlation of scores between test and criterion measure

Law (1987) has suggested that there are two ways of determining a test's responsiveness. The first is to determine the change over time in an attribute for two groups, one group in which the attribute is known to change and one in which it is considered to be stable. For example, comparing muscle strength in individuals who have been immobilized for a substantial period of time as compared with those individuals who have neither been immobilized nor changed their level of activity significantly. A second way of determining responsivity is to "evaluate the ability of the instrument to measure the effect of treatment that has been proven effective" (Law, 1987, p. 137).

To summarize, when the purpose of a test is to evaluate treatment efficacy, it is important to use a test that has been shown to detect change when change has occurred. This aspect of validity will become increasingly important as occupational therapists seek to demonstrate the efficacy of their treatment, necessitating the use of measures that will detect change.

▼ CULTURE FAIR EVALUATION

In many countries, cultural diversity is increasing. Occupational therapists may be required to evaluate an individual whose first language is not the official language of the country. The literature reviewed for this section of the chapter was concerned with tests developed in English, and the effect of their use with individuals whose first language is not English.

A number of issues are identified in the literature concerning the issue of evaluation when cultural diversity is a consideration. Probably the most significant issue is that of using a test developed in English, or for the North American culture, with an individual whose first language is not English or who is part of a culture other than the predominant culture in North America (Jensen, 1980; AERA, 1985; Lam, 1991). With that statement, it must be recognized that even within North America, among people whose first language is English, there is a disparity of culture (Jensen, 1980). The life experience of people living in remote areas of the Arctic is vastly different from that of individuals living in urban areas, and both are vastly different from the experience of many people of color. So, it is evident that the issue of cultural fairness in assessment is not a simple one to resolve. This section will discuss these issues and present some of the recommendations that have been made to minimize the influence of cultural diversity in the assessment situation.

Language can significantly confound the results obtained on an assessment. When the assessment requires a verbal response, or when the test items contain a substantial verbal component, the test may measure language ability more than whatever trait it purports to measure (AERA, 1985). Language ability affects the reliability of the test by increasing the error component. It is crucial to ascertain the intelligibility of the test items and instructions for individuals whose first language is not English (Jensen, 1980).

One seemingly obvious means to minimize the language issue is to provide a translation of the test. However, this approach is not as useful as it would appear. Many words or phrases do not have the same meaning when translated from one language to another. For example, *poser un lapin à quelqu'un* means "to stand someone up" in French. This phrase translates, in English, to "lay a rabbit on someone," which creates quite a different visual image than the French meaning. This direct translation then, does not take into consideration the effect of the idiosyncrasies of language on the content of the test and the subsequent influence on the established reliability or validity.

Behavioral expectations vary from one culture to another. Children in one culture may be discouraged from responding directly to an adult or from engaging in a detailed conversation (AERA, 1985). Such behavior would be considered rude. On an assessment during which children are expected to express their ideas, children of this culture would perform poorly, not because their ideas are ill-formed, but because their cultural expectations preclude them from engaging in a long conversation. The resulting score could not be said to reflect validly their actual performance.

Perception of time and the speed of completion of tasks may vary between cultures. People from cultures in which speed is not emphasized, as it is in North America, will not perform as well on a timed test. Again, scores achieved by these individuals may not reflect their actual ability.

Test content is another area affected by cultural diversity (Lam, 1991). The naming of common objects differs, even among English-speaking cultures. For example, in Britain, a nappy, petrol, and bonnet refer to a diaper, gasoline, and the hood of a car. British children who are asked to point to a diaper would not share the North American label for the item and may not be able to identify the target object. Similarly, concepts may differ between cultures. The Woodcock-Johnson Psychoeducational Test Battery (Woodcock, 1978), asks examinees to perform arithmetic calculations using Imperial measures. Canadian children learn the metric system of measurement and, thus, cannot correctly perform the calculations. It is clear how both the construct under consideration and the validity are affected by the lack of cultural commonality

The actual test situation may be unfamiliar for people from some cultures (Lam, 1991). The very act of placing people into a testing situation may put them at a disadvantage. Similarly, some persons may not be familiar with completion of computer-marked response cards or have limited experience using a paper and pencil or computer. The means of indicating a response, in this situation, requires skills or exposure to media that are not universal.

The foregoing discussion illustrates the complexity of the issue of performing assessments with individuals of a culture different from the one for which the instrument was standardized. The *Standards for Educational and Psychological Testing* (AERA, 1985), presents several standards to minimize the potential disadvantage to individuals of a diverse culture. These standards, and the recommendations from other writers, which follow, recognize that it is not generally feasible to create a test that may be considered free of cultural bias. It is the ethical responsibility of the examiner to ensure that measures have been taken to minimize the cultural bias (AERA, 1985, Jensen, 1980).

The *Standards for Educational and Psychological Testing* recommend that tests for non-English speakers, or those who speak certain English dialects, "should be designed to minimize the threats to test reliability and validity that may arise from language differences" (AERA, 1985, p. 74). The ability of non-English speakers to understand the test items or instructions should be ascertained, perhaps through the administration of practice items (Jensen, 1980). Test items should be reviewed, during the development phase, by representatives of minority groups to eliminate or modify those items with a cultural bias (Jensen, 1980). Where language modifications have been made to tests originally developed in English, information should be provided in the test manual to document those modifications and their influence on the psychometric properties of the test.

In both Canada and the United States, legislation exists to exert influence on the administration of assessments to children of diverse cultures for educational purposes. In Canada, where education is the jurisdiction of the provinces, the legislation differs by province. In the United States, these practices are governed by **Public Law (P.L.) 94-142**, *Education for all Handicapped Children Act* (1975), which was renamed *Individuals with Disabilities Education Act* (IDEA) in 1990 (Guernsey & Klare, 1993). In the province of Ontario, this legislation is part of *The Education Act* (Education Act, 1990). In Ontario, "the administration and interpretation of the assessment must be made carefully, recognizing the impact of the pupil's culture and language facility on the results of the assessment" (Ministry of Education, 1984, policy no. 59, p. 2). IDEA presents four criteria to effect fair and nondiscriminatory testing:

1. Assessments should be administered in the child's native language.
2. The assessment should be valid for its intended use.
3. A trained or licensed professional should administer the test.
4. The test should fit the child's educational level.

In summary, people of diverse cultures may be disadvantaged in the assessment situation because of the language differences and life experiences that may have afforded limited opportunity to experience a test situation, test materials, or means of response. It is crucial that the examiner understand how each of these factors may limit the client's performance on an assessment. The examiner should refer to the test manual for any suggested modifications and take into account the effect of these modifications on the psychometric properties of the test. If the examiner makes modifications to the test that have not been suggested in the manual, these modifications should be documented, and the threats to the psychometric properties of the test should be recognized.

▼ ISSUES IN THE EVALUATION OF PEOPLE WITH DISABILITIES

Because of the nature of our profession, the clients whom we evaluate have some form of **disability**. It is important to recognize the various ways in which a disability will limit performance on a test. It is equally important to understand how tests can be misused with this group of individuals. As with the use of tests with people of diverse cultures, the issues here are complex, and the solutions are often incomplete.

Many of the tests we use involve language ability. Individuals may be required to read instructions or test problems, comprehend auditory instructions, or provide a verbal response. Individuals with impairments in any of these skills are disadvantaged by the test. Persons with a hearing impairment who lost their ability to hear at a prelinguistic stage have particular difficulty with language skills (Baker, 1991). Their auditory deficit limits their ability to interact with the aural environment, which negatively affects their development in verbal areas (Baker).

Perception of the presentation of the test items raises difficulties for persons with a variety of disabilities. Auditory information is perceived with difficulty by those with a hearing impairment (Baker, 1991). Persons with a visual impairment cannot perceive information presented visually (Taylor, Sternberg, & Richards, 1995). A **learning disability** may interfere with the ability to process the information presented (Taylor, Sternberg, & Richards, 1995).

Those individuals with a disability affecting motor skills may have difficulty indicating a response when a movement is required (Hacker & Porter, 1987). They may have difficulty interacting with the test stimuli, maintaining a proper sitting position to facilitate taking the test, or may not have sufficient endurance to complete an assessment of 30 minutes, 60 minutes, or longer (Hacker & Porter, 1987).

Satisfactory performance on a test is dependent, in part, on the ability to engage in the testing situation. Individuals with behavioral or emotional problems, cognitive impairment, or a learning disability may have difficulty with engagement (Taylor et al., 1995). These individuals may need assistance to interact with the examiner and the test materials and to remain engaged in the testing situation for the duration of the test, when possible. Engagement in the testing situation may be limited also by an individual's behavioral or emotional disabilities (Taylor et al., 1995). Many individuals with disabilities have difficulty maintaining attention to a task for a prolonged time period (Taylor et al., 1995). Use of standardized tests may not be possible for

▼ **BOX 14-2**

An Example of a Test Evaluation

I. GENERAL INFORMATION

Title:	McCarthy Scales of Children's Abilities
Author:	Dorothea McCarthy
Publisher:	The Psychological Corporation
Time to Administer:	45–60 minutes
Materials Required:	Materials supplied with the test plus stopwatch, tape, paper, pencils, and book or toy, as identified in the manual.
Cost:	Variable over time—check with the publisher

II. BRIEF DESCRIPTION OF PURPOSE OF THE TEST

Purpose of test: Evaluation of young children's "general intellectual level as well as their strengths and weaknesses in important abilities" (McCarthy, 1972, p. 1)

Target Population: Children between the ages of 2 years 4 months and 8 years 7 months

Item Description: Children are evaluated on a variety of abilities involving general knowledge, verbal, quantitative, and motor skills, and memory. Items vary, dependent on the ability evaluated. Items are presented in a gamelike format.

Traits or Aptitudes Evaluated: Six scales are derived including verbal, perceptual–performance, quantitative, general cognitive index, memory, and motor.

III. PRACTICAL EVALUATION

Ease of Administration: Examiner should have experience with the age group. Items are arranged in such an order to maintain the child's engagement for the duration of the test.

Clarity of Directions: Instructions on administration are very clearly described.

Scoring Procedures: Scoring procedures require attention to detail and the method of deriving the scaled scores is somewhat difficult.

Examiner Qualifications and Training: No specific qualifications identified.

IV. TECHNICAL CONSIDERATIONS

A. NORMS

Type: Standardized scores are expressed as T-scores with a mean of 50 and SD of 10.

Standardization Sample: Standardized on 1032 children representing ages of the test and distribution of major U.S. population variables. Children not developing typically were not included in the standardization sample.

Standardization Procedures: These are considered to be exemplary by reviewers (Paget, 1985; Wodrich, 1985).

B. RELIABILITY

Split-Half: Corrected with Spearman–Brown formula. The average reliability coefficient for the general cognitive index is 0.93 with a range of 0.90 to 0.96 between different ages. The average reliability coefficient for the remaining scales ranges from 0.79 for memory and motor to 0.88 for verbal.

Stability: Reliability coefficient is reported for three ages. Range of reliability coefficient for general cognitive index is 0.89 to 0.91. For the remaining scales, the range is 0.69 for motor at 7.5 to 8.5 years to 0.89 for verbal at 3 to 3.5 years, quantitative at 5 to 5.5 years, and perceptual–performance for 7.5 to 8.5 years.

C. VALIDITY

Construct: Factor analyses confirms the structure of the scales, although each scale was not clearly established at each age (Paget, 1985).

Concurrent: Established with the Wechsler Preschool and Primary Scale of Intelligence. Results are clearly presented in the test manual.

Predictive: Established with the Metropolitan Achievement Tests. Results are clearly presented in the test manual.

D. TEST RESPONSIVENESS

Test responsiveness is not indicated in the test manual.

V. EXTERNAL REVIEWERS COMMENTS

NOTE: Only the major opinion of each reviewer is presented due to space limitations. Test has major strengths that "place it among the best of available broad-based diagnostic instruments for use with preschool children" (Paget, 1985, p. 922). The limitations of the test are the lack of 'exceptional children' in the standardization sample and the lack of sensitivity in the younger and older age ranges.

"All in all, [it] represents one viable clinical tool for assessing preschoolers" (Wodrich, 1985, p. 927). ". . . [it] must be considered a less desirable choice than the WISC-R because of that instrument's research base and its superior verbal items" (Wodrich, 1985, p. 927).

VI. SUMMARY OF STRENGTHS AND WEAKNESSES

The McCarthy scales have excellent psychometric properties, the standardization procedures were completed with stringent requirements, and it provides an excellent general evaluative instrument for older preschoolers and younger primary school children. It is less useful for evaluating the performance of the very young or very old children within the defined age range.

some individuals because of their extremely limited attention span.

A cognitive impairment may limit the person's ability to comprehend verbal or written instructions (Salvia & Ysseldyke; 1985; Taylor et al., 1995). Similarly, a person with an **aphasia** may have difficulty understanding instructions (Taylor et al., 1995). This brief review demonstrates that people with disabilities may have difficulties with any aspect of the testing process. It is important to ensure that the score reflects their ability and not their disability (Rehabilitation Act, 1973).

Modifications to the testing situation have been suggested. For persons with visual impairments, use of braille translations or auditory presentation of the stimuli may be possible (AERA, 1985). The use of sign language interpreters has been suggested for individuals with hearing impairments (Baker, 1991). Computer presentation of stimuli, assistive and augmentative communication devices, and modification of the means of response have been suggested for individuals with motor difficulties. (Hacker & Porter, 1987). Although all of these suggestions may enable people with disabilities to engage in a testing situation, unless satisfactory psychometric properties have been established with these modifications, the test scores cannot be interpreted with any degree of confidence (AERA, 1985). All of these modifications change the manner in which the test was standardized and, thereby, affect the reliability and validity. Unless these properties are specifically evaluated with these modifications, the obtained score can be used only for description or estimation of the individual's abilities.

As with modification of tests to minimize the influence of cultural diversity, there are no simple solutions in establishing a test that is fair for individuals with disabilities. The *Standards for Educational and Psychological Testing* (AERA, 1985), recommend that persons who modify any test for use with an individual with a disability do so with the assistance of an individual who is an expert in psychometrics. Furthermore, the test user should have knowledge about the manner in which the disability might affect the reliability and validity of the test. Test developers should report any modifications that they have made to the test for its use with persons with disabilities and report the effect of these modifications on the test's psychometric properties.

It is recommended that, where possible, empirical research be done to establish the influence of test modifications on the psychometric properties. For example, extending the amount of time has been suggested as a possible modification (AERA, 1985), yet there is little empirical evidence to indicate what influence such a modification might have. Indeed, extending the time limit introduces a further confounding factor, fatigue. Finally, the purpose of the testing must be considered in the determination of the norms used in the interpretation of the scores. When the purpose is to understand the individual's function relative to the population without disabilities, those norms should be used. If that is not the aim, the norms used should be those for persons with a similar disability (AERA, 1985).

Regulation 305 of the Ontario Education Act (1990), entitled *Special Education Identification, Placement and Review Committees and Appeals* provides for health, psychological, and educational assessment for identification and placement of "exceptional pupils." Guidelines for evaluating these students indicate that a variety of methods of assessment are necessary for identification of a disability (Ministry of Education, 1984). The results of these assessments are considered temporary, necessitating periodic review. It is not considered appropriate to use the results to predict future function.

The IDEA provides requirements for evaluation of individuals with disabilities similar to those that were indicated in the previous section concerning culture. In addition, no single criterion constitutes a satisfactory evaluation (IDEA, 1975). Individuals must be evaluated in all areas of suspected disability (IDEA). Provision must be made for a satisfactory means of communication when it is impaired. Under the Rehabilitation Act (1973) tests must be administered so that the results reflect the actual ability and not the effect of the disability. Tests are to be administered by a qualified professional who adheres to the standardization procedures (Rehabilitation Act). Adaptive behavior (which is not defined) must be considered in the evaluation process.

To summarize, individuals with sensory, physical, emotional, cognitive, or learning disabilities may be disadvantaged in the testing situation. Even though tests can be modified to accommodate, in some fashion, for these disabilities, unless reliability and validity have been established with these modifications, the score has little meaning. It is crucial for the test user to understand the effect that various disabilities will have on the individual's ability to engage in the testing situation, document any modifications that have been made, and be very conscientious in the interpretation and use of the scores that are derived from a test that has not been used in the standardized manner (Box 14-2).

▼ SOURCES OF PUBLISHED INFORMATION ON PUBLISHED TESTS

This chapter has provided an overview of issues with which an occupational therapist must be familiar to critique an assessment. A number of sources are available that provide reviews of published tests. The *Mental Measurements Yearbooks* (Conoley, 1995) provide reviews of most commercially available tests. Each successive edition reviews those tests published since the last edition and updates reviews of the major tests. *Test Critiques* (Keyser & Sweetland, 1987) provides information about test development, application, and psychometric properties of many tests. *Tests in Print* (Murphy, Conoley, & Impara, 1994) provides descriptive information and bibliographies.

There are several journals that publish reviews of a wide variety of tests, their reliability and validity, as well as theoretical discussions of these properties. Some of the more useful ones include *Educational and Psychological Measurement*, *Journal of Applied Psychology*, *Journal of Chronic Diseases* that evolved into *Journal of Clinical Epidemiology*, and *Psychological Assessment*.

▼ SUGGESTED BIBLIOGRAPHY

This chapter was meant to be an overview of the critical concerns in the critique of evaluations. It was not intended to include a detailed discussion of the various aspects, formulas, or calculations of test construction, item analysis, reliability, and validity. The asterisked (*) books on the reference list provide more detailed information, and frequently reviews of assessments commonly used in occupational therapy, for your further information.

Acknowledgments

Jennifer Landry and Linda Miller, School of Occupational Therapy, The University of Western Ontario provided valuable feedback on an earlier draft of this chapter. Joseph Hansen, Detroit Country Day School provided French language consultation.

▼ REFERENCES

American Educational Research Association, American Psychological Association, & National Council on Measurement in Education. (1985). *Standards for educational and psychological testing*. Washington, DC: American Psychological Association.*

Anastasi, A. (1982). *Psychological Testing*. (5th ed.). New York: Macmillan.*

Baker, R. M. (1991). Evaluation of hearing-impaired children. In K. E. Green (Ed.), *Educational testing: Issues and applications*. (pp. 77–107). New York: Garland.

Barclay, J. R. (1991). *Psychological assessment: A theory and systems approach*. Malabar, FL: Krieger.

Benson, J., & Clark, F. (1982). A guide for instrument development and validation. *American Journal of Occupational Therapy, 36* (12), 789–800.

Canadian Association of Occupational Therapists. (1991). *Guidelines for client-centred practice*. Toronto, Canada: Author.

Carmines, E. G., & Zeller, R. A. (1979). *Reliability and validity assessment*. Newbury Park, CA: Sage.*

Conoley, J. C. (Ed.). (1995). *Mental measurements yearbook*. New York: Buros Institute.

Cronbach, L. J. (1951). Coefficient alpha and the internal structure of tests. *Psychometrika, 16,* 297–334.

Cronbach, L. J. (1990). *Essentials of psychological testing* (5th ed.). New York: Harper-Collins.*

DePoy E., & Gitlin, L. N. (1993). *Introduction to research: Multiple strategies for health and human services*. St. Louis, MO: Mosby.

Education Act. (1990). Toronto, Canada: Queen's Printer for Ontario.

Ferguson, G. A. (1981). *Statistical analysis in psychology and education* (5th ed.). New York: McGraw-Hill.

Gowland, C., King, G., King, S., Law, M., Letts, L., MacKinnon, E., Rosenbaum, P., & Russell, D. (1991). *Review of selected measures in neurodevelopmental rehabilitation* (Neurodevelopmental Clinical Research Unit Rep. No. 91–2). Hamilton, Canada: Neurodevelopmental Clinical Research Unit.

Green, K. E. (1991). Reliability, validity, and test score interpretation.

In K. E. Green (Ed.). *Educational testing: Issues and applications* (pp. 27–38). New York: Garland.

Guernsey, T. F., & Klare, K. (1993). *Special education law*. Durham, NC: Carolina Academic Press.

Guyatt, G., Walter, S., & Norman, G. (1987). Measuring change over time: Assessing the usefulness of evaluative instruments. *Journal of Chronic Diseases, 40* (2), 171–178.

Hacker, B. J., & Porter, P. B. (1987). Use of standardized tests with the physically handicapped. In L. King-Thomas & B. J. Hacker (Eds.), *A therapist's guide to pediatric assessment* (pp. 35–40). Boston: Little, Brown & Company.

Individuals With Disabilities Education Act of 1990, 20 U.S.C.A. 1400 et seq. (West, 1996).

Isaac, S., & Michael, W. B. (1971). *Handbook in research and evaluation*. San Diego, CA: EdITS.

Jensen, A. R. (1980). *Bias in mental testing*. New York: The Free Press.

Kerlinger, F. A. (1973). *Foundations in behavioral research*. New York: Holt, Rinehart & Winston.

Keyser, D. J., & Sweetland, R. C. (Eds.). (1987). *Test critiques compendium: Reviews of major tests from the test critique series*. Kansas City, MO: Test Corporation of America.

King-Thomas, L., & Hacker, B. J. (Eds.). (1987). *A therapist's guide to pediatric assessment*. Boston: Little, Brown & Company.

Kirshner, B., & Guyatt, B. (1985). A methodological framework for assessing health indices. *Journal of Chronic Diseases, 38* (1), 27–36.

Kuder, G. F., & Richardson, M. (1937). The theory of the estimation test reliability. *Psychometrika, 2,* 151–160.

Lam, T. C. M. (1991). Testing of limited English proficient children. In K. E. Green (Ed.). *Educational testing: Issues and applications* (pp. 125–167). New York: Garland.

Law, M. (1987). Measurement in occupational therapy: Scientific criteria for evaluation. *Canadian Journal of Occupational Therapy, 54* (3), 133–138.

Messick, S. (1995). Validity of psychological assessment: Validation inferences from person's responses and performances as scientific inquiry into score meaning. *American Psychologist, 50* (9), 741–749.

Ministry of Education. (1984). *Special education information handbook*. Toronto, Canada: Author.

McCarthy, D. (1972). *McCarthy scales of children's abilities*. San Antonio, TX: The Psychological Corporation.

Murphy, L. L., Conoley, J. C., & Impara, J. C. (Eds.). (1994). *Tests in print IV: An index to tests, test reviews and the literature on specific tests*. Lincoln, NE: University of Nebraska Press.

Murphy, K. R., & Davidshofer, C. O. (1991). *Psychological testing: Principles and applications* (2nd ed.). Englewood Cliffs, NJ: Prentice-Hall.

Nunnally, J. C., & Bernstein, I. H. (1995). *Psychometric theory* (3rd ed.). Toronto, Canada: McGraw-Hill.*

Paget, D. (1985). Review of McCarthy scales of children's abilities. In J. V. Mitchell (Ed.). *Mental measurements yearbook*, (9th ed.). Lincoln, NB: University of Nebraska Press.

Pedhazur, E. J., & Schmelkin, L. P. (1991). *Measurement, design and analysis: An integrated approach*. Hillsdale, NJ: Lawrence Erlbaum Associates.

Rehabilitation Act of 1973, 29 U.S.C.A. 701 et seq. (West, 1996).

Rotter, J. (1966). Generalized expectancies for internal versus external control of reinforcement. *Psychological Monographs, 80,* 1–28.

Salvia, J., & Ysseldyke, J. E. (1985). *Assessment in special and remedial education* (3rd ed.). Boston: Houghton Mifflin.

Siegel, L. S. (1989). Evidence that infant test scores predict subsequent cognitive functioning. In M. Bornstein & N. A. Krasnegor (Eds.). *Continuity in development*. Hillsdale, NJ: Erlbaum.

Taylor, R. L., Sternberg, L., & Richards, S. B. (1995). *Exceptional children: Integrating research and teaching*, (2nd ed.). San Diego, CA: Singular Publishing Group.

Walsh, W. B., & Betz, N. E. (1990). *Tests and assessment* (2nd ed.). Englewood Cliffs, NJ: Prentice Hall.

Wiersma, W., & Jurs, S. G. (1990). *Educational measurement and testing* (2nd ed.). Needham Heights, MA: Allyn and Bacon.

Witt, J. C., Elliott, S. N., Gresham, F. M., & Kramer, J. J. (1988). *Assessment of special children.* Glenview, IL: Scott, Foresman & Company.

Wodrich, D. (1985). Review of McCarthy scales of children's abilities. In J. V. Mitchell (Ed.). *Mental measurements yearbook,* (9th ed.). Lincoln, NB: University of Nebraska Press.

Woodcock, R. (1978). *Woodcock-Johnson psycho-educational battery.* Hingham, MA: Teaching Resources Corporation.

Zeidner, M., & Most, R. (1992). *Psychological testing: An inside view.* Palo Alto, CA: Consulting Psychologists Press.

Chapter 15

Evaluation of Occupational Performance Areas

Section 1: Evaluation of Activities of Daily Living (ADL) and Home Management

Section 2: Evaluation of Work and Productive Activities: Work Performance Assessment Measures

Section 3: Evaluation of Work Performance and Productive Activities: Components of a Therapeutic Driving Evaluation

Section 4: Evaluation of Play and Leisure

Section 1

Evaluation of Activities of Daily Living (ADL) and Home Management

Joan C. Rogers and Margo B. Holm

The parameters of occupational therapy practice include **performance areas, performance components,** and **performance contexts.** This section focuses on **evaluation** of **activities of daily living (ADL)** and home management, which are classified as performance areas in the *Uniform Terminology for Occupational Therapy* [American Occupational Therapy Association (AOTA), 1994]. Dysfunctions in ADL and home management tasks are called **disabilities** in the model of disablement developed by the World Health Organization (World Health Organization, 1980). Evaluation is a key aspect of the occupational therapy process because it establishes the direction for therapeutic actions. Core questions to be addressed concerning the evaluation of ADL and home management tasks are:

- What use is to be made of the evaluation data?
- What tasks are to be evaluated?
- What parameters of task performance are to be evaluated?
- How are tasks to be evaluated?
- How are evaluation data to be integrated for clinical decision making?
- What instruments are available to aid data gathering?

These questions provide the organizational scheme for this section and each question will be addressed in sequence.

▼ PURPOSE OF EVALUATION OF ADL AND HOME MANAGEMENT ACTIVITIES

ADL and home management tasks may be evaluated for different purposes. At the level of individual client care, evaluation may be done to (1) screen for disability, (2) assess disability to plan occupational therapy intervention, or (3) facilitate decision making concerning actions such as discharge disposition or legal competence for independent living. At the programmatic level, evaluation may be done to document the need for program expansion or development and to appraise outcomes. Before starting an evaluation, the use that is to be made of the data gathered must be ascertained so that appropriate and sufficient data are obtained.

Screening

Screening involves a cursory evaluation to determine if a more intensive evaluation is needed. It is a case-finding procedure intended to separate individuals who have or are at risk for developing disability from those who do not have and are not at risk for developing disability. Because screening procedures are often applied to large groups of individuals, such as all applicants for an independent-living program, or all new clients in an outpatient clinic, they should be brief, easy to administer, and inexpensive. At the same time, they must have sufficient sensitivity to detect disability, so that individuals who have a disability are not incorrectly classified as not having one and, therefore, not needing further evaluation and help. Screening procedures do not need to be done by occupational therapy practitioners. They form the basis of any referral to occupational therapy and may be conducted by health care, social services and educational personnel, potential clients, or family members of potential clients.

Evaluation

Evaluation of ADL and home management tasks is more comprehensive and detailed than screening and must be conducted by an occupational therapy practitioner. Its purpose is to identify the ADL and home management tasks for which disability is present or may be developing. Evaluation data may be used to plan and monitor occupational therapy interventions or to assist in decision making relative to disposition, competency, conservatorship, or involuntary commitment. The extent of data gathering depends on the specific purpose for which the evaluation is being conducted.

PLAN AND MONITOR OCCUPATIONAL THERAPY INTERVENTIONS

Before practitioners intervene to improve performance of ADL or home management tasks, they must evaluate clients' baseline performance. When an evaluation is conducted to plan occupational therapy intervention, four types of data are needed (Rogers, Holm, & Stone, 1997). First, tasks in which performance is deficient need to be identified. To target intervention appropriately, the identification of deficits needs to be very precise. Knowing that clients have a disability in oral hygiene is insufficient for planning intervention. The evaluation needs to inform practitioners about the specific components of oral hygiene (eg, remove dentures, prepare denture solution) that clients can and cannot perform. Occupational therapy intervention can then be targeted to develop or compensate for the components that are

dysfunctional, while simultaneously maintaining and enhancing those that are functional.

The second type of data that is needed is data about the cause or causes of disability. For example, a disability in cooking might be caused by: (1) low vision, (2) a wheelchair inaccessible kitchen, (3) a lack of proficiency in cooking, or (4) poor motivation to cook. Occupational therapy intervention for a disability in cooking would be different for these different causes. Problems caused by low vision might be alleviated through assistive technology, such as a high-intensity light. Elimination of architectural barriers might remedy the inaccessible kitchen. Training might be initiated to improve cooking skills, and apathy may be approached through a structured program of activities meeting a client's interests and abilities. As these examples illustrate, to understand the etiology of disability, data about occupational areas (eg, ADL, home management) need to be supplemented with data about occupational performance components (eg, visual acuity) or occupational contexts (eg, physical structures).

Third, the occupational therapy evaluation should provide data about clients' capacities for modifying their task performance. These data also assist in establishing an overall approach to occupational therapy intervention. Interventions involving skill acquisition would be feasible for clients who demonstrate the ability to learn, whereas environmental modifications would be appropriate for those lacking this ability.

Fourth, the evaluation should yield data about the kinds of occupational therapy interventions that are most likely to develop or improve task performance. When an evaluation is conducted with the intent of providing intervention, it must go beyond describing disability, to providing data that enable practitioners to create a therapeutic situation that will likely move clients along the continuum of dysfunction to function. The practice of occupational therapy incorporates a broad array of restorative, compensatory, and preventive interventions that can be brought to bear on disabilities and their precursors. An essential yield of the evaluation process is a narrowing down of this array so that occupational therapy practitioners can select those interventions that are most likely to elicit positive outcomes within the projected time constraints for therapy.

The first two types of evaluation data—namely, identifying disabilities and their causes—are diagnostic. The last two types of evaluation data—determining clients' modifiability and ascertaining potential interventions—are therapeutically oriented. All four types of data are needed to devise adequate intervention plans. Once an intervention is implemented, its effects on task performance need to be monitored. Hence, re-evaluations need to be undertaken periodically to see if the intervention is alleviating disability; if not, a change of approach is needed.

FACILITATE DECISION MAKING

Clients may also be referred for evaluation of ADL and home management tasks to facilitate decision making about eligibility or disposition. The ability to care for oneself and one's home lies at the interface between independent and supported or assisted living. Supported living represents a continuum of options that includes in-home services (eg, chore services), personal care homes, assisted-living centers, foster homes, group homes, independent-living centers, supervised apartments, and transitional apartments. Within each setting a range of supports is offered to maintain or enhance daily-living skills. At the extreme dependency end of this continuum is institutionalization (eg, long-term care facility) where all ADL and home management needs can be met. Each point on this continuum, as well as each service or facility, has ADL and home management requirements that must be met for eligibility or admission. For example, depending on the site, residents may or may not need to manage their own medications or keep their rooms clean and tidy. When ADL and home management tasks are evaluated to serve these types of eligibility or disposition decisions, the evaluation may be less comprehensive and detailed than when it is done to plan individual interventions. The primary question to be answered through the evaluation is: Does the client meet the functional criteria? This question can generally be answered by identifying tasks in which disability is present.

A somewhat similar evaluation objective occurs when occupational therapy practitioners are asked to make recommendations about legal competence for independent living. This usually involves competence in caring for oneself or competence in managing one's property. Difficulties with the first type of competence lead to legal proceedings called guardianship, whereas difficulties with the second type of competence involve conservatorship (Uniform Probate Code, 1989). Evaluation may also be requested in conjunction with involuntary commitments to psychiatric facilities to appraise the influence of psychiatric status on daily living. Individuals are usually not competent or incompetent, rather competence is exhibited in some tasks, but not in others. When competence is used in the legal sense, the capacity to make judicious or responsible decisions usually takes precedence over the capacity to actually perform tasks. Individuals who have the ability to procure services and supervise caregivers in managing their personal care and living situation are viewed as competent, even though they may not be able to perform these tasks themselves. Thus, occupational therapy evaluations conducted with guardianship, conservatorship, or involuntary commitment in mind must take into account the decisional capacities and supervisory skills needed by clients.

Programmatic Uses

Although this section emphasizes evaluation for individual client care, it is important to recognize that data gathered about clients may be aggregated for programmatic purposes. For example, data about the ADL and home management characteristics of clients served in an occupational therapy clinic may be used to document the extent of particular disabilities and to support the development of new or expanded programs to manage them. In the current health care climate of cost effectiveness and cost containment, group data are increasingly being used to evaluate the outcomes of occupational therapy programs, occupational therapy interventions, and even the productivity of individual occupational therapy practitioners (DeJong & Sutton, 1995).

▼ CONTENT OF ADL AND HOME MANAGEMENT EVALUATION

One of the first decisions occupational therapy practitioners must make when approaching an ADL or home management evaluation concerns the specific tasks to be evaluated.. In making this decision, multiple conceptual and practical issues need to be taken into account. Terms, that is, concepts, used in reference to ADL and home management tasks need to be understood. The application of these concepts in practice through their operationalization, including task analysis, needs to be critically appraised. Most important, clients' needs must be recognized and the implications of terminology and its operationalization for their care must be carefully considered.

Differences in Terminology

Conceptually, ADL could apply to all tasks that individuals perform routinely. The term ADL was coined by Deaver to refer to a wide range of behavior patterns considered necessary for meeting the demands of daily living (U. S. Department of Education, 1982). In the *Uniform Terminology for Occupational Therapy* (AOTA, 1994), ADL is subtitled self-maintenance tasks, and includes 15 domains: grooming, oral hygiene, bathing or showering, toilet hygiene, personal device care, dressing, feeding and eating, medication routine, health maintenance, socialization, functional communication, functional mobility, community mobility, emergency response, and sexual expression. Home management is one of four domains listed under the work and productive area in the *Uniform Terminology for Occupational Therapy*, and is divided into: clothing care, cleaning, meal preparation and cleanup, shopping, money management, household maintenance, and safety procedures.

The *Uniform Terminology for Occupational Therapy* provides a nomenclature and organizational scheme for occupational therapy practitioners. Other health care and social services practitioners may be unfamiliar with this terminology and may use other terms to refer to these same ADL and home management concepts, or may use the same terms, but define them differently. For example, the term ADL is generally restricted to tasks involving functional mobility and personal care. Ambulation or wheelchair mobility, transfers, feeding, hygiene, toileting, bathing, and dressing are typically covered under ADL. Synonyms for ADL are basic ADL, physical ADL, basic self-maintenance, physical self-maintenance, and personal self-maintenance (Fillenbaum, 1988; Lawton & Brody, 1969; Lawton, 1972). Similarly, home management is generally classified as an **instrumental activity of daily living (IADL),** a term applied to tasks required for independent living. IADL usually includes telephone use, shopping, food preparation, housekeeping, medication management, financial management, and getting around one's community. Laundering and leisure may also be considered under IADL. Synonyms for IADL are independent-living skills, advanced ADL, and extended ADL (Lawton & Brody, 1969; Nouri & Lincoln, 1987). Occupational therapy practitioners need to be aware of these differences in terminology and usage when communicating with other professionals and when selecting evaluation instruments. We must know how to respond appropriately to a referral for an IADL evaluation. Table 15-1 lists specific tasks commonly found on measures of functional mobility, personal care, and home management.

Operationalization of Concepts

Before functional mobility, personal care, and home management tasks can be evaluated, they must be operationally defined, that is to say, the occupational therapy practitioner must know the precise meaning of each task. An operational definition is one that provides guidelines for measurement (Rothstein, 1985). It is an instructional tool that informs practitioners about the tasks that are to be evaluated and the components of tasks that are to be evaluated (Eakin, 1989). For example, because feeding is an abstract concept it cannot be observed. Feeding takes on concreteness and precision when it is operationalized as "moving solid and liquid food from dinnerware to the mouth." The movement of solid and liquid food from dinnerware to the mouth is observable and measurable.

The same concept may be operationalized in different ways, as is illustrated by the following definitions of feeding independence, which are on three widely used functional assessments:

On the Barthel Index (Barthel) (Mahoney & Barthel, 1965) independence in feeding is defined as:

The patient can feed himself from a tray or table when someone puts the food within his reach. He must put on an assistive device if this is needed, cut up food, use salt and pepper, spread butter etc. He must accomplish this in a reasonable time (p. 62).

On the Katz Index of ADL (Index of ADL) (Katz, Ford, Moskowitz, Jackson, & Jaffe, 1963), independence in feeding is defined as:

Gets food from plate or its equivalent into mouth; (precutting of meal and preparation of food, as buttering bread, are excluded from evaluation) (p. 915).

On the **Functional Independence Measure (FIM)** [Uniform Data System for Medical Rehabilitation (UDSMR), 1993], independence in feeding is defined as:

All of the tasks described as making up the activity are typically performed safely, without modification, assistive devices, or aids, within a reasonable amount of time (Page III-4). Subject eats from a dish, while managing all consistencies of food, and drinks from a cup or glass with the meal presented in the customary manner on a table or tray. The subject uses a spoon or fork to bring food to the mouth; food is chewed and swallowed. Performs safely (p. III-6).

Thus, Mr. Miles, who can perform hand-to-mouth actions, but cannot cut his food, would be dependent in feeding on the Barthel, but independent on the Index of ADL. Furthermore, because he needs to use feeding utensils with enlarged handles, he cannot be rated as fully independent on the FIM. His rating on the FIM would also be reduced because he tends to choke when swallowing liquids, a component of feeding that is not included on the Barthel or Index of ADL.

As might be expected because of their increased complexity, the operational definitions of home management tasks are more varied than those for ADL. The domain of meal preparation illustrates this point well. On the Instrumental Activities of Daily Living Scale (IADL Scale) (Lawton, 1972), which is generally considered to be the prototype instrument for IADL, the highest level of competence is described as, "plans, prepares, and serves adequate meals independently" (p. 133). Comparable items on the Nottingham Extended ADL Index (Nouri & Lincoln, 1987) inquire about the ability to make a hot drink and hot snack alone and easily. Thus, regardless of the scale used, Mrs. Stephen's independent performance of the cooking items would lead to a rating of independence in cooking, even though the subtasks on the Nottingham Extended ADL Index are much less complex than those on the IADL Scale.

Concepts are operationalized so that occupational therapy practitioners know what to look for in conducting an evaluation. The operationalization of concepts is similar to the process of task analysis in which tasks are broken down into the functional subtasks needed to complete them. In Table 15-2, we have analyzed the content of the Barthel, Index of ADL, and FIM definitions of independent feeding, and have added the task analysis from the Klein-Bell ADL Scale (Klein & Bell, 1979). Given the data previously presented about Mr. Miles' feeding abilities, his feeding performance is rated on the four instruments, using able or unable as the measurement scale. By reviewing the subtasks, the nature of Mr. Miles' eating disability and ability can be described very explicitly. The Barthel identified disabilities in cutting food and spreading butter, the FIM identified a swallowing dysfunction, and the Klein-Bell noted problems in cutting food and swallowing liquid without choking. However, only the scoring system of the Klein-Bell scale, which allows subtasks to be rated individually, yields evalua-

Table 15-1. Functional Mobility, Personal Care, and Home Management Tasks Included in Evaluation Tools

Functional Mobility	Personal Care	Home Management
Move in bed	Feeding or eating	Meal preparation
• Shift position	• Feed from dish	• Prepare cold food
• Turn	• Drink from cup, glass, straw	• Prepare hot food
• Sit	• Use utensils	• Use appliances/utensils
Transfer	• Cut food	• Use range
• Bed	• Manage finger food	• Use stove
• Chair	• Bite and chew	Housecleaning
• Bathtub	• Swallow	• Light housecleaning
• Shower	Hygiene	• Heavy housecleaning
• Car	• Clean teeth/dentures	Finances
Sit in chair	• Brush, comb hair	• Manage cash exchanges
Stand	• Shave	• Write checks
Walk	• Apply makeup	• Balance checkbook
• Level surface	• Groom nails	• Keep financial records
• Environmental terrain	Bathe	• Assemble tax records
• Ramps	• Upper body	Shopping
• Curbs	• Face	• For food
• Stairs	• Hands	• For clothing
Community mobility	• Arms	• For household necessities
• Get in or out of residence	• Trunk	Telephoning
• Cross street	• Lower Body	• Locate number
• Around neighborhood	• Groin	• Dial telephone
• To bus stop	• Buttocks	• Give messages
Work-related	• Upper legs	• Receive messages
• Bending, kneeling, stooping	• Lower legs/feet	Medication management
• Lifting and carrying	Dress	• Manage containers
• Reaching	• Upper body	• Take according to prescription
• Pushing and pulling	• Front opening garments	Laundry
• Manipulating	• Pull over garments	• Wash clothes
	• Brassiere	• Manage drying clothes
	• Corset/brace	Time management
	• Hearing aid/eye glasses	• Plan, organize, follow through
	• Lower body	• Keep track of appointments
	• Underclothing	Transportation
	• Slacks/skirt	• Drive car
	• Socks, stockings	• Public transportation
	• Shoes	
	• Brace, prosthesis	
	• Fasteners	
	Toileting	
	• Handle clothing	
	• Wipe	
	• Flush	
	• Control bladder	
	• Control bowels	
	Communicate	
	• Comprehend spoken language	
	• Comprehend written language	
	• Comprehend symbols	
	• Express Basic needs	
	• Speech	
	• Writing	
	• Sign or gesture	

Table 15-2. Task Analysis of Mr. Miles' Feeding on the Barthel, Index of ADL, FIM, and Klein-Bell subtasks, and Summarized as Able or Unable

Instrument	Mr. Miles' Performance	
	Able	Unable
Barthel Index (Mahoney & Barthel, 1965)		
• Put on assistive device	X	
• Feed self	X	
• Cut food		X
• Use salt and pepper	X	
• Spread butter		X
Katz Index of ADL (Katz et al., 1963)		
• Get food from plate (or its equivalent) into mouth	X	
FIM (Uniform Data System for Medical Rehabilitation, 1993)		
• Eats all food consistencies from a dish	X	
• Drinks from a cup/glass	X	
• Uses a spoon or fork to bring food to mouth	X, with device	
• Chews food	X	
• Swallows food		X, unsafe
Klein-Bell (Bell & Klein, 1979, p. 11)		
Eat solid food		
• Grasp fork/spoon	+	
• Cut food		+
• Spear food portion with fork	+	
• Place portion inside mouth	+	
• Chew	+	
• Swallow	+	
Eat semisolid food		
• Scoop food portion onto utensil	+	
• Place food inside mouth	+	
Eat liquid food		
• Scoop food portion from bowl	+	
• Place food portion inside mouth	+	
Drink		
• Grasp container	+	
• Bring container to mouth	+	
• Intake liquid without spilling	+	
• Swallow liquid without choking		+

ADL = Activities of Daily Living; FIM = Functional Independence Measure

tion data that enable occupational therapy interventions to be targeted precisely to the dysfunctional task components. The Barthel, Index of ADL, and FIM do not yield retrievable data about subtask performance because they are global scales. On global scales, task domains (eg, feeding or dressing) are rated as a unit, rather than by the subtasks comprising these domains. Although subtasks are taken into account in the operational definition of a task, this detail becomes lost (Settle & Holm, 1993). On the Barthel, for example, because of Mr. Miles inability to cut food and spread butter, he is rated as dependent in feeding; however, the instrument records only his overall dependency in feeding and not where this dependency occurred.

Clinical Guidelines: Content

Client-centered care requires that the occupational therapy evaluation responds to the unique needs and living situations of individuals. We can expect the tasks of concern for a 29-year-old female homemaker, caring for three young children, are very different from those of concern for a 49-year-old executive of a clothing business, and the evaluation needs to be tailored to take these life style differences into account. Occupational therapy practitioners need to give careful attention to the way in which they operationalize ADL and home management tasks, whether this operationalization occurs through the instruments they select to administer or the informal procedures they implement. Our review of several definitions of feeding and meal preparation has made it apparent that clients may be made more or less independent or dependent in a task depending on how the task is defined and measured by the practitioner. Because of the loss of descriptive data, global scales are less useful for planning occupational therapy interventions than scales that employ detailed task analyses. Global scales may be more useful when screening for disability than when evaluating with the intent to intervene. Because global scales are less sensitive to change, they are also less useful for documenting progress resulting from rehabilitation.

▼ PARAMETERS OF ADL AND HOME MANAGEMENT EVALUATION

The tasks classified as ADL and home management define the content of the occupational therapy evaluation for these areas. When planning an evaluation, decisions must be made about the parameters of task performance to evaluate as well as the content of the evaluation. What is it about task performance that practitioners want to know? Do we want to learn where a task is performed, when it is performed, or how it is performed? The parameters of task performance direct attention to the dimensions of ADL and home management tasks that are to be evaluated. Parameters of task performance are a part of the operational definition of a task (Eakin, 1989; Rothstein, 1985). In our previous review of the operational definitions of feeding on the Barthel, Index of ADL, and FIM scales, we considered not just feeding but *independence* in feeding. Independence was the parameter used to evaluate feeding. In general, ADL and home management evaluation provides data about those tasks that clients can do safely, independently, efficiently, and adequately, and those tasks for which supervision, assistance, or modification is required because of deficits in safety, independence, efficiency, or adequacy.

Evaluative Approaches

The parameters of task performance may be evaluated through qualitative or quantitative approaches. In the qualitative approach, task performance is described. In the quantitative approach, it is measured. Both approaches incorporate **clinical reasoning** to integrate evaluative data and ascertain its meaning.

QUALITATIVE APPROACH

In the qualitative approach to evaluation, the salient characteristics of clients' task performance are described. These descriptions are used to formulate inferences about clients' task performance on the evaluation parameters of interest. A practitioner might note, for instance, that a client named Mr. Brand could not bend (flex) at the waist sufficiently to reach his feet with his hands and could not bend (hip external rotation; knee flexion) his lower extremities sufficiently to move his feet closer to his hands. From these observations, the practitioner might infer that the client is unable to don socks and other lower extremity garments and, thus, is rated as dependent in lower extremity dressing. Both the data and the conclusions drawn from the data are managed qualitatively.

QUANTITATIVE APPROACH

In the measurement approach to evaluation, the evaluation parameters of interest are quantified through the assignment of numbers (Wade, 1992). Numbers can aid in determining the severity of dysfunction and the extent of improvement or deterioration. However, they can also lead to misinterpretations and erroneous conclusions, which is why it is important to understand the numbers that are generated by various measures and the mathematical procedures that can be appropriately applied to them. In this textbook, Polgar (see Chap. 14) discussed four levels of measurement: nominal, ordinal, interval, and ratio. Each of these levels is applicable to ADL and home management evaluation.

Nominal measurement involves the use of discrete categories. For example, a dressing disability might be diagnosed as 1 = dressing disability related to physical impairment; 2 = dressing disability related to cognitive impairment; or, 3 = dressing disability related to emotional impairment. The numbers 1, 2, and 3 merely indicate different types of dressing disability. There is no implication that a disability of emotional etiology, which is assigned a 3, is "better or worse" or "more or less" than a disability having a cognitive or physical basis, which are given a 2 and 1, respectively. Nominal measurement is essentially a process of grouping similar data and naming or labeling it (Fox, 1969; Wade, 1992). Nominal data cannot be added and subtracted because these manipulations have no numeric meaning.

Ordinal measurement entails a rank ordering of scores. A dressing disability, for example, may be rated as: 1 = requires minimal assistance; 2 = requires moderate assistance; 3 = requires maximal assistance. In this case, a 1 signifies less disability than a 3. However, the difference between requiring minimal and moderate assistance or between requiring moderate and maximal assistance, that is, between a 1 and 2 or a 2 and 3, are unknown. Hence, it cannot be stated that a client who receives a 2 has twice as much dressing disability than the one receiving a 1. To make such a comparative statement, the unit of measurement (eg, amount of assistance) must have the same quantitative meaning at each point on the scale. Thus, for example, caregivers must expend twice as much energy assisting clients scoring 2 than they do assisting clients scoring 1.

Ordinal measurement may also be devised using a task-descriptive approach. In this approach, each point on a scale is defined in terms of specific task behaviors. Dressing performance might be scaled as follows: 3 = locates, selects, and dons appropriate clothing; 2 = dons, but cannot locate or select appropriate clothing; and, 1 = cannot locate, select, or don appropriate clothing. In this example, dressing is scaled based on features that are inherent to, as well as essential to, task performance.

In interval measurement, the unit of measurement has the same quantitative meaning at any point on the scale. A 5-lb weight loss represents the same amount whether the weight loss occurs from 105 to 100 lb or from 350 to 345 lb. Because of this quality, comparative statements can be made because the difference between any two scores is equal. At this level of measurement, scores can be added and subtracted, but not multiplied or divided. Unfortunately, it is difficult to create equal-interval scales for ADL and home management because it is difficult to determine the weight to attach to individual tasks.

Ratio measurement is distinguished by having a definite or fixed zero point as well as an equal-interval scale. An example of ratio measurement would be measuring the time a client takes to complete dressing. Timing would begin when the first piece of clothing is picked up and would terminate when the last piece of clothing was donned. The time elapsed from start to finish would be the client's score. All arithmetic operations can be applied to ratio data.

Parameters of Task Performance for Description and Measurement

The parameters of task performance that occupational therapists are most interested in evaluating are: value, independence, safety, and quality (ie, efficiency, adequacy, or acceptability). Figure 15-1 provides an overview of the parameters discussed.

VALUE

When evaluating the meaning of task performance and task performance dysfunctions to clients, data about the value that they place on different tasks is essential. Value reflects the importance or significance of a task to the client. As an evaluation parameter, value is usually used in reference to the independent performance of tasks. Chiou and Burnett (1985), for example, ascertained that of 15 ADL, the ability to move indoors independently was most valued by clients with stroke. Similarly, Atwood, Holm, and James (1994) ascertained that nursing home residents reported higher capability in personal care tasks for which independence was most valued. Because our actions as humans are influenced by our values, ascertaining the relative value that ADL and home management tasks have for clients is useful for establishing intervention priorities and for negotiating target intervention outcomes with them.

INDEPENDENCE

The most common parameter used to measure disability is the level of independence clients exhibit when performing a task. A rating of independence or able means that clients are able to perform an activity by themselves. Conversely, a rating of dependence or unable means that clients are unable to perform a task by themselves; in other words, that help is required. When task performance is not totally independent, a more refined measurement scale may be used to quantify the extent of independence. For example, task performance may be rated as 75% independent, 50% independent, or 25% independent. Alternately, the reference point used to measure disability may be the effort exerted by caregivers, rather than by clients. For example, caregivers may provide no, minimal, moderate, or maximal assistance of one or more persons.

When assistance is required to complete an activity, the type of help needed may be added to the rating scale. Three general types of assistance are recognized and are rank ordered from least to most assistive as follows: assistive technology, nonphysical assistance, and physical assistance. Assistive technology, which is also referred to as assistive devices, adaptive equipment, and technical aids, qualifies as the least assistive type of help when it enables activity performance to be adaptive, but independent. Clients who can feed themselves using utensils with enlarged or elongated handles fit this definition. The use of assistive technology is treated differently on functional assessments. On some instruments, assistive technology is included in the definition of independent task performance, whereas on others it receives a lower rating (eg, FIM, UDSMR, 1993; Health Assessment Questionnaire, Fries, Spitz, Kraines, & Holman, 1980). Hence, even though assistive technology may enable clients to perform tasks by themselves, on some instruments they cannot receive the highest independence rating. Nonetheless, they would still be rated higher than clients requiring other kinds of assistance. The rationale behind using a lower score is that by using assistive technology, task performance is not done in a normative manner; that is, in the manner in which it is usually done by adults in this culture.

In terms of independence, the need for nonphysical help is considered to be less dependent than is implied by the need for physical, "hands-on" help. Nonphysical help takes into account an array of techniques, including task setup, supervision, standby assistance, and verbal and nonverbal encouragement and guidance. Task setup, also known as stimulus control, involves preparing task materials and the environment for task performance. Examples of task setup include opening milk cartons and sugar packets. Supervision means that the caregiver is available to monitor task performance and to intervene if problems arise. Standby assistance is similar to supervision, except that the caregiver must be physically present and in close proximity to the client at all times. A caregiver who is reviewing checks for accuracy after they have been written is an example of supervision, whereas walking alongside a client using a walker is an example of standby assistance. Verbal guidance means using words, either orally or in writing, to instruct clients about task performance or prompt them to initiate or continue it. Examples are reminding clients to brush their teeth or

VALUE

Independence is important _____ Independence is not important

INDEPENDENCE

Independent _____ Dependent

Able _____ Unable

100% Independent _____ 0% Independent

No assistance _____ Maximal assistance
• from 1 person
• from 2 persons

No assistance _____ Assistive technology _____ Nonphysical assistance
• Setup
• Supervision
• Standby assist
• Verbal assist
• Nonverbal assist
• Encouragement
• Instruction
_____ Physical assistance
• Physical guidance
• Physical assistance

I believe I can _____ I believe I cannot

SAFETY

Safe _____ Unsafe

No risk
• Client performance
• Environment _____ At risk
• Client performance
• Environment

QUALITY

Efficiency

No difficulty _____ Severe difficulty

Without difficulty _____ Unable to do

No pain _____ Severe pain

Pain does not interfere with performance _____ Pain prevents performance

Seconds/Minutes _____ Hours

Fatigue does not interfere with performance _____ Fatigue prevents performance

Adequacy/Acceptability

Meets normative standards _____ Does not meet normative standards

Satisfied _____ Dissatisfied

Satisfied 100% of the time _____ Satisfied 0% of the time

Previous experience _____ No previous experience

Recent experience _____ No recent experience

Frequent experience _____ Infrequent experience

Resources adequate to meet needs _____ Resources inadequate to meet needs

Absence of aberrant task behaviors _____ Presence of aberrant task behaviors

Figure 15-1. Parameters used to evaluate activities of daily living (ADL) and home management task performance.

telling them how to do a bathtub transfer. Nonverbal guidance involves the use of demonstration, which is also called modeling, or gestures to instruct clients about activity performance or prompt them to initiate or continue it. Examples include demonstrating a bathtub transfer or tapping on a client's foot to draw attention to the need to put socks on. Encouragement differs from guidance in that the intent is to motivate clients, rather than to teach them. "You are doing a great job," is an example of a motivational statement.

Although there is substantive consensus that the need for nonphysical help only implies greater independence than does the need for physical help, there is less consensus about the rank order of the techniques grouped under nonphysical help. For instance, is task setup less assistive than giving verbal cues or demonstrating how a task is to be done? Because of this lack of consensus, these techniques will be arranged differently on different scales.

Physical assistance includes physically guiding clients to do a task or part of a task and doing it for them. Although both of these techniques require direct "hands-on" contact with clients, when physical guidance is used the expectation is that clients will participate in the action once they understand what is to be done, whereas when physical assistance is used the only expectation for clients is that they cooperate with caregiving. Examples of physical guidance are inserting a client's hand into the armhole of a garment and positioning a client's hands on a walker. A practitioner putting a shirt on a client or lifting a client from a chair are examples of physical assistance.

Perceived self-efficacy is another facet of independent task performance. Perceived self-efficacy refers to clients' beliefs about their ability to perform tasks independently. If the distance between the bed and a wheelchair looks like the Grand Canyon to clients and they believe that they cannot execute a transfer successfully, it is likely that they will not perform the task. Self-perceptions of task performance capability influence task performance as significantly as actual capabilities (Gage, Noh, Polatajko, & Kaspar, 1994). Perceived self-efficacy is task-specific. Hence, it is measured only in relation to specific tasks. For example, clients may rate the extent to which they believe they can perform a bed-to-wheelchair transfer independently.

SAFETY

Safety refers to the extent to which clients are at risk when engaged in tasks. As used here, safety is applied to the way in which clients interact with objects and their environments to perform tasks. Safety is not a quality of the environment per se, but rather of the person–task–environment transaction. Although a bathtub safety rail is a safety feature, its presence in the bathroom will not improve clients' safety unless it is actually used, and used correctly, when bathtub transfers are executed. Unsafe features of a home, on the other hand, may be indicators of unsafe task performance or increased risk. A can of bacon grease on the stove or an electrical cord traversing a sink suggest that clients, or others in the home, have unsafe daily-living habits.

On some functional assessments (eg, FIM, UDSMR, 1993) safety is included in the judgment of independence. In other words, to be rated as independent, clients must perform a task safely. However, because clients may be able to execute tasks by themselves and yet do so unsafely, it is advantageous to rate safety separately from independence. This situation often occurs as ADL and home management abilities begin to decline owing to the progression of disease or the consequences of aging. Clients will continue to prepare meals, for example, but burn themselves or the food more often. Safety and independence are related but distinct evaluation parameters.

Safety may also include risks associated with poor judgment and decisions as well as those related to physical actions. Clients who take too much or too little medication may be acting in a manner that will lead to health risks. Those who leave the door unlocked at night or flash 20-dollar bills around while standing at the bus stop may also be acting unsafely. The risk to personal safety is the core factor being evaluated under safety.

Although safety has always been recognized as a critical evaluation parameter in occupational therapy, we are only beginning to devise scales to measure it separately from independence in task performance (Letts & Marshall, 1995). When working with clients, it is often difficult to decide where the line between safe and unsafe performance should be drawn, and when task performance is sufficiently unsafe that independence should be restricted. As occupational therapy practice moves more into clients' homes, interfaces more with the legal system for the purposes of guardianship, conservatorship, and involuntary commitment, and becomes more oriented toward prevention and health promotion, safety will increasingly move to the forefront of our evaluation technology.

ADEQUACY

Adequacy of task performance is a complex evaluation parameter that refers to the quality of the action used to execute tasks as well as the quality of the outcome or product of that action. When dressing, for example, movement may be efficient or inefficient. When dressing is completed, the individual may look neat or disheveled. Similarly, when paying bills, clients may take each bill in turn or shuffle them like a deck of cards. The checks written in payment for the bills may or may not correspond with the amount due, or the correct bill. The distinction between efficiency and the adequacy may be blurred on specific instruments. Parameters emphasizing the quality of action, or efficiency, usually come under the following headings: difficulty, **pain,** fatigue and dyspnea, and duration. Those emphasizing the outcome of action or adequacy, are generally categorized under: normative standards, satisfaction, experience, and aberrant task behaviors.

Difficulty

Difficulty refers to the perceived ease with which a task is accomplished. Rehabilitation theorist Verbrugge (1990) argued that difficulty is the most appropriate way to measure disability because ratings of difficulty come from clients, whereas ratings of the amount of assistance required to complete tasks come from clients' caregivers. Caregiver ratings of assistance may be more reflective of the assistance given than of the assistance that is actually needed. The Functional Status Index (FSI; Jette, 1980), a disability measure designed for use with adults with **arthritis,** uses a 4-point scale of no, mild, moderate, and, severe difficulty. The Health Assessment Questionnaire (HAQ; Fries et al., 1980), another disability instrument designed for clients with arthritis, also employs a 4-point scale that considers without any difficulty, with some difficulty, with much difficulty, and unable to do.

The level of difficulty experienced during task performance is increasingly being viewed as a marker of preclinical disability; that is, as a symptom that indicates that the individual is at risk for decline in function even though the precise nature of that decline is not yet apparent (Fried, Herdman, Kuhn, Rubin, & Turano, 1991). Unless the onset of pathology is sudden, such as that arising from a car accident or stroke, it is likely that clients will find it harder to perform tasks before they are unable to perform them. Along similar lines, an increase in perceived difficulty or the spread of difficulty from more difficult (eg, heavy housework) to easier (eg, oral hygiene) tasks may signal the progression of occult disability.

Pain

Pain is the discomfort or sensation of hurting that is experienced during task performance and may continue after performance has stopped (Jette, 1980). In relation to disability, the component of pain that is of most concern is the extent to which it interferes with task performance. Interference may be ascertained in relation to specific tasks, such as walking or dressing. Alternatively, interference may be gauged more globally in reference to clients' general activity level (McDowell & Newell, 1996). Because of pain, tasks may be modified, done at a slower pace, done less often or adequately, or eliminated from one's daily routine. In addition to interference with tasks, it may be useful to note: (1) the presence or absence of pain; (2) the location and distribution of pain; (3) the intensity of pain (eg, none, mild, moderate, severe); or, (4) the character of the pain experienced (eg, shooting, burning, dull).

Fatigue and Dyspnea

Fatigue is the discomfort or sensation of tiredness, weariness, or exhaustion that is experienced during or following task performance (Tack, 1991; Hart & Freel, 1982). When fatigued, clients describe themselves as tired and needing to rest (Freal, Kraft, & Coryell, 1984). Fatigue and dyspnea often occur together. Dyspnea is a sensation of difficult or labored breathing (Gift, 1987). Clients describe their symptoms of dyspnea as feeling short of breath, not getting enough air, chest tightness, and finding it hard to move air (Janson-Bjerklie, Carrieri, & Hudes, 1986). Fatigue and dyspnea may interfere with the ability to do tasks and may be exacerbated by task performance. Similar to pain, they may lead to modifications in the manner in which tasks are done, a slower pace, decreases in participation in tasks, and the transfer of responsibility to others. An interesting aspect of fatigue and dyspnea is that they can result from too much (eg, strenuous housework) as well as too little (eg, sedentary life style) physical activity (Gift & Pugh, 1993). They may be a component of both physical (eg, chronic lung disease) and mental (eg, anxiety) illness. As with pain, the fatigue/dyspnea-disability relation is generally approached by ascertaining the extent of interference with specific tasks and usual activity level. Scales may also record the presence or absence, the amount (eg, none, a lot), and the severity (ie, mild, severe) of pain (McDowell & Newell, 1996).

Duration

The duration of task performance—that is, the time needed to complete a task—is often used as a measure of efficiency. Less time is interpreted as meaning increased efficiency. In essence, time gives a measure of the speed of performance. Some functional assessments include a time criterion in the definition of independence. The FIM (UDSMR, 1993) specifies, for example, that tasks must be completed in "reasonable time." Practitioners often comment on tasks being completed "within normal limits." Interestingly, neither the average length of time adults take nor the minimum time they need to perform various ADL and home management tasks has been calculated.

Although time to task completion provides a ratio scale for measuring task performance, it is cumbersome data to collect in the clinical situation, because it requires the use of a stopwatch and the designation of precise beginning and ending points for each task. Furthermore, the time needed to complete tasks is highly dependent on the reason for engaging in the task. Dressing to do housecleaning is likely to take less time than dressing to go out to work. Time is also a poor marker of efficiency for clients who are impulsive or manic because they may rush through tasks with little consideration for safety or adequacy. Although they may prepare a meal in record time, for example, the food may be unappetizing and the kitchen cluttered with pots and cooking utensils when they are finished.

Societal Standards

In moving from looking at the quality of action to the quality of the outcome or product of that action, the question of adequacy or acceptability *to whom* must be addressed. One approach to evaluating the quality of task outcomes or products is to evaluate those results against the normative expectations of society. Accordingly, for example, humans are expected to maintain personal cleanliness and to not overdraw their checking accounts. Although there may be a wide, rather than a thin, line between what is acceptable and unacceptable, task performance that consistently goes outside the line, will be labeled unacceptable, inappropriate, or inadequate according to societal standards. In applying normative standards, practitioners must be careful to make allowance for cultural diversity.

Satisfaction

A second parameter of quality of task outcomes or products is satisfaction. Satisfaction refers to the experience of pleasure and contentment with one's task performance (Yerxa, Burnett-Beaulieu, Stocking, & Azen, 1988). As a parameter of performance, it is likely that satisfaction interacts with an individual's willingness to engage in a task. If clients fail to derive satisfaction from their task performance, they may restrict their participation. In relating satisfaction to task performance, a dichotomous scale may be used consisting of satisfied or dissatisfied, or satisfaction may be rated according to the proportion of time over a defined interval that clients experienced satisfaction (eg, 100%, 75%, and so on) (Yerxa et al., 1988; Pincus, Summey, Soraci, Wallston, & Hummon, 1983). Caregivers of clients may also be asked to rate the extent to which they are satisfied with the care recipient's task performance. This procedure has the potential for providing practitioners with information about the "normative expectations" for task performance within the family unit.

Experience

Experience refers to the direct participation in tasks that persons have accumulated. The assumption is that experience provides practice, which perfects performance and outcomes. Tasks classified under ADL are generally learned by all humans over the course of childhood and adolescence. As tasks basic to and essential for daily living, they are practiced regularly over adulthood. Possible exceptions to this norm include hair care being done by beauticians, fingernail care being done by manicurists, and toenail care being done by podiatrists. Nonetheless, the societal expectation is that all adults have a wide range of experience with these tasks and will perform them adequately. However, a similar expectation does not hold for home management tasks, for which humans have more options. Clients, therefore, may not have developed proficiency in home management tasks. Some may have no experience in preparing meals, doing the laundry, or managing finances. Clients' task performance history is essential for understanding their current performance level. A task performance dysfunction would be interpreted differently if clients had no or little prior experience performing the task than if they had been doing it immediately premorbidly.

In addition to past experience, recent or current experience must also be evaluated. When tasks are not performed regularly, the proficiency needed to do them can fall into disuse or become obsolete with technological advances. Inquiries about recency and frequency of task experience are generally approached by ascertaining clients' skills and habits in ADL and home management (Rogers & Holm, 1991a). Skill refers to the capability to do a task, whereas habit refers to usual or routine task performance. In our activity repertoires, we all have tasks that we usually do not perform, but that we can perform if situations arise where we have to do them or wanted to do them. For example, you may know how to cook, but prefer to let your spouse do this on a daily basis. However, if your spouse was away on a business trip, you could cook dinner for yourself. Inquiries about task skills are generally phrased in terms of "Can you (name the task)?" Inquiries about habits are generally phrased in terms of "Do you (name the task)?"

Resources

When an evaluation is conducted to assist in discharge decisions, the resources available to clients must be taken into account, as well as clients' skills. Consider, for example, Ms. Cross and Ms. Lum, who are unable to use the range and oven safely to prepare hot food. Ms. Cross has a niece who lives on the same city block as she does and is willing to assist her in preparing hot meals. Ms. Lum lives in a rural community, which does not have a meals-on-wheels program, and her neighbors are elderly themselves and unable to assist her. Although the meal preparation skills of both of these clients is the same, Ms. Lum is at greater risk for adverse outcomes than Ms. Cross because she has less supportive living resources available to her. Thus, when discharge decisions are at stake, the evaluation of ADL and home management skills becomes meaningful only when deficits are linked to resources (Williams et al., 1991).

Aberrant Task Behaviors

The task analyses used on ADL and home management instruments are based on the way in which tasks are usually, that is to say, normally, performed by individuals with disabilities. However, individuals with cognitive impairments, such as those associated with **dementia, traumatic brain injury, schizophrenia,** and **mental retardation** may exhibit task behaviors that are aberrant or abnormal. For example, they may pocket food in their cheeks or spit food out. In contrast to the subtasks derived from task analyses, which are to be encouraged during intervention, aberrant task behaviors are to be extinguished or reduced in frequency. Table 15-3 provides a listing of some common aberrant task-related behaviors. These behaviors are not well represented on available ADL and home management instruments, with the exception of the Routine Task Inventory, an instrument specifically devised for use with a psychiatric population (Allen, 1985).

Table 15-3. Aberrant Task Behaviors Observed During Task Performance Evaluations

Functional Mobility	Personal Care	Home Management
Move in bed • Drops onto bed • Rocks to gain enough momentum to get up from bed Transfer • Drops during standing pivot • Grabs onto clothing of caregiver Sit in chair • Drops down Stand • Falls deliberately Walk • Refuses to walk • Staggers • Weaves • Paces • Wanders Community mobility • Gets lost Work-related • Does not adhere to safety guidelines during mobility	Feeding/eating • Refuses to eat • Drools • Coughs, chokes, gags • Has delayed swallow; does not swallow • Has disturbing tongue movements • Eats too fast or too slow, or only certain foods • Spits food out of mouth • Stuffs food in mouth • Takes another person's food • Eats spoiled food Hygiene • Bites nails • Spits nails on floor Bathe • Refuses to bathe • Fear of water, hair washing • Neglects to wash some body parts • Fails to rinse soap Dress • Resists dressing • Sleeps in street clothes • Dons clothes inside out, backwards • Dons clothes on wrong body part • Dons underclothes on top of street clothes • Layers clothes • Takes clothes off at inappropriate times or places • Wears the same clothes everyday • Dons another person's clothes • Dons nonclothing items • Ignores weather conditions Toileting • Urinates in inappropriate places • Defecates in inappropriate places Communicate • Makes sexual gestures or advances • Is verbally aggressive • Is physically aggressive	Meal preparation • Burns food • Cooks food inadequately • Uses too much spice • Forgets to turn off stove, oven Housecleaning • Dusts inadequately • Leaves dirt on floor • Forgets to remove garbage • Cleans inadequately (eg, bathtub, stove) • Keeps spoiled food Finances • Forgets to pay bills • Makes errors in calculating costs • Throws out bills or money • Gives money away Shopping • Goes on a spending spree • Cannot remember what to buy Telephoning • Calls a person repeatedly thus being annoying • Calls police inappropriately • Neglects to give a message Medication management • Takes too much or too little • Stops taking • Takes at the wrong time Laundry • Stores soiled clothes Time management • Forgets appointments • Comes for appointments at wrong time Transportation • Forgets where car is parked • Gets lost • Gets on wrong bus • Confused about destination

Evaluation Parameters and Measurement Instruments

This discussion of evaluation parameters has emphasized individual items and the scores assigned to them. Item scores are often summed to obtain a total score. The total score provides a summary index of the client's overall status on the concept that is being evaluated (eg, ADL, home management). Several scoring systems may be used on measures. Most commonly, item scores are simply added, thus giving equal weight to all items on the scale. Bathing and grooming, for example, would make an equal contribution to the total score. On some instruments, items are differentially weighted to take into account the value or consequences that they have for disability or overall occupational status. Bathing, for example, might be given double the weight of grooming because it contributes twice as much to disablement. Item weights may be assigned through expert opinion or statistical methods. Intrinsic to each scoring system are assumptions about the relative value of each task item to the total score. Occupational therapy practitioners need to be aware of these scoring systems so that they can correctly interpret their clients' scores.

Most instruments used in professional fields, such as occupational therapy, medicine, rehabilitation, and education, do not have the precision required to qualify as interval measures. They are ordinal measures. Nonetheless, even though they do not meet the criteria for interval measures, they are often commonly treated and interpreted in this way (Eakin, 1989; Merbitz, Morris, & Grip, 1989; Wade, 1992). In other words, the unit of measurement is treated as equal from point to point (eg, minimal, moderate, maximal assistance) when it is not. Item ratings are added to obtain total scores, and statistical operations, such as means and standard deviations, are calculated. Occupational therapy practitioners need to be cautious about assuming that scales that appear to have equal measurement intervals are, in fact, interval scales. Rasch analysis, a relatively new mathematical method, has the capability of converting ordinal scales to interval ones (Wright & Linacre, 1989), thereby resolving the dilemma associated with nonequal interval scales. Rasch analysis has been applied to the FIM (UDSMR, 1993) and the **Assessment of Motor and Process Skills (AMPS)** (Fisher, 1993).

Clinical Guidelines: Parameters

The parameters for describing or measuring ADL and home management task performance are independence, safety, and quality. Although there are options in the ways in which these parameters may be operationalized, practitioners should evaluate them, regardless of the specific task or tasks being evaluated. They are essential to competent task performance. Task performance that is not independent indicates a need for assistance from technology or humans. Task performance that is independent, but unsafe, places clients at risk. Task performance that is independent, but marginal or inadequate in quality, restricts clients' role participation and may also place them at risk. Deficits in task independence, safety, and quality indicate a need for occupational therapy interventions or for supportive services for ADL or home management.

In view of the number of tasks involved in ADL and home management, practitioners need to devise "rules of thumb" or conceptual shortcuts to decide what tasks to include in the evaluation and the order in which they should be evaluated. Task hierarchies provide a basis for devising these conceptual shortcuts. Task hierarchies arrange tasks according to their level of difficulty. They enable practitioners to assume that clients passing items at an intermediate level would pass all easier items, but fail more difficult ones. Thus, by using background information about clients, practitioners would hypothesize about their functional level, start the evaluation with a task at a reasonable point on the hierarchy, and stop the evaluation after two or three items have been failed.

Development of the Index of ADL (Katz et al., 1963) was based on a Guttman scaling-type approach and ranked ADL, in order of increasing difficulty, as feeding, continence, transfers, toileting, dressing, bathing. Guttman scaling of the IADL Scale (Lawton & Brody, 1969) ranked the performance of older adults from least to most difficult as follows: uses telephone, takes care of all shopping needs, plans, prepares, and serves adequate meals independently, maintains light housework independently, does all laundry, travels by car or public transportation, takes medications with correct dosage at right time, and manages all financial tasks except major purchases or banking. Rasch analysis has provided a substantive boost to the delineation of task hierarchies, and practitioners can anticipate considerable advances in this area in the near future (Fisher, 1993; Velozo, Magalhaes, Pan, & Leiter, 1995).

By combining information from the different evaluation parameters practitioners can obtain information valuable for targeting intervention outcomes. Take for example, Mrs. Morris, a client with low vision, who indicates that independence in financial management is most important to her, and furthermore that this is the task for which she requires the most assistance. The practitioner would probably want to negotiate with her to intervene, at least initially, on an easier task—one in which she is also dependent, but for which less assistance is required, such as cooking. The reason for selecting an easier task is that the disparity between Mrs. Morris' current and desired performance is less, and the practitioner gauges her rehabilitation potential in cooking to be better than that of financial management. Client-centered practice is not violated when practitioners assist their clients in establishing feasible goals.

The occupational therapy evaluation yields data about clients' disabilities and abilities in task performance. Although the occupational therapy process focuses on preventing, remediating, or compensating for dysfunctions in task performance, practitioners need to document tasks that clients' can perform as well as those that they cannot perform. Clients' abilities are as significant as their disabilities for their adjustment to "living with a disability."

▼ ACTIVITIES OF DAILY LIVING AND HOME MANAGEMENT EVALUATION METHODS

Practitioners may use a combination of data-gathering methods to evaluate clients' ADL and home management tasks. The fundamental or basic methods are asking questions, observing, and testing. The specific procedures used to gather data within each of these methods range from unstructured to structured. When questions or observations about task performance are sufficiently structured, and when the questions or observations yield numerical scores, these methods are transformed into testing. Other methods of learning about clients task performance, such as client care conferences or record review (eg, medical, school, work) rely on these three basic methods.

Each data gathering method has advantages and disadvantages. The questioning method of data gathering is more subjective than observation, and this subjectivity may reduce reliability. Questioning is also less expensive and less labor-intensive. Interviews and questionnaires can be administered by less costly personnel than observational instruments because they require less skilled judgment on the part of the assessor. Moreover, clients are not placed at physical risk for injury when they talk about their task performance as they may be when they actually perform tasks. Hence, there is little need for skilled personnel to monitor risk. When observation is structured, it has the potential for increasing the reliability of evaluation results compared with questioning, because the meaning of items is clear. Item ambiguity is reduced because the items must be operationalized to be performed. In turn, increased reliability increases the ability to detect change, a critical factor for practitioners who seek to improve task performance through intervention. As we alluded to previously, the disadvantages of observation over questioning are that it is more time consuming, and more costly in terms of space, equipment, and personnel.

Although no data-gathering method is intrinsically superior to the others, a method may be better for some evaluation purposes than others or for some clinical situations than others. A practitioner's selection of a particular method, or a combination of methods, is largely determined by the overall purpose for conducting the evaluation in conjunction with practicalities, such as the time allowed for the evaluation and the equipment available (Holm & Rogers, 1989). However, practitioners need to be aware that the methods are not necessarily equivalent and do not always yield the same data about clients' ADL and home management performance (Sager et al., 1992).

Asking Questions

In the questioning method of data gathering, questions are posed about ADL and home management tasks. The questioning method may be implemented in an oral or a written format, using interviews or questionnaires, respectively. Neither format requires face-to-face contact. Interviews may be conducted over the telephone. Questionnaires may be completed while waiting for an appointment or mailed out in advance of a session. The degree of structure imposed on the interview or the questionnaire may vary considerably.

Table 15-4 provides data about the bathing performance of two clients that were obtained through questioning. The assessment of bathing consisted of five questions. The first question, "Can you bathe yourself?" was the most general and allowed clients the most leeway in interpreting the meaning of "bathe yourself." Questions 2 through 5 asked about specific components of bathing. These questions used task analysis to breakdown "bathe yourself" into four components—transferring in and out of the bathtub, lowering the body to the bottom of the bathtub, washing the body, and washing specific body parts. As these case data illustrate, the conclusion about bathing disability depends on the questions asked by the practitioner. If only the most general

question about bathing (question 1) had been asked, neither client would have been identified as having a bathing disability. By applying the task analysis approach, both clients were identified as having a bathing disability, but the site of the dysfunction was different. Further questioning of Ms. Beech about how she bathed, elicited the information that she showered in the bathtub. This information led the practitioner to reverse her conclusion about bathing disability because showering eliminates the need to sit in the bathtub. When Ms. Bern was questioned about how she washed her feet and back, she indicated that she soaked them while in the bathtub because she was unable to reach them. She also indicated that she felt that she bathed inadequately because her toes and back were constantly itchy and her back had a rash. Thus, the decision of bathing disability was retained for Ms. Bern.

It is preferable to have clients respond to questions about their task performance because they are the most knowledgeable about it. They have the opportunity for daily self-observation. However, if they have not performed tasks in a while, they may report their abilities inaccurately because they believe they can perform tasks that they actually can no longer perform. There are also numerous situations when clients are unable to respond on their own behalf. For example, they may be too physically ill or too depressed to participate in questioning. They may lack insight into their problems or be unable to respond reliably, as might occur with cognitive impairment, or they may refuse to respond, as might be the case with personality disorders or when clients fear that negative decisions will follow from giving the information (eg, institutionalization). In these situations, caregivers or other proxies may be asked to respond on behalf of clients. To a great extent, the usefulness of the information obtained from caregivers or proxies depends on their familiarity with a clients' ADL and home management performance and habits. For example, if the caregiver or proxy has not actually observed a client bathing, or has not done this for some time, the information given about bathing may be based more on opinion than data. Additionally, there are known biases in the reporting tendencies of caregivers and proxies. Family proxies are prone to perceive clients as more disabled than clients perceive themselves, and they perceive clients as more disabled than do professional caregivers (eg, nurses). In addition, spouses tend to be more negative in their evaluations of task performance than other family members (Rubenstein, Schairer, Wieland, & Kane, 1984). It is likely that caregiver responses are influenced by their own coping styles, which may lead them to minimize or magnify performance dysfunctions.

Evaluation parameters such as independence, safety, and aberrant task behaviors can be readily observed by caregivers and proxies. For some evaluation parameters, however, clients are the only appropriate respondents. Inquiries, for instance, about values, perceived self-efficacy, satisfaction, and activity-related pain are subjective and indices of these parameters are difficult for others to observe.

Table 15-4. Data Obtained about Bathing Performance from Questioning, Observing, and Testing

	Data Obtained from Questioning	
Question	Ms. Bern	Ms. Beech
1. Can you bathe yourself?	Yes	Yes
2. Can you get in and out of the bathtub by yourself?	Yes	Yes
3. Can you lower yourself to the bottom of the bathtub?	Yes	No
4. Can you wash yourself?	Yes	Yes
5. Can you wash your entire body including your feet and back?	No	Yes

	Data Obtained from Observing	
Bathing Step	Mr. Kline	Mr. Market
1. Move into tub	I, Instability when lifting foot to step into tub	I, Knelt on floor, "crawled" into tub
2. Lower to tub bottom	Dependent, physical assist—moderate, S	Crawling precluded this step
3. Fill tub with water	I, S, A	I, Filled tub with cool water, emptied hot water tank
4. Wash upper body	I, S, A	Dependent—verbal and manual guidance, S, A
5. Wash lower body	I, S, A	Dependent—verbal and manual guidance, S, A
6. Rise from tub bottom	Dependent, physical assist—moderate, S	I, S, Had difficulty getting feet under body—poor motor planning
7. Move out of tub	I, S, A	I, S, A
8. Dry upper body	I, S, A	Dependent—instruction not effective, S, neglected back
9. Dry lower body	I, S, A	I, S, A

	Data Obtained from Testing	
Test	Mr. Kline's Score	Mr. Market's Score
Functional Independence Measure (FIM)		
• Bathing	7	5
• Transfer	3	7

I = independence; S = safety; A = adequacy

The questioning method is particularly useful for screening for disability because a large number of tasks can be queried in a limited amount of time. However, it is less useful when evaluating disability for the purposes of intervention, because clients may not be able to describe their disability in sufficient detail to target the components of tasks that are problematic. Furthermore, they do not have the medical, rehabilitation, and occupational therapy knowledge to isolate the factors that may be causing disabilities. Nonetheless, questioning is usually the data-gathering method of choice when information is needed about daily-living **habits;** that is, about what clients usually do on a daily basis. Although it is theoretically possible to assess ADL and home management habits through observation, it is generally not practical to do so because this would require a series of observations, preferably in the natural setting (eg, home, nursing home, group home) and at the time of day that the task usually occurs. Consequently, habits are generally evaluated through questioning. Similarly, questioning is a primary mode of learning about clients' ADL and home management experience. The only other way to retrieve information about past performance is to examine existing records (medical, school, work, or other).

Observing

In the observation method, practitioners obtain data by watching clients as they perform ADL and home management tasks. Practitioners may observe task performance under natural or laboratory conditions. Under natural conditions, task performance is observed within the context that it usually takes place or is expected to take place. This includes the location (eg, home) and objects (eg, bathtub, soap) usually used for tasks and, if possible, the routine time that tasks take place. These conditions can often be met in long term-care settings and home care. For example, practitioners may observe clients bathe, groom, dress, and feed themselves as they perform their morning care tasks. When clients are seen when hospitalized or in outpatient clinics, observation of task performance takes places under laboratory conditions. The laboratory may be the occupational therapy clinic or the temporary space occupied by clients (eg, their hospital room).

Table 15-4 also provides data about the bathing performance of two clients that were obtained through observation. An advantage that the observation method has over the questioning method is the descriptive detail that it provides about task performance. When task performance is at risk for disability or when disability is already present, the characteristics of task performance exhibited by clients play an essential role in planning intervention. Mr. Kline's bathing performance, for example, is characteristic of motor impairment, whereas Mr. Market's is characteristic of cognitive impairment. Interventions would be planned with these impairments in mind. The descriptive detail gleaned through observation would be extremely difficult to elicit in an interview or through a questionnaire.

When clients engage in a task, they apply their abilities to accomplish it with available human and material resources, that is, within a specific context. The significance of context to task performance may be illustrated by thinking about the dysfunction that you would encounter if you prepared dinner this evening in your neighbor's house rather than your own. You would need to spend time locating food, cooking utensils, and pots and pans. You might be afraid of cutting yourself while paring carrots because the knife is not sharp. You may burn the chicken because you are accustomed to a gas rather than an electric range. You may forget to rotate the potatoes in the microwave because your appliance has a revolving tray. You may have difficulty expanding your recipes to provide for eight persons as opposed to the four in your family. As this scenario illustrates, the physical and social context in which task performance takes place has a strong influence on the quality of performance outcomes.

Regardless of where an evaluation is done, the influence of context on task performance must be taken into account so that valid conclusions about task performance can be drawn. Occupational therapy clinics are designed to promote function and have numerous adaptive features to compensate for impairments. These features may make it easier for clients to perform tasks in the clinic than in their own homes. Conversely, however, performance may be more difficult because clients are unfamiliar with the clinic. When an

evaluation is done in the home, clients have the advantage of using their own task objects in the confines of existing architecture. The social context is changed, however, because to conduct an evaluation practitioners oversee task performance, and their mere presence may affect the manner and the adequacy of the tasks performed.

As an objective data-gathering method, observation has the advantage of minimizing the subjective, distorting aspects associated with proxy and self-reports. However, the generalizability of clients' performance in laboratory settings to real-world situations is problematic. Research has suggested that evaluation results obtained in the laboratory differ from those obtained in clients' homes (Haworth & Hollings, 1979). Similar to proxy reports, observation is only appropriate for evaluation parameters that are observable. In contrast to both proxy and self-reports, however, observation provides practitioners with the opportunity to analyze impairments that may be interfering with task performance.

Testing

When questions and observations are systematically structured and when a numerical score or a category system is used to describe task performance, the questions or observations constitute a test (Cronbach, 1970). The traditional approach to testing has been norm-referenced. The purpose of norm-referenced testing is to compare a client's performance on a test with that of others on the same test (Popham, 1990). Norm-referenced tests are useful for answering questions such as: How do the home management skills of Mrs. Zone, who is 65 years old and has arthritis and cardiopulmonary disease, compare with those of others her age, who are living independently in the community? Norm-referenced testing requires evaluation under standardized conditions. Hence, the materials to be used in the test are specified, the instructions to be given to clients are detailed, the procedures for administering the test are outlined, and the manner of scoring clients' responses is designated. Standardization is needed to ensure the reliability and validity of test results. As Christiansen (1991) noted, standardization ". . . creates formidable difficulties if one is concerned with getting an accurate picture of the characteristic level of functional performance under everyday circumstances, which vary from one person to the next (p. 377)."

An alternative model of testing is provided by the criterion-referenced approach. The purpose of criterion-referenced testing is to compare a client's performance on a test with a performance standard (Popham, 1990). Criterion-referenced tests stress task mastery and address questions such as: Can Mrs. Zone perform all tasks, or procure the services, needed to live in the community by herself? Criterion referenced tests often incorporate task analyses, and the degree of structure imposed on testing is often more flexible than for norm-referenced testing.

In Table 15-4, data obtained on the FIM for Mr. Kline and Mr. Market are recorded. A score of 7 on the FIM, a criterion-referenced instrument, denotes complete independence, a score of 5 signifies the need for supervision or setup, and a score of 3 indicates the need for moderate assistance from a helper. Because Mr. Market's bathing dysfunction is likely due to cognitive impairment, the FIM may not be the most appropriate instrument to use, according to the instrument guidelines, for it is heavily oriented toward medical diagnoses.

Norm-referenced and criterion-referenced testing employ a static evaluation strategy. Clients' task performance is tested once to determine their task performance status at that point in time. A newer testing strategy, called dynamic, interactive, or process assessment, evaluates clients' performance, while interactively providing interventions to determine their potential for improving task performance (Haywood & Tzuriel, 1992; Missiuna, 1987). The outcomes of dynamic assessment are the identification and diagnosis of disability, the determination of effective intervention strategies for developing or restoring task performance or for compensating for deficits, and the determination of the potential for rehabilitation (Rogers et al., 1997). It provides answers to questions such as: What types of technological or human assistance does Mrs. Zone require to perform everyday tasks independently, safely, efficiently, and adequately? Does Mrs. Zone have the potential for improving her performance? Dynamic assessment focuses on measuring changes in task performance and the identification of interventions used during the assessment that effected those changes, so that they can be used during intervention. Hence, standardization is not necessary and practitioners can tailor the evaluation to the clients' needs. Dynamic assessment manages the formidable difficulties presented by standardization mentioned by Christiansen (1991).

Clinical Guidelines: Method

In conducting the occupational therapy evaluation, practitioners have a choice of data-gathering methods and options within each method. Perhaps the best data-gathering strategy is to use a combination of methods and sources relying on the convergence of data for the best profile of clients' abilities and disabilities. Discrepancies in the evaluation data would need to be clarified and reconciled. For example, when questioned about grocery shopping, clients may indicate independence, whereas caregivers state dependence. However, the two responses are not necessarily at variance, because clients may be responding in terms of their capacities (eg, I could do it if I had to. . .) and caregivers may be responding in reference to their habits (eg, she or he does not go shopping). Similarly, a practitioner may ascertain through performance testing that clients can execute bed to wheelchair transfers. Yet, clients may insist that they cannot. The inconsistency may arise because, although clients perform the transfer when the practitioner is present, they feel insecure about their abilities when they

have to execute transfers on their own. In both of these examples, the use of different data sources has identified a performance discrepancy between skill and habit (see Chap. 21, Section 1) that would not have been apparent through one source alone.

An effective strategy for combining data-gathering methods is to begin the evaluation with a questioning procedure. The primary purposes of the questioning procedure it to (1) provide an overall profile of clients' abilities and disabilities, (2) understand clients' priorities for learning how to manage their disabilities, and (3) target tasks requiring in-depth evaluation. Questioning is then followed by an observational procedure. The purpose of the observational procedure is to: (1) identify the deficit components of tasks already identified as dysfunctional or at risk for dysfunction through questioning; (2) hypothesize about the underlying cause of the performance deficit; (3) identify the most likely interventions for managing the deficit, which may be remedial, compensatory, or preventive; and (4) ascertain the clients' potential for improving their task performance. The evaluation is then completed because the practitioner has the data needed to intervene. If the observational procedure raises questions about the clients' task performance abilities previously delineated through questioning, these tasks would also be subject to observational procedures.

ADL and home management tasks are evaluated at entry to occupational therapy to provide a measure of clients' baseline performance status. An intervention to improve task performance may then be initiated. The intervention may be short-term and limited in scope, such as the prescription of a walker and training in using it correctly and safely, or it may be more long-term and intensive, such as homemaker training. Regardless of the extent and length of the intervention, re-evaluation of ADL and home management performance is needed to ascertain whether (1) the intervention is resulting in improvement; (2) the intervention should be continued or changed; or (3) maximal benefit from occupational therapy has been achieved, and task performance has reached a plateau. The best strategy for re-evaluation is to readminister the evaluations done at baseline. This involves using the same ADL and home management content, the same measurement parameters, and the same methods. By keeping all three factors constant at baseline and any subsequent reevaluations, the possibility of detecting change—attributable to intervention—in clients' performance is increased. If the evaluation content, parameters, or methods vary from one point in time to another, the same evaluative data are not available for comparison, and the potential for detecting change is reduced. For example, if task performance is evaluated in the occupational therapy clinic using observation immediately before discharge, and with a telephone survey following discharge, it is not possible to sort out if a decrease or increase in task performance is due to a client's deterioration or improvement, or the change in data-gathering methods (observation versus questioning).

▼ INTEGRATING EVALUATION DATA

The evaluation data obtained through observing, questioning, and testing methods must be analyzed, synthesized, and interpreted. Practitioners function as data processors and managers in grouping data that are similar into categories, resolving discrepancies, and finally, putting forth an occupational therapy diagnosis that integrates the findings into a cohesive problem statement that is simultaneously capable of functioning as the endpoint of the evaluation and the beginning point of intervention. This integration of data is accomplished through diagnostic reasoning, which is a component of clinical reasoning (Rogers, 1983; Rogers & Holm, 1991b). The clinical reasoning of practitioners resembles a dialectical process in which practitioners argue with themselves about the interpretation of the data. Evidence supporting one interpretation is weighed against evidence rejecting that interpretation. The pros and cons for each interpretation are summed—so to speak—and the interpretation is selected that has the most supporting or compelling evidence. If the evidence fails to sufficiently support one interpretation over another, more evaluative data are collected in an attempt to break the tie and make one interpretation more cogent than the others. Through this process the practitioner arrives at a cohesive understanding of the ADL and home management task performance of the client and of an appropriate therapeutic action (ie, direct intervention or recommendation). This understanding is presented to clients or their proxies for verification and collaborative decision making concerning the therapeutic action to be implemented.

▼ OCCUPATIONAL THERAPY AND REHABILITATION MEDICINE FUNCTIONAL ASSESSMENTS

Occupational therapy, similar to other health and rehabilitation professions, is moving out of the stage of relying on evaluation measures developed for facility-specific use, with little attention given to their psychometric properties. Genuine progress has been made over the past decade in addressing measurement issues concerning the conceptualization and operationalization of terms, standardization of measurement procedures, and reliability and validity of test results. The content of ADL and home management instruments may encompass only ADL, only home management, or it may combine both ADL and home management. The evaluation parameters and data-gathering methods used in these instruments vary substantively from instrument to instrument, with the purpose the instrument was designed for and the population it was intended to be applied to, as major factors contributing to these differences.

Instruments covering ADL and home management tasks may also contain impairment and handicap items (WHO, 1980). Whereas impairment is a deficit in the components of occupational performance—that is, in the motoric, cognitive, or emotional enablers of performance—disability is a deficit in task performance. **Impairments** tend to be characteristic of specific disorders or **diseases.** Clients with **chronic obstructive pulmonary disease** often experience fatigue, those with **stroke** exhibit motor control dysfunctions, those with **arthritis** have problems in muscle strength and range of motion, and those with **traumatic brain injury** have impairments in **memory,** problem-solving, and learning. In view of these and other known patterns, instruments constructed for clients with specific diseases tend to incorporate impairment items so that ADL and home management dysfunctions can be related to identified impairments.

Similarly, handicap items also tend to be found on ADL and home management instruments. Whereas **disability** refers to difficulty performing tasks, **handicap** refers to deficits in performing social **roles** (WHO, 1980). The performance of social roles, however, is dependent on the performance of the tasks that comprise them. For example, to be a successful homemaker, clients must be able to accomplish the array of home management tasks expected of them. The distinction between disability and handicap is often blurred on functional assessments.

Our presentation of occupational therapy and rehabilitation medicine instruments is highly selective. A list of resources that give a more comprehensive review of functional assessments is provided at the end of this section. Key words to be used when searching for ADL and home management instruments are the following: functional assessment, disability evaluation, functional disability, health status, ADL scales, IADL scales, physical function, and quality of life. In selecting instruments for use in clinical practice, psychometric quality as well as practical considerations must be taken into account. Matching the content, parameters, and methods of the instrument to the practitioner's informational needs is the most essential practical concern.

Descriptions of Specific Instruments

For each instrument, the following information is given: purpose, description, method, psychometric properties. Instruments are presented in alphabetical order.

ÁRNADÓTTIR OT-ADL NEUROBEHAVIORAL EVALUATION (A-ONE)

Purpose

The A-One evaluation (Arnadóttir, 1990) has a dual purpose: (1) to assess independence in selected ADL and the types of assistance needed to complete them, and (2) to identify the types and severity of neurobehavioral impairment. These data are to be used to assist in setting goals and planning treatment. The A-One was designed for use with adults with central nervous system dysfunctions having cortical origin.

Description

Part I of the A–One encompasses the Functional Independence Scale and the Neurobehavioral Specific Impairment Scale. The former scale covers five ADL domains:namely, dressing, grooming and hygiene, transfer and mobility, feeding, and communication. The latter scale accompanies each of the ADL domains and includes 11 impairments (eg, motor apraxia, ideational **apraxia,** perseveration), except when applied to feeding and communication, for which it is modified. The ADL and neurobehavioral impairments are rated on a 5-point ordinal scale, ranging from 0 to 4. The high point of the functional scale connotes independence and the ability to transfer the task to other situations, whereas the low point connotes an inability to perform the task, that is, being totally dependent on assistance. The neurobehavioral scale ranges from no-observed impairment, to client needs maximum physical assistance related to severe neurobehavioral impairment. The intent of Part II of the A–One, the Neurobehavioral Scale Summary Sheet, is to assist practitioners in identifying the most likely lesion site for the identified neurobehavioral deficits. Part II is not meant to be a diagnostic tool, but rather, to foster understanding of the central nervous system deficit so that an appropriate intervention plan can be formulated. Completion of Part II is optional.

Method

Data for Part I are gathered through informal observation. Part II relies on the practitioner's clinical reasoning about the underlying cause or causes of task performance deficits.

Psychometric Properties

Interrater reliability for the Functional Independence Scale achieved a kappa coefficient of 0.83 and for the Neurobehavioral Specific Impairment Scale 0.86. Test-retest reliability for items in part 1 with a 1-week interval was at least $r_s = 0.85$. Content validity of the A–One is based on literature reviews and expert judgment. In a sample of normal individuals no ADL disabilities or neurobehavioral impairments were evidenced. Persons with cerebral vascular accident scored lower than normal persons on both scales. The instrument appears to have the capability of detecting ADL improvement.

ASSESSMENT OF LIVING SKILLS AND RESOURCES (ALSAR)

Purpose

The ALSAR was developed (Williams et al., 1991) to assess IADL as well as to identify needs, assign risk, and prioritize intervention. A unique feature of the instrument is the consideration of IADL skills in relation to the resources available to mitigate skill deficits. Although skills are intrinsic to clients, and represent their ability to perform tasks or procure services, resources are extrinsic to clients, and represent

human or technical, formal or informal supports for task accomplishment. Conceptually, IADL deficits must not be interpreted solely in terms of skills, but rather, from the perspective of the environmental resources available to compensate for these deficits. Thus, a client with arthritis who was unable to do laundry, housekeeping, or home maintenance would not be at risk if a sibling were available to do these tasks.

Description

The eleven IADL included on the ALSAR are telephoning, reading, leisure task, medication management, money management, transportation, shopping, meal preparation, laundering, housekeeping, and home maintenance. For each task, skill is rated as independent, partially independent, or dependent, and resources are rated as consistently available, inconsistently available, and not available or in use. The 3-point skill and resources scales range from a high of 0 to a low of 2. The skill and resources scores are combined to obtain a risk score for each IADL. Risk is designated as low (combined score of 0 or 1), moderate (combined score of 3), or high (combined score of 4). The risk score assists in setting priorities for intervention.

Method

The ALSAR is an interview measure, and questions are provided to assist in data gathering.

Psychometric Properties

Internal consistency using Cronbach's alpha was calculated as 0.91. Interrater percent agreement ranged from 72% to 94% for skills and 78% to 100% for resources. Content validity of the ALSAR is based on the expert judgment of geriatric practitioners from occupational and physical therapy and social work. Evidence of criterion-related validity was obtained from significant correlations between the risk score and the following changes at 6-month follow-up: move to a more structured living situation; move to a more supportive living situation; nursing home placement; hospitalization; and death. The risk score also correlated with measures of mental status and ADL status, but not with depression and caregiver burden.

ASSESSMENT OF MOTOR AND PROCESS SKILLS (AMPS)

Purpose

The AMPS (Fisher, 1994) is used to examine the relation between motor and process skills and task performance, to establish the current level of task competence, and to predict performance in IADL. It is useful for treatment planning and has been used with children, adolescents, and adults with a variety of underlying impairments.

Description

The AMPS consists of 56 calibrated tasks, such as sweep the floor, repot a plant, and change sheets on a bed. Tasks are rated on 16 motor skills (eg, reaches, lifts, paces) and 20 process skills (initiates, searches, adjusts). Each motor and process skill item is rated on a 4-point ordinal score, ranging from 1, which signifies that the deficit is severe enough to result in damage, danger, or task breakdown; to 4, which signifies that there is no evidence of a deficit that affects performance; that is, competence. AMPS item scores are then transformed from ordinal to an interval scale with a many-faceted Rasch analysis program (Linacre, 1989), which allows them to be adjusted based on rater leniency and task difficulty. This analysis also makes it possible to predict a client's performance on the other calibrated task (Doble, Fisk, Fisher, Ritvo, & Murray, 1994). The AMPS takes 30 to 60 minutes to administer.

Method

Clients' normal routines are identified through interview. Subsequently, the practitioner suggests five or six tasks for clients to perform, asks them to select several from these options, and observes and rates their performance.

Psychometric Properties

Of the 300 trained raters, 95% have achieved Rasch goodness-of-fit statistics that indicate adequate interrater reliability (Doble et al., 1994). For tasks to be considered valid, they must fit a pre-established Rasch measurement model. The AMPS has undergone extensive validity testing, including comparisons between settings (Nygård, Bernspång, Fisher, & Winblad, 1994) and across cultures (Fisher, Liu, Velozo, & Pan, 1992)

FUNCTIONAL INDEPENDENCE MEASURE (FIM)
Purpose

The FIM (UDSMR, 1993) measures disability associated with physical impairments. It is a part of the Uniform Data System for Medical Rehabilitation and, as such, provides a mechanism for standardizing data collection nationwide for clients entering medical rehabilitation. The FIM was devised to provide a more comprehensive measure of disability than was previously available on functional assessments, such as the Barthel and the Index of ADL, by expanding functional mobility and personal self-care and including communication and cognitive function. It is not intended to provide a comprehensive disability evaluation covering all occupational areas.

Description

Eighteen critical tasks are included on the FIM. Of these, 13 have a motor emphasis and are related to self-care (ie, feeding, grooming, bathing, dressing upper body, dressing lower body, toileting), sphincter control (ie, bladder and bowel management), mobility (bed, chair, wheelchair, toilet, and tub or shower transfers) and locomotion (walk or wheelchair, stairs). The remaining five have a cognitive emphasis and involve communication (ie, comprehension, expression) and social cognition (ie, social interaction, problem solving,

memory) (Linacre, Heinemann, Wright, Granger, & Hamilton, 1994). The type and amount of assistance required to perform tasks is used to measure disability severity and care burden. Tasks are scored using a 7-point or 4-point scale. A score of 7 reflects complete independence; 6, modified independence, which implies some delay, safety risk, or device usage; 5, supervision; 4, minimal assistance with clients exerting 75% plus effort; 3, moderate assistance with clients exerting 50% plus effort; 2, complete dependence with clients exerting 25% plus effort; and 1, total assistance with clients exerting less than 24% effort. The 7-point scale converts to a 4-level one as follows: 4 = independence (7); 3 = modified independence (6); 2 = modified dependence (5,4,3); and 1 = dependence (2,1). The potential for detecting change in disability is greater with the 7-point than with the 4-point scale. The rationale underlying the rating scale is that the amount of assistance needed by clients to complete tasks is an index of the social and the economic costs of disability.

Method

The FIM requires observation of task performance and rating by trained observers, who may be practitioners, clients, or family members. A telephone version is available (Jaworski, Kult, & Boynton, 1994).

Psychometric Properties

With the 4-point scale, the intraclass correlation for total FIM scores was 0.86 at admission and 0.88 at discharge from rehabilitation. The average kappa statistic for each of the 18 items was 0.54 (Hamilton, Granger, Sherwin, Zielezny, & Tashman, 1987). The FIM has been transformed from an ordinal to an interval scale through Rasch analysis and the structures of the motor and cognitive scales have been shown to be stable at admission and discharge (Linacre et al, 1994). This gives the FIM an advantage over other disability measures because it can be used more accurately to measure clinical change and for research purposes. FIM admission scores can predict discharge status and length of stay in rehabilitation, although predictive power varies with impairment type. Function in motor tasks emerged as a more important predictor of length of stay than function in cognitive tasks. Shorter stays were associated with greater cognitive capability for clients with traumatic brain injury and lesser cognitive capability for those with stroke and neurologic impairments (Heinemann, Linacre, Wright, Hamilton, & Granger, 1994).

KLEIN-BELL ACTIVITIES OF DAILY LIVING SCALE (KLEIN-BELL)
Purpose

The Klein-Bell scale (Klein & Bell 1979, 1982) was designed to measure ADL independence in children and adults. It is useful for determining current status, change in status, and the subtasks to focus on during intervention.

Description

The Klein-Bell has 170 items in six domains: dressing, mobility, elimination, bathing and hygiene, eating, and emergency communication. Task analysis was used to identify critical and observable subtasks in the tasks included in these domains. Each subtask is scored as able to perform, unable, or not applicable. An expert panel of rehabilitation professionals was used to establish subtask weights and weights of 1, 2, or 3 were assigned to each subtask. In weighting the items four factors were considered: its importance to health, its difficulty for a nondisabled person, the time required to perform it, and, the associated burden of caregiving. The total points achieved within each domain are added to give an overall independence score. These scores can range from 0 to 313, but are expressed as percentages of the total points possible.

Method

The Klein-Bell Scale is an observational instrument.

Psychometric Properties

Interrater agreement across all items was estimated as 92%. Evidence of predictive validity was obtained from correlations between Klein-Bell scores and the hours clients required assistance per week for a 5- to 10-month period following discharge (Klein & Bell, 1982). Use of the Klein-Bell to examine bathing training, suggests that it is capable of measuring change (Shillam, Beeman, & Loshin, 1983).

KOHLMAN EVALUATION OF LIVING SKILLS (KELS)

Purpose

The KELS (McGourty, 1979, 1988) was designed to aid in discharge planning for clients with psychiatric diagnoses. It evaluates the ability to live independently and safely in the community and has also been used with geriatric clients and those with mental retardation, brain injury, and cognitive impairment.

Description

The 18 tasks included on the KELS are grouped into five categories: self-care, safety and health, money management, transportation and telephone, and work and leisure. Hence, the tasks span all occupational areas. Task performance is scored as 0, signifying independent, and 1 or ½ signifying needs assistance. Independence means safe and healthy performance without the assistance of others. Assistance in six or more tasks is indicative of a need for a supportive living situation. Information about impairments influencing clients' performance, such as attention span, visual figure-ground, and comprehension, is included in a summary note. The KELS can be administered and scored in 30 to 45 minutes.

Method

The KELS combines interview and performance-based methods and tends to emphasis the knowledge component of tasks.

Psychometric Properties

Percent rater agreement ranged from 74% to 94% in one study (Ilika & Hoffman, 1981a) and 84% to 94% in another (Tateichi, as cited in McGourty, 1988). The higher scores of residents of sheltered-living situations compared with individuals living independently in the community were used to establish construct validity (Tateichi, as cited in McGourty, 1988). Evidence of concurrent validity was obtained from correlations between scores on the KELS and Bay Area Functional Performance Evaluation ($r = -0.84$; p<0.0001) and the Global Assessment Scale (between $r = 0.78$ and 0.89; p<0.0001) in samples of inpatient mental health clients (Ilika & Hoffman, 1981b; Kaufman, 1982). The results of predictive validity studies were inconclusive (McGourty, 1988; Morrow, as cited in McGourty, 1988).

MILWAUKEE EVALUATION OF DAILY LIVING SKILLS (MEDLS)

Purpose

The MEDLS (Leonardelli, 1988a,b) was designed to establish baseline behaviors necessary to develop treatment objectives and guide intervention relative to daily living skills for clients with chronic mental health problems.

Description

The MEDLS consists of 20 subtests covering the following: communication, personal care, clothing care, safety in the home and community, money management, personal health care, medication management, telephone use, transportation usage, and time awareness. The subtests can be administered individually or in combination. A screening form is used to ascertain the specific items to be examined for each client. The screening form can be employed as a tool for obtaining information from clients and their families, the health care team, and the medical record. Each subtest is scored according to the number of skills completed for that task. No summary score is calculated for the MEDLS because the administration of subtests varies from client to client. Subtests have a specified time for completion, and when this time is exceeded, the practitioner makes a clinical judgment about the cause of the delay (eg, comprehension, motivation).

Method

For testing, some activities are performed (eg, dressing); others are simulated (eg, bathing); and others are described (eg, transportation).

Psychometric Properties

Interrater reliability coefficients for most subtests were greater than $r = 0.80$. Content validity is based on the literature and other similar instruments (Leonardelli, 1988a).

PERFORMANCE ASSESSMENT OF SELF-CARE SKILLS, VERSION 3.1 (PASS)

Purpose

The PASS, designed (Rogers & Holm, 1989, 1994) to evaluate the independent living skills of adults, is a criterion-referenced instrument. It has been used with healthy, older adults as well as those with osteoarthritis, dementia, depression, cardiopulmonary disease, schizophrenia, bipolar affective disorder, mental retardation, and low vision. It can be used to assess baseline status and change over time following intervention or age-associated or disease-related changes. Additionally, it provides data useful for planning intervention or the support needed at discharge.

Description

The 26 items included on the PASS encompass functional mobility, personal care, and home management. For each task, the PASS yields three summary scores: independence, safety, and outcome. Each of these measurement parameters is rated on a 4-point ordinal scale, with 0 representing dysfunction and 3 representing function. Independence ratings are applied to subtasks (ie, lower self to tub bottom), rather than a task as a whole (ie, tub transfer). This procedure enables the practitioner to identify the specific point or points in a task sequence where breakdown occurs. Furthermore, the number and types of assists necessary for safe and adequate task performance are recorded, thereby furnishing information useful for planning intervention, including supportive services. There are two protocols for the PASS: one for use in the home and the other for use in a client's living situation. The two protocols are identical in terms of the tasks included and the performance criteria. However, in the home, clients use their own task materials.

Method

The PASS is a performance-based observational tool.

Psychometric Properties

Percent agreement between two observers, whether done in the clinic or the home, ranged between 96% and 99%. Content validity of the PASS is based on four interview instruments for evaluating independent living skills: the Physical Self-Maintenance and Instrumental Self-Maintenance Scales (Lawton & Brody, 1969), the Activities of Daily Living Scale of the OARS Multidimensional Functional Assessment Questionnaire (Fillenbaum, 1988), the Comprehensive Assessment and Referral Evaluation (Gurland et al., 1977-1978), and the Functional Assessment Questionnaire (Pfeffer, Kurosaki, Harrah, Chance, & Filos, 1982). Construct validity is based on the performance of the instrument on groups with different medical and psychiatric diagnoses or level of acuity and on ADL and IADL categories. Thus, healthy adults score higher than those with depression, and those with depression score higher than those with dementia. Inpatients with depression score lower at admission than at discharge, but even at discharge they score lower than depressed outpatients. Outpatients with early dementia score lower in IADL than ADL skills.

SATISFACTION WITH PERFORMANCE SCALED QUESTIONNAIRE (SPSQ)

Purpose

The SPSQ was designed (Yerxa, Burnett-Beaulieu, Stocking, & Azen, 1988) to operationalize satisfaction experienced in the performance of independent living skills. Satisfaction is defined as perceived pleasure or contentment. The SPSQ is useful for identifying intervention goals for community-based persons with disabilities because areas of low satisfaction may be targeted for independent living skills training.

Description

The SPSQ contains two subscales involving independent living skills. Subscale I, Home Management, contains 24 items relevant to this occupational area. Typical items are scrape and stack dishes, use stove-top elements, clean bathtub or shower, handle a milk carton, and stir against resistance in a bowl. Subscale II, is titled Social/Community, and contains 22 items. Some of these items are typically included under home management (eg, pay bill and balance account, budget your income), whereas others are more oriented toward interpersonal, educational, vocational, and leisure skills. Each item is scored on a 5-point scale using the percentage of time over the past 6 months that clients felt satisfied with their performance as the reference point. The percentage scale ranges from all (100%) of the time to none (0%) of the time.

Method

The SPSQ is a self-report questionnaire.

Psychometric Properties

Split-half reliability coefficients were 0.97 and 0.93 for the Home Management and Social/Community Problem Solving scales, respectively. Evidence suggestive of construct validity was obtained from a small study in which clients with spinal cord injury scored lower than nondisabled subjects on the Home Management and Social/Community scales.

ROUTINE TASK INVENTORY-2 (RTI-2)

Purpose

The RTI-2 (Allen, Earhart, & Blue, 1992) is designed to establish the level of functional status and document change in status based on the Allen Cognitive Levels (ACL) (Allen,

1985, 1990). Thus, it relates cognitive impairment to task performance.

Description

The content of the RTI is based on the disability categories of the model of disablement proposed by the World Health Organization (1980). The 32 items encompass self-awareness disability (eg, grooming, dressing, bathing), situational awareness disability (eg, housekeeping, spending money, shopping), occupational role disability (eg, planning/doing major role tasks, pacing and timing actions, speaking); and social role disability (eg, communicating meaning, following instructions, caring for dependents). The behaviors that would be indicative of functioning at each of the six ACL levels are defined and described for each of the items. There are no standardized procedures or directions for administration or scoring. The practitioner matches descriptions or observations of performance with the operational definitions for each level of functioning. A 3-point to 6-point ordinal scale is used for each item, with lower scores indicating lower abilities and higher scores indicating higher abilities. For example, the highest score for grooming, which is a 5, means that clients can initiate and complete grooming without assistance; the lowest score for the same item, which is a 3, means that clients ignore personal appearance and may not cooperate with caregiving actions. For less complex behaviors in the self-awareness and situational awareness categories, the ACL levels defined for scoring range from 1 to 6 or 2 to 5; for more complex behaviors in the occupational and social role categories, the lowest ACL level defined for scoring is level 3 and the highest is level 6. The RTI-2 can be administered in either a clinic or a home setting.

Method

The RTI may be rated through observing or questioning, and clients or proxies may be respondents. Self-report is not recommended for clients at ACL levels 1 through 4.

Psychometric Properties

Interrater reliability (r = 0.98), test-retest reliability (r = 0.91), and internal consistency (r = 0.94) were established on the original version of the instrument. Evidence of validity was obtained from correlating RTI scores with those on the Mini-Mental State Examination. The obtained correlation of r_s = 0.61 supported the relationship between functional decline and cognitive impairment (Allen, Kehrberg, & Burn, 1992). Correlations between the RTI and the ACL levels were calculated as r_s = 0.54 to 0.56 (Heimann, Allen, & Yerxa, 1989; Wilson, Allen, McCormack, & Burton, 1989).

▼ RESOURCES FOR ADL AND HOME MANAGEMENT INSTRUMENTS

Asher, I. A. (1996). *An annotated index of occupational therapy evaluation tools.* Rockville, MD: American Occupational Therapy Association.

Cole, B., Finch, E., Gowland, C., & Mayo, N. (1994). *Physical rehabilitation outcome measures.* Toronto, Ontario: Canadian Physiotherapy Association.

Ernst, M., & Ernst, N.S. (1984). Functional capacity. In D. J. Mangen and W. A. Peterson (Eds.), *Health, program evaluation, and demography, Vol. 3*, (pp. 9-84). Minneapolis, University of Minnesota.

Kane, R. A., & Kane, R. L. (1981). *Assessing the elderly.* Lexington, MA: D. C. Heath.

Kidd, T., & Yoshida, K. (1995). Critical review of disability measures: Conceptual developments. *Physiotherapy Canada, 47*, 108–119.

Law, M., & Letts, L. (1989). A critical review of scales of activities of daily living. *American Journal of Occupational Therapy, 43*, 522-528.

McDowell, I., & Newell, C. (1996). *Measuring health: A guide to rating scales and questionnaires.* New York: Oxford University Press.

Spiker, B. (1990). *Quality of life assessment in clinical trials.* New York: Raven Press.

ter Steeg, A. M., & Lankhorst, G. J. (1994). Screening instruments for disability. *Critical Reviews in Physical & Rehabilitation Medicine, 6*, 101-112.

Section 2

Evaluation of Work and Productive Activities: Work Performance Assessment Measures

Sherlyn Fenton and Patricia Gagnon

Historical Overview
Evaluation Process
   Intake Interview
   Physical Capacity Evaluation
   Standardized and Nonstandardized Tests
   Report
Americans With Disabilities Act (ADA)
   Job Site Analysis
Preplacement Screenings
Ergonomic Consultation
Work Evaluation Conclusion

▼ HISTORICAL OVERVIEW

Occupational therapy practitioners have been using work tasks to evaluate and rehabilitate persons with mental and physical impairments since the 1920s. "Employment therapy" and treatment programs involving activities, such as printing and construction, were common in the 1930s with the work evaluations of the time consisting of: (1) client interview; (2) job analysis defining duties, requirements, and conditions of the job; and (3) organization of tasks in a hierarchy of levels (Marshall, 1985).

Despite the acceptance of work evaluations in occupational therapy practice throughout the 1940s, these evaluations were not considered a necessary component of practice in the 1950s. Occupational therapists opting to continue administering work evaluations joined vocational evaluators and work adjusters within the vocational rehabilitation realm. Occupational therapists became increasingly involved in acute care settings in the 1960s. However, the interest in the role of work in occupational therapy reemerged throughout the next decade (Marshall, 1985).

Occupational therapists of the 1980s demonstrated an interest in work and work assessments that continues among therapists even now. "Reductions in rehabilitation funding have provided incentive to improve accuracy and efficiency of assessments" (Jacobs, 1991, p. 23). Today the number of injured workers is on the rise and the existence of a comprehensive evaluation is essential. "Occupational therapy can play an important and unique role in linking work evaluations to psychosocial and environmental variables and in formulating comprehensive theoretical models of work that should improve and refine present evaluations" (Velozo, 1993, p. 203). As professionals with a sound understanding of occupation and its relevance to injured workers, we can be instrumental in future research and development relative to work assessments.

▼ EVALUATION PROCESS

Administered by an occupational therapist, the **Functional Capacity Evaluation (FCE)** is a comprehensive battery of tests that yields objective measures regarding clients' current levels of functioning and their abilities to perform work-related tasks. FCE tests often include, but are not limited to, a Physical Capacity Evaluation (PCE), standardized testing, and nonstandardized testing to assess activities of daily living (ADL) and job-simulated tasks. The data collected and integrated from these test results are used to predict clients' work capacities. The administration procedures for these evaluations must meet five criteria established by the National Institute of Occupational Safety and Health (NIOSH) (1981): safety of administration, reliability, job relatedness, practicality, and predictiveness (Iserhagen, 1990, p. 15).

Intake Interview

Before the actual client assessment, the appropriate documentation for referral, physician orders, and insurance approval must be obtained. Once all operational issues are clarified and a client is considered an appropriate candidate for evaluation, the intake interview occurs. This interview focuses on the client's past history, present medical condition, vocational status, and psychosocial history. Information on previous or reoccurring injuries, results of diagnostic procedures, and medical interventions is reported to determine whether special testing methods are indicated.

During this initial intake interview, clients complete a functional job description to identify the physical, functional, and psychological demands of their work day. The daily vocational tasks are defined in terms of frequency, duration, and methods of work. Lifting, carrying, pushing, pulling, walking, climbing, sitting, standing, driving, and key-stroking are just a few of the demands considered and described. It is beneficial to compare the worker's **job description** with that submitted by the client's employer and that listed in the *U. S. Department of Labor's Dictionary of Occupational Titles* (U. S. Department of Labor, 1991). This comparison provides a comprehensive view of the job's demands, which helps the therapist establish effective treatment programs and discharge plans.

The initial intake also addresses clients' subjective perceptions of their ability to perform ADL such as bathing, dressing, homemaking, sleeping, and driving. Performance limitations may include medical restrictions, but more commonly are due to clients' pain experiences. Therefore, self-reporting methods are used to determine clients' perceptions of pain. Some commonly used pain scales are the Ransford Pain Drawing (Ransford, Cairns, & Mooney, 1979), the Borg Numerical Pain Scale (Borg, 1982), The Visual Analog Scale (Huskisson, 1974), the McGill Pain Questionnaire (Melzack, 1983, 1987), and the Oswestry (Fairbanks, Davies, Cooper, & O'Brien, 1980). (See Chap. 20, Section 8 for additional information about pain evaluation.) Comparison of similar scales can support a clinical diagnosis or demonstrate inconsistencies that may indicate abnormal illness behavior. A thorough intake interview provides the therapist with insight into the potential needs of clients' and ideas about possible treatment approaches.

Physical Capacity Evaluation

The Physical Capacity Evaluation (PCE) assesses the physical and biomechanical aspects of the client's level of function. The musculoskeletal portion of assessment involves objective measurements of the client's active range of motion, muscle strength, posture, and gait. Volumetric measurements, sensation, and cardiopulmonary status are also included in the PCE. The Canadian Aerobic Fitness Test ("step test"), the modified Bruce Treadmill Test, upper body ergometer, or the YMCA bicycle ergometer tests are all methods for cardiovascular screening to assess the client's tolerance for a given load. The client may also be referred to a specialized laboratory if more structured stress testing is indicated. Additional examination techniques may be incorporated for clients with lower back pain to identify nonorganic physical signs.

To identify nonorganic signs, a group of nine physical tests were developed and used in studies performed by Waddell, McCulloch, Kummel, and Venner (1980). The tests are superficial tenderness, nonanatomic tenderness, axial loading, simulated rotation, muscle testing in comparison with available active range of motion, straight-leg raising, muscle weakness, sensory disturbance, and overreaction. Abnormalities in three of these tests is clinically significant in suggesting the client is experiencing a pattern of abnormal illness behavior (Waddell et al., 1980).

Documentation received from the client's physician and other medical professionals in conjunction with the results of the PCE provide a baseline of the client's current physical capacity and any performance discrepancies. This information helps the therapist determine if the client requires further medical or psychological intervention, or if the client is appropriate to continue with the FCE.

The reliability and validity of physical evaluations are often questioned by the third-party payers. Performing Maximum Voluntary Efforts Tests (MVE) in a serial fashion allows the therapist to determine the client's intratask consistency. Many instruments are available for MVEs, but only a select few are appropriate in an industrial rehabilitation setting. Recommended instrumentation and test procedures for MVE include: Jamar Dynamometer Endurance Test, Jamar Dynamometer Rapid Exchange Grip (Hildreth, Breidenbach, Lister, & Hodges, 1989), **Baltimore Therapeutic Equipment (BTE)** Work Simulator using a sequence of tool attachments of varying sizes requiring upper extremity pronation and supination and flexion and extension tasks (Niemeyer, Matheson, & Carlton, 1989), and the West 4 Upper Extremity Strength for Torquing.

The most frequently used MVE tests are those performed with the Jamar Dynamometer. Individuals are instructed to apply maximal gross strength with each trial. For the Jamar Dynamometer Endurance Test, clients complete three trials in each of the five dynamometer handle positions. Readings can be either graphed or calculated for two methods of scoring. Graphing should depict a bell-shaped curve if maximal force is exerted; a straight line can be representative of submaximal effort. A statistical analysis of the readings that yields a coefficient of variation (CV) that exceeds experimentally derived values may also indicate a submaximal effort. Therapists should also observe the client's grasping patterns and displayed effort. Noted contraction of muscle groups in the forearm, neck, or jaw, and visible tightening of tendons typically indicate strong effort, whereas cocontraction of the hand and forearm muscles causing tremors is often observed in individuals who are not putting forth MVE (Stokes, 1983).

In addition to these instruments and tests, several tool activity sorts are used to provide further information on perceived ability and effort. The West Tool Sort, Loma Linda Activity Sort, and Spinal Functions Sort are all means by which the evaluator can compare the client's responses to demonstrated functioning during clinical testing. For example, clients who rate themselves as disabled from lifting a 20-lb bag of groceries on the Spinal Function Sort can be evaluated during a lifting evaluation for intratasks consistency. Isolated use of effort testing can result in inaccurate assessments and documentation (Jacobs, 1991; Niemeyer et al, 1989). Fear of injury, anticipation of pain, lack of clarity during test procedure instructions, and anxiety, all may produce test results erroneously illustrating submaximal effort. Therefore, therapists should refrain from subjective conclusions while maintaining objectivity by documenting actual test results.

Standardized and Nonstandardized Tests

A therapist also has additional standardized and nonstandardized evaluation tools from which to chose. These tools are chosen based on the client's diagnosis, job description, and discharge plan. Standardized tests that are work task oriented such as the Bennett Hand Tool Dexterity Test, the Minnesota Rate of Manipulation, Purdue Peg Board, Nine-Hole Peg Test, O'Connor Finger Dexterity Test, and the Jebsen Hand Function Test, all relay information about the client's capabilities and physical tolerances for fine and gross motor skills, standing, reaching, bending, and tool handling in comparison with a standardized population. "Standardized evaluation implies uniformity of procedures in administering and scoring the test, afford comparison to test results with a normative group and assumes that validity and reliability have been established" (Jacobs, 1991, p. 24). Nonstandardized tests allow the therapist to assess the client during specific tasks and ADL.

The therapist's ability to attain a baseline of a client's ability to perform job-simulated tasks is facilitated by several commercially developed work samples. The Valpar Component Work Samples numbers 1 to 19 and 202 to 205, the Skills Assessment Module (SAM), the Baltimore Therapeutic Equipment Box, and the West 2A, 3, 4A, and 7, all are used in work evaluations owing to their systematic methods of simulating work activities while adhering to NIOSH standards. Both the Valpar and SAM work samples use a methods time measurement (MTM) approach.

MTM is an example of a criterion-referenced procedure which analyzes any manual operation or method into basic motions required to perform it and assigns to each motion a predetermined time standard which is determined by the nature of the motion and the conditions under which it is made (Jacobs, 1991, p. 24).

An example of the application of a work sample would be to evaluate a parcel delivery worker's ability to complete essential job functions, as defined by the job description and the U.S. Department of Labor's *Dictionary of Titles*, after a low back injury. The Valpar Work Sample No. 19 requires the client to read invoices, fill, lift, and move various weighted trays from various heights. The SAM would require the client to complete three written tests and 12 hands-on modules. The SAM written tests include a learning style inventory, a revised Beta Examination, and an Auditory Directions Screen (ADS). Mail sorting, alphabetizing cards, payroll computation, ruler reading, pipe assemble, Etch a Sketch Maze, patient information memo, small parts, O-rings, block design, color sort, and circuit board are the 12 hands-on modules (Jacobs, 1991; Rosinek, 1985). The outcomes of these samples demonstrate the client's affective, cognitive, and manipulative abilities and relate the findings to vocational performance. The therapist's ability to choose the most appropriate work sample for the client's job demands is the key to attaining beneficial information for future vocational recommendations.

There are numerous tests available to evaluate clients' capabilities for material handling. Maximal and repetitive lift tests are performed to evaluate strength, knowledge of proper body mechanics, and to determine a client's current physical demand level, as categorized according to the U. S. Department of Labor. Free-weighted tests as well as high-technology evaluating equipment, such as the BTE, both have advantages and drawbacks when attempting to assess the client's strength and job simulation skills. Free-weighted tests include, but are not limited to, the Maximum Isoinertial Effort Test, West 2 Lifting Protocol, and the Progressive Isoinertial Lifting Evaluation (PILE). These tests are described in this text for reference purposes only. Therapists need to refer to the actual testing protocols to familiarize themselves with the individual procedures and objectives of each assessment tool.

The Maximum Isoinertial Lift Test measures the maximum weight the client can tolerate for a single trial. Maximum weight levels are determined for three levels of lifting (floor to waist, waist to shoulder, and shoulder to overhead), as well as for pushing and pulling. Test methods may need to be adjusted for some clients to prevent reinjury. For example, overhead lifting may be limited for a client with a neck injury, whereas a floor-to-waist lift may be modified for a client with a knee injury. The client determines the physical endpoint, but the therapist may terminate the test before a client signals if poor body mechanics or pain behaviors are evident.

The Progressive Isoinertial Lifting Evaluation (PILE) is an evaluation tool that assesses a client's "frequent" lifting capacity. The test requires the client to repetitively lift within a designated time frame from the lumbar and the cervical levels. These results are then compared with the maximum isoinertial lift results, and the numerical values are adjusted and extrapolated to determine the client's Physical Demand Level (PDL) (Mayer et al., 1988; Mayer, Gatchell, Barnes, Mayer, & Mooney, 1990).

The use of highly technological versions of work capacity evaluation devices has paralleled the growth of functional capacity evaluations. The devices simulate and evaluate a wide variety of physical demands, such as lifting, pushing, pulling, and gripping. The BTE Work Simulator, the BTE Dynamic Lift, the Lido Work Set, and ERGOS are all examples of commonly used devices. The BTE Dynamic Lift, for example, tests a client's ability to lift, lower, push, and pull in various planes, at various heights, in either a dynamic or **isometric** mode. The trials are computerized to document test procedures and results, calculate coefficients of variation, and compare performance with NIOSH standards.

The results of material-handling tests are related to the client's job description and extrapolated into a PDL as described by the U. S. Department of Labor in the DOT, (U. S. Department of Labor, 1991). The numeric values achieved during the individual tests are translated into work classifications according to the force (sedentary, light, medium, heavy, and very heavy), frequency, and duration (occasional, frequent, and constant), of lifts achieved during testing.

Report

Once the FCE is complete and the results have been documented, the therapeutic recommendations are communicated to the client, attending physician, and all authorized case management members. Recommendations may range from immediate return to work, without modification or limitation, to the client being recommended for a full-time functional restoration program to address limitations in current physical demand levels. In the middle of the continuum would be the need for vocational counseling or retraining or return to work at adjusted or light-duty status. It is imperative that comprehensive recommendations are conveyed to all involved parties through clear and concise documentation.

▼ AMERICANS WITH DISABILITIES ACT (ADA) AND JOB SITE ANALYSIS

The Rehabilitation Act of 1973 had been the only legislation that addressed the civil rights of persons with disabilities in the United States before the passing of the **Americans With Disabilities Act (ADA)** on July 29, 1990. The advent of the ADA guarantees Americans with disabilities access to employment, local and state services, transportation, telecommunications, and public accommodations equal to that of Americans without disabilities (Bowman, 1992). Title I: Employment, was written to prevent employers from discrimination practices against applicants and employees with disabilities.

An individual with a disability who can perform the essential functions of a job with or without **reasonable accommodations** cannot be discriminated against. An employer must provide reasonable accommodations to a qualified person with a disability unless it will cause undue hardship (Bowman, 1992, p. 411).

Historically, occupational therapists have played a significant role in assisting and guiding individuals with disabilities toward independence at home and in the work place. Under the employment provision of the ADA, occupational therapists can have extended influence in the work place. The comprehensive background of the occupational therapist is a tremendous resource to both employees and employers in the following: (1) creating ADA compliant interviewing procedures; (2) creating postoffer, preplacement work screenings; (3) facilitating the development of functional job descriptions; and (4) recommending reasonable accommodations. A **job site analysis** is the first step in familiarizing oneself with a work setting seeking occupational therapy consultation relative to ADA compliance.

Job Site Analysis

Before analyzing a job process, it is important for the therapist to have a good understanding of anthropometrics and ergonomics. Anthropometrics describes the physical dimensions and properties of the body, in terms of functional arm, leg, and body movements, made by a worker performing a task. Matching the job to the person is ergonomics. By improving the interaction of the worker with the equipment, work process, and work station, design therapists can contribute to workers' well-being.

The tools most often used in a job site analysis (JSA) include a stopwatch, tape measure, video camera, tripod, yard stick, and a variety of force gauges. These tools provide straightforward methods of assessing physical heights, distances, and work cycles in order to consider the requirements of force, repetition, and awkward postures. A review of job descriptions in conjunction with worker and employer interviews gives information concerning job practices, duration of jobs, and the specific equipment and materials used in jobs. Observation during different work phases, shifts, and seasons is also essential in realizing both the physical and psychologic demands of the work environment. Moreover, work practices and safety procedures need to be considered, as well as adhered to by the therapist while at the site.

The choice of JSA methods depends on the goal of the analysis or the type of job being evaluated. A manual material handling (MMH) task, such as stocking shelves in a grocery store, may be approached in four ways: psychophysics, static biomechanical models, the NIOSH lifting guidelines, and the dynamic biomechanical model.

PSYCHOPHYSICS

Snook's tables have been used since the 1970s as a means to evaluate MMH from a psychophysics base. This approach depicts maximum acceptable values for lifting, carrying, pushing, and pulling that are perceived as acceptable by percentages of the working population (Snook & Ciriello, 1991).

STATIC BIOMECHANICAL MODELS

Compression of the spine has been considered a limiting factor for material handlers since the 1970s. Today, computer programs exist that provide spinal compression force based on posture information entered into the system. These programs have been an important contribution to the static biomechanical model in assessing the stress of MMH

NIOSH LIFTING GUIDELINES

The NIOSH lifting guidelines, first published in 1981 and updated in 1991, provide a recommended lifting (weight) limit defined for a set of task conditions over a period of time that will not increase the risk of developing low back pain. The equation used to determine the recommended weight limit takes into consideration disc compression force (static biomechanics), maximum energy expenditures (physiologic studies), and maximum acceptable weight (psychophysical data). The appeal of this method is the ease with which the required data can be collected.

DYNAMIC BIOMECHANICAL MODEL

Lastly, the dynamic biomechanical theory suggests that torsional forces combined with compression increase the risk factors of occupational low back injuries (Buttle, 1995). Occupational therapists could observe job motions for examples of torsion and compression, (eg, lifting a heavy load and twisting around with feet planted to place the load on a shelf).

The completed JSA should yield information that will allow the employer to determine the essential functions of the job. "The essential functions of a job are the job duties a person must be able to perform unaided or with reasonable accommodations. The essential functions are not marginal function" (Rybski, 1992, p. 412). Once the functions are determined, a job description that accurately depicts the requirements can be written. This job description is the mechanism by which the employer can either reinstate an injured worker with reasonable accommodation, or decide on the need for screening new employees.

When the worker's capabilities do not meet the physical demands, as defined by the essential functions of the job, recommendations may include a full FCE with a functional restoration program, a change in jobs, or a reasonable accommodation. "Reasonable accommodations are modifications or adjustments that enable persons with disabilities to perform a job they are otherwise qualified to perform" (Rybski, 1992, p. 412). Reasonable accommodations may include modifying a work schedule, job reassignment, restructuring the work station, and providing more appropriate tools. Accommodations that strain the financial resources of the employer or fundamentally alter the nature of the job are considered to be undue hardship. An organization's entire resources are evaluated when determining if a reasonable accommodation is an undue hardship. Most reasonable accommodations, however, can be made inexpensively, allowing workers to return to their original duties.

▼ PREPLACEMENT SCREENINGS

Emphasis by regulatory agencies, such as the Occupational Safety and Health Administration (OSHA), on accommodations at the work place, job placement, and ergonomics support the need for preplacement assessments. Preplacement screenings under the ADA state that employment testing must be job-related and consistent with business necessity. Screenings can be performed after a conditional offer of employment has been made, but before the offer has been finalized, and must test the job's essential functions to be consistent with business necessity. Essential functions that should be included in the preplacement-testing protocol are those tasks involving high risk. OSHA has identified three factors as significant contributors to risk: force, distance (awkward posture), and frequency. Tasks that have previously recorded injuries may also be included in the protocol.

In screening, it is important to remember it is the outcome of the task, not the manner in which the task was performed that matters. We do not want to disqualify persons with disabilities who are able to perform the job tasks in an alternative fashion. Therapists administering preplacement screenings must be prepared to offer reasonable accommodation to applicants in the testing situation as well as post-screening to assist the employer in addressing possible accommodations for the applicant unable to perform an essential function.

Although preplacement screenings can assess the fit between worker and work, they cannot predict future injuries or worker productivity. In addition, the issues surrounding preplacement screenings, such as accuracy, validity, disclosure, and discrimination, are of ongoing concern. Employers who use preplacement screens must administer the testing to all applicants in a job category and must not screen out individuals with disabilities.

▼ ERGONOMIC CONSULTATION

Although health care reform may affect the future reimbursement rate and services offered by occupational therapists, the legislative changes brought on by the ADA, OSHA, and **Workers' Compensation** have created a demand for ergonomic **consultation** and training. Industries are searching for effective means of preventing injuries at work, and they are turning to occupational therapists as consultants to implement company programs. Industries are looking at their bottom line and are finally seeing the value of injury prevention programs and industrial rehabilitation. A successful ergonomic or injury prevention program will be reflected in decreased workers' compensation costs, increased productivity and efficiency, and improved morale. Ergonomic programs should involve everyone from the front-line employees to the executive officers. Employers who care about the safety and well-being of their employees and take the initiative to implement prevention programs are bound to reap the benefits from a healthier bottom line.

▼ WORK EVALUATION CONCLUSION

Although many functional evaluations and work assessment techniques exist, the limitations of these evaluations need to be recognized. For example, there are questions about how well some FCE procedures predict occupational performance. In addition, our present work assessments do not consider the meaning of work from the employee's perspective. This arena of work assessment is fertile ground for development within the realm of occupational therapy. "Improved measurements of work-related constructs, such as work capacity and worker role identity, and the determination of the relevance of their measurements to actual work performance are needed" (Velozo, 1993, p. 208). There is need for a comprehensive evaluation that address both the physical and the psychosocial variables involved in work, allowing therapists to more effectively relate an individual's capabilities or limitations to the workplace. The role of occupational therapy in functional and work assessments continues to hold bright promise for the future.

Section 3

Evaluation of Work and Productive Activities: Components of a Therapeutic Driving Evaluation

Sherlyn Fenton and Wendy Kraft

> Evaluation
> Clinical Component
> Road Practicum
> Driving Report

▼ EVALUATION

A comprehensive driving evaluation consists of a clinical component, a road practicum, and a report that documents the individual's performance on clinical and road tests, and provides therapeutic recommendations about driving, including suggestions for equipment resources. The ultimate objective of a driving evaluation is to provide the client with a comprehensive plan for community mobility at the individual's highest level of functioning.

As a result of the emphasis on mobility in our society, the Commission for Accreditation of Rehabilitation Facilities now requires a rehabilitation center to provide a driver rehabilitation service either directly or through a qualified referral source in the community. Given their medical background and expertise in activity analysis and adaptive technology, occupational therapists have been in the forefront of the development of a specialty area in driver rehabilitation. (Pierce, 1993, p. 1)

Clinical Component

Occupational therapists begin therapeutic driving evaluations in the structured setting of the clinic, gathering information about the client's medical history, social situation, vocational status, physical status, visual abilities, and cognitive and perceptual functioning, all as related to driving. Information about medical history, social situation, and vocational status is obtained through interview and medical record review. The therapist should request the individual's medical records and all pertinent therapeutic documentation to facilitate the clinical driving evaluation (Latson, 1987). The initial interview also investigates the client's previous driving experience, future requirements for driving frequency, road conditions, and the client's current access to a vehicle.

The physical examination includes active range of motion, tone, strength, coordination, and sensation throughout the client's head, neck, trunk, upper and lower extremities. Static and dynamic sitting balance, general endurance, and the client's ability to transfer to and from the vehicle are also addressed. Finally, the physical evaluation requires the client to display simulated driving skills, such as manipulation of a (modified) steering wheel and brake reaction time.

"Driver rehabilitation specialists should become familiar with their state's visual requirements for driving" (Strano, 1993, p. 4). To assess clients' abilities to meet state visual standards, the occupational therapist administers a comprehensive visual evaluation that may include, yet not be limited to, the following tests: visual acuity for distance, visual fields, convergence, peripheral vision, saccades, color discrimination, and scanning. Vision testing technology is available and recommended to minimize testing variability and subjectivity while maximizing validity and reliability.

Perceptual skills tested may include depth perception, form constancy, figure ground, spatial relations, and the presence of neglect. For cognitive testing, one may consider the following: attention or concentration, insight into disability, visual or verbal memory, sequencing, problem solving, judgment, processing time, and knowledge and integration of driving laws. The therapist should also be able to identify other limiting factors, such as impulse control and anxiety. At the conclusion of the clinical portion of the driving evaluation, the occupational therapist makes a recommendation about whether or not the client is ready to pursue the road practicum evaluation.

Road Practicum

When deemed appropriate to continue in the driving evaluation process, the client is evaluated for safe-driving skills within the functional setting of an on-the-road practicum. For the road practicum, a rehabilitation program has the choice of using a local commercial driving school instructor in conjunction with a specialized occupational therapist, or providing the service in-house with facility-owned equipment and an occupational therapist who has completed the required courses to become a driving evaluator or instructor. In either case, the first consideration is to establish a predetermined driving route that encompasses the following driving environments: parking lot, quiet residential streets, busy roadways, city congestion, and highway traffic.

A driving test route should give opportunities for drivers to demonstrate their ability to search for hazards, immediate and potential, using perceptual skills. Decision making ability can be indicated by appropriate direction and speed control in relation to traffic and environmental situations. The timing of each to various situations is an indication of proper attitudinal reaction. (Smith, 1987, p. 4)

The final test route must allow for quick and safe modification options during the actual practicum to assure client and community safety.

The road practicum evaluates the client's ability to operate the systems of the vehicle. These are inclusive but not limited to: positioning, steering, braking, maneuvering, and integrating the visual–perceptual and cognitive demands of the road. Traffic symbol knowledge is also assessed in the course of the road practicum.

Driving Report

Following the clinical and road practicum evaluations, the therapist must interpret all of the data to devise client-specific recommendations. The worst-case scenario would be that the therapist identifies areas of dysfunction that exclude the client from driving. In this situation, other mobility options should be investigated and discussed.

When the client displays potential, yet lacks readiness, the recommendation may be to refrain from current driving and either continue with therapy or follow with a home program to strengthen deficient areas. Another plan for the slightly higher-functioning client could consist of the client's participation in a professional driver-training program while practicing with family and friends before repeating another therapeutic evaluation. If all goes well throughout the clinical and road practicum, the therapist will recommend that the client complete his or her state's registry of motor vehicles competency test to reestablish driving status and re-enter the community as a skilled driver. Client assistive aids and vehicle equipment modifications may be evaluated and implemented at this time (Fig.

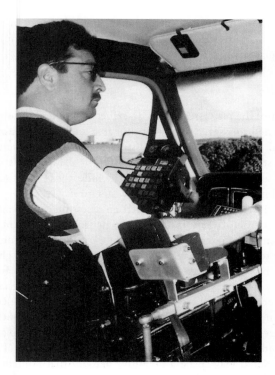

Figure 15-2. Some vehicle adaptations that can be made for drivers with limited arm and no functional leg movements.

15-2). "Mobility in the community is paramount for a person to achieve daily and life goals" (Pierce, 1993, p. 1).

For more information contact:

The Association of Driver Educators for the Disabled
P.O. Box 49
Edgerton, WI 53534

The National Mobility Equipment Dealers Association
909 E. Skagway Ave.
Tampa, FL 33604

Section 4

Evaluation of Play and Leisure

Susan H. Knox

Occupations are "the chunks of culturally and personally meaningful activity in which humans engage" (Clark et al., 1991, p. 310). People create or orchestrate their daily experiences through planning and participating in occupations (Yerxa et al., 1989). Occupational therapy generally considers work, self-care, **leisure,** play, and rest to be the major occupations of people. Since the inception of the profession, occupational therapy has always valued a balance of these occupations. However, it is not always clear what is work or play or what constitutes a balance. Often activities that one person might consider work, another might consider play. There often is an overlap of work and play or leisure, or a person can be involved in more than one activity at a time.

The purpose of this section is to provide an overview of assessments that are designed to examine play and leisure. To apply these assessments appropriately, one needs to understand the theories behind them. Therefore, this section also discusses the play, work, leisure relationship and suggests a way to consider the balance.

▼ THE PLAY, WORK, LEISURE RELATIONSHIP

Reilly (1974) described play along a continuum leading to work and leisure. Children learn skills and develop interests through play that affect later choices and success in work and leisure. Play is the arena for the development of sensory integration, physical abilities, cognitive and language skills, and interpersonal relationships. In their play, children practice adult and cultural roles and learn to become productive members of society (Bergen, 1988; Levy, 1978; Reilly, 1974).

In adults, the word play is seldom used. Instead, adults are said to engage in leisure activities or in recreation. Leisure is usually differentiated from work. This is unfortunate in that there is not always a clear distinction between the two. Also, do adults play? If so, do they play only during leisure time? What distinguishes work, play, and leisure? Much of the problem stems from the definitions of the three words, for they all have been defined in four ways: (1) as activity, (2) by degree of time pressure associated with them, (3) as having certain characteristics, and (4) as experience or state of mind.

Work has been defined as activity done for production or reward as well as nonsalaried activity that contributes to subsistence, such as homemaking, or reproduction, such as child care. It is usually done within time constraints, provides satisfaction, a livelihood, and goal achievement. Work is usually driven by external motivation. Characteristics that distinguish work are (1) extrinsic rewards, (2) formal duties and obligations, (3) performance within specified structure or time constraints, (4) task determined, and (5) predictability (Anderson, 1961; Brook & Brook, 1989; Neulinger, 1981; Parker, 1983).

Leisure or play usually occurs outside of the obligations of one's work and provides opportunities for enjoyment, relaxation, recreation, personal growth, and goal achievement. Leisure is driven by internal motivation, implies freedom of choice, and is not usually done within time constraints. The functions or characteristics of leisure or play can be described as (1) personal development, (2) enjoyment, (3) entertainment, (4) interaction with others, (5) relaxation, (6) free choice, (7) challenge, and (8) goal achievement (Dumazedier, cited in Anderson, 1961; Brook & Brook, 1989; Iso-Ahola, 1979; Kelly, 1983).

Recently, the emphasis has been more on play and leisure as an experience or state of mind, and this seems more helpful when considering a balanced life. Csikszentmihalyi (1975, 1990) has contributed a great deal to understanding how people experience and give meaning to their daily activities through the concept of optimal experience and **flow.** Optimal experience occurs when the challenge of an activity is congruent with a person's skills and abilities. This state of psychic energy is described as flow. Flow is a state of deep concentration in which consciousness is well ordered. Elements present during flow are a feeling of control, loss of self-consciousness, transformation of time, and concentration on the task at hand. Csikszentmihalyi states, "people become so involved in what they are doing that the activity becomes spontaneous, almost automatic; they stop being aware of themselves as separate from the actions they are performing" (1990, p. 53). Flow can occur in almost any type of activity, be it work or nonwork, and it provides motivation, satisfaction, and inner rewards.

The way a person approaches the activities in his or her daily life may be more important to health and life satisfaction than the activities themselves. If a person really enjoys and is challenged by a task, be it work or play, satisfaction and a feeling of well-being ensues.

Primeau (1996) states:

One's affective experience while participating in an occupation is as important as participation in the occupation itself. Thus, what may be more crucial to health and well-being than a balance of work and leisure occupations is a balance of affective experiences that may be achieved as people engage in their customary round of occupations within daily life and throughout their life span. (p. 576)

▼ PLAY EVALUATION

Play assessments can generally be considered in three types: (1) those that assess skills in a particular area through play;

(2) those that assess developmental competencies; and (3) those that assess the way a child plays, including playfulness and play style.

Skills

Most of the play assessments described in the literature were designed to assess a particular skill area, such as cognition or social interaction. These assessments use either structured play settings, materials and activities, or play observations. The assessments described here include those most often cited in the occupational therapy literature.

Kalverboer (1977) developed an assessment to examine the relation of play organization to neurologic function. His assessment relied on descriptions of the child's behavior, relative to the physical and social environments, and the child's own behavior. Levels of complexity of play were defined, and consistency and duration of play were designated. Kalverboer videotaped play observations with preselected play materials in a structured setting with a preset sequence.

Several assessments have stressed the relation of play to cognition and language development. Rosenblatt (1977) considered play to be a cognitive activity that contributed to childrens' knowledge of their relation to the world about them. Play and language were part of a continuum in the development of the meaning of symbols outside the child. She observed children from 9 to 24 months of age in their homes, with a standard set of toys, using time sampling, and classified the child's responses to toys in terms of types of play and quality of play.

Hulme & Lunzer (1966) were also interested in the relationship of play, language, and reasoning. They observed the free play of children, age 2 to 6 years, using an observation rating scale. The behavior was rated on each of two subscales: adaptiveness in the use of materials and integration of behavior. Adaptiveness in the use of materials considered the degree to which the child used the material appropriately and the extent that the child adapted materials in other than obvious ways using his own constructive or imaginative purpose. Integration of behavior was a measure of complexity of behavior.

The Piagetian stages of cognitive development formed the basis of a number of play assessments. Smilanski (1968) elaborated on the stages of play development discussed by Piaget and others in her examination of sociodramatic play. She developed an assessment of six elements of sociodramatic play: (1) imitative role play; (2) make-believe in regard to objects; (3) make-believe in regard to actions and situations; (4) persistence; (5) interaction; and (6) verbal communication.

Rubin, Maioni, and Hornung (1976), Rubin, Watson, and Jambor (1978), and Sponseller (1974) developed similar observation models that featured the social play categories of Parten and the cognitive play categories described by Piaget and Smilanski. Behaviors were coded along the dimensions of social and cognitive play categories. These scales were used for observing toddler and preschool children.

Wolfgang and Phelps (1983) used children's preferences for play materials as reflecting cognitive development. They developed an inventory based on Piaget's categories of play that used pictures of play, and children were asked about play preferences.

The classic assessment of the social aspects of play was that of Parten (1933). She assessed social participation in play of preschool children by examining two dimensions: degree of participation and degree of leadership. Degree of participation included the social interaction during play and was rated as unoccupied, solitary, onlooker, parallel, associative, and organized supplementary play. Degree of leadership included how much the child depended on or directed others in play. The child was rated as independent, following some and directing others, sharing leadership with others, and directing alone.

Developmental

A few assessments attempt to assess the developmental skills of the child through play. Linder's (1993) transdisciplinary play-based assessment evaluates the child in cognitive, social-emotional, language, and physical and motor development. The child is evaluated through a questionnaire filled out by the parents and through observation of play in structured and unstructured settings, alone, with a play facilitator, parents, and a peer. Observation worksheets are filled out during the observation and summarized in terms of strengths, abilities, and recommendations.

Two assessments developed by occupational therapists explore play developmentally: the Play History (Takata, 1969, 1971, 1974) and the Preschool Play Scale (Knox, 1968, 1974, 1997a; Bledsoe & Shephard, 1982). Takata (1969, 1971, 1974) looked at play as a developmental phenomenon, bounded by time and space, reflecting the interaction between the individual and the external environment. She identified two elements of play: form and content. Form includes the choice of play materials, amount and nature of playfulness and organization in play, and parallels changes in development. Content is the expression of the child's immediate needs, impulses, physical, and emotional state, and reflects life's situations. The Play History developed from these ideas is a semistructured interview and play observation that yields information on the child's daily activity schedule. The interview and play observation are analyzed according to a taxonomy of play epochs, and behaviors are classified as evident, not evident, encouraged, and not encouraged. A play prescription can be developed from this analysis. Behnke and Fetokovich (1984) conducted reliability and validity studies on the Play History and found it to be a reliable and valid instrument for assessing children's play behavior.

Knox (1968, 1974, 1997a) developed an observational assessment designed to give a developmental description of normal play behavior through the ages birth to 6 years. This assessment was revised by Bledsoe and Shephard (1988) and most recently by Knox (1997a). The assessment describes play in terms of 6-month increments through age 3 and yearly increments through age 6. Four dimensions are examined: space management, material management, pretense or symbolic, and participation. Space management is the manner in which children learn to manage their body and the space around them. Material management is the way the child manages material surroundings. The pretense or symbolic dimension is the way the child learns about the world through imitation and the development of the ability to understand and separate reality from make-believe. Participation is the amount and manner of social interaction. Children are observed indoors and outdoors and rated on all four dimensions. Bledsoe and Shephard (1982) examined reliability and validity on the first revision with normal children. Harrison and Kielhofner (1986) did the same with a population with disabilities. Both found the scale to be highly reliable and valid.

Experience

Play can also be evaluated in terms of the child's experience or state of mind when playing. This category includes assessments of playfulness and play style.

Barnett (1990, 1991) devised a rating scale, based on Liebermann's (1977) playfulness concepts. Children are rated on items representing the five playfulness traits: physical spontaneity, manifest joy, sense of humor, social spontaneity, and cognitive spontaneity.

Bundy (1997) developed the Test of Playfulness (ToP), designed to assess the individual's degree of playfulness. The scale contains 68 items representing four elements of playfulness: intrinsic motivation, internal control, ability to suspend reality, and framing, and the child is rated on scales of extent, intensity, and skill. The ToP can be scored from videotapes of children engaged in free play.

Advantages and Disadvantages of Play Evaluation

Watching children play is like looking through a window into their lives. Analysis of children's play tells us much about their physical and cognitive abilities, social participation, imagination, independence, coping mechanisms, and environment (Brown & Gottfried, 1985; Bruner, Jolly, & Sylva, 1976; Ellis, 1973; Garvey, 1977; Hartley & Goldenson, 1963; Bergen, 1988). Evaluation of play and of the child's abilities as seen through play are necessary to provide the therapist with tools to analyze play and plan treatment.

The advantages of testing play are that one sees the child performing routine, self-chosen, familiar activities in naturalistic settings, and this gives us a picture of everyday competencies. It is important not only to test the abilities of the child, but also to see what is routine. Play assessments also focus on the abilities of the child and not as much on the disabilities.

Some of the disadvantages to play assessments have been summarized by Kielhofner and Barris (1984), Knox

(1997b), and Bundy (1993). Play is an interaction between the child and the environment, and there can be a tremendous difference in a child's play depending on the human and physical factors in the environment (Knox, 1997b). Most assessments are designed to take place in standardized settings with standardized toys. This in itself alters the play, and often inhibits true play.

Additionally, since play specifies its own purpose, observed behaviors may have different meanings and serve different purposes for different people. It is difficult for an observer to evaluate the meaning of play to the participant.

Another limitation is in the amount of time one observes the child. Is the sample behavior sufficient, typical, or is it even play? Knox (1997b) found that over a prolonged time, a child's play could be vastly different at different times. Also, children engaged in play episodes for prolonged times (up to 1 hour in some cases). To capture a variety of play, one needs to observe a child multiple times and in a variety of settings.

▼ LEISURE EVALUATION

There are measures of leisure activity in terms of time, money, or both; activities and interests; characteristics; and as experience, including the meaning of leisure. Most of the assessments reviewed measure a combination of these areas.

Leisure as Time

Most assessments include some indication of how much time a person spends doing a variety of activities. Two assessments use history taking. Potts' (1969) leisure history contains questions on leisure and on use of leisure time. Activities are divided into five areas: (1) manipulative-exploratory, (2) practical-inventive, (3) reflective-epistemonic, (4) social, and (5) communal. Florey and Michelman's (1982) screening device, the Occupational Role History, explores the following areas: (1) sequence and continuity of occupational roles and components; (2) satisfaction with interests, people, tasks, and environments; (3) occupational roles and expressed comfort, satisfaction, and competence in each; (4) areas of skill and problem areas; and (5) degree of balance between work, chores, and leisure.

Medrich, Roizen, Rubin, and Buckley's (1982) questionnaire describes children's activities when out of school. The instrument examines opportunities and constraints on time use and explored attitudes, purposes, and meanings for non-school-time use.

Leisure Activities and Interests

Matsutsuyu's (1969) Interest Check List examines the intensity of a person's interest in 80 different activities. Interests are classified in five categories: (1) manual skills, (2) physical/sports, (3) social recreation, (4) activities of daily living, and

(5) cultural or educational. This check list was revised to allow factor analysis by Rogers, Weinstein, and Figone (1978).

McCree's (1993) Leisure/Play Interest Survey determines past participation, interest, and skill in a variety of leisure activities. McKechnie's (1975) Leisure Activity Blank is a self-report that provides information on past leisure activity and future intentions to participate. Kautzmann's (1984) self-assessment of leisure interests provides information on skill or interest in activities, importance to the individual, and priority for future participation.

Leisure as Activity and Meaning

Nystrom's (1974) questionnaire measures active participation and includes questions about the definition of leisure; this questionnaire was derived from Nystrom's study of the activity patterns, leisure concepts, and meaning of leisure time activity among a group of elderly residents in a low-income urban housing development. Gregory (1983) adapted Nystrom's Activity Check List to include questions related to the meaning of the activities and also asked questions related to life satisfaction; this change was based on Gregory's study of the activities of a group of retirees in relation to life satisfaction.

Tickle and Yerxa's (1981) Need Satisfaction of Activity Interview examines an individual's two most important activities, the frequency of participation in them, and the type of need in Maslow's hierarchy each activity primarily satisfied. Neulinger's (1981) leisure attitude questionnaire contains questions on leisure, work, sex, and background information. Neulinger has identified five factors influencing leisure choices: (1) amount of work or vacation desired, (2) society's role in leisure planning, (3) self-definition through work or leisure, (4) amount of perceived leisure, and (5) affinity to leisure.

Some assessments focus on the meaning of activity. Csikszentmihalyi and Larson (1984) used experience sampling methods to examine activities and their meanings in adolescents. The experience sampling method consisted of using electronic pagers to send random signals to individuals. On receiving the signals, the individual fills out a self-report related to current activities, companions, emotional feelings, and mood. This method enabled in-depth examination of personal experiences (activities) and of thoughts and feelings about those.

Qualitative methods have also been used to study the meaning of leisure. Glancy (1986) used participant observation of sport-group membership. She felt the method was useful in developing grounded theory associated with freedom, expressiveness, meaning, and motivation in leisure. Howe (1988) used structured interviews to explore the role of leisure with subjects in a senior adult fitness program and used case study design to describe emergent patterns. Krefting and Krefting (1991) described how ethnographic approaches may be applied to the understanding of leisure activity among disabled populations.

▼ INTERPRETING PLAY AND LEISURE ASSESSMENTS

Occupational therapists need to evaluate play and leisure in order to (1) obtain a complete picture of an individual's competence in **occupational behavior** and (2) adequately plan intervention that focuses on helping that person participate in meaningful and self-satisfying occupations. Such assessments provide the therapist with a picture of how individuals use play and leisure activities in their daily lives. In the child, analysis of play also provides the therapist with a picture of the child's skills in motor, cognitive, and social areas. This is especially helpful when assessing a child who does not respond well to standardized developmental testing. In the adult, leisure assessment provides not only a picture of a person's abilities and interests, but also an indication of the meaning certain activities hold for that person.

Some of the newer assessments of affect, playfulness, or play style indicate how the individual approaches and gives meaning to the gamut of activities during the day. These instruments hold much promise in helping determine how an individual balances his or her daily occupations in a meaningful way.

Assessment in occupational therapy leads to treatment planning. Knowledge of the individual's skills, interests, and play style assists in this planning and guides treatment. Bundy (1993) offers a number of considerations when observing an individual's play that are useful in developing treatment goals.

(a) in what activities the client becomes totally absorbed; (b) what the client gets from these activities; (c) whether or not the client engages routinely in activities in which he or she feels free to vary the process, product, and outcome in whatever way he or she sees fit; (d) whether or not the client has the capacity, permission, and support to do what he or she chooses to do; and (e) whether or not the client is capable of giving and interpreting messages that "this is play; this is how you should interact with me now." (p. 219)

These considerations, when asked as questions, guide the treatment-planning process. Treatment through play and leisure is addressed in Chapter 19, Section 5.

▼ REFERENCES

Allen, C. K. (1985). *Occupational therapy for psychiatric diseases: Measurement and management of cognitive disabilities.* Boston: Little, Brown & Co.

Allen, C. K. (1990). *Allen cognitive level test manual.* Colchester, CT: S & S Worldwide.

Allen, C. K., Earhart, C. A., & Blue, T. (1992). *Occupational therapy treatment goals for the physically and cognitively challenged.* Rockville, MD: American Occupational Therapy Association.

Allen, C. K., Kehrberg, K., & Burns, T. (1992). Evaluation instruments, In C. K. Allen, C. A. Earhart, & T. Blue (Eds.), *Occupational therapy treatment goals for the physically and cognitively challenged* (pp. 31–68). Rockville, MD: American Occupational Therapy Association.

American Occupational Therapy Association (AOTA). (1994). Uniform terminology for occupational therapy, third edition. *American Journal of Occupational Therapy, 48,* 1047–1054.

Anderson, N. (1961). *Work and leisure.* New York: Free Press.

Árnadóttir, G. (1990). *The brain and behavior: Assessing cortical dysfunction through tasks of daily living.* St. Louis: C.V. Mosby.

Atwood, S., Holm, M. B., & James, A. (1994). ADL capabilities and values of long-term care facility residents. *American Journal of Occupational Therapy, 48,* 710–716.

Barnett, L. (1990). Playfulness: Definition, design, and measurement. *Play and Culture, 3,* 319–336.

Barnett, L. (1991). The playful child: Measurement of a disposition to play. *Play and Culture, 4,* 51–74.

Behnke, C., & Fetokovich, M. (1984). Examining the reliability and validity of the play history. *American Journal of Occupational Therapy, 38,* 94–100.

Bergen, D. (1988). *Play as a medium for learning and development.* Portsmouth, NH: Heinemann Educational Books.

Bledsoe, N., & Shepherd, J. (1982). A study of reliability and validity of a preschool play scale. *American Journal of Occupational Therapy, 36,* 783–788.

Borg, G. (1982). Psychophysical bases of perceived exertion. *Medicine & Science in Sports and Exercise, 14,* 377–381.

Bowman, J. (1992). Nationally speaking Americans have a shared vision: Occupational therapists can help to create the future reality. *American Journal of Occupational Therapy, 46,* 409–418.

Brook, J., & Brook, R. (1989). Exploring the meaning of work and nonwork. *Journal of Organizational Behavior, 10,* 169–178.

Brown, C., & Gottfried, A. (Eds.) (1985). *Play Interactions.* New Jersey: Johnson & Johnson Baby Products.

Bruner, J.S., Jolly, A., & Sylva, K (Eds.) (1976). *Play—its role in development and evolution.* New York: Basic Books.

Bundy, A. (1993). Assessment of play and leisure: Delineation of the problem. *American Journal of Occupational Therapy, 47,* 217–222.

Bundy, A. (1997). Play and playfulness: What to look for. In D. Parham & L. Fazio, (Eds.), *Play in occupational therapy for children,* (pp. 52–66). St. Louis, MO: Mosby Yearbooks.

Buttle, C.S. (1995). Ergonomic job analysis. *Rehab Management, 8* (2), 63–66.

Chiou, I. L., & Burnett, C. N. (1985). Values of activities of daily living: A survey of stroke patients and their home therapists. *Physical Therapy, 65,* 901–906.

Christiansen, C. (1991). Occupational performance assessment. In C. Christiansen & C. Baum (Eds.), *Occupational therapy: Overcoming human performance deficits.* (pp. 375–424). Thorofare, NJ: Slack.

Clark, F., Parham, D., Carlson, M., Frank, G., Jackson, J., Pierce, D., Wolfe, R., & Zemke, R. (1991). Occupational science: Academic innovation in the service of occupational therapy's future. *American Journal of Occupational Therapy, 45,* 300–310.

Cronbach, L. J. (1970). *Essentials of psychological testing* (3rd ed.). New York: Harper & Row.

Csikszentmihalyi, M. (1975). *Beyond boredom and anxiety.* San Francisco: Jossey-Bass.

Csikszentmihalyi, M. (1990). *Flow.* New York: Harper & Row.

Csikszentmihalyi, M., & Larson, R. (1984). *Being adolescent.* New York: Basic Books.

DeJong, G., & Sutton, J. P. (1995). Rehab 2000: The evolution of medical rehabilitation in American health care. In P. K. Landrum, N. D. Schmidt, & A. McLean (Eds.), *Outcome-oriented rehabilitation* (pp. 3–42). Gaithersburg, MD: Aspen.

Doble, S. E., Fisk, J. D., Fisher, A. G., Ritvo, P. G., & Murray, T. J. (1994). Functional competence of community-dwelling persons with multiple sclerosis using the Assessment of Motor and Process Skills. *Archives of Physical Medicine and Rehabilitation, 75,* 843–851.

Eakin, P. (1989). Problems with assessments of activities of daily living. *British Journal of Occupational Therapy, 52,* 50–54.

Ellis, M.J. (1973). *Why people play.* Englewood Cliffs, NJ: Prentice-Hall.

Fairbanks, J., Davies, J., Cooper, J., & O'Brien, J. (1980). The Oswestry low back pain disability questionnaire. *Physiotherapy, 66*, 271–273.

Fillenbaum, G. G. (1988). *Multidimensional functional assessment of older adults: The Duke older Americans resources and services procedures.* Hillsdale, NJ: Lawrence Erlbaum Associates.

Fisher, A. G. (1993). The assessment of IADL motor skills: An application of many-faceted Rasch analysis. *American Journal of Occupational Therapy, 47*, 319–329.

Fisher, A. G. (1994). *Assessment of Motor and Process Skills manual* (research edition 7.0). [Unpublished test manual]. Fort Collins, CO: Colorado State University.

Fisher, A. G., Liu, Y., Velozo, C. A., & Pan, A. W. (1992). Cross-cultural assessment of process skills. *American Journal of Occupational Therapy, 46*, 876–885.

Florey, L., & Michelman, S. (1982). Occupational role history: A screening tool for psychiatric occupational therapy. *American Journal of Occupational Therapy, 36*, 301–308.

Fox, D. J. (1969). *The research process in education.* New York: Holt, Rinehart & Winston.

Freal, J., Kraft, G., & Coryell, J. (1984). Symptomatic fatigue in multiple sclerosis. *Archives of Physical Medicine and Rehabilitation, 65*, 135–138.

Fried, L. P., Herdman, S. J., Kuhn, K. E., Rubin, G., & Turano, K. (1991). Preclinical disability: Hypotheses about the bottom of the iceberg. *Journal of Aging and Health, 3*, 285–300.

Fries, J. F., Spitz, P., Kraines, R. G., & Holman, H. R. (1980). Measurement of patient outcomes in arthritis. *Arthritis and Rheumatism, 23*, 146–152.

Gage, M., Noh, S., Polatajko, H. J., & Kaspar, V. (1994). Measuring perceived self-efficacy in occupational therapy. *American Journal of Occupational Therapy, 48*, 783–790.

Garvey, C. (1977). *Play.* London: Fontana/Open Books Publishing.

Gift, A. G. (1987). Dyspnea: A clinical perspective. *Scholarly Inquiry in Nursing Practice, 1*, 73–85.

Gift, A. G., & Pugh, L. C. (1993). Dyspnea and fatigue. *Nursing Clinics of North America, 28*, 373–384.

Glancy, M. (1986). Participant observation in the recreation setting. *Journal of Leisure Research, 18*, 59–80.

Gregory, M. D. (1983). Occupational behavior and life satisfaction among retirees. *American Journal of Occupational Therapy, 37*, 548–553.

Gurland, B., Kuriansky, J., Sharpe, L., Simon, R., Stiller, P., & Birkett, P. (1977–78). The Comprehensive Assessment and Referral Evaluation (CARE). *International Journal of Aging and Human Development, 8*, 9–42.

Hamilton, B. B., Granger, C. V., Sherwin, F. S., Zielezny, M., & Tashman, J. S. (1987). A uniform national data system for medical rehabilitation. In M. J. Fuhrer (Ed.), *Rehabilitation outcomes: Analysis and measurement* (pp. 137–147). Baltimore, MD: Paul H. Brooks.

Harrison, H., & Kielhofner, G. (1986). Examining reliability and validity of the preschool play scale with handicapped children. *American Journal of Occupational Therapy, 40*, 167–173.

Hart, L., & Freel, M. (1982). Fatigue. In C. Norris (Ed.), *Concept clarification in nursing* (pp. 251–262). Rockville, MD: Aspen.

Hartley, R., & Goldenson, R. (1963). *The complete book of children's play.* New York: Cornwall Press.

Haworth, R. J., & Hollings, E. M. (1979). Are hospital assessments of daily living activities valid? *International Rehabilitation Medicine, 1*, 59–62.

Haywood, H. C., & Tzuriel, D. (Eds.) (1992). *Interactive assessment.* New York: Springer-Verlag.

Heimann, N. E., Allen, C. K., & Yerxa, E. J. (1989). The Routine Task Inventory: A tool for describing the functional behavior of the cognitively disabled. *Occupational Therapy Practice, 1*, 67–74.

Heinemann, A. W., Linacre, J. M., Wright, B. D., Hamilton, B. B., & Granger, C. (1994). Prediction of rehabilitation outcomes with disability measures. *Archives of Physical Medicine and Rehabilitation, 75*, 133–143.

Hildreth, D., Breidenbach, W., Lister, G., & Hodges, A. (1989). Detection of submaximal effort by use of rapid exchange grip. *Journal of Hand Surgery, 14A*, 742–745.

Holm, M. B., & Rogers, J. C. (1989). The therapist's thinking behind functional assessment, II. In C. Royeen (Ed.), *Assessment of function: An action guide* (pp. 1–36). Rockville, MD: American Occupational Therapy Association

Howe, C. (1988). Using qualitative structured interviews in leisure research: Illustrations from one case study. *Journal of Leisure Research, 20*, 305–324.

Hulme, I., & Lunzer, E. A. (1966). Play, language and reasoning in subnormal children. *Journal of Child Psychology and Psychiatry, 7*, 107–123.

Huskisson, E. (1974). Measurement of pain. *Lancet, 2*, 1127–1131.

Ilika, J., & Hoffman, N. G. (1981a). *Reliability study on the Kohlman Evaluation of Living Skills.* Unpublished manuscript.

Ilika, J., & Hoffman, N. G. (1981b). *Concurrent validity study on the Kohlman Evaluation of Living Skills and the Global Assessment Scale.* Unpublished manuscript.

Iserhagen, S. (1990). Pre-work screening. *Industrial Rehabilitation Quarterly, 3* (1), 7–47.

Iso-Ahola, S. E. (1979). Basic dimensions of definitions of leisure. *Journal of Leisure Research, 11*, 28–39.

Jacobs, K. (1991). *Occupational therapy—work related programs and assessments.* (pp. 23–59; 255–357). Boston, MA: Little, Brown & Co.

Janson-Bjerklie, S., Carrieri, V. K., & Hudes, M. (1986). The sensations of pulmonary dyspnea. *Nursing Research, 35*, 154–159.

Jaworski, D. M., Kult, T., & Boynton, P. R. (1994). The Functional Independence Measure: A pilot study comparison of observed and reported ratings. *Rehabilitation Nursing Research,* Winter, 141–147.

Jette, A. M. (1980). Functional Status Index: Reliability of a chronic disease evaluation instrument. *Archives of Physical Medicine and Rehabilitation, 61*, 395–401.

Kalverboer, A. (1977). Measurement of play: Clinical applications. In B. Tizard & D. Harvey (Eds.). *Biology of play* (pp. 100–122). Philadelphia: J. B. Lippincott.

Katz, S., Ford, A. B., Moskowitz, R. W., Jackson, B. A., & Jaffe, M. A., (1963). Studies of illness in the aged: The Index of ADL. *Journal of the American Medical Association, 185*, 914–919.

Kaufman, L. (1982). *Concurrent validity study on the Kohlman Evaluation of Living Skills and the Bay Area Functional Performance Evaluation.* Unpublished master's thesis, University of Florida, Gainesville.

Kautzmann, L. (1984). Identifying leisure interests: A self assessment approach for adults with arthritis. *Occupational Therapy in Health Care, 1*, 45–52.

Kelly, J. R. (1983). *Leisure identities and interactions.* London, George Allen & Unwin.

Kielhofner, G., & Barris, R. (1984). Collecting data on play: A critique of available methods. *The Occupational Therapy Journal of Research, 4*, 150–180.

Klein, R. M., & Bell, B. (1979). *The Klein-Bell ADL Scale Manual.* Seattle, WA: Educational Resources. University of Washington.

Klein, R. M., & Bell, B. (1982). Self-care skills: Behavioral measurement with Klein-Bell ADL scale. *Archives of Physical Medicine and Rehabilitation, 63*, 335–338.

Knox, S. (1968). *Observation and assessment of the everyday play behavior of the mentally retarded child.* Unpublished master's thesis, University of Southern California, Los Angeles, CA.

Knox, S. (1974). A play scale. In M. Reilly, (Ed.). *Play as Exploratory Learning* (pp. 247–266). Beverly Hills: Sage Publications.

Knox, S. (1997a). Development and current use of the Knox Preschool Play Scale. In D. Parham & L. Fazio (Eds.), *Play in occupational therapy for children.* (pp. 35–51). St. Louis, MO: Mosby Yearbooks.

Knox, S. (1997b). *Play and play styles of preschool children.* Unpublished doctoral dissertation. University of Southern California, Los Angeles, CA.

Krefting, L., & Krefting, D. (1991). Leisure activities after a stroke: An ethnographic approach. *American Journal of Occupational Therapy, 45,* 429–436.

Latson, L. (1987). Overview of disabled drivers' evaluation process. *Physical Disabilities Special Interest Section Newsletter, 10* (4), 1–7.

Lawton, M. P. (1972). Assessing the competence of older people. In D. P. Kent, R. Kastenbaum, & S. Sherwood (Eds.), *Research planning and action for the elderly: The power and potential of social science* (pp. 122–143). New York: Behavioral Publications.

Lawton, M. P., & Brody, E. M. (1969). Assessment of older people: Self maintaining and instrumental activities of daily living. *Gerontologist, 9,* 179–186.

Leonardelli, C. A. (1988a). *The Milwaukee Evaluation of Daily Living Skills.* Thorofare, NJ: Slack.

Leonardelli, C. A. (1988b). The Milwaukee Evaluation of Daily Living Skills (MEDLS). In B. J. Hemphill (Ed.), *Mental health assessment in occupational therapy* (pp. 151–162). Thorofare, NJ: Slack.

Letts, L., & Marshall, L. (1995). Evaluating the validity and consistency of the SAFER tool. *Physical & Occupational Therapy in Geriatrics, 13,* 49–66.

Levy, J. (1978). *Play behavior.* Malabar, FL: Robert E. Krieger.

Liebermann, J. (1977). *Playfulness: Its relationship to imagination and creativity.* New York: Academic Press.

Linacre, J. M. (1989). *Many-facet Rasch measurement.* Chicago: MESA Press.

Linacre, J. M., Heinemann, A. W., Wright, B. D., Granger, C. V., & Hamilton, B. B. (1994). The structure and stability of the Functional Independence Measure. *Archives of Physical Medicine and Rehabilitation, 75,* 127–132.

Linder, T. (1993). *Transdisciplinary play-based assessment.* Baltimore: Paul H. Brooks.

Mahoney, F. I., & Barthel, D. W. (1965). Functional evaluation: The Barthel Index. *Maryland State Medical Journal, 14,* 61–65.

Marshall, E. (1985). Looking back. *American Journal of Occupational Therapy, 39,* 297–299.

Matsutsuyu, J.S. (1969). The interest check list. *American Journal of Occupational Therapy, 23,* 323–334.

Mayer, T., Baines, D., Kishiro, N., Nichols, G.M., Gatchel, R., Mayer, H., & Mooney, V. (1988). Progressive isoinertial lifting evaluation: A standardized protocol and normative database. *Spine, 13,* 933–997.

Mayer, T., Gatchell, R., Barnes, D. Mayer, H., & Mooney, V. (1990). Progressive isoinertial lifting evaluation erratum notice. *Spine, 15,* 5.

McCree, S. (1993). *Leisure and play in therapy.* Tucson, AZ: Therapy Skill Builders.

McDowell, I., & Newell, C. (1966). *Measuring health: A guide to rating scales and questionnaires,* 2nd ed. New York: Oxford University Press.

McGourty, L. K. (1979). *Kohlman Evaluation of Living Skills.* Seattle, WA: KELS Research.

McGourty, L. K. (1988). Kohlman Evaluation of Living Skills. In B. Hemphill, (Ed.), *Mental health assessment in occupational therapy* (pp. 133–146). Thorofare, NJ: Slack.

McKechnie, G. (1975). *Leisure activities blank.* Palo Alto, CA: Consulting Psychologists Press.

Medrich, E.A., Roizen, J., Rubin, V., & Buckley, S. (1982). *The serious business of growing up: A study of children's lives outside school.* Berkeley: University of California Press.

Melzak, J. (1983). The McGill pain questionnaire: Major properties and scoring methods. *Pain, 1,* 227–229.

Melzak, J. (1987). Short form McGill pain questionnaire. *Pain, 30,* 191–197.

Merbitz, C., Morris, J., & Grip, J. C. (1989). Ordinal scales and foundations of misinference. *Archives of Physical Medicine and Rehabilitation, 70,* 308–312.

Missiuna, C. (1987). Dynamic assessment: A model for broadening assessment in occupational therapy. *Canadian Journal of Occupational Therapy, 54,* 17–21.

National Institute for Occupational Safety and Health. (1981). *Work practices guide for manual lifting* [Technical Report 81–122]. Cincinnati, OH: Division of Biomedical and Behavioral Science, NIOSH.

Niemeyer, L., Matheson, L., & Carlton, R. (1989). Testing consistency of effort: BTE work simulator. *Industrial Rehabilitation Quarterly, 2,* 5–32.

Neulinger, J. (1981). *The psychology of leisure* (2nd ed.) Springfield, IL: Charles C. Thomas.

Nouri, F. M., & Lincoln, N. B. (1987). An extended activities of daily living scale for stroke patients. *Clinical Rehabilitation, 1,* 301–305.

Nygård, L., Bernspång, B., Fisher, A. G., & Winblad, B. (1994). Comparing motor and process ability of persons with suspected dementia in home and clinic settings. *American Journal of Occupational Therapy, 48,* 689–696.

Nystrom, E.P. (1974). Activity patterns and leisure concepts among the elderly. *American Journal of Occupational Therapy, 28,* 337–345.

Parker, S. (1983). *Leisure and work.* London: Allen & Unwin.

Parten, M. (1933). Social play among pre-school children. *Journal of Abnormal and Social Psychology, 28,* 136–147.

Pfeffer, R. I., Kurosaki, T. T., Harrah, C. H., Chance, J. M., & Filos, S. (1982). Measurement of functional activities in older adults in the community. *Journal of Gerontology, 37,* 323–329.

Pierce, S. (1993). Legal considerations for a driver rehabilitation program. *Physical Disabilities Special Interest Section Newsletter, 16* (1), 1.

Pincus, T., Summey, J. A., Soraci, S. A., Wallston, K. A., & Hummon, N. P. (1983). Assessment of patient satisfaction in activities of daily living using a modified Stanford Health Assessment Questionnaire. *Arthritis and Rheumatism, 26,* 1346–1353.

Popham, W. J. (1990). *Modern educational measurement: A practitioner's perspective* (2nd ed.). Englewood Cliffs, NJ: Prentice Hall.

Potts, L (1969). *Toward a developmental assessment of leisure patterns.* Unpublished master's thesis, University of Southern California, Los Angeles, CA.

Primeau, L. (1996). Work and leisure: Transcending the dichotomy. *American Journal of Occupational Therapy, 50,* 569–577.

Ransford, A., Cairns, D., & Mooney, V. (1979). The pain drawing as an aid to the psychological evaluation or patients with low back pain. *Spine, 1,* 127–134.

Reilly, M. (1974). *Play as exploratory learning.* Beverly Hills: Sage Publications.

Rogers, J. C. (1983). Eleanor Clarke Slagle Lectureship—1983; Clinical reasoning: The ethics, science, and art. *American Journal of Occupational Therapy, 37,* 601–616.

Rogers, J. C., & Holm, M. B. (1989). *Performance Assessment of Self-Care Skills-Revised (PASS-R)* [Unpublished functional performance test]. Pittsburgh, PA: University of Pittsburgh.

Rogers, J. C., & Holm, M. B. (1991a). Older persons with depression: Educational issues. *Topics in Geriatric Rehabilitation, 6,* 27–44.

Rogers, J. C., & Holm, M. B. (1991b). Occupational therapy diagnostic reasoning: A Component of clinical reasoning. *American Journal of Occupational Therapy, 45,* 1045–1053

Rogers, J. C., & Holm, M. B. (1994). *Performance Assessment of Self-Care Skills (PASS)* (version 3.1). [Unpublished functional performance test]. Pittsburgh, PA: University of Pittsburgh.

Rogers, J. C., Holm, M. B., & Stone, R. G. (1997). Assessment of daily living activities: The home care advantage. *American Journal of Occupational Therapy, 51,* 410–422.

Rogers, J., Weinstein, J., & Figone, J. (1978) The interest check list. *American Journal of Occupational Therapy, 32,* 628–630.

Rosenblatt, D. (1977). Developmental trends in infant play. In B. Tizard & D. Harvey, (Eds.). *Biology of play* (pp. 33–44). Philadelphia: J. B. Lippincott.

Rosinek, M. (1985). *Skills assessment module.* Athens, GA: Piney Mountain Press.

Rothstein, J. M. (1985). Measurement and clinical practice: Theory and application. In J. M. Rothstein (Ed.), *Measurement in physical therapy* (pp. 1–46). New York: NY: Churchill Livingstone.

Rubenstein, L. A., Schairer, C., Wieland, G. D., & Kane, R. (1984). Systematic biases in functional status assessment of elderly adults. *Journal of Gerontology, 39,* 686–691.

Rubin, K., Maioni, T. L. & Hornung, M. (1976). Free play behaviors in middle and lower-class preschoolers: Parten and Piaget revisited. *Child Development, 47,* 414–419.

Rubin, K., Watson, K., & Jambor, T. (1978). Free play behaviors in preschool and kindergarten children. *Child Development, 49,* 534–536.

Rybski, D. (1992). A quality implementation of Title I of the Americans With Disabilities Act of 1990. *American Journal of Occupational Therapy, 46,* 409–418.

Sager, M. A., Dunham, N. C., Schwantes, A., Mecum, L., Halverson, K., & Harlowe, D. (1992). Measurement of activities of daily living in hospitalized elderly: A comparison of self-report and performance-based methods. *Journal of the American Geriatric Society, 40,* 457–462.

Settle, C., & Holm, M. B. (1993). Program planning: The clinical utility of three activities of daily living assessment tools. *American Journal of Occupational Therapy, 47,* 911–918.

Shillam, L. L., Beeman, C., & Loshin, P. M. (1983). Effect of occupational therapy intervention on bathing independence of disabled persons. *American Journal of Occupational Therapy, 37,* 744–748.

Smilanski, S. (1968). *The Effects of Sociodramatic Play on Disadvantaged Preschool Children.* New York: John Wiley & Sons.

Smith, D. (1987). Evaluation of disabled drivers: An instructor's perspective. *Physical Disabilities Special Interest Section Newsletter, 10* (4), 4.

Snook, S., & Ciriello, V. (1991). The design of material handling tasks: Revised tables of maximum acceptable weights and forces. *Ergonomics, 34,* 1197–1213.

Sponseller, D. B. (1974). *Play as a learning medium.* Washington, DC: Association for the Education of Young Children.

Stokes, H. (1983). The seriously uninjured hand-weakness of grip. *Journal of Occupational Medicine, 25,* 683–684.

Strano, C. (1993). Visual deficits and their effects on driving. *Physical Disabilities Special Interest Section Newsletter, 16* (1), 4.

Tack, B. B. (1991). *Dimensions and correlates of fatigue in older adults with rheumatoid arthritis.* Unpublished doctoral dissertation, University of California at San Francisco.

Takata, N. (1969). The play history. *American Journal of Occupational Therapy, 23,* 314–318.

Takata, N. (1971). The play milieu—a preliminary appraisal. *American Journal of Occupational Therapy, 25,* 281–284.

Takata, N. (1974). Play as a prescription. In M. Reilly (Ed.), *Play as exploratory learning,* (pp. 209–246). Beverly Hills: Sage Publications.

Tickle, L., & Yerxa, E. (1981). Need satisfaction of older persons living in the community and in institutions, part 2: Role of activity. *American Journal of Occupational Therapy, 35,* 650–655.

Uniform Data System for Medical Rehabilitation (UDSMR) (1993). *Guide for the uniform data set for medical rehabilitation* (adult FIM) Version 4.0. Buffalo, NY: UB Foundation Activities.

Uniform Probate Code (1989). Chicago: National Conference of Commissions on Uniform State Laws.

U. S. Department of Education (1982). *Annual report of the National Council on the Handicapped.*

U.S. Department of Labor. (1991). *Dictionary of Occupational Titles,* revised fourth edition. Washington, DC: Author.

Velozo, C. (1993). Work evaluations: Critique of the state of the art of functional assessment of work. *American Journal of Occupational Therapy, 47,* 203–209.

Velozo, C. A., Magalhaes, L. C., Pan, A., & Leiter, P. (1995). Functional scale discrimination at admission and discharge: Rasch analysis of the Level of Rehabilitation Scale-III. *Archives of Physical Medicine and Rehabilitation, 76,* 705–712.

Verbrugge, L. M. (1990). The iceberg of disability. In S. M. Stahl (Ed.), *The legacy of longevity: Health and health care in later life* (pp. 55–75). Newbury Park, CA: Sage

Waddell, G., McCulloch, J., Kummel, E., & Venner, R. (1980). Nonorganic physical signs of low back pain. *Spine, 5,* 117–125.

Wade, D. T. (1992). *Measurement in neurological rehabilitation.* Oxford: Oxford University Press.

Williams, J. H., Drinka, T. J. K., Greenberg, J. R., Farrel-Holtan, J., Euhardy, R., & Schram, M. (1991). Development and testing of the Assessment of Living Skills and Resources (ALSAR) in elderly community-dwelling veterans. *Gerontologist, 31,* 84–91.

Wilson, D. S., Allen C. K., McCormack, G., & Burton, G. (1989). Cognitive disability and routine task behaviors in a community based population with senile dementia. *Occupational Therapy Practice, 1,* 58–66.

Wolfgang, C., & Phelps, P. (1983). Preschool play materials preference inventory. *Early Child Development and Care, 12,* 127–141.

World Health Organization (WHO). (1980). *International classification of impairments, disabilities, and handicaps: A manual of classification relating to the consequences of disease.* Geneva: World Health Organization.

Wright, B., & Linacre, J. M. (1989). Observations are always ordinal; measurements, however, must be interval. *Archives of Physical Medicine and Rehabilitation, 70,* 857–860.

Yerxa, E. J., Burnett-Beaulieu, S., Stocking, S., & Azen, S. P. (1988). Development of the satisfaction with scaled performance questionnaire (SPSQ). *American Journal of Occupational Therapy, 42,* 215–222.

Yerxa, E., Clark, F., Frank, G., Jackson, J., Parham, D., Pierce, D., Stein, C., & Zemke, R. (1989). An introduction to occupational science, a foundation for occupational therapy in the 21st century, *Occupational Therapy in Health Care, 6* (4), 1–17.

Chapter 16

Evaluation of Performance Components

Section 1: Evaluation of Sensory and Neuromuscular Performance Components
Section 2: Evaluation of Perception and Cognition
Section 3: Evaluation of Psychosocial Skills and Psychological Components

---

Section 1

Evaluation of Sensory and Neuromuscular Performance Components

Kirsten Kohlmeyer

E valuation is a process to gather data, formulate hypotheses, and make decisions to guide action. It is necessary to do the following:

1. Establish treatment goals and interventions
2. Demonstrate efficacy of therapeutic interventions
3. Determine independent living status
4. Document need for a specific program
5. Facilitate educational or vocational placement
6. Substantiate insurance claims
7. Support litigation

Evaluation is an ongoing process of collecting and interpreting the data necessary for treatment planning, treatment modification, and discharge planning (Christiansen, 1991; Opacich, 1991). Assessment refers to specific tools or instruments used in the evaluation process (Commission on Practice, 1995).

The primary objective of evaluation is to select that combination of data collection approaches that provide the clearest and most complete picture of the individual's level of function, with the least expenditure of time, energy and cost. To be an effective evaluator, a therapist must be (1) knowledgeable about the dysfunction—its causes, course, and prognosis; (2) familiar with a variety of evaluation methods, their uses, and proper administration; and (3) able to select evaluation methods that are suitable to the client. The evaluation process includes collecting data from the client, medical record, other professionals, and family members. The process continues with administration of assessment tools, and it concludes with an analysis and summary of results, specifically how performance deficits affect function. (Christiansen, 1991; Opacich, 1991, Pedretti, 1996d, Smith, 1993, Trombly, 1995c).

When choosing an assessment instrument or strategy, the practitioner should be well informed and discriminative. Many types of assessments are available: informal, formal, standardized, nonstandardized, nonreferenced, and criterion-referenced. Box 16–1 lists several considerations when determining strategies for evaluation. Chapter 14 provides additional background for choosing assessments. This section will focus on assessments of sensory, neuromuscular, and neuromotor performance components. It provides a general overview; references refer to other texts that give more specific information.

A *performance component* can be defined as a specific skill or subsystem that affects one's ability to function. Performance components include neuromuscular skills, processing skills, communication skills, and interaction skills. Other influences that affect performance include one's physical, social, political, and cultural environments (Christiansen, 1991).

The medical diagnosis may guide a therapist toward specific assessment tools and may provide tentative expectations about the nature of performance deficits. However, diagnosis alone is not an accurate predictor of the factors most influencing occupational performance. Clinical observation of how performance components affect function is key. In today's health care environment there are shorter lengths of stay, increased managed care, and community-based programs. Evaluation and treatment areas need to be prioritized based on those programs with the most influence on functional performance areas that are of priority to the client. For example, an individual cannot raise his arm and wants to be able to brush his hair. Is it because he lacks passive range of motion? Strength? Does he lose his balance with only one or no upper extremity support? Does he know where his arm is in space? Is it a motor-planning problem? The therapist observes other areas of self-care and deter-

---

▼ **BOX 16-1**

Sample Questions for Critical Analysis of Assessment Instruments or Strategies

1. Are the philosophy, rationale, and frame of reference used in constructing the instrument evident and accessible?
2. Are guidelines set forth for potential examiners in terms of training, credentials, or theoretical background?
3. Is adequate information available regarding the method of standardization (or formalization), the standardization sample, or field testing?
4. Are the statistics and statistical methods appropriate and understandable?
5. What evidence exists for the instrument's validity?
6. Are reliability values acceptable?
7. Is the training process explicitly presented or offered to insure interrater reliability?
8. Do test scores reasonably lend themselves to interpretation?
9. Is the instrument under consideration designed and/or standardized for the population on which you wish to use it?
10. Is the manual complete, well organized, and easy to use?
11. Is the complexity of administration congruent with the levels of required training and potential clinical decisions?
12. Are administration procedures clear and precise?
13. Does the assessment take a reasonable amount of time to conduct?
14. Is the test format organized, logical, and appealing?
15. Is all the necessary equipment included? Is it safe, durable, manageable, and replaceable?
16. Would you consider this a cost effective assessment strategy?
17. Is this test or strategy of a quality that would be respected by other health professionals?
18. Were references and corollary studies cited or conducted?
19. Does the assessment represent the highest state of the art in its target area?

(Developed by K. J. Opacich, Department of Occupational Therapy, Rush University. Reprinted with permission from Opacich, K. [1991]. Assessment and informed decision-making. In C. Christiansen & C. Baum (Eds.). *Occupational therapy. Overcoming human performance deficits.* [p. 369]. Thorofare, NJ: Slack.)

---

mines that the client has limited shoulder flexion and external rotation. Given those observations, the clinician (1) checks the medical record for previous injury (ie, rotator cuff tear), (2) interviews the client for any recent trauma to the area, and (3) initially evaluates passive range of motion, muscle tone, muscle strength, glenohumeral and scapular soft tissue integrity, scapular mobility, and scapulohumeral rhythm.

Although additional information is important, significant time is not spent on sensory examination (the individual can feel and manipulate items safely), specific muscle test of C6, 7, 8 myotomes (the client's upper extremity strength appears normal distal to the elbow), sitting balance, or coordination tests. Clinical evaluation of the following performance components are described below: **sensation**, **range of motion**, **muscle tone**, **muscle strength**, soft tissue integrity, **reflexes**, **endurance**, and **coordination**.

▼ SENSORY TESTING

Purpose

Sensation supplies our nervous system with information that allows us to develop accurate and reliable maps of ourselves and the environment. Problems with the peripheral nervous system diminish transmission to the brain. Damage to the brain interferes with perception, interpretation or integration of sensory information. Occupational therapists use sensory testing to detect deficits that may interfere with safety, motor control, motor retraining, speed of performance, and most importantly, function. Evaluation of sensation is appropriate for persons with peripheral or central nervous system disorders. Typical diagnoses include burn injury, peripheral nerve injury, spinal cord injury, cerebral vascular accident, brain injury, and complex upper-extremity fracture. Results of the sensory evaluation determine the need for teaching precautions against injury, compensatory techniques (personal and environmental), or **sensory re-education**. They can also document neural recovery, as in a peripheral nerve injury (Bentzel, 1995; Dunn, 1991; Pedretti, 1996c).

Professional Roles

Occupational therapists' roles in sensory testing vary slightly, depending on the facility where they work. Areas typically evaluated by occupational therapy include the primary and discriminative somatic systems, which convey sensory information from skin, joints, and skeletal muscles. Other areas that may be evaluated by an occupational therapist or other professionals include:

Vision: Light perception, conjugate movement, visual field, visual activity, visual range of motion, saccade. Professionals involved include the occupational therapist, optometrist, ophthalmologist, neurologist, neurophthalmologist, or some combination thereof.

Hearing: Responsiveness to auditory stimulation, recognition of auditory stimulation, localization to auditory stimulation, and acuity. Professionals involved include an audiologist, speech and language pathologist, ear, nose, and throat (ENT) physician.

Olfaction: Ability to detect, identify various odors, and make bilateral comparisons. Professionals involved include the occupatioinal therapist, speech and language pathologist, and ENT physician.

Gustation: As it relates to taste, salivation trigger, and swallowing. Professionals involved include the occupational therapist, speech and language pathologist, and ENT physician.

By having a knowledge of data collected by other professionals and its relation to occupational therapy data, therapists can create more cohesive intervention strategies (Dunn, 1991). Table 16–1 summarizes sensory components of tests frequently used by occupational therapists and other professionals.

Somatic Sensation Testing

GENERAL METHODOLOGY PRINCIPLES

The following principles apply to all somatic sensation testing.

1. Explain the procedure to the client. Ask for feedback or questions.
2. Give instructions when the client's eyes are not occluded. Demonstrate on noninvolved extremity if there is one.
3. Test nonaffected area to
   a. Determine client's understanding.
   b. Establish what is normal for that individual.
4. Occlude client's vision (eg, with a manila folder, screen, eyes closed). Have client open eyes in between tests to avoid dizziness or disorientation.
5. Apply stimuli.
   a. Proximal to distal.
   b. Randomly interspersed with nonpresentation trials.
   c. On dorsal and ventral surfaces.
6. If client cannot respond verbally, he or she can point to a duplicate stimulus or picture or replicate movement if appropriate.
7. Enter results on form; date and sign it.
8. Scoring, definitions, and recording methods should be consistent (Smith, 1993; Bentzel, 1995)

The environment should be conducive to testing. The client should understand the general purpose and specific procedure and be able to actively participate and communicate responses. Specific testing procedures for primary and discriminative somatic sensation are delineated below.

PRIMARY SOMATIC SYSTEM

1. *Light touch* (ability to feel light touch)
   Stimulus: Light touch on a small area of the client's skin with a cotton swab, eraser tip, or therapist's fingertip.
   Response: Client gives an indication when stimulus is felt with a response of "now," "yes," describe or point to location (Bentzel, 1995; Dunn, 1991; Pedretti, 1996c)

Fine gradations of light touch can be evaluated using the Semmes-Weinstein Calibrated Monofilament Test. This test

TABLE 16-1. Summary of Sensory Components of Tests Used by Occupational Therapists

Test Name	Sensory/Perceptual Subtest	O	G	A	Vis	S
Balcones Sensory Integration Screening	Finger to nose					
	Standing balance				X	
	Visual motor forms				X	
	Arm postures					
	Stereognosis					
	Tactile graphics					X
Beery Developmental Test of Visual Motor Integration					X	X
DeGangi-Berk Test of Sensory Integration	Postural control items					
Marianne Frostig Developmental Test of Visual Perception	All subtests				X	
Miller Assessment for Preschoolers	Foundations Index				X	X
	Coordination Index					
	Complex Task Index				X	
	Behaviors and Observations					X
Motor free Visual Perception Test	All subtests				X	
Sensory Integration and Praxis Tests	Visual subtests				X	
	Somatosensory subtests					X
Quick Neurological Screen Test	Figure recognition and production				X	
	Palm form recognition					X
	Sound patterns			X		
	Double simultaneous stimuli					X
	Arm and leg extension					
	Stand on one leg			X	X	X
	Behavior irregularities					
Southern California Postrotary Nystagmus Test						
Southern California Sensory Integration Tests	Visual subtests				X	
	Somatosensory subtests					X
Test of Visual Motor Skills					X	
Test of Visual Perceptual Skills (non-motor)	All subtests				X	

*O = olfactory; G = gustatory; A = auditory; Vis = visual; S = somatosensory; Ves = vestibular; P = proprioceptive; LD = learning disabled

This information was compiled from the following sources: Keyser, D.J. & Sweetland, R.C. (Eds.) (1984) Test critiques. Test Corporation of America, Kansas City; Sweetland, R.C. & Keyser, D.J. (1986) Tests. Test Corporation of America, Kansas City; Mitchell, J.V. (Ed.) (1985). The Ninth mental measurement yearbook. The Buros Institute of Mental Measurements, Lincoln, NB; King-Thomas, L. & Hacker, B.J. (Eds.) (1987). A therapist's guide to pediatric assessment. Little, Brown & Co., Boston; Compton, C. (1984). A guide to 75 tests for special education. Fearon Education, Belmont, CA; Sattler, J.M. (1982). Assessment of children's intelligence and special abilities (2nd Ed.). Allyn and Bacon, Inc., Boston; Ayres, J. (1989). Sensory integration and praxis tests manual. Los Angeles: Western Psychological Services. Test manuals were used when they could be obtained. (Reprinted with permission from Cnristiansen & Baum (Eds.) (1991). Dunn, W. (1991). Assessing sensory performance enablers. In C. Christiansen & C. Baum (Eds.). Overcoming human performance deficits (pp. 474–475). Thorofare, NJ: Slack.)

Ves	P	Age Group	Diagnosis	Validity	Reliability	Norms
	X	Primary grades	Learning			130
X	X		Neurological behavior			Children 6–9 yr
	X					
		2–15 yr	Developmental Neurological LD	Construct	Interrater	1039 Normal
X	X	3–5 yr	Developmental delays	Construct	Test–retest	101 Normal; 38 delayed
		4–8 yr	Learning problems	Predictive	Test–retest	100 Normal
	X	2 yr 9 mo–5 yr	Developmental at-risk	Criterion–relation	Test–retest	1200 Normal
	X					
	X					
X	X					
		4–8 yr	All types	Construct	Test–retest	881 Normal 22 states
	X	4–9 yr	Learning and behavior problems	Construct Criterion Content	Test–retest Interrater	1997 Children
		5 yr+	Neurological	Interrater	Test–retest	1231 normal; 1008 LD
X	X					
	X					
X		5–9 yr	Learning problems		Interrater	226 normal
	X	4–8 yr 11 mo for sensory tests	Learning problems		Test–retest	Somato 953; normal visual 240; normal
		4–12 yr 11 mo	Learning problems	Content Criterion	Internal consistency	1000+ normal
		4–12 yr 11 mo	Learning problems	Content Criterion	Internal consistency	962 normal

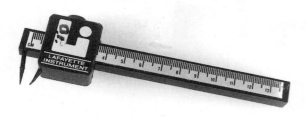

▲
Figure 16-1. Aesthesiometer. (Photo courtesy of the Rehabilitation Institute of Chicago.)

controls the amount of force applied to the client's hand by a calibrated, handheld instrument. This type of evaluation is particularly important for clients with peripheral nerve involvement. The Semmes–Weinstein Monofilament Test has intra- and interinstrument and intra- and interrater reliability as well as administration and interpretation guidelines (Fess, 1993).

2. *Pain* (ability to feel pain)
   Stimulus: Safety pin with one sharp, one blunt end. Therapist applies mixed sharp and dull stimuli randomly with same degree of pressure.
   Response: Client gives an indication when and which stimulus is felt by answering "sharp" or "dull."
   Note. Pin should be cleaned with an alcohol swab before and after testing (Bentzel, 1995; Dunn, 1991; Pedretti, 1996c).
3. *Temperature* (ability to distinguish variations in temperature)
   Stimulus: Capped test tubes (metal conducts better than glass); one filled with ice water, one with hot tap water tolerable to normal touch. Randomly alternate use of each stimulus, keeping on body surface long enough to allow a temperature change to occur on the skin (approximately 1 second).
   Response: Client gives an indication of which stimulus is felt by answering "hot" or "cold" to each stimulus (Bentzel, 1995; Dunn, 1991; Pedretti, 1996c).

DISCRIMINATIVE SOMATIC SYSTEM

1. **Tactile localization (ability to localize touch)**
   Stimulus: Therapist touches client's skin with eraser tip or fingertip. Stimulus intensity and duration significantly influence accuracy of response.
   Response: After each stimulus, client opens eyes and places finger on or describes area touched (Bentzel, 1995).

2. *Two point discrimination* (ability to perceive two distinct stimuli when touched with two stimuli simultaneously)
   Stimulus: Aesthesiometer (Fig. 16–1), Boley Gauge, or paper clip. Two points are applied simultaneously along the longitudinal axis in the center of the zone to be tested, with equal light pressure to the palmar surface of the forearm, hand, and fingers. Therapist adjusts the distance between the double stimuli during testing to identify the amount of distance needed between the two stimuli before the client perceives that two stimuli are present. One point application trials are interspersed with test trials.
   Response: Client identifies stimulus with an answer of "one" or "two" points. A score is recorded for each skin area examined. Several normative values exist for distance between the double stimuli felt (Bentzel, 1995; Dunn, 1991).
3. *Stereognosis* (ability to identify objects tactually)
   Stimulus: Common object is placed in individual's hand (ie, pen, key, quarter, cotton ball). Individual is asked to manipulate and identify the object. The test is not appropriate if client is unable to manipulate object on own.
   Response: Client names object(s) as it is identified, describes properties if unable to name object, or points to a choice from a photograph or display of identical objects (Bentzel, 1995; Dunn, 1991; Pedretti, 1996c).
4. *Proprioception* (ability to identify limb position in space without vision)
   Stimulus: Therapist holds body part being tested laterally to avoid cutaneous input and slowly, passively positions the joint being tested. Joints are tested singly and in combination.
   Response: Client is asked to reproduce the position with the opposite extremity. If unable to copy limb position, a verbal response may be given such as "up" or "down," or the client may use a gesture or point to directional arrows (Bentzel, 1995; Dunn, 1991; Pedretti, 1996c).
4. *Kinesthesia* (movement sense)
   Stimulus: Therapist holds body part being tested laterally to reduce **tactile** input and moves the joint up or down. Level of detection of kinesthesia is influenced by velocity. It is easier to detect brisk movement.
   Response: After each stimulus, the client indicates in which direction the body part was moved (Pedretti, 1996c).

Recording Results

Recorded results should be specific enough to enable future comparison of progress and to communicate useful information to others. Sensation could be recorded as intact, impaired, or absent. Recording options include graphic methods (Fig. 16–2), diagrams, peripheral nerve distribution, dermatome distribution (Fig. 16–3), or the number correct, or the number of trials (such as stereognosis).

Pain/Temp				Proprioception			Two Point Discrimination			
L	R			L	R		N: .3–.6 cm	P: .6–1.2 cm	S: 1.2....cm	
	C4			Shoulder						
	C5			Elbow						
	C6			Wrist				L		R
	C7			Hand				C6		
	C8							C7		
	T1							C8		

Figure 16-2. Sensory record for pain/temperature and two-point discrimination by dermatome and for proprioception by joint. (Reprinted with permission from the Rehabilitation Institute of Chicago.)

Note. N=no apparent deficit; P=partial deficit; S=severe deficit; NE=not examined. Recordings made in unshaded areas.

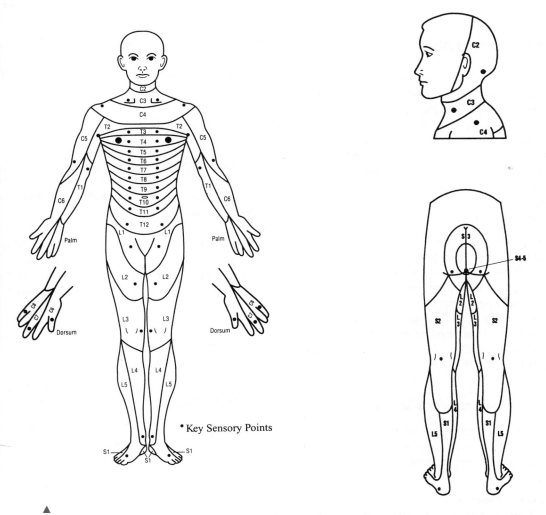

• Key Sensory Points

Figure 16-3. Dermatome chart for recording results of sensory testing. (© American Spinal Injury Association. From *International standards for neurological and functional classification of spinal cord injury*. Revised 1996.)

Interpreting Results

Therapists must be alert to the influence of cognitive, perceptual, psychosocial, and motor deficits on sensory performance. Some clients may not be able to attend to or appreciate the abstract nature of tests used to evaluate sensation. They may have difficulty comprehending instructions, may guess at responses, or may find the procedure irrelevant and not fully participate. It is important to ask the client to describe (if able) what he or she feels. Observe clients during functional activities. Do they use proper force when grasping an object? Do they acknowledge or feel uncomfortable when touched? Are they aware of the position of their extremities when getting dressed? Do they drop items when not looking directly at the item? If sensation appears to be a contributing source to performance problems, accurately identify which deficits contribute to the problems. Educate the client, team members, and caregivers to the deficits and potential functional ramifications, such as safety issues, compensatory techniques, and environmental adaptations to facilitate sensory awareness and processing (Dunn, 1991; Okkema, 1993a).

▼ RANGE OF MOTION

Range of motion (ROM) is the arc of motion through which a joint passes. Passive range of motion (PROM) is the arc of motion through which the joint passes when moved by an outside force. Active range of motion (AROM) is the arc of motion through which the joint passes when moved by muscles acting on the joint. Joint structure and the integrity of surrounding tissues determine the directions and limits of motion for any given joint (Pedretti, 1996a; Trombly, 1995a).

The occupational therapist evaluates ROM to

1. Determine limitations that affect function
2. Determine limitations that may produce deformity
3. Determine additional range needed for function
4. Keep a record of progression or regression
5. Determine appropriate treatment goals
6. Determine the need for splints, assistive devices, or both
7. Select appropriate treatment modalities, positioning techniques, and other strategies to decrease limitations (Pedretti, 1996a; Trombly, 1995a).

Goniometric Measurement Tools

A goniometer is the instrument used to measure joint ROM. Goniometers can be metal or plastic, come in several sizes, and are available from medical and rehabilitation equipment companies.

Goniometer Parts and Functions

Protractor: A half-circle, attached to the stationary bar, printed with a scale of degrees from zero to 180° in each direction, permits measurement of motion in both directions (ie, flexion and extension) without reversing the tool.

Stationary bar: Attached to the axis.

Movable bar: Also attached to the axis.

Axis: Where the two arms are riveted together. Acts as the fulcrum; it must move freely, yet be tight enough to remain where it was set when the goniometer is removed from the body segment following joint measurement (Figs. 16–4 and 16–5).

A neutral zero method for measuring and recording is recommended by the Committee on Joint Motion of the American Academy of Orthopedic Surgeons. Most clinics use this 180-degree system where:

1. 0 degrees is the starting position for all joint motions.
2. Anatomic position is the starting position.
3. 180 degrees is superimposed as a semicircle on the body in the plane in which the motion will occur.
4. The axis of the joint is the axis of the semicircle or arc of motion.
5. All joint motions begin at 0 degrees and increase toward 180° (Pedretti, 1996a; Trombly, 1995a).

Other measurement systems used include the 360-degree system where 180 degrees is a starting position and motion occurs toward 0 degrees (Pedretti, 1996a; Trombly, 1995a).

General Principles

Formal joint measurement is not necessary with every client, especially when limited ROM is not anticipated. Typical diagnoses that may necessitate closer attention include **arthritis**, fractures, **cerebrovascular accident (CVA)**, and **spinal cord injury**. AROM can be visually observed during activities of daily living (ADL) or by having the client move through various positions. All joints can be put briefly through PROM (Pedretti, 1996a).

Normal ROM varies from one person to the next. Ranges are listed in the literature and on most recording

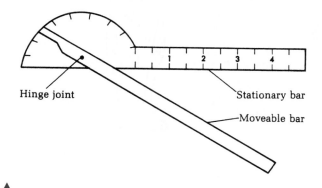

▲

Figure 16-4. Goniometer.

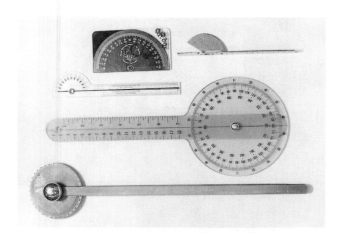

▲
Figure 16-5. Goniometers. (Photo courtesy of the Rehabilitation Institute of Chicago.)

forms. One could also measure the uninvolved extremity as a normal comparison. A medical history should be noted for any previous joint injury or secondary diagnosis affecting ROM. The ROM can be limited by pain. Joints should not be forced beyond the point of resistance during PROM (Pedretti, 1996a).

When evaluating ROM, the therapist may need to provide outside support or stability so the individual is free to concentrate and attempt the desired movement, as opposed to "fixing" in order to even sit upright. One should also evaluate scapular mobility, thoracic spinal extension, head and neck positioning before proceeding with shoulder joint measurements, as these all affect glenohumeral joint motion (Pedretti, 1996a).

Finally, before actual evaluation, the therapist needs to know the average normal ROM, how the joint moves, and how to position himself or herself, the client, and the joints for measurement. One should think about comfort as well as body mechanics to protect oneself and the client while placing the goniometer and providing support to the joint being tested.

ROM Evaluation Procedure
1. Position client comfortably.
2. Explain and demonstrate to client what you are doing and why.
3. Stabilize joint proximal to joint being measured.
4. Observe available movement by having client move joint or examiner move joint passively to get a sense of joint mobility.
5. Place goniometer axis over joint axis in starting position. Stationary bar goes over stationary bone proximal to the joint, parallel to the longitudinal axis of the bone. Movable bar goes over movable bone distal to the joint, parallel to the longitudinal axis of the bone. Face top of goniometer protractor away from the direction of movement to avoid goniometer dial (end of movable bar) going off the measurement scale.

6. Record the number of degrees at starting position.
7. Hold the body part securely above and below the joint being measured. Gently move the joint through the available PROM. Do not use excessive force. Note any **crepitus**. Stop at any point of pain or end of range. The axis of motion for some joints coincides with bony landmarks. Other joint axes are found by observing the movement of the joint to determine the point around which the motion occurs.
8. Return limb to resting position.
9. Record the number of degrees at the final position. Note in which position the joint measurement was taken when more than one position can be used (ie, shoulder internal or external rotation). Date and sign.

Figures 16–6 through 16–11 show examples of goniometer measurements for shoulder abduction elbow flexion and wrist extension. Things that influence accuracy and reliability of goniometer measurement include the type of support given to the body part, bulky clothing, environmental factors, such as temperature, time of day, client fatigue, reaction to pain, and examiner experience (LaStays & Wheeler, 1994; Pedretti, 1996a; Riddle, 1992; Wei, McQuade, & Smidt, 1993).

Recording Results

When using the 180-degree system, the evaluator should record the number of degrees at the starting position and

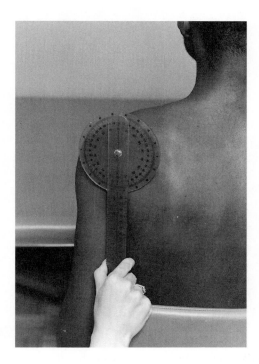

▲
Figure 16-6. Goniometric measurement of shoulder abduction—starting position. (Photo courtesy of the Rehabilitation Institute of Chicago.)

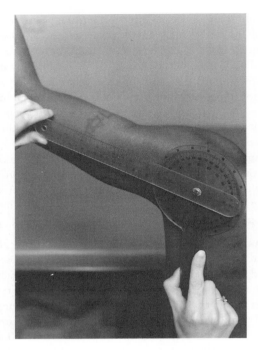

▲

Figure 16-7. Goniometric measurement of shoulder abduction. (Photo courtesy of the Rehabilitation Institute of Chicago.)

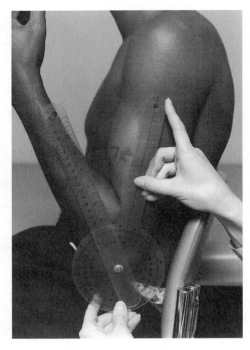

▲

Figure 16-9. Goniometric measurement of elbow flexion. (Photo courtesy of the Rehabilitation Institute of Chicago.)

the number of degrees at the final position after the joint has passed through the maximal possible arc of motion. Normal ROM starts at 0 degrees and increases toward 180 degrees. A limitation can be indicated at either end of the scale; for example, for the elbow:

0–140 degrees	Normal
20–140 degrees	Limited extension
0–100 degrees	Limited flexion
(Pedretti, 1996a)	

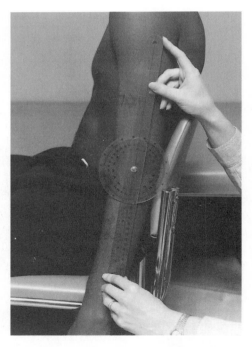

▲

Figure 16-8. Goniometric measurement of elbow flexion—starting position. (Photo courtesy of the Rehabilitation Institute of Chicago.)

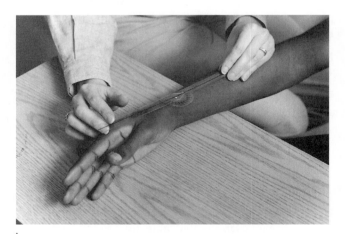

▲

Figure 16-10. Goniometric measurement of writst extension—starting position. (Photo courtesy of the Rehabilitation Institute of Chicago.)

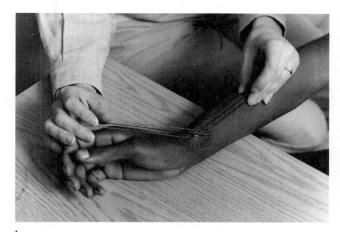

▲
Figure 16-11. Goniometric measurement of wrist extension. (Photo courtesy of the Rehabilitation Institute of Chicago.)

A sample form for recording ROM measurements is shown in Figure 16–12.

Interpreting Results

A therapist should focus on ranges that fall below functional limits; that is, the amount of joint range necessary to perform ADL without the use of special equipment. Evaluate what is causing the decreased range. Is it pain, edema, muscle weakness, skin adhesions, **spasticity**, bony obstruction or destruction, or soft tissue **contracture**? Is the cause changeable? Can you increase active range or prevent further loss with stretching, strengthening, orthotic management, casting, or modalities? Treatment goals should reflect the identified problem. If the available range is not expected to change, one should focus on adaptive techniques or use of adaptive equipment to perform the desired task (Pedretti, 1996a; Trombly, 1995a).

▼ MUSCLE TONE

Definitions

Muscle tone can be defined in several ways. Barrows (1980) defines it as resistance offered by a muscle to a stretch when a joint is passively moved. Brooks (1986) defined muscle tone as resistance to stretch that is generated by lower motor neuron activity, viscoelastic properties of muscles and joints, and sensory feedback. Chusid and DeGroot (1988) state that tone is a continuous mild contraction of the muscle tissue in its resting state. Undzis, Zoltan, and Pedretti (1996) add that muscle tone is dependent on the integrity of the peripheral and central nervous system mechanisms as well as muscle contractility, elasticity, ductility, and extensibility. Normal muscle tone varies from person to person and can be dependent on age, sex, and occupation. Normal tone can be

characterized by the ability to move against gravity, shift between stability and mobility, use muscles in groups or selectively, and balance between agonist and antagonists (Undzis, Zoltan, & Pedretti, 1996).

The level of tone in a muscle can be increased or decreased by damage to the nervous system. Figure 16–13 exhibits this continuum.

HYPOTONIA

Hypotonia is characterized by decreased muscle tone resulting from hyporesponsiveness to sensory stimulation and efferent commands. Clinically, muscles appear soft, flabby, and lax. This, in addition to weak cocontraction around proximal joints, may result in a wider range for passive ROM. Deep tendon reflexes are diminished or absent. Hypotonia occurs in primary muscle diseases, cerebellar lesions, **lower motor neuron** disorders, and the initial phases of **cerebral vascular accident** and **spinal cord injury** (Undzis et al, 1996; Warren, 1991).

SPASTICITY

Spasticity is a motor disorder characterized by a velocity-dependent increase in tonic stretch reflexes, with exaggerated tendon jerks, resulting from hyperexcitability of the stretch reflex as one component of the **upper motor neuron** syndrome (Katz & Rymer, 1989; Katz, Rovai, Brait, & Rymer, 1992). The selective nature of spasticity results in a disruption of synergistic movement caused by an imbalance between muscle groups. Clinically, characteristics of spasticity include hypertonic muscles, hyperactive deep tendon reflexes, clonus, abnormal spinal reflexes, increased resistance to passive movement, and decreased motor coordination. Spasticity occurs in upper motor neuron disorders such as **multiple sclerosis**, **cerebral palsy**, spinal cord injury, cerebral vascular accident, and **traumatic brain injury** (Undzis et al, 1996; Warren, 1991).

Spasticity is influenced by postural reflex mechanisms as well as extrinsic factors such as contracture, anxiety, temperature extremes and emotional or physical pain. It can be characterized as mild, moderate, or severe (Table 16–2).

RIGIDITY

Rigidity is the simultaneous increase of muscle tone in agonistic and antagonistic muscles that results in increased resistance to passive movement in any direction throughout the ROM. "Lead pipe" rigidity is characterized by a feeling of constant rigidity throughout the available ROM. "Cogwheel" rigidity is characterized by a tremor superimposed on rigidity causing alternate contraction and relaxation throughout the ROM. Rigidity occurs in extrapyramidal system lesions such as **Parkinson's disease**, encephalitis, or tumors. Rigidity and spasticity may both be present in a muscle group (Mathiowetz & Haugen, 1995; Undzis et al, 1996).

Name:									
RIC #:									
Physician:									

				JOINT RANGE MEASUREMENTS						
AROM	AROM	PROM	PROM				PROM	PROM	AROM	AROM
Date	Date	Date	Date				Date	Date	Date	Date
				< - Left	Right - >					
				Flexion	0-180					
				Extension	0-60					
				Abduction	0-180					
				External Rotation	0-90	Shoulder				
				Internal Rotation	0-70					
				Horiz. Abduction	0-90					
				Horiz. Adduction	0-45					
				Flexion	0-150					
				Supination	0-80	Elbow				
				Pronation	0-80					
				Flexion	0-80					
				Extension	0-70	Wrist				
				Ulnar Dev.	0-30					
				Radial Dev.	0-20					
				M.P. Flexion	0-50	Thumb				
				I. P. Flexion	0-80					
				Abduction	0-70					
				M. P. Flexion	0-90					
				M. P. Extension	0-45	Index F.				
				P. I. P. Flexion	0-100					
				D. I. P. Flexion	0-80					
				M. P. Flexion	0-90					
				M. P. Extension	0-45	Long F.				
				P. I. P. Flexion	0-100					
				D. I. P. Flexion	0-90					
				M. P. Flexion	0-90					
				M. P. Extension	0-45	Ring F.				
				P. I. P. Flexion	0-100					
				D. I. P. Flexion	0-90					
				M. P. Flexion	0-90					
				M. P. Extension	0-45	Little F.				
				P. I. P. Flexion	0-100					
				D. I. P. Flexion	0-90					

◄

Figure 16-12. Form for recording range of motion measurements. (Reprinted with permission from the Rehabilitation Institute of Chicago.)

Hypotonia (Floppy; Flaccid)	Normal Muscle Tissue	Hypertonia (Spasticity; Rigidity)
LESS ◄ - - - -	- - - - - - - - - - - - - -	- - - - ► MORE

▲

Figure 16-13. Muscle tone changes possible with central nervous system changes.

Purpose of Muscle Tone Evaluation

The occupational therapist evaluates muscle tone to

1. Establish a baseline
2. Plan treatment and select treatment methods
3. Train client in special methods or use of assistive devices to accomplish functional tasks
4. Structure environmental factors to minimize negative effects of abnormal tone (Undzis et al, 1996)

Methods of Measurement

To date, it has been difficult to achieve both reliability and validity when measuring muscle tone. There is no standardized procedure. Various electromyographic, biomechanical, and myotonometric methods have varying degrees of success. Often, evaluation equipment is expensive and more suited to research than to clinical applications (Undzis et al, 1996; Worley et al, 1991).

Clinically, numerous methods exist. The most common method of measuring tone is by grasping the body part gently, firmly, and moving it briskly through the desired movement pattern. The Ashworth (1964) scale grades tone from a 0 (no increase in tone) to a 4 (limb is rigid in flexion or extension). Bohannan and Smith (1987) modified Ashworth's scale by adding an additional level, incorporating the angle at which resistance appeared, and controlling the speed of passive movement with a 1-second count (Table 16–3).

Brennan (1959) measured ROM that is possible before resistance to movement is felt. King (1987) established a five-point rating scale for each of four functions: presence of tone, AROM, alternating movement, and resistance to passive movement. Bobath (1978) described a method of evaluating the combined effects of tone and primitive reflexes. Clients' limbs are moved in normal patterns of usage, and the adaptation of the different muscle groups to changes in position are noted. Fugl-Meyer, Jaasko, Leyman, Olson, and Steglind (1975) established an objective method to measure function as well as movement in hemiparetic clients (Table 16–4).

Recording Results

When recording results, one should note the position in which testing was done, the presence of abnormal reflexes, as well as any external factors that may influence results. This may include environmental temperature, time of day, and medications. One should note the presence, degree, distribution, and type of abnormal tone, as well as its effect on the client's ability to perform ADL. This can be done graphically, with a table, or in narrative form.

Interpreting Results

If a client has abnormal tone, one should ask several questions. First, does it affect function? What influences the

TABLE 16-2. Categories of Spasticity

Mild Spasticity	Moderate Spasticity	Severe Spasticity
Stretch reflex occurs in last 1/4 of range	Stretch reflex occurs midrange	Stretch reflex occurs in initial 1/4 range
Slight imbalance in tone between agonist and antagonist	Marked imbalance of tone between agonist and antagonist	Severe imbalance of tone between agonist and antagonist
Mild increased resistance to passive stretch	Considerable resistance to passive stretch; able to move through full PROM	Marked resistance to passive movement unable to complete full PROM
May exhibit slight decreased mobility and ability to perform fine, selective movements	May exhibit slow gross movements that require increased effort and show decreased coordination	Significant decreased or lack of active movement, may exhibit joint contractures

PROM = passive range of motion
(Mathiowetz & Haugen, 1995; Undzis et al, 1996)

TABLE 16-3. Modified Ashworth Scale

Grade	Description
0	No increase in muscle tone
I	Slight increase in tone, manifested by a catch and release or by minimal resistance at the end of the range of motion (ROM) when the affected part is moved in flexion or extension
+I	Slight increase in muscle tone, manifested by a catch, followed by minimal resistance throughout the remainder (less than half) of the ROM
2	More marked increase in muscle tone through most of the ROM, but affected part easily moved
3	Considerable increase in muscle tone, passive movement difficult
4	Affected part rigid in flexion or extension

(Reprinted from Physical Therapy, *Bohannon, R.W. & Smith, M.B. Interrater reliability of a modified Ashworth scale of muscle spasticity, 1987; 67, 207, with permission of the American Physical Therapy Association.)*

tone—position of the head, hips, or trunk? Does a combination of muscle tones exist? Do medications have a pharmacological effect? Do facilitation or inhibitory techniques have any short- or long-term effect?

If low tone is present, a muscle test can determine the degree of weakness. If recovery from low tone is expected, graded exercise and therapeutic activity is appropriate. Adaptive equipment may be necessary on a short- or long-term basis. Positioning should protect weak muscles from overstretching.

High muscle tone necessitates techniques to maintain ROM, perform ADL, and position in patterns opposite the spastic patterns. Inhibitory techniques depend on the nature and severity of the disability, abnormal tone distribution, and other concomitant problems (Undzis et al, 1996; Warren, 1991; Mathiowetz & Haugen, 1995)

▼ MUSCLE STRENGTH

Definition and Purpose

Muscle strength can be defined as "the capacity of a muscle to produce the tension necessary for maintaining posture, initiating movement or controlling movement during conditions of loading on the musculoskeletal system" (Markos,

1977). Clinical evaluation of muscle strength examines the maximal contraction of a muscle or muscle group when apparent weakness or difficulties with function exist. Muscle weakness is typically seen in lower motor neuron disorders, primary muscle diseases, and neurological diseases. Disabilities that cause disuse or immobilization, such as burn, arthritis, and amputation, can also cause weakness (Pedretti, 1996b; Trombly, 1995a).

Evaluation of muscle strength can

1. Facilitate diagnosis in some neuromuscular conditions (ie, spinal cord injury, peripheral nerve lesion)
2. Establish a baseline for treatment
3. Determine if weakness is limiting performance
4. Determine the need for compensatory measures or assistive devices on a temporary or long-term basis, depending on the nature of the disability
5. Make evident a muscle imbalance that may require strengthening if possible or orthotic intervention to prevent deformity
6. Evaluate the effectiveness of treatment

Muscle strength can be measured by spring scales, tensiometers, dynamometers, weights, or manual resistance. The evaluation of muscle strength does not measure endurance, coordination, or performance capabilities (Pedretti, 1996b).

TABLE 16-4. FuGL–Meyer Scale of Functional Return after Hemiplegia

Grade	Movement of the Shoulder, Elbow, Forearm, and Lower Extremity
I	Muscle stretch reflexes can be elicited
II	Volitional movements can be performed within the dynamic flexor–extensor synergies
III	Volitional motion is performed mixing dynamic flexor and extensor synergies
IV	Volitional movements are performed with little or no synergy dependence
V	Normal muscle stretch reflexes

General Principles

Gross muscle testing evaluates the strength of groups of muscles that perform specific movements at each joint (ie, elbow flexors). Manual muscle testing evaluates individual muscles (ie, biceps, brachialis, brachioradialis). A therapist might first observe functional performance and then decide to focus on a certain muscle group based on the outcome of the observation. Certain diagnoses, such as spinal cord injury, Guillan Barré syndrome, and peripheral nerve injury, may necessitate specific muscle testing as opposed to a diagnosis of generalized weakness, lower extremity amputee, or hip replacement, which lend themselves to gross muscle testing.

To perform muscle testing, a therapist needs to know muscles and their functions, anatomic position and direction of muscle fibers, and angle of pull on joints. Substitution patterns (ie, when a muscle or muscle group attempts to compensate for lack of function in a weak or paralyzed muscle) should be expected and targeted (ie, shoulder external rotation and eccentric lengthening of biceps versus triceps elbow extension in gravity-eliminated position).

Muscle testing cannot be used accurately with clients who have upper motor neuron disorders. In these clients, hypertonicity muscle tone and movement tend to occur in gross synergistic patterns and may be influenced by primitive reflexes (Pedretti, 1996b). Note that in spinal cord injury, which is an upper motor neuron disorder, the muscles being tested are those innervated by spinal cord segments above the level of the injury.

Gravity influences muscle function. Gravity-eliminated positions are used with (O-P+ or 0-2+) grades. Movements against gravity are used with (F-N or 3-5) grades. Definitions for muscle grades are relatively standard (Table 16–5).

Assignment of muscle grades depends on clinical judgment, knowledge, and examiner experience. The amount of resistance given (ie, slight, moderate, or full) is determined by the client's age, sex, body type, and occupation. The amount of resistance given also varies from one muscle group to the next. One must consider the size and relative muscle power and leverage used when giving resistance. That is, one would not apply the same force to finger flexors as to shoulder flexors (Daniels & Worthingham, 1986; Kendall, McCreary, & Provance, 1993; Pedretti, 1996b; Rancho, 1978; Trombly, 1995a).

In individual cases, positioning for muscle testing in the correct plane may not be possible due to medical precautions, immobilization devices, trunk instability, or weakness. Modifications in positioning and grading are cited for individual tests in muscle-testing manuals (Daniels & Worthingham, 1986; Kendall et al, 1993). Lamb (1985) discusses various aspects of manual muscle testing, including variables of testing procedures, reliability, and validity issues. Differences in methods (ie, force application, stabilization, and positioning) and strength determination during controlled studies are discussed by Smidt and Roger (1982).

Procedure for Muscle Testing

Whether performing gross or manual muscle testing, certain general procedures apply.

1. Determine available PROM of the joint associated with muscles being examined.
2. Position and stabilize the body part proximal to part being tested.
3. Demonstrate or describe test motion.
4. Ask client to perform movement.
5. Palpate by placing fingerpads firmly and gently over muscle tendon or belly.
6. Observe client's movement.
7. Ask client to hold position.
8. For grades above fair or 3, resist
   a. In the opposite direction of test movement

TABLE 16-5. Muscle Testing Grades

Number Grade	Word or Letter Grade	Definition
0	Zero (0)	No muscle contraction can be seen or felt.
1	Trace (T)	Contraction can be felt, but there is no motion.
1−	Poor minus (P−)	Part moves through an incomplete ROM with gravity eliminated.
2	Poor (P)	Part moves through a complete ROM with gravity eliminated.
2+	Poor plus (P+)	Part moves through incomplete ROM (less than 50%) against gravity or through complete ROM with gravity eliminated against slight resistance.
3−	Fair minus (F−)	Part moves through an incomplete ROM (more than 50%) against gravity.
3	Fair (F)	Part moves through complete ROM against gravity.
3+	Fair plus (F+)	Part moves through a complete ROM against gravity and slight resistance.
4	Good (G)	Part moves through a complete ROM against gravity and moderate assistance.
5	Normal (N)	Part moves through complete ROM against gravity and full resistance.

(Reprinted with permission from Pedretti, L.W. [1996]. Evaluation of muscle strength. In L.W. Pedretti (Ed.), Occupational therapy. Practice skills for physical dysfunction, [4th Ed.] [p. 113]. St. Louis: C.V. Mosby.)

TABLE 16-6. Suggested Sequence for Muscle Testing

Backlying (supine)

Grades N to F
Scapula abduction and upward rotation
Shoulder horizontal abduction
All tests for forearm, wrist, and fingers can be given in the
   backlying position if necessary

Grades P to O

Shoulder abduction	Hip external rotation
Elbow flexion	Hip internal rotation
Elbow extension	Foot inversion
Hip abduction	Foot eversion
Hip adduction	

Facelying (prone)

Grades N to F

Scapula depression	Shoulder horizontal
Scapula adduction	abduction
Scapula adduction and	Elbow extension
downward rotation	Hip extension
Shoulder extension	Knee flexion
Shoulder external rotation	Ankle plantar flexion
Shoulder internal rotation	

Grades P to O

Scapula elevation	Scapula adduction
Scapula depression	

Sidelying

Grades N to F

Hip abduction	Foot inversion
Hip adduction	Foot eversion

Grades P to O

Shoulder flexion	Knee flexion
Shoulder extension	Knee extension
Hip flexion	Ankle plantar flexion
Hip extension	Ankle dorsiflexion

Sitting

Grades N to F

Scapula elevation	Hip flexion
Shoulder flexion	Hip external rotation
Shoulder abduction	Hip internal rotation
Elbow flexion	Knee extension
All forearm, wrist, finger, and	Ankle dorsiflexion with
thumb movements	inversion

Grades P to O
All forearm, wrist, finger, and thumb movements
Ankle dorsiflexion with inversion

N = normal; F = fair; P = poor; O = zero. See Table 16-5 for more detailed information.

(Reprinted with permission from Pedretti, L.W. [1996]. Evaluation of muscle strength. In L.W. Pedretti [Ed.]. Occupational therapy. Practice skills for physical dysfunction [4th ed.] [p. 117]. St Louis: C.V. Mosby.)

b. At the end of available ROM
c. On the distal end of the moving bone
d. As close to a perpendicular direction as possible (Pedretti, 1996b)

Table 16–6 suggests a sequence of muscle testing that streamlines the clinical evaluation process:

Figures 16–14 through 16–19 illustrate specific muscle testing techniques in both gravity-eliminated and against gravity positions for (1) shoulder abduction (middle deltoid; see Figs. 16–14 and 16–15), (2) elbow flexion (biceps; see Figs. 16–16 and 16–17), and (3) wrist extension (extensor carpi radialis longus; see Figs. 16–18 and 16–19).

Comparison of Rancho–Kendall–Daniels and Worthingham

There are primarily three dominant philosophies and methods for clinical evaluation of muscle strength proposed by (1) Rancho Los Amigos Hospital in Downey, California (1978); (2) Kendall (Kendall et al, 1993); and Daniels and Worthingham (1986). Each philosophy defines muscle grades slightly differently.

RANCHO PHILOSOPHY

The muscle grades in Table 16–7 are described in comparison with a normal muscle. It is important to keep in mind that muscles of normal strength vary in strength tremendously within the body, owing to the size of the muscle and to the work each muscle is normally required to perform. Normal strength likewise varies between individuals, owing to differences in age and body types. Therefore, in grading muscles higher than "fair," the degree of objectivity increases with the therapist's increasing knowledge of normal strength for various age groups and for that particular muscle, previous to the illness or injury.

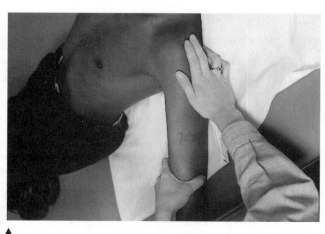

▲
Figure 16-14. Muscle testing for shoulder abduction (middle deltoid) in gravity-eliminated position. (Photo courtesy of the Rehabilitation Institute of Chicago.)

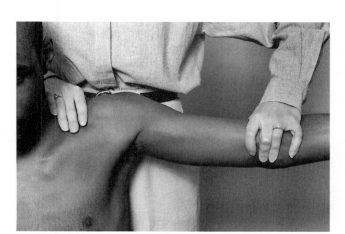

▲
Figure 16-15. Muscle testing for shoulder abduction (middle deltoid) in against-gravity position. (Photo courtesy of the Rehabilitation Institute of Chicago.)

KENDALL PHILOSOPHY

The Kendall philosophy uses isometric "hold" or break tests. The muscle strength required to hold the test position, with few exceptions, is considered equivalent to the muscle strength required to complete the test movement. It also recommends using assistive movements into antigravity positions, rather than frequent position changes, and uses percentage values. Table 16–8 shows the Kendall muscle grades and their definitions.

DANIELS AND WORTHINGHAM PHILOSOPHY

According to Daniels and Worthingham (1986), grading is based on the following three factors:

1. Amount of resistance that can be given manually to a contracting muscle

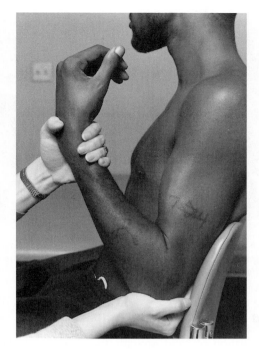

▲
Figure 16-17. Muscle testing for elbow flexion (biceps) in against-gravity position. (Photo courtesy of the Rehabilitation Institute of Chicago.)

2. Ability of muscle to move a part through complete ROM
3. Evidence of the presence or absence of contraction

Table 16–9 shows the Daniels and Worthingham muscle grades and their definitions.

Tables 16–10 and 16–11 describe examples of test position for serratus anterior and rhomboids, respectively, using the three muscle testing methods.

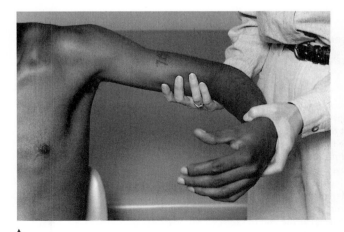

▲
Figure 16-16. Muscle testing for elbow flexion (biceps) in gravity-eliminated position. (Photo courtesy of the Rehabilitation Institute of Chicago.)

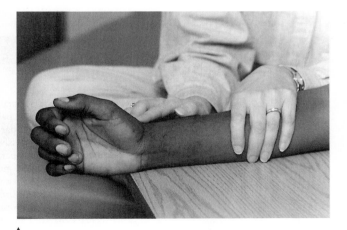

▲
Figure 16-18. Muscle testing for wrist extension (extensor carpi radialis longus) in gravity-eliminated position. (Photo courtesy of the Rehabilitation Institute of Chicago.)

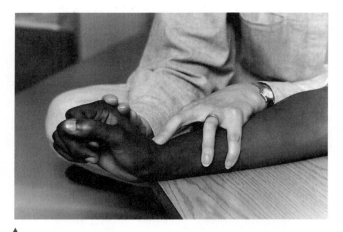

▲
Figure 16-19. Muscle testing for wrist extension (extensor carpi radialis longus) in against-gravity position. (Photo courtesy of the Rehabilitation Institute of Chicago.)

Hand Strength

For evaluation of hand strength, the American Society of Hand Therapists (ASHT) recommends standard methods of measurement on which norms are based. Standardized positioning and instructions are also recommended by Mathiowetz, Volland, Kashman, and Weber (1984). Grip strength is measured by a standard adjustable handle dynamometer. The subject is seated, shoulder adducted, elbow flexed at 90 degrees and forearm in neutral position. An average of three successive forceful grips is taken (Fig. 16–20) (Pedretti, 1996b; Trombly, 1995a; Smith, 1993)

Pinch strength is tested on a standard pinch dynamometer in three ways:

1. Palmar pinch—thumb tip to index finger
2. Lateral pinch—thumb pulp to lateral aspect of middle phalanx of index finger

3. Three-point pinch—thumb tip to tips of index and long fingers

An average of three successive trials is taken (Pedretti, 1996b; Smith, 1993; Trombly, 1995a). Figures 16–21 and 16–22 are illustrations of a pinch dynamometer.

Oral Motor Control

Some occupational therapists evaluate and treat oral motor control problems. This can be done alone or in conjunction with a speech and language pathologist. In some work settings occupational therapists do not address this area at all.

Dysphagia is defined as difficult in swallowing. Swallowing is a multistage sequence that, when normally elicited, momentarily blocks the opening to the respiratory tract as food or beverage is passed through the pharynx and into the esophagus. Swallowing can occur either by willful cortical initiation or by a reflex, elicited independently from higher brain centers (Miller, Groher, Yorkston, & Rees, 1988).

Swallowing has three phases: (1) oral—preparation of the bolus or mass of chewed food; (2) pharyngeal—bolus is propelled through the pharynx away from the airway, and (3) esophageal—a primary peristaltic wave that propels the bolus through the lower esophageal sphincter and into the stomach.

When dysphagia is recognized or a swallowing complaint registered, the examination should include the following: (1) a complete medical history, (2) a description of the complaint and associated symptoms, (3) a physical examination of the peripheral deglutitive motor and sensory system, and (4) motion radiographic studies (Miller et al, 1988).

Nasal regurgitation is a symptom associated with weakness of the palatopharyngeal mechanism. Aspiration of food or liquid into the "windpipe" is a common complaint of clients with neurological impairment of the swallowing

TABLE 16-7. Rancho Muscle Grades		
Letter Grade	**Word Grade**	**Definition**
0	Zero	No movement of part; contraction cannot be palpated.
T	Trace	Contraction can be palpated; no movement of part.
P–	Poor minus	Gravity eliminated, part moves through only a *portion* of the range of *available* (not necessarily normal) passive range of motion.
P	Poor	Gravity eliminated, part moves through complete available range of motion.
F	Fair	Against gravity, part moves through complete available range of motion.
F+	Fair plus	Part moves through complete available range of motion against gravity with "slight" resistance (for that muscle) at end of range.
G	Good	Part moves through complete available range of motion against gravity and takes "good" resistance (for that muscle) at the end of range.
N	Normal	Part moves through complete available range of motion against gravity and takes "normal" resistance (for that muscle) at the end of the range.

Note: *Because some body parts cannot be positioned to work against gravity, the grading of some muscles is modified.*

TABLE 16-8. Kendall Muscle Grades

Letter (% Grade)	Definition
N (100%)	Can hold against gravity and maximal resistance, which is defined as sufficient resistance to displace body weight proximal to tested part.
G, G+ (80%–90%)	Can hold against gravity and moderate resistance.
F+, G– (60%–70%)	Can hold against gravity and slight resistance.
F (50%)	Ability to hold test position.
F– (40%)	Gradual release from test position or ability to complete ROM with gravity eliminated.
P+ (30%)	Ability to move through moderate arch of ROM with gravity eliminated, or can move into test position with moderate assistance.
P (20%)	Ability to move through minimal arch of ROM with gravity eliminated; can move into test position with maximum assistance.
P–/T (10%–5%)	Muscle can be seen or palpated, but no visible movement.

Note N = 100%

TABLE 16-9. Daniels and Worthingham Muscle Grades

Letter Grade	Definition
N	Able to move part through full ROM against gravity, and hold against maximal resistance at end of range (Break Test).
G	Able to move part through full ROM against gravity and take good resistance at end of range.
F+	Able to move through full ROM against gravity and take minimal resistance at end of range.
F	Able to move part through full ROM against gravity, but are not able to take any resistance at end of range.
F–	Able to move part through more than one-half the ROM against gravity.
P+	Able to move part through less than one-half the ROM against gravity.
P	Able to move part through full ROM in a gravity-eliminated position.
P–	Able to move part through more than one-half the ROM in a gravity-eliminated position.
T+	Able to move part through less than one-half the ROM in a gravity-eliminated position.
T	Contraction can be palpated—no movement of the part.

TABLE 16-10. Serratus Anterior Testing: Comparison of Three Methods

Testing Element	Rancho	Kendall	Daniels & Worthingham
Client position			
• Above fair	Sitting, arm abducted, elbow extended		
	Sitting	Sitting	Supine (stabilize arm)
• Below fair			
Palpitation	Does not depend on	Does not address	Does not address
Motion	Raise arm to 90–120 degrees scapula should rotate and abduct. Scapula does not collapse with resistance.	Abduction and lateral rotation of inferior angle of scapula through maintaining humerus between 120–130 degrees flexion.	Abduction and lateral rotation of interior angle of scapula (humerus flexed to 90 degrees).
• Above fair			
• Below fair	90 degrees shoulder flexion. Push forward. Scapula does not collapse with motion.		
Resistance	Push humerus into extension	Against lateral border of scapula, rotating inferior angle medially and against shoulder in direction of extension.	Grasp around forearm and elbow; pressure is downward and inward toward table.
Substitution	Scapular elevation, lateral trunk flexion or extension.	Does not address	Does not address

TABLE 16-11. Rhomboids Testing: Comparison of Three Methods

Testing Element	Rancho	Kendall	Daniels & Worthingham
Client Position			
• Above fair	Prone: humerus internally rotated, abducted, with hand on opposite buttock.	Prone	Prone: head rotated to opposite side
• Below fair	Prone: arm supported by therapist.	Prone	Sitting: arm internally rotated, adducted across back (shoulder relaxed)
Palpitation	Vertebral border of scapula along spine	Does not address	Angle formed by vertebral border of scapula and internal fibers of lower trapezius
Motion	Lift hand off buttock. Adduct and downwardly rotate scapula.	Elbow flexed, humerus adducted in slight extension and lateral rotation.	Adduction and medial rotation of inferior angle of scapula.
Resistance	Push forearm into abduction and upward rotation	Examiner attempts to rotate inferior angle of scapula laterally with one hand at the shoulder, pushing in the direction of shoulder depression and scapula lateral rotation.	On vertebral border of scapula outward and slightly downward.
Substitution	Middle trapezius (no inferior angle rotation).	Does not address	Does not address

muscles. In dysphagia for solids, a feeling of blockage is common.

Occupational therapy examination (Miller et al, 1988; Nelson, 1996) includes evaluation of

1. Mental status
2. Strength of muscles of the face, mouth, neck, and trunk
3. Oral sensation
4. Primitive reflexes
5. Intraoral mucosa
6. The adequacy of swallowing

Recording Results

A sample form is presented for recording results of muscle strength testing. The timing of re-evaluation may depend on the expected recovery rate, length of stay in therapy, and department protocol. Keep in mind, the focus of therapy, should be an increase in function, not necessarily an increase in the component area of strength (Table 16–12).

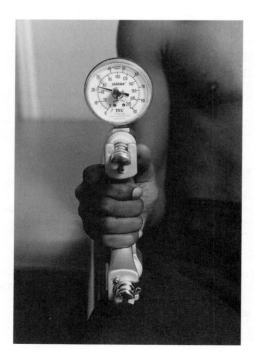

▲
Figure 16-20. Dynamometer. (Photo courtesy of the Rehabilitation Institute of Chicago.)

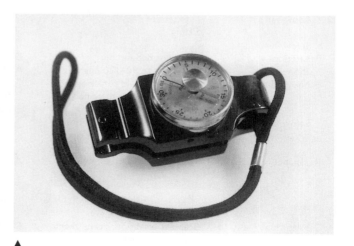

▲
Figure 16-21. Pinch meter. (Photo courtesy of the Rehabilitation Institute of Chicago.)

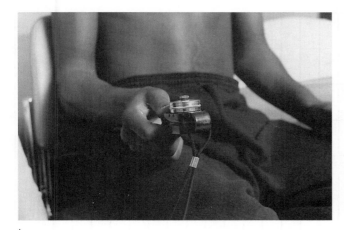

Figure 16-22. Pinch meter measurement of lateral pinch. (Photo courtesy of the Rehabilitation Institute of Chicago.)

Interpreting Results

Performing a muscle test is only one component of an evaluation. How a therapist interprets and uses the information is more important. Some considerations are as follows:

1. Is the problem one of strength, endurance, or a combination thereof? Endurance is the number of repetitions of muscle contraction before fatigue. If endurance is the issue, the therapist needs to emphasize repetitive movements (at less than maximal contraction) to increase endurance.
2. Is the result of your evaluation influenced by impaired tactile sensation or proprioception?
3. What is the diagnosis or expected course of the disease? Is there an expected recovery period? Progression of decline? Periods of exacerbation or remission?
4. The degree of weakness, distribution, and pattern of weakness (ie, generalized or specific) and the muscle imbalance between agonists and antagonists suggest the type of intervention (ie, resistive exercises, active assistive activities, orthotic intervention).
5. Coordinate the therapy program with other professionals so that timing and type of appointments and goals are in line with other interventions (Pedretti, 1996b).

▼ SOFT TISSUE EVALUATION

Soft tissue comprises the matrix of the body and is of four primary types:

1. Epithelial tissue serves to protect, secrete, and absorb
2. Muscular tissue contracts
3. Nervous tissue conducts
4. Connective tissue provides support, nutrition, and defense

Connective tissue can be further broken down into several types:

1. Fascia—specialized tissues enveloped in connective tissue sheaths
2. Tendons—bundles of heavy collagen fibers that run parallel to one another and connect muscles to bones
3. Ligaments—similar to tendons, but the fibers are not as regularly arranged; usually connect bone to bone
4. Cartilage—fibrous connective tissue with an abundant, firm matrix
5. Muscle—smooth or striated
6. Bone—modified form of collagen; a harder bundle of connective tissue in which large amounts of calcium make up a solid matrix of fibrous connective tissue (Adams & Hamblen, 1990).

Normal movement depends on the force exerted by muscles as they act on a joint, the shape of articular surfaces, atmospheric pressure within a joint, and the restraining influences of soft tissue, particularly ligaments. When any of these factors are dysfunctional because of trauma, infection, or immobilization, irritation can develop which, in turn, can cause pain, muscle tension, tissue damage, inflammation, and ultimately, functional disability (Fig. 16–23) (Cailliet, 1978).

Part of the musculoskeletal evaluation involves soft tissue evaluation. Initially, a therapist may do a general or scan evaluation of the upper quadrant, cervical spine, ROM, reflexes, strength, and sensation. When a client has a more specific orthopedic or pain complaint the therapist can focus on a more localized area, but not rule out the possibility of referred pain or a multifaceted problem (eg, wrist pain caused by incorrect posture and work station setup, in addition to repetitive motion). The interview process should include identification, location, duration, and intensity of the problem. The time(s) of day the pain occurs, things that make the pain better or worse, and most importantly, how the pain affects the person's ability to perform daily activities should also be noted (Cailliet, 1978; Edwardson, 1992).

Careful palpation can detect abnormality in the texture of tissues, visual and tactile asymmetry, difference in movement and quality throughout ROM, type of end feel on completion of available range, and ultimately, a change in findings over time. The following information provides a brief overview of soft tissue examination of the upper extremity, particularly the shoulder, elbow, wrist, and hand.

Shoulder

Examination of soft tissue structures of the shoulder can be divided into four clinical zones:

1. Rotator cuff
2. Subacromial and subdeltoid bursa
3. Axilla
4. Prominent muscles of the shoulder girdle

A common abnormality of the rotator cuff is degeneration and subsequent tearing of the tendon of insertion. The supraspinatus, infraspinatus, and teres minor (SIT) muscles insert into the greater tuberosity of the humerus and can be

TABLE 16-12 Form for Recording Results of Strength Testing

REHABILITATION INSTITUTE OF CHICAGO OCCUPATIONAL THERAPY DEPARTMENT
FUNCTIONAL SKILLS/MOTOR FUNCTION

Name:
RIC #:
Physician:

MANUAL MUSCLE EXAMINATION OF THE UPPER EXTREMITIES
GROSS / SPECIFIC (circle one)

			Date	Date
Date	Date			
Abd/up rotation	Serratus anterior	C5-7		
Elevation	Upper trapezius	C2-4		
Add/Depression	Lower trapezius	C2-4		
Adduction	Middle trapezius	C2-5		
Add/down rotat.	Rhomboids	C5		
SHOULDER				
Flexion	Anterior deltoid	C5-6		
Extension	Latissimus dorsi	C7-8		
Abduction	Middle deltoid	C5-6		
Horiz. abd.		C5-6		
Horiz. add. Pect major (clavicular)		C5-7		
Horiz. add. Pect major (sternal)		C7-T1		
External rotator group		C5-6		
		C5-T1		
ELBOW/FOREARM				
Flexion	Biceps brachii	C5-6		
	Brachioradialis	C5-6		
Extension		C(6)7-8		
Supination		C5-6(7)		
Pronation		C6-T1		
WRIST				
Flexion	Flexor carpi ulnaris	C7-8		
	Flexor carpi radialis	C6-8		
	Palmaris longus	C6-7		
Ext.	Extensor carpi radialis longus	C6-7		
	Extensor carpi radialis brevis	C6-7		
	Extensor carpi ulnaris	C7-8		

JOINT RANGE MEASUREMENTS

			AROM	AROM	PROM	PROM			AROM	PROM	PROM	AROM	AROM
	< - Left	Right - >	Date	Date	Date	Date			Date	Date	Date	Date	Date
Shoulder	Flexion	0-180											
	Extension	0-60											
	Abduction	0-180											
	External Rotation	0-90											
	Internal Rotation	0-70											
	Horiz. Abduction	0-90											
	Horiz. Adduction	0-45											
Elbow	Flexion	0-150											
	Supination	0-80											
	Pronation	0-80											
Wrist	Flexion	0-80											
	Extension	0-70											
	Ulnar Dev.	0-30											
	Radial Dev.	0-20											
Thumb	M.P. Flexion	0-50											
	I. P. Flexion	0-80											
	Abduction	0-70											

FINGERS

MP Extension-Ext. digitorum communis	1	
	2	C7-8
	3	"
	4	"
DIP Flexion-Flex. digitorum profundus	1	
	2	C7-T1
	3	"
	4	"
PIP Flexion-Flex digit. superficialis	1	
	2	C6-8
	3	"
	4	"
MP Flexion Lumbricales	1	C8-T1
Lumbricales	2	
Lumbricales	3	
Lumbricales	4	
Adduction - Palmar Interoscous	1	
"	2	C8-T1
"	3	
Abduction - Dorsal Interoscous	1	
"	2	C8-T1
"	3	
"	4	

THUMB

MP Flexion	Flex. Poll. brevis	C8-T1
IP Flexion	Flex. poll. longus	C8-T1
MP Extension	Ext. poll. brevis	C7-8
IP Extension	Ext. poll. longus	C7-8
Abduction	Abd. poll. brevis	C8-T1
	Abd. poll. longus	C7-8
Adduction	Adductor pollicis	C8-T1
Opposition	Opponens policis	C8-T1

Grade: N=Normal; G=Good; F=Fair; P=Poor; T=Trace; 0=Zero

(Range of Motion)

Index F.	
M. P. Flexion	0-90
M. P. Extension	0-45
P. I. P. Flexion	0-100
D. I. P. Flexion	0-80

Long F.	
M. P. Flexion	0-90
M. P. Extension	0-45
P. I. P. Flexion	0-100
D. I. P. Flexion	0-90

Ring F.	
M. P. Flexion	0-90
M. P. Extension	0-45
P. I. P. Flexion	0-100
D. I. P. Flexion	0-90

Little F.	
M. P. Flexion	0-90
M. P. Extension	0-45
P. I. P. Flexion	0-100
D. I. P. Flexion	0-90

PREHENSILE STRENGTH

	Date	Left	Right	Norm
Cylindrical Grasp				
3-Point Pinch				
Lateral Pinch				
9 Hole Peg Test				

Therapist _____ Date _____

02-300275-10

(Reprinted with permission from the Rehabilitation Institute of Chicago.)

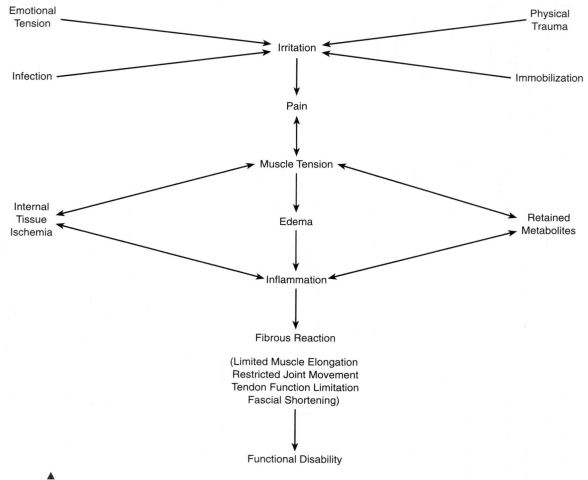

Figure 16-23. Factors leading to functional disability. (From Cailliet, R. [1978]. *Soft tissue pain and disability* [p. 23]. Philadelphia: F. A. Davis Co., reprinted with permission.)

palpated when the shoulder is passively extended. The subscapularis muscle cannot be palpated. Portions of the subacromial and subdeltoid bursa can be palpated just below the edge of the acromion. The axilla is a quadrilateral pyramidal structure within the pectoralis major, latissimus dorsi, and ribs 2 through 6 (covered by the serratus anterior), and the bicipital groove of the humerus. The glenohumeral joint is the apex of the pyramid and major vessels that pass through the area are the axillary artery and brachial plexus. Shoulder girdle muscles that can be palpated are the sternocleidomastoid; pectoralis major; biceps; anterior, middle, and posterior deltoid; and trapezius (Hoppenfeld, 1976). Special tests that can be performed on soft tissue structures associated with the shoulder complex are as follows:

Drop arm test—detects partial tear of the rotator cuff. The client is instructed to abduct the arm to 90 degrees, then the therapist applies gentle pressure. If the client is unable to hold the arm up at all or is unable to lower the arm slowly, rotator cuff damage is indicated (Edwardson, 1992; Hoppenfeld, 1976).

Impingement sign—detects supraspinatus tendinitis. The therapist forces the forward flexed arm of the client against the anteroinferior surface of the acromion, jamming the supraspinatus against the acromion. Pain indicates a positive result (ie, inflammation of the supraspinatus tendon) (Edwardson, 1992).

Speed's test—detects tendinitis of the long head of the biceps. The client extends the elbow and supinates the forearm, then forward flexes the extended arm against therapist resistance. A painful response is a positive sign of biceps tendon inflammation. Tendon palpation would also confirm the finding (Edwardson, 1992).

Apprehension (crank) test for anterior shoulder dislocation—detects anterior instability of the shoulder. The client's arm is abducted to 90 degrees and then slowly placed in external rotation. The client will demonstrate apprehension and resist the movement if instability is present (Edwardson, 1992).

Posterior apprehension test—detects posterior instability of the shoulder. Client's arm is placed in forward flexion to 90 degrees, adducted, and then internally rotated. Posterior pressure is applied on the tip of the elbow. A positive sign is the client's apprehension and opposition to movement (Magee, 1992).

The upper limb tension test (ULTT) was developed by Elvey (1979) in an attempt to differentiate between the cervical spine and the glenohumeral joint as the cause of the client's shoulder problem. During the performance of the Elvey test the upper nerve roots of the brachial plexus are put on stretch and in the presence of a cervical spine disorder the client's pain will be produced. Component movements of the test are taken to the end of the pain-free range only to avoid stretching structures other than the nerve root. A positive ULTT result indicates a cervical spine abnormality involving the nerve root. A negative ULTT result does not rule out other problems in the cervical spine area. The test is performed and client's pain evaluated in three sequential steps:

1. Abduction, extension, and lateral rotation of the shoulder, with elbow kept flexed
2. Full supination followed by elbow extension
3. Wrist and finger extension

The test is described for the right side.

Client position: Supine with the side to be tested close to the edge of the mat.

Therapist position: Sit on the mat at the side of and facing the client, close to the right shoulder. Therapist's right hand embraces the top of client's right shoulder girdle with the palm on top of the shoulder and the fingers bent down behind the shoulder girdle's posterior aspect.

Movement 1: With the left hand, the therapist abducts the arm to approximately 110 degrees, or to where maximum tension is exerted. The arm is then extended to about 10 degrees beyond the coronal plane and laterally rotated to approximately 60 degrees. The position should be comfortable for the client and not pushed to the limit to avoid unnecessary stretch on shoulder structures. The client is questioned about any shoulder pain.

Movement 2: While maintaining the end position for movement 1, the therapist supinates the forearm and slowly extends the elbow. The client's arm is supported by the therapist's thigh just proximal to the elbow. The client is questioned about any shoulder pain.

Movement 3: If the client has not complained of pain, the therapist's right hand supports the client's elbow as the left hand gently extends the wrist and fingers.

When movement 3 has been performed there is maximum stretch on the peripheral nerve or nerve roots. The client is asked again about shoulder pain. If pain has not been reproduced, the test can be repeated with side flexion of the cervical spine to the left (making the test more sensitive). Certain stretch responses, such as across the anterior aspect of the shoulder, elbow, and tingling in C_6 and C_7 dermatomes in the hand are normal. The ULTT is positive only

if the client's shoulder pain is reproduced by the test positions (Edwardson, 1992).

Elbow

The elbow is a hinge joint with three articulations: humeroulnar, humeroradial, and radioulnar. One should inspect for swelling, scars, carrying angle, and perform bony palpation. Soft tissue palpation of the elbow can be divided into four clinical zones:

1. *Medial aspect*
   a. Ulnar nerve—located in the sulcus between the medial epicondyle and olecranon process; feels soft, round tubular
   b. Wrist flexors—flexor carpi radialis longus, palmaris longus, and flexor carpi radialis brevis. The pronator teres is not distinctly palpable
   c. Medial collateral ligament
2. *Posterior aspect*
   a. Olecranon bursa
   b. Triceps—long, lateral, and medial heads
3. *Lateral aspect*
   a. Wrist extensors—extensor carpi radialis longus, brevis, and ulnaris
   b. Lateral collateral ligament—not palpable
   c. Annular ligament—not palpable
4. *Anterior aspect*: cubital fossa—triangular space bordered by pronator teres and brachioradialis. Structures passing through include:
   a. Biceps tendon
   b. Brachial artery
   c. Median nerve
   d. Musculocutaneous nerve (not palpable)

Ligamentous tests that can be performed on the elbow include:

Tinel sign—designed to elicit tenderness over a neuroma within a nerve by tapping the ulnar nerve in the groove between the olecranon and medial epicondyle. A positive result is a tingling sensation.

Tennis elbow test—with the forearm stabilized in pronation and the elbow in flexion, the client makes a fist with extended wrist. Therapist applies pressure to the dorsum of hand to push wrist into flexion. A positive sign is sudden, severe pain at the lateral epicondyle (Edwardson, 1992; Hoppenfeld, 1976).

Wrist and Hand

Detailed examination of the wrist and hand is beyond the scope of this text. Observations should include swelling (local or general), atrophy, discoloration, deformity, resting position, normal tenodesis, normal alignment, and rotational alignment. Tables 16–13 and 16–14 summarize the clinical zones for soft tissue palpation of the wrist and hand.

TABLE 16-13. Soft Tissue Zones for Wrist

Zone	Tunnels (#) and Muscle Tendons in Them	Anatomical Landmark(s)	Clinical Significance
I. Radial Styloid Process	1. Abductor pollicis longus Extensor pollicis brevis	Anatomical snuffbox (radial side)	Site for stenosing tenosynovitis (DeQuervain's disease)
II. Lister's Tubercle	2. Extensor carpi radialis longus Extensor carpi radialis brevis	Radial side of Lister's tubercle	
	3. Extensor pollicis longus (EPL)	Ulnar side of Lister's tubercle	EPL may rupture due to Colles fracture or rheumatoid arthritis
	4. Extensor digitorum communis Extensor indicis	Ulnar to tunnel 3; radial to radioulnar articulation	
III. Ulnar Styloid Process	5. Extensor digit; minimi (EDM)	Indentation lateral to the ulnar styloid process	EDC may be irritated by rheumatoid arthritis, subject to attrition by friction or from synovitis
	6. Extensor carpi ulnaris	Groove between apex of ulnar styloid process and the ulnar head	ECU may tear in Colle's fracture; may be displaced or tear in rheumatoid arthritis
IV. Pisiform (palmar aspect)		Flexor carpi ulnaris (FCU)	Calcium deposits can cause pain in FCU
		Tunnel of Guyon (depression between pisiform and hook of Hamate)	Contains ulnar nerve and artery—site for compression injuries
		Ulnar artery pulse proximal to pisiform	
V. Palmaris Longus and carpal tunnel	Carpal tunnel: Median nerve finger flexor tendons from the forearm to the hand	Bisects the anterior aspect of wrist Lies deep to palmaris longus defined proximally by pisiform and tubercle of navicular, distally by hook of Hamate and tubercle of trapezium	Absent in 7% of population Site of carpal tunnel syndrome due to dislocation of lunate; swelling due to Colle's fracture; synovitis due to rheumatoid arthritis or long-term repetitive motion
	Not in tunnel: Flexor carpi radialis	Radial to palmaris longus; crosses navicular before inserting into base of 2nd metacarpal	

(Hoppenfeld, 1976)

Swelling, which is caused by edema (increased interstitial fluid), can be measured with a volumeter or with circumferential measurements taken with a tape measure. The volumeter measures the amount of water displaced by the hand and is useful for measuring generalized edema (Fig. 16–24). The uninvolved hand can be measured as a normal comparison. For clients with open wounds or infections, the volumeter may be contraindicated (Fess, 1993). Circumferential measurements are useful for more localized edema, for example, around a specific joint (Fig. 16–25).

Functional Tests for the Wrist and Hand

Functional tests for the wrist and hand involve passive movements to test the inert joint structures, resisted isometric contractions to test the integrity of muscles involved in joint movements, accessory movements to test the small articular movements, and special tests used to detect or con-

firm abnormalities. Table 16–15 describes some of these tests.

Special Tests

The following tests are commonly used in the evaluation of the hand:

THE ALLEN TEST

Purpose: To determine efficacy of blood flow in radial and ulnar arteries.

Procedure: Client makes a fist and releases it several times. Next, he or she is instructed to make a fist and hold it so that the venous blood is forced from the palm.

The therapist locates the radial artery with his or her thumb and the ulnar artery with the index and middle fingers. Pressure is exerted on these arteries to occlude them and the client then opens the hand. The therapist releases

TABLE 16-14. Soft Tissue Zones for Hand

Zone	Structures or Muscles Within	Anatomical Landmark(s)	Clinical Significance
I. Thenar eminence	Abductor pollicis brevis Opponens pollicis Flexor pollicis brevis	Situated at base of thumb in palm	Compression of median nerve can cause atrophy of thenar eminence
II. Hypothenar eminence	Abductor digiti quinti Opponens digiti Flexor digiti quinti	Lies proximal to little finger and extends longitudinally to the pisiform	Compression of ulnar nerve can cause atrophy of hypothenar eminence
III. Palm	Structures not distinctly palpable due to thick muscular padding (thenar and hypothenar eminences) and palmar fascia that cover them	Palmar aponeurosis Finger flexor tendons	Nodules can cause a flexion deformity of fingers (Dupuytren's contracture) Trigger finger or trigger thumb (sudden palpable and audible snapping often caused by a nodule in the flexor tendon that catches on an annular ligament over the metacarpal head)
IV. Dorsum	Extensor tendons		Extensor tendons become displaced ulnarly in rheumatoid arthritis and cause ulnar drift of fingers
V. Phalanges	Flexor and extensor tendons		Abnormal fusiform enlargement at joints can indicate synovitis If central slip of extensor digitorum communis tendon is avulsed from its insertion, Boutonniere deformity results Nodules on dorsal and lateral surfaces of DIP (Heberden's nodes) may indicate osteoarthritis If distal insertion of extensor digitorum communis has been torn away from distal phalanx with an avulsion of a bony fragment, a "mallet finger," deformity results
VI. Tufts of the fingers	Contain most of the hand's sensory nerve endings		Pathology affects hand function

(Hoppenfeld, 1976)

the pressure on one artery at a time, looking for immediate flushing. If flushing is slow to occur, or does not occur, there is interference with the normal blood supply of the hand (Edwardson, 1992; Hoppenfeld, 1976).

THE BUNNEL-LITTLER TEST

Purpose: Tests the tightness of the intrinsic muscles of the hand (lumbricals and interossei) and determines if flexion limitation in the proximal interphalangeal (PIP) joint is due to tight intrinsics or joint capsule contractures.

Procedure: To test the tightness of intrinsic muscles, hold the metacarpophalangeal joint in a few degrees of extension and try to move the PIP joint into flexion. If, in this position, the PIP joint can be flexed, the intrinsics are not tight and are not limiting flexion. If the PIP joint cannot be flexed, either the intrinsics are tight or joint capsule contractures exist.

To determine intrinsic muscle versus joint capsule tightness, flex the involved finger a few degrees at the metacarpophalangeal joint and move the PIP joint into flexion. If the joint is now capable of full flexion, the intrinsics are probably tight. If the joint does not flex completely, the limitation is probably due to PIP joint capsule contractures (Edwardson, 1992; Hoppenfeld, 1976).

FINKLESTEIN'S TEST

Purpose: To determine if pain in the radial styloid area is due to DeQuervain's disease (inflammation of the synovial sheath surrounding the extensor pollicis brevis and abductor pollicis longus).

Procedure: Client flexes the thumb across the palm and deviates hand ulnarly. A painful response indicates sheath involvement (Edwardson, 1992; Hoppenfeld, 1976).

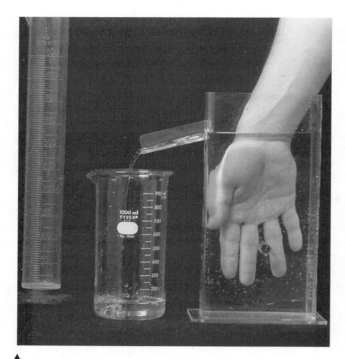

▲
Figure 16-24. Volumeter.

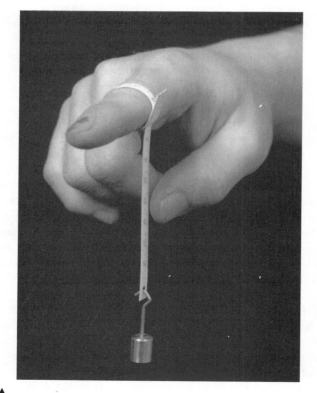

▲
Figure 16-25. Circumferential measurement of edema with a tape measure.

THE RETINACULAR TEST

Purpose: To determine if restricted distal interphalangeal (DIP) flexion is due to a tight oblique retinacular ligament or a tight capsule.

Procedure: The PIP joint is flexed a few degrees to relax the oblique retinacular ligament. If the restriction of flexion still remains, the restriction in flexion at the DIP is due to a tight capsule. If DIP flexion is complete with the PIP flexed, but restricted with the PIP extended, the limitation is due to tightness in the oblique retinacular ligament (Edwardson, 1992; Hoppenfeld, 1976).

▼ REFLEX TESTING

"A reflex is an involuntary, stereotyped response to a particular stimulus" (Mathiowetz & Haugen, 1995; p. 170). Reflex responses develop in utero and are clearly apparent in infancy. In normal development, primitive spinal and brainstem reflexes gradually become less obvious, and higher-level righting and equilibrium reactions become more obvious. Reflexes are the foundations of normal motor function (Farber, 1991a,b; Undzis et al, 1996; Mathiowetz & Haugen, 1995).

Following central nervous system injury or disease, the nervous system may exhibit more exaggerated reflexes. A reflex assessment is necessary to determine the status of the primitive reflex integration and of the righting and equilibrium reactions. The following principles should be noted when testing primitive reflexes:

1. Reflexes and responses should be tested in several developmental postures.
2. Any stress can release elements of primitive postural reflexes in both the neurologically intact as well as neurologically impaired population.
3. Clients with chronic neuromotor disorders will rarely demonstrate a primitive postural reflex in its pure form. Most often, reflexes are combined so that clients demonstrate elements of several reflexes in one behavioral response (Farber, 1991a,b).
4. Reflexes are usually tested in developmental sequence.

See Tables 16–16 through 16–21 for an overview of various levels of reflex testing.

Innate Primary Reactions

Innate primary reactions are primitive reflexes found in newborns that involve total patterns of flexion and extension (Table 16–16).

Automatic Movement Reflexes

Automatic movement reactions are produced by changes of the head's position in space (Table 16–17). *(text continues on page 253)*

TABLE 16-15. Functional Tests for the Hand

Joint	Passive Movement	Resisted Isometric Contractions	Accessory Movements
Inferior radioulnar	Pronation Supination		Dorsal–volar glide
Radiocarpal (the wrist joint)	Flexion Extension Radial deviation Ulnar deviation	Flexion Extension Radial deviation Ulnar deviation	Traction Ventral glide Dorsal glide Radial deviation
1st carpometacarpal	Extension	Flexion Extension Abduction Adduction	Ulnar deviation
Fingers (metacarpal phalangeal (MP); proximal interphalangeal (PIP); distal interphalangeal (DIP)		Flexion Extension Abduction } MPs only Adduction } MPs only	

(Edwardson, 1992)

TABLE 16-16. Innate Primary Reactions

Reflex/Reaction	Reflex/Reaction age range	Test position	Stimulus	Response
Reflex stepping	Birth–3 mo	Supported in upright position with some weight-bearing on feet	Lean client forward; pressure of feet on supporting surface	Rhythmic, alternating stepping
Grasp reflex	Birth–3 to 4 mo	Any—usually supine	Pressure in palm of hand or ulnar side	Flexing of fingers, grasping of stimulus object
Placing reaction	Birth–2 mo	Sitting or supine	Brush dorsum of one of the client's hands against the under edge of a table or edge of a stiff cardboard	Flexion of the arm with placement of the hand on to the tabletop
Sucking reflex	Birth–2 mo	Any	Stimulation to lips, gums, or front of tongue	Sucking, swallowing motions
Rooting reflex	Birth –4 mo	Any	Touch or stroke outward on corner of lips or on cheek	Lower lip, tongue, and head more toward stimulus

(Mathiowetz & Haugen, 1995: Simon & Daub, 1993; Sroufe, Cooper, & Deltart, 1992)

TABLE 16-17. Automatic Movement Reflexes

Reflex	Reflex age range	Test position	Stimulus	Response
Moro reflex	Birth–5 mo	Semireclining or supine	Dropping head backward from a semisitting position or a loud noise near the head	Extension or flexion and abduction of arms and spreading of fingers
Landau reflex	4 mo–12 to 24 mo	Prone, suspended in space with support under the chest	Passive or active neck extension	Back and legs extend
Protective extensor thrust	6 mo–remainder of life	Sitting or prone	Displace body forward, sideways and backward (separately)	Protective extension of limb to protect head

(Mathiowetz & Haugen, 1995: Simon & Daub, 1993; Sroufe, Cooper, & Deltart, 1992)

TABLE 16-18. Spinal Level Reflexes

Reflex	Reflex age range	Test position	Stimulus	Response
Flexor withdrawal	Birth–2 mo	Supine or sitting with head in midposition, legs extended	Stimulation to sole of foot	Uncontrolled flexion of stimulated leg
Extensor thrust	Birth–2 mo	Supine or sitting with head in midposition. One leg is in extension and the other leg is fully flexed	Pressure to the ball of the foot of the flexed leg	Uncontrolled extension of the stimulated leg
Crossed extension	Birth–2 mo	Supine with head in midposition. One leg is in extension and the other leg is fully flexed	Passively flex the extended leg	Extension of the opposite leg, with hip internal rotation and adduction

(Mathiowetz & Haugen, 1995: Simon & Daub, 1993; Sroufe, Cooper, & Deltart, 1992)

TABLE 16-19. Brainstem Reflexes

Reflex	Reflex age range	Test position	Stimulus	Response
Asymmetrical tonic neck reflex (ATNR)	Birth–4 to 6 mo	Supine or sitting, with arms and legs extended. Clients with minimal reflexes responses can be tested in quadruped.	Passively or actively turn the head 90 degrees to one side	Increase of extensor tone of limbs on the face side and flexor tone of limbs on the skull side
Symmetrical tonic neck reflex (STNR)	Birth–4 to 6 mo	Sitting or quadruped	1. Flex client's head and bring chin toward chest 2. Extend client's head	1. Flexion of upper extremities and extension of lower extremities 2. Extension of upper extremities and flexion of lower extremities
Tonic labyrinthine reflex (TLR)	Birth–4 mo	Prone with head in midposition	Test position is the stimulus	Flexion of the extremities or increase in flexor tone
Tonic labyrinthine reflex: Supine	Birth–4 mo	Supine with head in midposition	Test position is the stimulus	Extension of the extremities or increase in extensor tone
Positive supporting reaction	Birth–6 mo	Standing, supine, or sitting	Firmly contact the ball of the foot to the floor; or footboard of the bed and dorsiflex the foot	Rigid extension of lower extremity due to co-contraction of flexors and extensors of knee and hip joints
Associated reactions	Associated movements are normal throughout life when attempting strenuous activities. Associated reactions are stereotyped tonic reactions by which one extremity influences the posture of another extremity.	Any position	Resist any motion or have client squeeze an object with unaffected hand	The motion used as a stimulus will be mimicked by the other hand.

(Mathiowetz & Haugen, 1995: Simon & Daub, 1993; Sroufe, Cooper, & Deltart, 1992)

Spinal Level Reflexes

Reflexes mediated at the spinal level are phasic and are basic to mobility motor patterns (Table 16–18).

Brainstem Level Reflexes

Reflexes mediated at the brain stem level are static, postural reflexes that cause a change in muscle tone throughout the body. The changed tone is in response to a change of the head's position in space or in relation to the body, which activates the vestibular system; the changed tone is maintained as long as the stimulus is present (Table 16–19).

Midbrain Level Reactions

A reaction is a stereotyped, nonobligatory response to a particular stimulus. Midbrain reactions permit the development of maturationally acquired motor milestones. **Righting reactions** are integrated at this level and interact with one another to effect the normal head-to-body relation in space and to each other (Table 16–20).

Cortical Reactions

Cortical level reactions are the result of the efficient interaction of the cerebral cortex, basal ganglia, and the cerebellum. Equilibrium reactions occur when muscle tone is normalized and enable the adaptation to changes in the body's center of gravity. They are the integration of vestibular, visual, and tactile inputs (Table 16–21).

Recording Results

Test position(s) should be noted. Results are usually recorded as to whether the client's response is positive or negative. Intensity (ie, the speed of response and degree of change) as well as quality (ie, which components of the response are present under which conditions) of responses should be documented.

Interpreting Results

Obligatory reflexive responses, such as domination of a postural reflex, indicates severe central nervous system abnormality. Disturbance of higher-integrating centers manifests by evidence of a reflex, but not complete domination (Farber, 1991a,b). For example, a weak reflex response would be tonal changes in the extremities as opposed to actual movement. This should not be confused with tonal changes in a stimulus-neutral condition. Problems with reflex integration result in decreased (1) trunk segmentation, (2) ability to perform isolated movement, (3) adaptation of muscles to postural change, (4) function of antigravity muscles, and (5) increased synergistic movement. Formal assessment should always be accompanied by observing how reflexes affect motor and functional performance. For example, a positive **asymmetric tonic neck reflex** (ATNR) can prevent rolling from supine to prone owing to scapular retraction on the skull side extremity (which prevents bringing that arm across) and an extended arm on the face side (Trombly & Scott, 1989).

TABLE 16-20. Midbrain Reactions

Reaction	Reaction age range	Test position	Stimulus	Response
Neck righting	Birth–6 mo	Supine with arms and legs extended	Passively turn head to one side and hold it there	Body rotates as a whole in the direction to which the head was turned
Labyrinthine righting acting on the head	2 mo–throughout life	Prone, supine, or vertical positions in space. Subject's vision is occluded	Prone or supine positions are test stimuli, or in vertical position body is tilted laterally	Head seeks vertical position in space
Body righting acting on the head	6 mo–5 years	Client is blindfolded 1. Prone 2. Supine	Asymmetric stimulation of the pressure sense organs on the anterior of the body surface	Head is brought into a face-vertical position that orients it to the surface that the client is in contact with
Body righting on the body	6 mo–18 mo	Supine with arms and legs extended	Passively or actively turn the head to one side	Segmental rotation around the body axis toward the direction of the head

(Mathiowetz & Haugen, 1995; Simon & Daub, 1993: Sroufe, Cooper, & Deltart, 1992: Trombly & Scott, 1989)

Reaction	Reaction age range	Test position	Stimulus	Response
Optic righting	2 mo–throughout life	Prone or supine on a raised mat sitting with the head laterally flexed. Eyes are open	Position of the head in relation to landmarks in space	Head is raised upright in space
Equilibrium reaction	Depends on test position (see next column)—throughout life	Supine (7–8 mo) Prone (5 mo) Quadruped (9–12 mo) Sitting (6 mo) Kneel–standing (15 mo) Standing (15 mo)	Rocking client or supporting surface sufficiently to disturb balance	Automatic movements to maintain balance, right head and body; protective reactions

TABLE 16-21. Cortical Reactions

(Mathiowetz & Haugen, 1995: Simon & Daub, 1993; Sroufe, Cooper, & Deltart, 1992; Trombly & Scott, 1989)

▼ ENDURANCE

Endurance can be defined as the ability to sustain a given activity over time. It is related to cardiopulmonary, biomechanical, and neuromuscular function (Asmussen, 1979; Farber, 1991a,b; Lunsford, 1978; Trombly, 1995a). Endurance is a measure of stamina and fitness that can be compromised by inactivity, immobilization, cardiorespiratory deconditioning, muscular deconditioning, and diminished flexibility.

Endurance is related to intensity, duration, and frequency of activity. It can be reported as a percentage of maximal heart rate, a number of repetitions over time, or the amount of time a contraction can be held (Trombly, 1995a).

Cardiorespiratory Endurance

Cardiorespiratory endurance is defined by the American College of Sports Medicine (1991) as "the ability to perform large-muscle, dynamic, moderate-to-high intensity exercises for prolonged periods" (p. 39). Cardiorespiratory endurance depends on the functional states of the respiratory, cardiovascular, and musculoskeletal systems. Maximal oxygen uptake (abbreviated VO$_2$max) is a standard measure of cardiorespiratory endurance. It is a measure of the maximal amount of oxygen that a person can take in and dispense during exercise and is related to a person's maximal metabolic equivalent (MET) capacity (American College of Sports Medicine, 1991). "One MET is equivalent to an oxygen uptake of 3.5 [milliliters per kilogram body weight per minute]. It is conventional in exercise testing to express VO$_2$max in METS (eg, VO$_2$max of 35 [milliliters per kilogram body weight per minute] is equivalent to 10 METS)" (American College of Sports Medicine, 1991, p. 16). The VO$_2$max measurements require sophisticated equipment; occupational therapists are not qualified to make these measurements, but can use other indicators of cardiorespiratory endurance related to VO$_2$max—MET levels of activity and heart rate responses to activity.

To measure MET levels of activities, an occupational therapist can consult a MET table that indicates the average number of METS expended for given activities (Table 16–22). These tables report MET levels that have been established by exercise physiology research; the MET level values reported represent the average number of the METS expended by a 150 lb person. Heavier people will expend more METS and lighter people will expend fewer METS than the values indicated on a MET table for any given activity. Additionally, MET levels vary with stress and environmental conditions (American College of Sports Medicine, 1991). Therefore, a MET table figure represents only an approximate range of MET expenditure for any given activity and should be reported as such. For example, an occupational therapist could report that a client who was able to dress without experiencing shortness of breath or an increase in heart rate of more than 20 beats per minute could tolerate activities of approximately 2.5 to 3.5 METS (Trombly, 1989).

Clients' specific heart rate responses to activity need to be recorded in addition to MET levels. Heart rate quantifies the physiological demand of an activity; in healthy individuals higher heart rates correspond to higher oxygen consumption. This is not true for persons with cardiopulmonary diseases, because these diseases disrupt normal physiological responses to activity. Heart rate responses to treatment activities can be related to a person's maximal heart rate as a percentage of maximum. For persons without cardiopulmonary disease, maximum heart rate can be determined by the formula: 220 − age. In persons with cardiopulmonary disease, maximum heart rate should be determined by an exercise stress test administered by a cardiologist (American College of Sports Medicine, 1991).

Biomechanical and Neuromuscular Endurance

Biomechanical neuromuscular endurance refers to the capacity of a muscle or muscle group to sustain a contrac-

TABLE 16-22. Metabolic Equivalent (MET) Values for Some Occupational Performance Areas

MET Levels (Oxygen consumed) [Level of Activity]	Self-care Activities	Work and Productive Activities	Play and Leisure Activities
1.5–2.0 METS (4–7 mL/kg/min) [Very light/minimal]	Eating Shaving, grooming Getting in and out of bed Standing Walking (1.6 km or 1 mph)	Desk work Typing Writing	Playing cards Sewing Knitting
2–3 METS (7–11 mL/kg/min) [Light]	Showering in warm water Level walking (3.25 km or 2 mph)	Ironing Light woodworking Riding lawn mower	Level bicycling (8 km or 5 mph) Billiards Bowling Golfing with power cart
3–4 METS (11–14 mL/kg/min) [Moderate]	Dressing, undressing Walking (5 km or 3 mph)	Cleaning windows Making beds Mopping floors Vacuuming Bricklaying Machine assembly	Bicycling (10 km or 6 mph) Fly fishing (standing in waders) Horseshoe pitching
4–5 METS (14–18 mL/kg/min) [Heavy]	Showering in hot water Walking (5.5 km or 3.5 mph)	Scrubbing floors Hoeing Raking leaves Light carpentry	Bicycling (13 km or 8 mph) Table tennis Tennis (doubles)
5–6 METS (18–21 mL/kg/min) [Heavy]	Walking (6.5 km or 4 mph)	Digging in garden Shoveling light earth	Bicycling (16 km or 10 mph) Canoeing (6.5 km or 4 mph) Ice or roller skating (15 km or 9 mph)
6–7 METS (21–25 mL/kg/min) [Very heavy]	Walking (8 km or 5 mph)	Snow shoveling Splitting wood	Bicycling (17.5 km or 11 mph) Light downhill skiing Ski touring (4 km or 2.5 mph)

Note: mL/kg/min = milliliters of oxygen consumed per kilogram body weight per minute; km = kilometer; mph = miles per hour
(Atchison, 1995; Brannon, Foley, Starr, & Black, 1993; Trombly, 1989)

tion over time. In normal muscle, only a few of available motor units are needed at any one time as active and resting units take turns. "However, if a person sustains a contraction that exceeds 15% to 20% maximum voluntary contraction (MVC) for the muscle group involved, blood flow to the working muscles will decrease, causing a shift to anaerobic metabolism which limits duration" (Dehn, 1980; cited in Trombly, 1995a, p. 153). Anaerobic metabolism can lead to an accumulation of lactic acid and slowed conduction velocity to muscle fibers, resulting in muscle fatigue, reduced tension development, and eventual inability to hold a contraction (Basmajian & DeLuca, 1985). Persons with poor neuromuscular endurance will experience muscle fatigue sooner than those with good neuromuscular endurance.

Static endurance refers to the measure of sustained contractions. Isometric testing times how long an individual can maintain the tension of a maximum voluntary contraction, by using strain gauges, dynamometers, and some isokinetic equipment. Normally, a person can hold 25% MVC for 5 to 6 minutes, 50% MVC for 1 to 2 minutes, and 100% MVC only momentarily (Dehn & Mullins, 1977; Minor, 1991). Persons being tested should talk while doing an iso-

metric contraction to preclude breath holding and a significant increase in **blood pressure** or additional stress to the cardiopulmonary system.

Clinical Functional Endurance

Perhaps the most pertinent clinical information on muscular endurance comes from monitoring client progress through a treatment program, as opposed to comparing scores to population norms. One can evaluate and quantify endurance performance by applying the principles of the timed test of repetitions at a submaximal workload. Another method is to time how long a client can participate in activities, such as dressing or light homemaking, before requiring a rest. Another method that is clinically applicable to evaluating changes in activity tolerance is to monitor the client's perception of how hard he or she is working, or how tired he or she is after a given amount of time at a specified workload. One accepted such scale is the Borg Scale of Rating of Perceived Exertion (RPE) which ranges from "no work at all" (0 on the scale) to "very very heavy work" (10 on the scale) (Brannon, Foley, Starr, & Black, 1993; Minor, 1991).

▼ GROSS COORDINATION

Coordination is the combined activity of many muscles into smooth patterns and sequences of motion. Coordinated movement is characterized by rhythm, appropriate muscle tension, postural tone, refinement to the minimal number of muscle groups necessary to produce the desired movement, and equilibrium. Coordination is an automatic response that is monitored primarily through proprioceptive sensory feedback. Visual and tactile sensory feedback, body scheme, and ability to judge and move the body through space also affect overall coordination (Undzis et al, 1996; Mathiowetz & Haugen, 1995; Smith, 1993).

Incoordination is a broad term for extraneous, uneven, or inaccurate movements. Many types of lesions can produce disturbances of coordination. Cerebellar lesions, muscle or peripheral nerve disease or injury, lesions of the posterior column of the spinal cord, and lesions of the frontal or post-central cortex can all cause incoordination.

The occupational therapist evaluates aspects of coordination that appear to interfere with function by using standardized tests and clinical observation. The neurologist or physiatrist usually perform the neurological examination. The physical therapist evaluates coordination as it relates to mobility. Occupational and physical therapy may compliment each other in so far as evaluating how gross coordination affects functional mobility, such as standing at the sink to perform oral–facial hygiene, gathering items and preparing a meal in the kitchen, bathing, and numerous other ADL (Mathiowetz & Haugen, 1995; Smith, 1993; Undzis et al, 1996).

Several standardized tests exist to evaluate coordination (Table 16–23).

Cerebellar Dysfunction

Types of cerebellar dysfunction and methods of evaluating them are as follows:

Intention tremor: Intention tremor occurs during voluntary movement, is less apparent or absent during rest, and intensifies at the termination of the movement. To test for this, the therapist can ask the client to alternately touch his or her own nose and then the therapist's finger, held in front of the client in various positions. Tremor can also be observed during performance of daily activities, or during the finger-to-finger test. Similar to the finger-to-nose test, the client is asked to touch one of the examiner's fingers, then another held a distance away. Distance and target points are changed as the therapist notes tremor level, speed of response, and success rate.

Dysdiadochokinesia: Dysdiadochokinesia is a decreased ability to perform rapid alternating movements smoothly. Tests include having the client supinate and pronate the forearm, flex and extend the elbow, or grasp and release. Other tests include alternate rotation of fully extended arms or tapping the table with extended fingers. Tests are performed bilaterally. The number of alternations within a given time period and any differences between extremities are noted.

Dysmetria: Dysmetria is the inability to control muscle length, which results in overshooting or pointing past an object. The finger-to-nose or finger-to-finger test are used to evaluate this. Functionally, clients may hit themselves in the face with a comb in an attempt to comb their hair, or overshoot and miss picking up the comb from the nightstand.

TABLE 16-23. Standardized Tests of Gross Motor Coordination

Test	Age Level	Description
Bruininks–Oseretsky Test of Motor Proficiency	4 1/2–14 1/2 yr	Assesses gross and fine coordination, dexterity, upper limb speed, visual motor control, muscle strength running, balance
Devereux Test of Extremity Coordination	4–10 yr	Assesses static balance, motor attention span, body image, fine motor activity, and sequential motor activity
Lincoln–Oseretsky Motor Development Scale	6–14 yr	Assesses 36 motor tasks, such as one-foot standing, tapping rhythms, walking backwards, speed of movement, eye–hand coordination
Miller Assessment for Preschoolers	Preschool	Assesses 27 items, such as walking a line, stepping, hand-to-nose test, gross motor assessment
The Quick Neurological Screening Test	5 yr–adult	Screens neurological integration: attention, balance, spatial organization, rate and rhythm of movement, motor planning, coordination
The Rail-Walking Test	6 yr–adult	Assesses balance and locomotor coordination
The Riley Motor Problem Inventory	4–9 yr	Screens gross and fine motor coordination
The Test of Motor Impairment	5–14 yr	Assesses motor deficits: static and dynamic balance, manual dexterity, speed of movement, eye–hand coordination, problem-solving ability

(Farber, 1991a,b)

Dyssynergia: Dyssynergia is a decomposition of movement. The lack of synergistic action between agonists and antagonists produces jerky movements. Dyssynergia can be observed in the alternating movement, finger-to-nose, and finger-to-finger tests.

Ataxic gait: Ataxic gait is often unsteady and wide-based; clients with this gait show a tendency to veer or fall toward the side of the lesion. The therapist can observe the client walking or ask the client to walk and turn quickly or walk heel to toe along a straight line.

Rebound phenomenon of Holmes: Rebound phenomenon of Holmes is a lack of a "check reflex" to stop a motion to avoid striking something in the path of motion. To test, the examiner resists the elbow flexion at the forearm and unexpectedly releases the resistance; the client's hand may hit his or her own chest, shoulder, or face if he or she is unable to check the motion.

Hypotonia: Hypotonia is decreased muscle tone and decreased resistance to passive movement due to the loss of the cerebellum's facilitory influence on the stretch reflex. The therapist can observe hypotonia clinically and perform a quick stretch.

Posterior Column Dysfunction

The types of posterior column dysfunction and methods of evaluating them are as follows:

Ataxia: In this type of ataxia the wide-based gait results from loss of proprioception. The client's ability to self-correct if he or she visually compensates as he or she watches the floor and the placement of the feet differentiates posterior column from cerebellar dysfunction.

Romberg sign: The Romberg sign is the inability to maintain standing balance with feet together and eyes closed. In posterior column deficit, dysmetria in the finger-to-nose test is exacerbated with the eyes closed.

Basal Ganglia Dysfunction

Types of basal ganglia dysfunction and methods of evaluating them are as follows:

Athetosis: Athetosis is a movement disorder characterized by slow, writhing, twisting, continuous, and involuntary movements, particularly of the neck, face, and extremities. These movements are not present during sleep. Muscles may have either increased or decreased tone. The therapist should note proximal or distal involvement, involved extremities, pattern of motions, and what stimuli increase or decrease the abnormal movements.

Dystonia: Dystonia is a form of athetosis that causes twisting movements of the trunk and proximal muscles of the extremities, distorted postures, and torsion spasms.

Chorea: Choreiform movements are irregular, purposeless, coarse, quick, jerky, and dysrhythmic. Muscles are hypotonic. Chorea may occur in sleep.

Hemiballism: Hemiballism is a rare, unilateral chorea that involves violent, forceful, sudden flinging movements of the extremities on one side of the body.

Tremors at rest: Resting tremors stop at the initiation of voluntary movement, but resume during the holding phase of a motor task, particularly when the client is tired or attention is diverted. An example is the pill-rolling tremor seen in Parkinsonism.

Bradykinesia: Bradykinesia means poverty of movement. Automatic movements, such as arm swinging during gait and facial expressions, are diminished (Mathiowetz & Haugen, 1995; Smith, 1993; Undzis et al, 1996).

▼ POSTURAL CONTROL

Before evaluation of postural control, one needs to do an examination of posture. Posture is a composite of the positions of all the joints of the body at any given time. It is the static position assumed by any body part or by the body in general that requires muscular effort (Brooks, 1986; Farber, 1991a,b; Kendall et al, 1993). Kinesiologically, one needs to evaluate spinal alignment and curves, pelvis, trunk, head and neck, and upper extremity posture alone and in relation to each other in positions of standing, sitting, and lying down if appropriate. Good body alignment occurs when the center of gravity of each body segment is located over the supporting base of the body. Structural problems and muscle strength deficits or imbalances can have a mechanical effect on postural control.

Postural control, or balance, refers to the ability to maintain the center of body mass or a body part over a stable or moving base of support (Crutchfield, Shumway-Cook, & Horak, 1989). There are several prerequisites for "normal" internal postural control. Clients need to be able to:

1. Produce movement through adequate ROM in the trunk and extremities.
2. Differentiate body parts from one another (for example, rotate the head independently of the shoulders).
3. Stop and hold movement at midrange of motion to stabilize against gravity. This is critical for transitional movement.
4. Distribute normal postural tone in the body segments to support movement.
5. Function symmetrically.
(Gilfoyle, Grady, & Moore, 1981).

One difficulty in identifying the specific determinants of balance deficits is that balance behavior can be influenced by the somatosensory (proprioceptive, cutaneous, and joint), visual, and **vestibular** systems. Clients may show deficits in balance control during expected and unexpected perturbations, voluntary postural adjustments, or postural adjustments preceding voluntary limb movements. Valid conclusions about balance dysfunction require tests that differentiate among conditions that modify sensory inputs (Difablo & Badke, 1990).

The therapist should note clinical observations of the client's ability to acquire and maintain the following developmental positions: prone, supine, sitting, crawling, standing, and walking, noting automatic responses in sagittal, frontal, and transverse body planes. Balance during various functional activities, such as reaching in the kitchen, tying shoes, and bathing, should be noted as well. Lastly, there are several clinical assessment tools that evaluate postural control (Table 16–24).

▼ FINE COORDINATION AND DEXTERITY

Coordination can be defined as the smooth and harmonious action of groups of muscles working together to produce a desired motion. Dexterity is a type of fine coordination usually demonstrated in the upper extremity. There are several standardized tests that evaluate aspects of dexterity such as speed of object manipulation, accuracy of movement, grasp and release, prehension patterns, writing skills, and hand posture (Farber, 1991a,b; Mathiowetz & Haugen,

1995; Smith, 1993; Undzis et al, 1996). These tests are usually administered with the individual sitting with the arm supported. However, it is important to observe fine motor functioning in a variety of positions, with the arm supported and unsupported, as they occur in ADL.

Functional tasks such as buttoning, using scissors, handling coins, and writing should be observed for the ease, accuracy, and timing of performance. The tests listed in Table 16–25 can be used to specifically identify as well as monitor progress with dexterity difficulties in a more standardized fashion.

Recording Results

Observation of functional abilities can be recorded directly on the initial evaluation. Results of standardized tests should be recorded according to the directions of each test.

Interpreting Results

Irregularity in rate of movement, excessive force, incorrect sequencing, and sudden corrective movements may indicate problems with coordination. Scores on standardized dexter-

TABLE 16-24. Postural Control Assessments

Assessment	Description	Source
Sensory Organization Test (SOT)	Defines six different sensory conditions or environments to measure postural sway. Assesses influence of vision, somatic and vestibular sensory information.	Nashner, 1993a
Sensory Integration Test	A foam surface is used to disrupt somatic sensation; a visual conflict dome with dots or lines is used to disrupt vision; measures client's ability to maintain balance under six conditions.	Horak & Shupert, 1994
Functional reach	Measures the distance between the anatomical reach and the maximal reach without slipping.	Duncan, Weiner, Chandler, & Studenski, 1990
Mobility skills assessment	Variety of tasks such as maintenance of unsupported sitting, standing, reach, transfer, are scored using a three-point descriptive scale.	Studenski, Duncan, & Hogue, 1989
Tinetti's balance and gait evaluation	Client is asked to do a variety of tasks, such as move from sitting to standing, ambulate. Has high predictive validity for frail elderly at risk for falls.	Tinetti, 1986
Berg balance scale	Client asked to complete 14 different tasks. Each task is scored using a four-point scale.	Berg, Wood-Dauphinee, & Williams, 1989
SMART Balance Master	Equipment performs posturography testing and training of postural control.	Neuro Com International Clackamas, OR
Limits of Stability Test	Client stands and a computerized forceplated center of gravity is calculated. The client volitionally shifts weight toward a series of targets. Monitors movement for smoothness and accuracy of postural movements.	Nashner, 1993b
Fugl–Meyer Sensorimotor Assessment	Balance subtest measures the amount of assistance and time tolerated during static standing balance and tilting reactions.	Fugl–Meyer, 1980

TABLE 16-25. Fine Motor Coordination Tests

Dexterity Assessment	Description–Features	Source
Crawford Small Parts Dexterity Test	Measures eye–hand coordination and manipulation of small hand tools. Designed for teenagers and adults. Pins, collars, screws, tweezers, screwdriver. Examinee is timed on tasks such as inserting pen in hole in metal plate with tweezers, covering with collar, threading screws	Psychological Corporation 304 East 45th St. New York, NY 10017
The Erhardt Developmental Prehension Assessment	Part of text by Rhoda P. Erhardt *Developmental Hand Dysfunction: Theory, Assessment, Treatment.* Measures components and skills of hand function development. Designed for birth–6 yr. Uses variety of objects, such as small suitcase, plastic pail, toy hammer, key, beads, tin can, rubber ball, stacking rings, to measure grasp and reflex, manipulation skills	RAMSCO Publishing Co. PO Box N Laurel, MD 20707
Fine Dexterity Test	Assesses fine finger movements of adults.	Educational and Industrial Test Services Ltd. 83 High St. Hemel Hempstead, Heas. HPI 3AH, England
The Grooved Pegboard Test	Measures eye–hand coordination and finger dexterity. Placing grooved pegs in 25-hole pegboard, in various random positions.	Lafayette Instrument Co. PO Box 5729 Lafayette, IN 47903
Moore Eye–Hand Coordination and Color Matching Test	Measures speed of eye–hand coordination and color matching for all age groups.	Joseph E. Moore and Assoc. Perry Drive, RFD 12, Box 309 Gainesville, GA 30501
Purdue Pegboard Test	Measures movements of arms, hands, fingers, and fingertip dexterity. Normed for adults and children 5–15 years, 11 months. Placing pins in pegboard; assembly of pins, washers, and collars.	Science Research Assoc. 259 E. Erie St. Chicago, IL 60611
Box and Block Test	Tests manual dexterity. Normed for children 7–9 yr, adults and adults with neuromuscular involvement. Picking up one block at a time and placing it in attached compartment.	Mathiowetz, Volland, Kashman, & Weber, 1985
Nine Hole Peg Test of Fine Motor Coordination	Measures fine dexterity. Normed for adults older than 20 yr. Timed score to place nine 1 1/4″ pegs in a 5x5″ board and remove them.	Mathiowetz, Weber, Kashman, & Volland, 1985
Jebsen-Taylor Hand Function Test	Evaluates functional capabilities. Subtests include writing, card-turning, picking up small objects, simulated feeding, stacking checkers, picking up light and heavy objects.	Jebsen, Taylor, Trieschmann, Trotter, & Howard, 1969
Minnesota Rate of Manipulation Test	Measures dexterity. Placing, turning, displacing, one-hand turning and placing, and two-hand turning and placing round blocks.	American Guidance Service Publishers Bldg. Circle Pines, MN 55014

(Farber, 1991, a, b; Mathiowetz & Haugen, 1995; Smith, 1993; Undzis et al, 1996)

ity tests below norms also signal fine motor coordination problems. Determining the root(s) of the problem leads to a treatment plan. Several considerations should include sensory, specifically proprioceptive deficits, problems with body scheme, coordination of agonist and antagonist muscles, and ability to accurately judge space; cerebellar, spinal cord, posterior column, frontal, and postcentral cerebral cortex lesions also affect coordination. Again, the focus of treatment should be the functional implications of the performance deficit (Undzis et al, 1996).

►SENSORY AND NEUROMUSCULAR PERFORMANCE COMPONENTS CONCLUSION

Evaluation is an ongoing process to gather data, formulate hypotheses, and guide clinical decisions. Although it is important to understand mechanics, such as administration protocols and diagnostic implications, evaluation is more than a compilation of technical information. Today's health care environment necessitates that evaluation provide an overview and be prioritized based on how performance deficits affect function. The occupational therapist must integrate the information and focus on performance deficits that are of most concern to the client. Those performance deficits, as well as social, emotional, and environmental factors, affect functional outcomes.

Section 2

Evaluation of Perception and Cognition

Kathleen M. Golisz and Joan Pascale Toglia

▼ WHY EVALUATE COGNITIVE-PERCEPTUAL COMPONENTS?

Cognition can be defined as the person's capacity to acquire and use information to adapt to the environment (Lidz, 1987). It consists of interrelated processes including the ability to perceive, organize, assimilate, and manipulate information to enable the individual to process information, learn, and **generalize** (Abreu & Toglia, 1987). Cognitive impairments may be seen as a result of developmental or learning problems, brain injury or disease, psychiatric dysfunction, or sociocultural conditions (American Occupational Therapy Association [AOTA], 1991). Cognitive impairments can result in significant disability in all aspects of the client's life: self-care, independent-living skills, work, leisure, and social or interpersonal skills.

▼ DIFFERENCES IN CONCEPTUALIZATION AND IMPLICATIONS FOR EVALUATION APPROACHES

Deficit-Specific Approach

The conceptualization of cognition determines how one approaches the evaluation process. Cognition has traditionally been conceptualized in terms of higher cortical skills divided into hierarchically arranged distinct subskills. This view of cognition is derived from psychometric models of intelligence testing and localization approaches (Toglia, 1992). In this conceptual framework a perceptual motor- or deficit-specific approach is used in the evaluation process. This reductionist approach identifies the impairments from an impaired performance on tests of the cognitive skill. For example, difficulty performing a figure-ground task (ie, differentiating foreground objects or figures from background objects, such as picking up a white sock off a white sheet) would lead to the client being identified as having a "figure-ground impairment" (Siev, Freishtat, & Zoltan, 1986).

This approach does not consider the quality of the client's performance or look for patterns of failure among several tests. For example, a client may perform poorly on assessments of both figure-ground and constructional skills because of a tendency to overattend to the details. On the figure-ground task the client may attend to a small portion of an overlapping object and attempt to identify the object from this limited information. On the constructional task, which requires the client to build a structure with blocks of different lengths, the client may attend to only one portion of the structure and not realize that additional blocks are needed on a different portion of the structure. In this evaluation approach the client is classified as have impairments in both figure-ground and constructional praxis, although the cause of failure can actually be the same (ie, the overattention to details). In the clinical setting, one rarely sees isolated cognitive impairments. Cognitive problems overlap and are interrelated to one another, leading one to question the benefit of applying a reductionist approach to the evaluation process (Toglia & Golisz, 1990).

Dynamic Interaction Approach

In recent cognitive psychology work, cognition is conceptualized in terms of a dynamic interaction between the person, the task, and the **environment** (Toglia, 1991b). Figure 16–26 displays the components of the dynamic interactional model. This model suggests that to understand cognitive function and dysfunction, one must analyze the interaction between external task parameters, the environment, and internal processing strategies (ie, the person's **metacognitive** abilities, and individual characteristics) (Toglia, 1991b). Processing strategies and behaviors are organized approaches, routines, or tactics that operate to select and guide the processing of information (Toglia, 1989a). Metacognitive skills involve both an awareness of one's cognitive abilities and an ability to monitor performance of cognitive tasks through recognizing and correcting errors and regulating task performance. Cognition is not viewed as static, but as a dy-

namic interaction between the internal and external worlds. This conceptual framework leads an occupational therapist to use a dynamic interactional evaluation approach and a dynamic treatment approach, such as Toglia's Multicontext Approach (1991a) (see Chap. 26). Dynamic approaches place little emphasis on performance outcomes for specific assessment tasks because various different factors can influence performance outcome. Information from the evaluation includes an analysis of the strategies used in task performance as well as the conditions that influence performance. Deficient cognitive functions represent areas of weakness and vulnerability. The extent to which symptoms are observed depends on the characteristics of the task, such as the amount, the familiarity, the predictability, the number of decisions, or the spatial arrangement. These task parameters determine the cognitive strategies necessary for task performance.

▼ CHARACTERISTICS OF DIFFERENT TYPES OF ASSESSMENTS

Static and Quantitative Assessments

Static assessments have rigid administration guidelines and compare the client's performance to norms. They are quantitative, product-oriented assessments that help the occupational therapist identify impairments and quantify the severity of those impairments. Scores obtained from quantitative assessments are summary statements about the observed behavior or performance (Lezak, 1983), and the test score is often viewed as most important. The occupational therapist should be wary in interpreting the functional meaning of a particular static assessment score. Clients with relatively in-

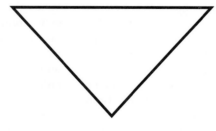

INDIVIDUAL
- Structural Capacity
- Processing Strategies & Behaviors
- Metacognition
- Individual Characteristics (knowledge, motivation, emotions, personality, coping style, experience)

TASK
- Number of items
- Complexity
- Familiarity
- Arrangement
- Movement

ENVIRONMENT
- Social Interaction (e.g. cues)
- Physical
- Multiple Contexts
- Cultural
- Familiarity and predictability

▲

Figure 16-26. The dynamic interactional model. (From Toglia, J. P. [1992]). A dynamic interactional approach to cognitive rehabilitation. In N. Katz [Ed.], *Cognitive rehabilitation: Models for intervention in Occupational Therapy.* Boston: Andover Medical Publisher. Reprinted with permission.)

tact scores on static quantitative assessments can be severely limited in functional performance, whereas clients with very poor scores on quantitative assessments can often perform functional tasks fairly well.

Dynamic and Qualitative Assessments

Qualitative assessments focus on observing and analyzing the process of task performance. Dynamic evaluation is a qualitative evaluation that investigates a person's ability to learn certain tasks and identifies the conditions that facilitate such learning. The aim is not normative comparison or diagnosis of dysfunction. The objective is to discover what the person is capable of doing with assistance or under favorable conditions. This may be useful in predicting a client's response to treatment and in discriminating differences in abilities not typically identified using conventional methods.

The client's learning potential is evaluated through investigating the client's response to cues: Does the client detect errors or, if errors are pointed out, does the client's performance improve? What happens if the therapist focuses the client's attention on a particular component of the assessment task? If provided with a strategy to approach the task, does performance improve? To use strategies effectively, the client must have an awareness of his or her current skills, be able to evaluate the level of task difficulty, and recognize the need to use a strategy. The client must then choose the appropriate strategy and monitor its effectiveness.

The client's use of strategies is investigated through clinical interview techniques that reflect or repeat the client's answers back to him or her for clarification, or present a hypothesis for verification. This interview reveals the client's cognitive style and strategies.

Toglia (1992) describes a systematic cuing process used in a dynamic interactional assessment that moves from general to specific cuing. In this cuing sequence the client may first be cued to check his or her answer. Next the therapist might provide the client with more specific feedback that an error exists and follow up with a cue that provides an approach to the task. If cues appear to be ineffective in improving task performance, the occupational therapist may investigate the effect of a modification of the task (eg, the number of items or the arrangement of the stimuli). Both qualitative and quantitative information gathered from the client's performance with the alteration of the task can help the therapist gain insight into the client's impairments.

Toglia (1992) evaluates metacognitive skills by asking the client to predict performance before the initiation of the task. Does the client's estimation match his or her performance on the task? The occupational therapist is not aiming for the client to predict perfect performance, but rather, for the client to have a clear understanding of his or her limitations and the need to monitor strategy use and task performance. The occupational therapist is interested in whether the client (1) knows the types of tasks that are most difficult

for him or her, (2) identifies when strategy use will be required, (3) monitors his or her performance by checking for errors, and (4) progresses towards the task goal. After completing the task, the therapist investigates the metacognitive skills by asking the client to rate his or her performance. Does the client have an accurate perception of how he or she performed?

The dynamic assessment approach is relatively new and needs further research to determine if dynamic assessments really measure learning potential and if standardized protocols for cuing procedures are needed (Campione & Brown, 1987; Jensen & Feuerstein, 1987). Assessments using this method are currently limited in number and traditional psychometric-testing models do not easily accommodate for cuing, greater client-therapist interaction, or measurement of change within the testing session.

▼ COGNITIVE-PERCEPTUAL EVALUATION: PRINCIPLES

Defining the Evaluation Objective

There are numerous assessments in the area of cognition and perception that an occupational therapist may choose to administer to better understand the client. How does a therapist choose from this vast array and use the evaluation time most effectively? An occupational therapist must first decide what questions he or she has that need to be answered. The therapist then must select an assessment that will address these questions. Does the therapist want to identify the presence of impairments, understand the effect of impairments on performance of functional tasks, gather information to establish a baseline for treatment, or measure change and rehabilitation outcomes?

IDENTIFYING IMPAIRMENTS

When the occupational therapist questions if impairments exist, **mental status examinations** or cognitive screenings may be used to compare the client's performance to normative data. The mental status examinations and screenings outlined in Table 16–26 focus primarily on the skills of **orientation**, **attention**, and **memory**. Cognitive-screening assessments are global and are designed to identify problems that need special or further attention. Many of the cognitive-screening assessments were designed for specific populations, such as clients with strokes (Hajek, Rutman, & Scher, 1989), multiple sclerosis (Rao, Leo, Bernardin, & Unverzagt, 1991), dementia (Mattis, 1976), traumatic brain injury (Ansell & Keenan, 1989), or elderly clients (Golding, 1989).

Occupational therapists should note that mental status examinations rely heavily on verbal skills, may not pick up subtle impairments, and have substantial false-negative rates. The deficits of clients with focal lesions, particularly right hemisphere lesions or mild diffuse cognitive disorders, are

TABLE 16-26. Cognitive Screening Assessments and Mental Status Exams

Assessment	Subtests
Mental Status Examinations	
Mini Mental State Exam (MMSE) (Folstein, Folstein, & McHugh, 1975)	Orientation (time and place), memory for three objects, attention and calculation (Serial 7s or spelling "world" backward), and language skills (naming objects, phrase repetition, following a 3-step oral command and 1-step written command, writing a sentence, and copying a design). Has been used with a variety of populations.
Test of Orientation for Rehabilitation Patients (TORP) (Deitz, Beeman, & Thorn, 1993)	Questions are either open-ended or recognition–multiple choice. Orientation to person and personal situation (*"How old are you?"*), place (*"What is the name of the state we are in right now?"*), time (*"What year is it?"*), schedule (*"What is the first therapy you usually have in the morning?"*), and temporal continuity (*"What season comes after spring?"*). Designed for adults with brain injury or adolescents in a rehabilitation setting.
Galveston Orientation and Amnesia Test (GOAT) (Levin, O'Donnell, & Grossman, 1979)	Orientation to person, place, and time, and recall of events before (retrograde amnesia) and after (anterograde amnesia) the injury (*"What is the first event you can remember after the injury?"*). Designed for use with post-coma patients.
Cognitive Screening Assessments	
Middlesex Elderly Assessment of Mental State (MEAMS) (Golding, 1989)	Consists of 12 subtests: orientation questions, recall of a name, recognition of pictures, comprehension, verbal fluency, arithmetic ability, spatial construction (line drawing), naming of objects, perception of fragmented letters and photos of objects from usual and unusual views, and motor perseveration. Designed for ages 65 and older.
Neurobehavioral Cognitive Status Screening Examination (NCSSE) (Kieman, Mueller, Longston, & VonDyke, 1987)	Assesses intellectual functioning in the areas of: language (spontaneous speech, comprehension, repetition, and naming), construction (involves concentration, visual memory, and constructional ability), memory, calculations, and reasoning (similarities and judgments). Attention, level of consciousness, and orientation are independently scored. Norms available on ages 20–92.
Cognitive Assessment of Minnesota (CAM) (Rustad et al., 1993)	Consists of 17 subtests covering a wide range of skills, such as attention span, memory, orientation, mathematics, visual neglect, following directions, object identification, judgment, reasoning, and safety. Tasks arranged to test the fund of knowledge, manipulation of knowledge, social awareness and judgment, and abstract thinking. Normed on ages 17–70.

(Adapted from Toglia, J.P. [1996, June]. A Multicontext Approach to Cognitive Rehabilitation. Supplemental manual to workshop conducted at New York Hospital-Cornell Medical Center, New York.)

often missed (Nelson, Fogel, & Faust, 1986). Cognitive-screening assessments may also miss the deficits of clients with more subtle impairments displayed by higher-level clients as the breadth and depth of item content is limited.

Occupational therapists also use cognitive–perceptual batteries, such as the Lowenstein Occupational Therapy Cognitive Assessment (LOTCA) (Katz, Itzkovich, Averbuch, & Elazar, 1989) to detect impairments. The LOTCA is a standardized, reliable, and valid battery that has a series of subtests for orientation, perception, visuomotor organization, and thinking skills. Attention and concentration are observed for all subtests.

DETERMINING IMPACT OF DEFICITS ON FUNCTIONAL PERFORMANCE

An occupational therapist may choose to use a functional assessment to either determine the functional tasks with

which the client has difficulty, or to identify specific cognitive–perceptual impairments that interfere with functional task performance. When the therapist wants to determine the functional tasks with which the client has difficulty, performance is usually rated on a numerical or descriptive scale, such as the Functional Independence Measure (FIM) (Granger, Cotter, Brown, & Fiedler, 1993). Most standardized functional assessments used in physical disabilities focus on the amount of physical assistance needed to perform the task. These assessments do not identify the cognitive and perceptual impairments that contribute to poor performance on the functional task, but they do contribute concrete information on potential safety problems and need for cues, assistance, or both. Research is currently being conducted on a modification of the FIM that will grade both physical and verbal levels of assistance and document interfering factors and the need for specific adaptive equipment, compensatory techniques, or increased amount of time to perform the task (Dellarosa, Chan, Toglia, & Finkelstein, 1991).

Functional assessments have also been developed to identify the cognitive–perceptual components that are interfering with successful performance of tasks. Arnadottir's OT-ADL Neurobehavioral Evaluation (A-ONE) (1990), is an assessment that attempts to relate the results of an occupational therapy activities of daily living (ADL) evaluation to specific neurobehavioral impairments and to generate a hypothesis about the localization of cerebral dysfunctions. For example, the task of putting on a shirt is analyzed for the possible behavioral indications of spatial-relation difficulties, unilateral spatial or body neglect, comprehension problems, ideational or ideomotor apraxia, tactile **agnosia,** organization and sequencing difficulties, attention impairments, and motivational impairments.

Other assessments such as the Cognitive Performance Test (CPT) (Allen, Earhart, & Blue, 1992), and the Rabideu Kitchen Evaluation–Revised (RKE-R) (Neistadt, 1992) also identify cognitive–perceptual components interfering with function. Fisher's Assessment of Motor and Process Skills (AMPS) (1993a,b) is an attempt to more systematically analyze the process skills involved in the performance of functional activities. Process skills, such as the client's ability to initiate, inquire, notice and respond, pace, sequence, organize, and terminate, are evaluated through the client's performance of functional activities. Functional tasks require integration of all performance components, so it may be difficult to isolate specific problems interfering with function. These assessments tend to identify broad areas of cognitive and perceptual strengths and weaknesses by identifying the underlying processes that contribute to difficulty performing functional tasks.

ESTABLISHING BASELINES FOR TREATMENT

The evaluation and treatment approach embraced by a given therapist will determine that therapist's choice of baseline measures. An occupational therapist who takes a functional approach to cognitive rehabilitation uses baseline assessments that determine the disability or handicap (ie, the amount of assistance needed to perform a specific task or task components). The underlying skills or impairments are not the focus of this approach to evaluating cognition and perception.

Occupational therapists who take a deficit-specific approach use client scores on tests of cognitive skills as baseline measurements. The occupational therapist who uses a dynamic approach to evaluation and treatment evaluates a client's strategy use, response to cues, and awareness of impairments for baseline measurements. Occupational therapists embracing the dynamic approach to evaluation and treatment often use investigative techniques and modifications to specific skills assessments (Toglia, 1992).

MEASURING CHANGE OR REHABILITATION OUTCOMES

The increasing demands of third-party payers and a need to be accountable for the effectiveness of our services have encouraged occupational therapists to include measuring change and rehabilitation outcome as a goal of cognitive–perceptual evaluation. This requires a definition of success and a determination of what expectations were established based upon the initial evaluation. Is success improved performance on normative tests, greater functional independence, improved vocational outlook, or improved quality of life? When the occupational therapist needs to evaluate the change in the underlying impairment, specific cognitive perceptual or neuropsychological assessments provide the needed information. Functional assessments will rate the changes in functional task performance that have occurred as a result of treatment. Changes in the perception of functional disability by the client or the family are growing in use as are assessments of vocational outcome. Changes in the quality of life and psychosocial variables measured by time usage and daily activity patterns also provide valuable information on cognitive–perceptual improvements. Any measure of outcome on its own may show little change, but the combination of several outcome measures may hold key information on the effectiveness of treatment.

Performance Contexts

It is important to remember the client's individual history and his or her natural social **context** and physical environment when performing a cognitive–perceptual evaluation (Diller, 1993). Cognitive–perceptual performance components cannot be evaluated or interpreted in isolation from the temporal and environmental performance contexts. The client's age, developmental stage, employment, and educational history may influence the client's response to the evaluation process and performance on certain assessments. Therapists should ensure that the assessments being administered are appropriate for the client's age and educational level; otherwise, the results may be invalid. The acuteness or chronicity of the client's cognitive impairments should also be considered during the evaluation process. Will there be a need to frequently monitor the client for recovery of cognitive–perceptual functions (during the acute phase of recovery) or is the disability considered stable?

Environmental contexts may also influence the client's performance on cognitive–perceptual assessments. Physical aspects of the environment, such as the room selected for testing (lighting, noise level, and such) may have an influence, but the social expectations and the cultural background of the client also need to be considered during interpretation of the assessment results. What was the client's previous quality or standard of work? Is the client from a different culture than the normative group of the assessment? Is the client of such a different cultural background than the occupational therapist that there is potential for misinterpretation of responses and performance? What is "normal" within this client's culture?

▼ THE ROLE OF THE OCCUPATIONAL THERAPIST WITHIN A MULTIDISCIPLINARY TEAM

Currently, there is no single discipline responsible for the evaluation and treatment of cognitive–perceptual impairments. Neurologists, neuropsychologists, speech language pathologists, occupational therapists, special educators, and cognitive therapists (specialists with 2- to 4-year degrees), all have the potential to make valuable contributions to understanding the client with a cognitive–perceptual impairment. Because of this overlapping responsibility for cognitive–perceptual performance components there can be confusion and duplication of evaluation and intervention procedures. Treatment team members should discuss the philosophy of their respective disciplines and how their individual approaches to cognition and perception might complement each other, rather than fragment the rehabilitation provided for the client. Although some cognitive assessments, such as mental status examinations, can be administered by a variety of rehabilitation team members, other tests require specialized training or advanced degrees (typically relegated to team members with doctorates). Formal training in the test administration, advanced or continuing education, and supervision are necessities to provide quality cognitive–perceptual evaluation and intervention. Administration of cognitive assessments or any assessment by an untrained health professional is unethical and can invalidate the results (Stringer, 1996).

Neuropsychologists have doctorate level training in the areas of cognitive, educational, clinical, and experimental psychology and often head the cognitive rehabilitation team. The neuropsychologist's approach to cognitive–perceptual assessment is typically diagnostic. Psychometric-based assessments that are quantitative and compare the client's performance with established norms are typically administered by neuropsychologists. Speech language pathologists have training in the higher cognitive functions that are related to language: deductive and inductive reasoning, memory, and organizational skills. The speech language pathologist typically takes an educational perspective toward the cognitive problems.

Occupational therapists provide a unique contribution to the evaluation and rehabilitation of cognitive perceptual performance components owing to their educational background, training in activity analysis, and ability to analyze how cognitive–perceptual symptoms change with different task conditions. The role of the occupational therapist in evaluating cognition and perception is to provide clear, comprehensive information about the effect of cognitive–perceptual impairments on functional tasks of self-care, work, leisure, and community skills. The work environment in which the therapist practices may determine the depth of the occupational therapist's involvement owing to the nature of the practice setting and the client's length of stay. In acute care settings, the occupational therapist may focus on screening for potential impairments that should be followed up in rehabilitation settings or outpatient treatment. In rehabilitation settings, the occupational therapist may perform in-depth assessments and treatment. A **certified occupational therapy assistant (COTA)** can contribute to the evaluation process by administrating standardized cognitive screenings, providing clinical observations, and completing behavioral checklists. These tasks should be carried out under the supervision of the certified **occupational therapist** once the occupational therapy assistant has demonstrated service competency.

▼ EVALUATION OF SPECIFIC COGNITIVE AND PERCEPTUAL COMPONENTS

Orientation

Orientation is the ability to understand the self and the relation between the self and the past and present environment. Orientation depends on the integration of several mental activities that are represented in different areas of the brain. Disorientation indicates that there are significant impairments in attention and memory (Lezak, 1983). Disoriented clients may think they are home in their own house, rather than in a hospital. They may confuse the hospital staff with relatives, and they may believe each time they wake up from a short nap that it is a new day.

Evaluation of orientation traditionally includes the client's orientation to person, place, and time. Orientation to person involves both the self and others. Is the client able to report personal facts and events and describe his or her previous lifestyle? Does the client recognize people and associate them with their role and name? Orientation to place is demonstrated by the client's ability to understand the type of place he or she is in (eg, a hospital), to report the name and location of the place, as well as to appreciate distance and direction. Orientation to time requires an ability to report the current point in time (month, year, date, day), the continuity and sequence of time (estimation), and to associate events with time.

Topographical orientation is often considered a component of orientation to place. It is the ability to follow a familiar route or a new route once given an opportunity to become familiar with it. This skill involves the ability to describe the relation between one place and another, as well as visuospatial skills (Benton, 1985; Bouska, Kauffman, & Marcus, 1985). Topographical orientation also incorporates components of memory. Difficulties with the visual–spatial and memory components of topographical orientation need to be distinguished during evaluation (Okkema, 1993b). Can the client provide a verbal description of the location of the target site, but become confused and lost when attempting to follow a route to the site?

Orientation assessments are traditionally covered in mental status examinations. The Galveston Orientation Amnesia Test (GOAT) (Levin, O'Donnell, & Grossman, 1979) and the Test of Orientation for Rehabilitation Clients (TORP) (Deitz, Beeman, & Thorn, 1993) are two standardized screening tools for orientation. Both of these assessments are described in Table 16–26.

Occupational therapists frequently use nonstandardized measures of orientation such as interviews with open-ended questions asked in a conversational or informal manner. Most therapists use cues to determine the severity of the disorientation. If the client is unable to answer the questions independently, the therapist may offer the client a multiple choice array or offer verbal cues. Cues usually move from general or abstract cues initially to more concrete cues as the severity of disorientation requires (eg, "Today is the beginning of the work week." versus "Today is the day after Sunday."). The number and type of cues offer a method of scoring and monitoring progress. Fluctuations in orientation during the day should be noted as clients may experience "**sundowning**" during which they become confused in the evening because of fatigue.

Insight and Awareness

Insight refers to the degree of awareness one has of his or her own physical or cognitive-perceptual disability. Decreased ability to recognize one's strengths and weaknesses results in poor judgment or a tendency to attempt activities that are beyond one's capabilities. For example, clients with poor insight may attempt to independently transfer themselves to the toilet, despite dense hemiplegia and the need for physical assistance from a health care worker. Lack of insight or awareness differs from denial, which is a psychological defense mechanism characterized by overrationalization. When a client is in denial, the client is aware, but unwilling to confront problems. He or she may become increasingly agitated when confronted with denied reality.

Crosson and coauthors (1989) described different types of awareness, including intellectual, emergent, and anticipatory awareness. In the neurological literature implicit knowledge of impairments has also been identified as a type of awareness. The client's awareness of his or her impairments has implications for rehabilitation and the client's ability to function independently.

Intellectual awareness, according to Crosson and associates (1989), is present when the client has knowledge that a particular function is impaired, but does not use this knowledge to monitor performance. The client may report he or she has difficulty remembering things, but when asked to bring certain items to the next treatment session does not attempt to initiate any strategy that could assist recall (eg, writing the items down in a notebook or pocket calendar). Clients with only intellectual awareness of their impairments show significant safety risks as they do not perform within their limitations.

Implicit knowledge of impairments is observed when clients deny the existence of an impairment, but behave as though they have some knowledge of it. The client may deny memory problems, but consistently write notes in a notebook. When questioned about the behavior the client reports, "I just need to do this." Safety issues can exist with clients with this type of awareness, for they may be inconsistent in initiating compensatory strategies that demonstrate awareness. The client may not admit to memory problems, but be fairly consistent in double checking that he or she turned off the stove. However, one slip in this behavior can threaten life and property.

A client who has the ability to recognize a problem only when it is actually happening has emergent awareness. For example, a client may estimate that a task requiring significant organizational and problem-solving skills (both observed areas of difficulty for this individual) will "be easy." When faced with difficulty during the performance of the task, the client with emergent awareness might state, "Everything is all messed up. I guess this is harder than I thought. Maybe I do have problems." For clients to be able to initiate use of strategy, they must have a minimum level of emergent awareness to be able to recognize problems and the need for compensatory strategies (Bruce, 1993). Clients with emergent awareness may not demonstrate a significant safety risk if they work within their limitations, and recognize and correct errors. However, if they attempt tasks significantly outside their limits, they may end up in a situation where they are incapable of recognizing errors and making necessary corrections to ensure safety.

Anticipatory awareness is the ability to anticipate that a problem will likely occur as the result of an impairment, before performing the task (Crosson et al., 1989). Before beginning a task of higher-level organizational and problem-solving skills, a client with anticipatory awareness might state, "This is my weaker area. I should use a checklist to make sure I get all the information and stay organized. I also need to leave time to check my work for mistakes." Clients with this type of awareness are excellent candidates for rehabilitation, for they comprehend the extent and implications of their impairments. Safety is typically not a major concern for these clients because they have the ability to determine which tasks may be risky and to self-monitor their performance during tasks.

The occupational therapist needs to understand the client's level of awareness during the evaluation process to make recommendations for treatment. The client and family members also need to understand the accuracy of the client's perception of his or her current abilities and the potential safety risks the client's current insight level presents.

Interview and rating scales for insight and awareness generally evaluate (1) a client's awareness of his or her limitations and strengths, (2) the ability to generalize the effect of the limitations on functional tasks, (3) concern about disability, and (4) judgment. A nonstandardized insight interview typically asks the client questions about reason for hospitalization, physical and cognitive difficulties, and functional implications in a conversational or informal manner. Because awareness is not an all-or-nothing phenomenon, the occupational therapist offers cues if the client is unable to answer independently. The questions should move from awareness of the limitations impairments impose on general abilities (anticipatory awareness) to more specific questioning if the client does not appear to understand the functional implications of his or her impairments (eg, "Why are you in the hospital?" to "Do you have difficulty writing?"). Reality testing, during which the client is asked to perform the activity, would be used to evaluate whether awareness emerges when the client experiences difficulty with a particular task requiring skills that are deficient.

The occupational therapist may use a formal assessment that focuses entirely on a client's awareness of his or her impairments such as Prigatano's (1986) Competency Rating Scale, which consists of 30 items in which the client is asked to rate on a 5-point scale how easy or difficult it is to carry out a specific activity. The client and a caregiver fill out separate forms to provide the therapist with information on each person's perspective of the functional influence of the impairments. The Contextual Memory Test (Toglia, 1993b) and the Toglia Category Assessment (Toglia, 1994) are two tests that evaluate the cognitive skills of memory and organization, respectively, but also include a format of test prediction to evaluate the client's awareness on Crosson's continuum. The client is asked general questions concerning his or her awareness of impairments, then asked to predict performance before, and estimate performance immediately after completion of the test. The difference between the scores is an estimate of the client's level of awareness.

Attention

Attention is a multidimensional capacity that involves several components: alertness (detection and reaction), selective attention, sustained attention, shifting of attention, and mental tracking. It incorporates far more than the quantitative measure of the length of time a client can concentrate. A client may be able to perform the lower-level tasks within each component of attention. However, this same client may have difficulty if requested to perform a task that incorporates several different attentional components. Table 16–27 provides examples of basic and complex tasks for each component of attention.

A task may emphasize the detection and reaction component of attention through orienting responses. This component includes the ability to respond discretely to specific visual, auditory, or tactile stimuli, with emphasis on speed and reaction time. Impairments in the detection and reaction component of attention present clinically as insufficient mental alertness or mental lethargy and result from a impairment in the tonic arousal mechanism of the brain. Impairments in the arousal component of attention are most commonly seen in clients who have sustained traumatic brain injuries and are emerging from comas.

The selection component of attention involves the ability to attend to one stimulus while inhibiting other irrelevant stimuli. As the number of irrelevant stimuli increases,

---

TABLE 16-27. Assessment of The Components of Attention

Component	Basic and Complex Tasks
Detect/react	*Basic:* detect and react to a gross change in the environment (eg, telephone ringing or name being called). *Complex:* detect with increasing amounts of stimuli with emphasis on speed (eg, find the spelling errors on a page as quickly as possible).
Selection	*Basic:* maintain visual fixation on a brightly colored pencil eraser while ignoring another pencil moved in visual field. *Complex:* attend to target and inhibit competing distraction (eg, attending to work task and ignoring music playing, or people talking).
Sustain	*Basic:* persist with a repetitive activity, such as bouncing a ball, over time. *Complex:* persist and keep track of information (eg, empty dishwasher top and bottom shelves, stuff envelopes and keep track of the number completed).
Shifting attention	*Basic:* follow one change in an activity (eg, add numbers then subtract numbers). *Complex:* shift back and forth between two tasks–sequences (eg, stop and answer telephone while filing and typing).
Mental tracking	*Basic:* immediate recall (eg, remembering a phone number just given on the telephone). *Complex:* keep track of two or more stimuli simultaneously (eg, cooking while listening to the radio).

(Adapted from Toglia, J.P. [1996, June]. A Multicontext Approach to Cognitive Rehabilitation. Supplemental manual to workshop conducted at New York Hospital–Cornell Medical Center, New York.)

the difficulty level will also increase (eg, finding items in a crowded store). When the differences between the target and distracters are subtle, the competition to inhibit an automatic response is higher. Clinically, the client with impaired selective attention may exhibit extreme distractibility during which attention is easily captured by any stimuli, and the client is unable to inhibit an orienting response. Goal-directed behavior is diminished, and responses are either too fast (impulsive) or too slow. The client displays impaired ability to engage his or her attention or focus on relevant information, especially with increasing amounts of stimuli.

Attention span or vigilance is the ability to persist or sustain attention over time. The longer the task, the more persistence that is required. The more novel the distracting stimuli the more difficult it is to sustain attention to the task at hand.

Shifting attention is the ability to alternate between stimuli or tasks. Tasks used to evaluate ability to shift attentional sets should also follow a continuum of simple to complex (see Table 16–27).

Mental tracking refers to the ability to simultaneously attend to multiple pieces of the task while keeping track of the stimuli or associated ideas. It has also been termed divided attention or simultaneous attention. This component of attention is akin to immediate recall. Standardized tests, such as the Digit Span (Lezak, 1983) and the Knox Cube Test (Stone & Wright, 1980), evaluate attention span and immediate recall of auditory and visual information, respectively. The Paced Auditory Serial Addition Test (PASAT) (Gronwall, 1977) detects subtle impairments in attention and speed of processing. Scores on the PASAT are predictive of outcome after a traumatic brain injury (Gronwall, 1977). Functionally, mental-tracking tasks are needed in everyday activities. Each time we complete a multiple component cooking task, or drive and carry on a conversation we test our mental-tracking abilities. Which of us have not become immersed in a conversation while driving and missed our exit or turn?

The Test of Everyday Attention (TEA) (Robertson, Ward, Ridgeway, & Nimmo-Smith, 1994) was designed to tap the different aspects of attention. It consists of eight subtests that use familiar, everyday materials, such as map and telephone book searching (ie, selective visual attention and divided attention), counting elevator "beeps" on tape (ie, sustained attention and auditory selective attention), visual elevator floor counting (ie, flexibility and switching attention), and lottery ticket reviews (ie, sustained attention). There are three parallel versions of the TEA for test-retest and norms for ages 18 to 80.

Visual Processing: Visual Discrimination

Clinical vision evaluation for oculomotor dysfunction should be performed before a visual-processing evaluation to screen out visual problems that will interfere with the accuracy of perceptual testing. Several clinical observations during functional tasks can alert occupational therapists to the need for a formal visual assessment: compensatory head movements and tilting, squinting, shutting of one eye, or a tendency to lose one's place while reading.

Whenever possible the input of a neuro-ophthalmologist should be sought in the clinical evaluation of vision; however, a basic screening can be performed by the occupational therapist. Visual acuity should be measured for both near and distant vision with any corrective lens the client uses. Pupillary functions of size at rest, response to light, and **visual accommodation** need to be evaluated. The occupational therapist should evaluate the ROM of the eyes and ocular alignment. Visual field impairments are common after brain injuries or strokes and are best evaluated by an ophthalmologist or optometrist through perimeter testing. When this test is unavailable, the visual fields can be grossly evaluated using a confrontation method, described later, under unilateral inattention. Lastly, visual pursuits (ie, smooth tracking of moving objects), saccades (ie, quick eye movements to place an object of interest in view), and visual-scanning functions should be evaluated. Any disruptions of these foundational skills, which are vulnerable to a wide range of neural injuries, will affect all interpretations of higher-level visual-processing assessments (Warren, 1993).

The deficit-specific approach to visual processing categorizes visual perception into specific areas, such as figure-ground, position in space, form constancy, spatial relations, and visual recognition. An information-processing perspective conceptualizes visual perception as a process involving the reception, organization, and assimilation of visual information. Visual perception in the information-processing model, is viewed on a continuum from simple to complex processing in each specific area. When we process a simplistic visual scene (such as a familiar object or shape) we process the information globally at a fast speed with minimal effort. However, when processing a more complex visual array, with unfamiliar stimuli or the need for more subtle discriminations, our processing is slower and requires maximal effort. In this conceptualization a visual-processing dysfunction is defined as a decrease in the amount that the visual system is able to assimilate at any one time (Toglia, 1989b). To understand the client's visual perceptual skills and the effect of impairments on functioning we need to look at the task conditions (complexity, amount, familiarity, and predictability), rather than the type of task (visual spatial, visual discrimination, visual motor, or visual gestalt).

Simple visual-processing dysfunction may include (1) difficulty in visual discrimination between objects, pictures of objects, colors, and basic shapes; (2) difficulty in detecting gross differences in size, position, direction, angles, and rotations; (3) decreased ability to visually locate single visual targets in space or to judge gross distances between two objects; (4) decreased ability to detect simple part–whole relations in objects or basic shapes; and (5) decreased ability to draw simple shapes or objects (eg, geometric shapes or flower). Let us take, for example, an assessment of a client's ability to recognize objects.

CASE STUDY

Mr. J is having difficulties locating objects in his bathroom closet and his bedside stand drawer. He will name what he wants to pick up, but then reach for a different object. Mr. J's ability to recognize objects was tested in the treatment room with him sitting at a table covered with a white cloth. He was initially presented with single objects that were self-related and presented in a vertical arrangement. Mr. J demonstrated no difficulty when asked to "Tell me what this object is." His ability remained constant regardless of the number of objects (up to eight) presented in a horizontal line. When objects were presented in a scattered overlapping format Mr. J had a tendency to miss objects and misperceive components of objects as separate items. This tendency was even stronger when he was given unconventional objects and increasing amounts. For example, he thought the handle of a small magnifying glass was an allen wrench. He only identified it as a magnifying glass when the overlapping object was removed. With all object identification tasks Mr. J demonstrated slow visual-processing time. With further testing Mr. J's ability to imagine what an object looked like was intact. He was able to verbally describe the critical features of various objects that could help in identifying them.

Prerequisites to visual object evaluation should include a visual screening, a discussion with the speech language pathologist to rule out language impairments, and visual imagery questioning. A deficit-specific approach to object identification presents clients with actual objects or pictures of objects and asks the client to identify each object. The person is labeled as demonstrating visual **agnosia** when unable to accurately identify the objects presented.

The dynamic interactional approach to evaluating visual object perception conceptualizes object recognition on a continuum and evaluates both conventional and unconventional objects under a variety of different task conditions (eg, environment, amount, and arrangement). Table 16–28 illustrates how an occupational therapist using this approach would analyze and systematically manipulate task parameters and cue responses to investigate use of strategies and to fully analyze why a client is having difficulty recognizing objects. Cues are used to facilitate object recognition when the client encounters difficulty.

Lets revisit Mr. J, discussed above. The occupational therapist has formed the hypothesis that Mr. J overfixated on individual features or parts of objects and misidentified objects based on salient characteristics without integrating the elements (eg, Mr. J's focus on the handle of the magnifying glass and subsequent misidentification of the object). The therapist initiates the cuing process by providing a cue of repetition ("Look again Mr. J.") which provides Mr. J with the general feedback that his response was incorrect. Because this cue did not appear to assist Mr. J in identifying previous misperceived objects a deeper analysis cue might be tried which asks Mr. J to describe properties of the object (weight, size, material, and such). This type of cue analyzes the effect of focusing on components of the object. This cuing is not expected to aid Mr. J, for he already over-

TABLE 16-28. Dynamic Assessment of Object Identification

			Task Parameters			
Task Grading	Environment	Familiarity of Objects	Directions	Number of Objects Present	Spatial Arrangement	Response Rate per Object
Least difficult	Normal context	Self-related (eg, toothbrush)	"What is this?"	1–5	Linear, nonrotated	<0.8 seconds
Moderately difficult	Associated context	Non–self-related (eg, pen)	"Find the [object]."	10	Scattered, rotated	1.1 seconds
Most difficult	Out of context	Unconventional (eg, pen shaped like a candycane)	"Tell me what you see."	20	Scattered, rotated, overlapping	1.3 seconds

(With permission from Toglia, J. P. [1989]. Visual perception of objects: An approach to assessment and intervention. American Journal of Occupational Therapy, 43, 587–595.)

focuses on features of the objects. The occupational therapist next provides Mr. J with specific perceptual cues to focus his attention on a critical detail of the object that should aid in identification, such as pointing to the lens of the magnifying glass and asking Mr. J to "Look here." Additional items that overlap the target item may be removed to enable Mr. J to see the target item as a continuous whole. Specific semantic cues that provide a multiple choice array of possible categories that the object may belong to (eg, "Mr. J, does this item belong to the category of tool, jewelry, or grooming items?") narrow the range of possible objects when combined with visual cues and aid in identification.

Complex **visual perceptual** skills require a high degree of integration and analysis and typically involve visually confusing environments; abstract, unfamiliar, or detailed visual information; or conditions under which the distinctive visual features are partially obscured (eg, constructing a three-dimensional object that cannot be rotated). Dysfunction of complex visual perceptual skills may include decreased ability to detect subtle differences in abstract shapes and objects, or of angles, size, distance, and position. A client may have difficulty making sense out of ambiguous, incomplete, fragmented, or distorted visual stimuli. As with Mr. J, the complexity of object recognition increased when distinctive features of objects were partially obscured (eg, unconventional views, silhouettes, figures concealed in a complex pattern, or targets masked by extraneous lines, shading, and so forth). One might expect Mr. J to also have difficulty performing functional tasks, such as finding items on a crowded refrigerator shelf, closet, or supermarket shelf, or locating key information on a bill or map. Safety risks may be present if Mr. J misperceives items in the kitchen (eg, carving knife and spatula) or bathroom (eg, razor and toothbrush).

Visual Processing: Visual Motor

Visual motor skills may include drawing tasks (eg, drawing a map to a specific location) or construction of three-dimensional figures (eg, assembling a coffee pot or making a flower arrangement). These skills involve visual discrimination, motor planning abilities, and other cognitive–perceptual skills. Clients may demonstrate difficulty on these types of tasks for many reasons. For example, a client may have difficulty constructing a block design because of (1) poor scanning of the complete design; (2) decreased planning and organization; (3) unilateral inattention; (4) impaired discrimination of size, angles, and rotations; or (5) constructional apraxia. The client is labeled as having "constructional apraxia" when he or she has difficulty performing drawing tasks or activities in which parts are put together to form a single entity or object, when this difficulty cannot be attributed to perceptual impairments, ideomotor apraxia, organizational impairments, or primary motor or sensory impairments (Benton, 1985). Constructional impairments may be seen in clients following damage to either parietal lobe, but the clinical presentation differs in spatial aspects based on the hemisphere involved. Clients with right hemisphere damage typically lose the overall configuration and perform the task in a piecemeal approach with disorganization and additions. Clients with left hemisphere damage maintain the overall configuration, but lose the details and miss individual features; they simplify the design and reduce the number of pieces used (Kramer, Kaplan, & Blusewicz, 1991; Robertson & Lamb, 1991). Several authors have found a close correlation between constructional abilities and ADL performance (Bernspang, Asplund, Eriksson, & Fugl-Meyer, 1987; Neistadt, 1992; Warren, 1981).

Tasks used to evaluate visual motor skills are diverse and methods of test administration differ. Both two-dimensional graphomotor tasks and three-dimensional object assembly have been used. The sample task may or may not be presented as a model, and the tasks themselves may vary in complexity. Two-dimensional free-drawing and copying tasks (eg, draw a person, house, clockface, flower, or bicycle) are frequently used. There is little standardization of scoring in these drawing tasks. The Benton Constructional Praxis Test (Benton, Hamsher, Varney, & Spreen, 1983) is a classic standardized assessment of three-dimensional visual motor and constructional skills. The client is shown each of three block or photographic models, which are increasingly more complex, and asked to reproduce the construction. The Benton Constructional Praxis Test correlated with performance in self-care activities in clients who sustained strokes (Titus, Gall, Yerxa, Roberson, & Mack, 1991). Nonstandardized construction tasks are also frequently used by occupational therapists in the evaluation of visual motor and constructional praxis. Reproducing matchstick or toothpick designs, block designs, puzzles, and parquetry blocks (Neistadt, 1989) have all been used.

Unilateral Inattention

Unilateral inattention is one of the most dramatic disorders seen in the clinic. Unilateral inattention (also commonly called neglect) is a failure to orient to, respond to, or report stimuli presented on the side contralateral to the cerebral lesion in clients who do not have primary sensory or motor impairments (Heilman, Watson, & Valenstein, 1985). Mr. Y, described in the following, presents with many of the typical clinical symptoms of unilateral inattention.

In the acute phase, unilateral inattention is often characterized by a marked deviation of the head, eyes, and trunk away from the left hemispace. The client appears to be magnetically drawn toward those stimuli and activities located on the right side. It is not uncommon to see a bewildered client looking for the voice coming from the person sitting on his or her left, under his or her wheelchair on the right. In severe cases, clients may fail to recognize their contralateral extremities as their own and attempt to fling the "unknown person" out of their beds.

The term *neglect* connotes a volitional component to the disorder, but this is a misnomer. The client with unilateral

Mr. Y recently sustained a right-hemisphere stroke. He requires cues in the dining room to locate items on the left side of his food tray. If not cued Mr. Y eats only the food on the right side of his plate. During morning self-care Mr. Y shaves only the right side of his face and combs the right side of his hair. He gropes for his left arm when dressing and needs cues to straighten his shirt on his left shoulder. When pushing his wheelchair he constantly veers toward the left and bumps into walls.

inattention is unaware of the incompleteness of his or her perception and responses to the environment.

Unilateral inattention can be a major disability in the acute phases of recovery from stroke and can impede later attempts to rehabilitate the client. Unilateral inattention has been identified as a major factor impeding functional recovery in clients who have sustained strokes (Chen Sea, Henderson, & Cermak, 1993). It is also the important variable related to the difference in improvement of ADL between right- and left-lesioned subjects (Kinsella & Ford, 1985). Left hemisphere-lesioned clients with severe handicaps owing to language dysfunction make a better functional recovery than right hemisphere-lesioned clients with unilateral inattention.

Occupational therapists evaluating clients with unilateral inattention must first distinguish between hemianopsia and unilateral inattention. Visual field cuts (hemianopsia) are hemiretinal, whereas neglect is hemispatial. Clients with visual field cuts typically have awareness of their visual field loss and make compensatory head movements and turns. Unilateral inattention may exist with or without hemianopsia. One syndrome does not cause the other. A complete visual screening is needed to document the presence or absence of hemianopsia.

Unilateral inattention varies with stimulus characteristics. Clients may display asymmetry in functional activities, drawing tasks, reading, and writing, depending on the task characteristics: sensory, motor, distance of task from body, spacial size of task, and arrangement of the task stimuli. For example, studies have found significant differences between right- and left-lesioned subjects on a small-space task. No significant differences were found with the same subjects on large-space tasks (Rizzolatti & Berti, 1993). Many of the clients with unilateral inattention exhibit anxiety or flattened affect and appear to deny the presence of their impairments. This lack of awareness can result in a display of anger when challenged about the presence of difficulties.

Traditional evaluation of unilateral inattention has involved tasks of extinction and confrontation, line bisection, cancellation, and drawing tests. Tests of extinction and confrontation evaluate the sensory component of unilateral inattention (ie, when two stimuli are presented at the same time the client attends only to the right-sided stimuli). For example, the occupational therapist may evaluate visual extinction by holding both arms at shoulder height in the client's intact visual fields and moving a finger on one or both hands. Clients with visual extinction will report the single stimulus in each visual field, but only the right-sided stimulus when simultaneous stimuli occurs. Before beginning tests for extinction the examiner must ensure that basic sensation for each modality is intact bilaterally.

Line bisection tasks require the client to estimate and mark the midpoint of lines. A deviation toward the ipsilesional side is considered a demonstration of unilateral inattention. Testing should be done with lines in horizontal and vertical orientations, for differences can be seen. There are numerous variations of line bisection tasks that manipulate the task demands or stimulus parameters: length of the line (usually the longer the line, the greater the inattention), anchors at the end of the line (eg, a red line drawn down the left-sided margin), direction of visual scanning, different orientations of the lines, and different positions in space.

Researchers have also explored the performance of clients with unilateral inattention on line extension and line erasure tasks (Ishiai, 1994). In line extension tasks the client is asked to extend a horizontal line leftward to double its original length. This task directs attention toward the left not the right and thus clients display less neglect than on traditional line bisection tasks. Line erasure tasks require the client to erase the line to midpoint. The gradual decrease in the amount of right stimuli leads to less demonstration of unilateral inattention.

Cancellation tests have been traditionally used to detect the presence of neglect. These tasks require the ability to locate and cancel, or mark, target stimuli from among a series of stimuli. The stimuli may be arranged in random or structured, linear formation and include lines, letters, numbers, and stars or other shapes such as bells (Gauthier, Dehaut, & Joanette, 1989). Cancellation tasks may vary in how easily the targets can be discriminated from the background stimuli. For example, it is simpler for a client to select the red socks from a table scattered with white socks, than to select dinner forks of a particular silverware pattern from a tabletop scattered with four or more silverware patterns. The second task requires focal attention and subtle discriminations. Search time would be expected to increase with increases in amount or display size owing to the slow, analytical search which must be conducted.

Drawing tests have been traditionally used to evaluate unilateral inattention. Clients with unilateral inattention typically have difficulty producing symmetric drawings of objects such as butterflies, daisies, clocks, and bicycles. The type and distribution of errors have been scored and analyzed, but there is no reported normative date, reliability, or validity. The Parietal Lobe Test of the Boston Diagnostic Aphasia Examination (Goodglass, & Kaplan, 1972) is an example of an assessment that provides standardized procedures and specifies criteria for scoring drawings for neglect. Copying asymmetric nonsense figures may be more sensitive than copying well-known symmetric objects.

The Behavioral Inattention Test (BIT) (Wilson, Cockburn, & Halligan, 1987) was designed to include both conventional tests of neglect and tests of everyday skills, to provide more comprehensive information for developing rehabilitation programs. It includes the conventional subtests of line crossing, letter cancellation, star cancellation, figure and shape copying, line bisection, and representational drawing. Behavioral subtests include picture scanning, telephone dialing, menu reading, telling and setting time, coin sorting, address copying, and map following.

A study by Hartman-Maeir and Katz (1995) explored the validity of the behavioral subtests of the BIT. Seven of the nine behavioral subtests differentiated significantly between subjects with visual neglect and those without neglect. The article-reading and time-telling subtests appear to lack sufficient sensitivity to detect neglect, and educational background influenced performance on the article reading. Six of the nine subtests correlated significantly with parallel performance tasks or an ADL checklist items. Picture scanning and map navigation did not correlate significantly with parallel functional measures, suggesting that they are not valid measures of eating and mobility. The authors provide a framework for analyzing qualitative aspects of performance and suggest that the client's response to cuing has potential implications for treatment planning. Further studies are needed on the cuing aspect of this version of the BIT.

Functional performance measures have also been used to evaluate unilateral inattention. Reading tests such as the Caplan Indented Paragraph Test (1987), checklists, and semistructured ADL scales have been used to examine the relation between scores on traditional tests of neglect and ADL performance. Reliability and validity of these ADL measures have not been examined.

Hartman-Maeir and Katz's study of the BIT support Toglia's argument that it is not enough to know that unilateral inattention is present or absent on different tasks; we need to understand which task characteristics change the magnitude of neglect (Toglia, 1991b). Toglia's dynamic interactional assessment model attempts to differentiate symptoms of unilateral inattention by exploring the tasks and activities that the client can or cannot perform along with the client's awareness of his or her unilateral inattention.

After a baseline performance is established, cues are used to explore and facilitate performance. Cues question the client's awareness or detection of errors by providing the client with feedback on his or her performance. "How do you think you did? Was the task difficult? Do you think you got all the information on the left side of the paper?" Cues may also direct the client's attention to the essential features of the task (eg, "I want you to look over to where your left hand is on the edge of the paper. See if you find any other information that you may have missed.") or probe strategy use to gain insight into the client's cognitive style and task approach (eg, "What did you do to make sure you were looking over to your left?").

Cues may present a hypothesis for verification (eg, "It seems you had a hard time bringing your eyes and attention over toward the left.") or provide the client with strategies for performing the task (eg, "Let's try this again, but this time I want you to make sure you touch your left hand as you look towards that left side of the paper to make sure you are all the way over on the left.").

When using a dynamic approach to evaluating unilateral inattention, the occupational therapist makes a hypothesis about the individual's performance and tests the hypothesis by repeating the task with modifications. Some task components will be held constant while one task component is varied. For example, if it is hypothesized that the client is neglecting greater information because of the arrangement of the information (scattered versus linear), then the arrangement of the information is changed while the amount and complexity of the material stay the same.

Motor Planning

Motor planning or praxis is the ability to figure out how to make your body do what you want it to do (Lane, 1991). **Apraxia** is a narrower component of motor-planning impairments that is defined as a disorder of skilled movement that cannot be adequately accounted for by incoordination, sensory loss, visual spatial problems, language comprehension difficulties, or cognitive problems alone (Heilman & Rothi, 1985). Mrs. H in the following case study illustrates a typical client with apraxia.

Motor planning has been viewed as a broad skill that involves the integration of many different processes: vision and perception, cognition, tactile-kinesthetic sensation, language, and selection and organization of movements. Motor planning involves the cognitive formulation of the intention to move, selection of a goal, planning the movement, and anticipating the end result. Knowledge of the functional properties of objects, actions, and action sequences is necessary, as are attentional processes that enable the individual to analyze the task demands and attend to relevant environmental task cues. Skilled movement also requires the integration of tactile–kinesthetic information such as where the body is in space, how the parts of the body relate to each other during movement, and how the body and limbs are positioned. Vestibular functions provide a sense of body position and movement in space that help in making postural

CASE STUDY

Mrs. H sustained a burst cerebral aneurysm in the left parietal region and, although she sustained no gross language, physical, or cognitive impairments, she appears to be having problems in the performance of functional tasks. During a meal preparation activity of making a grilled cheese sandwich Mrs. H is able to verbally describe the sequence to completing the task, but when she attempts the task she is observed placing the cheese on the toaster oven tray without the bread. The bread is on the countertop. Mrs. H states "I know that's wrong." During the task of making muffins she has significant difficulty assembling the rotary blades into the mixer. She appears frustrated and states "This shouldn't be so difficult." When asked to stop and pantomime the sequence of making the muffins Mrs. H tends to verbally report her intended actions, rather than physically demonstrate them. When encouraged to act out the procedure Mrs. H is observed using her hand as the motion of the mixer and many of her motor acts appear to be clumsy and perseverative (repetitive). If she was not verbally reporting what she was pantomiming an observer would not be able to identify the act of baking.

adjustments during the execution of movement. Visual–spatial information about size, spatial position, orientation, shape, and texture of objects helps guide the selection of motor patterns. Linguistic skills aid the individual in translating verbal commands into action or using action and movement to convey meaning. The sequencing of the movement requires selection and pretuning of the order and configuration of muscles to be activated as well as the speed and amplitude of both the initial movement and the transition from one movement to another.

Apraxia is thought to be due to damage to the areas of the brain involved with the cognitive aspects of motor control: the association areas (Kertesz, 1982). Apraxia is commonly seen in clients who have sustained a left hemisphere lesion (Heilman & Rothi, 1985) and who often display related impairments of aphasia, gesture recognition, and sequencing impairments (Harrington & Haaland, 1992). The related impairments, however, do not appear to be the primary cause of the client's inability to produce skilled movement.

Roy (1978) identified two major subsystems in apraxia: the conceptual and the production subsystems. The symptoms of apraxia may reflect disorders in one of these subsystems or in both. The production aspect of motor planning concerns generating the action plan, sequencing and organizing the appropriate elements, and carrying out the plan (eg, reaching for a glass of water to take a drink). This is thought of as the executive aspect of movement. The traditional term used to describe production errors is ideomotor apraxia. Production errors may be spatial (eg, reaches with right hand to the left side of the glass) or temporal (eg, perseverative or repetitive). The greatest difficulty is observed when the client is asked to perform transitive pantomimes that are pretended use of a tool or object (eg, "Show me how you use a toothbrush.") or to perform intransitive limb gestures (eg, "Show me how you wave goodbye."). Perseveration or repetition of component movements may be seen,

or the client may use a body part as the object (eg, use a finger as the toothbrush). Some improvement may be seen when the client is asked to imitate the motion or to perform the motion with the actual object, but the movement is still imprecise. The client makes spatiotemporal errors when required to perform a series of actions (eg, pour coffee into a cup, add sugar and milk, stir, and drink it).

The conceptual aspect of motor planning includes knowledge about the functional properties of an object, the object action, and the sequence of action. Conceptual errors, traditionally called ideational apraxia, involve object function (eg, using a knife as a spoon), action knowledge (eg, match demonstrated gesture to picture or object), and knowledge of sequence (eg, brushing one's teeth). Some authors (Belanger, Duffy, & Coelho, 1994) question if ideomotor and ideational apraxia are distinct disorders representing unique underlying neuropsychological impairments or a single underlying disorder along a continuum of severity.

The clinical evaluation of apraxia has varied greatly and is primarily subjective. Evaluation typically involves observation of the client's performance of different types of movements (Table 16–29), the method of evocation (eg, command, imitation, or object use) (Belanger, Duffy, Coelho, 1994), and the type of errors made (eg, position, orientation, target, body-part-as-object, **perseveration**, delay, or clumsiness [Haaland, 1993]). The evaluation of apraxia is difficult to score reliably because item difficulty and familiarity, as well as sequential requirements, vary with each assessment.

The evaluation of apraxia has broadened recently to include the recognition and discrimination of gestures by having the client observe videotapes of gestures and select a picture of the pantomimed object or to discriminate between well-performed and poorly performed pantomime acts (Heilman, Rothi, & Valenstein, 1982; Rothi, Heilman, & Watson, 1985). York and Cermak (1995) found differences in impairments between clients with left versus right hemi-

TABLE 16-29. Categories of Motor Planning Tasks	
Category of Movement	**Verbal Command**
Proximal transitive	Show me how you would bounce a basketball.
Proximal intransitive	Show me how you stop traffic.
Distal transitive	Show me how you dial a phone.
Distal intransitive	Show me how you snap your fingers.
Oral nonrespiratory	Show me how you lick a lollipop.
Oral respiratory	Show me how you sniff a flower.

Note: *Transitive = movements pantomiming use of an object; Intransitive = movements involving limb gestures without objects.*
(From Helm-Estabrooks, 1992)

sphere strokes. Clients with right hemisphere damage exhibited the most difficulty on tests of gesture discrimination, whereas clients with left hemisphere damage demonstrated difficulty with tests of gesture comprehension.

When evaluating the client for motor-planning abilities it is important to conduct a thorough neurological assessment because apraxia is defined by exclusionary criteria. Clients may display motor-planning problems owing to significant sensory loss or incoordination, but clients with apraxia display motor-planning problems when free of significant sensory or motor impairments and incoordination. Because many apraxic clients are also aphasic (both disorders are typically seen following left hemisphere dysfunction) information on the client's language skills should be obtained from the speech language pathologist or screened for by testing for yes or no comprehension and the ability to follow one-step commands. Many clients with right hemiparesis and apparent apraxia will attribute their "clumsiness" to the use of their nondominant hand. There are many standardized assessments of gesture use available, but these assessments are narrow and restrictive. They should be supplemented with evaluation of whole-body movements, and functional movements both on request and within an automatic context. Some static assessments focus on localizing and diagnosing apraxia, which is not the major priority of an occupational therapist. Assessments for apraxia typically ask the client to perform or imitate a gesture, use an actual object, or imitate the examiner using an object. The movements are either performed by using a limb or the face (buccofacial).

The Test of Oral and Limb Apraxia (TOLA) (Helm-Estabrooks, 1992) was designed to evaluate ideomotor, limb, and oral apraxia. Limb apraxia tasks distinguish between distal and proximal gestures and intransitive and transitive (pretend object use) gestures. Table 16–29 describes some of the movements requested in the TOLA. All tasks are evaluated both to command and imitation. In addition, a gestured pictures subtest probes the ability to produce a gesture appropriate for a pictured object. Borod, Fitzpatrick, Helm-Estabrooks, and Goodglass (1992) found that there was a significant relation between praxis performance and gestural communication in naturalistic settings.

A broader approach to kinematic analysis has been developed using videotapes of client's movements (Poizner, Mack, Verfaellie, Rothi, & Heilman, 1990). Some researchers have used videotapes of ADL performance to code a client's movements quantitatively and qualitatively (Schwartz, Mayer, FitzpatrickDeSalme, & Montgomery, 1993). The concept of video analysis of movement holds promise for the evaluation of apraxia. Occupational therapists may ask the client or family if there are any videos of the client's movement before the injury that can help the therapist select familiar movement subroutines at rates and rhythms that approximate the client's typical movement patterns. It may be helpful to visit work sites and home when possible to be sure to evaluate movements in the contexts in which the client typically performs them.

Fisher (1993a,b) suggests the use of the Assessment of Motor and Process Skills (AMPS) to observe the actions a person uses to move the body or task objects during the performance of all daily living tasks. The AMPS simultaneously evaluates motor and process skills involved in motor-planning functional tasks. Abreu (1994) has a broader view of motor planning and recommends including evaluation of gestures, timing of movement, object manipulation, and block construction in her assessment of apraxia.

An occupational therapist employing a dynamic assessment method would attempt to identify the task conditions under which the limb apraxia symptoms emerge. The task conditions, the response to cuing, and the client's awareness of his or her task performance, all are evaluated in a dynamic interactional assessment model. The client would be asked to predict performance and then to perform a variety of movement tasks. A series of cues (ie, visual, verbal, or tactile) may be used if the client experiences difficulty performing a requested movement. The cues are not arranged in any particular order. The degree to which the cue is effective depends on the nature of the error and the underlying difficulty. For example, returning to the case of Mrs. H, the occupational therapist might bypass verbal cuing because

Mrs. H's narration of the sequence does not appear to be improving her performance. The therapist would evaluate the effectiveness of visual and tactile cues on improving her task performance. Mrs. H may be cued by asking her to visually imagine the sequence or to watch a demonstration of the correct action sequence. Tactile cues, such as performing hand over hand through the task, may be attempted to evaluate the effect of tactile cues on Mrs. H's motor performance.

Memory

Memory gives us the ability to draw on past experiences and learn new information (Toglia, 1993a). This provides us with a sense of continuity in the environment and frees us from dependency in here-and-now situations. Memory is conceptualized in several models. The stage model views memory as a multistep process involving encoding, storage, and retrieval (Squire & Butters, 1984). Memory has also been described in terms of sensory memory (impairments appear as perceptual impairments), working or immediate memory, and long-term memory. Table 16–30 defines types

of memory, typical assessment tasks, and functional implications. Working memory temporarily holds information in mind, internalizes information, and uses that information to guide behavior without the aid of external cues (Goldman-Rakic, 1993). Long-term memory holds an unlimited amount of information in a permanent state for hours or years. Long-term memory is usually divided into categories of semantic or episodic (see Table 16–30). Long-term memory may also be classified into categories of declarative memory (ie, information can be verbally stated and the instance in which it was learned can be recalled) (Squire & Cohen, 1982) or procedural memory (ie, performance of a task displays learning occurred, but there is no recall of how the information was acquired or how the task was learned) (Baddeley, Harris, Sunderland, Watts, & Wilson, 1987).

Typical clinical manifestations of clients with memory dysfunction include rapid forgetting, normal short-term capacity, and preserved skill acquisition. There is frequently greater ability in recognition tasks than in tasks requiring free recall and improved performance when provided with retrieval cues. Table 16–31 describes the different types of retrieval tasks a client may be asked to perform.

TABLE 16-30. Types of Memory Tasks

Types of Memory	Definitions	Typical Assessments	Functional Implications
Immediate memory	Recall of information immediately after presentation or exposure (within 60 sec after stimulus presentation).	Client is asked to recall a list of words just read to him/her. Client is asked to recall 10 objects just shown to him or her.	Loses track of instructions or rules of the task or activity.
Delayed memory (Declarative long-term memory) Semantic vs. episodic	Recall of previously presented material anytime minutes to hours after presentation. (2 types) Semantic: recall of knowledge, such as major world events, famous people, and general facts. Episodic: recall of personally experienced events.	Client is asked to perform the above tasks after a delay of 20 mins. Semantic: client is asked to recall historical facts (eg, London is in England). Episodic: client is asked autobiographical information (eg, how did he/she spend his or her last birthday?).	Forgets conversation that took place 1/2 hr ago. Forgets dates of wedding anniversary, birthdays of family members, and such. Knows date of wedding anniversary, but unable to relate personal experience of the event.
Skill or procedural learning	The ability to remember "how to" perform a task or procedure. Memory for an action sequence, rather than a set of facts.	Client is shown a magic trick and asked to demonstrate it immediately and after a delay.	Knows how to ride a bicycle or perform the correct sequence of ambulation with a walker.
Prospective memory	The ability to respond to cues, such as an alarm that reminds a person to perform particular activity at a future time.	Client is asked to remember to bring a specific object to next session, to mail a letter when he or she passes a mailbox, or to return a phone call in 20 min.	Forgets appointments, dates to pay bills, phone calls to make, and such.

(Adapted from Toglia, J. P. [1996, February]. Application of the Multicontext Treatment Approach to Disorders in Attention, Memory and Executive Function. Supplemental manual to workshop held at Rehabilitation Institute of Chicago. New York: private publication.)

TABLE 16-31. Types of Memory Retrieval

Types of Recall	Definitions	Sample Assessment Tasks
Free recall	Ability to recall information when no specific retrieval cues are provided.	Remember a list of words read or an array of objects shown (may be increasing amounts of information).
Cued recall	Ability to recall information when provided with cues (first letter, category, context, and such) either during the encoding or retrieval phase.	Client is shown photos of musical instruments and cued to think about the category the items fit into.
Recognition	Ability to recognize previously presented information.	Multiple-choice format in which the client is shown 10 photos of faces then asked to pick the faces he or she saw before from an array of 20 faces.
		Client is read a sentence then asked to pick the sentence he or she heard from a choice of three sentences.

(Adapted from Toglia, J. P. [1996, June]. A Multicontext Approach to Cognitive Rehabilitation. Supplemental manual to workshop conducted at New York Hospital–Cornell Medical Center, New York.)

A comprehensive evaluation of memory, whether static or dynamic, must address the different types of memory and methods of retrieval. Verbal and visual representations of events are thought to be independently coded, and both need to be evaluated. Evaluation of memory impairments should explore performance on the different aspects of memory as well as modality-specific impairments and the presence of retrograde and anterograde amnesia (see GOAT, Table 16–26). Memory assessments must take into consideration the qualitative aspects of performance such as the effects of associated cognitive impairments, task demands, rate of forgetting, and amount and type of information that can be retained. The demands of the assessment task itself may influence memory and should be considered during evaluation: (1) the modality in which the information is presented (auditory or visual), (2) the type of instructions (general or specific), (3) the amount of stimuli presented, (4) the familiarity and meaningfulness of the information, (5) the presence of contextual cues during the storage and recall phases, (6) the type of information to be remembered (factual or skill related), and (7) the length of retention.

Memory questionnaires and ratings of memory problems in everyday life, such as Sunderland and Harris' (1984) Everyday Memory Questionnaire, explore a client's general awareness of memory capabilities and knowledge about the functioning of memory and memory strategies. These questionnaires also examine the frequency and type of forgetting. The Rivermead Behavioral Memory Test (RBMT) (Wilson, Cockburn, & Baddeley, 1985) tests both visual (mainly recognition) and verbal memory (mainly recall). The RBMT was designed to predict everyday memory tasks that will be difficult for clients with memory impairments. Tasks include (1) remembering a name, a hidden belonging, an appointment, a paragraph, a route, and to deliver a message; (2) recognizing pictures and faces; and (3) answering orientation questions. There are four equivalent versions for retesting and norms on ages 16 to 96.

Dynamic assessment of memory incorporates assessment of awareness of memory capabilities, knowledge of and spontaneous use of strategies. Toglia's (1993b) Contextual Memory Test (CMT) was designed to evaluate awareness of memory capacity, recall, strategy use, and performance with induced encoding. The CMT begins by having the client answer general questions about his or her memory functioning and estimate his or her score before and immediately following task performance. Recall of a page of 20 line-drawn objects related to a common theme are tested immediately after a 90-second exposure and after a 15- to 20-minute delay under various conditions (free recall, cued recall, and recognition). The client's use of strategies for encoding and retrieval are probed. If the client has difficulty, an alternative version is given and the client is provided a cue during the encoding phase to facilitate recall (eg, "When you look at the pictures think about what happens when you go to a restaurant"). The CMT is not intended to be a comprehensive memory assessment, but is a test to screen for memory impairments and provide information for treatment planning. Data is being collected to expand the normative base.

Executive Functions, Organization, and Problem Solving

Executive functions are a broad band of skills that allow a person to engage in independent, purposeful, self-directed behavior. Organization and problem-solving skills are specific higher-level cognitive functions that fall under the umbrella of executive functions. Impairments in executive functioning are often seen after frontal lobe injuries and involve a cluster of deficiencies of which one or two may be especially prominent (Lezak, 1995). Lezak identifies four primary components of executive functions: volition, planning, purposeful action, and self-awareness and self-monitoring. Volition is the capacity to formulate an intention or goal and to initiate action. The planning component of executive functioning involves the ability to efficiently organize the steps or elements of the behavior or task. Planning also requires the ability to look ahead, anticipate consequences, weigh and make choices, conceive of alternatives, sustain attention, and sequence the task. Purposeful action is the translation of an intention or plan into the activity, the carrying out of plans. This requires the ability to initiate, switch, and stop sequences (flexibility), as well as self-regulation. The individual's understanding of impairments and how they affect functioning (self-awareness) and the ability to monitor, self-evaluate, and correct performance (self-monitoring) are also considered executive functions.

Executive dysfunction syndromes may significantly influence performance of ADL no matter how well preserved the individual's other cognitive skills may be (Lezak, 1983). Detailed in the following is a case of a young client with brain injury exhibiting executive function impairments.

Chris shows many of the typical difficulties seen in clients with executive function disorders. Clients with executive skill dysfunction may demonstrate decreased initiation, decreased ability to carry out established plans, poor planning and organizational skills, and poor self-awareness. With problems in initiation, the client may appear passive, disinterested, apathetic, or unmotivated. This needs to be distinguished from psychological causes (ie, depression) that clinically look similar. Clients with poor initiation require prompts to engage in activities, for they may not recognize the need for action.

Clients with poor planning and organizational skills have a tendency to develop unrealistic goals and to underestimate the time required for task completion. Impairments in other cognitive skills, such as attention and memory, may affect the ability to perform organizational tasks. For example, a client may sort items incorrectly because of an inability to attend to critical details, or to an inability to recall the sort-

ing principle. Concrete thinking may also be seen when the client overfocuses on one aspect of the object or situation and has difficulty gathering, consolidating, or sorting information. For example, when asked to sort a grocery list to make shopping easier, the client with concrete thinking might place the lemons separately from other produce items because "they are sour."

Clients displaying executive dysfunction may demonstrate their greatest difficulty in problem-solving tasks. Decreased ability to carry out established plans may be clinically seen as decreased flexibility or impulsivity in carrying out tasks. Often the client's approach is perseverative, concrete, or rigid. Poor self-awareness, as we have discussed earlier in this chapter, may need to be addressed early in the treatment process because the client with poor self-awareness shows an inability to profit from feedback and may have significant safety risks owing to poor detection of errors.

Problem-solving tasks may be graded on a continuum that considers the demands of the task and the environment to determine the amount of effort and the extent to which different cognitive and perceptual skills are needed. In basic tasks, the problem is clear and readily identified. All the relevant information is present and limited in amount. Irrelevant information, the number of factors that can influence outcome, and possible choices and solutions are also limited. The solutions typically involve only one to three steps and incorrect solutions are readily apparent, for they may prevent success in resolution of the problem.

Complex problem-solving tasks require sorting out information to determine where the real problem exists (eg, the checking account statement does not match your personal records). Analysis of the problem requires searching large amounts of information for additional information needed to solve the problem. This searching requires sorting out the irrelevant information, and keeping track of a large number of factors that can influence outcome. Solving the complex problem requires the ability to plan, test, and reject

CASE STUDY

Chris is 26 years old and sustained a closed head injury from a car accident approximately 6 months ago. Before the accident Chris was employed as a certified public accountant. Chris is presently receiving outpatient therapy and has not returned to work. Physical impairments are subtle balance problems and, cognitively, the neuropsychologist reports Chris scores within normal ranges on all cognitive–perceptual tests except in the area of executive functions. Chris' parents, with whom he lives, report that Chris' personality has changed

dramatically. Before the accident Chris was an active, friendly person with a good sense of humor. He was a "self-starter," who was well organized and able to handle many different tasks. Now Chris spends most of his day watching television. He does not shower or participate in family activities unless pushed to do so. He appears very passive, rarely initiates conversation, appears to have lost his sense of humor, is disorganized, and is unable to get things done once cued to start tasks. Chris' parents are afraid to let him drive or leave the house on his own.

different hypotheses, and formulate alternatives to the problem. Execution of the plan requires carrying out several steps and incorrect solutions are not readily apparent. Verification that the problem has been solved requires actively comparing the solution with the original problem. Clients with executive dysfunction syndromes appear to have difficulty with complex problem-solving tasks owing to the more abstract and ambiguous nature of these tasks.

Bransford and Stein (1984) identified the components of the *IDEAL* problem solver. The *IDEAL* problem solver (1) *I*dentifies the problem, (2) *D*efines the problem precisely, (3) *E*xplores possible strategies, (4) *A*cts on the chosen strategy, and (5) *L*ooks at the effects to determine if the problem has been solved. Adults with brain injury tend to show typical patterns of breakdown at different stages of the problem-solving process, often caused by impairments in executive functions. Identification of the problem involves attention and awareness of the environment and an exploration of the environment and task. Some clients do not recognize that a problem or obstacle exists; thus, they do not engage in a problem-solving process. Clients who have difficulty understanding cause and effect may be unable to predict the consequences of an obstacle or action.

Defining the problem precisely requires analyzing the conditions of the problem and constructing a meaningful internal representation of it. How one defines the problem is important in determining how the problem-solving process proceeds. Often clients perform an incomplete analysis of the problem and omit critical details. They may overattend to one aspect of the problem or engage in concrete thinking in which they interpret the issues literally and fail to see the whole picture.

Exploring possible strategies involves the ability to formulate a plan, try alternative strategies, and test hypotheses. Clients with executive dysfunction syndromes caused by brain injury tend to approach problems in a haphazard, trial-and-error manner. Often they will have difficulty deciding how to approach the problem and will choose inefficient strategies. When their chosen strategy is obviously ineffective, they may still have difficulty letting go of a hypothesis and generating an alternative one.

When required to carry out the strategy or plan, some clients have difficulty initiating, persisting, or remembering and following the plan owing to executive skill dysfunction. Looking at the end results of completion of the strategy or plan requires that one compare the final solution with the original conditions of the problem. Some clients with brain injury forget this vital step of self-monitoring because of problems in executive functions.

Disorders in executive functions are most apparent in situations that are novel and require a deviation from the routine or when the tasks are unstructured and the client has to initiate, plan, and prioritize. Most standardized cognitive assessments are structured and do not adequately examine the area of executive functions; therefore, impairments in executive functions can easily be missed. Several assessments for executive functions have recently been developed, but research data on the reliability and validity of these assessment tools is minimal.

The Executive Function Route Finding Task (EFRT) (Boyd & Sautter, 1993) requires a client to find his or her way from a starting point to a predetermined location within the building. The client is required to provide his or her own plan and structure and modify it according to feedback from the environment. While accompanying the client, the examiner rates that client on the following areas: (1) understanding the task, (2) seeking information, (3) remembering instructions, (4) detecting errors, (5) correcting errors, and (6) ability to stick with the task (or task behavior). General or specific cues are provided if needed. PRO-EX—Profile of Executive Control System (Branswell et al., 1992) is a rating scale that rates behaviors in seven areas: goal selection, planning and sequencing, initiation, time sense, awareness of impairments, and self-monitoring while the client is performing an unstructured task (eg, organize contents of a desk drawer; find out how to register to vote).

The Toglia Category Assessment (TCA; 1994) evaluates a client's categorization skills and deductive-reasoning abilities. The first subtest uses 16 plastic utensils of different sizes and colors to evaluate category flexibility. Once the utensils are grouped according to one attribute the client is asked to sort the items again in a different way. This is repeated a third time, with the examiner asking the client after each trial to explain how the groups differ. The deductive-reasoning component is a questioning task that investigates the client's ability to formulate and test different hypotheses. The client must determine which of the utensils the examiner is thinking of with the fewest number of yes or no questions and the least amount of guessing possible. The examiner uses a set of standard sequential cues with each subtest if the client encounters difficulty identifying the target item in the minimum number of questions that should be needed.

Nonstandardized evaluation of executive function, organizational, and problem-solving skills may include unstructured functional tasks. For example, the client can be asked to organize and sequence a day filled with multiple errands, state the time he or she would leave home, and the sequence in which the errands would be completed (Toglia, 1991a). The client can be given tasks within the hospital environment that require seeking information (eg, find out the location of the client library, billing department, or client recreation area). Information-seeking tasks can also involve use of the telephone (eg, call three local banks to find out their hours and fees for checking and use of an automatic teller machine [ATM] card; or prepare a price comparison list). Functional problem-solving tasks that require identifying the lack of necessary information (eg, "You just bought a new hat for $12.60. When you received your change you realized that you did not receive the correct amount. How much change should you have received?") or organizing and planning (eg, "You are organizing a breakfast meeting for 14 people. Coffee is 50 cents each, tea is 35 cents each, bagels are 65 cents each, doughnuts are 75 cents each, and danishes are 1 dollar each. You have 22 dollars. What could you buy?") should also be used.

An occupational therapist who uses a dynamic interactional approach to the evaluation of executive functions, organizational, and problem-solving skills would pose questions to investigate the client's executive skill performance on all cognitive–perceptual assessments, not just those deemed as problem-solving or executive function assessments. The questions should explore the client's (1) awareness; (2) ability to perform new versus rote, routine tasks; (3) need for prompts to start or complete simple activities (eg, brushing teeth, eating, getting a snack); (4) ability to deal with the unexpected in simple, everyday tasks (eg, does the client take action if the toothpaste tube is empty?); and (5) ability to stay on task and not get sidetracked by irrelevant information.

▼ FACTORS THAT MAY AFFECT EVALUATION

Psychosocial Components

Occupational therapists need to consider not only their clients' cognitive status, but also their coping capacities and the changing context of their lives as a result of the injury or disease (Fine, 1993). The reaction to a brain injury may be immediate, with changes in personality and behavior as well as cognitive–perceptual abilities. These changes affect the client's perception of himself or herself and relationships with others. The psychosocial response to brain damage and cognitive impairments is a major life transition that involves stages of adjustment (Diller, 1993). One of the most common secondary emotional responses to brain injury is depression. Occupational therapists need to understand the cognitive changes that may result from depression because many depressed clients display behavior patterns that appear similar to dementia. Depression may be exhibited in perseverative thoughts, poor initiation, slowed reaction times, and poor ability to predict the quality of task performance. There are differences in clinical presentation; depressed clients are more likely to be aware of their impaired cognitive skills and have a tendency to significantly underestimate performance both before and after the task. Clients with brain injury will overestimate task performance and show limited awareness (Squire & Zouzounis, 1988).

The client's poor performance on cognitive-based testing may be greatly influenced by psychological factors. The secondary depression may make the cognitive impairments appear greater and prevent the client from initiating use of coping strategies. Cognitive deficits can also exacerbate depression. Recognizing and appraising the situation requires attention, memory, and self-awareness. Coping with the situation requires initiative, decision making, flexibility, persistence, self-control, and self-regulation. These are the very skills that may be limited by the cognitive or executive skill dysfunction and, thereby, make the depression more evident and difficult to treat (Fine, 1993).

Language Impairments

Occupational therapists working with clients with language impairments will need to use keen observational skills and deductive reasoning to understand clients' cognitive–perceptual strengths and weaknesses. Information is often needed on the cognitive and perceptual abilities of clients with aphasia to determine the extent to which any impairment may interfere with the ability to successfully use an alternative communication system. To use a basic communication board requires the client to have awareness that an alternative communication system is needed as well as skills in visual attention, visual scanning, object identification, matching of line drawing or words to real objects, and association or categorization.

Whenever possible the occupational therapist should consult with the speech language pathologist to gain a better understanding of the client's level of comprehension and the most reliable method of expression. If information on the client's receptive and expressive language skills is not available the occupational therapists should first gain an understanding of "yes and no" reliability by evaluating the client's ability to follow simple commands. Such reliability is demonstrated when the client responds accurately to a series of single statement questions (eg, "Are you a woman?", "Is it snowing?", and so on). The client may be able to handle multiple choice questions with four or five choices if there is established yes and no reliability.

The ability to comprehend simple written commands can be screened by having the client read and follow one-to two-step directions. It will be important for the occupational therapist not to provide any gestural cues during this assessment to accurately determine if the client can follow the written direction. If the client cannot read, the command may be presented auditorily. Motor-planning impairments frequently coexist with language impairments and need to be ruled out as an interfering factor. The ability to imitate or follow gestural directions needs to be evaluated if the client cannot follow verbal one-step commands. Tactile cues may be necessary during this assessment.

If the client cannot demonstrate yes or no reliability and is unable to follow one-step commands, cognitive–perceptual skills cannot be accurately evaluated through formal methods. Most occupational therapists faced with this situation will take a functional approach to both evaluation and treatment. When basic communication skills of yes and no reliability and following simple commands are intact, cognitive–perceptual testing should still be adapted to minimize speech and language requirements. Tests that can be answered by a yes or no response or multiple choice questions are recommended. In all tests the directions should be brief, accompanied by gestures, and have at least three trials with corrections and assistance before actual testing to ensure that the client understands the directions.

Sensory Impairments

Evaluating a client with primary sensory loss (vision or hearing) will be a challenge to the occupational therapist. Therapists will need to focus their evaluation on the sensory modality that is intact by modifying existing assessments or selecting assessments that do not tap the impaired sensory modality. For example, the client who has a hearing impairment may be provided with written directions to follow, and the client with visual impairments may be presented with enlarged stimuli. Qualitative analysis along with clinical observations will be needed to interpret the client's performance. Documentation of the results should clearly describe the modifications and means of evaluation.

▼ INTERPRETATION AND DOCUMENTATION OF RESULTS

Differences In Evaluation Purpose Are Reflected in Documentation

The approach an occupational therapist takes to the process of evaluating cognitive-perceptual dysfunction will guide the documentation process. When the evaluation method incorporates primarily static cognitive screening tools, or a deficit-specific approach, the documentation will typically include a statement concerning the purpose of the evaluation, the name, and a brief overview of the assessment or battery administered, the results, and the recommendations (Box 16–2).

When a dynamic interactional assessment has been conducted the documentation will reflect the focus on reporting the task conditions that influenced cognitive-perceptual symptoms and the client's awareness of the impairments and use of processing strategies. The documentation will describe (1) each task and the conditions that either increased or decreased the symptoms; (2) the response to cuing; (3) the client's awareness or ability to detect, predict, monitor, explain, or correct errors; and (4) a summary that establishes relations to ADL, work, leisure, and social skills (Box 16–3).

Relating Results To Function

Relating the cognitive-perceptual impairments to functional abilities is the unique domain of occupational therapists. We are able to link the potential effect of the identified cognitive-perceptual impairments with the demands of task performance. The present and future performance contexts should be considered when relating the observed impairments to performance areas. The therapist should consider

▼ **BOX 16-2**

Documentation Example

Mr. B was given the Middlesex Elderly Assessment of Mental State (MEAMS) which was designed to screen for gross impairment of specific cognitive skills in elderly clients (aged 65 and older). Subtests include orientation, name learning, naming, comprehension, remembering pictures, arithmetic, spatial construction, fragmented letter perception, unusual views, usual views, verbal fluency, and motor perseveration. Client scored 6 out of a possible score of 12 on the pass or fail screening format. This indicates the need for more detailed investigation and evaluation of cognitive perceptual functioning. Subtests that were performed with 100% accuracy included: orientation, arithmetic, comprehension, and motor persistence. Subtests that the client had the most difficulty with included unusual views of objects, fragmented letter perception, and spatial construction. *Recommendations:* Further testing in the areas of difficulty. Follow-up and education to caregivers regarding possible difficulties.

that the structured, yet unfamiliar, hospital environment may either facilitate or impede performance. Documentation of the functional implications of the cognitive-perceptual impairments is vital for occupational therapists to demonstrate their valuable contribution to the health care team in the evaluation and rehabilitation of cognitive and perceptual dysfunction, and to ensure that third-party payers recognize this contribution.

Goal Setting

Goals addressing cognitive-perceptual areas require the same components as any goal. The goal should describe the behavior that is targeted for treatment, the conditions under which the behavior should be displayed, and the expected level of performance. Cognitive goals that address improved safety awareness and safe, independent performance of functional activities should be documented. Long-term cognitive-perceptual goals should address the general cognitive-perceptual areas and the functional level of performance (eg, "Client will demonstrate increased awareness of impairments so that the client can successfully use compensatory strategies for independence in self-care by discharge.") Short-term goals typically target more specific components of cognitive-perceptual skills that are necessary steps to achieving improved functional performance (eg, "As a prerequisite to independence in basic self-care skills, the client will demonstrated the ability to use an organized scanning approach to locate target items in a crowded array [refrigerator shelf, drawer, telephone book, or other] five times during a 30-minute session." or "As a prerequisite to independence in the community, the client will demonstrate increased simultaneous attention, as evidence by ability to perform mul-

BOX 16-3

Documentation Example

Terry demonstrates no difficulty in attentional or visual discrimination tasks that involve eight to ten items. When presented with tasks that involve greater amounts of information, she demonstrates increasing disorganization and difficulty keeping track of the information. Terry has no difficulty sorting items into self-established categories when the task involves eight to ten items. However, when presented with more items (25 picture cards) Terry required assistance to structure categories to complete the task. She appeared to lose track of her categories and changed her sorting principle. On the Contextual Memory Test (20 line drawings of items related to a restaurant) Terry initially recalled only seven items and did not appear to use any strategy to group the information. She did not identify that the items were related to a restaurant. When provided with the theme of the items in part II of the test (a morning scene), Terry's performance improved to 14 out of 20 items. *Summary:* Throughout all tasks Terry did not consistently check her work for errors, although when questioned she did report that since her accident she was experiencing problems in memory and concentration. Despite this vague understanding of her problems, Terry frequently overestimated her task performance before beginning tasks. Terry had the most difficulty with tasks that required attention to detail, tracking, and organizing larger quantities (greater than 10 items) of information. Performance generally improved when provided with one to two cues to structure the information or when the information was limited (fewer than 10 items). Terry appears to have the ability to successfully use strategies when they are provided. Terry will be vulnerable to performance breakdown in tasks such as organizing monthly bills or performing a multiple step cooking task that requires use of two or more cooking appliances and three or more foods.

---

tiple step cooking tasks with only one or two verbal cues"). Cognitive goals, similar to all goals, should be behavioral and clearly written so if given to another therapist he or she will know when the goal you have established has been achieved.

▶EVALUATION OF PERCEPTION AND COGNITION CONCLUSION

The American Occupational Therapy Association states that "occupational therapy practitioners have an important role in promoting maximal levels of performance in persons with cognitive impairments." (AOTA, 1991, p. 1067). Our unique educational background in biological and behavioral sciences, activity analysis, and human components of performance allows us to understand how daily-living task performance is affected by cognitive and perceptual impairments. With a particular client in mind, the occupational therapist can select an approach and assessments to evaluate the influence of cognitive perceptual impairments on functional performance and use this information to plan and carry out an intervention plan.

Section 3

Evaluation of Psychosocial Skills and Psychological Components

Susanne Garred Seymour

Why Evaluate Psychosocial Skills and Psychological
  Components?
    Occupational Therapy is Holistic
    Building the Therapeutic Alliance
    Setting Treatment Goals and Choosing Appropriate Treatment Activities
Types of Evaluations
    Formal Assessments
    Informal Evaluation
Choosing an Assessment
Psychosocial Evaluation by Occupational Therapy
  Within the Interdisciplinary Team
Implications of Psychosocial Evaluation
Evaluation of Psychosocial Skills and Psychological
  Components Conclusion

Psychosocial skills and psychological components are described as the ability to interact in society and to process emotions (American Occupational Therapy Association, 1994). To provide appropriate occupational therapy services, it is essential to evaluate these components in all occupational therapy clients, regardless of the client's primary diagnosis or treatment setting. The occupational therapy practitioner's ability to help clients maximize function within their environments depends in part on how well the therapist understands the clients' psychosocial skills and psychological components.

The Uniform Terminology breaks this area of performance down into three categories:

1. Psychological skills:
  a. *Values*—Identifying ideas or beliefs that are important to self and others.
  b. *Interests*—Identifying mental or physical activities that create pleasure and maintain attention.
  c. *Self-concept*—Developing the value of the physical, emotional, and sexual self.

2. Social skills:
   a. *Role performance*—Identifying, maintaining, and balancing functions one assumes or acquires in society (eg, worker, student, parent, friend, religious participant).
   b. *Social conduct*—Interacting by using manners, personal space, eye contact, gestures, active listening, and self-expression appropriate to one's environment.
   c. *Interpersonal skills*—Using verbal and nonverbal communication to interact in a variety of settings.
   d. *Self-expression*—Using a variety of styles and skills to express thoughts, feelings, and needs.
3. Self-management:
   a. *Coping skills*—Identifying and managing **stress** and related factors.
   b. *Time management*—Planning and participating in a balance of self-care, work, leisure, and rest activities to promote satisfaction and health.
   c. *Self-control*—Modifying one's own behavior in response to environmental needs, demands, constraints, personal aspirations, and feedback from others.
   (AOTA,1994; pp. 1047–1054)

▼ WHY EVALUATE PSYCHOSOCIAL SKILLS AND PSYCHOLOGICAL COMPONENTS?

Occupational Therapy is Holistic

Health care has traditionally followed the medical model, which is reductionist. Reductionism separates a person into various, measurable component parts and views the client as the sum of his or her various component parts (Kielhofner, 1978). This model assumes that normalization of the parts will result in health and restoration of function (Mathiowetz, 1993). The medical model is problem oriented. For example, if a client had fallen and fractured a hip, according to the medical model, the hip would be the focus of treatment. However, since its beginnings, occupational therapy has been holistic, considering the whole person, rather than just the component parts of a person (Engelhardt, 1977; Howard, 1991). Occupational therapy is a process that focuses not on the skill deficits that result from illness and injury, but on maximizing the person's remaining capabilities (Rogers, 1982). Under a holistic model, health care professionals treating the same client would consider not only the fractured hip, but the overall effects of the injury on the client's life, including quality of life. Occupational therapy recognizes that quality of life is an essential theme in human performance (Fidler, 1996). Quality of life is directly related to personal satisfaction; this satisfaction comes from participation in personally relevant activities that focus on and maximize individual strengths and interests (Fidler, 1996). An occupational therapist treating the client would recognize that the client's hip fracture will affect the entire person. This includes values and interests, which are psychoso-

cial performance components. For example, the therapist would consider the influence of the injury on the client's self-concept. A fractured hip may result in ambulation with a cane or walker; use of these devices may affect how the client views himself or herself. The therapist would consider whether the injury would affect role performance. The fractured hip may interfere with some of the client's usual roles, such as homemaker or worker. The therapist would also consider whether the client has the self-management skills to cope with changes brought about by the injury. For example, a client who has difficulty with time management may have difficulty allocating extra time for adapting activities of daily living (ADL), such as dressing with adaptive equipment, or allowing extra time to travel from place to place. A client may lack the coping skills or self-control to manage feelings of frustration generated by a decrease in his or her independence. Evaluating a client's psychosocial skills and psychological components helps the therapist understand possible implications of disease or disability for that specific client, across all areas of the client's life. This helps the therapist treat the whole person, rather than treating just the disability or dysfunction.

Building the Therapeutic Alliance

The therapeutic alliance is a special relationship the occupational therapist develops with the client. The nature of this relationship is just what the name implies, that the therapist and client are *allies*. (Unit IV: Establishing the Therapeutic Alliance provides a more detailed explanation of this relationship.) This partnership makes the client an active participant in the treatment process, rather than a passive recipient of treatment. To develop this alliance, the therapist must know who the client is, which includes learning about the person's interests, values, self-concept, and roles. The therapist gathers this information through evaluation of psychosocial skills and psychological components. This information can then be integrated with information about other performance areas into the client's treatment.

Setting Treatment Goals and Choosing Appropriate Treatment Activities

Once the therapist has completed an evaluation that includes the client's psychosocial skills and psychological components, he or she can collaborate with the client to create an individualized treatment plan. Evaluating the client's psychological, social, and self-management skills helps the therapist and client focus on the client's priorities for treatment. Together the therapist and client set treatment goals that reflect those priorities. Payton, Nelson, and Ozer found that when clients are actively involved in establishing their treatment goals, they are more likely to have interest in and work toward those goals (as cited in Northern, Rust, Nelson, & Watts, 1995). Increased client investment and participation are not the only reason to involve the client in goal setting. Incorporating the client's interests, values, and experiences into treatment communicates caring to the client, which is of great importance to the healing process (Borg & Bruce, 1991).

After setting goals collaboratively, the occupational therapist chooses activities the client will find meaningful and purposeful to achieve those goals. Intrinsic motivation is elicited and maintained when the activity chosen is consistent with the biopsychosocial characteristics of the person (Fidler, 1996). The therapist should choose treatment activities that correspond with the client's values, interests, and roles. For example, a client who dislikes cooking, but enjoys gardening, will likely be more highly motivated to participate in gardening. Research suggests that, in addition to improving motivation, choosing activities that the client finds purposeful helps organize client's behavior (Trombly, 1995b); the more organized the client's behavior, the more likely the activity will be successful. Knowing about the client's social and self-management skills will help the therapist structure activities in ways that help the client succeed. For example, someone who has weak interpersonal skills will probably perform best when interpersonal demands are kept at a minimum. A client who lacks coping skills or has difficulty with self-control may perform best in a situation where possible distractions are limited or eliminated. By the same token, a client with strong interpersonal and self-expression skills may benefit from an activity that provides opportunities for socialization, allowing the client to draw on his or her strengths. Knowing about the person's psychosocial skills and psychological components will help the therapist provide the client with a "just right" challenge (Rogers, 1982, p. 713).

▼ TYPES OF EVALUATIONS

Formal Assessments

Many formal assessment tools are available for occupational therapists to evaluate clients' psychosocial performance components. Formal assessments can be especially useful for beginning therapists; they provide a place for the therapist to begin, and a structure to guide the evaluation process. These can be divided into two types: objective and subjective.

OBJECTIVE ASSESSMENTS

Objective assessments focus on the client's observable behavior. Some specific behaviors that may be observed and evaluated are self-conduct and self-expression, interpersonal skills, social conduct, coping skills, self-control, and time management. These assessments provide the therapist with information about the client's performance in specific areas. They are not designed to elicit information about clients' priorities, or about how they feel about their current level of functioning. These assessments rely on performance cri-

teria; the assumption is that using specific, predetermined criteria will increase the likelihood that two or more evaluators will arrive at similar conclusions (Borg & Bruce, 1991).

In some treatment environments, several occupational therapists work with the same clients; objective assessments can be helpful, as the therapists will be using the same performance criteria and will be interpreting the results of the assessments in a similar way. Most objective assessments used in occupational therapy measure performance in ADL, rather than psychosocial performance components. However, some address both ADL and psychosocial performance components. One frequently used objective assessment is the Allen Cognitive Level Test (Allen, 1985), which is described in Chapter 26. The Bay Area Functional Performance Evaluation (Bloomer & Williams, 1982) is an objective assessment that allows the evaluator to observe performance in goal-oriented tasks and in social interactions. The Comprehensive Occupational Therapy Evaluation (COTE) (Brayman & Kirby, 1982) defines 25 observable behaviors, and divides them into three categories: general behavior, interpersonal behavior, and task behavior.

SUBJECTIVE ASSESSMENTS

Subjective assessments do not give the therapist specific behaviors to observe; they rely on the client's point of view for information. Evaluation from the client's perspective helps the therapist gain an understanding of the client's personal experience, and helps provide a means for the client to take responsibility for the therapy process (Borg & Bruce, 1991). This type of evaluation can also assist the client to better understand his or her own personal experiences. Subjective assessments do not provide specific measurements of clients' performance; they provide information about which performance areas are important to clients, and how they feel about their current level of functioning. Some subjective assessments are the Adolescent Role Assessment (Black, 1976), the Occupational Case Analysis Interview and Rating Scale (OCAIRS) (Kaplan & Kielhofner, 1989), the Assessment of Occupational Functioning (AOF) (Watts, Brollier, Bauer, & Schmidt, 1988), the Occupational Performance History Interview (Kielhofner, Henry, & Walens, 1989), the Role Activity Performance Scale (Good-Ellis, Fine, Spencer, & DiVittis, 1987), the Worker Role Interview (Velozo, Kielhofner, & Fisher, 1992), and the Canadian Occupational Performance Measure (COPM) (Law et al, 1994). These assessments are described in detail in Chapter 13.

Informal Evaluation

The method most often used by occupational therapists to evaluate psychosocial components is informal evaluation. This is the process of gathering information during interaction with, or observation of, clients without using the structure of a specific assessment tool. Whenever a therapist is with clients, he or she has an opportunity to gather both objective and subjective information about their psychosocial component skills. The therapist uses conversation to gather information about clients' self-concept, roles, values, and interests. "How are you doing today?" is a simple question, but it can elicit a wide variety and depth of responses. This opening gives clients an opportunity to express any concerns they may have; listening carefully to the answer gives the therapist clues about the clients' psychosocial skills. Observation is another tool the therapist uses informally. The therapist can evaluate clients' psychosocial skills by observing their behavior within almost any context or activity. Observing clients with others gives the therapist information about social skills. Observing clients during activities can help the therapist to evaluate their self-management skills.

After the client's initial evaluation, the occupational therapist will continue to informally evaluate the client's skills throughout the course of treatment. Experienced therapists do this constantly as a part of the **clinical reasoning** process. This helps the therapist adjust treatment to meet clients' changing needs, and monitor their progress. This process is explained in detail in Chapter 9.

There are several advantages to this type of evaluation. One advantage is that the more casual style of informal evaluation is less stress-producing for clients than a formal evaluation. If clients are relaxed, the information elicited is more likely to be an accurate representation of their skills, than if they are nervous about the evaluation. Another advantage is that informal evaluation can be done anytime, anywhere. It requires no testing kit, special forms or equipment; therapists rely on their own interpersonal and observation skills to gather information. It requires no special training; however, experience is helpful. This type of evaluation can be difficult for inexperienced therapists, because there is no framework or structure to guide it. The therapist can take advantage of this lack of structure to guide the conversation or manipulate the environment to elicit specific information from a client, tailoring the evaluation to that person's specific needs.

▼ CHOOSING AN ASSESSMENT

The type of assessment a therapist chooses depends on several factors. One is the type and extent of psychosocial needs of the client. It is the role of the occupational therapist to emphasize whether a client can do what is necessary and fulfilling, not to give a psychiatric diagnosis. Occupational therapy is concerned with psychosocial skills and psychological components not in and of themselves, but as they relate to functional performance (Bonder, 1993). The therapist should choose assessments that measure those psychosocial and psychological components that have a direct bearing on the individual client's functional capabilities. It is important for the therapist to understand the uses and limitations of the assessment tools he or she has chosen. For example, an interest checklist may be helpful in determining client preferences and priorities and in choosing meaningful treatment activities. However, it does not tell the therapist anything about the client's level of functional performance (Bonder, 1993). The therapist needs information about both preferences and priorities (subjective) and about the client's current level of functional performance (objective).

The therapist's choice of evaluation will also depend on the theoretical frame of reference being used and how much treatment time is available. The therapist should know whether assessments being used are standardized, valid for the characteristics being evaluated, and reliable. These concepts are explained in detail in Chapter 14.

The therapist's choice of assessment also depends on the setting or environment where the treatment is taking place. Most treatment environments specialize in evaluation and treatment of certain performance areas, and minimize the importance of others. Most facilities have an evaluation protocol, a set of steps for therapists to follow when evaluating clients. The protocol differs from setting to setting. In settings that follow the medical model, the protocol typically focuses on the evaluation of the performance components directly affected by the primary diagnosis. Often the protocol places little emphasis on other aspects of the person, such as how the primary diagnosis affects the rest of the person's life. This raises a conflict between the occupational therapy value of respect for the whole person, and the medical model within which therapists frequently practice. Occupational therapy's respect for the whole person is an ethical guideline for practice; to truly practice occupational therapy, we must incorporate our clients' experiences, beliefs, values, and motives within the treatment (Wood, 1995). In practice settings that do not emphasize psychosocial components, occupational therapists frequently use informal methods to evaluate and treat those aspects of the person. This has been referred to as "underground practice" (Mattingly & Fleming, 1994). This underground practice allows the therapist to treat the whole person, addressing any performance area that will help the client achieve his or her treatment goals. This does not mean that the therapist operates in secret; it simply means that the therapist, while evaluating and treating the areas emphasized in a particular practice setting, evaluates and treats the rest of the person as well.

▼ PSYCHOSOCIAL EVALUATION BY OCCUPATIONAL THERAPY WITHIN THE INTERDISCIPLINARY TEAM

The occupational therapist plays a vital role in psychosocial evaluation within the interdisciplinary team. Because of occupational therapy's holistic point of view, the occupational therapist has a unique contribution to make to the client's treatment. An important part of that contribution may be helping other members of the team look at the client as a whole person. One way the therapist does this is through his or her actions. The therapist's interactions with the client are a powerful example for others. Focusing on the client as a whole person, and respecting his or her choices and priorities, helps others to view them in a similar way.

The therapist may also help other members of the team view the client as a whole person by sharing information about the client with them. The information shared must be relevant to treatment. For example, the therapist may want to share information about a client's love of fishing with the recreation therapy department to give them a basis for engaging the client. Some of the information gained by the therapist is more personal; the therapist must consider carefully whether sharing it is likely to benefit the client. Some information may actually bias other team members against the client, and interfere with treatment. If information is not likely to enhance treatment and benefit the client, it is best not to share it. Any information that is given should only be shared with the client's permission; failing to ask permission is a violation of confidentiality, and of the client's trust. The therapist may want to ask, "Is it okay if I share this information about you with the other therapists? I think it would help them with your treatment."

The occupational therapist may also learn about the client from assessments completed by others. Often clients' records arrive at the treatment setting with documentation concerning their psychosocial histories. It is important for the therapist to review this information. Knowing that a certain assessment has already been done keeps the therapist from repeating it and, thereby, wasting the client's treatment time and money. If the information in the client's record gives a different picture than the client is currently presenting, the therapist knows changes may have taken place since the information was compiled. Often psychiatric diagnoses and scores from specific psychometric tests are included. Taking the time to review records can pay off in a greater understanding of the client and may give valuable information that the therapist can use to apply to the client's current treatment.

Although being familiar with clients' records is important, it is also important to keep an open mind about the information they contain. Reports of the clients' previous behavior may not take into account the context of the behavior; they may not tell the whole story. Most assessments give information about skills a client is able to display or express at the time the assessment was given. This does not mean that the client will demonstrate exactly the same level of skills over time. Most assessments tell what is happening at the time they are completed. But most people function at a variety of levels at different times, depending on how they are feeling physically and emotionally, and on their environment. When reading evaluations of clients' previous behaviors, it is important to realize that although clients may exhibit similar behaviors in the future, they may also exhibit different ones. Clients are greatly influenced by therapists' expectations, even if these expectations are not directly stated. Clients tend to live up, or down, to therapists' expectations. If therapists give even subtle, unintentional cues to a client that a particular behavior is expected, they may elicit that behavior. Being aware of the influence of their expectations on the client allows therapists to consciously encourage more functional behaviors, and discourages those that do not contribute to function.

Evaluating psychosocial skills and psychological components is an integral part of occupational therapy. It helps the therapist look at the client as a whole person, and aids in the setting of goals and the choice of treatment activities. However, some clients may have more extensive psychosocial needs than others. These clients may benefit from a more comprehensive psychological evaluation. The occupational therapist may need to refer clients that require additional evaluation to other members of the team, such as a psychologist, social worker, or psychiatrist. They have specialized training in evaluating psychosocial factors. Their specific training is required to administer some types of assessments, such as personality inventories, intelligence tests, and projective tests. Use of those restricted assessments without the appropriate training and credentials will invalidate the results, and could jeopardize the occupational therapist's license.

▼ IMPLICATIONS OF PSYCHOSOCIAL EVALUATION

Before initiating an evaluation, it is the therapist's responsibility to consider how the evaluation will affect the client. The process of evaluating clients' functional skills creates a power relationship in which the therapist has the capacity to affect the life of the client (Kielhofner, 1993). Because of this inherent imbalance of power, it is critical for the therapist to handle the relationship sensitively, fostering the therapeutic alliance. Giving the client choices, respecting his or her priorities, and making him or her an active participant in therapy helps to balance the relationship.

Every evaluation has the potential to have a psychosocial effect on the client. Clients are likely to interpret the evaluation, not as a measure of skills they have or values they hold, but a measure of them as individuals. The feeling that they are being measured may cause them to feel inadequate or defective in some way. This may be compounded by the fact that, in some settings, many professionals may be performing evaluations with the same client, causing the client to feel "under the microscope." When administering assessments, it is important for the therapist to convey to clients that the purpose of the assessment is to gather information, and not to judge them; and that above all else, the therapist values them as individuals, regardless of the results of any assessment. Sharing evaluation results with the client in an open, positive way will help them feel less under the microscope and more a part of the collaborative process.

Every time a therapist completes an evaluation, the results become a part of the client's medical or psychosocial history. This can have an effect on how other medical or psychosocial professionals view the person. This is particularly true of psychosocial evaluations; professionals are not immune to the social stigma our culture still attaches to psychosocial evaluation and treatment. It is important to keep this in mind when considering whether and how to evaluate someone's skills. The recording of results should be descriptive; therapists need to avoid judgmental statements. Results of any psychosocial evaluation should be accompanied by contextual information to help the reader interpret the results, and should include anything that is likely to have affected the results.

▶ EVALUATION OF PSYCHOSOCIAL SKILLS AND PSYCHOLOGICAL COMPONENTS CONCLUSION

Psychosocial skills and psychological performance components give people the ability to interact in society and to process emotions. These skills are important to evaluate in all occupational therapy clients, across all types of practice settings. Some settings have evaluation and treatment protocols that do not emphasize psychosocial components. However, evaluating these components helps the therapist address any performance area more effectively.

Evaluation of Psychosocial Skills and Psychological Components Acknowledgments

I would like to thank the following people for their help with this section: Danielle Amero, Judith Churchill, Ardythe Eaton, and Ann D. Ury.

▼ REFERENCES

Abreu, B. C. (1994). Perceptual motor skills: Assessment and intervention strategies. In C. B. Royeen (Ed.), *AOTA self-study series: Cognitive rehabilitation.* (lesson 8). Rockville, MD: American Occupational Therapy Association.

Abreu, B., & Toglia, J. P. (1987). Cognitive rehabilitation: A model for occupational therapy. *The American Journal of Occupational Therapy, 41,* 439–448.

Adams, J. C., & Hamblen, D.L. (1990). *Outline of orthopaedics* (11th ed.). Edinburgh: Churchill Livingstone.

Allen, C. (1985). *Occupational therapy for psychiatric diseases: Measurement and management of cognitive disabilities.* Boston: Little, Brown & Co.

Allen, C. K., Earhart, C. A., & Blue, T. (1992). *Occupational therapy treatment goals for the physically and cognitively disabled.* Rockville, MD: American Occupational Therapy Association.

American College of Sports Medicine (1991). *Guidelines for exercise testing and prescription* (4th ed.). Philadelphia: Lea & Febiger.

American Occupational Therapy Association (AOTA) (1991). Statement: Occupational therapy services management of persons with cognitive impairments. *The American Journal of Occupational Therapy, 45,* 1067–1068.

American Occupational Therapy Association (1994). Uniform terminology for occupational therapy-third edition. *American Journal of Occupational Therapy, 48,* 1047–1054.

Ansell, B. J., & Keenan, J. E. (1989). The Western Neuro Sensory Stimulation Profile: A tool for assessing slow-to-recover head injured patients. *Archives of Physical Medicine and Rehabilitation, 70,* 104–108.

Arnadottir, G. (1990). *The brain and behavior: assessing cortical dysfunction through activities of daily living.* St. Louis, MO: C.V. Mosby.

Ashworth, B. (1964). Preliminary trial of carisoprodol in multiple sclerosis. *Practitioner, 192,* 540–542.

Asmussen, E. (1979). Muscle fatigue. *Medical Science and Sports, 11,* 313–321.

Atchison, B. (1995). Cardiopulmonary diseases. In C.A. Trombly (Ed.), *Occupational therapy for physical dysfunction* (4th ed.) (pp. 875–892). Philadelphia: Williams & Wilkins.

Baddeley, A., Harris, J., Sunderland, A., Watts, K. P., & Wilson, B. (1987). Closed head injury and memory. In H. Levin, J. Grafman, & H. Eisenberg (Eds.), *Neurobehavioral recovery from head injury.* New York: Oxford University Press.

Barrows, H. (1980). *Guide to neurological assessment.* Philadelphia: J. B. Lippincott.

Basmajian, J.V., & DeLuca, C. J. (1985). *Muscles alive: Their functions revealed by electromyography* (5th ed.). Baltimore: Williams & Wilkins.

Belanger, S. A., Duffy, R. J., & Coelho, C. A. (1994). An investigation of limb apraxia regarding the validity of current assessment procedures. *Clinical Aphasiology, 22,* 191–201.

Benton, A. L. (1985). Visuoperceptual, visuospatial, and visuoconstructive disorders. In K. M. Heilman and E. Valenstein (Eds.), *Clinical Neuropsychology* (pp. 151–185). New York: Oxford University Press.

Benton, A. L., Hamsher, K., Varney, N., & Spreen, O. (1983). *Contributions to neuropsychological assessment: Clinical manual.* New York: Oxford University Press.

Bentzel, K. (1995). Evaluation of sensation. In C.A. Trombly (Ed.), *Occupational therapy for physical dysfunction* (4th ed.) (pp. 187–199). Philadelphia: Williams & Wilkins.

Berg, K., Wood-Dauphinee, S., & Williams, J. (1989). Measuring balance in the elderly. Preliminary development of an instrument. *Physiotherapy Canada, 41,* 304–311.

Bernspang, B., Asplund, K., Eriksson, S., & Fugl-Meyer, A. R. (1987). Motor and perceptual impairments in acute stroke patients: Effects on self care ability. *Stroke, 18,* 1081–1086.

Black, M. M. (1976). Adolescent role assessment. *American Journal of Occupational Therapy, 30,* 73–79.

Bloomer, J., & Williams, S. (1982). The Bay Area Functional Performance Evaluation. In Hemphill, B. J. (Ed.) . *The evaluative process in psychiatric occupational therapy* (pp. 255–308). Thorofare, NJ: Slack.

Bobath, B. (1978). *Adult hemiplegia: Evaluation and treatment* (2nd ed.). London: William Heinemann Medical Books.

Bohannon, R., & Smith M. (1987). Interrater reliability of a modified Ashworth scale of muscle spasticity. *Physical Therapy, 87,* 206–207.

Bonder, B. R. (1993). Issues in assessment of psychosocial components of function. *American Journal of Occupational Therapy, 47,* 211–216.

Borg, B., & Bruce, M. A. (1991). Assessing psychological performance factors. In C. Christiansen & C. Baum, *Occupational therapy: Overcoming human performance deficits,* (pp. 540–586). Thorofare, NJ: Slack.

Borod, J. C., Fitzpatrick, P. M., Helm-Estabrooks, N., & Goodglass, H. (1989). The relationship between limb apraxia and the spontaneous use of communicative gesture in aphasia. *Brain and Cognition, 10,* 121–131.

Bouska, M. J., Kauffman, N. A., & Marcus, S. (1985). Disorders of the visual perceptual system. In D. Umphred (Ed.), *Neurological Rehabilitation.*. Philadelphia: F. A. Davis.

Boyd, T. M., & Sautter, S. W. (1993). Route-finding: A measure of everyday executive functioning in the head-injured adult. *Applied Cognitive Psychology, 7,* 171–181.

Brannon, F. J., Foley, M.W., Starr, J.A., & Black, M.G. (1993). *Cardiopulmonary rehabilitation: Basic theory and application* (2nd ed.). Philadelphia: F. A. Davis.

Bransford, J. D., & Stein, B. S. (1984). *The ideal problem solver.* New York: W. H. Freeman & Co.

Branswell, D., Hartry, A., Hoornbeek, S., Johansen, A., Johnson, L., Schultz, J., & Sohlberg, M. M. (1992). *The profile of executive control system.* Puyallup, WA: Association for Neuropsychological Research and Development.

Brayman, S. J., & Kirby, T. (1982). The Comprehensive Occupational Therapy Evaluation. In Hemphill, B. J. (Ed.). *The evaluative process in psychiatric occupational therapy* (pp. 211–226). Thorofare, NJ: Slack.

Brennan, J. (1959). Clinical method of assessing tonus and voluntary movement in hemiplegia. *British Medical Journal, 1,* 767–768.

Brooks, V.B. (1986). *The neural bases of motor control.* New York: Oxford University Press.

Bruce, M. G. (1993). Cognitive rehabilitation: Intelligence, insight, and knowledge. In C. B. Royeen (Ed.), *AOTA self-study series: Cognitive rehabilitation* (lesson 5). Rockville, MD: American Occupational Therapy Association.

Cailliet, R. (1978). *Soft tissue pain and disability.* Philadelphia: F. A. Davis.

Campione, J. C., & Brown, A. L. (1987). Linking dynamic assessment with school achievement. In C. Lidz (Ed.), *Dynamic assessment.* New York: Guilford Press.

Caplan, B. (1987). Assessment of unilateral neglect: A new reading test. *Journal of Clinical and Experimental Neuropsychology, 9,* 359–364.

Chen Sea, M. J., Henderson, A., & Cermak, S. A. (1993). Patterns of visual spatial inattention and their functional significance in stroke patients. *Archives of Physical Medicine and Rehabilitation, 74,* 355–360.

Christiansen, C. (1991). Occupational therapy: Intervention for life performance. In C. Christiansen & C. Baum (Eds.), *Occupational Therapy. Overcoming human performance deficits* (pp. 3–43). Thorofare, NJ: Slack.

Chusid, J.G., & DeGroot, J. (1988). *Correlative neuroanatomy* (20th ed.). East Norwalk, CT: Appleton & Lange.

Commission on Practice (1995). Clarification of the use of the terms assessment and evaluation. *American Journal of Occupational Therapy, 49,* 1072–1073.

Crosson, C., Barco, P. P., Velozo, C., Bolesta, M. M., Cooper, P.V., Werts, D., & Brobeck, T. C. (1989). Awareness and compensation in post-acute head injury rehabilitation. *Journal of Clinical and Experimental Neuropsychology, 2,* 355–363.

Crutchfield, C., Shumway-Cook, A., & Horak, F. (1989). Balance and coordination training. In R. Skully & M. Barnes (Eds.). *Physical Therapy* (825–843). Philadelphia, PA: J. B. Lippincott.

Daniels, L., & Worthingham, C. (1986). *Muscle testing—techniques of manual examination* (5th Ed.). Philadelphia: W. B. Saunders.

Dehn, M.M. (1980, March). Rehabilitation of the cardiac patient: The effects of exercise. *American Journal of Nursing, 80,* 435–440.

Dehn, M.M., & Mullins, C.B. (1977, April). Physiologic effects and importance of exercise in patients with coronary artery disease. *Cardiovascular Medicine, 2,* 365–371; 377–387.

Deitz, T., Beeman, C., & Thorn, D. (1993). *Test of Orientation for Rehabilitation Patients.* Tucson, AZ: Therapy Skill Builders.

Dellarosa, D., Chan, S., Toglia, J.P., & Finkelstein, N. (1991). ADL assessment in acute care: Simultaneous grading of physical and verbal levels of assistance. *Occupational Therapy Practice, 2* (2), 38–45.

DiFablo, R. P., & Badke, M. B. (1990). Relationship of sensory organization to balance function in patients with hemiplegia. *Physical Therapy, 70,* 342–548.

Diller, L. (1993). Introduction to cognitive rehabilitation. In C. B. Royeen (Ed.), *AOTA self-study series: Cognitive rehabilitation* (lesson 1). Rockville, MD: American Occupational Therapy Association.

Duncan, P., Weiner, D., Chandler, J., & Studenski, S. (1990). Functional reach: A new clinical measure of balance. *Journal of Gerontology: Medical Sciences, 45* (6), 192–197.

Dunn, W. (1991). Assessing sensory performance enablers. In C. Christiansen & C. Baum (Eds.), *Occupational Therapy. Overcoming human performance deficits* (pp. 471–505). Thorofare, N.J.: Slack.

Edwardson, B. (1992). *Musculoskeletal assessment—an integrated approach.* San Diego: Singular Publishing Group.

Elvey, R.L. (1979). Brachial plexus tension tests and the pathoanatomical origin of arm pain. Aspects of manipulative therapy. *Proceedings of a Multidisciplinary International Conference on Manual Therapy,* Melbourne, Australia.

Engelhardt, H. T. (1977). Defining occupational therapy: The meaning of therapy and the virtues of occupation. *American Journal of Occupational Therapy, 31,* 666–672.

Farber, S.D. (1991a). Assessing neuromotor performance enablers. In C. Christiansen & C. Baum (Eds.), *Occupational therapy. Overcoming human performance deficits* (pp. 507–521). Thorofare, N.J.: Slack.

Farber S.D. (1991b). Neuromotor dimensions of performance. In C. Christiansen & C. Baum (Eds.), *Occupational therapy. Overcoming human performance deficits* (pp. 259–282). Thorofare, N.J.: Slack.

Fess, E.E. (1993). Hand rehabilitation. In H.L. Hopkins & H.D. Smith (Eds.), *Willard & Spackman's Occupational Therapy* (8th ed.) (pp. 674–690). Philadelphia: J. B. Lippincott.

Fidler, G. S. (1996). Life-style performance: From profile to conceptual model. *American Journal of Occupational Therapy, 50,* 139–147.

Fine, S. (1993). Interaction between psychological variables and cognitive function. In C. B. Royeen (Ed.), *AOTA self-study series: Cognitive rehabilitation* (lesson 3). Rockville, MD: American Occupational Therapy Association.

Fisher, A. G. (1993a). Functional measures: Part 1: What is function, what should we measure and how should we measure it? *American Journal of Occupational Therapy, 46,* 183–185.

Fisher, A. G. (1993b). Functional measures: Part 2: Selecting the right test, minimizing the limitations. *American Journal of Occupational Therapy, 46,* 278–281.

Folstein, M. F., Folstein, S. E., & McHugh, P. R. (1975). Mini-mental state: A practical method for grading the cognitive state of patients for the clinician. *Journal of Psychiatric Research, 12,* 189–198.

Fugl-Meyer, A.R. (1980). Post-stroke hemiplegia assessment of physical properties. *Scandinavian Journal of Rehabilitation Medicine, 7* (suppl), 85–93.

Fugl-Meyer, A., Jaasko, L., Leyman, I., Olson, S., & Steglind, S. (1975). The post-stroke hemiplegic patient: A method for evaluation of physical performance. *Scandinavian Journal of Rehabilitation Medicine, 7,* 13–31.

Gauthier, L., Dehaut, F., & Joanette, Y. (1989). The Bells Test: A quantitative and qualitative test for visual neglect. *International Journal of Clinical Neuropsychology, 11,* 49–54.

Gilfoyle, E. M., Grady, A. P., & Moore, J. C. (1981). *Children adapt.* Thorofare, NJ: Slack.

Golding, E. (1989). *The Middlesex Elderly Assessment of Mental State.* England: Thames Valley Test Co.

Goldman-Rakic, P. S. (1993). Specification of higher cortical functions. *Journal of Head Trauma Rehabilitation, 8,* 13–23.

Good-Ellis, M. A., Fine, S. B., Spencer, J. H., & DiVittis, A. (1987). Developing a role activity performance scale. *American Journal of Occupational Therapy, 41,* 232–241.

Goodglass, H., & Kaplan, E. (1972). *Assessment of aphasia and related disorders.* Philadelphia: Lea & Febiger.

Granger, C., Cotter, A. C., Brown, B. B., & Fiedler, R. C. (1993). Functional assessment scales: A study of persons after stroke. *Archives of Physical Medicine and Rehabilitation, 74,* 133–138.

Gronwall, D. M. A. (1977). Paced Auditory Serial Addition Task: A measure of recovery from concussion. *Perceptual and Motor Skills, 44,* 367–373.

Haaland, K.Y. (1993, March). *Assessment of limb apraxia.* Presentation at the AOTA Neuroscience Institute Treating Adults with Apraxia, Baltimore, MD.

Hajek, V. E., Rutman, D. L., & Scher, H. (1989). Brief assessment of cognitive impairment in patients with stroke. *Archives of Physical Medicine and Rehabilitation, 70,* 114–117.

Harrington, D. L., & Haaland, K.Y. (1992). Are some cognitive deficits specific to limb apraxia? *Brain, 115,* 857–874.

Hartman-Maeir, A., & Katz, N. (1995).Validity of the Behavioral Inattention Test (BIT): Relationships with functional tasks. *The American Journal of Occupational Therapy, 49,* 507–516.

Heilman, K. M., & Rothi, L. J. (1985). Apraxia. In K. M. Heilman & E. Valenstein (Eds.), *Clinical Neuropsychology.* New York: Oxford University Press.

Heilman, K. M., Rothi, L. G., & Valenstein, E. (1982). Two forms of ideomotor apraxia. *Neurology, 32,* 342–346.

Heilman, K. M., Watson, R. T., & Valenstein, E. (1985). Neglect and related disorders. In K. M. Heilman & E. Valenstein (Eds.), *Clinical Neuropsychology.* New York: Oxford University Press.

Helm-Estabrooks, N. (1992). *Test of oral and limb apraxia (TOLA).* Chicago: Riverside Publishing.

Hoppenfeld, S. (1976). *Physical examination of the spine and extremities.* New York: Appleton-Century-Crafts.

Horak, F., & Shupert, C. (1994). Role of the vestibular system in postural control. In S. Herdman (Ed.), *Vestibular Rehabilitation* (pp. 22–46). Philadelphia, PA: F. A. Davis.

Howard, B. S. (1991). How high do we jump? The effect of reimbursement on occupational therapy. *American Journal of Occupational Therapy, 45,* 875–881.

Ishiai, S. (1994). Unilateral spatial neglect. *Neuropsychological Rehabilitation, 4,* 143–146.

Jebsen, R. H., Taylor, N., Trieschmann, R. B., Trotter, M. J., & Howard, L. A. (1969). An objective and standardized test of hand function. *Archives of Physical Medicine and Rehabilitation, 50,* 311–319.

Jensen, M. R., & Feuerstein, R. (1987). The learning potential assessment device: From philosophy to practice. In C. S. Lidz (Ed.), *Dynamic assessment.* New York: Guilford Press.

Kaplan, K., & Kielhofner, G. (1989). *Occupational case analysis interview and rating scale.* Thorofare, NJ: Slack.

Katz, N., Itzkopvich, M., Averbuch, S., & Elazar, B. (1989). Lowenstein Occupational Therapy Cognitive Assessment (LOTCA) battery for brain-injured patients: Reliability and validity. *The American Journal of Occupational Therapy, 43,* 184–192.

Katz, R. T., Rovai, G. P., Brait, C., & Rymer, W. Z. (1992). Objective quantification of spastic hypertonia: Correlation of clinical findings. *Archives of Physical Medicine and Rehabilitation, 73,* 339–347.

Katz, R., & Rymer, W. (1989). Spastic hypertonia: Mechanisms and measurement. *Archives of Physical Medicine and Rehabilitation, 70,* 144–155.

Kendall, F. P., McCreary, E. K., & Provance, P. G. (1993). *Muscles testing and function* (4th ed). Baltimore: Williams & Wilkins.

Kertesz, A. (1982). *Western Aphasia Battery.* Psychological Corporation, Harcourt Brace Jovanovich.

Kielhofner, G. (1978). General systems theory: Implications for theory and action in occupational therapy. *American Journal of Occupational Therapy, 31,* 637–645.

Kielhofner, G. (1993).The issue is—functional assessment: Toward a dialectical view of person-environment relations. *American Journal of Occupational Therapy, 47,* 248–251.

Kielhofner, G., Henry, A. D., & Walens, D. (1989). *A user's guide to the occupational performance history interview.* Rockville, MD: American Occupational Therapy Association.

Kiernan, R. J., Mueller, J., Langston, J. W., & Von Dyke, C. (1987).The Neurobehavioral Cognitive Status Examination: A brief but differentiated approach to cognitive assessment. *Annals of Internal Medicine, 107,* 481–485.

King, T. (May 6,1987). A scale for more definitive measurement of hypertonicity. *Occupational Therapy Forum, 2,* 9–12.

Kinsella, G., & Ford, B. (1985). Hemi-inattention and the recovery patterns of stroke patients. *International Rehabilitation Medicine, 7,* 102–106.

Kramer, J. H., Kaplan, E., & Blusewicz, M. J. (1991).Visual hierarchical analysis of block design configural errors. *Journal of Clinical and Experimental Neuropsychology, 13,* 455–465

Lamb, R. (1985). Manual muscle testing. In Rothstein (Ed.), *Measurement in Physical Therapy* (pp. 47–55). New York: Churchill Livingstone.

Lane, S. (1991). Motor planning. In C. B. Royeen (Ed.), *AOTA self-study series: Neuroscience Foundations of human performance.* (lesson 8). Rockville, MD: American Occupational Therapy Association

LaStays, P., & Wheeler, D. (1994). Reliability of passive wrist flexion and extension goniometric measurements: A multicenter study. *Physical Therapy, 74,* 162–174.

Law, M., Baptiste, S., Carswell, A., McColl, M. A., Polatjko, H., & Pollock, N. (1994). *Canadian occupational performance measure.* (2nd ed.). Toronto: Canadian Association of Occupational Therapists.

Levin, H. S., O'Donnell, V. M., & Grossman, R. G. (1979). The Galveston Orientation and Amnesia Test: A practical scale to assess cognition after head injury. *Journal of Nervous and Mental Diseases, 167,* 675–684.

Lezak, M. D. (1983). *Neuropsychological assessment.* (2nd edition) New York: Oxford University Press.

Lezak, M. D. (1995). *Neuropsychological assessment.* (3rd edition) New York: Oxford University Press.

Lidz, C. (1987). *Dynamic assessment.* New York: Guilford Press.

Lunsford, B. R. (1978). Clinical indicators of endurance. *Physical Therapy, 58,* 704–709.

Magee, D. J. (1992). *Orthopedic physical assessment* (2nd ed.). Philadelphia: W. B. Saunders.

Markos, P. (1977). *Comparison of hold-relax and contract-relax and contralateral effects.* Unpublished master's thesis. Boston University.

Mathiowetz, V. (1993). The role of physical performance component evaluations in occupational therapy functional assessment. *American Journal of Occupational Therapy, 47,* 225–230.

Mathiowetz, V., & Haugen, J. B. (1995). Evaluation of motor behavior: Traditional and contemporary views. In C. A. Trombly (Ed.), *Occupational therapy for physical dysfunction* (4th ed.) (pp. 157–185). Philadelphia: Williams & Wilkins.

Mathiowetz, V., Volland, G., Kashman, N., & Weber, K. (1985). Adult norms for the box and block test of manual dexterity. *American Journal of Occupational Therapy, 39,* 386–391.

Mathiowetz, V., Volland, G., Kashman, N., & Weber, K. (1984). Reliability and validity of grip and pinch strength evaluations. *Journal of Hand Surgery, 9A,* 222.

Mathiowetz, V., Weber, K., Kashman, N., & Volland, G. (1985). Adult norms for the nine hole peg test of finger dexterity. *Occupational Therapy Journal of Research, 5,* 24–38.

Mattingly, C., & Fleming, M. H. (1994). *Clinical reasoning: Forms of inquiry in a therapeutic practice.* Philadelphia: F.A. Davis.

Mattis, S. (1976). Mental status examination for organic mental syndromes in the elderly patient. In L. Ballak & T. E. Karasu (Eds.), *Geriatric Psychiatry.* New York: Grune & Stratton.

Miller, R., Groher, M., Yorkston, K. & Rees, T (1988). Speech, language, swallowing and auditory rehabilitation. In J. DeLisa (Ed.), *Rehabilitation medicine principles and practice* (pp. 116–139). Philadelphia: J. B. Lippincott.

Minor, M. (1991). Assessing the physiological enablers of performance. In C. Christiansen & C. Baum (Eds.), *Occupational therapy. Overcoming human performance deficits* (pp. 455–468). Thorofare, NJ: Slack.

Nashner, L. (1993a). Computerized dynamic posturography. In G. Jacobson, C. Newman, & J. Kartush (Eds.), *Handbook of balance function testing* (pp. 280–307). St. Louis, MO: C.V, Mosby.

Nashner, L. (1993b). Practical biomechanics and physiology of balance. In G. Jacobson, C. Newman, & J. Kartush (Eds.), *Handbook of balance function testing* (pp, 261–279). St. Louis, MO: C.V. Mosby.

Neistadt, M. E. (1989). Normal adult performance on constructional praxis training tasks. *American Journal of Occupational Therapy, 43,* 448–455.

Neistadt, M. E. (1992). The Rabideau Kitchen Evaluation—Revised: An assessment of meal preparation skill. *The Occupational Therapy Journal of Research, 12*, 242–255.

Nelson, A., Fogel, B. S., & Faust, D. (1986). Bedside cognitive screening instruments: A critical assessment. *Journal of Nervous and Mental Disease, 174*, 73–83.

Nelson, K.L. (1996). Dysphagia: Evaluation and treatment. In L. W. Pedretti (Ed.), *Occupational therapy. Practice skills for physical dysfunction* (4th ed.) (pp. 165–191). St. Louis, MO: C.V. Mosby.

Northern, J. G., Rust, D. M., Nelson, C. E., & Watts, J. H. (1995). Involvement of adult rehabilitation patients in setting occupational therapy goals. *American Journal of Occupational Therapy, 49*, 214–220.

Okkema, K. (1993a). *Cognition and perception in the stroke patient.* Gaithersburg, MD: Aspen Publishers.

Okkema, K. (1993b). Factors influencing cognitive and perceptual evaluation. In K. Okkema (Ed.), *Cognition and perception in the stroke patient—a guide to functional outcomes in occupational therapy* (pp. 13–20). Gaithersburg, MD: Aspen Publishers.

Opacich, K. (1991). Assessment and informed decision-making. In C. Christiansen & C. Baum (Eds). *Occupational therapy. Overcoming human performance deficits* (pp. 355–372). Thorofare, NJ: Slack.

Pedretti, L.W. (1996a). Evaluation of joint range of motion. In L. W. Pedretti (Ed.), *Occupational therapy. Practice skills for physical dysfunction* (4th ed.) (pp. 79–107). St. Louis, MO: C.V. Mosby.

Pedretti, L. W. (1996b). Evaluation of muscle strength. In L. W. Pedretti (Ed.), *Occupational therapy. Practice skills for physical dysfunction* (4th ed.) (pp. 109–149). St. Louis, MO: C.V. Mosby.

Pedretti, L. W. (1996c). Evaluation of sensation and treatment of sensory dysfunction. In L. W. Pedretti (Ed.), *Occupational therapy. Practice skills for physical dysfunction* (4th ed.) (pp. 213–230). St. Louis, MO: C.V. Mosby.

Pedretti, L. W. (1996d). Occupational therapy evaluation and assessment of physical dysfunction. In L. W. Pedretti (Ed.), *Occupational therapy. Practice skills for physical dysfunction* (4th ed.) (pp. 35–42). St. Louis, MO: C.V. Mosby.

Poizner, H., Mack, L., Verfaellie, M., Rothi, L. J., Heilman, K. M. (1990). Three dimensional computergraphic analysis of apraxia: Neuronal representation of learned movement. *Brain, 113*, 85–101.

Prigatano, G. P. (1986). *Neuropsychological rehabilitation after brain injury.* Baltimore, MD: Johns Hopkins University Press.

Rancho (1978). *Guide for muscle testing of the upper extremity.* Rancho Los Amigos Hospital Occupational Therapy Department. Downey, CA: Professional Staff Association of Rancho Los Amigos Hospital.

Rao, S. M., Leo, G. J., Bernardin, L., & Unverzagt, F. (1991). Cognitive dysfunction in multiple sclerosis. *Neurology, 41*, 684–691.

Riddle, D. (1992). Measurement of accessory motion: Critical issues and related concepts. *Physical Therapy, 72*, 865–874.

Rizzolatti, G., & Berti, A. (1993). Neural mechanisms of spatial neglect. In I. H. Robertson & J. C. Marshall (Eds.), *Unilateral neglect: Clinical and experimental studies.* Hillsdale, NJ: Lawrence Erlbaum Associates.

Robertson, L., & Lamb, M. R. (1991). Neuropsychological contributions to theories of part/whole organization. *Cognitive Psychology, 23*, 299–230.

Robertson, I., Ward, T., Ridgeway, V., & Nimmo-Smith, I. (1994). *The Test of Everyday Attention (TEA).* England: Thames Valley Test Company.

Rogers, J. C. (1982). The spirit of independence: The evolution of a philosophy. *American Journal of Occupational Therapy, 36*, 709–715.

Rothi, L. G., Heilman, K. M., & Watson, R. T. (1985). Pantomime, comprehension and ideomotor apraxia. *Journal of Neurology, Neurosurgery, and Psychiatry, 48*, 207–210.

Roy, E. A. (1978). Apraxia: A new look at an old syndrome. *Journal of Human Movement Studies, 4*, 191–210.

Rustad, R. A., DeGroot, T. L., Jungkunz, M. L., Freeberg, K. S., Borowick, L. G., & Wanttie, A. M. (1993). *The Cognitive Assessment of Minnesota.* Tucson, AZ: Therapy Skill Builders.

Schwartz, M. F., Mayer, N. H., FitzpatrickDeSalme, E. J., & Montgomery, M. W. (1993). Cognitive theory and the study of everyday action disorders after brain damage. *Journal of Head Trauma Rehabilitation, 8*, 59–72.

Siev, E., Freishtat, B., and Zoltan, B. (1986). *Perceptual and cognitive dysfunction in the adult stroke patient.* Thorofare, NJ: Slack.

Simon, C. J., & Daub, M. M. (1993). Human development across the life span. In H. L. Hopkins & H. D. Smith (Eds.), *Willard & Spackman's Occupational Therapy* (8th ed.) (pp. 95–130). Philadelphia: J. B. Lippincott.

Smidt, G. & Roger M. (1982). Factors contributing to the regulation and clinical assessment of muscle strength. *Physical Therapy, 62*, 1283.

Smith, H. (1993). Assessment and evaluation: An overview. In H. L. Hopkins & H. D. Smith (Eds.), *Willard & Spackman's Occupational Therapy* (8th ed.) (pp. 169–191). Philadelphia: J. B. Lippincott.

Squire, L. R., & Butters, N. (Eds.) (1984). *Neuropsychology of memory.* Hillsdale, NJ: Lawrence Erlbaum Associates.

Squire, L. R., & Cohen, N. J. (1982). Remote memory, retrograde amnesia, and the neuropsychology of memory. In L. S. Cermak, I. Grant, & K. M. Adams (Eds.), *Human memory and amnesia.* Hillsdale, NJ: Lawrence Erlbaum.

Squire, L. R., & Zouzounis, J. A. (1988). Self-ratings of memory dysfunction: Different findings in depression and amnesia. *Journal of Clinical and Experimental Neuropsychology, 10*, 727–738.

Sroufe, L.A., Cooper, R.G., & Deltart, G.B. (1992). *Child development* (2nd ed.). New York: McGraw-Hill.

Stone, M. H., & Wright, B. D. (1980). *Knox Cube Test.* Chicago: Stoelting.

Stringer, A. Y. (1996). *A guide to adult neuropsychological diagnosis.* Philadelphia: F. A. Davis.

Studenski, S., Duncan, P., & Hogue C. (1989). *Progressive mobility skills.* Paper presented at the American Geriatrics Society annual meeting, Boston, MA., May 12, 1989.

Sunderland, A., & Harris, J. (1984). Failures in everyday life following severe head injury. *Journal of Clinical Neuropsychology, 6*, 127–142.

Tinetti, M. E. (1986). Performance oriented assessment of mobility problems on elderly patients. *Journal of the American Geriatrics Society, 34*, 119–126.

Titus, M. N. D., Gall, N. G., Yerxa, E. J., Roberson, T. A., & Mack, W. (1991). Correlation of perceptual performance and activities of daily living in stroke patients. *American Journal of Occupational Therapy, 45*, 410–418.

Toglia, J. P. (1989a). Approaches to cognitive assessment of the brain injured adult: Traditional methods and dynamic investigation. *Occupational Therapy Practice, 1*, 36–57.

Toglia, J. P. (1989b). Visual perception of objects: An approach to assessment and intervention. *American Journal of Occupational Therapy, 43* (9), 587–595.

Toglia, J. P. (1991a). Generalization of treatment: A multicontext approach to cognitive perceptual impairment in adults with brain injury. *American Journal of Occupational Therapy, 45*, 505–516.

Toglia, J. P. (1991b). Unilateral visual inattention: Multidimensional components. *Occupational Therapy Practice, 3* (1), 18–34.

Toglia, J. P. (1992). A dynamic interactional approach to cognitive rehabilitation. In N. Katz (Ed.), *Cognitive rehabilitation: Models for intervention in Occupational Therapy.* Boston: Andover Medical Publisher.

Toglia, J. P. (1993a). Attention and memory. In C. B. Royeen (Ed.), *AOTA self-study series: Cognitive rehabilitation.* (lesson 4). Rockville, MD: American Occupational Therapy Association.

Toglia, J. P. (1993b). *The Contextual Memory Test.* Tucson, AZ: Therapy Skill Builders.

Toglia, J. P. (1994). *Toglia Category Assessment (TCA).* Paquannock, NJ: Maddak.

Toglia, J.P. (1996, February). *Application of the multicontext treatment approach to disorders in attention, memory and executive function.* Supplemental manual to workshop held at Rehabilitation Institute of Chicago.

Toglia, J.P. (1996, June). *Cognitive rehabilitation: A dynamic interactional approach.* In Supplemental manual to workshop held at New York Hospital-Cornell Medical Center.

Toglia, J. P., & Golisz, K. (1990). *Cognitive rehabilitation: Group games and activities.* Tucson, AZ: Therapy Skill Builders.

Trombly, C. A. (1989). Cardiopulmonary rehabilitation. In C. A. Trombly (Ed.), *Occupational therapy for physical dysfunction* (43rd ed.) (pp. 581–603). Baltimore: Williams & Wilkins.

Trombly, C. A. (1995a). Evaluation of biomechanical and physiological aspects of motor performance. In C. A. Trombly (Ed.), *Occupational therapy for physical dysfunction* (4th ed.) (pp. 73–156). Baltimore: Williams & Wilkins.

Trombly, C. A. (1995b). Occupation: Purposefulness and meaningfulness as therapeutic mechanisms. Eleanor Clarke Slagle Lecture. *American Journal of Occupational Therapy, 49,* 960–972.

Trombly, C. A. (1995c). Planning, guiding, and documenting therapy. In C. A. Trombly (Ed.), *Occupational therapy for physical dysfunction* (4th ed.) (pp. 29–40). Baltimore: Williams & Wilkins.

Trombly, C. A., & Scott, A. D. (1989). Evaluation of motor control. In C. A. Trombly (Ed.) (1989). *Occupational therapy for physical dysfunction* (3rd ed.) (pp. 55–71). Baltimore: Williams & Wilkins.

Undzis, M. F., Zoltan, B., & Pedretti, L. W. (1996). Evaluation of motor control. In L. W. Pedretti (Ed.), *Occupational therapy. Practice skills for physical dysfunction* (4th ed.) (pp. 151–164). St. Louis, MO: C. V. Mosby.

Velozo, C., Kielhofner, G., & Fisher, G. (1992). *A user's guide to the worker role interview.* (Research version.) Department of Occupational Therapy, University of Illinois at Chicago.

Warren, M. (1981). Relationship of constructional apraxia and body scheme disorders to dressing performance in CVA. *American Journal of Occupational Therapy, 35,* 431–442.

Warren, M. (1991). Strategies for sensory and neuromotor remediation. In C. Christiansen & C. Baum (Eds.), *Occupational therapy. Overcoming human performance deficits* (pp. 633–662). Thorofare, NJ: Slack.

Warren, M. (1993). A hierarchical model for evaluation and treatment of visual perceptual dysfunction in adult acquired brain injury, part 1. *American Journal of Occupational Therapy, 47,* 42–54.

Watts, J. H., Brollier, C., Bauer, D., & Schmidt, W. (1988). The assessment of occupational functioning: The second revision. *Occupational Therapy in Mental Health, 8* (4), 7–27.

Wei, S, McQuade, K., & Smidt, G. (1993). Three dimensional joint range of motion measurements from skeletal coordinate data. *Journal of Physical Therapy, 18,* 687–691.

Wilson, B., Cockburn, J., & Baddeley, A. (1985). *The Rivermead Behavioral Memory Test.* England: Thames Valley Test Company.

Wilson, B., Cockburn, J., & Halligan, P. (1987). *Behavioral Inattention Test (BIT).* England: Thames Valley Test Company.

Wood, W. (1995). Weaving the warp and weft of occupational therapy: An art and science for all times. *American Journal of Occupational Therapy, 49,* 44–52.

Worley, J., Bennett, W., Miller, G., Miller, M., Walker, B., & Harmon, C. (1991). Reliability of three clinical measures of muscle tone in the shoulders and wrists of post-stroke patients. *American Journal of Occupational Therapy, 45,* 50–58.

York, C. D., & Cermak, S. A. (1995). Visual perception and praxis in adults after stroke. *The American Journal of Occupational Therapy, 49,* 543–550.

Chapter 17

Evaluation of Performance Contexts

Jean Cole Spencer

▼ MEANINGS OF CONTEXT

Performance contexts are defined in the Uniform Terminology for Occupational Therapy as "situations or factors that influence an individual's engagement in desired and/or required performance areas" (American Occupational Therapy Association [AOTA], 1994, p. 1047). The term context is derived from the Latin word *contexere* meaning "to weave together," suggesting a holistic view of "the whole situation, background, or environment relevant to some happening or personality," including its location in both time and space (*Webster's New World Dictionary,* 1957, p. 319).

Emphasis on the context of occupational performance represents a shift in perspective away from the historical view that problems of persons with disabilities are solely due to some defect or malfunction within the individual. In the last several decades there have been a number of social movements that contested this individual-centered view of disability, including the normalization movement (Wolfensberger, 1972), the independent-living movement (DeJong, 1979), and the movement for inclusion of children with disabilities in regular school settings (Gliedman & Roth, 1980). Each of these movements is based on the premise that the environmental context is at least as powerful a determinant of the lives and functioning of persons with disabilities as their individual impairments.

▼ ASSESSMENT TOOLS IN THE CONTEXT OF THEORY AND RESEARCH

This chapter will provide a variety of practical approaches and tools that can be used in clinical practice to evaluate various aspects of the temporal and environmental contexts of occupational therapy clients. However, rather than providing an exhaustive listing of all available tools and their dimensions, the chapter will examine connections between selected tools and the "contexts" from which they came. This involves considering theoretical perspectives that identify factors to which one should pay attention, as well as methods by which various domains of context can be studied. The focus is on conceptualization of evaluation goals and strategies, rather than on critiques of the measurement properties of particular tools, which are available elsewhere (Asher, 1989; Forer, 1996; Letts, et al., 1994; Mitchell, 1985). The assessments cited have been selected to illustrate four major traditions of evaluation. Central features of these four traditions are briefly summarized in Table 17–1 as a reference that may be useful to readers as they examine particular tools throughout the chapter.

TABLE 17-1. Four Major Traditions of Evaluation

Type	Description
Experimental tradition	Based on performance of standardized tasks; high degree of examiner control over testing situation
Behavior observation tradition	Documentation of natural behavior in "real-world" settings, usually on a time-sampling basis
Survey tradition	Use of written or oral questionnaires that document self-reported practices or opinions of respondents
Ethnographic tradition	Participant observation and interviews with open-ended questions designed to capture an "insider's view" of activity and its meanings to participants

▼ TEMPORAL CONTEXTS

Alternative Perspectives

Temporal context refers to the location of occupational performance in time. In the Uniform Terminology this includes chronological age, developmental stage, life cycle phase, and disability status. Historically in occupational therapy, consideration of temporal aspects of context emphasized how specific points in an individual's maturation or particular life events were defined from the "outsider's perspective" of society. For example, there is common social agreement on the meaning of terms such as a 29-year-old person, a child who is in "the terrible twos," an adult in midlife crisis, or a disability that is chronic, because these designations are based on commonly accepted theories and beliefs about how human life unfolds over time. More recently, occupational therapy practitioners and other clinical professionals have begun to consider temporal context from the "insider's perspective" as lived by the individual. This trend is represented by a growing interest in disability experience and in life history and by growing consideration of the relevance of these insider perspectives for occupational performance and adaptation.

Chronological Age

Chronological age is a relatively straightforward term, referring to the length of time a person has lived measured in calendrical units such as days, weeks, months, or years. Age is frequently used in developmental assessments to compare the performance of a particular individual with that of his or her age peers. This seems to be particularly important in the early years of life and in old age, when substantial biological changes related to the age of the human organism are expected. In research, age has been shown to be an important predictor of the extent of recovery from injury and disease, with younger persons generally recovering more quickly and more extensively. Age at onset of various disabilities often influences the effectiveness of treatment and the effects of the disability on the life of the individual.

Age is usually reported in years from birth for adults. For young children it is commonly reported in months and, for newborns, in weeks. For example, in the Miller Assessment for Preschoolers, age is calculated in months, whereas in the Bayley Scales of Infant Development it is calculated in weeks. Practitioners may encounter cultural variability in how age is calculated and reported by clients. For example, among Koreans the age of a child is reportedly often calculated by families from the time of conception rather than from the time of birth as is common in the United States (Carruth, 1994). In this system, a child considered to be 6 months old by a family in the United States might be considered 15 months old by a Korean family who were including the 9-month gestation period in their reckoning of age. In situations for which differences in calculating age are possible, it is wise to ask families how they determine age and to identify actual date of birth if possible.

Developmental Stage

Developmental stage is defined in the Uniform Terminology as "stage or phase of maturation" (AOTA, 1994, p. 1054). This refers to internal maturation of the individual organism as an unfolding biological, cognitive, and psychosocial process. Use of a developmental perspective is common in many areas of occupational therapy practice (see Chapters 25 and 35). Research on developmental stages has employed both laboratory methods and naturalistic methods that study human development in daily life settings.

In the classic instrument-development tradition that is based on an experimental approach, data are gathered on the performance of a large sample of normal children performing a set of standardized tasks to identify the range of capabilities exhibited by children of different ages. Through this process norms are developed that allow a clinician to compare the performance of any particular child with that of other children of the same chronological age. In occupational therapy this type of developmental assessment is represented by the Miller Assessment for Preschoolers (Miller, 1983).

The *Miller Assessment for Preschoolers* (MAP) is a screening tool for children 2 years 9 months to 5 years 8 months of age to determine developmental status and identify moderate developmental delays (this tool is not intended for severely disabled children). The MAP contains 27 core items that evaluate sensory and motor abilities, yielding a foundations index and coordination index; cognitive abilities, yielding a verbal and a nonverbal index; and combined abilities, which yields a complex tasks index. There is also a format for supplemental observations to document observations of clinically trained examiners. Subscale and combined total scores allow a therapist to compare the performance of a particular child with established norms and thus to identify any areas in which that child may be functioning at a lower level than his or her age peers. Studies are underway to evaluate the ability of this test to allow early prediction of children who are at-risk for later school-related difficulties so that intervention can be initiated in specific areas in which the child is delayed.

Naturalistic research on human development emerged in response to the concern that persons in laboratory or testing settings may not behave as they ordinarily behave in daily life. Early researchers in this area studied the natural or free play of children and observed developmental progression of physical and social skills (Parten, 1932; Bronfenbrenner, 1979). A more recent example of naturalistic research on human development is the work of Gilligan (1982), who used interviews and observations of girls and young women in daily life situations to discover that their moral development typically follows a different progression than that posited by Kohlberg, which was based on studies of males (1981, 1984). A naturalistic approach to evaluation of developmental levels of children is illustrated by the Preschool Play Scale developed by Knox (1974) and refined by Bledsoe and Shepard (1982).

In the *Preschool Play Scale* the free play of children is observed for a specified period (30 minutes recommended) in a setting that has toys that allow various forms of play to occur spontaneously. Sixteen kinds of play behavior are documented in four major areas, including space management, material management, imitation, and participation. A grid indicates types of play activities within each of these areas that are typical for children of specified ages. Comparison of the actual play of a particular child with the age-graded list of play behaviors allows the therapist to judge the developmental play age of the child in the four major domains, as well as an overall play age. This tool has been used with normal preschoolers (Bledsoe & Shephard, 1982), as well as with children with disabilities (Harrison & Kielhofner, 1986). Children who do not demonstrate forms of play that would be expected for a child of that age would be likely to receive intervention designed to cultivate lacking play skills or underlying abilities that would support particular types of play.

Life Cycle Phase

Life cycle phase is defined in the Uniform Terminology as "place in important life phases, such as career style, parent-ing cycle, or educational process" (AOTA, 1994; p. 1054). In contrast with a developmental perspective, which emphasizes internal maturation of the individual, life cycle phase refers to the involvement of the person in social roles and life tasks that are common for persons of that age and social status in the culture in which the individual lives. The life course perspective that underlies this view emphasizes the importance of **major life events** that cumulatively shape the evolving life history of the individual (Abeles & Riley, 1977; Baltes, 1979). In this perspective, major life changes are generally viewed not as isolated experiences, but as events that occur in the context of competing demands from a variety of areas, such as work, family life, physical development, and people significant to the individual (Danish, Smyer, & Nowak, 1980).

Research on life cycle phases has employed two major methods. One involves cohort studies that examine the roles and experience of large groups of individuals who are at similar points in the life cycle (Vaillant, 1977). The second emphasizes ways in which individuals adapt to various kinds of major life transitions or life cycle changes (Schlossberg, 1982).

In occupational therapy, life cycle approaches emphasize the involvement of the individual in social roles, such as those of preschooler, student, sibling, sports team member, spouse, parent, worker, volunteer, or friend, and in the life tasks or occupations commonly associated with those roles. These approaches also emphasize the importance of past experience as groundwork that shapes the future of the individual. For example, Reilly (1974) and many of her students studied the play of children as precursors to work roles in adulthood. The early work of Kielhofner (1977) identified temporal adaptation as an evolving process that involves both hindsight, or looking back at past life experience, and foresight, through which the individual seeks to imagine future possibilities and take actions to make those possibilities happen.

There are several clinical tools in occupational therapy that examine engagement in a broad range of roles. These are exemplified by the Role Checklist (Oakley, Kielhofner, Barris, & Reichler, 1986).

The *Role Checklist* documents past, present, and projected future engagement in a list of ten productive roles of adults. The checklist can be presented in written or oral form. Respondents indicate whether they have past, present, or expected future engagement in each role, and also the extent to which each role is valued. Points are totaled for continuous roles, disrupted roles, role changes, past roles, present roles, future roles, and whether each role is not valuable, somewhat valuable, or very valuable. Research has shown that role loss is common with both physical and psychosocial disabilities, indicating that retention of valued roles or engagement in new roles is often an important clinical issue for therapists to consider in working with clients.

In addition to general tools that examine a broad range of roles, there are also various specialized tools designed for clients who are in particular life cycle phases, such as adolescence (Black, 1976), or particular roles, such as that of worker. These are exemplified by the Worker Role Interview (Velozo, Kielhofner, & Fisher, 1990).

The *Worker Role Interview* is a semistructured interview based on the Model of Human Occupation. Content areas include (1) personal causation (evaluates abilities and limitations, expects job success, takes responsibility); (2) values (committed to work, has work-related goals); (3) interests (enjoys work, interests consistent with work); (4) roles (identifies with being a worker, appraises work expectations, influence of other roles); (5) habits (has work habits, has daily routine, adapts routine); and (6) environment (physical setting, family and peers, boss, coworkers). Scoring is done on a four-point scale. This tool is intended for use as part of an initial evaluation of injured workers to evaluate psychosocial and environmental factors that may influence an individual's ability to return to work successfully (Biernacki, 1993).

Clinical tools that evaluate perceptions of life changes and the influence of personal history in shaping future life cycle phases are exemplified by the Occupational Performance History Interview (Henry & Kielhofner, 1989) and the Play History developed by Takata (1969) and modified by Behnke and Menarchek-Fetkovich (1984).

The *Occupational Performance History Interview* is based on the Model of Human Occupation, but also has a version designed for use with other models of practice. This assessment identifies five domains in which the individual is asked to describe current functioning compared with level of functioning before some demarcation point that is a major life change identified by the individual. The domains include (1) organization of daily living routines, (2) life roles, (3) interests, values, and goals, (4) perception of ability and responsibility, and (5) environmental influences. In addition to documenting narrative information about past and current functioning in these content areas, the therapist also rates the client on a five-point scale for each area, ranging from highly adaptive to maladaptive. A rating is also made of the individual's overall life history pattern using ratings that indicate how periods of adaptation and maladaptation have typically occurred. This evaluation process, based on a life course perspective, allows therapist and client to collaborate in identifying areas in which performance has declined following some major life change and to identify future goals based on the past life experience of the individual.

The *Play History* is an interview format to gather information from a child's parent or caretaker on four elements of the play situation, including materials, action, people, and settings. It is organized according to five major epochs through which children move, including (1) sensorimotor play, (2) symbolic and simple constructive play, (3) dramatic and complex constructive play, and (4) game play, with a fifth area (recreational play) not included in the tool. This tool is described as a semistructured qualitative questionnaire aimed at identifying "play experiences, interactions, environments, and opportunities" (Behnke & Menarchek-Fetkovich, 1984; p. 94). Some research has been done that indicates children with disabilities may lack opportunities for kinds of play that are expected among their peers and which may have implications for later life experiences of these individuals (Gralewicz, 1973). A life cycle perspective would prompt therapists working with families of children with disabilities to foster opportunities for life experiences that are typical for children in the culture in which the family lives as groundwork for later life opportunities as the child grows up.

Disability Status

Disability status is defined in the Uniform Terminology as "place in continuum of disability, such as acuteness of injury, chronicity of disability, or terminal nature of illness" (AOTA, 1994; p. 1054). This area emphasizes the history of the problem that has brought the client to therapy. Factors to be considered in examining disability status include (1) whether the problem began recently or some time ago (**acute** or **chronic** onset); (2) the expected duration of functional limitations resulting from the problem (acute or chronic effects); (3) the expected course of limitations over time which may include recovery, stability, or progressive loss of abilities; and (4) the point in the individual's life cycle at which the problem began (at birth, early childhood, or later in life).

Acute illnesses are generally considered to be those of recent onset, the effects of which are expected to be temporary, as exemplified by a hand injury that can be successfully repaired by surgery. After a period of healing and rehabilitation, the client would be expected to be able to return to previous life occupations and level of performance. In addition to physical injuries, an acute problem from which good recovery is expected might also be exemplified by clients who exhibit depression for the first time in response to a major loss such as death of a spouse or loss of a job.

In contrast to this form of temporary disability, practitioners frequently work with clients shortly after onset of acquired disabilities (those occurring after a some period of "normal" development) that are expected to have long-term functional consequences and from which full recovery is typically not expected, as exemplified by spinal cord injury, head injury, or stroke. Frequently, once the client has been medically stabilized and has undergone a period of rehabilitation to maximize functional potential, he or she is expected to return home with changed methods of performing some major occupations, including possible use of assistance from technology or other persons.

In addition to disabilities that are acquired through traumatic injury, acquired chronic disabilities may also be due to onset of progressive illnesses, such as muscular dystrophy, multiple sclerosis, or arthritis, which typically occur at various chronological ages (muscular dystrophy during childhood, multiple sclerosis in middle age, and arthritis in middle or older age). However, onset may occur at atypical times for a particular individual. Progressive disabilities are those for which functional consequences are expected to become more disabling over time. Some progressive disabilities have a long course, marked by up and down periods, with remissions and exacerbations of symptoms, as is often true with multiple sclerosis, whereas others such as amyotrophic lateral sclerosis are expected to have a relatively rapid downhill course. These expectations for the future clearly have major implications for kinds of treatment goals established with clients, as well as important implications for the psychosocial issues involved in treatment.

There are also many psychosocial disabilities that are considered chronic in the sense that, although there may be periods in which clients function relatively well followed by those in which functioning declines, the underlying problems are not expected to disappear; hence, the potential for difficult periods is always present. Examples include schizophrenia and manic-depressive illness. Although consistent use of medications and support systems can minimize fluctuations in level of functioning, full recovery and disappearance of the disorder is usually not a realistic expectation. Psychosocial disabilities can also be progressive, as exemplified by Alzheimer's disease and vascular dementia.

Finally, in contrast to acquired disabilities that occur during the life course, there are many disabilities that occur before birth or shortly thereafter, which mean that an individual does not have a period of "normal" development before onset. Growing up with a disability can have major implications for the life experiences and occupational history of the person, as well as for growth and development of the human organism. Examples of such disabilities include **cerebral palsy**, congenital limb deficiencies, fetal alcohol syndrome, or **autism**. For persons who grow up with disabilities the goals of services are typically thought of as being habilitative, rather than rehabilitative, indicating that the purpose is to foster as many opportunities for growth and life experience as possible for the individual.

Research on the significance of disability status has employed several approaches. One approach involves stage theories based on the premise that adaptation to onset of disability typically includes certain emotional stages that occur in a usual sequence. Various authors identify different numbers of stages such as shock, anxiety, depression, internalized anger, externalized hostility, acknowledgment, and adjustment (Bray, 1978; Kerr & Thompson, 1972; Livneh & Antonak, 1990, 1991). This tradition is exemplified by a tool developed by Livneh and Antonak (1990).

The *Reactions to Impairment and Disability Inventory* is a multidimensional rating instrument consisting of 90 randomly arranged items scored as eight subscales measuring personal reactions to the onset of physical disability. The eight subscales, in their hypothesized sequence, include Shock (8 items), Anxiety (11 items), Denial (10 items), Depression (14 items), Internalized Anger (8 items), Externalized Hostility (12 items), Acknowledgment (12 items), and

Adjustment (15 items). Each item is rated on a four-point scale indicating the frequency with which the stated reaction is experienced (never, rarely, sometimes, or often). Research indicates that the sequence in which these stages are experienced may differ from that originally hypothesized by the authors, as well as indicating that the overall duration of the adaptation process appears to be variable for different individuals (Livneh & Antonak, 1991). This tool could be used by therapists to assist clients in articulating many of the psychosocial issues associated with onset of physical disabilities. An approach based on stage theory would suggest that temporary negative reactions to disability, such as anxiety, denial, or depression, are a normal part of a healthy adaptation process that evolves over time.

Another approach to consideration of disability status is the notion of disability trajectory developed by Corbin and Strauss (1987) in their research on persons with chronic disabilities. A trajectory refers to the "course of an illness and the work of all those involved in managing it, plus the impact of that on the workers' relationships, which in turn affects their work of managing the illness" (Corbin & Strauss, 1987; p. 280). This approach suggests that individuals with disabilities and persons with whom they have significant relationships develop changing adaptations over time. Incorporation of disability experience into one's life is referred to by these authors as "biographical accommodation." The disability trajectory perspective emphasizes continuity as well as change over time, as illustrated by the work of Becker (1993), who studied ways in which elders sought to maintain continuity in life following major disruptions caused by strokes.

Nosek and Fuhrer (1992) used the construct of independence as a way to conceptualize a process by which individuals can gain increasing control over the consequences of disability over time, a notion that can be viewed as being grounded in a disability trajectory perspective. The Personal Independence Measure (Nosek, Fuhrer, & Howland, 1992) is based on this construct.

The *Personal Independence Measure* was developed to provide a comprehensive measure that could be used by independent living programs and other service delivery systems to document "consumers' progress toward becoming more independent" (Nosek, Fuhrer, & Howland, 1992; p. 21). On the basis of careful prior analysis of the construct of independence (Nosek & Fuhrer, 1992), this tool has four subscales including Control (10 questions based on a five-point Likert Scale), Psychological Independence (34 items based on a five-point Likert scale), Physical Functioning (25 items addressing mobility, physical activity, dexterity, social role, and activities of daily living), and Environmental Resources (16 questions about housing, education, income, employment, and transportation). Initial research using this tool indicates that there is little relation between the degree of independence on psychological and control scales and degree of functional (physical) independence. This finding strongly suggests that measures of physical functioning alone are inadequate indicators of independence, as defined by the independent-living movement. Therapists could use this tool to provide a holistic view of clients' "independent mindedness" and thus incorporate psychosocial as well as physical aspects of independence into treatment goals.

A third way of considering issues related to disability status is to use individual narratives or life stories. Narratives have been used in medicine to advocate for a clinical practice that takes into account the illness experience of clients (meaning the consequences of disability as experienced in daily life by the individual), as well as treating the disease, which is typically the focus of treatment (Kleinman, 1988). Kleinman argued that managing chronic illnesses should be a collaborative process between clients and health care providers in which the daily life experience of clients is central. Use of life history and narratives is receiving growing attention in occupational therapy as a way to understand the meaning of occupations and relationships to clients and as a way to direct therapy toward future hopes valued by clients (Clark,1993; Helfrich, Kielhofner, & Mattingly, 1994; Frank, 1996).

The *Life History Approach* generally uses open-ended interviews in which the individual is asked to tell about his or her life and allowed to select events and stories about it to elicit an "insider's view" of what is important and why it is significant for the overall life story (Frank, 1996). This approach allows one to identify what is meaningful to an individual and how he or she views factors that shape the overall course of life. This perspective lets the therapist direct treatment toward goals that matter to the individual and to use treatment strategies that are congruent with the person's beliefs about how life change occurs. These clinical uses of narratives are exemplified by the work of Clark (1993) in physical disabilities practice and by Helfrich, Kielhofner, and Mattingly (1994) in mental health practice.

Summary of Strategies for Evaluating Temporal Context

This section has reviewed several approaches for evaluating aspects of temporal context, ranging from highly structured measurement tools, grounded in the experimental research tradition, to relatively unstructured qualitative approaches that emphasize the insider's perspective of the individual client. Structured measurement tools offer the advantage of gathering highly consistent types of data in which the performance of one individual can readily be compared with that of a normative sample (in norm-referenced tools) or with identified standards of acceptable performance (in criterion-referenced tools). Unstructured tools allow greater individualization in understanding what shapes the performance of a specific person and what factors can be used clinically to improve performance. Both types of information are very important in establishing goals and treatment plans that are reasonable and meaningful for clients (Neis-

tadt, 1995) and in doing the kinds of clinical reasoning that are required for effective practice (Mattingly & Fleming, 1994).

▼ ENVIRONMENTAL CONTEXTS

Alternative Perspectives

Environmental context refers to the location of occupational performance in space. Space in this sense does not refer to physical territory alone, but also incorporates the social and cultural systems that are attached to particular places. The notion of behavior settings has frequently been used to conceptualize the connections between physical spaces and the occupations that regularly occur there. According to Roger Barker (1978), who developed this idea in the field of ecological psychology, behavior settings are locations in which a standing pattern of behavior occurs, irrespective of the inhabitants of the setting. Barker used the classic example that in the post office, people behave "post office," indicating that the physical arrangement of counters and post boxes, the social roles of staff and customers, and the culturally patterned occupations of picking up mail or sending packages are closely interwoven.

In this chapter the organizing framework, as illustrated in Table 17–2, will be used to compare alternative tools for evaluating physical, social, and cultural environmental contexts, as distinguished in the Uniform Terminology. The distinction between these environmental domains is somewhat artificial because virtually all environments used by humans have all three aspects, which are usually thought of as integrated wholes by users of the setting. However, this distinction highlights particular aspects singled out for "foreground" attention. Physical, social, and cultural environments will be considered at four different scales, moving from those closest to the individual to those that are more remote. These scales are defined in ways that "make sense" as recognized entities by persons who inhabit environments at each level. These scales are important not only because they draw our attention to different kinds of influences on occupational performance, but also because they have important implications for who controls the environment and, therefore, the processes through which environmental change might occur.

Immediate scale environments include surroundings that are in close and direct contact with the individual (such as one's computer workstation), or direct personal interactions (such as those between a caregiver and care recipient or between client and practitioner). Typically evaluation at this level involves close examination of a single occupation. Usually clients or their advocates are able to exert relatively direct influence to make changes in their immediate scale environments.

Proximal scale environments include surroundings at the level of single-behavior settings, such as a kitchen, office,

TABLE 17-2. Framework for Comparing Environmental Assessments and Environmental Dimensions

Scales	Physical	Social	Cultural
Immediate	Work capacity evaluation Assistive technology evaluation Fine motor tasks	Mother–child interaction Cost of care index	Ethnographic assessment Caregiver intervention
Proximal	Accessibility checklists Negotiability rating Interview-in-place	Family assessment Work environment scale	Classroom observation guide Home observation format
Community	Community accessibility Neighborhood mobility	Sociospatial support Resources and services	Handicap assessment Community integration
Societal	Disability rights guide	Social distance scale	Media representation models

playground, or occupational therapy clinic, which can typically be traversed by walking or simple mobility devices. Typically such settings include interactive occupations of several individuals. Clients may have substantial influence in making decisions about proximal scale environments, but these settings are often shared with other persons who also influence decisions.

Community scale environments are geographic neighborhoods or communities, as defined and known personally by inhabitants, which may be traversed by walking along paths or streets, but that often are traversed by more complex modes of transportation. Typically, such environments would include the overall constellation of occupations that are part of an individual's usual daily routine. Clients may have difficulty altering environments at this scale, but they can choose to move to a more compatible environment or participate in social processes to advocate for community change.

Societal scale environments include public policies, widely held beliefs and attitudes, and major social institutions, such as transportation, health care, or educational systems. Clients have little direct control over environments at this scale, but they can participate actively in social or public policy processes to advocate for change in environments at this level.

Physical Environments

Physical environments are defined in the Uniform Terminology as "nonhuman aspects of contexts; includes the accessibility to and performance within environments having natural terrain, plants, animals, buildings, furniture, objects, tools, or devices" (AOTA, 1994, p. 1054). Theories that have shaped views of physical aspects of environments in occupational therapy have come both from social science disciplines, such as ecological psychology and geography, and applied fields, such as architecture and urban planning, rehabilitation engineering, and ergonomics. Some of these fields are concerned with how physical settings shape naturally occurring activity and social interaction and with the symbolic meanings attached to places. Others are concerned with how buildings and public spaces should be designed to

facilitate movement of people and performance of activities, or how objects and tools should be designed to make them easier to manipulate.

IMMEDIATE SCALE PHYSICAL ENVIRONMENTS

Studies of immediate scale physical environments include work in ergonomics and industrial design which examines the usability of particular tools and equipment. Experimental methods are typically used in these disciplines to determine ability to perform tasks with particular tool designs. For example, such methods have been employed in usability testing of various types of computer programs that involve presentation of specific tasks and careful documentation of kinds of errors and problems encountered by subjects (Chapanis, 1991). Similar experimental testing of whether persons have the strength and endurance to use particular types of tools and equipment is common in Work Capacity Evaluations in occupational therapy (Velozo, 1993). Such evaluations are exemplified by the Baltimore Therapeutic Equipment (**BTE**) Work Simulator (Neimeyer, Matheson, & Carlton, 1989).

The *Baltimore Therapeutic Equipment Work Simulator* is designed to evaluate upper extremity performance. Various devices, such as a knob, screwdriver, lever, or steering wheel, are attached to an electrically controlled brake assembly that permits adjustment of resistance to simulate specific work demands and, thereby, measure the amount of force produced during simulated tasks. This equipment allows therapists to determine whether clients have the capabilities required to return to work tasks they have done previously or to perform simulated tasks that may have lesser demands. If increased strength is required for task performance, the simulator allows therapists to pinpoint specific upper extremity areas in which improved performance is needed.

Experimental methods also underlie rehabilitation engineering evaluations of how individuals with disabilities perform when using special kinds of assistive technology, such as seating and positioning equipment, various kinds of switches, or alternative computer interface technologies. Cook and Hussey (1995) have developed a comprehensive framework for organizing an assistive technology evaluation process.

The *Assistive Technology Evaluation Process* is based on a Human Activity Assistive Technology Model the elements of which include the human, an activity, assistive technology, and the context in which the person seeks to function. Formats for structuring the evaluation process include a Background Information Questionnaire that documents demographic information; referral information; medical and health information; sensory and perceptual abilities; activities of daily living; social interaction, learning, and behavior; functional abilities; motor skills; mobility and positioning; and communication skills. Evaluation forms provide standardized tasks for evaluating: (1) motor abilities (grasp, hand range, body part movement and control, foot range, and head control); and (2) symbol location, type, and size (symbol location and symbol size verification). Formats are also provided for a Communication Prosthesis Payment Review Summary and a Seating/Wheeled Mobility Payment Review Summary. Use of this holistic evaluation process can allow therapists to consider assistive technology as an "extrinsic enabler" that allows an individual to maximize efficient performance of selected activities; it can also provide a rationale for the selection of particular devices to justify reimbursement.

In contrast to the experimental approach, naturalistic methods have been used to document how persons use naturally occurring objects and spaces. The naturalistic approach is illustrated by studies of infant free play with objects in home or playground settings. In these studies tightly structured behavior observation based on time sampling is used to document infants' manipulation of various kinds of toys, allowing inferences about development of hand skills and other more abstract capabilities, such as understanding of cause-effect relations (Yarrow, Rubenstein, & Pederson, 1975). Observational methods using behavior checklists and time-sampling procedures borrowed from these studies can be used by occupational therapists to evaluate how persons interact with naturally occurring objects and tools and how they organize and use space in their immediate physical setting, including things such as sitting posture in different desk and chair arrangements. The behavior observation tradition is illustrated by a format used to study fine motor tasks in classroom settings (McHale & Cermak, 1992).

The *Fine Motor Task Assessment* was developed to document fine motor requirements of work in regular elementary school classrooms. Tasks are grouped into four categories, including (1) fine motor tasks (require major use of hands), (2) integrated fine motor tasks (fine motor and other academic tasks occur simultaneously), (3) other academic tasks (frequent use of hands not required), and (4) nonacademic activities (functional or transitional, rather than instructional). The duration of time spent on specific tasks is recorded during an established observation period. Fine motor tasks are described in detail (the academic subject, the precise task, and materials used), which facilitates task

analysis in terms of kinds of tools required (pencil-and-paper versus manipulative tasks), degree of student control (eg, copying versus creative drawing), or other dimensions. This assessment yields a detailed picture of kinds of interactions expected of children with tools and objects in their immediate physical environment that can be used by therapists to cultivate required skills in children or to provide consultation with teachers on how to make environmental demands more manageable for students with fine motor problems.

In addition to studies focusing on the effect of physical environments on task performance, symbolic aspects of immediate scale physical environments have also received some attention in occupational therapy. Bates, Spencer, Young, and Rintala (1993) used in-depth qualitative interviews as well as chart review to examine the process by which a young iron worker, disabled by spinal cord injury, adapted during his rehabilitation to use of a wheelchair that would become a lasting part of his immediate physical environment. Initially, this young man hated the wheelchair as a symbol of disability and helplessness, in dramatic contrast to the views of staff who considered it a useful tool to allow him greater mobility. This study, which identified both pragmatic (performance oriented) and emotional adaptation processes, indicates that assistive technology may have many meanings to users, many of which are quite different from those of occupational therapy practitioners. Research indicates that assistive devices quite frequently are discarded by persons with disabilities after they return home from clinical facilities, for a variety of reasons, ranging from lack of acceptability or failure of the device, to improved function of the individual (Brooks, 1991; Garber & Gregorio, 1990). Attention to the meaning of devices and equipment to clients can have important implications for their acceptance and use over time.

PROXIMAL SCALE PHYSICAL ENVIRONMENTS

In studying physical environments of proximal scale behavior settings, much attention has been directed toward wheelchair accessibility of various home and work settings. In the early years of advocacy for accessibility for persons with disabilities, emphasis was given to development of special standards that focused on ability of persons in wheelchairs to maneuver in various spaces (American National Standards Institute [ANSI], 1980). However, a more recent concept that guides current research in this area is the notion of universal design which is based on the premise that ordinary physical spaces and objects can be designed and built to be usable by persons with a wide range of capabilities so that individuals who have mobility impairments are not excluded. Several accessibility checklists, which sometimes also address safety issues, have been developed for use in home settings, such as the Home Modification Workbook (Adaptive Environments Center, 1988) or Source Book (Kelly & Snell, 1989), as well as in workplace or public settings, such as the Workplace Workbook (Mueller, 1990) or the American With Disabilities Act Accessibility

Guidelines Checklist for Buildings and Facilties (U.S. Architectural & Transportation Barriers Compliance Board, 1992). These checklists address features such as doorway widths or ramp slopes in terms of their usability by "the average" wheelchair user.

In occupational therapy, accessibility and safety issues in home environments have commonly been addressed through activities of daily living (ADL) assessments to help rehabilitation clients anticipate how they will be able to perform specific self-care or housekeeping activities in the physical spaces of their home bathrooms or kitchens (Christiansen, 1994). Historically there have been many activities of daily living checklists designed by therapy staff of particular facilities, rather than a few well-developed standardized assessment tools that are widely used. Frequently, these activities of daily living assessments are performed in clinic settings designed to simulate the kitchen or bathroom spaces of clients' homes. However, the assumption that performance in a simulated clinic setting will be a good indicator of performance in the real proximal environment of home has been questioned in recent research (Park, Fisher, & Velozo, 1994). Bates (1994) has advocated that instead of standardized activities of daily living checklists based on the concept of accessibility, practitioners should adopt the concept of negotiability. This idea was developed through research using behavior observation of how effectively particular individuals can use various environmental features in their own settings (Norris-Baker & Willems, 1978). Negotiability refers to "ability to access a feature of the environment and use it for its intended purpose with only one's usual adaptive equipment" (Bates, 1994; p. 426). Negotiability thus involves a functional interaction between a specific individual with particular capabilities, an environment with particular features, and specific adaptive equipment regularly used by the individual. Bates (1994) has described how this approach can be used by therapists during home visits.

The *Negotiability Rating Process* involves making a careful inventory of all features of the home environment. The client is then asked to try to use each environmental feature for its intended purpose, with only his or her usual adaptive equipment. Notes are made on those features that are negotiable. For features that cannot be used by the client, factors that limit negotiability are documented (such as shelves that are 12 inches above the client's reach). From this list, a negotiability rating may be obtained by computing the percentage of all features that are negotiable. This calculation is useful for documenting measurable changes in negotiability as a result of occupational therapy intervention through provision of new adaptive equipment or environmental modification.

Although much of the research on the effect of proximal scale physical environments has focused on concrete observations of activity performance, some authors have recognized the symbolic importance of behavior settings for users. For example, Bates (1994) cites the circumstances of a woman who chose not to make her recently redecorated bathroom wheelchair accessible despite the fact that it would have made performance of self-care tasks much easier. This choice reflected her personal value of appearance over function, a values priority that should be respected by practitioners. The geographer, Graham Rowles, eloquently urged practitioners to recognize the meaning of place as a component of occupational therapy (1991), a view that is consistent with the growing emphasis in the profession on understanding the great importance of the meaning of occupations as well as their performance requirements (Trombly, 1995). The architect Raymond Lifchez (1987) addressed these issues in examining how designers of the built environment can come to understand what he called the "quality of experience" of persons with disabilities through use of an Interview-in-Place.

Lifchez's *Interview-in-Place* is based on ethnographic methodology. The client is asked to select a place (a room at home, a cafe, his or her workplace) in which he or she feels comfortable speaking about that place as a physical and social setting. The setting itself will generate a variety of topics for discussion. What physical and social factors make the setting noteworthy for you? How do you feel being in that setting and going to and from it? Additional questions allow generalization of these findings to other spaces. What places outside your home do you regularly visit? How do you get there? What sorts of activities do you need help with in those settings? What places would you most like to visit that you have not been able to visit, and what prevents you from going there? This methodology hinges on the premise that being in the client's commonly used settings will prompt the individual to articulate personal environmental meanings and priorities in ways that will not be evoked in the foreign setting of an architect's office or an occupational therapy clinic, a premise that has been supported by Lifchez's research on interactions between architectural students and persons with physical disabilities (1987). This assessment approach could be particularly usable for therapists in community-based practice for which being in the client's "territory" is a natural occurrence to develop understanding of how environmental features and symbolic meanings shape occupational performance.

COMMUNITY SCALE PHYSICAL ENVIRONMENTS

Surprisingly, although community scale physical environments are frequently studied in fields such as architecture and urban planning, they have received relatively little attention in occupational therapy. This is surprising because many clients have mobility impairments that may limit their ability to move easily around the neighborhood and community; thus, their access to spaces and resources, which are available to others, are unavailable to them. Some therapists have become involved in surveying the accessibility of neighborhood and community scale environments for features such as curb cuts and reasonable slope of ramps that potentially influence use of these spaces by persons with disabilities. Various accessibility checklists for evaluating community scale environments are available, such as the Readily Achievable Checklist (Cronburg, Barnett, & Goldman, 1991) and The Accessibility Checklist (Goltsman, Gilbert, & Wohlford, 1992).

Beyond surveys of specific features that limit the capacity of persons with disabilities to use neighborhood spaces, there has been some research that examines actual use of neighborhood and community spaces by elderly persons. Cantor (1979) conducted an extensive survey of white, black, and Hispanic senior citizens in inner city neighborhoods in New York City and mapped their mobility spheres and use of resources, such as grocery stores. Rather than being isolated and homebound, Cantor found that many older persons frequently traveled within a 10-block radius by walking to visit valued destinations. Her study methodology forms the groundwork for the Neighborhood Environment Survey (Cantor, 1979).

The *Neighborhood Environment Survey* was designed for research, rather than for clinical use, but it contains a framework for evaluating how far and by what methods people travel on a regular basis to reach important resources in the environment. A list of resources is provided, which includes grocery stores and other shops, banks, restaurants and bars, health services, churches and synagogues, and recreational facilities such as parks. Respondents are asked how often they visit these resources, how far they travel in blocks (which could be converted to miles), and what methods of mobility or transportation they use. The findings are portrayed by use of concentric circles representing commonly used distances—such as 1 to 2 blocks, 2 to 6 blocks, or 6 to 10 blocks—depending on use patterns of the particular individual. At each level of the person's mobility sphere, frequently used resources are listed. Evaluating these issues has important implications for therapists working with clients who are planning where to live, shop, and work following onset of disabilities. Having resources within walking or wheelchair-rolling distance can minimize the need for formal transportation services that generally remain inadequate in most communities for persons with disabilities, despite progress in recent decades to improve availability of this service.

SOCIETAL SCALE PHYSICAL ENVIRONMENTS

Societal scale physical environments are generally not evaluated by occupational therapists as part of routine clinical practice. However, it is important for practitioners to be knowledgeable about broad social policies and their influence on the lives of clients. These policies can have major implications for the usability of the physical environment by persons with disabilities. Two examples include public policies concerning accessibility of transportation systems (Bowe, 1978, 1980) and policies concerning availability of housing and assistive technology (Frieden, Frieden, & Laurie, 1981).

The *Disability Rights Guide* is a tool designed to identify problems affecting persons with disabilities in accessing community and broader-scaled resources (Goldman, 1991). The guide is a self-report questionnaire that is contained within a textbook with content based on the Americans With Disabilities Act. The questionnaire is useful for community planning and advocacy for public policies that support the rights of persons with disabilities—activities that are identified in the Occupational Therapy Code of Ethics as appropriate concerns for practitioners who are committed to improving the lives of clients in ways beyond hands-on intervention at an individual level.

Social Environments

Social environments are defined in the Uniform Terminology to include "availability and expectations of significant individuals, such as spouse, friends, and caregivers. Also includes larger social groups which are influential in establishing norms, role expectations, and social routines" (AOTA, 1994, p. 1054). Theories from the social sciences, including social psychology, sociology, and anthropology about how human interaction is organized and patterned, have been borrowed in occupational therapy to evaluate the kinds of social interaction that shape occupational performance. Role theory has been particularly influential from this tradition as a way in which occupational practitioners have conceptualized how occupations are selected and their performance organized by individuals. The Occupational Performance Model outlined by Christiansen and Baum (1992) and the Model of Human Occupation developed by Kielhofner (1985, 1995) are two models that view roles as central organizing ideas.

IMMEDIATE SCALE SOCIAL ENVIRONMENTS

In social environments of immediate scale, attention is focused in depth on social interactions between dyads of two individuals. The application of these approaches in occupational therapy often involves evaluation of the nature of interaction between a client and his or her caregivers. Several different methods have been used to study these close human interactions, including behavior observation, as illustrated by studies of interaction between mothers and children with disabilities (Barrera & Vella, 1987); qualitative interviews, as illustrated by research of Hasselkus (1989) on ethical dilemmas and decision-making between elders and their caregivers; and textual analysis of interactions between therapists and clients used in studies of clinical reasoning (Crepeau, 1991; Mattingly & Fleming, 1994). These studies show that caregivers can have a powerful effect on occupational performance that is encouraged or allowed for persons with disabilities and, likewise, that the behavior of care recipients influences the interaction in significant ways. McCuaig and Frank's (1991) research on ways in which a woman with cerebral palsy managed independent living indicated that a central focus of her efforts was convincing persons with whom she interacted that she was an intelligent and competent person, in spite of major mobility and speech impairments. These issues are of great importance to occupational therapy practitioners, who are often in a position to influence the ways in which families interact with children or adults with disabilities, or ways in which persons with disabilities learn to interact with personal care assistants. Clinical assessments, reviewed in the following, that focus on interaction at the scale of immediate social environments are the Mother-Child Interaction Checklist based on a behavior observation approach (Barrera & Vella, 1987), and an interview format called the Cost of Care Index (Kosberg & Cairl, 1986).

The *Mother-Child Interaction Checklist* provides a structured format for detailed observations of interactions between mothers and children that has been used in comparisons of children with disabilities and those without disabilities and their mothers (Barrera & Vella, 1987). The observation format specifies (1) maternal behaviors, including vocalization, verbalization, question, command, praise, regard, and interactive play; (2) infant behaviors, including vocalization, negative response, regard, en face (visual orientation toward the face of another), interactive play, independent play, and looking away; and (3) reciprocal behaviors that involve particular sequences of maternal and child behaviors. Research has indicated that mothers of disabled infants exhibited more controlling behaviors than mothers of nondisabled infants, and physically disabled infants engaged in less eye contact and vocalizations than their nondisabled peers (Barrera & Vella, 1987). Assessment of interaction patterns between mothers and infants with disabilities could be used by therapists to encourage parents to behave in ways that promote optimal participation of infants in their proximal social environments.

The *Cost of Care Index* was developed as a case management tool to help health professionals identify issues in families in which care is being provided to elders (Kosberg & Cairl, 1986). There are 20 items that address five domains including personal and social restrictions, physical, and emotional health; value placed on caregiving; characteristics of the care recipient that may evoke negative responses; and economic costs of caregiving. Client responses to statements range from "strongly agree" to "strongly disagree." Scores for each domain highlight potential problem areas that can be addressed in intervention with caregivers or care recipients.

PROXIMAL SCALE SOCIAL ENVIRONMENTS

Social environments of proximal scale have been studied using the concept of social roles attached to particular behavior settings, such as classrooms, workplaces, or clinical settings. The concept of role refers to defined social positions that have attached expectations for behavior. Roles organize the ways in which persons with different social positions interact in a particular setting, as illustrated by the roles of stu-

dents and teachers organizing ways in which they interact in classroom settings, or the roles of clients and practitioners organizing who does what in clinic environments. An assessment that examines roles and interaction patterns within families, the Family Assessment Device, illustrates use of this conceptualization of proximal social environments (Epstein, Baldwin, & Bishop, 1983).

The *Family Assessment Device* is based on the McMaster model of family functioning. It is a self-administered questionnaire that includes 53 items that make up seven subscales, including general family functioning, problem solving, communication, roles, affective responsiveness, affective involvement, and behavior control (Epstein, Baldwin, & Bishop, 1983). This tool has been used to evaluate methods of adaptation to the demands and stresses associated with having a child with head injury (Rivara et al, 1996). Research on families that include children with disabilities indicates that strong support systems, involvement in outside activities, good communication and problem solving skills, low levels of family conflict and stress, and positive belief systems are predictors of positive adjustment over time (Beavers, Hampson, Hulgas, & Beavers, 1986; Hauser et al, 1986; Rivara et al, 1992). These are resources and skills that therapists can seek to cultivate in families that include a child with a disability.

The term "social climate" was developed by Moos and his associates to convey the expectations associated with roles in various settings (1974). His initial work (1974) on this concept involved development of a measure called the Ward Atmosphere Scale in which he had staff and clients rate ten dimensions of psychiatric clinic settings including areas such as order, initiative, anger, and autonomy. In occupational therapy Kannegeiter (1987) used the work of Moos in developing an Environmental Assessment Scale for evaluating psychiatric clinical settings. This method for evaluating social climate of proximal scale social environments has been applied to many other kinds of settings, including workplaces, as illustrated by the Work Environment Scale (Moos, 1981).

The *Work Environment Scale* provides a list of statements about the interpersonal environment of a workplace that address a variety of dimensions in three broad areas, including relationships, personal growth, and system maintenance and change. Employers and workers indicate their agreement or disagreement with a set of statements about these dimensions, which can be used to compare the perceptions of different participants in the setting. Similar to previous scales by the same author, designed initially for evaluating treatment environments (Moos, 1974), this scale can also be rated according to perceptions of the actual environment in contrast to perceptions of what employers and workers feel would be an ideal environment. Differences between actual and ideal can be used as a stimulus for planning change in the work setting (Moos, 1981)

An additional method that has been used to study roles and social climate in clinical settings is ethnography, which was developed in the discipline of anthropology. Rather than using rating scales or structured instruments, this qualitative method uses the researcher as a participant observer, who takes part in the interaction within the setting, and documents both how persons interact and how various participants understand social processes. A classic study using this method was completed by Caudill on The Psychiatric Hospital as a Small Society (1958) in which he found many social mechanisms that distanced the roles of clients from those of various kinds of staff. A recent study in occupational therapy examined the social relationships among clients and between clients and staff in a rehabilitation hospital; important differences were found in how these groups thought about the purposes and methods of rehabilitation (Spencer, Young, Rintala, & Bates, 1995). The social systems of proximal scale environments have major implications for ways in which persons with disabilities are incorporated into, or distanced from, the usual rounds of activity; thus, they become an important focus for occupational therapy practitioners who see their role as fostering engagement of clients in daily life opportunities.

COMMUNITY SCALE SOCIAL ENVIRONMENTS

Community scale social environments involve human interaction over wider distances than particular behavior settings, such as homes, workplaces, or clinical settings. Social network analysis has frequently been used to study social environments at this scale, with detailed examination of the kinds of social support that are exchanged by network members (Gottlieb, 1981). Social support, including both instrumental and emotional assistance, is frequently a key factor in adapting to a broad variety of illnesses and disabilities (McCubbin, Cauble, & Patterson, 1982; Moos, 1986). There are many measures of social support that use structured questionnaires to gather information on types of assistance received and kinds of persons who provide assistance to the respondent. The social support assessment cited here also incorporates analysis of geographical factors that shape how social support exchanges operate at a community level. In an extensive study of the ways in which elders functioned within the social system of a small community in Appalachia, Rowles (1983) found that different types and intensities of support were derived from different spatial zones. This finding led to the concept of sociospatial support systems.

The *Sociospatial Support Inventory* identifies a spatial hierarchy of seven zones, including home, surveillance zone, vicinity, community, subregion, region, and nation. Rowles used space-time diaries, in which respondents recorded trips outside of home, all visits, and telephone calls made and received, to identify kinds of support received within these zones. The home was a major source of assistance with daily activities for persons who lived with a companion, although many elderly persons and those with disabilities lived alone. The surveillance zone that can be seen from the respondent's home was an important source of "watchful reciprocity" with neighbors, who monitored daily routines and de-

partures from routine, which served as a signal of potential trouble. Within the vicinity (up to half a mile radius), neighbors and family members provided frequent functional support, such as buying groceries, providing a ride to church, or completing minor home repairs. At the level of community the senior citizens interacted frequently with fellow members of "the society of the old," used many formal resources, such as stores, banks, and medical services, and exchanged frequent telephone calls to provide information, reassurance, and help with decision making. The subregion (up to 25 miles radius) defined the outer boundaries of territory known personally and of formal resources used regularly (such as a hospital). Family members living within this zone often visited frequently. At the level of region (250 mile radius) and nation, support is provided almost exclusively by family members on a relatively infrequent basis, although these contacts are potentially important in crisis situations. The concept of sociospatial support systems allows evaluation of not only the kinds of assistance received, but also examination of the logistic issues (such as transportation) involved in provision of support. Therapists could use this assessment tool to help elders or persons with disabilities examine alternative ways they might manage community-living support arrangements under the circumstances of a particular geographic context in which a person currently lives or to which he or she might move.

In contrast with an emphasis on informal social support, another view of community scale social environments conceptualizes the community as a network of formal (organizationally based) resources and services. This view is illustrated by the Older Americans Resources and Services model developed by researchers at Duke University to study community support "service packages" that could be coordinated to prevent unnecessary institutionalization of elders (Duke University Center for the Study of Aging and Human Development, 1978). The Multidimensional Functional Assessment Questionnaire developed through this project has been widely used for clinical program intake, population surveys, and longitudinal studies.

The *Multidimensional Functional Assessment Questionnaire* is a structured interview consisting of part A, which examines the functional level of the individual, and part B, which examines community service use and the client's perceived need for services. Dimensions evaluated in part A include mental health, physical health, economic resources, social resources, and activities of daily living of the client, which are rated on a six-point scale, ranging from excellent to totally impaired. Part B documents actual use of, and perceived need for, a list of 24 community services, including transportation; social and recreational services; various kinds of employment, education, and training services; mental health services, including psychotropic drugs; personal care, nursing, medical, and physical therapy services; supportive devices and prostheses; supervision; homemaker-household and meal preparation services; checking services; legal protection services; financial assistance; assistance with food and groceries; housing or relocation services; and information and referral. Although designed for use with senior citizens, this structured questionnaire could be used by therapists to evaluate service use and needs of a variety of clients with physical or mental disabilities in many service-delivery settings to plan optimal community-living arrangements. The ways in which elders and persons with disabilities make decisions about when to use formal service delivery systems and how these decisions are related to their informal support systems is an important issue (Soldo, Agree, & Wolf, 1989).

SOCIETAL SCALE SOCIAL ENVIRONMENTS

At a societal scale, various methods have been used to study ways in which persons with disabilities are included, or excluded, from social systems. There is a long history of studies of attitudes toward persons with disabilities that use survey questionnaire methods (Antonak, 1981; Yuker, 1988). One approach within this tradition, uses the concept of social distance to examine levels of social interaction that people would find acceptable or unacceptable with specific types of other individuals, rather than examining attitudes toward people with disabilities in general (Tringo, 1970).

The *Disability Social Distance Scale* (Tringo, 1970) was developed to determine whether attitudes toward persons with disabilities are affected by the type of disability. A list is provided that includes 21 disabilities or "anomalous social conditions," such as having a criminal record. The list includes hidden disabilities, such as diabetes or ulcers; potentially visible physical disabilities, such as cerebral palsy or stroke; or mental retardation, mental illness, alcoholism, or a criminal record. For each of these social groups respondents are asked to specify one of nine levels of social interaction that they would find acceptable. These levels include "would marry, would accept as a close kin by marriage, would have as a next door neighbor, would accept as a casual friend, would accept as a fellow employee, would keep away from, would keep in an institution, would send out of my country, and would put to death." Studies using this tool have found that occupational therapy students do not differ substantially from other students in their preferences for social interaction with persons who have hidden disabilities, followed by visible physical disabilities, with least preferred groups being those who have "disorders of the mind" such as mental retardation, psychiatric disorders, alcoholism, or a criminal record (Lyons & Hayes, 1993). Such findings about how students view persons with disabilities have important implications for socialization of students to values of the profession (Eberhardt & Mayberry, 1995).

Social processes involving persons with disabilities have also been studied using ethnographic methods, including participant observation to examine their interactions with other members of society. The anthropologist Robert Murphy who himself became disabled by a spinal cord tumor (Murphy, 1990) used the concept of **liminality** (meaning an in-between state) to describe the lack of a clear social status and consequent uncertain social processes surrounding persons with physical disabilities in our society (Murphy, Scheer, Murphy, & Mack, 1988). Although usually not evaluated in structured ways, such social processes are often observed by practitioners who go with clients into community settings where they interact with the general public on outtrips to restaurants or recreational activities. Informal evaluation of such experiences with clients can become useful avenues for discussion of strategies clients can use to interact successfully in society.

Cultural Environments

Cultural environments are defined in the Uniform Terminology as "customs, beliefs, activity patterns, behavior standards, and expectations accepted by the society of which the individual is a member. Includes political aspects, such as laws that affect access to resources and affirm personal rights. Also includes opportunities for education, employment, and economic support." (AOTA, 1994; p. 1054). Although there are many definitions of culture, in general this term refers to the shared way of life of a group of people. The group may be a small as a family, or as large as an ethnic group. Increasing attention is being given in occupational therapy to the importance of culture in shaping human occupational life (Krefting & Krefting, 1992). Current definitions of culture emphasize its importance both in providing established patterns for how things are done, and belief systems for interpreting the meanings of what is done by various participants in the action (Geertz, 1973, 1983). This attention to meaning makes the concept of culture particularly useful in occupational therapy because of growing emphasis on understanding occupations as meaningful units of activity and the belief that engagement in human occupation is therapeutic in part because of its meaning (Clark, 1993; Trombly, 1995). The concept of culture provides a way to examine meanings that are shared within a group, in contrast to personal meanings based on individual experience. The medical anthropologist and psychiatrist Arthur Kleinman (1992) coined the term "local worlds" to describe the shared culture attached to local settings in which people live their daily lives, such as the culture of the large household of an extended family, the culture of a workplace, the culture of a school, or of a neighborhood. In these settings there are established patterns of activity and agreed-on ways of understanding the motivations that prompt people to do things that shape the meaning of activity for members of the group. The concept of culture thus expands the notion of behavioral settings to include the beliefs and values that shape how experience is interpreted by participants. For example, in a small-town restaurant the children of strangers might be greeted enthusiastically by fellow diners who interpret this action as a friendly gesture, whereas in the local world of a city restaurant this same action might be interpreted as a hazard to the safety of the children.

Cultures have typically been studied using the classic anthropological methods of participant observation, in-depth interviews, and sometimes document review. These methods, which rely heavily on the perceptiveness and skill of the researcher as the main instrument of study, have been used quite frequently in occupational therapy to study environments and their effects on occupational performance at several levels. Ethnographic methods were originally designed for use by full-time researchers who visited "remote" cultures and spent months or years conducting research. Adapting them for applied use in health care professions has required some modification. However, the essence of the traditional methods designed to capture the insiders perspective of participants in the culture, rather than the mindset of outside researchers has continued in ethnographic studies of the influence of culture on occupational life (Krefting & Krefting, 1992). An ethnographic assessment process for use in occupational therapy has been developed in a way that can be applied to a variety of local worlds to study cultural environments at various levels (Spencer, Krefting, & Mattingly, 1993).

The *Ethnographic Assessment Process* involves a sequence of four steps: (1) define the unit of study (which could be a single behavior setting, such as a workplace or day care environment, or which could be the community in which an individual's entire constellation of routine occupations are conducted); (2) describe the culture of this unit, including the material domain (how occupations are regularly performed), the social domain (the roles and relationships that organize performance of these occupations), and the ideological domain (the meaning and value of occupations to participants); (3) analyze the functioning of the individual according to expectations within the context; and (4) develop individual intervention goals for the person or the context. Methods for gathering and interpreting data are described. This assessment allows therapists to evaluate occupational performance according to standards and expectations within the local world of the client and, thereby, avoid imposing personal goals valued by therapists on clients who may value other ways of organizing their occupational lives. For example, in a local world that values interdependence and cooperative performance of tasks, emphasis on independence by the occupational therapist may be incongruent.

IMMEDIATE SCALE CULTURAL ENVIRONMENTS

In occupational therapy the general methods of ethnography have been applied to a number of particular evaluation problems. Studies of immediate scale cultural environments have demonstrated the usefulness of this approach for understanding how culture shapes interaction between a practitioner and client (Crepeau, 1991), or how cultural beliefs about independence shape a how a woman with cerebral palsy manages her attendant assistance in order to live independently (McCuaig & Frank, 1991). Evaluation of cultural contexts at this immediate level will be represented here by a Home-Based Intervention for Caregivers of Elders With Dementia developed by Corcoran and Gitlin (1992) for use in understanding the culture of the family and how it can shape intervention designed to fit the context of each families' needs, goals, preferences, and resources.

The *Home-Based Intervention for Caregivers of Elders With Dementia* involves a series of five home visits and an evolving process of evaluation and intervention centered on caregiver use of the environment to manage behavioral problems common among persons with dementia. Visit 1 involves building rapport, identifying problem areas, and establishing goals. Visit 2 involves specification of environmental influences on problems identified previously, introduction of information on dementia management, and development of a plan to address specific problem behaviors of the elderly person with dementia. Visit 3 involves review of the plan and initial implementation by the caregiver and refinement or modification of planned management strategies. Visit 4 involves transfer of greater decision-making and problem-solving to the caregiver and generalization of the problem-solving process to other problems. Visit 5 includes final review of the problem-solving process, final modifications of specific strategies, and discussion of applying environmental management strategies to future problems. Use of this process can be thought of as a strategy for modifying the culture of the household to support optimum occupational performance of both elderly persons and caregivers.

PROXIMAL SCALE CULTURAL ENVIRONMENTS

The concept of culture is well-suited to studying the "local worlds" of proximal behavior settings of living environments, classroom and work settings, and clinical environments. For example, Suto and Frank (1994) examined the culture of board and care homes for persons with schizophrenia and how their occupational routines and belief systems shaped the time use and future time perspective of residents. Dyck (1992) studied the effects of the culture within a fish-packing work setting on the ways in which a Chinese woman managed her arthritis, and Griswold (1994) studied the cultures of classroom settings that shaped occupational performance of students. Evaluation of cultural environments at this level is illustrated by the Classroom Observation Guide developed by Griswold (1994) for use in school-based practice.

The *Classroom Observation Guide* examines three domains of classroom settings, including activities, people, and communication. Dimensions of activities include purpose, objects used, time required, space required, and type of learning. The dimensions of people include roles and interaction. Those of communication include who is giving information, to whom information is given, purpose, context, words used, nonverbal communication, and consequences of communication (Griswold, 1994). Griswold's study provides examples of contrasting classroom cultures that have important implications for how children with disabilities are able to function. Use of this tool can allow therapists to suggest activities and strategies to enhance the development and functioning of children with special needs.

An additional clinical tool, the Home Observation for Measurement of the Environment (HOME), illustrates use of a more highly structured interview and observation format to examine the culture of home settings, including both the physical space and social interaction patterns and how they shape the experience of young children(Caldwell & Bradley, 1979).

The *Home Observation for Measurement of the Environment (HOME)* is intended to evaluate the stimulation potential of a child's early home environment by examining daily transactions and activities. A checklist is used to gather information by observation and interview concerning the quality and quantity of social, emotional, and cognitive support available to the child. There is an Infants and Toddlers Scale which has 45 items and six subscales, and a Preschool Scale with 55 items and eight subscales. Subscale scores help pinpoint the presence or absence of specific kinds of environmental support believed to influence the healthy development of children. Identification of "at-risk" homes can allow intervention designed to teach parents ways they can change the culture of their home setting to make it more conducive to healthy child development.

COMMUNITY SCALE CULTURAL ENVIRONMENTS

The cultures of community scale environments have also been studied in occupational therapy in terms of their effects on the life experience of persons with disabilities. Kielhofner (1981) examined the community experience of de-institutionalized adults with mental retardation and found that, although these individuals were living in community settings, they were excluded from many of the routine activities and taken-for-granted meanings of events that went on there. Similarly, Krefting (1989) studied the experience of persons with head injury living in the community and found that they worked very hard to conceal their disabilities and to revise the generally accepted meanings of key terms such as work or independence. Such research clearly suggests that the cultures of community scale environments may not readily incorporate persons with disabilities, findings that have major implications for the lives of many occupational therapy clients. A striking exception to the commonly found isolation or "liminality" of persons with disabilities (Murphy, Scheer, Murphy, & Mack, 1988) was studied by Groce (1985) in a remarkable community on the island of Martha's Vineyard in which congenital deafness was historically very prevalent. Because persons with hearing impairments were a taken-for-granted part of the community, use of sign language by everyone was a part of the shared culture on this island, which allowed individuals with disabilities to participate fully in the family, school, work, recreational, and social life of the community. Groce's work provides striking evidence for the cultural influence of a local world on the lives of persons with disabilities.

Two assessments that examine the involvement of persons with disabilities in community scale environments are the Craig Handicap Assessment and Report Technique (CHART) (Whiteneck, Charlifue, Gerhart, Overholser, & Richardson, 1988, 1992) and the Community Integration Questionnaire (CIQ) (Willer, Rosenthal, Kreutzer, Gordon, & Rempel, 1993).

The *Craig Handicap Assessment and Report Technique* is based on the model of disablement developed by the World Health Organization (WHO) to evaluate the concept of handicap. In contrast with impairments and disabilities that occur at a person level, handicap involves disadvantages that limit or prevent the fulfillment of a role that would be considered normal for an individual in his or her culture. Six dimensions of handicap identified by the WHO include (1) orientation, (2) physical independence, (3) mobility, (4) occupation, (5) social integration, and (6) economic self-sufficiency. The CHART is an interview tool that addresses each of these dimensions except orientation. CHART items identify behaviors, rather than perceptions or attitudes, such as hours per day someone provides physical assistance to the individual (physical independence); time out of home and use of transportation (mobility); time spent in employment, schooling, home-making, recreation, and self-improvement activities (occupation); family, friends, and associates with whom the individual interacts (social integration); and household income (economic self-sufficiency). The instrument is intended to make it possible for an individual to "demonstrate the absence of handicap" in a number of ways on each subscale, with a maximum score of 100 on each subscale, combining to yield an overall index of handicap. "Absence of handicap" can be interpreted to mean the individual's active engagement in the culture of the community and in roles expected within that culture.

The *Community Integration Questionnaire*, also intended to measure "reduced handicap," was specifically designed as a simple and efficient tool for use with persons who have brain injury, who are living in the community. It contains 15 items that evaluate participation in household activities, shopping, errands, leisure activities, visiting friends, social events, and productive activities that are grouped into three dimensions, including home integration, social integration, and productive activities. This tool, which takes 10 to 15 minutes to complete, has been used as a measure of community integration in the Model Traumatic Brain Injury Systems funded by the National Institute for Disability and Rehabilitation Research. Therapists could use the CHART or CIQ to help clients examine the extent of their community participation and to identify goals and problem-solving strategies to increase involvement in the local world of the community.

SOCIETAL SCALE CULTURAL ENVIRONMENTS

Finally, cultural environments have been studied at a societal level in terms of their effect on persons with disabilities. Shapiro (1993) has traced historic changes in how persons with disabilities have been viewed in our society, articulating a general trend from a cultural view of such persons as objects of charity and pity to a view that emphasizes their civil rights as citizens who make important contributions to society. Research has used media images as ways of examining how persons with disabilities are viewed culturally (Biklen, 1986; Clogston, 1990; Haller, 1995; Zola, 1985). Although not designed as a clinical assessment, eight models of media representation identified by Haller (1995) can provide a strategy for evaluating aspects of cultural context, at a societal level, that have important implications for how practitioners think about and relate to clients.

The framework of *Models of Media Representation of Disability* categorizes eight models as traditional or progressive (Haller, 1995). Traditional models include (1) the medical model in which disability is presented as an illness or malfunction, (2) the social pathology model in which people with disabilities are presented as disadvantaged and needing support, which is regarded as a gift, rather than a right, (3) the "superscrip" model in which a person with a disability is portrayed as deviant because of superhuman feats in spite of disability, and (4) the business model in which people with disabilities are costly to society. Progressive models include (5) the minority–civil rights model in which people with disabilities are seen as members of a disability community that has legitimate political grievances based on denial of civil rights, (6) the legal model in which it is illegal to treat people with disabilities in certain ways, (7) the cultural pluralism model in which people with disabilities are seen as multifaceted individuals and their disabilities do not receive undue attention, and (8) the consumer model in which people with disabilities are seen as an untapped consumer group. These models could be used by therapists to identify subtle ways in which general societal beliefs about persons with disabilities shape their own views. They could also be used to help clients anticipate and deal with how they may be viewed when they reenter society following onset of a new identity as a person with a disability.

Summary of Environmental Evaluation Strategies

An array of clinical tools have been provided that illustrate alternative ways of evaluating environments at an immediate, proximal, community, and societal scale. These tools employ a variety of methods, ranging from formal measurement of variables, such as distance or rates of performance, behavior observation using coding checklists, and time-sampling procedures that document how environments are naturally used in daily life; self-report of how various aspects of environments are perceived by users; and interpretive judgment of the qualities of environments by experts trained in particular perspectives such as anthropology or occupational therapy. Some assessments have been designed to be applicable in a variety of environmental settings, such as the Negotiability Rating Process (Bates, 1994) or the Ethnographic Assessment Process (Spencer, Krefting, & Mattingly, 1993). Others have been designed for use in quite specific settings such as the HOME (Caldwell & Bradley, 1979), the Work Environments Scale (Moos, 1981), or the Classroom Observation Guide (Griswold, 1994). Each of these methods offers strengths and weaknesses, and collectively, they can be viewed as complementary approaches to understanding relevant features of environmental contexts. As many others have pointed out, having a clear sense of what questions one wants to ask should precede decisions about the best tools to use for a particular purpose (Davidson, 1992; Letts et al, 1994; Ottenbacher, 1992).

▶ CONCLUSION

The studies reported in this chapter indicate that performance contexts indeed have a powerful effect on occupational performance; therefore, wise use of tools for evaluating context can become important aspects of a practice grounded in the daily life experience of clients. Yerxa (1994) asserted that occupational therapy practitioners are particularly well-equipped to help clients bridge the gap between their experience in health care or other service delivery settings and their daily life settings, which Kleinman (1988) would call their "local worlds." Practitioners are beginning to examine in greater depth how evaluation and intervention in the domains of performance context can be used clinically (Dunn, Brown, & McGuigan, 1994). In an era in which there are many pressures to standardize treatment, practitioners are challenged to maintain the relevance of therapy to the lives of clients as individuals and to maintain our beliefs in the personal, social, and cultural meaning of human occupation as a major aspect of its therapeutic potential.

Acknowledgments

My ideas about the significance of environmental contexts in occupational therapy have been shaped by professional interactions and collaborative research with many colleagues and students. Most significant among these has been my ongoing work with Harriett Davidson, beginning when I was a professional master's degree student and continuing when we became faculty colleagues at Texas Woman's University. In preparation of this chapter I have drawn on literature reviews completed by Megan Montgomery and Alison Young. I am also grateful for assistance from June Long and Colleen Rice in collecting evaluation tools and references.

▼ REFERENCES

American National Standards Institute (1980). *Specifications for making buildings and facilities accessible to and usable by physically handicapped people.* New York: Author.

American Occupational Therapy Association (AOTA) (1994). Uniform terminology for occupational therapy—third edition. *American Journal of Occupational Therapy, 48,* 1047–1054.

Abeles, R., & Riley, M. (1977). A life-course perspective on the later years of life: Some implications for research. *Social Science Research Council Annual Report, 1976–1977* (pp. 1–16).

Adaptive Environments Center (1988). *Home Modification Workbook.* Boston: Author.

Antonak, R. (1981). Prediction of attitudes toward disabled persons: A multivariate analysis. *The Journal of General Psychology, 104,* 119–123.

Asher, I. (1989). *An annotated index of occupational therapy evaluation tools.* Rockville, MD: American Occupational Therapy Association.

Baltes, P. (1979). Life span developmental psychology: Some converging observations on history. In P. Baltes & O. Brim (Eds.), *Life-span development and behavior,* (Vol 2). (pp. 256–279). New York: Academic Press.

Barker, R. (1978). *Habitats, environments, and human behavior.* San Francisco: Jossey-Bass.

Barrera, M., & Vella, D. (1987). Disabled and nondisabled infants' interactions with their mothers. *American Journal of Occupational Therapy, 41,* 168–172.

Bates, P. (1994). The self-care environment: Issues of space and furnishings. In C. Christiansen (Ed.), *Ways of living: Self-care strategies for special needs.* (pp. 423–451). Rockville, MD: American Occupational Therapy Association.

Bates, P., Spencer, J., Young, M. & Rintala, D. (1993). Assistive technology and the newly disabled adult: Adaptation to wheelchair use. *American Journal of Occupational Therapy, 47,* 1014–1021.

Beavers, J., Hampson, R., Hulgas, Y., & Beavers, W. (1986). Coping in families with a retarded child. *Family Process, 25,* 365–378.

Becker, G. (1993). Continuity after stroke: Implications of life-course disruptions in old age. *The Gerontologist, 33,* 148–158.

Behnke, C., & Menarchek-Fetkovich, M. (1984). Examining the reliability and validity of the play history. *American Journal of Occupational Therapy, 38,* 94–100.

Biernacki, S. (1993). Reliability of the worker role interview. *American Journal of Occupational Therapy, 47,* 797–803.

Biklen, D. (1986). Framed: Journalism's treatment of disability. *Social Policy, 16,* 45–51.

Black, M. (1976). Adolescent role assessment. *American Journal of Occupational Therapy, 30,* 73–79.

Bledsoe, N., & Shepard, J. (1982). A study of reliability and validity of a preschool play scale. *American Journal of Occupational Therapy, 36,* 783–788.

Bowe, F. (1978). *Handicapping America: Barriers to disabled people.* New York: Harper & Row.

Bowe, F. (1980). *Rehabilitating America: Toward independence for disabled and elderly people.* New York: Harper & Row.

Bray, G. (1978). Rehabilitation of spinal cord injured: A family approach. *Journal of Applied Rehabilitation Counseling, 9,* 79–88.

Bronfenbrenner, U. (1979). *The ecology of human development.* Cambridge: Harvard University Press.

Brooks, N. (1991). Users' responses to assistive devices for physical disability. *Social Science and Medicine, 32,* 1417–1424.

Caldwell, B., & Bradley, R. (1979). *Home Observation for Measurement of the Environment (HOME).* Little Rock: University of Arkansas.

Cantor, M. (1979). Life space and social support. In Byerts, T., Howell, S., & Pastalan, L. (Eds.), *Environmental context of aging: Lifestyles, environmental quality, and living arrangements* (pp. 33–61). New York: Garland STPM Press.

Carruth, L. (1994). *An illness experience involving the Ilizarov external fixator.* Unpublished manuscript, School of Occupational Therapy, Texas Woman's University.

Caudill, W. (1953). *The psychiatric hospital as a small society.* Cambridge: Harvard University Press.

Center for Research on Women With Disabilities.(undated). *Personal Independence Profile.* Houston: Author.

Chapanis, A. (1991). *Human factors for informatics usability.* New York: Cambridge University Press.

Christiansen, C., & Baum, C. (Eds.). (1992). *Occupational therapy: Overcoming human performance deficits.* New York: McGraw Hill.

Christiansen, C. (Ed.). (1994) *Ways of living: Self-care strategies for special needs.* Rockville, MD: American Occupational Therapy Association.

Clark, F. (1993). Occupation embedded in real life: Interweaving occupation science and occupational therapy. 1993 Eleanor Clarke Slagle Lecture. *American Journal of Occupational Therapy, 47,* 1067–1078.

Clogston, J. (1990). *Disability coverage in 16 newspapers.* Louisville: Advocado Press.

Cook, A., & Hussey, S. (1995). *Assistive technologies: Principles and practice.* St. Louis: C.V. Mosby.

Corbin, J., & Strauss, A. (1987). Accompaniments of chronic illness: Changes in body, self, biography, and biographical time. In J. Roth & P. Conrad (Eds.), *Research in the sociology of health care, Vol 6, The experience and management of chronic illness* (pp. 249–282). Greenwich, CT: JAI Press.

Corcoran, M., & Gitlin, L. (1992). Dementia management: An occupational therapy home-based intervention for caregivers. *American Journal of Occupational Therapy, 46,* 801–808.

Crepeau, E. (1991). Achieving intersubjective understanding: Examples from an occupational therapy treatment session. *American Journal of Occupational Therapy, 45,* 1016–1026.

Cronburg, J., Barnett, J., & Goldman, N. (1991) *Readily achievable checklist: A survey for accessibility.* Washington DC: National Center for Access Unlimited.

Danish, S., Smyer, M., & Nowak, C. (1980). Developmental intervention: Enhancing life event processes. In P. Baltes & O. Brim (Eds.), *Life-span development and behavior, (Vol 3).* (pp. 340–366). New York: Academic Press.

Davidson, H. (1992). Assessing environmental factors. In C. Christiansen & C. Baum (Eds.), *Occupational therapy: Overcoming human performance deficits* (pp. 427–452). New York: McGraw Hill.

DeJong, G. (1979). Independent living: From social movement to analytic paradigm. *Archives of Physical Medicine and Rehabilitation, 60,* 435–446.

Duke University Center for the Study of Aging and Human Development. (1978). *Multidimensional functional assessment: The OARS methodology.* Durham, NC: Author.

Dunn, W., Brown, C., & McGuigan, A. (1994). The ecology of human performance: A framework for considering the effect of context. *American Journal of Occupational Therapy, 48,* 595–607.

Dyck, I. (1992). Managing chronic illness: An immigrant woman's acquisition and use of health care knowledge. *American Journal of Occupational Therapy, 46,* 696–705.

Eberhardt, K., & Mayberry, W. (1995). Factors influencing entry-level occupational therapists' attitudes toward persons with disabilities. *American Journal of Occupational Therapy, 49,* 629–636.

Epstein, N., Baldwin, L., & Bishop, D. (1983). The McMaster family assessment device. *Journal of Marital and Family Therapy, 9,* 171–180.

Forer, S. (1996). *Outcome management and program evaluation made easy: A toolkit for occupational therapy practitioners.* Bethesda MD: American Occupational Therapy Association.

Frank, G. (1996). Life histories in occupational therapy clinical practice. *American Journal of Occupational Therapy, 50,* 251–264.

Frieden, L., Frieden J., & Laurie, G. (1981). *Living independently: Three views of the European experience with implications for the United States.* New York: World Rehabilitation Fund.

Garber, S., & Gregorio, T. (1990). Upper extremity assistive devices: Assessment of use by spinal cord injured patients with quadriplegia. *American Journal of Occupational Therapy, 44,* 126–131.

Geertz, C. (1973). *The interpretation of cultures.* New York: Basic Books.

Geertz, C. (1983). *Local knowledge: Further essays on interpretive anthropology.* New York: Basic Books.

Gilligan, C. (1982). *In a different voice: Psychological theory and women's development.* Cambridge: Harvard University Press.

Gliedman, J., & Roth, W. (1980). *The unexpected minority: Handicapped children in America.* New York: Harcourt Brace Jovanovich.

Goldman, C. (1991). *Disability rights guide: Practical solutions to problems affecting people with disabilities.* Lincoln NE: Media.

Goltsman, S., Gilbert, T., & Wohlford S. (1992). *The accessibility checklist: An evaluating system for buildings and outdoor settings.* Berkeley, CA: M. I. G. Communications.

Gottlieb, B. (Ed.). (1981). *Social networks and social support.* Beverly Hills, CA: Sage Publications.

Gralewicz, A. (1973). Play deprivation in multihandicapped children. *American Journal of Occupational Therapy, 27,* 70–72.

Griswold, L. (1994). Ethnographic analysis: A study of classroom environments. *American Journal of Occupational Therapy, 48,* 397–402.

Groce, N. (1985). *Everyone here spoke sign language: Hereditary deafness on Martha's Vineyard.* Cambridge: Harvard University Press.

Haller, B. (1995). Rethinking models of media representation of disability. *Disability Studies Quarterly, 15* (2), 26–30.

Harrison, H., & Kielhofner, G. (1986). Examining reliability of the preschool play scale with handicapped children. *American Journal of Occupational Therapy, 40,* 167–173.

Hasselkus, B. (1989). The meaning of daily activity in family caregiving for the elderly. *American Journal of Occupational Therapy, 43,* 649–656.

Hauser, S., Jacobsen, D., Wertlieb, B., Weiss, P., Follansbee, D., & Wolfselorf, J. (1986). Children with recently diagnosed diabetes: Interactions with their families. *Health Psychology, 5,* 273–276.

Helfrich, C., Kielhofner, G., & Mattingly, C. (1994). Volition as narrative: Understanding motivation in chronic illness. *American Journal of Occupational Therapy, 48,* 311–317.

Henry, A., & Kielhofner, G. (1989). *The occupational performance history interview.* Rockville, MD: American Occupational Therapy Association.

Kannegeiter, R. (1987). The development of the environmental assessment scale. *Occupational Therapy in Mental Health, 6,* 67–83.

Kelly, C., & Snell, K. (1989). *The source book: Architectural guidelines for barrier free design.* Toronto, ON: Barrier-Free Design Centre.

Kerr, W., & Thompson, M. (1972). Acceptance of disability of sudden onset in paraplegia. *Paraplegia, 10,* 94–102.

Kielhofner, G. (1977). Temporal adaptation: A conceptual framework for occupational therapy. *American Journal of Occupational Therapy, 31,* 235–242.

Kielhofner, G. (1981). An ethnographic study of deinstitutionalized adults: Their community settings and daily experiences. *Occupational Therapy Journal of Research, 1,* 125–142.

Kielhofner, G. (1985). *A model of human occupation: Theory and application.* Baltimore: Williams & Wilkins.

Kielhofner, G. (1995). *A model of human occupation* (2nd ed.). Baltimore: Williams & Wilkins.

Kleinman, A. (1988). *The illness narratives: Suffering, healing, and the human condition.* New York: Basic Books.

Kleinman, A. (1992). Local worlds of suffering: An interpersonal focus for ethnographies of illness experience. *Qualitative Health Research, 2,* 127–134.

Knox, S. (1974). A play scale. In M. Reilly (Ed.), *Play as exploratory learning.* (pp. 247–266). Beverly Hills, CA: Sage Publications.

Kohlberg, L. (1981). *The philosophy of moral development.* New York: Harper & Row.

Kohlberg, L. (1984). *The psychology of moral development.* New York: Harper & Row.

Kosberg, J., & Cairl, R. (1986). The cost of care index: A case management tool for screening informal care providers. *The Gerontological Society of America, 26,* 273–278.

Krefting, L. (1989). Reintegration into the community after head injury: The results of an ethnographic study. *Occupational Therapy Journal of Research, 9,* 67–83.

Krefting, L., & Krefting, D. (1992). Cultural influences on performance. In C. Christiansen & C. Baum (Eds.), *Occupational therapy: Overcoming human performance deficits.* (pp. 101–122). New York: McGraw-Hill.

Letts, L., Law, M., Rigby, P., Cooper, B., Stewart, D., & Strong, S. (1994) Person-environment assessments in occupational therapy. *American Journal of Occupational Therapy, 48,* 608–618.

Lifchez, R. (1987). *Rethinking architecture: Design students and physically disabled people.* Berkeley, CA: University of California Press.

Livneh, H., & Antonak, R. (1990). Reactions to disability: An empirical investigation of their nature and structure. *Journal of Applied Rehabilitation Counseling, 21,* 13–21.

Livneh, H., & Antonak, R. (1991). Temporal structure of adaptation to disability. *Rehabilitation Counseling Bulletin, 34,* 298–319.

Lyons, M., & Hayes, R. (1993). Student perceptions of persons with psychiatric and other disorders. *American Journal of Occupational Therapy, 47,* 541–548.

Mattingly, C., & Fleming, M. (1994). *Clinical reasoning: Forms of inquiry in a therapeutic practice.* Philadelphia: F. A. Davis.

McCuaig, M., & Frank, G. (1991). The able self: Adaptive patterns and choices in independent living for a person with cerebral palsy. *American Journal of Occupational Therapy, 45,* 224–234.

McCubbin, H., Cauble, A., & Patterson, J. (1982). *Family stress, coping, and social support.* Springfield, IL: Charles C. Thomas.

McHale, K., & Cermak, S. (1992). Fine motor activities in elementary school: Preliminary findings and provisional implications for children with fine motor problems. *American Journal of Occupational Therapy, 46,* 898–903.

Miller, L. (1983). The Miller Assessment for Preschoolers (MAP): A review. *American Journal of Occupational Therapy, 37,* 333–340.

Mitchell, J. (Ed.) (1985). *The ninth mental measurements yearbook.* Lincoln NE: University of Nebraska Press.

Moos, R. (1974). *Evaluation of treatment environments: A sociological approach.* New York: Wiley.

Moos, R. (1981). *Work environment scale manual.* Palo Alto, CA: Consulting Psychologists Press.

Moos, R. (Ed.) (1986) *Coping with life crises: An integrated approach.* New York: Plenum Press.

Mueller, J. (1990). *The workplace workbook: An illustrated guide to job accommodation and assistive technology.* Washington, DC: The Dole Foundation.

Murphy, R. (1990). *The body silent.* New York: W. W. Norton.

Murphy, R., Scheer, J., Murphy, Y., & Mack, R. (1988). Physical disability and social liminality: A study in the rituals of adversity. *Social Science and Medicine, 26,* 235–242.

Neimeyer, L., Matheson, L., & Carlton, R. (1989). Testing consistency of effort: BTE work simulator. *Industrial Rehabilitation Quarterly, 2,* 5–32.

Neistadt, M. (1995). Methods of assessing clients' priorities: A survey of adult physical dysfunction settings. *American Journal of Occupational Therapy, 49,* 428–436.

Norris-Baker, C., & Willems, E. (1978). Environmental negotiability as a direct measurement of behavior-environment relationships: Some implications for theory and practice. In A. Seidel & S. Danford (Eds.). *Proceedings of the Tenth Annual Conference of the Environmental Design Research Association* (pp. 209–214). Houston, TX.

Nosek, M., & Fuhrer, M. (1992). Independence among people with disabilities: A heuristic model. *Rehabilitation Counseling Bulletin, 36* (1), 6–19.

Nosek, M., Fuhrer, M., & Howland, C. (1992). Independence among people with disabilities: Personal independence profile. *Rehabilitation Counseling Bulletin, 36* (1), 21–36.

Oakley, F., Kielhofner, G., Barris, R., & Reichler, R. (1986). The role checklist: Development and empirical assessment of reliability. *Occupational Therapy Journal of Research, 6* , 157–169.

Ottenbacher, K. (1992). Nationally speaking—confusion in occupational therapy research: Does the end justify the method? *American Journal of Occupational Therapy, 46,* 871–874.

Park, S., Fisher, A., & Velozo, C. (1994). Using the assessment of motor and process skills to compare occupational performance between clinic and home settings. *American Journal of Occupational Therapy, 48*, 697–709.

Parten, M. (1932). Social participation among pre-school children. *Journal of Abnormal & Social Psychology, 27*, 243–269.

Reilly, M. (1974). *Play as exploratory learning.* Beverly Hills, CA: Sage.

Rivara, J., Jaffe, K., Polissar, N., Fay, G., Liao, S., & Martin, K., (1996). Predictors of family functioning and change three years after traumatic brain injury in children. *Archives of Physical Medicine and Rehabilitation, 77*, 754–764.

Rowles, G. (1983). Geographical dimensions of social support in rural Appalachia. In G. Rowles & R. Ohta (Eds.), *Aging and milieu: Environmental perspectives on growing old* (pp. 111–130). New York: Academic Press.

Rowles, G. (1991). Beyond performance: Being in place as a component of occupational therapy. *American Journal of Occupational Therapy, 45*, 265–272.

Soldo, B. J. Agree, E. M., & Wolf, D. A. (1989). The balance between formal and informal care. In J. Ory & K. Bond (Eds.), *Aging and health care: Social science and policy perspectives*, (pp. 193–216). New York: Routledge.

Schlossberg, N. (1982). A model for analyzing human adaptation to transition. The *Counseling Psychologist, 9* (2), 2–18.

Shapiro, J. (1993). *No pity: People with disabilities forging a new civil rights movement.* New York: Times Books/Random House.

Spencer, J., Krefting, L., & Mattingly, C. (1993). Incorporation of ethnographic methods in occupational therapy assessment. *American Journal of Occupational Therapy, 47*, 303–309.

Spencer, J., Young, M., Rintala, D., & Bates, S. (1995). Socialization to the culture of a rehabilitation hospital: An ethnographic study. *American Journal of Occupational Therapy, 49*, 53–62.

Suto, M., & Frank, G. (1994). Future time perspective and daily occupations of persons with chronic schizophrenia in a board and care home. *American Journal of Occupational Therapy, 48*, 586–589.

Takata, N. (1969). The play history. *American Journal of Occupational Therapy, 23*, 314–318.

Tringo, J. (1970). The hierarchy of preference toward disability groups. *The Journal of Special Education, 4*, 295–306.

Trombly, C. (1995). Occupation: Purposefulness and meaningfulness as therapeutic mechanisms. 1995 Eleanor Clarke Slagle Lecture. *American Journal of Occupational Therapy, 49*, 960–972.

U.S. Architectural & Transportation Barriers Compliance Board. (1992). *Americans With Disabilities Act accessibility guidelines checklist for buildings and facilities.* Washington, DC: Author.

Vaillant, G. (1977). *Adaptation to life.* Cambridge: Harvard University Press.

Velozo, C. (1993). Work evaluations: Critique of the state of the art of functional assessment of work. *American Journal of Occupational Therapy, 47*, 203–208.

Velozo, C., Kielhofner, G., & Fisher, A. (1990) *A user's guide to the Worker Role Interview.* University of Illinois at Chicago, College of Associated Health Professions, Department of Occupational Therapy.

Webster's New World Dictionary (1957). Cleveland: The World Publishing Company.

Whiteneck, G., Charlifue, S., Gerhart, K., Overholser, J., & Richardson, G. (1988). *Guide for use of the Craig Handicap Assessment and Report Technique (CHART).* Englewood, CO: Craig Hospital.

Whiteneck, G., Charlifue, S., Gerhart, K., Overholser, D., & Richardson, G. (1992). Quantifying handicap: A new measure of long-term rehabilitation outcomes. *Archives of Physical Medicine and Rehabilitation, 73*, 519–526.

Willer, B., Rosenthal, M., Kreutzer, J., Gordon, W., & Rempel, R. (1993). Assessment of community integration following traumatic brain injury. *Journal of Head Trauma Rehabilitation, 8* (2), 75–87.

Wolfensberger, W. (1972). *Normalization: The principle of normalization in human services.* Toronto, Canada: National Institute on Mental Retardation.

Yarrow, L., Rubenstein, J., & Pederson, F. (1975). *Infant and environment: Early cognitive and motivational development.* New York: Wiley.

Yerxa, E. (1994). Dreams, dilemmas, and decisions for occupational therapy practice in a new millennium: An American perspective. *American Journal of Occupational Therapy, 48*, 586–589.

Yuker, H. (1988). *Attitudes toward persons with disabilities.* New York: Springer.

Zola, I. (1985). Depictions of disability—metaphor, message, and medium in the media: A research and political agenda. *Social Science Journal, 22* (4), 5–17.

UNIT VI
CLIENT APPLICATIONS

Maureen E. Neistadt

In Chapter 3, you met Mary Weber and her occupational therapist, Anna Deane Scott. Anna Deane's evaluation process was exactly what Mary needed. Let us look at why in light of what you have read in this evaluation unit.

Anna Deane did not choose to use any formal, standardized tests of occupational performance, performance components, or performance contexts with Mary. There were two reasons for this. First, for the first 6 months that Anna Deane worked with her, Mary was crying too much and having too many seizures to participate in formal testing. Mary was grieving the loss of her life as she had known it before her injury. Her activity tolerance was also severely restricted by the seizure disorder and mental fatigability that resulted from her traumatic head injury. When she became mentally fatigued, she could not process information to engage in conversation or activity. Under these conditions, formal evaluations of occupational performance would have to be done in incremental pieces over several testing sessions. The end result of that testing would have been to tell Anna Deane what she already knew from Mary's friend, Sally—that Mary was having tremendous difficulty in her day-to-day activities. Mary was already at home, and often unsafe due to her occupational performance problems. Time spent on formal evaluation would be time lost from helping Mary problem-solve strategies for safer day-to-day functioning. So, Anna Deane chose to use observation and activity analysis as her primary evaluation tools.

Second, when Anna Deane began working with Mary in the late 1970s, there were no standardized occupational therapy assessments available for Mary's primary component skill deficit areas, perception and cognition. Anna Deane felt she needed more in-depth information about Mary's perceptual and cognitive deficits than non-standardized assessments could provide. So, when Mary was able to participate in testing, Anna Deane arranged for her to have neuropsychology testing at home. This neuropsychology testing confirmed the hypotheses Anna Deane had formed about Mary's deficits, based on her observations of Mary's functional performance. This testing provided additional information as well. For example, the neuropsychology testing indicated that Mary was experiencing right frontal and left parietal lobe dysfunction. This information helped Anna Deane think of additional strategies Mary might use to perform her daily activities more safely.

During the first session, Anna Deane interviewed Mary. That interview started with Mary "sitting in the dark on a couch, crying" (see Chap. 3, p. 28). Anna Deane took her cues from this situation; she understood that Mary might need the darkness to keep her sensory stimulation to a minimum and prevent a seizure. She respected Mary's sadness and the darkness, and sought to talk with Mary about something clearly of value to her—her dogs. When you go to visit Mary, you cannot miss her dogs and cats. They are numerous and friendly. As a dog owner, Anna Deane understood how important one's pets can be. So she talked of dogs to form a bond that might help ease Mary's sadness. And in the process, she would have been able to evaluate Mary's ability to engage in a conversation, to concentrate on a topic, to recall dog stories, to talk abstractly about people's attachments for their pets. When Mary called Anna Deane after their first meeting, Anna Deane was genuine and empathetic, telling Mary she "felt sad" during their first meeting. This genuineness and empathy led Mary to feel she could trust Anna Deane; therapeutic collaboration is built on trust.

After the first meeting, Anna Deane would spend each session listening to Mary identify day-to-day problems, and observing Mary try the activities she identified. By listening to Mary describe her problems and watching how Mary attempted activities, Anna Deane was able to hypothesize component skill deficits and suggest solutions to overcome those deficits, solutions that tapped Mary's remaining assets. Sometimes the solutions needed to be modified. Here again, Anna Deane used the processes of listening, observation, and activity analysis to figure out how failed solutions could be modified to make them work.

In Mary's case, observation and activity analysis were the primary occupational therapy evaluation tools. Evaluation was an ongoing part of treatment and progress was measured in Mary's increased independence in her daily activities. Although the occupational therapy evaluation in this story was informal, nonetheless, it was rigorous and successful. The therapist in this story also sought consultation from other professionals (neuropsychologists), as needed, to supplement her evaluation information. This sharing of evaluation information among the professionals involved in a client's care yields a rich composite picture of client's strengths and deficits, and avoids costly duplication of assessments.

Some of your future clients will, like Mary, need informal evaluation procedures. Others may need more formal evaluations, especially at the beginning, midpoint, and end of treatment. All practitioners should be using Anna Deane's evaluation methods of listening, observation, and activity analysis throughout the treatment process to fine tune treatment programs in response to clients' changes.

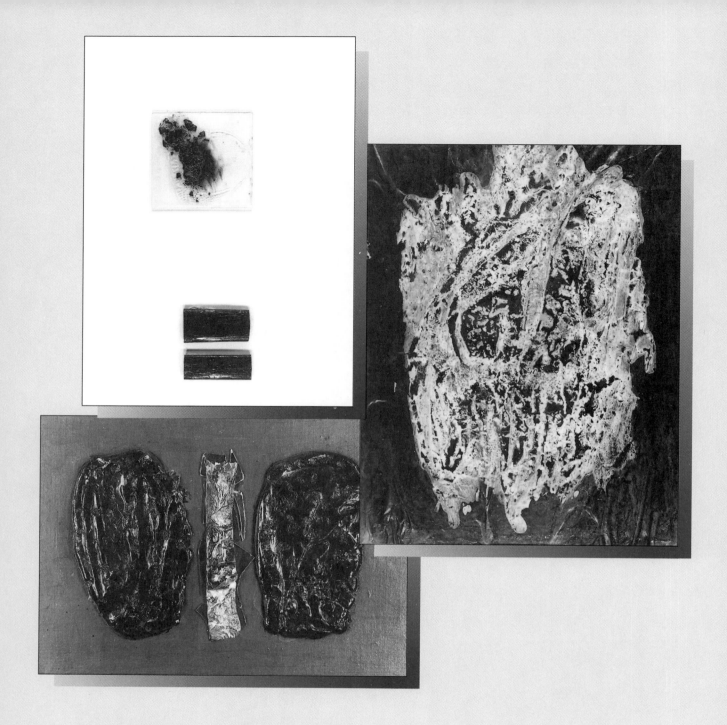

(top) When I Think of Dying: As I got better, I realized how much I had lost. It was at this time that I thought about suicide. This picture was what I imagined the soul might look like upon leaving the dying body (Courtesy of Mary Feldhaus-Weber).

(right) White Brain: At a certain point I began to make my brain pictures more "decorative," artistic. I was no longer so obsessed with understanding the damage. I think I was trying to integrate my feelings about the head injury (Courtesy of Mary Feldhaus-Weber).

(bottom) Hemispheres: Someone told me that the injured brain had to learn to communicate again, find new pathways that worked, that the right side had to take up what the left side used to do. I put broken mirrors between the two hemispheres—it all seemed so very difficult. Painful. Terrible. (Editor's note: This photo does not adequately represent this painting. When you stand in front of it, your image is fractured by the broken mirrors). (Courtesy of Mary Feldhaus-Weber).

UNIT VII

Occupational Therapy Treatment

LEARNING OBJECTIVES

After completing this unit, readers will be able to:

▶ Describe several adaptive techniques that can be taught to improve activities of daily living (ADL) performance.

▶ Explain how specific pieces of adaptive equipment can enhance ADL functioning.

▶ Explain how various disorders can affect sexual functioning.

▶ Describe the role of the occupational therapist in home and family management.

▶ Identify specialized services that may be offered by an industrial rehabilitation program.

▶ Differentiate between play and leisure as treatment goals and as treatment modalities.

▶ Describe treatment techniques used in sensory re-education.

▶ Describe the inhibition and facilitation techniques of neuromuscular treatment approaches.

▶ Apply the principles of muscle strengthening to a treatment plan for strength deficits that affect occupational performance.

▶ Identify client performance problems appropriate for motor control intervention.

▶ Identify the purposes and rational for splinting clients with upper extremity dysfunction.

▶ Discuss methods for treating cognitive–perceptual deficits in orientation, attention, memory, visual processing, organization, problem solving, and executive functions.

▶ Delineate a treatment plan for a client with psychosocial dysfunction.

▶ Formulate a minimum of three approaches for pain intervention.

▶ Describe twelve stress management techniques.

▶ Explain the principles of environmental adaptation.

▶ Describe the assessment, selection, and application of various assistive devices with a variety of clients.

This unit describes the variety of treatment techniques occupational therapy practitioners use to address client problems identified during an occupational therapy evaluation. The ultimate goal of occupational therapy treatment is to help clients become as proficient as possible in their valued life activities. The methods practitioners use to achieve that goal fall into three general categories: (1) training in actual or simulated occupational performance area activities, (2) exercises to improve the component skill deficits interfering with occupational performance, and (3) environmental adaptation to make performance of occupational activities easier. A practitioner might use some techniques from each category with any given client. The mix of treatment techniques will depend on (1) the client's particular problems, treatment preferences, prognosis for recovery, and anticipated length of treatment; (2) the knowledge of the practitioner; and (3) the resources available in any given treatment setting. No one treatment technique or combination of techniques is appropriate for all clients. Later units on treatment theories and diagnostic conditions in children and adults will provide guidelines for individualizing treatment. (*Note*: Words in **bold** type are defined in the Glossary.)

Chapter 18

Overview of Treatment

Maureen E. Neistadt

The purpose of occupational therapy treatment is to help clients learn or relearn the activities of daily living (ADL), work, and leisure routines that they need to live as independently as possible—routines that have been disrupted by illness or disability. For example, a young adult with schizophrenia, who has never held a full-time job because of his or her mental health problems, has never developed a work routine and will have to learn work behaviors, such as showing up on time, paying attention to work tasks, following multiple step tasks, interacting with coworkers, responding to supervision, and dressing and grooming appropriately, to be able to earn a living. In contrast, an adult with a back injury, who has worked full time in a grocery store for 15 years, knows these work behaviors well, but will now have to relearn the physical part of his or her job to prevent reinjury. That is, this person will have to learn to do his or her job tasks with better techniques for lifting and reaching.

Occupational therapy treatment is paid for either privately by clients or by clients' insurance companies. Both private payers and insurance companies want to see results from occupational therapy treatment; they will be willing to pay only for treatment that leads to improvements in occupational performance (ADL, work, leisure). Clients want to be able to do more for themselves so that their lives will be more satisfying and fulfilling. Insurance companies want to see behavior changes in clients that will result in decreased health care costs. That is, insurance companies want to see occupational therapy treatments result in clients who will need either decreased or no assistance. For an elderly client with multiple diagnoses, for example, the best outcome from an insurance company perspective would be for the client to return home completely independent so that no further money needs to be spent on rehabilitation for this particular health crisis. A lesser, but still positive outcome for the insurance company would be for the client to become independent enough to return home with continued, home-based rehabilitation and home health aide services, for these services cost less than hospitalization in a rehabilitation facility.

Occupational therapy treatment that helps clients learn or relearn their preferred occupational behaviors improves quality of life and decreases health care costs. The number and length of treatment sessions you will have to teach clients their preferred occupational behaviors will be limited by the amount of money the client or the insurance company is willing to spend on treatment. You need to be aware of how much time you will have to work with a given client so that you can set realistic goals for treatment. This means that you will not necessarily be working with clients until they have reached their maximal level of occupational performance. The rehabilitation hospital practitioner working with the client above who went home with home-based rehabilitation services, for instance, would be working with that client through only part of the client's total rehabilitation course. The last part of that client's services would be delivered at home by a different set of practitioners. Your treatment goals, then, will sometimes be only high enough for the client to reach the next, less costly, level of health care services. For example, for the client slated to receive home-based rehabilitation and home health aide services, your discharge ADL goal may be: "Client will be able to perform all ADLs with minimal physical assistance, given adaptive equipment," instead of "client will be able to perform all ADLs independently, given adaptive equipment."

▼ FOCUS OF TREATMENT

The focus of occupational therapy treatment is derived from the client priorities and problems identified in the occupational therapist's initial evaluation. To illustrate, let us look at two possible case scenarios involving two 10-year-old children with **cerebral palsy**, a congenital problem with brain functioning that typically results in problems in movement and can also affect perception and thinking or cognition skills. A school-based occupational therapist has been asked to evaluate the grooming skills of these two 10 year olds— Tim and John. Both are in wheelchairs and have spasticity or extra tightness in all of their muscles. The therapist picks toothbrushing as one of the evaluation tasks because the parents of both boys say they would like their sons to be able to do this task by themselves. The therapist finds that Tim can identify the toothbrush, toothpaste, cup, and towel, and can recite all the steps for brushing his teeth, in proper order. However, his movement problems are so pronounced that he cannot actually perform the steps without assistance. John, on the other hand, has less severe movement problems and can manipulate the toothbrushing objects, but does not seem to know what to do with them. He cannot describe the steps of this task and needs step-by-step instructions to brush his teeth. Both boys have an occupational performance deficit in toothbrushing. Both have deficits in performance components related to movement (eg, muscle tone, postural control, motor control). John also has a deficit in performance components related to cognition (eg, initiation, sequencing, concept formation).

Toothbrushing training for these two boys would be different because their problems are different. With Tim, the focus could be on helping him with positioning his body better at the sink. The size of his toothbrush handle could be increased to make it easier for him to hold it. For Tim, the focus would be on trying both to improve his movement skills and to make the task easier to compensate for his movement problems. With John, a focus on movement problems would not be enough. For John, time would also have to be spent on teaching the steps of toothbrushing. If you were to spend time teaching Tim the steps of the activity, he would be insulted and bored because he already knows how toothbrushing is done. If you focused only on movement problems with John, he would never learn to brush his teeth.

▼ OCCUPATIONAL PERFORMANCE AND PERFORMANCE COMPONENT TREATMENTS

Traditionally, occupational therapy treatment has been geared toward either occupational performance or performance components. More recently, occupational therapy practitioners have begun to consider clients' performance contexts, both physical and social, as equally important in the treatment process (American Occupational Therapy Association [AOTA], 1994). Chapter 21 discusses treatment of performance contexts.

Chapters 19 and 20 provide details about how practitioners provide treatment for occupational performance areas and performance components, respectively. Here, I will briefly compare occupational performance and performance component foci for treatment. Performance component training can be done either during occupational task training, or outside the context of those tasks. In general, treatment geared toward occupational performance aims to help clients compensate for their deficits, whereas treatment geared toward performance components aims to help clients recover from their deficits. Performance component training should always be used to help prepare clients to perform their preferred occupational performance activities in their anticipated performance contexts.

An occupational performance focus for Tim and John would mean working with both of them on the task of toothbrushing, adapting or altering the task as needed to make it possible for them to brush their teeth more independently. A performance component focus for Tim's movement problems during toothbrushing training might include giving him exercises in his wheelchair to help him position his trunk better before he starts trying to brush his teeth at the sink; exercises intended to improve his postural control. A performance component focus for John's cognitive problems during toothbrushing training might include having him tell you the steps to the task as he is doing them, to help him remember the steps in their proper order or sequence; an attempt to improve John's cognitive skills.

Outside the context of the toothbrushing task, a performance component focus for Tim's movement problems might include working with him on a therapy mat to help him position his trunk better; a performance component focus for John's cognitive problems might include working with him on putting pictures of the steps of a toothbrushing task in the right order. These treatments would be seeking to improve Tim's movement problems and John's cognitive problems, respectively. Performance component treatment outside the context of actual occupational tasks is helpful only for those clients who understand how to use the skills they learn in component treatment during occupational task performance (Neistadt, 1994a). Tim, for example, with his intact cognitive skills, may try, during toothbrushing, to practice the postural skills you taught him on the mat. John, on the other hand, may not connect the toothbrushing pictures with the actual task owing to his cognitive problems and may be able to learn to brush his teeth only by practicing the actual task over and over again. Even clients who understand how to use skills learned outside the context of actual occupational tasks need to practice their component skills in the context of occupational tasks, just as a basketball player needs to ultimately practice his or her basketball shooting, not just during drills, but also during an actual game. Motor-learning research suggests that it is difficult for people to use movement skills learned in one activity in other situations (Jarus, 1994; Mathiowetz & Haugen, 1994). That is why a basketball player who wants to become proficient at basketball practices basketball, not baseball. Similarly, a client who wants to develop competency at ADL, work, and leisure activities needs to practice those specific activities.

Ideally, occupational therapy practitioners use a combination of occupational performance and performance component training, with a minimum of the latter being performed outside the context of occupational performance activities. As insurance companies continue to decrease the treatment time for which they will pay, it is important that the bulk of occupational therapy treatment time be dedicated to the practice of clients' preferred occupational performance area activities, so that clients learn to be competent in these activities and become more independent as quickly as possible.

▼ TREATMENT AS LEARNING

For occupational therapy treatment to be effective, clients need to learn the skills practitioners are trying to teach them. Therefore, it is important for practitioners to structure their treatments to facilitate maximal client learning. Clients are helped to learn when they (1) work on activities that are important to them, (2) know their baseline performance (ie, their performance at the beginning of treatment) on those activities, and (3) have concrete, measurable goals to work toward. If you were treating Tim and John, for instance, would want to check and be sure these boys were interested in brushing their own teeth and willing to work on that activity. If this activity was important to the boys' parents, but not to the boys themselves, then a practitioner insisting on toothbrushing training would very likely be working with two very uncooperative gentlemen. If the boys and their parents share this toothbrushing priority, then before training begins, Tim and John would need to know how much help and what kinds of help they need with toothbrushing. They would also need to know how much help you anticipated they would need after treatment, so that they knew how much improvement they had to make. As an occupational therapy practitioner, you would have information about Tim and John's priorities and baseline behaviors from the initial evaluation. You would also have measurable treatment goals from that evaluation.

Clients are also helped to learn by practitioner feedback during treatment. To stay motivated, Tim and John, for instance, would have to receive periodic feedback from you about their performance (ie, you would have to tell them how much progress they were making). As a practitioner, you will be writing periodic notes about client progress; sharing these notes with your clients is one way to give them feedback. By sharing the results of interim evaluations

you will also help clients know how much progress they have made. Another way to give feedback is to tell clients at the end of each session how far they have come since your last treatment session with them. Development of a graph or chart of progress might be another way to keep clients informed of how they are progressing. It is important not to give too much feedback during treatment sessions. If you are saying "good!" every 2 minutes, then your clients may either become dependent on this level of praise or start to discount your praise as automatic and irrelevant to their performance.

Clients are also helped to learn by a practitioner's cuing during treatment. Tim and John, for example, would need cues or verbal prompts from you during their treatment to help them perform better. These cues are much like the advice a coach gives to an athlete during practice. Some clients will not be able to understand your verbal prompts because they either do not speak a language you know, or have damage to the parts of their brains that control language comprehension. For these clients your coaching may have to be in the form of gestures, or sometimes, hand-over-hand instruction.

Clients are also helped to learn when they feel challenged during treatment. That is, you need to **grade** treatment tasks, or to make them a little more difficult, as clients become competent at certain steps. For example, during your first treatment sessions with Tim you might squeeze the toothpaste onto the toothbrush for him, letting him concentrate on mastering the manipulation of the toothbrush. Once he begins to feel comfortable with using the toothbrush, you would want to have him try to put the toothpaste on the brush himself. Once Tim becomes comfortable with all steps of the toothbrushing task after you set up his toothbrush, toothpaste, cup, and towel at the sink, you would want to work with him on gathering and setting up his own toothbrushing supplies. This method of grading, during which you gradually withdraw assistance for the last to the first steps, in that order, is called backward chaining (Trombly, 1989). The rate at which you withdraw your assistance will depend on how quickly a client develops a degree of competency at the later steps of the task. For example, you would not ask Tim to start trying to put his toothpaste on his brush until he had become capable at manipulating the toothbrush.

Although it is important for clients to feel challenged by treatment, it is also important for them to be and feel successful with treatment tasks before we start asking them to do more. If you make treatment tasks too difficult too soon, clients will become frustrated and discouraged. If you asked Tim to start trying to put his toothpaste on his brush before he had developed some skill at manipulating the toothbrush, for instance, he might well start to feel as if he will never get any of this task right. Clients will also feel discouraged if you do not celebrate their small victories with them. If Tim is successful with independently manipulating his toothbrush in his mouth during one session, you need to tell him how well he has done and give him a few minutes to be excited and proud of his accomplishment. You also need to ask him if he is ready to try the toothpaste step the next time. That is, you need to give your clients some control over how fast you present additional challenges to them. Tim may feel that he needs another session or two doing things the same way to be sure he has this toothbrush manipulation thing down pat. The amount of leeway you can give someone will depend on how many treatment sessions the payer will allow. In grading treatment, then, you need to walk a fine line between client frustration and client boredom, always keeping in mind the total number of treatment sessions you have to work with this particular client. Finally, clients are helped to learn by receiving summary feedback from you about their overall progress. At the end of your treatment course with Tim, for example, you would want to reevaluate his toothbrushing performance and let him know how far he has come from his initial evaluation. Your discharge evaluation should give you this information.

Hence, for occupational therapy treatment to be an effective learning experience for clients, you need to have (1) information about what activities are important to clients (*clients' priorities*), (2) record of clients' *baseline performances (ie, performances before treatment)*, (3) *measurable treatment goals*, (4) a system of providing *feedback* to clients about their performance, (5) a system for giving *cues* to clients during treatment, (6) a systematic way to *grade the treatment tasks* in difficulty to keep your clients challenged, (7) *recognition of clients' treatment successes* as they happen, and (8) a *measure of treatment outcome*, or clients' performances at the end of treatment. The following guidelines for training in the occupational performance area of meal preparation illustrates how these learning factors can be systematically incorporated into treatment.

▼ MEAL PREPARATION GUIDELINES

These guidelines were developed for young adults and adults having trouble with meal preparation because of thinking or cognitive problems. The guidelines were tested in a research study and were found to be effective in improving meal preparation skill and cognitive-perceptual processing within 6 weeks in adult men with long-term diffuse brain injury. The treatment task used with these guidelines is preparation of a hot beverage (coffee, tea, hot chocolate) and a snack, which could include toast with a choice of toppings (lightly salted butter, lite margarine, lite cream cheese, peanut butter, low sugar jelly or jam, cinnamon, marshmallow fluff, or cheese spreads), fruit salads, frozen dough rolls, gelatin, or low-fat puddings. The snacks are relatively low fat, nutritious, and reasonable to complete in a 30-minute treatment session (Neistadt, 1994b). The guidelines include the learning factors listed in the preceding paragraph.

Clients' Priorities

Clients' priorities for this occupational performance activity could be assessed as part of the initial occupational therapist's evaluation, with an interview tool such as the Canadian Occupational Performance Measure (COPM) (Pollock, 1993). Chapter 13 includes more detail about the COPM and other interview instruments.

Baseline Information

Baseline information about clients' meal preparation abilities could be gathered by using the Rabideau Kitchen Evaluation—Revised (RKE-R) (Fig. 18–1),

---

Rating Scale

0—Subject requires no assistance. He or she initiates and performs the component step independently.
1—Subject requires one verbal cue or instruction to perform the component step.
2—Subject requires more than one verbal cue or instruction to perform the component step.
3—Subject is unable to perform the component step and requires direct intervention from the supervisor to complete the step.

Component Steps of the Activities

Rating   *Preparation of a Hot Instant Beverage*

1. Initiates beverage preparation procedure (exhibits intent/awareness of goal by picking up beverage box, asking appropriate questions, seeking appropriate items)

2. Scans directions on beverage box

3. Selects appropriate container for boiling water on stovetop (heat resistant, with handles, large enough)

4. Brings container to sink for filling

▲

Figure 18-1. Rabideau Kitchen Evaluation-Revised (RKE-R) (From Neistadt M.E. [1994]. A meal preparation treatment protocol for adults with brain injury. *American Journal of Occupational Therapy, 48,* p. 437. © The American Occupational Therapy Association, Inc. Reprinted with permission.)

5.	Reaches and operates faucet
6.	Fills container with adequate amount of water (sufficient to provide for minimum 1 cup of beverage)
7.	Brings container to stove
8.	Places container on stovetop burner
9.	Turns on appropriate burner
10.	Turns burner to appropriate heat setting (medium to high)
11.	Selects adequate cup for beverage (large enough, heat resistant)
12.	Opens beverage box, selects and opens individual beverage packet
13.	Pours contents of packet into cup
14.	Safely determines if water on stove is adequately heated (waits for signs—steam, bubbles forming, does not touch water, does not touch burner)
15.	Turns proper burner off
16.	Removes container of water safely from stove (uses handles)
17.	Transports hot container safely (uses handles)
18.	Pours hot water into cup safely (uses handles, does not overflow cup, does not touch hot portions of container)
19.	Returns hot container to safe location on stove
20.	Stirs hot beverage (uses appropriate, heat resistant utensil, does not touch hot liquid, does not spill beverage while stirring)

Total score for beverage: _____

Rating	*Preparation of a Cold Sandwich With Two Items*
21.	Initiates sandwich preparation procedure (exhibits intent/awareness of goal by asking appropriate questions, seeking appropriate items)
22.	Locates loaf of bread and transports safely to counter
23.	Opens bread wrapper
24.	Selects only two slices of bread

Rating	*Preparation of a Cold Sandwich With Two Items*
25.	Reseals bread wrapper
26.	Arranges slices on flat surface to prepare sandwich
27.	Locates item #1 only and transports safely to counter
28.	Opens container for item #1
29.	Applies item #1 to slice of bread
30.	Reseals container for item #1
31.	Returns item #1 to original location
32.	Locates item #2 only and transports safely to counter
33.	Opens container for item #2
34.	Applies item #2 to slice of bread

▲

Figure 18-1. (Continued)

35.	Reseals container for item #2	
36.	Returns item #2 to original location	
37.	Uses appropriate utensil to apply items (knife for spreading)	
38.	Closes sandwich properly (items inside between slices of bread)	
39.	Cuts sandwich safely (selects knife, knife below hand with blade down, stabilizes item when cutting)	
40.	Initiates kitchen clean-up activity (exhibits intent/awareness of goal by asking appropriate questions relating to cleanup, places dirty items in sink, wipes counters)	

Total score for sandwich: _____ Total score for beverage and sandwich: _____ Total time preparation of meal: _____

▲

Figure 18-1. (Continued)

. . . a valid and reliable test of the functional sequencing ability of adults with brain injury. Preliminary standards about the performance of adult men with diffuse brain injury on this instrument are available (Neistadt, 1992). The RKE-R requires subjects to prepare a simple meal: a cold sandwich with two fillings and a hot, instant beverage. On the evaluation form, the sandwich and beverage tasks are broken down into 40 component steps. These steps are listed in the order they are most commonly performed, but subjects are not required to follow this exact order [see Fig. 18–1].

Each component step on the evaluation form is scored on a scale of 0 to 3, with 0 being no assistance and 3 being total assistance (see [Fig.] 18–1). The minimum possible score is zero which indicates total independence. The maximum possible score is 120

Client Name: _____ Date: _____ Therapist: _____ Level: _____

Setup:
_____ _____ Choose beverage and snack   _____ _____ Collect foodstuffs, kettle, utensils, dishware

Start beverage:
_____ Fill kettle with water   _____ Put kettle on stove   _____ Turn burner on to medium-high

Prepare snack:
_____ Take bread slice(s) out of package **or** _____ Peel fruit **or** _____ Open packages
_____ Close package   _____ Slice fruit   _____ Mix ingredients
_____ Toast bread   _____ Mix fruit   _____ Put gelatin or pudding in refrigerator
_____ _____ _____ _____ Open spreads
_____ _____ _____ _____ Put spreads on toast
_____ _____ _____ _____ Close spreads
                    or
_____ Preheat oven   _____ Open dough   _____ Place on cookie sheet _____
_____ Remove from oven   _____ Remove from cookie sheet

Finish beverage:
_____ Turn off stove when water boils   _____ _____ Pour water into cups
_____ _____ Add milk, sugar, marshmallows, as desired
_____ _____ Stir beverages   *Time:* _____

Eating snack:
_____ _____ Take beverages and snack to table (beverage only with gelatin or pudding)
_____ Have beverage and snack   *Time:* _____

Clean up:
_____ Clear table
_____ Wipe table
_____ Put foodstuffs away
_____ Wash and dry dishes and utensils
_____ Put dishes and utensils away
_____ Wipe counters   *Time:* _____   *Total Time:* _____

Scoring: Number the steps in the sequence performed. Note whether performance was:
I—Independent
VC(#)—Verbal cues needed to complete step safely (/S) or within time limits (/T)
A/S—physical assist needed to complete step safely (/S) or within time limits (/T)

▲

Figure 18-2. Meal preparation scoring sheet. (From Neistadt M.E. [1994]. A meal preparation treatment protocol for adults with brain injury. *American Journal of Occupational Therapy, 48,* p. 436. © The American Occupational Therapy Association, Inc. Reprinted with permission.)

which indicates a need for physical assistance with all steps of the sandwich and beverage tasks. Exact instructions for test administration can be found elsewhere (Neistadt, 1992). (Neistadt, 1994b; p. 433).

Measurable Treatment Goals

Measurable treatment goals could be written from the first evaluation with the RKE-R.

In my study of adult men with head injury, 23 clients showed an average improvement of 7.9 points on the RKE-R after 6 weeks of 30 minute sessions, 3 times a week using these meal preparation treatment guidelines (Neistadt, 1991). These clients also showed an average 20% decrease in the amount of time they needed to complete the RKE-R after treatment (Neistadt, 1991, unpublished data). (Neistadt, 1994b, p. 435).

A measurable treatment goal for this activity then, could be that the client would improve his or her RKE-R score by 7.9 points after treatment. This goal could be translated into functional terms by generally describing the level of assistance a client who achieved that score would need.

Feedback

Feedback about clients' performance with meal preparation tasks could be given from the scoring sheet in Figure 18–2. A practitioner who filled out one of these score sheets during each treatment session and kept all of the scoring sheets would have very precise information to give a client on any given treatment day about how much progress he or she had made relative to previous sessions.

Graded Levels of Task Difficulty

The light meal activity has been broken down into six levels of difficulty [Box 18–1], with Level 1 being the easiest and Level 6 the most difficult. For each successive level, the number of steps required to complete the activity increases, thereby increasing the demand on the client's visual perceptual, sequencing, and organizational skills. Level 1—preparation of a single cup of hot beverage—is an appropriate starting level for clients who are unable to initiate a kitchen activity at all or score above 20 on the pretest RKE-R. Level 6, with more involved snacks like fruit salads, is an appropriate starting level for clients who score 5 or less on the pretest RKE-R. (Neistadt, 1994b, p. 433)

Within each level, clients' would have a choice about the ingredients they wanted for their snacks and which hot beverages they wanted to make.

Cuing

Cuing for this treatment activity is meant to promote problem solving. The practitioner starts the treatment session with a general cue, such as, "Let's get started." If the client does not initiate or begin the activity after that cue, then the

▼ **BOX 18-1**

Meal Preparation Treatment Protocol Grading

The task difficulty will be increased by increasing the number of steps, and, consequently the amount of planning needed in the snack preparation. The levels of difficulty from least to most, are:

Level 1: Tea, hot chocolate, or coffee—1 serving
Level 2: Tea, hot chocolate, or coffee, toast with one topping—1 serving
Level 3: Tea, hot chocolate, or coffee, toast with two toppings—1 serving
Level 4: Tea, hot chocolate, or coffee, toast with one topping—2 servings
Level 5: Tea, hot chocolate, or coffee, toast with two toppings—2 servings
Level 6: Fruit salads using variety of fresh fruits (the greater the number of different fruits, and the greater the number of pieces of fruit to be cut up, the more difficult the salad), or frozen cinnamon rolls, or other frozen pastries, and 2 hot beverages, or low-fat puddings or gelatin with fruit.

(From A Meal Preparation Treatment Protocol for Adults with Brain Injury by M.E. Neistadt. *American Journal of Occupational Therapy, 48,* pp. 436–437. © 1994 by the American Occupational Therapy Association, Inc. Reprinted with permission.)

practitioner could ask the following set of questions to guide the client's perceptual analysis and cognitive planning of the activity: (1) What do you see?, (2) Does anything that you see suggest what you have to do next?, (3) What steps are you going to take to complete your task?

Recognition of Client's Treatment Successes and Treatment Outcomes

The practitioner can acknowledge the client's successes in treatment by giving the feedback described in the foregoing and by sitting down with the client at the end of the treatment activity while the client eats and enjoys what he or she has prepared. Treatment outcomes could be measured by administering the Rabideau Kitchen Evaluation—Revised at the end of treatment.

► CONCLUSION

Occupational therapy treatment is a learning process for clients. Therefore, to deliver effective treatment, practitioners need to be good teachers, incorporating basic learning principles into their treatment sessions. These learning principles include a focus on (1) clients' priorities, (2) clients' baseline performances, (3) measurable treatment goals, (4) feedback, (5) cuing methods, (6) task grading, (7) clients' successes, and (8) treatment outcomes. These principles can be applied to the planning and implementation of any treatment session, for any treatment activity, to promote optimal client learning and outcomes.

▼ REFERENCES

American Occupational Therapy Association (1994). Uniform terminology for occupational therapy—third edition. *American Journal of Occupational Therapy, 48*, 1047–1054.

Jarus, T. (1994). Motor learning and occupational therapy: The organization of practice. *American Journal of Occupational Therapy, 48*, 810–816.

Mathiowetz, V., & Haugen, J.B. (1994). Motor behavior research: Implications for therapeutic approaches to central nervous system dysfunction. *American Journal of Occupational Therapy, 48*, 733–745.

Neistadt, M. E. (1991). *Occupational therapy treatments for constructional deficits.* Doctoral dissertation, Boston University, 1991.

Neistadt, M. E. (1992). The Rabideau Kitchen Evaluation—Revised: An assessment of meal preparation skill. *Occupational Therapy Journal of Research, 12*, 242–255.

Neistadt, M. E. (1994a). The neurobiology of learning: Implications for treatment of adults with brain injury. *American Journal of Occupational Therapy, 48*, 421–430.

Neistadt, M. E. (1994b). A meal preparation treatment protocol for adults with brain injury. *American Journal of Occupational Therapy, 48*, 431–438.

Pollock, N. (1993). Client-centered assessment. *American Journal of Occupational Therapy, 47*, 298–302.

Trombly, C. A. (1989). *Occupational therapy for physical dysfunction,* (3rd ed.). Baltimore: Williams & Wilkins.

Chapter 19

Treatment of Occupational Performance Areas

Section 1: Treatment of Activities of Daily Living

Section 2: Treatment of Activities of Daily Living: Sexuality and Disability

Section 3: Treatment for Work and Productive Activities:
Home and Family Management

Section 4: Treatment of Work and Productive Activities: Functional
Restoration, An Industrial Rehabilitation Approach

Section 5: Treatment Through Play and Leisure

Section I

Treatment of Activities of Daily Living

**Margo B. Holm, Joan C. Rogers, and
Anne Birge James**

Parameters Used for Establishing Target Intervention Outcomes

  The Influence of Task Parameters on Treatment
    Planning

  Client's Capacity for Learning

  Prognosis for Performance Components

  Time for Intervention

  Expected Performance Context: Discharge Setting

  Projected Follow-Through with Home Program

Treatment Implementation

  Selection of a Treatment Approach

  Grading the Treatment Program

Treatment of ADL Conclusion

The occupational therapy practitioner must carefully craft a treatment program to meet the individual needs of clients. The specific treatment strategies available to the occupational therapy practitioner are endless and many of these are described in detail in subsequent chapters of this book. Before selecting treatment strategies, however, the practitioner must determine the appropriate treatment ap-

proach for each client. Several approaches are available to select from, and they may be used singly or in combination. Because of the complexity of human behavior, the employment of standardized, that is, nonindividualized, treatment strategies will likely fail to meet the needs of most clients. Similar to the ubiquitous "one size fits all" dress, which may be donned by all, but fits no one well, standardized treatment strategies may make treatment planning easier and faster for the occupational therapy practitioner, but this may be at the expense of the client whose potential may not be realized. In a health care era when occupational therapy practitioners must meet high demands for productivity, it is easy to fall into treatment planning "ruts." These ruts may be adopting standardized protocols or following the same treatment-planning strategies with all clients, because they have worked well in the past and the practitioner is efficient and comfortable in using them. This section is designed to assist practitioners in planning client-centered treatment for deficits in activities of daily living (ADL) and, hence, to prevent them from falling into planning ruts.

This section is divided into two major subsections. In the first subsection, the parameters used to describe and measure task performance in occupational areas introduced in Chapter 15, are revisited and discussed in relation to establishing target intervention outcomes. Target intervention outcomes are a necessary prerequisite to planning treatment because, as the old adage says, "if you don't know where you are going, you will not know how to get there or when you have arrived." In the second subsection, three approaches to treating ADL disabilities—namely, **remediation**, **compensation**, and education—are presented and, under each of these approaches, strategies for promoting independent, safe, and adequate task performance are outlined.

323

▼ PARAMETERS USED FOR ESTABLISHING TARGET INTERVENTION OUTCOMES

The critical first step in planning treatment is establishing reasonable, attainable, functional outcomes, or goals, that are to be achieved through occupational therapy. This requires analysis of the evaluation data in conjunction with additional factors influencing outcome: namely, the client's ability to learn, the client's prognosis, the time allocated for treatment, the client's discharge disposition, and the client's ability to follow through with new routines or techniques. Synthesizing this vast amount of information into a meaningful, individualized treatment plan is a complex cognitive task and can be overwhelming for the student or new occupational therapy practitioner. A closer look at the implications for treatment of the multiple factors influencing outcomes may help guide novice practitioners in clinical reasoning and structure the problem-solving process for more experienced practitioners, when they are managing particularly complex or challenging clients.

The Influence of Task Parameters on Treatment Planning

In Chapter 15, evaluation of performance areas was described relative to four parameters: (1) value of the task to the client, (2) level of independence in performing the task, (3) safety of task performance, and (4) adequacy of task performance. Adequacy of task performance involved difficulty, pain, fatigue and dyspnea, duration (efficiency), societal standards, satisfaction, experience, resources, and aberrant task behaviors. A comprehensive evaluation addresses all these parameters, and each is viewed from the perspective of the known or anticipated performance context before decisions concerning outcomes and treatment strategies are finalized.

VALUE

Identification of a client's role deficits and the tasks that comprise these roles is an essential component of the occupational therapy evaluation and should be the first consideration in establishing outcomes. Evaluation using a top-down approach (Trombly, 1993) begins with the identification of the client's life roles, including the relative value each role has in the client's life, the roles that are most disabled, and the client's priorities for working on roles during rehabilitation (Clark, 1993; Pollock et al, 1990; Trombly, 1995a). Because the specific tasks that make up a role vary considerably from individual to individual, these tasks must also be identified by clients (Canadian Association of Occupational Therapists, 1991). For example, two young men with similar **spinal cord injuries** may both identify being the father of a young son as a significant life role. However, tasks that define the role of father may be very different for each of them. For one father, coaching little league, hiking, and camping are essential tasks, whereas for the other father, teaching computer skills and going to the science museum assume priority. The treatment strategies for these two fathers need to be quite different if each is to successfully return to his role of "father."

The value clients place on a given task influences the motivation for participation in any treatment aimed at improving performance for that task. Because many occupational therapy treatments require the acquisition of new skills through practice, motivation can greatly influence the ultimate functional outcome. Clients who put little value on the task being addressed in treatment are unlikely to follow through with the home program necessary for improving skill in that task.

Values are difficult to change, so whenever possible, occupational therapy practitioners should work within the values defined by clients. This requires a collaborative approach between the client and occupational therapy practitioner as the details of the treatment plan are established. Priorities for tasks to be included in treatment must be established by the client under the guidance of the practitioner, who needs to elicit sufficient data about a client's values and preferences to devise an individualized plan. One life role commonly omitted by clients is the self-care role. The role of "self-carer," typically developed by the age of 6, becomes so habituated by adulthood that adults often neglect to mention it as a valued role. Self-care is highly valued by most adults because of the dependency on others that accompanies role dysfunction. However, persons with severe disabilities may need or desire to accept assistance from others in ADL, so that they can conserve energy to perform other tasks. This was the situation with Mr. Fritz, a 32-year-old man with a recently sustained spinal cord injury resulting in C6 quadriplegia. He is married with three small children and self-employed as a tax accountant. His wife works part-time as a nurse and takes care of their children before and after school. The family is very dependent on Mr. Fritz's income. He has no disability insurance coverage. Although outcomes in ADL were initially established for Mr. Fritz, it soon became apparent that attempts at self-care retraining were being met with resistance and frustration. Further discussion of the targeted treatment outcomes revealed that Mr. Fritz was anxious to return to work and that he could do this if he could use the computer in his home office. Although he expressed an interest in becoming independent in self-care, he felt that the best option for him was to return to work as quickly as possible to minimize the financial burden on his family from his current inability to work. His wife is able and willing to help him with self-care tasks when he returns home. The couple feels that self-care retraining can be delayed until the family business is again operational. With treatment outcomes refocused on tasks most valued by Mr. Fritz—namely computer access and home mobility—he became well motivated for therapy.

Some clients may identify reasonable intervention outcomes, but establish priorities that make the treatment process inefficient and potentially ineffective. Particularly when dealing with severe disability of sudden onset (eg, stroke, traumatic injury), self-care training often helps clients develop abilities and problem-solving skills that can later be applied to tasks that are more complex than self-care. For example, if Mr. Fritz had needed to drive to get to work, an ultimately realistic goal for his injury, different treatment priorities might have been established. Initiating treatment with driver training would have been impractical because he lacks the prerequisite functional mobility skills. Functional mobility skills must be developed to an adequate level before driver training can begin. ADL training, involving bathing, dressing, transferring, and wheelchair mobility would facilitate the development of functional mobility skills. Such training, therefore, logically precedes driver training. In this situation, having someone assist Mr. Fritz with financial planning and educating him about the relationship between self-care and driving skills, may best meet his needs. This plan recognizes his valued roles and progresses him to the desired outcome in the most efficient way possible.

When the most valued tasks and roles are beyond the potential skill level of clients, the occupational therapy practitioner helps clients refocus their priorities so that the treatment plan is realistic and outcomes are achievable. If Mr. Fritz were the owner-cook of a small restaurant, for example, it would be unlikely that he could meet the essential job requirements of a short-order cook, even if the kitchen were adapted for wheelchair accessibility and use, because tasks must be done quickly. It is possible, however, that he could perform the tasks of "restaurant owner." For example, he could manage personnel, handle the finances, operate the cash register, and seat customers. In this and similar situations, occupational therapy practitioners assist clients in establishing realistic outcomes for treatment by offering expertise in task analysis and functional adaptation.

INDEPENDENCE

The parameter most commonly focused on in occupational therapy intervention is independence in task performance. The targeted outcome is generally to increase the level of independence (Evans, Small, & Ling, 1995). This may be accomplished in various ways, including changing task materials (eg, using overhead instead of cardigan-type garments), teaching adapted techniques (eg, dressing an impaired extremity before a nonimpaired one), and prescribing assistive technology (eg, providing a shoehorn with an extended handle). The occupational therapy practitioner may also structure task performance so that progressively less human assistance is given as recovery of function occurs. For example, as muscle strength increases, the amount of physical assistance provided by the practitioner to perform a task is decreased. Alternatively, rather than changing the amount of assistance, the type of human assistance may change, with less powerful assists replacing more powerful ones. For example, as muscle strength increases verbal cuing may replace physical assistance.

Task performance may be divided into two phases: initiation, or beginning a task; and maintenance, or continuing a task to completion. Initiation is an aspect of task performance that is frequently overlooked when intervention outcomes are established, partly because it is difficult to evaluate and treat. The very presence of the occupational therapy practitioner may be a cue to initiate a task, and certainly a greeting, such as, "Good morning Mrs. Smith, today we will work on dressing," serves as a prompt for action. Adults are typically expected to initiate self-care and home management tasks independently. Expectations for children also exist and vary depending on their age, skills, and the division of task responsibilities among family members. Impairments in task initiation may occur as a result of many injuries and diseases, such as **dementia**, **depression**, **schizophrenia**, brain injury from **trauma** or **stroke**, **multiple sclerosis**, and **Parkinson's disease**. Family members generally find it very frustrating to have to cue (ie, constantly nag) each aspect of a daily routine for a family member with an initiation impairment. Additionally, lack of initiation severely limits a client's ability to find and retain employment, engage in leisure, and participate in meaningful social roles and relationships. Training in the use of memory aids, such as, memory notebooks, checklists, cue cards, and electronic cuing devices may be viable for these clients (Parenté & Herrman, 1996).

Perceived self-efficacy, that is, clients' beliefs about their ability to perform tasks, influences both the initiation and performance of self-care tasks (Gage, Noh, Polatajko, & Kaspar, 1994). Clients may overestimate or underestimate their skill level. The primary concern with clients who overestimate their skill level is safety, and this is addressed subsequently. Those who underestimate their skill level may impose a disability on themselves, even though they have the capability to be safe, independent, and adequate in performing in a task. For example, Mrs. Jasper slipped on the ice last winter and fractured her left hip. Surgery was required to stabilize the fracture, but she recovered well and returned to her home where she lives alone. Before her fall, she was independent in shopping, which she did in a small grocery store 1 block from her home. The physical therapy discharge summary from home health care indicated that Mrs. Jasper could ambulate independently without a walking aid on a variety of indoor and outdoor walking surfaces. She was advised to use a cane if it made her feel more secure. However, since her accident Mrs. Jasper has had a persistent fear of falling and believes that she cannot walk safely outdoors. Hence, she continues to be dependent in shopping, relying on her daughter to shop for her. In this case, task disability in shopping is caused by a perceived inability to walk safely outdoors, not on actual walking ability. This client is unlikely to meet the otherwise realistic intervention outcome of independence in shopping, unless treatment includes strategies to alleviate her fear of falling and her contingent perceived incompetence.

Caregiver training may be implemented to maximize a client's functional outcome while minimizing the efforts of the caregiver (Watts, 1990). For example, Mr. Ford, sustained a left **cerebrovascular accident (CVA)** and required minimal physical assistance with verbal cuing from the occupational therapy practitioner for wheelchair transfers. Mrs. Ford was physically able to help her husband, but had no previous experience in transferring individuals with hemiparesis. One day she decided to help her husband move from his hospital bed to the chair. Because she did not block his right knee or tell him to wait for her cue before standing, they both fell onto the bed while attempting to execute the transfer. Fortunately, no one was hurt. As a consequence of this experience, Mrs. Ford was convinced she could not care for her husband at home. At the same time, she was distressed by the thought of having to admit him to a long-term care facility. She was very receptive to receiving transfer training from the occupational therapy practitioner and was delighted to find that by using the proper physical and verbal techniques, she could easily and safely assist her husband. In this example, caregiver training increased the client's level of independence and the probability that he could go home at discharge.

SAFETY

During the occupational therapy evaluation, it is recommended that the parameters of task performance—safety and independence—be rated independently to assure that deficits in safety are clearly identified. Because safety is a quality of the person–task–environment transaction, however, it cannot be observed or treated in isolation from independence. Although, the intervention outcomes of safety and independence are inextricably linked, it is often advisable to list them as separate outcomes, because clients can be independent, but not safe. A comparison of two clients with T4 paraplegia, secondary to spinal cord injury, who are learning independent transfers illustrates this point. Ted and Ryan were both recently injured and are learning sitting balance and mobility skills. Ted demonstrates good judgment and a realistic perception of his skills. He has learned to transfer safely by following certain guidelines (eg, position wheelchair at a 45 degree angle to the bed; secure brakes on wheelchair; ascertain that bed height is level with the wheelchair); he follows these guidelines consistently; hence, he is allowed to do bed–chair transfers independently. Ryan's spinal cord injury is similar to Ted's, but he also suffered a mild brain injury. Although Ryan's motor skills are comparable to Ted's, Ryan has difficulty recalling the guidelines for transfers. Hence, he is not considered independent in transfers because his performance is inconsistent and, when he fails to implement the guidelines, he places himself at risk for falling out of his wheelchair. Both Ted and Ryan have the motor capability to perform transfers independently, however, Ted consistently performs them safely, whereas Ryan does not meet this criterion. Ryan continues to require supervision and occasional verbal cuing for safety. Ryan's treatment outcomes may need to be adjusted to realistically reflect his capacity for safe, as well as independent, transfers.

Although occupational therapy practitioners agree that "safety" is a treatment priority, there is less consensus about specific task behaviors that are safe or unsafe. A wide range of behaviors fall into a questionable zone, where tasks may be rated as safe by some and unsafe by others. For example, few people would disagree that it is unsafe to drive on an urban interstate at 110 miles/hour, even when traffic is light and road conditions are excellent. With a posted speed limit of 65 miles/hour, however, most would agree that driving 70 miles/hour is still within the safety margin. So, what speed would mark the transition from safe to unsafe? Ask ten people and you would probably get ten different answers. Occupational therapy practitioners must frequently address questions of safe and unsafe behaviors. The attitudes of clients, caregivers, and families may be helpful in determining the level of risk that is viewed as acceptable.

When determining acceptable risk, it is useful to consider the client's comfort level with risk, the ability to analyze the risks associated with a particular task and devise a plan for managing them, and most importantly, the ability to implement the plan expeditiously despite impairments. For example, rock climbing has obvious inherent risks, but the skilled mountaineer knows how to analyze situations to minimize the potential for accidents and has a repertoire of rescue and emergency skills that facilitate a safe outcome, even when things go wrong. Novices who opt to climb without this "bag of tricks" may find themselves more frequently in difficulty. Occupational therapy clients have varying abilities to adapt to situations that have inherent risks or present unexpected hazards. At times, the level of independence in task performance may need to be sacrificed for safety. An individual who is independent in ambulation, but has delayed and impaired balance reactions, may need to restrict walking to smooth, level walking surfaces. This restriction may significantly limit independence in community mobility. The inability to adapt to unexpected events (eg, regain balance after being bumped) makes it necessary to limit independence to maximize safety.

Analysis of a client's risk orientation can provide valuable insight into the tendency to engage in risky behaviors before disability. Many clients find themselves in need of occupational therapy services because of risky behaviors: for example, the client with traumatic brain injury from a motor vehicle accident that occurred while driving under the influence of drugs or alcohol; the client with acquired immunodeficiency syndrome (**AIDS**) who reported having multiple sexual partners without protection; or the teenager with multiple fractures and skin abrasions who rode a skateboard through rush hour traffic in downtown Manhattan. Treatment goals aimed at identifying the potential risks inherent to specific behaviors and the consequences of risky behavior may be appropriate to establish for these clients.

Clients who tend to overestimate their abilities may present occupational therapy practitioners with challenging safety issues. Tasks that were previously performed by clients may continue to be perceived as "do-able," despite newly acquired limitations that make such tasks unsafe. The nature of the task itself and the consequences of limited capacity in performing the task are important considerations. Tasks that require mobility, including walking and transferring, are common examples of tasks that may be unsafe when attempted by those with insufficient skill. A likely consequence of the skill deficit, in this instance, is a fall. For other tasks, skill deficit may lead to unsuccessful performance, but present no hazard to clients or others. For example, disability in eating may result in soiled clothing, but clients are unlikely to injure themselves attempting this task, unless the food is very hot or swallowing is impaired.

The task performance context must also be taken into account when considering safety. Clients with reasonable judgment may be forced to engage in risky behavior if the performance context does not accommodate alterations in task performance to ensure safety. For example, Mrs. Ethridge has **rheumatoid arthritis** and requires a walker for safe ambulation since her recent hospitalization for an acute flare-up. She was discharged to her home where she lives alone. When she returned home, she discovered that her walker did not fit into her bathroom. Thus, she had to walk the length of the bathtub to get to the toilet, while holding onto the shower curtain to help maintain her balance. Although she recognized that this was unsafe, she saw no other options.

Treatment for limitations in safe task performance is often aimed at adapting the task or the environment so that performance can be improved as soon as possible. In contrast, improvement in independence can occur over time, as long as adequate assistance is available. Education for clients and their caregivers should be a component of treatment for safety, because clients relearn familiar tasks with reduced levels of ability, and often within new and unfamiliar performance contexts.

ADEQUACY

Several aspects of task performance contribute to the adequacy or quality of the action or outcome. Most standardized assessment tools do not include measures of adequacy, although these parameters may be instrumental in motivating clients to follow through with tasks. This may be particularly important for clients who are "independent" and "safe" with their performance, but feel dissatisfied with the process or the outcome. Without measurement of these qualitative deficits and the establishment of outcomes that include adequacy parameters, the justification for funding additional treatment is lacking. Nine adequacy parameters will be discussed: difficulty, pain, fatigue and dyspnea, duration, societal standards, satisfaction, experience, resources, and aberrant task behaviors. Some of these parameters may be interdependent in a client. For instance, pain may lead to changes in duration of task performance (eg, takes longer), as well as the ability to meet normative standards and personal satisfaction.

Difficulty

The perceived ease with which a client completes a task, as well as the projected difficulty that will remain following treatment, are important to incorporate into treatment outcomes (Fried, Herdman, Kuhn, Rubin, & Turano, 1991; Verbrugge, 1990). The occupational therapy practitioner, with skill in activity analysis and knowledge of pathology and impairment, must determine the prognosis for "functional difficulty." This prognosis must then be communicated to clients so that decisions about "acceptable levels of difficulty" can be made collaboratively. Clients set treatment priorities, in part, by weighing the projected level of difficulty within the context of value; that is, how much difficulty are they willing to tolerate to be independent in a task? For example, Mrs. Hernandez lives alone in an apartment in a retirement community. Her sister and brother-in-law also reside in the community and she has many close friends there. She has had multiple sclerosis for many years, with some weakness and **spasticity**, but she remained independent in her daily living activities until a recent exacerbation which required hospitalization. An increase in lower extremity spasticity and decrease in strength left her dependent on a wheelchair for mobility and requiring physical assistance in self-care. Strength, endurance, and balance may improve somewhat over time; however, it is anticipated that she will need a wheelchair indefinitely. The retirement community requires Mrs. Hernandez to be independent in self-care and able to prepare breakfast and a light evening snack. A hot meal is provided at midday. The occupational therapy practitioner explained to Mrs. Hernandez that, although independence in self-care is a reasonable goal, completing her self-care activities will likely be time-consuming and may leave her little energy for other tasks. Mrs. Hernandez is enthusiastic about beginning treatment, indicating that she is willing to face the difficulty associated with these tasks because independence will enable her to remain in the retirement community with family and friends.

A different scenario plays out with Mrs. McKay, who also has multiple sclerosis. Similar to Mrs. Hernandez, she had a recent exacerbation causing a similar functional decline and prognosis for independent functioning. Mrs. McKay works full-time as a programmer for a local radio station and is the mother of two young children. Mrs. McKay perceived her role as a self-carer to be important, along with those of worker and mother. However, when it became apparent that independence in self-care would significantly interfere with her ability to perform her work and parenting roles, she opted to hire a personal care attendant.

The frequency with which a task is performed should also be considered when establishing intervention outcomes that reflect the level of difficulty. In general, for tasks that need to be done routinely, a higher level of proficiency or ease of performance is needed, whereas for tasks that are done only occasionally a lower level of proficiency or ease of performance may be acceptable. However, the risk associated with a lower performance standard also needs to be taken into account. For example, Mr. James has a spinal cord injury resulting in C8 quadriplegia. He has a neurogenic bladder and requires intermittent catheterization. He identified self-catheterization as a critical task for fulfilling roles as self-carer as well as being a worker because he is away from home for 9 hours daily. The occupational therapy practitioner is working with Mr. James and the nursing staff to adapt this task so he can complete it accurately and efficiently. Repetition is a critical treatment strategy, as is completing the task in both a bed and in a wheelchair. Another client, Mr. Frank also has a C8 quadriplegia from spinal cord injury. He can typically achieve adequate emptying of his bladder without self-catheterization and wears a condom catheter. On rare occasions, however, Mr. Frank has episodes of urinary retention, requiring catheterization within about an hour of experiencing symptoms. Mr. Frank lives alone and works at home. He worked with the occupational therapy practitioner and nursing staff to learn self-catheterization. The task is very tedious for him and must be done in bed. The process he uses is safe and clean and the outcome—bladder emptying—is met. Although the task remains extremely difficult for him, his skill level is adequate for meeting his needs because he does not have to catherize himself very often.

Pain

Pain, either during or following a task, can also negatively influence performance, even if the task is completed independently. The source of pain as well as the prognosis for it must be carefully considered when establishing intervention outcomes and selecting a treatment approach. Task modification to minimize or eliminate pain is an obvious first choice for treatment, although the cause of the pain or the nature of the task may not make this feasible. Clients may use a variety of modalities for pain management. These modalities may include medication, massage, transcutaneous electrical nerve stimulation (TENS), visual imagery, relaxation techniques, yoga, and chiropractic care, to name a few. The role of the occupational therapy practitioner is to integrate successful pain management modalities with the performance of ADL to minimize pain during task performance, thereby enhancing the adequacy of performance. Collaboration with the professional(s) who prescribed the pain treatment modalities is essential so that safe and effective follow-through with that modality is maintained. Intervention outcomes must include an index of pain so that treatment remains focused on achieving the projected level of independence while simultaneously reducing the influence of pain. Chapter 20, Section 8, provides more information about pain management strategies.

For clients with certain disorders, pain is a signal to stop or restrict a movement or task. For example, for individuals with rheumatoid arthritis who have erosion of the joint capsule, pain may indicate that action is causing further destruction of the bony surfaces and hastening joint deformity. Task modification is an important treatment strategy with these clients, for treatment aimed only at pain reduc-

tion may enable clients to participate in potentially harmful tasks. Additionally, outcomes must be established that reflect the client's capability to follow through with tasks while respecting pain, by altering performance to minimize further impairment (Lorig & Fries, 1990).

Fatigue and Dyspnea

Fatigue, the sensation of tiredness experienced during or following a task, and dyspnea, difficult or labored breathing, may interfere with task performance. Both fatigue and dyspnea are likely to be exacerbated by task performance. Task analysis takes into account the effort required to perform a task and its typical duration. Additionally, the client's entire daily routine must be examined so that the energy demands of one task can be weighed in relation to the client's other tasks. Assisting clients to examine the physical demands of their preferred tasks can help them prioritize tasks so that appropriate outcomes can be established. Similar to budgeting money, clients must be encouraged to look at their "energy dollars" and decide how they wish to spend them. The occupational therapy practitioner consults in this decision-making process by bringing valuable information about options for task adaptation that may reduce the endurance demands of tasks, thereby "saving" clients' energy dollars for additional tasks.

Diagnosis is important to consider when treatment outcomes are formulated relative to fatigue and dyspnea. Overexertion may exacerbate symptoms, or even the disease process itself, for conditions such as cardiac disease and multiple sclerosis. Prognosis is another important diagnostic consideration, especially when deciding on specific task adaptations or the advisability of treating performance component deficits. Clients with chronic obstructive pulmonary disease are likely to become worse; therefore, task adaptations that accommodate a decline in function are appropriate. With paraplegia secondary to spinal cord injury, however, fatigue from poor endurance is likely a result of having to use and develop the smaller muscles of the upper extremity for wheelchair mobility to compensate for the loss of the lower extremity muscles previously used for functional mobility. With this condition, endurance is likely to improve, and treatment activities should be graded to require increasing endurance to facilitate progress (Gift & Pugh, 1993; McDowell & Newell, 1996; Tack, 1991).

Duration

The length of time required to complete tasks is typically thought of as a reflection of efficiency. Although measuring performance time may be a relatively simple task, interpreting time data in a meaningful way is often difficult. The duration of daily living tasks is highly dependent on the nature of the task and the task objects individuals choose to use in performing them. It takes longer to prepare dinner than it does to fix a light snack. Most of us spend more time dressing when we are going out to dine in an elegant restaurant than we do when we are going to a fast-food place. Thus, it is difficult to establish meaningful norms for daily-living tasks. Establishing acceptable time frames for specific ADL must be done with clients and their significant others and should be reflected in the functional outcomes. For example, Dan, a 12 year-old-boy with **cerebral palsy (CP)**, is independent in dressing, but dressing takes almost 90 minutes to complete. He needs to be on the school bus at 7:15 AM It is not practical for Dan or his parents to arise at 5:00 AM to enable Dan to dress independently. Instead, Dan's parents assist him with dressing on school days. To increase efficiency for some dressing components, on school days, Dan is expected to manage his clothing during toileting and donning and doffing his jacket, because these skills are needed in school. To increase efficiency for the entire task, however, he is encouraged to dress independently on nonschool days. This schedule enables Dan to increase his dressing efficiency in a way that best meets his and his family's needs. By taking into account a client's diagnosis, impairments, disabilities, and treatment options, the occupational therapy practitioner can offer expertise in functional rehabilitation by predicting a likely outcome for the duration of a specific task.

When analyzing task performance that seems too short, safety, independence, and adequacy, all come into play. Clients may be at increased risk when they rush through tasks. Professional caregivers may limit the independence of task performance by giving "overcare" to meet their own productivity requirements. Clients may also neglect performance standards just to get tasks done quickly. Task performance that seems too long also needs to be evaluated in reference to safety, independence, and adequacy. Clients with swallowing deficits, for example, may need to eat slower than those without such deficits, to avoid choking. Individuals with poor fine motor coordination or sensory deficits may need to slow down when using a sharp knife, to improve control of the knife and prevent injury. However, slower task performance is not necessarily safer. Crossing a street, for example, must occur within the time allowed by the traffic light, or safety is compromised.

Societal and cultural standards also need to be taken into consideration when establishing outcomes for task duration. In the United States, timeliness is highly valued, and efficient performance in community skills is expected. Shoppers generally become irritated when they are standing in a checkout line behind a customer who takes several minutes to identify and count currency. In other countries, this delay may go unnoticed. An American with cognitive deficits that interfere with the ability to count currency may need to decrease the time required for this task, to reduce embarrassment when shopping. The intervention outcome, then, needs to include an efficiency measure to reflect this task parameter. A client from a culture that measures time in hours, rather than minutes, may feel that treatment focused on increasing speed is unnecessary.

Societal Standards

Performance standards, determined by the society and culture in which one lives, are likely to exist for outcomes in terms of both the end result and the process through which this is achieved. As discussed in the evaluation section, the line between acceptable and unacceptable performance is likely to be thick, rather than thin, and may vary considerably depending on characteristics, such as age, gender, and cohort (ie, generational) membership. Societal norms exist, for example, for neatness. A client may dress safely and independently, but if the color of clothing clashes and appearance is disheveled (ie, end product), the client's dressing may or may not meet societal standards. If the client is a teenager, who is going out to "hang out" with friends, it would likely be considered acceptable. However, if the client is a public relations manager going to work, it would likely be labeled unacceptable and could well put the client's job in jeopardy. An example of varied societal standards for process is evident in expectations for eating behavior. "Wolfing down" a hot dog in record time while waiting for a subway would be unlikely to draw attention from fellow passengers, as long as the individual did not choke, spill food on clothing or on others, and disposed of litter properly. Displaying this same process as a bridal attendant seated at the head table at the wedding reception would be considered ill mannered.

Evaluation of societal standards must take into account who established the standards and the context in which specific performance behaviors are to occur. It is critical to identify the most relevant societal standards for inclusion in intervention outcomes, and when planning treatment, to keep the focus manageable. Although consideration of societal standards may seem subjective and difficult, the use of indicators of these standards is critical for establishing outcomes, justifying treatment, establishing treatment strategies, and documenting a change in performance. From the foregoing example, the treatment outcome may be that when eating during a social event, Ms. Lee will demonstrate appropriate pacing as evidenced by completing a meal in no less than 15 minutes, swallowing each bite before putting additional food into her mouth, and conversing between bites of food.

Satisfaction

In addition to societal standards, clients have their own standards of acceptable performance, and these standards also need to be incorporated into functional outcomes. Mr. Bruce, for example, is always losing things. He never seems to know where his wallet and keys are, and he is always searching for something. Nonetheless, items seem to turn up and he sees no reason to go to the trouble of organizing his apartment better to help him keep track of his belongings. Mr. John, however, has always been meticulously neat and could put his hands on items the minute he wanted them. Recently, he sought medical attention for memory problems. He complained that he needs to search for items because he has failed to put them in their usual place. He is particularly concerned about his memory problem because of a family history of Alzheimer's disease. He was referred to occupational therapy to learn strategies to help him remember where items are placed. Objectively, Mr. John is not performing any worse than Mr. Bruce; however, he interprets his performance as negative, and furthermore, he is dissatisfied with his performance.

Individuals with acquired impairments may set very high standards for satisfaction in the performance of tasks that they performed well before becoming disabled. In a study (Taylor & McGruder, 1996) that surveyed the significance of sea kayaking in individuals with spinal cord injuries, one female participant identified its significance in terms of it being a new skill. Because sea kayaking was new to her, she did not have preconceived ideas about how well she should perform. Before injury, she had been a basketball player. Although she had tried wheelchair basketball, she found it extremely dissatisfying because she could not meet her preinjury standards. Hence, she chose to abandon basketball and exchange it for a new sport, sea kayaking, because of the satisfaction it gave her.

When establishing client satisfaction, it is necessary to elicit this objectively from the client. During the evaluation as well as treatment, keep questions open-ended and focused on clients' feelings about task performance. When trying to understand the satisfaction or dissatisfaction that clients experience from tasks, occupational therapy practitioners should refrain from giving their observations about clients' performance as well as their projections about the extent to which performance might be improved through training.

Experience

Information gathered in the evaluation of a client's past and recent experience with a task is important to consider so that relevant and attainable outcomes are established, and effective treatment strategies for attaining them are identified. Recent experience may facilitate progress in reestablishing independence in a task, because the client is learning a new way to do the task, rather than developing a new skill. For example, Mrs. McCarthy needs to relearn cooking skills following a CVA. She uses a wheelchair for mobility and has minimal use of her right, dominant, hand. Her cognitive skills are intact and she can easily follow a recipe. Furthermore, she demonstrates good problem-solving abilities in adapting cooking tasks to improve her performance. Similar to Mrs. McCarthy, Miranda, a 12-year-old girl with spastic hemiplegia caused by cerebral palsy, has limited use of one hand and uses a wheelchair for mobility. She wants to cook simple meals and bake cookies. Her treatment is likely to require more time and guidance than Mrs. McCarthy's treatment, because she has to learn basic cooking skills along with the task adaptations required to compensate for her impairments. At times, adults are also confronted with needing to learn new tasks. Some of these tasks relate to skills needed to manage disability, such as performing self-catheterization, donning pressure garments, or learning to operate an environmental control unit. New learning may also be needed when new roles are assumed; for example, when a spouse becomes disabled or dies and the partner has to take on new responsibilities. Whenever a skill is unfamiliar to clients, additional treatment time and instruction from the occupational therapy practitioner may be needed for basic skill acquisition.

Resources

Established functional outcomes must be achievable within the client's available resources, including social and financial. The social environment is particularly salient to consider when human assistance is needed for the performance of essential ADL. Some families may be able to provide the level and type of assistance needed, wheras other families may be unable or unwilling to do this. When task adaptations or assistive devices are beneficial, the client's ability to pay for them must be appraised. Some task adaptations and assistive devices are expensive and may not be covered by the client's insurance carrier. If the client does not have the financial resources to pay for needed items, treatment outcomes may need to be appropriately adjusted.

Aberrant Task Behaviors

Functional outcomes and treatment must address any aberrant task behaviors that interfere with task performance. Criterion-referenced measures are often the easiest to use when aberrant task behaviors are a problem, because they can include criteria that require the reduction or elimination of the aberrant task behaviors if outcomes are to be reached. Treatment strategies to eliminate such behaviors vary greatly, depending on the nature of the target behavior. Behavior modification techniques may be useful for aberrant behaviors under volitional control, such as stuffing food into the mouth. Unwanted movements, such as athetoid movements, are typically involuntary, and modification of the environment through proper seating and positioning may be required for their reduction or elimination. Exploration of the underlying cause of the aberrant task behavior facilitates the establishment of realistic outcomes and the selection of effective treatment strategies.

Client's Capacity for Learning

The client's capacity for learning must be evaluated because treatment often requires learning new methods of completing tasks (Cahill, 1987). Fewer treatment options exist for clients with limited learning capacity and the duration of treatment may need to be longer. Clients with a good capacity for learning and an openness to alternative methods may be able to address more task deficits because of increased treatment options and the reduced time required for learning. It is important for one to view capacity for learning on a continuum, because clients may fall between the extremes, and capacity may be better for some tasks than for others. A client may be capable of learning the relatively simple task adaptation of using a joystick to drive a wheelchair, but unable to master a more complex environmental control system, even one that relies on the same movements used to control the joystick.

Prognosis for Performance Components

The client's potential for improvement in the performance areas must be examined within the context of any existing disease or abnormalities and resulting performance component deficits (Hansen & Atchison, 1993). First, the practitioner must consider any precautions or contraindications pursuant to the diagnosis that may preclude the use of certain treatment strategies. Compare, for example, two clients whose endurance significantly limits their performance. Mr. Bell has multiple sclerosis, a disorder that may worsen if he becomes overfatigued. An aggressive program to increase endurance is contraindicated for him, so alternative treatment strategies should be explored. Mr. Jones, who sustained multiple injuries in a motor vehicle accident, has had several surgical operations and has been primarily confined to bed for 7 weeks. Although his medical problems have been resolved, he is very deconditioned. A program to extend the limits of his endurance may be an efficient way to increase endurance, thereby enhancing performance of functional tasks.

Second, the prognosis for improvement of performance component deficits given the client's diagnosis (ie, disorder) must be considered. Increasing impairment is expected in progressive disorders, such as Alzheimer's disease, **amyotrophic lateral sclerosis**, and rheumatoid arthritis. Hence, treatment outcomes must be established with these potential declines in mind, so that they are realistic. Occupational therapy practitioners must examine each performance component deficit separately, however, because progressive diseases may not affect all components directly. This point is illustrated by Jonathan, a teenager who has muscular dystrophy. He has significant muscle weakness in the trunk and all four extremities and has developed some limitations in pelvic and ankle range of motion (ROM) that preclude maintaining an optimal position for functioning from his wheelchair. His muscle strength is expected to decline, even with treatment. His ROM deficits, however, are secondary to the muscle weakness, not a direct result of the muscular dystrophy. Treatment gains can be expected in ROM despite the overall prognosis. In turn, increased ROM can enhance function through improved positioning.

Stable or diminishing impairments may be anticipated in many disorders and injuries. Pharmacological treatment, for example, may improve the impairments associated with depression, so that occupational therapy treatment can be focused on transferring gains made in cognitive and psychological performance components into the performance areas. Typically, clients who have had CVAs can expect some spontaneous return of motor function in the early stages of recovery. Projected treatment outcomes take into account the "typical" improvements for this diagnosis.

Time for Intervention

The projected timeline for occupational therapy may be influenced by multiple factors, including the functional prognosis, the client's motivation for improvement, and the client's finances. In managed health care, it is becoming common for health insurance carriers to set the number of visits or length of treatment (DeJong & Sutton, 1995; Johnston, Keith, & Hinderer, 1992). To a considerable extent, the occupational therapy treatment program must be tailored to meet the client's needs as much as possible within the time allotted. Nonetheless, it must also be recognized that best practice takes into account all the client's needs. Often, with clear and complete documentation of adequate progress toward established outcomes, additional occupational therapy visits can be approved by third-party payers. Occupational therapy practitioners need to be aware of their professional responsibility to clients to request treatment extensions and to support these requests through their documentation.

Expected Performance Context: Discharge Setting

Clients' expected discharge environments must be considered when establishing outcomes and selecting treatment that is to be relevant to the environment in which clients will ultimately perform tasks (Dunn, 1993; Dunn, Brown, & McGuigan, 1994; Law et al., 1996, Rogers & Holm, 1989). The human environment is critical for clients who require assistance from others following discharge. Clients' needs vary broadly in terms of the type and duration of assistance required. Some clients need only supportive services, such as help with shopping or housecleaning. Those with significant physical dysfunction and intact cognition may require considerable physical assistance, but can be left alone once they are toileted, bathed, dressed, mobile in their wheelchairs, and have had something to eat. Clients with cognitive deficits generally need little physical assistance, but may need verbal cuing to maintain task performance, and this assistance may need to be constant. Inadequate support in the client's expected environment may necessitate an alteration in the discharge plan.

The physical environment must also be considered in treatment planning (Hagedorn, 1995). For example, Mr. Flora has been progressing with his bathing skills during his hospital-based rehabilitation and is now independent with a bath bench, hand-held shower hose, and a grab bar. The occupational therapy practitioner wants to order this equipment for him. However, Mr. Flora reports that he must shower in a 3 ft by 3 ft shower stall because the only bathtub is on the second floor and he cannot manage stairs. This shower will not accommodate the transfer tub bench he requires for safe transfers and balance during showering. An alternative approach to bathing should have been explored at the beginning of treatment so that Mr. Flora's program focused on developing skills he could use at home, such as sponge bathing at the sink.

The actual adaptability of the discharge environment must also be explored. A house that is high above the street with 21 steps to the front door makes the installation of a properly graded ramp extremely difficult. Wall grab bars cannot be installed on fiberglass tub surrounds, making a safety rail placed on the side of the bathtub the only feasible option, regardless of where the client really needs the most support. Clients living in rental units may be unable to make structural alterations as desired because they do not own the unit.

Lastly, the client's expected discharge environments must be explored if tasks are likely to be performed in more than one place. Clients in a hospital-based setting may be primarily focused on returning home, but most individuals do not confine themselves to a single environment. Hence, at some point, treatment must address performance of tasks across environments. Adaptations for toilets, such as raised toilet seats and toilet armrests, are commonly used for persons with limited mobility. Home adaptations are easily made, but clients may often be in environments that have not been adapted, such as public buildings, friends' homes, airplanes, hotels, and porta-potties at the local fair. If clients are likely to be in these environments, treatment must incorporate the varied features of these environments if independence is to be enhanced.

Projected Follow-Through with Home Program

Efforts to contain health care costs have led to increasingly shorter lengths of stay in hospitals and rehabilitation centers and a reduction in community-based and home care visits. Clients are expected to take a more active role in their therapy programs and to supplement formal treatment with self-directed treatment (eg, home programs). Treatment outcomes, therefore, need to be established with some estimate of the client's capacity to follow through with a self-directed program in mind, as this will greatly influence the success of treatment (Cope & Sundance, 1995).

Several of the task parameters previously delineated can give the occupational therapy practitioner guidance in this area. Clients have more motivation for programs aimed at tasks that they value highly than for those they value less highly, making a client-centered approach critical for success. Additionally, task parameters such as difficulty, fatigue, pain, and satisfaction must be graded so that self-directed programs are manageable within the context of the client's daily routines. "Manageable" must be established by clients in consultation with the occupational therapy practitioner and should take into consideration their daily tasks and responsibilities, tolerance for frustration, and perseverance.

Many clients require some assistance to practice tasks, and the occupational therapy practitioner must be sure that these resources are available. This assistance may include setting up a task, providing assistance for specific task compo-nents, and allowing ample time, as prescribed, for effective practice. It is important to remember that many diseases and disabilities influence the ability to initiate tasks. For these clients, assistance is needed for initiation and follow-through in the home program. This responsibility often falls on family members, and occupational therapy practitioners need to interact with and educate family members for this critical role (DaCunha & Tackenberg, 1989).

▼ TREATMENT IMPLEMENTATION

The selection of specific treatment strategies is largely guided by the frame(s) of reference selected by the occupational therapy practitioner for each client. Specific frames of reference are beyond the scope of this chapter and can be found in Unit VIII. The following section focuses on broader treatment approaches and strategies. It includes a discussion of grading activities to progress clients toward the established outcomes, and it concludes with outlines of treatment strategies for several prototypic functional problems.

Selection of a Treatment Approach

Treatment approaches for limitations in task performance fall into three broad categories: (1) remediation, (2) compensation, and (3) education (Tables 19–1 through 19–9). Frames of reference tend to focus on either remediation or compensation. The biomechanical and sensory integrative frames of reference are remediation approaches because they focus on restoring skills at the performance component level, with the assumption that gains made in performance components will be transferred into performance areas. The rehabilitation frame of reference relies on compensatory techniques to accommodate or compensate for performance component deficits that hinder task performance, and this is a compensatory approach. The remedial and compensatory approaches need to be combined with an educational approach to ensure carryover of the program to functional tasks (Trombly, 1995b).

REMEDIATION (RESTORATIVE OR ESTABLISH)

A remediation approach typically focuses treatment at the performance component level to restore or establish the deficit performance components that are needed for functional tasks (Dunn et al., 1994; Trombly, 1995a). Treatment may be used to restore component skills such as strength, endurance, ROM, short-term memory, visual figure-ground, and interests. More information on specific techniques may be found in the chapters that follow. Regardless of the specific frame of reference or techniques used, however, one must always establish the link between the performance component deficit(s) and the resulting functional task deficits. Careful documentation of the evaluation assists other health professionals and third-party payers to understand the connection between the treatment being given and the established functional outcomes. Clients must also be educated in the relation between performance components and performance areas so that they understand how the treatment will ultimately lead to improved task performance.

All treatment programs designed to restore or establish performance component skills must provide clients with a structured opportunity to transfer the gains made in these skills to relevant functional tasks. This ensures that the treatment outcome is functional, and helps maintain gains made in component skills, by providing an opportunity for practice within the daily routine. For example, treatment resulting in increased right shoulder flexion should be accompanied by functional tasks that require movement into the newly acquired range, such as using the right upper extremity to reach into kitchen cabinets or resuming swimming or yoga practice.

Treatment aimed at remediation is often most efficient for clients for whom a few impairments affect many tasks and for whom performance component deficits can be expected to improve. For example, Mr. Stapinski, has had circumferential second-degree burns to both upper extremities. The resulting bilateral limitations in elbow flexion prevent him from completing most self-care tasks, due to an inability to reach his face, head, or trunk. Tasks can be easily adapted by using long-handled devices, but extended tools would likely be needed for all self-care tasks (eg, eating utensils, toothbrush, comb, brush, bath sponge). Because clients with burns can be expected to increase elbow flexion with exercise and scar management, treatment will be most efficient if it is aimed at increasing ROM. This one performance component gain will enhance function across many different tasks.

A restorative approach may be appropriate for some clients with progressive disorders. The focus with these clients is to slow the decline of specific component skills that are expected to deteriorate, given the typical course of the disease. For example, clients with Parkinson's disease may slow the progression of bradykinesia and difficulty in initiating and ceasing movement through the use of a movement exercise program.

For several performance component deficits, carefully structured tasks can restore or establish component skills while permitting practice of the tasks. Clients who are severely deconditioned may find their activity level limited by poor endurance. For example, treatment could be aerobic exercise to increase cardiopulmonary endurance. This would leave the client unable to participate in functional tasks until an adequate increase in cardiopulmonary capacity was achieved. Instead, treatment that graded the intensity and duration of daily living activities could be as effective in increasing cardiovascular fitness while enabling the client to participate in desired tasks. Additionally, gains made in endurance are immediately transferred into functional tasks.

The nature of the specific performance component that needs remediation warrants attention, for the remediation of some performance components does not result in generalization of the skills to functional tasks. Visual–perceptual skills, such as visual scanning, figure-ground perception, right-left discrimination, and topographical orientation are often treated with "exercises" outside of the context of daily tasks. Few studies have been done to support the efficacy of this approach for improving functional performance (Quintana, 1995). In one study, Ross (1992) examined the effect of computer-based treatment to enhance visual-scanning skills on the ability to locate items on a grocery shelf. She found that clients demonstrated improvement in scanning skills during the computer task, but that these skills did not improve the grocery store scanning task. Higher-level cognitive skills also require practice within the context of a task because clients must learn to interpret and use relevant contextual cues for problem solving, and these cues are task-dependent.

Recent studies in motor learning support the treatment of sensorimotor skills within the context of functional tasks because of the importance of contextual cues and the task-specificity of motor control (Horak, 1991; Mathiowetz & Bass Haugen, 1995; Shumway-Cook & Woollacott, 1995). It is important for tasks to be structured to challenge the client's motor skills, so careful grading of functional tasks is critical. Although some task adaptations may be made to compensate for motor skills the client does not yet possess, it is crucial that the client not compensate for skills he does have. For example, a built-up handled spoon may be used by clients with limited grasp in the dominant hand who could not eat successfully with a regular spoon. Compensation with the uninvolved nondominant hand may facilitate task performance, but would not be consistent with the remediation approach for improving motor control.

Depending on the nature of the performance component deficit and the degree of impairment, the length of treatment needed when using remedial approaches may be longer than that required for compensatory approaches. This increased time must be taken into consideration, particularly in managed care settings. In addition, clients must recognize that the rehabilitation period may be longer and that follow-through with a home program is vital if gains are to be made.

COMPENSATION

Task performance can be enhanced through compensation for performance component deficits, rather than remediation of the deficits themselves. This is often necessary when remediation is not an option; a client with a complete C5 quadriplegia will not regain normal hand function, regardless of the remedial approach used. Compensation for deficits is needed. Even in clients for whom remediation is possible, a compensatory approach may be more appropriate if time limitations or client motivation would lead to less than optimal outcomes. Compensatory strategies may also be war-

(text continues on page 338)

TABLE 19-1. ADL Treatment Approaches and Examples of Treatment Strategies for Task Disabilities Associated With Visual Impairments

Impairment: Low vision, absence of vision, or visual-perceptual impairment
Common pathologies: Macular degeneration, glaucoma, cataracts, diabetic retinopathy, corneal disease, retinitis pigmentosa, stroke, trauma, and congenital blindness

Broad treatment approaches	Remediation	Compensation
Treatment strategies	*Restore/Establish*	*Alter the task method*
ADL tasks: Grooming, oral hygiene, bathing, and showering *Task Disabilities* • Client may walk into open drawers and doors left ajar • Client may have difficulty with sharp objects (eg, razors, fingernails scissors) • Client may have difficulty locating or discerning among bathing, grooming, and oral hygiene task objects • Client may have difficulty applying makeup accurately, or shaving evenly • Client may neglect aspects of task performance not in visual field (eg, one side, peripheral visual field) • Client may experience fatigue and decreased endurance during task performance • Task outcomes may not meet acceptable societal standards • Client may express dissatisfaction with task outcomes • Client may initially demonstrate aberrant task behaviors (eg, spray deodorant on hair)	• Sensory training to enhance tactile sensibility • Establish routines • Develop memory aids (eg, 2 rubber bands indicates the container holds shampoo) • Train client to visually scan through total range (one-sided neglect) • Train client to use peripheral vision • Recommend evaluation by low-vision specialist	• Always close drawers and return doors to open or closed positions immediately after use • Rely on tactile cues in addition, or in lieu of, visual cues • Store task objects in the same place • Adhere to routines and patterns that make grooming, hygiene, and bathing tasks more efficient • Use only the level of assistance that is needed; do not remove the client's right to participate in the task if it is not harmful • Do not rush the task • Simplify hairstyle • Use electric razor • Grow beard • Simplify makeup • Use clippers
ADL task: Toileting *Task Disabilities* • Client may walk into open drawers, and doors left ajar • Client may have difficulty positioning self onto toilet seat • Client may have difficulty determining if cleansing is adequate after a bowel movement • Task outcomes may not meet acceptable societal standards (eg, fecal matter on cuff of sleeve after cleansing) • Client may initially demonstrate aberrant task behaviors (eg, inadequate cleansing of hands after toileting)	• Sensory training	• Replenish supplies on a routine basis • Use toilet paper, moistened wipes, and then toilet paper to ensure adequate cleansing after a bowel movement

Compensation		Education	Sample Target Outcomes
Adapt task objects *Assistive devices*	*Adapt the task environment*	*Client/Caregiver Education*	

• Replace overhead incandescent lights with fluorescent lights
 • Label like containers with large black letters for easier identification by those with low vision, or with tactile labels (eg, raised print letters, braille, or special glue dots) for those without vision
 • Use pump-action containers of different shapes for soap, toothpaste, and shampoo
 • Use plastic tape of a contrasting color to the countertop to mark small items (eg, clippers), so that they are easier to see
 • Float bright-colored object in tub to see water height
 • Use soap-on-a-rope
	• Increase the amount of light available (eg, fluorescent lights overhead, incandescent lights or halogen lights for near tasks related to grooming)
	 • Decrease glare with amber tint on overhead light fixture or by installing a dimmer switch in the bathroom
	 • Keep task materials in the same place on the counter and keep materials for like tasks together (eg, caddy)
	 • Install tap water overflow alarm
	 • Mount magnifying mirror on wall with an extension arm
	 • Reset water temperature below 120°F
	 • Install wall-to-wall or indoor–outdoor carpeting in bathroom to prevent slipping on spills that cannot be seen
	 • Install grab bars around tub or shower
	 • Place contrasting bathmat over tub edge to increase its visibility
	 • Use nonskid mat of contrasting color so foot placement is accurate
		• Instruct family members about the necessity of closing drawers/opening doors, and returning task objects to a designated place
		 • Demonstrate restorative/adaptive strategies (eg, sample marking systems for memory aids), and have client do a return demonstration
		 • Provide a handout or other resources with drawings or pictures of the strategies (eg, suggestions for lighting) as well as directions and a number to call for assistance
		 • Provide a videotape of suggested treatment strategies, with the client as the subject, if possible, and the practitioner demonstrating the caregiver's role, if applicable
			• Increased level of independence
			 • Improved safety
			 • Improved adequacy of performance, as indicated by
			   Decreased difficulty
			   Decreased fatigue
			   Increased task endurance
			   Increased approximation to acceptable societal standards for task performance
			   Increased satisfaction
			   Decrease in aberrant task behaviors

• Use color-contrasting tissue	• Provide storage space for toilet paper and moistened wipes within arm's reach if seated on the toilet
	 • Use color-contrasting toilet seat
	 • Toilet seat frame with arms if client also has difficulty lowering or raising self or has balance problems
		• Instruct family members about the necessity of closing drawers/opening doors, and returning task objects to a designated place (eg, supplies)
		 • Provide a handout with enlarged drawings or pictures of the technique or adaptations, as well as sequential directions and a number to call for assistance
		 • Provide an audiotape of suggestions that the client can listen to, including telephone numbers for vendors and items numbers for any assistive equipment (eg, toilet frame with arms)
			• Increased level of independence
			 • Improved safety
			 • Improved adequacy of performance, as indicated by
			   Decreased difficulty
			   Increased approximation to acceptable societal standards for task performance
			   Decrease in aberrant task behaviors

(continued)

TABLE 19-1. (Continued)

Broad treatment approaches	Remediation	Compensation
Treatment strategies	*Restore/Establish*	*Alter the task method*
ADL task: Dressing *Task Disabilities* • Client may have difficulty selecting clothing that matches • Client may walk into open drawers, and doors left ajar • Client may experience fatigue and decreased endurance during task performance • Task outcomes may not meet acceptable societal standards (eg, client may not see stains on front of work clothing) • Client may express dissatisfaction with task outcomes (eg, client may have difficulty differentiating like outfits of different colors) • Client may initially demonstrate aberrant task behaviors (eg, not notice necktie is label-side out)	• Sensory training • Establish routines • Develop behavioral memory aids • Recommend evaluation by low-vision specialist	• Hang "go-together" outfits on the same hanger, or on adjacent hangers with clothes pins connecting them • Ask another person to spot check clothing for stains on a routine basis
ADL tasks: Feeding and Eating *Task Disabilities* • Client may not know what is on the plate if someone else has served the food • Task outcomes may not meet acceptable societal standards (eg, client may bump and spill items when reaching) • Client may initially demonstrate aberrant task behaviors (eg, spoon sugar onto table instead of coffee cup)	• Sensory training • Develop behavioral memory aids	• Place food groups in the same place on the plate consistently • Use systematic approach to the arrangement and placement of food and tableware • Use the "clock" method to identify where food is located if serving the client, and the same method if client is serving self
ADL task: Medication management routine *Task Disabilities* • Client may not be able to see directions on medication container • Client may have difficulty determining time for taking medication • Client may have difficulty telling pills apart if they are spilled, or out of the container • Client may demonstrate unsafe aberrant task behaviors (eg, distribute wrong medication into organizer)	• Sensory training • Develop behavioral memory aids	• Organize medications so that they are always in the same place (eg, alphabetical order) • Organize medicine cabinet so other health supplies and over-the-counter medications are always in the same place • Use medication syringe for liquids instead of spoon for both client and caregiver administration

Compensation		Education	Sample Target Outcomes
Adapt task objects **Assistive devices**	**Adapt the task environment**	**Client/Caregiver Education**	

• Keep upper body clothing buttoned except at the neck, for easier one-step overhead donning as well as ease of keeping them on hangers
• Use washable textile puff paints to put color system dots or letters on clothing items
	• Have client arrange drawers, closets, and cupboards based on own system, so that it is logical for the client
	• Install automatic, or pull-chain wall lights inside closets and cupboards in a position that casts the least amount of shadows or glare
		• Instruct family members about the necessity of closing drawers/opening doors, and returning task objects to a designated place (eg, clothing after laundering)
		• Help client decide on a memory aid system that will work to distinguish among like clothing items, etc.
		• Provide an audiotape of suggested organization strategies and memory aids that the client may find helpful, as well as a number to call for assistance
			• Increased level of independence
			• Improved safety
			• Improved adequacy of performance, as indicated by
			  Decreased difficulty
			  Decreased fatigue
			  Increased task endurance
			  Increased approximation to acceptable societal standards for task performance
			  Increased satisfaction
			  Decrease in aberrant task behaviors

• Use contrasting dinnerware if the food is primarily light or dark in color
• Use small separate dishes for food items
	• Set the table consistently, with glasses, cups, and other spillable items always located in the same place	• Demonstrate restorative/adaptive strategies (eg, clock method), and have client/caregiver do a return demonstration
		• Provide a handout with enlarged drawings or pictures of the technique (eg, suggested position of tableware to avoid bumping, spilling) or adaptations as well as sequential directions and a number to call for assistance
		• Provide an audiotape of suggested adaptations
			• Increased level of independence
			• Improved adequacy of performance, as indicated by
			  Decreased difficulty
			  Increased approximation to acceptable societal standards for task performance
			  Decrease in aberrant task behaviors

• Have pharmacist put only non–child-proof lids on pill bottles
• Use a medication organizer, acceptable to the client, for chronic condition medications and distribute them into organizer on the first or last day of the month
• Use Daytimer™ appointment alarm to signal medication schedule (can set up to 31 alarms per day)
• Label pill bottle with a black marker and a single large letter for easy identification (eg, P for Prozac™)
	• Place medications out in a logical place where they are easy to retrieve at the time they are to be taken (eg, kitchen counter, bedside table) if client is responsible for medication management	• Demonstrate medication management routines and have client/caregiver do a return demonstration
		• Provide audiotape with adaptive strategies
			• Increased level of independence
			• Improved safety
			• Improved adequacy of performance, as indicated by
			  Decreased difficulty
			  Decrease in aberrant task behaviors

(continued)

TABLE 19-1. (Continued)

Broad treatment approaches	Remediation	Compensation
Treatment strategies	*Restore/Establish*	*Alter the task method*
ADL task: Functional mobility *Task Disabilities* • Client may walk into open drawers, and doors left ajar • Client may be unsafe when ambulating (eg, unable to avoid clutter left in traffic areas or on stairs) • Client may be unsafe at top and bottom of stairs • Client may experience fatigue and decreased endurance • Client may be unable to find way around home or community • Client may express dissatisfaction with task performance • Client may demonstrate aberrant and unsafe behaviors during task performance (eg, bump into things, hesitant gait, walk into wrong room, walk wrong direction, become disoriented)	• Sensory training • Develop behavioral memory aids • Recommend evaluation by mobility specialist for individuals with low or no vision	• Have client wear sturdy, low, and broad-heeled shoes if gait is unsteady • Have client walk next to and slightly behind caregiver, holding onto caregiver's elbow (especially in the community or on uneven ground) • Have caregiver accompany client until way-finding is mastered

ranted when some, but not full, remediation is achieved. Generally, compensatory strategies require less treatment time for achieving functional outcomes compared with remediation strategies.

Three treatment strategies may be employed in the compensatory approach. The task method may be altered, the task objects may be adapted, or the environment may be adapted (see Tables 19–1 through 19–9). Combinations of these methods may be used to maximize client performance.

Alter the Task Method

When the task method is altered, the same task objects are used in the same environment, but the method of performing the task is altered to make the task feasible given the performance deficits. Many one-handed techniques for tasks that are normally done with two hands use this strategy, including one-handed dressing, one-handed shoe tying (Fig. 19–1), and one-handed typing techniques. To successfully master an altered task method, clients require learning capability. The level of learning capability required depends on the complexity of the method that is to be learned. Practice is a necessary component of learning, so good follow-

through with a training program is needed to meet adequacy parameters, such as difficulty, satisfaction, and duration. Lengthy practice is required if the desired outcome is habituation of the skill for routine performance.

Adapt the Task Objects or Prescribe Assistive Devices

The objects used for the task may be altered to facilitate performance, for example, built-up handled utensils may be used for clients with decreased finger ROM. For many tasks, adaptation of the task objects does not significantly alter the task method, so the need for learning is less than when the method is altered. When this is the case, the need for practice is reduced. Examples of simple adaptations include utensils with enlarged or extended handles, a cutting board with nails to stabilize food while cutting, and elastic shoe laces. The prescription of assistive devices must simultaneously take into account the client's capabilities and the features of the device. The proliferation of assistive devices, however, has not been accompanied by a corresponding proliferation of good information about the features of the devices, including weight of the model and exact dimensions (Rogers & Holm, 1991). The prescription of an assistive device is frequently

Compensation		Education	Sample Target Outcomes
Adapt task objects *Assistive devices*	*Adapt the task environment*	*Client/Caregiver Education*	

• Use cane holder to keep cane near and easy to locate (eg, for client with low-vision and mobility impairment)
 • Use tape of contrast color to make cane easy to locate (eg, for client with low-vision and mobility impairment)
	• Locate furniture that can be used as a tactile guide near natural traffic routes
	 • Remove low coffee tables
	 • Repair walking surfaces so they are even and remove tripping hazards
	 • Provide a lighted pathway from bedroom to bathroom (eg, night light) so client does not need to turn on/off a bright light and wait for eyes to accommodate
	 • Make stairways safe
	    Sturdy handrails on both sides
	    Uniform stair height and tread widths
	    Clearly discernible tread edges
	    Top and bottom landings marked with a different color or surface
	 • Add lighting to area at top and bottom of stairways
		• Instruct family members about the necessity of closing drawers/opening doors, returning furniture to a designated place, and keeping traffic areas free of clutter
		 • Provide a catalog with relevant assistive devices marked
		 • Provide handouts with enlarged drawings or pictures of the technique or adaptations (eg, stair safety guidelines) and a number to call for assistance
		 • Provide an audiotape of suggested adaptations
			• Increased level of independence
			 • Improved safety
			 • Improved adequacy of performance, as indicated by
			    Decreased difficulty
			    Decreased fatigue
			    Increased task endurance
			    Increased satisfaction
			    Decrease in aberrant task behaviors

oversimplified. Figure 19–2 (see p. 362) emphasizes the complexity of the decision–making process by highlighting the potential decisions involved in prescribing an adapted spoon. Although many assistive devices prescribed by occupational therapy practitioners are quite simple mechanically, some are very sophisticated and include complex electronics, circuits, and microprocessors, such as environmental control units that interact with smart houses.

Just as the prescription of assistive devices seems deceptively simple, so do task adaptations. Some task adaptations, however, significantly alter task performance, and they require consider– *(text continues on page 347)*

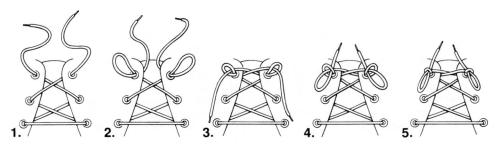

1. Lace laces in usual way.
2. Put both lace ends back through the holes they exited until the loops formed are small.
3. Put the lace ends through the opposite loops and pull to tighten loops, allowing just enough room to put the lace end back through the loop.
4. Put lace ends back through the loops, forming another loop.
5. Pull on these loops alternately to tighten.

▶

Figure 19-1. One-handed shoe-tying method. (From Jan Davis, OTR, NDT, Certification Course, 1977, Harmarsville, PA.)

TABLE 19-2. ADL Treatment Approaches and Examples of Treatment Strategies for Task Disabilities Associated With Unilateral Impairments

Impairment: One upper extremity or one upper extremity and lower extremity (one body side) passive and active range-of-motion (ROM) or strength impairment, with or without sensory loss

Common pathologies: Cerebrovascular accident, traumatic brain injury, unilateral amputation, cerebral palsy (hemiplegia), peripheral nerve injury, tendon laceration

Broad treatment approaches	Remediation	Compensation
Specific treatment strategies	*Restore/Establish*	*Alter the task method*
ADL tasks: Grooming, oral hygiene, bathing, and showering *Task Disabilities* • Client may be unable to reach, hold, manipulate, adjust, open, or close task objects that require the use of both hands, or bilateral coordination, thus preventing task initiation, continuation, or completion • Client may be unable to sustain grooming or oral hygiene actions long enough to complete tasks adequately (eg, decreased endurance) • Task performance may be unsafe (eg, tub transfers, use of a straight-edge razor with non-dominant hand) • Client may experience pain, fatigue, or lack of satisfaction with task performance • Task outcomes may not meet acceptable societal standards	• Passive ROM • Active assistive, active, or resistive exercises for strengthening • Continuous passive motion • Inhibitory or facilitatory treatment • Motor learning • Transfer of dominance training • Splinting • Casting • Desensitization program • Sensory reeducation • Prosthetic training	• Use unaffected extremity to assist or compensate for affected or missing extremity • Use affected extremity to stabilize objects, unaffected extremity to manipulate objects • Use mouth to stabilize or open containers • Stabilize task objects on nonskid surfaces or on towels • Stabilize task objects between knees • Rest elbow of affected extremity on counter edge so unaffected hand is free to apply deodorant, shave armpit • Use electric razor • Simplify hairstyle • Use a beauty salon • Grow a beard
ADL task: Toileting *Task Disabilities* • Client may be unable to lower self, raise self, or transfer onto a toilet safely • Client may have difficulty doffing and donning clothing associated with toileting • Client may be unstable (ie, unsafe) when reaching for toilet paper or reaching to cleanse • Client may have difficulty manipulating toilet paper roll, or separating paper from roll • Client may experience pain or fatigue during task performance	• Postural stability • Weight shifting exercises • Balance exercises • Transfer of dominance training • Motor learning • Passive ROM • Active assistive, active, or resistive exercises for strengthening • Inhibitory or facilitatory treatment • Motor learning	• Use unaffected upper extremity to assist or compensate for affected or missing extremity • Use extra-wide base of support to prevent slacks, underpants from dropping to floor • Position head against wall to maintain balance while pulling up clothing with one hand • Wrap end of toilet paper stream around dispenser edge or nearby towel rack to make it easier to rip off paper • Maintain extra-broad base of support while seated on toilet to prevent imbalance or falls while reaching for toilet paper for cleansing self

Compensation		Education	Sample Target Outcomes
Adapt task objects **Assistive devices**	**Adapt the task environment**	**Client/Caregiver Education**	

• Use pump-action containers for soap, toothpaste, and shampoo
• Use suction devices to hold soap in place
• Use suction brushes for nails and dentures
• Use soap-on-a-rope or make it by dropping soap into an old nylon and securing it to shower head or faucet
• Stabilize fingernail clipper to board, and extend lever arm of clipper for easier use with one hand
• Fliptop lipsticks
• Use mirror that can be hung around neck
	• Clear a shelf or counter so that all items for each task can be stored on counter or shelf in a basket or plastic container that can be transported to the task site with one hand (eg, handle over forearm)
	• Remove a cupboard door for easier access
	• Make space for a stool or chair near a counter so that surfaces (counter, lap) can be used
	• Mount the hairdryer on the wall so that it does not have to be held
	• Install mirror with extension arm on wall
	• Install grab bars around tub/shower area for safety and stability when entering and exiting or turning
	• Install a bath bench that extends over the tub edge for safer transfers
	• Install a shower caddy for holding items
	• Install a hand-held flexible shower hose with an on/off switch that can be controlled at the shower head
		• Demonstrate restorative strategies (eg, self-ranging, passive ROM by caregiver before grooming, bathing, etc.), and have client/caregiver do a return demonstration
		• Demonstrate adapted methods and have client/caregiver do a return demonstration
		• Demonstrate proper use of adapted task objects and have client/caregiver do a return demonstration
		• Provide a handout with drawings or pictures of the strategies or adaptations as well as sequential directions and a number to call for assistance
		• Provide a videotape of suggested treatment strategies, with the client as the subject, if possible, and the practitioner demonstrating the caregiver's role
		• Teach caregiver how to compensate for client's loss of protective sensibility
			• Increased level of independence
			• Improved safety
			• Improved adequacy of performance, as indicated by
			    Decreased difficulty
			    Decreased pain
			    Decreased fatigue
			    Increased task endurance
			    Increased approximation to acceptable standards for task performance
			    Increased satisfaction

• Substitute a free-standing toilet roll holder that positions the roll vertically rather than horizontally
• Put tissue in a basket next to the toilet instead of toilet paper on a roll
• Use reacher to get clothes up from the floor
• Attach suspender to slacks on affected side to bring lower body clothing up while coming to stand and while securing fasteners
• Use slacks with elastic in the waist band or with hook closures for easier manipulation with one hand
	• Install grab bars for raising and lowering from toilet if stability is a problem
	• Install floor-to-ceiling pole for transfer, as well as to lean into while adjusting clothing with one hand (see Fig. 19-3)
	• Install waist-high bar that client can lean into while doffing and donning clothing
	• Install commode at bedside for night use
	• Place urinal next to bed for night use
		• Demonstrate restorative strategies (eg, weight-shifting exercises, balance exercises), and have client/caregiver do a return demonstration
		• Demonstrate adapted methods and have client/caregiver do a return demonstration (eg, positioning and repositioning the wheelchair by the toilet)
		• Demonstrate proper use of adapted task objects and assistive devices and have client/caregiver do a return demonstration
			• Increased level of independence
			• Improved safety
			• Improved adequacy of performance, as indicated by
			    Decreased difficulty
			    Decreased pain
			    Decreased fatigue
			    Increased task endurance

(continued)

TABLE 19-2. (Continued)

Broad treatment approaches	Remediation	Compensation
Specific treatment strategies	*Restore/Establish*	*Alter the task method*

ADL task: Dressing
Task Disabilities

• Client may be unsafe during task performance (eg, unable to simultaneously maintain balance and reach or manipulate task items) • Client may have difficulty donning and doffing clothing items on unaffected side • Client may be unstable when reaching to don or doff lower body clothing items • Client may have difficulty manipulating and securing fasteners • Client may be unable to tie laces on shoes • Client may experience pain or fatigue during task performance • Client may express lack of satisfaction with results of task performance or time necessary to complete task performance • Task outcomes may not meet acceptable societal standards (eg, fasteners not secured) • Client may demonstrate aberrant task behaviors (eg, tries to dress only unaffected side)	• Passive ROM • Active assistive, active, or resistive exercises for strengthening • Continuous passive motion • Inhibitory or facilitatory treatment • Motor learning • Transfer of dominance training • Splinting • Casting • Desensitization program • Sensory reeducation • Prosthetic training	• Use unaffected upper extremity to assist or compensate for affected or missing extremity • Don and doff clothing using methods suggested in Tables 19-3–19-5 • Sit on bed with pillows on either side for added stability when dressing • Lie on bed to don lower body garments and bridge using unaffected lower extremity to pull up garments • Lie on bed to don lower body garments and roll from side to side while pulling up • Use extra-wide base of support to prevent slacks, underpants from dropping to floor while donning in a standing position • Position head against wall, if unsteady when standing, to achieve stability while pulling up clothing with one hand • Use one-handed shoe-tying method

ADL tasks: Feeding and Eating
Task Disabilities

• Client may have difficulty swallowing liquids and solids • Client may aspirate liquids and solids • Client may have difficulty cutting food • Client may have difficulty scooping up food • Client may experience pain, fatigue, and inadequate endurance to complete task performance • Task performance may not meet societal standards (eg, client may drool) • Client may express lack of satisfaction with task performance (eg, food does not taste good, takes too much effort to eat)	• Oral motor stimulation • Recommend a swallowing evaluation • Fine-motor dexterity exercises for nondominant hand • Transfer of dominance training • Motor learning • Sensory reeducation	• Position the client with chin slightly tucked, trunk aligned and upright, hips and knees and ankles flexed at 90°, and feet supported • Use unaffected upper extremity to assist or compensate for affected or missing extremity • Support affected extremity • Have caregiver cut food • Prepare food of optimal consistency (eg, thickened; cold versus room temperature; ground beef versus steak)

Compensation		Education	Sample Target Outcomes
Adapt task objects *Assistive devices*	*Adapt the task environment*	*Client/Caregiver Education*	
		• Provide a handout with drawings or pictures of the technique or adaptations as well as sequential directions and a number to call for assistance • Provide a catalog with relevant assistive devices • Provide a videotape of suggested treatment strategies, with the client as the subject, if possible, and the practitioner demonstrating the caregiver's role	

• Keep upper body clothing buttoned except at the neck, for easier overhead donning
• Use elastic on buttoned cuffs to allow hands to move through easily
• Use button hook with suction at end for buttons on sleeve on unaffected side
• Trap button hook in drawer or between knees for stability while using it to button sleeve on unaffected side
• Use reacher to get clothes up from the floor or to pull on pant loops
• Attach suspender to slacks on affected side to bring lower body clothing up, while coming to stand and while securing fasteners
• Use slacks with elastic in the waist band or with hook closures for easier manipulation
• Use clothing items that stretch (eg, knits)
• Elastic shoelaces or shoes with Velcro™ closures
	• Place stable chair with arms near bed to use for dressing
	• Install floor-to-ceiling pole by the bed to transfer, as well as to lean into while adjusting clothing with one hand
		• Demonstrate restorative techniques (eg, weight-shifting exercises), and have client/caregiver do a return demonstration
		• Demonstrate adapted dressing methods and have client/caregiver do a return demonstration
		• Demonstrate proper use of adapted task objects and assistive devices and have client/caregiver do a return demonstration
		• Provide a handout with drawings or pictures of the technique (eg, one-handed shoe-tying method) or adaptation as well as sequential directions and a number to call for assistance
		• Provide a catalog with relevant assistive devices
		• Provide a videotape of suggested treatment strategies, with the client as the subject, if possible, and the practitioner demonstrating the caregiver's role
			• Increased level of independence
			• Improved safety
			• Improved adequacy of performance, as indicated by
			  Decreased difficulty
			  Decreased pain
			  Decreased fatigue
			  Increased task endurance
			  Increased approximation to acceptable societal standards for task performance
			  Increased satisfaction
			  Decrease in aberrant task behaviors

• Add Thickit™ or similar thickening agent to liquids
• Change food consistency so that a bolus is easily formed
• Provide straw for liquids to enable easy handling of liquids in an upright position
• Use Knifork with unaffected side
• Use rocker knife
• Use plate guard, soup bowl, or plate with raised edge to enable easier scooping
	• Provide stable chair that accommodates positioning devices
	• Adjust table height to accommodate wheelchair
	• Install wall-mounted jar opener
	• Install jar opener under cupboard
		• Demonstrate restorative techniques (eg, stimulation of the tongue), and have client/caregiver do a return demonstration
		• Demonstrate feeding methods and have client/caregiver do a return demonstration (eg, to ensure that caregiver is not using "bird"-feeding techniques
		• Demonstrate proper use of adapted task objects and assistive devices and have client/caregiver do a return demonstration
			• Increased level of independence
			• Improved safety
			• Improved adequacy of performance, as indicated by
			  Decreased difficulty
			  Decreased pain
			  Decreased fatigue
			  Increased task endurance
			  Increased approximation to acceptable societal standards for task performance
			  Increased satisfaction

(continued)

TABLE 19-2. (Continued)

Broad treatment approaches	Remediation	Compensation
Specific treatment strategies	*Restore/Establish*	*Alter the task method*
• Client may initially demonstrate aberrant task behaviors (eg, food may accumulate in cheek of affected side)		

ADL task: Medication management routine
Task Disabilities

• Client may have difficulty opening pill bottles, removing lids from liquid medication containers, and removing pills from medication organizer compartments • Client may have difficulty opening medication patch packaging, and separating patch from protective liner • Client may have difficulty pouring liquid medication onto a spoon without spilling • Client may express dissatisfaction with task performance (eg, time needed to complete task; number of errors made)	• Fine-motor dexterity exercises for non-dominant hand • Transfer of dominance training • Active assistive, active, or resistive exercises for strengthening • Inhibitory or facilitatory treatment • Motor learning • Prosthetic training	• Use unaffected extremity to assist or compensate for affected or missing extremity • Stabilize bottles on nonskid surfaces or between knees to open lids • Use medication syringe for liquids instead of spoon • Sort medications into nut cups that can be easily picked up and emptied

ADL task: Functional mobility
Task Disabilities

• Client may be unable to move safely, efficiently, or without difficulty or pain during
  • Bed mobility
  • Wheelchair transfers to/from
    Bed
    Toilet
    Bathtub bench
    Easy chair
    Car
• Client may be unable to transfer objects while ambulating
• Client may be unable to manipulate objects while standing
• Client may experience pain, fatigue, and inadequate endurance for task performance (eg, transferring in and out of bathtub)
• Client may experience dissatisfaction with performance (eg, "feels unsteady or unsafe")
• Client may demonstrate aberrant task behaviors (eg, forget to lock knee before beginning to ambulate)
	• Postural control exercises
	• Weight-shifting exercises
	• Balance exercises
	• Active assistive, active, or resistive exercises for strengthening
	• Inhibitory or facilitatory treatment
	• Motor learning
	• Transfer of dominance training
		• Standing pivot transfer
		• Standing pivot transfer with assistance
		• Bobath transfers

Compensation		Education	Sample Target Outcomes
Adapt task objects *Assistive devices*	*Adapt the task environment*	*Client/Caregiver Education*	
• Place nonslip placemat under plate to prevent the plate from moving, or consider dishes with nonslip surfaces underneath • Provide lap board for wheelchair • Consider suspension sling for affected extremity to remove the effect of gravity		• Provide a handout with drawings or pictures of the technique (eg, suggested position of tableware to avoid bumping, spilling) or adaptations as well as sequential directions and a number to call for assistance • Provide a catalog with relevant assistive devices marked • Provide a videotape of suggested treatment strategies, with the client as the subject, if possible, and the practitioner demonstrating the caregiver's role (eg, positioning client who needs to be fed)	Decrease in aberrant task behaviors
• Have pharmacist put only non–child-proof lids on pill bottles • Put liquid medicine into a squeeze bottle and relabel the squeeze bottle • Use rubber circle to increase resistance on liquid medicine bottles • Stabilize liquid medicine bottle between knees and use jar opener • Use Daytimer™ appointment alarm to signal medication schedule (can set up to 31 alarms per day)	• Place medications out in a logical place where they will be constantly noticed and easy to access (eg, kitchen counter) if client is responsible for medication management • Install wall-mounted jar opener • Install jar opener under cupboard	• Demonstrate one-handed methods for manipulating containers and bottles and have client/caregiver do a return demonstration • Demonstrate proper use of adapted task objects and assistive devices and have client/caregiver do a return demonstration • Provide a catalog with relevant assistive devices marked	• Increased level of independence • Improved safety • Improved adequacy of performance, as indicated by Decreased difficulty
• Insert rail on one side of bed so client can use it to pull against when positioning self in bed, lowering into and raising up from bed • Attach overhead trapeze bar on bed • Use denser foam cushion in wheelchair to raise the seat for easier transfers • Use a portable dense foam cushion to place in easy chairs to make them the same height as the wheelchair • Use plastic garbage sacks on car seats to ease shifting and turning • Use a wheeled cart to transport task objects if ambulatory • Use a walker bag or tray to transport task objects • Use a wheelchair bag or lapboard to transport task objects	• Ensure that the distance from the floor to all surfaces for transfers (toilet seat, tub bench, easy chair, etc.) is no greater than the distance between the floor and 2 in. below the midpoint of the client's patella when client is seated • Install grab bars by toilet and in tub area as needed • Install floor-to-ceiling pole by bed on client's unaffected side	• Demonstrate restorative techniques and have client/caregiver do a return demonstration • Demonstrate proper use of adapted task objects and assistive devices (eg, bed rail) and have client/caregiver do a return demonstration • Provide a catalog with relevant assistive devices marked • Provide handouts with drawings or pictures of the technique or adaptations as well as sequential directions and a number to call for assistance • Provide a videotape of suggested treatment strategies (eg, use of floor-to-ceiling pole, car transfers), with the client as the subject, if possible, and the practitioner demonstrating the caregiver's role	• Increased level of independence • Improved safety • Improved adequacy of performance, as indicated by Decreased difficulty Decreased pain Decreased fatigue Increased task endurance Increased satisfaction Decrease in aberrant task behaviors

TABLE 19-3. Alternative Methods of Putting on and Taking Off Upper Body Clothing for Clients With Impairments in Passive and Active Range of Motion in Upper Extremities

Method 1

1. Place shirt (over-head or cardigan) face down on lap, with sleeves and collar near knees.
2. Slide arms through shirt into sleeves, and push sleeves over elbows.
3. Gather shirt back and lift over head (may rest elbows on knees or table and bend head down to push through shirt collar).
4. Protract and retract and elevate and depress shoulders to get shirt over shoulders, or push shirt over one shoulder, then the other, with opposite upper extremity.
5. Retract shoulder while leaning forward slightly to get shirt down in back.
6. Pull shirt front panels near bottom to straighten and bring down fully (cardigans).
7. Place hands inside shirt front and pull slightly away from body, down and toward sides, to bring shirt down fully (over-head clothing).
8. To remove garment over head, place hand inside shirt toward opposite sleeve, and pull sleeve opening over elbow. Repeat for other sleeve and remove over head.
9. To remove cardigan garment, push collar area back over shoulders, extend upper extremity, and retract shoulders to help sleeve drop below elbow, pull arm from sleeve. *Or,* push one sleeve off shoulder, reach opposite upper extremity to sleeve hole, and hold while elevating shoulder, extending arm and flexing elbow to remove arm from sleeve. Then, pull shirt around back to other side with arm still in sleeve and slide arm out.
10. Unbutton using hand to stabilize shirt against body and thumb or knuckle to push button through hole while opposite thumb pushes fabric up over bottom.

Method 2

This method is available for patients with good trunk and lower extremity mobility, but limited upper extremity strength and or range of motion (eg, upper-extremity amputees, burn patients).

1. Place cardigan garment face up on bed.
2. Place one upper extremity in sleeve, and lie down using friction of shirt against bed to hold garment while sliding arm in.
3. Once one arm is all the way in and collar is up over shoulder, start other arm in sleeve and sit up to work arm into sleeve (garment must be loose for this method).

Method 3

This method is for use with over-head clothing.
1. Put head through neck hole first.
2. Place hand in sleeve, and push arm all the way into sleeve.

TABLE 19-4. Alternative Methods of Putting on and Taking Off Upper Body Clothing for Clients With Impairments of One Upper Extremity or Body Side

Method 1

1. Place cardigan garment on lap with front up, collar toward knees, and affected side sleeve opening exposed between legs.
2. Place affected upper extremity into sleeve, leaning forward to drop into sleeve as far as possible.
3. Pull sleeve up arm, at least above the elbow.
4. With unaffected hand, grasp collar and sleeve that are to be put on that side.
5. Lift unaffected arm over head, pulling shirt around back.
6. While pulling shirt around back, slip unaffected arm in sleeve, letting shirt fall onto arm, and pushing arm into sleeve as shirt is pulled around.

Method 2

1. Place cardigan garment on lap with front up, collar near thighs, and sleeve opening of affected side exposed between legs.
2. Place affected upper extremity in sleeve opening, leaning forward to drop it in as far as possible.
3. Pull sleeve up affected arm, at least above elbow, preferably up to axilla.
4. Place unaffected upper extremity in its sleeve.
5. Grasp collar, gather up back material, and lift over head.

Method 3

This method is used for over-head clothing.
1. Place shirt collar down on lap, and open bottom of shirt to expose sleeve openings.
2. Place affected upper extremity in its sleeve opening, and pull garment on to above elbow.
3. Place unaffected upper extremity in its sleeve opening.
4. Grasp back collar, gather back fabric with unaffected upper extremity, and lift over head.

Removing Cardigan Garment

1. Pull fabric toward unaffected side to make it as loose as possible.
2. Grasp unaffected side of unbuttoned cardigan garment, reach back and to the side to get it off shoulder, then pull it down and wriggle elbow out of shirt. *Or,* grasp sleeve of unaffected side with that hand, and gradually pull it down until elbow can be worked out of sleeve.
3. Pull fabric to affected side, and remove affected upper extremity.

Removing Over-head Garment

1. Pull fabric toward unaffected side to loosen.
2. Pull bottom of shirt on unaffected side down, squeeze elbow through sleeve hole, and remove unaffected upper extremity from sleeve.
3. Gather fabric, and grasp collar to lift garment over head. *Or,* grasp collar near nape of neck, gather back fabric with hand, and pull back over head.
4. Remove unaffected upper extremity from sleeve.
5. Remove sleeve from affected upper extremity.

TABLE 19-5. Alternative Methods of Putting on and Taking Off Clothing for Clients With Impairments of One Upper Extremity or Body Side

Putting on Clothing

1. Sit on bed at side or in chair or wheelchair that allows feet to be firmly positioned on the floor. Sitting on bed is preferable if unable to stand to pull up pants because patient can lie back down in bed to roll and pull pants over hips.
2. Cross affected leg over nonaffected leg.
3. Place garment over foot, and pull up to or over knee, making sure foot is through bottom of leg opening.
4. Replace foot on floor.
5. Hold garment near waist with unaffected upper extremity, and reach down to allow lifting of unaffected lower extremity into opening.
6. Pull garment up over thighs as far as possible while sitting.
7. Use affected upper extremity if possible to hold pants up while coming to stand, or hold pant waist with unaffected hand while using affected upper extremity as support while coming to stand.
8. Stand to pull pants over hips, leaning against wall, bed, or other stable object if necessary.
9. Attach fasteners while standing because clothing is looser if this can be done safely; if not, wear looser clothing and fasten while sitting.

Removing Clothing

1. Unfasten in seated position.
2. Allow garment to drop from hips while coming to stand.
3. Remove unaffected leg first, then affected leg by letting garment drop to floor and lifting affected leg out while holding garment on floor with unaffected leg, or by crossing affected leg over unaffected leg.

Putting on Socks and Shoes

1. Put on loose socks by putting unaffected hand in sock opening and spreading fingers to start sock over toes.
2. Place affected foot on a footstool or lift to the opposite knee to stabilize it during sock donning.
3. Once socks are over the toes, pull up using the unaffected upper extremity.
4. Put shoes on the unaffected side without adaptation.
5. Put shoes on the affected side by lifting the foot to the opposite knee or crossing the affected leg over the nonaffected leg, then using the nonaffected upper extremity to place the shoe on the foot. Some shoes may be able to be put on the affected lower extremity by placing the shoe on the floor and lifting the foot into the shoe, then pushing on the affected knee to push the heel into the shoe.

Putting on and Taking off Angle–Foot Orthoses*

To put on orthosis:
1. Open the laces wide, and fold the tongue back over the laces.
2. Lay the brace on the floor between feet with shoe directly under knees.
3. Lift affected foot into shoe.
4. Pick up brace by calf band or metal upright, and slide shoe onto foot while moving it into position flat on the floor. Use the unaffected foot to prevent the heel of the affected foot from slipping backward out of the shoe.
5. Push on the knee of the affected leg to slide the heel into the shoe.
To remove orthosis:
1. Loosen straps and laces.
2. Hold heel of shoe down with unaffected foot while lifting affected heel out, then push on calf band to push shoe off. Or, cross affected leg over unaffected, and lever shoe off foot by pushing on calf band.

*Other methods are suggested by Trombly (1987) and Malick and Almasy (1983, p. 261).

---

able learning on the part of clients. For example, a system of Morse Code may be used with a sip-and-puff switch for typing on a computer. Clients need to have good cognitive skills and considerable practice to master this task adaptation efficiently.

One disadvantage of adapting task objects is that the adaptive equipment must be available to clients whenever and wherever they engage in the task. This may or may not pose a problem, depending on the task and the adaptation. Clients who use a memory book at work to compensate for cognitive deficits may incorporate the structure and cues needed into a daily schedule and calendar system that was routinely carried before disability. If a client requires built-up utensils for eating, however, and the plan is to eat at a restaurant, the utensils must be taken along. This is cumbersome and some clients find it embarrassing.

Finally, some clients find that the use of adaptive equipment reduces satisfaction with task performance. To enhance personal satisfaction with task performance, they may be willing to cope with the increased difficulty of doing a task without adapted tools. For example, a female client with multiple sclerosis found that her mobility was safer and easier in a wheelchair, but she preferred to walk when out in the community. Her dissatisfaction with the wheelchair overrode other considerations.

Adapt the Task Environment

Adaptation of the environment itself may be used to facilitate task performance (Dunn et al, 1994). Typically, when the environment is adapted, the demand for learning and (text continues on page 355)

TABLE 19-6. ADL Treatment Approaches and Examples of Treatment Strategies for Task Disabilities Associated With Upper and Lower Body Impairments

Impairment: Upper and lower extremity passive and active range-of-motion (ROM) or strength impairment, with or without sensory loss

Common pathologies: Quadriplegia, arthritis, multiple sclerosis, burns, cerebral palsy, multiple amputations, traumatic brain injury, orthopedic trauma

Broad treatment approaches	Remediation	Compensation
Specific treatment strategies	*Restore/Establish*	*Alter the task method*
ADL tasks: Grooming, oral hygiene, bathing, and showering *Task Disabilities* • Client may be unable to safely initiate, continue, or complete all aspects of task performance (eg, transfers) • Client may be unable to reach, hold, manipulate, adjust, lift, open, or close task objects, thus preventing task initiation, continuation, or completion • Client may be unable to sustain grooming or oral hygiene actions long enough to complete tasks adequately • Client may be unable to get into or out of tub/shower • Client may be unable to reach all body parts for grooming or bathing • Client may experience pain, fatigue, or inadequate endurance for task performance • Client may express dissatisfaction with effort and time necessary to complete task performance	• Passive ROM • Continuous passive motion • Splinting • Casting • Prosthetic training • Active assistive, active, or resistive exercises for strengthening • Inhibitory or facilitatory treatment • Motor learning • Sensory reeducation	• Use one extremity to assist another • Use tenodesis action to pick up small items • Use both hands to hold objects • Use mouth to stabilize or open containers • Stabilize task objects on damp towels • Stabilize task objects between knees • Rest elbows on counter edge to apply deodorant, shave armpits • Use electric razor • Simplify hairstyle • Use a beauty salon • Grow a beard • Use terry cloth robe as towel
ADL task: Toileting *Task Disabilities* • Client may not always be able to reach bathroom in time • Client may be unable to lower self, raise self, or transfer self onto a toilet safely • Client may have difficulty managing catheter valve • Client may have difficulty doffing and donning clothing associated with toileting • Client may be unstable or have difficulty when reaching for or manipulating toilet paper roll, or separating paper from roll • Client may be unstable when reaching to cleanse body parts • Client may need assistance with catheterization or bowel program	• Passive ROM • Postural stability • Weight-shifting exercises • Balance exercises • Active assistive, active, or resistive exercises for strengthening • Training in self-catheterization, bowel stimulation	• Maintain extra broad-base of support while seated on toilet to prevent imbalance or falls while reaching for toilet paper, cleansing self, or being cleansed • Wrap end of toilet paper stream around dispenser edge or nearby towel rack to make it easier to rip off paper • Wrap toilet paper around hand/stump • Eliminate underwear • Plan ahead for adequate hydration • Plan ahead for incontinence emergencies

Compensation		Education	Sample Target Outcomes
Adapt task objects **Assistive devices**	**Adapt the task environment**	**Client/Caregiver Education**	

• Use splints for wrist stability and functional hand position
• Use pump-action containers for soap, toothpaste, and shampoo
• Use adapter for spray deodorant
• Use nonskid materials to stabilize items (eg, nail file, dentures)
• Use soap-on-a-rope
• Stabilize fingernail clipper to a board, and extend lever arm
• Use fliptop lipsticks
• Use adapted or loop handles, special holders, universal cuffs, or extended handles on brushes, razors, and so on
• Use electric toothbrush or Water-pik™
• Use wash mitt
• Use sponge with dorsal hand band
• Use long-handled lightweight sponge with loop handle for back, feet
• Suction long-handled sponge to wall or wedge in grab bars to wash underarms
• Use long-handled mirror for skin inspection
	• Store task items on counter or shelf in a basket or plastic container that can be transported to the task site easily (eg, handle over forearm)
	• Remove a cupboard door for easier access
	• Make sink area wheelchair accessible (eg, remove cupboard bottom, recess or insulate plumbing)
	• Mount the hairdryer on the wall
	• Install mirror with extension arm on wall
	• Install single-lever faucets
	• Install grab bars around tub/shower area
	• Install a bath bench that extends over the tub edge for safer transfers
	• Install a shower caddy for holding items
	• Install a hand-held flexible shower hose with an on/off switch that can be controlled at the shower head
	• Install nonskid surface/mat on tub or shower bottom
	• Use portable shampoo basin
		• Demonstrate restorative strategies (eg, self-ranging, passive ROM by caregiver before grooming, bathing), and have client/caregiver do a return demonstration
		• Demonstrate adapted methods (eg, bathing strategies) and have client/caregiver do a return demonstration
		• Demonstrate proper use of adapted task objects (eg, deodorant adapter) and have client/caregiver do a return demonstration
		• Provide a handout with drawings or pictures of the strategies or adaptations as well as sequential directions and a number to call for assistance
		• Provide a videotape of suggested treatment strategies (eg, bathtub transfers), with the client as the subject, if possible, and the practitioner demonstrating the caregiver's role
			• Increased level of independence
			• Improved safety
			• Improved adequacy of performance, as indicated by
			    Decreased difficulty
			    Decreased pain
			    Decreased fatigue
			    Increased task endurance
			    Increased satisfaction

• Substitute a free-standing toilet roll holder that positions the roll vertically, rather than horizontally
• Put tissue in a hanging basket next to the toilet
• Use reacher to get clothes up from the floor
• Use slacks with elastic in the waist band for easier donning/doffing
• Use slacks with Velcro™ leg seams for easy access to catheter and quick removal
• Wear rings on fingers to create friction on catheter tubes, etc.
• Use incontinence garment
	• Install grab bars for raising and lowering from toilet if stability is a problem
	• Install elevated toilet seat
	• Install elevated toilet seat that client or caregiver can reach under for bowel program
	• Install toilet frame that can provide security for client with poor trunk control
	• Install a bidet
	• Install commode near bed for night use
	• Provide space to store urinal near bed for night use
		• Demonstrate restorative strategies (eg, weight shifts), and adaptive strategies (eg, applying condom catheter) and have client/caregiver do a return demonstration
		• Demonstrate proper use of adapted task objects and assistive devices and have client/caregiver do a return demonstration
			• Increased level of independence
			• Improved safety
			• Improved adequacy of performance, as indicated by
			    Decreased difficulty
			    Decreased pain
			    Decreased fatigue
			    Increased task endurance
			    Increased satisfaction

(continued)

TABLE 19-6. (Continued)

Broad treatment approaches *Specific treatment strategies*	Remediation *Restore/Establish*	Compensation *Alter the task method*
• Client may experience pain, fatigue, or inadequate endurance for task performance • Client may express dissatisfaction with effort required and time necessary to complete task performance • Client may initially demonstrate aberrant task behaviors (eg, inadequately seal condom catheter)		
ADL task: Dressing *Task Disabilities* • Client may be unable or have difficulty lifting clothing items or body parts • Client may be unable or have difficulty donning and doffing clothing items • Client may be unable to reach all body parts (eg, feet, back) • Client may be unstable when reaching to don or doff lower body clothing items • Client may have difficulty manipulating and securing fasteners • Client may be unable to tie laces on shoes • Client may not be able to stand or sit unsupported while dressing • Client may experience pain, fatigue, or inadequate endurance for task performance • Client may express dissatisfaction with effort required and time necessary to complete task performance	• Postural stability • Weight-shifting exercises • Balance exercises • Fine-motor dexterity exercises • Train client in use of tenodesis action • Prosthetic training	• Dress in bed • Dress in wheelchair • Don and doff clothing using methods suggested in Tables 19-7, 19-8 • Position bed against two walls and wedge self into corner for stability when dressing • Place clothing for next day next to bed • Alter dressing sequence to accommodate donning/doffing of upper body and lower body prosthetics, ankle–foot orthoses, and splints • Lick palm for friction when donning socks • Wear slip-on shoes (eg, nonambulator)
ADL tasks: Feeding and Eating *Task Disabilities* • Client may be unable or have difficulty grasping utensils • Client may have difficulty cutting food	• Oral motor stimulation • Recommend a swallowing evaluation • Training in use of tenodesis action	• Position the client with chin slightly tucked, trunk aligned and near upright, and feet supported

Compensation		Education	Sample Target Outcomes
Adapt task objects **Assistive devices**	**Adapt the task environment**	**Client/Caregiver Education**	

• Use long-handled toilet aid or tongs
• Use assistive devices for bowel/bladder care
    Catheter insertion device
    Devices to prepare and apply external catheter
    Adapted urinary drainage bag valve
    Labia spreader
    Suppository inserter
    Digital stimulator
		• Provide a handout with drawings or pictures of the strategies (eg, changing catheter from bed bag to leg bag) or adaptations as well as sequential directions and a number to call for assistance
		• Provide a catalog with relevant assistive devices marked
		• Provide a videotape of suggested treatment strategies, with the client as the subject, if possible, and the practitioner demonstrating the caregiver's role	

• Keep upper body clothing buttoned except at the neck, for easier overhead donning
• Use elastic on buttoned cuffs to allow hands to move through easily
• Use clothing items that stretch (eg, knits)
• Order special clothing designed to meet the needs of clients in wheelchairs or with range of motion restrictions
• Use baggy over foot to decrease friction when donning pants
• Sew loops on clothing for better grasp
• Wear rings on fingers for friction when changing catheter tubes, etc.
• Use assistive devices for dressing
    Reacher
    Dressing stick
    Long shoe horn
    Clothing ladder
    Sock aid
    Zipper pull
    Velcro™ closures
    Button hook
    Elastic shoelaces
    Shoes with Velcro™ closures
    Rubber palm for friction
    Leg lifters
• Use splints for wrist stability or functional hand position
	• Place stable chair, with arms, near bed, to use for dressing
	• Install trapeze bar or rope ladder to shift body weight and position self
	• Install bed rails
	• Order bed with elevating head
	• Install floor-to-ceiling pole
		• Demonstrate restorative strategies (eg, weight-shifting exercises), and have client/caregiver do a return demonstration
		• Demonstrate adapted dressing methods (eg, dressing in wheelchair) and have client/caregiver do a return demonstration
		• Demonstrate proper use of adapted task objects (eg, loops on clothing) and assistive devices (eg, rope ladder) and have client/caregiver do a return demonstration
		• Provide a handout with drawings or pictures of the strategies (eg, baggies on socks) as well as sequential directions and a number to call for assistance
		• Provide a catalog with relevant assistive devices marked
		• Provide a videotape of suggested treatment strategies (eg, dressing in wheelchair), with the client as the subject, if possible, and the practitioner demonstrating the caregiver's role
			• Increased level of independence
			• Improved safety
			• Improved adequacy of performance, as indicated by
			    Decreased difficulty
			    Decreased pain
			    Decreased fatigue
			    Increased task endurance
			    Increased satisfaction

• Add Thickit™ or similar thickening agent to liquids	• Provide stable chair that accommodates positioning devices	• Demonstrate restorative strategies (eg, tenodesis action), and have client/caregiver do a return demonstration	• Increased level of independence • Improved safety

(continued)

TABLE 19-6. (Continued)

Broad treatment approaches	Remediation	Compensation
Specific treatment strategies	*Restore/Establish*	*Alter the task method*
• Client may have difficulty scooping up food and reaching to get food to mouth • Client may aspirate liquids or solids • Client may be unable or have difficulty grasping finger foods • Client may be unable to lift a drink • Client may experience pain, fatigue, or inadequate endurance for task performance • Client may express dissatisfaction with effort and time necessary to complete task performance	• Prosthetic training • Active assistive, active, or resistive exercises for strengthening • Passive ROM	• Support extremities • Use one extremity to assist the other • Weave utensil handles through fingers • Use tenodesis action to pick up light objects and larger finger foods • Use both hands to hold objects • Cut finger foods so they can be eaten with utensils
ADL task: Medication management routine *Task Disabilities* • Client may be unable to open pill bottles, remove lids from liquid medication containers, and remove pills from medication organizer compartments • Client may be unable to open medication patch packaging, or separate patch from protective liner • Client may have difficulty pouring liquid medication onto a spoon without spilling • Client may be unable or have difficulty getting spoon with medication to mouth • Client may experience pain trying to open medication containers • Client may express dissatisfaction with effort required and time needed for task performance	• Use of tenodesis action • Prosthetic training • Fine-motor dexterity training • Active assistive, active, or resistive exercises for strengthening • Passive ROM	• Use medication syringe for liquids instead of spoon • Sort medications into nut cups that can be easily picked up and emptied into mouth

ADL task: Functional mobility
Task Disabilities
• Client may be unable to move safely, efficiently, or without difficulty or pain during
  • Bed mobility
  • Wheelchair transfers to or from
    • Bed
    • Toilet
    • Bathtub/bench
    • Easy chair
    • Car
• Client may experience fatigue or inadequate endurance during task performance
	• Postural control exercises
	• Weight-shifting exercises
	• Balance exercises
	• Prosthetic training
	• Active assistive, active, or resistive exercises for upper extremity strengthening
		• Dependent transfer
		• Standing pivot transfer
		• Stand by assist
		• Independent transfer

Compensation		Education	Sample Target Outcomes
Adapt task objects **Assistive devices**	**Adapt the task environment**	**Client/Caregiver Education**	

• Place nonslip placemat under plate to prevent the plate from moving, or consider dishes with nonslip surfaces underneath
• Use mobile arm supports
• Use suspension sling or other antigravity device to support weight of upper arm and enable hand-to-mouth motion
• Use splints for wrist stability or functional hand position
• Use universal cuff for utensils if grasp is absent or inadequate
• Use built-up handles if grasp is incomplete or weak
• Use swivel utensils or extended utensils if excursion is inadequate
• Use plate guard, soup bowl, or plate with raised edge to enable easier scooping
• Use Swedish™ knife
• Use extra long straw and straw holder
	• Add lapboard to wheelchair
	• Add water bottle set up and straw to wheelchair to encourage hydration
		• Demonstrate feeding methods and have client/caregiver do a return demonstration (eg, to ensure that caregiver is not using "bird"-feeding techniques)
		• Demonstrate proper use of assistive devices (eg, utensils) and have client/caregiver do a return demonstration
		• Provide a handout with drawings or pictures of the strategies (eg, position mobile arm support) as well as sequential directions and a number to call for assistance
		• Provide a catalog with relevant assistive devices marked
		• Provide a videotape of suggested treatment strategies (eg, use of mobile arm support for eating), with the client as the subject, if possible, and the practitioner demonstrating the caregiver's role
			• Improved adequacy of performance, as indicated by
			  Decreased difficulty
			  Decreased pain
			  Decreased fatigue
			  Increased task endurance
			  Increased satisfaction

• Use splints for wrist stability or functional hand position
• Have pharmacist put only non–child-proof lids on pill bottles
• Use rubber circle to increase resistance on liquid medicine bottles
• Stabilize liquid medicine bottle between knees and use jar opener
• Use Daytimer™ appointment alarm to signal medication schedule (can set up to 31 alarms per day)
	• Place medications out in a logical place—where they will be used (eg, kitchen table if medications are taken at mealtime, bathroom or bedside if medications are taken at bedtime), if client is responsible for medication management	• Demonstrate system for organizing medications and have client/caregiver do a return demonstration
		• Demonstrate proper use of adapted task objects and assistive devices and have client/caregiver do a return demonstration
		• Provide a catalog with relevant assistive devices marked
			• Increased level of independence
			• Improved safety
			• Improved adequacy of performance, as indicated by
			  Decreased difficulty
			  Decreased pain
			  Increased satisfaction

• Sliding board transfer
• Standing pivot
• Insert rail on one side of bed so client can use it to pull against when positioning self in bed, lowering into bed, and raising self up from bed
• Use gel or foam cushion in wheelchair to raise the seat for easier transfers
• Use a portable cushion to place in easy chairs to make them the same height as the wheelchair
	• Ensure that the distance from the floor to all surfaces for transfers (toilet seat, tub bench, easy chair, etc.) is no greater than the distance between the floor and 2 in. below the midpoint of the client's patella when client is seated
	• Attach overhead trapeze bar on bed
	• Attach rope ladder to bed to help with positioning
		• Demonstrate restorative strategies and have client/caregiver do a return demonstration
		• Demonstrate proper use of adapted task objects and assistive devices (eg, rope ladder) and have client/caregiver do a return demonstration
		• Provide a catalog with relevant assistive devices marked
			• Increased level of independence
			• Improved safety
			• Improved adequacy of performance, as indicated by
			  Decreased difficulty
			  Decreased pain
			  Decreased fatigue
			  Increased task endurance
			  Increased satisfaction

(continued)

TABLE 19-6. (Continued)

Broad treatment approaches	Remediation	Compensation
Specific treatment strategies	*Restore/Establish*	*Alter the task method*
• Client may become fatigued during task performance • Client may express dissatisfaction with the effort required and time needed to complete task performance		

TABLE 19-7. Alternative Methods of Putting on and Taking Off Pants for Clients With Impairments in Passive and Active Range of Motion in Upper and Lower Extremities

Method 1
1. Sit with legs extended in bed, with or without back support, with clothing nearby on bed or chair.
2. Use weak grasp or drape garment over hand to hold it in preparation for putting it over foot.
3. Pull leg with forearm, lift under knee to bend leg, and bring foot up to opposite knee.
4. Drape garment over foot through leg opening, and pull it up to knee.
5. Lift leg and push on knee to extend.
6. Pull trousers over the foot and up to the knee during the same step as underwear, or use the same method for trousers as for underwear *after* underwear are pulled to the waist.
7. Once garment is pulled to the knees, pull it partly over the thighs by pulling on crotch of pants with forearm and pulling with hand in pocket of pants, or use both hands together to grasp and pull.
8. Lie down and roll side to side, pulling pants up over hip that is on top with each roll. Pull pants up using hand in pocket, thumb in belt loop, or hand inside pants under waistband.
9. Elastic waist bands can eliminate the need to use equipment to fasten the garment.
10. Reverse the process to remove the clothing.

Method 2
This method uses a different approach to get the clothing started over the feet and up to the knees, but is otherwise the same as method 1.
1. Leave the legs extended in bed, separated slightly.
2. Reach forward to the feet, and place one wrist under the ipsilateral heel.
3. Drape the garment leg opening over the toes, and pull the garment over the heel while lifting the upper extremity under the heel slightly.

Method 3
This method offers another way to get the pants over the feet and up to the knees.
1. Place pants face up with the waist just above the knees and under the legs.
2. Lift legs up with the forearm one at a time, and place feet in leg openings.
3. Exert pressure on the knee to cause the leg to extend into the trouser.

Compensation		Education	Sample Target Outcomes
Adapt task objects **Assistive devices**	**Adapt the task environment**	**Client/Caregiver Education**	
• Use plastic garbage sacks on car seats to ease shifting and turning • Order wheelchair with removeable armrests	• Install grab bars by toilet and in tub area as needed • Arrange spaces so that the wheelchair can be placed in an optimal position for transfers	• Provide handouts with drawings or pictures of the strategies or adaptations (eg, transfers) as well as sequential directions and a number to call for assistance • Provide a videotape of suggested treatment strategies (eg, car transfers), with the client as the subject, if possible, and the practitioner demonstrating the caregiver's role	

practice is less than that required for learning an alternative method or using adapted task objects. Environmental adaptations are often fixed in place so clients do not need to "remember" to bring along the necessary adaptations, and the adaptations cannot be easily displaced (eg, they cannot be dropped out of reach). Usually, the task method is unchanged, or only minimally changed, so that clients can rely on previous experience. Examples include installing a wheelchair ramp, installing grab bars and a floor-to-ceiling pole (Fig. 19–3) in the bathroom, recessing plumbing under the sink to accommodate a wheelchair user, increasing available light, removing cupboard doors for easy access, and installing a toilet seat frame.

The biggest drawback of environmental adaptations is that clients become very limited in terms of performance context. They must do the task in the adapted environment or in one that has been similarly adapted, because the adaptations are not easily transportable and may be custom designed for a specific environment.

INTEGRATING TREATMENT OF PERFORMANCE COMPONENT DEFICITS AND TASK DEFICITS

At first glance, it may seem that remediation and compensation are mutually exclusive treatment approaches; that is, the outcome is either to correct the performance component deficit or compensate for it. Use of both approaches simultaneously may seem a bit like using a belt and suspenders. A carefully crafted program, however, enables clients to be more functional through the use of compensatory strategies while, at the same time, working to remediate performance component deficits. It is critical that the occupational therapy practitioner reduce the use of compensatory strategies as clients make gains in the performance component skills. For example, Mr. Stapinski, the

client with burns resulting in bilateral limitations in elbow flexion, may benefit from utensils with extended handles. With the extended handles on the utensils he can feed himself independently during the 2 to 3 weeks that it takes to increase his elbow flexion sufficiently for him to feed himself without these utensils. The extended handles should be fabricated to require him to flex fully within his available range and should be shortened as ROM gains are made so that the new range is incorporated into the feeding task. Whenever task or environmental adaptations are anticipated to be temporary, it is necessary to consider cost in relation to the anticipated time the equipment will be needed and the potential benefit to clients. Thermoplastic or wood extensions can be added to the handles of regular

(text continues on page 360)

TABLE 19-8. Method of Dressing From the Wheelchair for Clients with Mobility Impairments

1. Sit on low bed, wheelchair, or standard chair with feet firmly on floor.
2. Cross one leg over the other to start garment and put on socks and shoes.
3. To pull garment over hips in wheelchair or bed (if unable to stand), lean far to one side to pull garment over opposite thigh and buttock; repeat for opposite side. Or, in wheelchair, support weight on elbows and lean on back of chair, bridging to lift buttocks from chair, and pull pants up.
4. To stand to pull up garment, stabilize with one upper extremity on ambulation aide or grab bar while pulling up garment with the other upper extremity, alternating sides. Or, stabilize against wall, bed, or grab bar while pulling garment up.

TABLE 19-9. ADL Treatment Approaches and Examples of Treatment Strategies for Task Disabilities Associated With Cognitive Impairments

Impairment: Cognitive (e.g., attention span, memory, sequencing, problem solving, generalization, initiation and termination of task)
Common pathologies: Cerebrovascular accident, traumatic brain injury, dementia, mental retardation

Broad treatment approaches	Remediation	Compensation
Specific treatment strategies	*Restore/Establish*	*Alter the task method*
ADL tasks: Grooming, oral hygiene, bathing, and showering *Task Disabilities* • Client may use poor judgment with sharp objects (eg, razors, fingernail scissors) • Client may fear or resist bathing, grooming, and oral hygiene tasks or insist the tasks were just completed • Client may use poor judgment around water (turn on faucet and leave it running, run water that is too hot) • Client may have difficulty getting into and out of the bathtub • Client's dentures may become loose and cause mouth sores after weight loss • Client may lose dentures or retainers • Client may be at risk for falls due to poor judgment • Task outcomes may not meet acceptable societal standards (eg, body odor from inadequate bathing) • Client may demonstrate aberrant task behaviors (eg, client may swallow toothpaste rather than spit it out)	• Cognitive retraining • Establish routines • Observe for client preferences so that these can be built on • Develop behavioral memory aids for use until routines and habits are established	• Adhere to routines and patterns that reinforce the timing and occurrence of grooming, hygiene, and bathing tasks • Use only the level of assistance that is needed; do not remove the client's right to participate in the task if it is not harmful • Explain each step with client before proceeding so that there are no surprises • Do not rush the task • Change to the client's preferred time if possible • Monitor bathing/showering at all times • Partially fill tub before entering bath area with client so there is no waiting • State that "bath is ready" if client tends to think bath has already been completed • Bathe at the sink • Let client hold washcloth and scrub one area while caregiver washes another • Provide toothpaste that can be swallowed • Use electric razors • Use clippers • Make nail care into a time to be pampered

ADL task: Toileting
Task Disabilities
• Client may be incontinent of bladder and bowel
• Client may not make it to the bathroom in time
• Client may not remember what to do when brought in to the bathroom
• Client may not want to stay seated on toilet
• Client may forget to cleanse self after toileting
• Client may have difficulty doffing and donning clothing associated with toileting
• Client may be at risk for falls due to poor judgment
• Task outcomes may not meet societal standards (eg, client may soil self in the toileting process)
• Client may demonstrate aberrant task behaviors (eg, stuff toilet paper into toilet, leave water running in sink)
	• Cognitive retraining
	• Establish routines
	• Develop behavioral memory aids for use until routines and habits are established
		• Adhere to routines and patterns that reinforce the timing and occurrence of toileting
		• Take client to the bathroom; do not ask
		• Within a task, explain next step to client before proceeding so that there are no surprises
		• Do not rush the task
		• Remove items that client tends to urinate in
		• Help to initiate toileting by
		  Pulling down client's clothing
		  Having client sit on toilet
		  Running water in sink
		  Giving water to drink
		  Rubbing lower back
		  Pouring warm water over perineum into the toilet
		  Giving magazine to hold

Compensation		Education	Sample Target Outcomes
Adapt task objects *Assistive devices*	*Adapt the task environment*	*Client/Caregiver Education*	

• Use handheld shower if caregiver is assisting
• Mark dentures and retainers with client's name
• Place rubber mesh in sink bottom when client brushes dentures in case denture is dropped
• Use foaming gel spray on washcloth if client gets agitated with the water running
• Place a checklist in the bathroom to be marked when each task is completed
	• Keep task materials in the same place and keep materials for like tasks together
	• Install nonskid bath mat in tub or shower
	• Install grab bars around tub or shower
	• Reset water temperature below 120°F
	• Install tap water overflow alarm
	• Keep sharp, toxic (eg, nail polish) items in a locked cabinet, if necessary
	• Label drawers/cupboards with contents inside
	• Remove clutter from task performance area
		• Demonstrate restorative/adaptive strategies (eg, hierarchies of assistance) and have caregiver do a return demonstration
		• Demonstrate proper use of distraction to avoid confrontation and have caregiver do a return demonstration
		• Provide a handout with drawings or pictures of the strategies or adaptations as well as sequential directions and a number to call for assistance
		• Provide a videotape of suggested treatment strategies, with the client as the subject, if possible, and the practitioner demonstrating the caregiver's role
			• Increased level of independence
			• Improved safety
			• Improved adequacy of performance, as indicated by
			  Decreased difficulty
			  Decreased pain
			  Increased approximation to acceptable societal standards for task performance
			  Decrease in aberrant task behaviors

• Use clothing and underwear that is easy to remove
• Use incontinence garments
• Use protective sheet on bedding
• Use foaming gel spray to cleanse fecal matter and urine from client if bathing is not possible
• Place checklist in front of toilet with reminders about flushing and washing hands
	• Keep task materials stocked and within arm's reach so one hand can be on the client while the other is reaching for wipes, etc.
	• Use raised toilet seat if client has difficulty lowering or raising self
	• Use padded toilet seat if client needs to sit for extended periods
	• Label drawers and cupboards with contents inside
		• Demonstrate restorative/adaptive strategies (eg, hierarchies of assistance; behavioral signs that client needs to use the toilet), and have caregiver do a return demonstration
		• Demonstrate proper use of distraction to avoid confrontation and have caregiver do a return demonstration
		• Provide a handout with drawings or pictures of the strategies or adaptations as well as sequential directions and a number to call for assistance
		• Provide a videotape of suggested treatment strategies, with the client as the subject, if possible, and the practitioner demonstrating the caregiver's role
			• Increased level of independence
			• Improved safety
			• Improved adequacy of performance, as indicated by
			  Decreased difficulty
			  Increased approximation to acceptable societal standards for task performance
			  Decrease in aberrant task behaviors

(continued)

TABLE 19-9. (Continued)

Broad treatment approaches	Remediation	Compensation
Specific treatment strategies	Restore/Establish	Alter the task method
ADL task: Dressing *Task Disabilities* • Client may be unable to select appropriate clothing • Client may wear same outfit day after day • Client may have difficulty sequencing the donning and doffing of clothing items • Client may have difficulty manipulating and securing fasteners • Client may have difficulty attending to the task • Client may be unable to tie laces on shoes • Client may be unstable when donning or doffing clothing • Task outcomes may not meet societal standards (eg, client may layer clothing inappropriately—don dress over coat) • Client may demonstrate aberrant task behaviors (eg, may remove clothing at inappropriate times)	• Cognitive retraining • Establish routines • Develop behavioral memory aids for use until routines and habits are established	• Force clothing options by limiting clothing available in client's closet or drawers • Buy several outfits that are alike if client has distinct preference • Remove extra clothing from closets and drawers if client layers • Ascertain if client is warm enough if layering persists • Keep only seasonally appropriate clothing in closet/drawers • Have client sit while dressing • Arrange clothing in a stack, in the order that clothing is to be donned • Use clothes that are difficult to remove if client doffs clothing in inappropriate places • Use clothing items that stretch (eg, knits) • Use clothing that is easy to don/doff • Use shoes with Velcro™ closures
ADL tasks: Feeding and Eating *Task Disabilities* • Client may forget to eat or drink • Client may not initiate self-feeding, or may not continue • Client may have difficulty managing utensils • Client may have difficulty cutting food • Client may have difficulty scooping up food • Client may forget to chew • Client may eat nonfood items • Client may choke on liquids • Client may be distracted or inattentive during mealtime • Task outcomes may not meet acceptable societal standards (eg, client may drool) • Client may demonstrate aberrant task behaviors (eg, may refuse to open mouth, or may stuff food in cheeks)	• Cognitive retraining • Oral stimulation • Develop behavioral memory aids for use until routines and habits are established • Recommend a swallowing evaluation	• Set alarm to remind client it is time to fix food or to eat or drink • Position the client upright, with feet supported • Monitor fluid intake • Place only small amounts of food in front of client at one time • Provide food that smells appetizing • Point out each type of food and put a small amount of food on client's lips to stimulate opening of mouth • Ask client to say "ah" and demonstrate, instead of "open your mouth" • Cut food into small bites • Use finger foods and tolerate finger feeding • Tolerate declining table manners • Remind client to chew • Remind client to swallow after each bite and stroke client's throat gently • Demonstrate chewing • Serve soft foods • Avoid sticky food and food that is hard • Put hand on client's arm to block movement if client is stuffing food in mouth and remove extra food • If client is living alone, check refrigerator for spoiled food
ADL task: Medication management routine *Task Disabilities* • Client may not remember to take medications	• Cognitive retraining • Develop behavioral memory aids for use until routines and habits are established	• Use medication syringe for liquids instead of spoon for both client and caregiver administration

Compensation		Education	Sample Target Outcomes
Adapt task objects Assistive devices	**Adapt the task environment**	**Client/Caregiver Education**	

• Keep upper body clothing buttoned except at the neck, for easier one-step overhead donning
• Use elastic on buttoned cuffs to allow hands to move through easily
• Adapt clothing for easier donning/doffing (eg, Velcro™ fasteners, zipper pulls, large buttons)
• Develop checklists for donning/doffing clothing (eg, hang up or put in laundry basket)
	• Place stable chair with arms, near bed, to use for dressing
	• Label drawers/cupboards, closets with contents inside
		• Demonstrate restorative/adaptive strategies (eg, routines, use of memory aids), and have client/caregiver do a return demonstration or explain how they would be used
		• Provide a handout with drawings or pictures of the strategies (eg, setting up clothing for donning) or adaptations as well as sequential directions and a number to call for assistance
		• Provide a videotape of suggested treatment strategies, with the client as the subject, if possible, and the practitioner demonstrating the caregiver's role
			• Increased level of independence
			• Improved safety
			• Improved adequacy of performance, as indicated by
			   Decreased difficulty
			   Increased approximation to acceptable societal standards for task performance
			   Decrease in aberrant task behaviors

• Place nonslip placemat under plate to prevent the plate from moving, or consider dishes with nonslip surfaces underneath
• Use small plastic glasses or cups and then refill
• Use Thickit™ or other thickening agent in liquids
• Develop checklists for using the microwave, putting away food, etc.
	• Provide suitable stable chair
	• Label drawers/cupboards, closets with contents inside
	• Lock cupboards that contain sharps or nonedible item (eg, detergent) if necessary
		• Demonstrate restorative strategies (eg, oral stimulation), and have client/caregiver do a return demonstration
		• Demonstrate feeding methods and have client/caregiver do a return demonstration (eg, to ensure that caregiver is not using "bird"-feeding techniques)
		• Demonstrate proper use of adapted task objects and assistive devices and have client/caregiver do a return demonstration
		• Provide a handout with drawings or pictures of the strategies (eg, suggested position of tableware to avoid bumping, spilling) or adaptations as well as sequential directions and a number to call for assistance
		• Provide a videotape of suggested treatment strategies, with the client as the subject, if possible, and the practitioner demonstrating the caregiver's role (eg, managing the client during mealtime)
			• Increased level of independence
			• Improved safety
			• Improved adequacy of performance, as indicated by
			   Decreased difficulty
			   Increased task endurance
			   Increased approximation to acceptable societal standards for task performance
			   Decrease in aberrant task behaviors

• Have pharmacist put only non–child-proof lids on medication bottles if client is managing medications	• Lock medications in cupboard if client is likely to take medications inappropriately	• Demonstrate medication management routines and have client/caregiver do a return demonstration	• Increased level of independence • Improved safety

(continued)

TABLE 19-9. (Continued)

Broad treatment approaches	Remediation	Compensation
Specific treatment strategies	*Restore/Establish*	*Alter the task method*
• Client may not interpret medication directions correctly • Client may not remember that medications were taken and take extra doses • Client may have difficulty opening medication containers • Client may refuse "medication" • Client may demonstrate aberrant task behaviors (eg, may spit out pills)	• Recommend a swallowing evaluation	• Check with nurse or pharmacist about which medications can be crushed and mixed into applesauce or other soft foods • Sort medications into nut cups, envelopes, or saucers that are labeled with day and time so that client knows when to take medications and if medications were not taken
ADL task: Functional mobility *Task Disabilities* • Client may be unable to find way around home or community • Client may move in an unsafe and awkward manner (eg, bump into things, unsteady gait, trip over items) • Client may have difficulty getting up from a bed or chair • Client may pace and wander • Client may not remember limitations, precautions, or how to use assistive device for ambulation and thus be at risk for falls, especially if client has concomitant physical impairment • Client may demonstrate aberrant task behaviors (eg, pick up walker and carry it around)	• Postural control exercises • Balance exercises • Cognitive retraining • Develop behavioral memory aids for use until routines and habits are established • Practice way-finding with client	• Have client wear sturdy, low and broad-heeled shoes if gait is unsteady • Have client walk beside caregiver, holding onto arm • Have caregiver accompany client until way-finding is mastered • Write out directions for community wayfinding and provide an easy-to-follow map

utensils temporarily, rather than prescribing the more costly commercially available utensils with elongated handles. For some tasks, safety concerns supersede cost considerations. Use of a collapsible lawn chair in the shower would be an inexpensive alternative to a shower chair, but it would fail to provide adequate stability.

CLIENT OR CAREGIVER EDUCATION

Instructional Methods

A variety of instructional methods are available for client and caregiver education (Cahill, 1987; DaCunha & Tackenberg, 1989). Methods should be selected that best meet the needs of the individual (see Tables 19–1 through 19–9). When a facility has a homogeneous client population, group instruction can be an efficient and effective method for providing basic education. Many arthritis centers provide group instruction in proper lifting techniques. Teaching a group is cost-effective and, when well structured, can fa-

cilitate learning through peer interaction. For caregiver groups, the contact with others who are experiencing similar problems in their caregiving roles, can provide valuable emotional support and an opportunity for constructive group problem solving. Some type of individualized instruction is typically needed to complement group instruction so that information can be tailored to meet the specific and unique needs of each person. If group instruction has preceded the individualized instruction, the client-specific sessions can be relatively short and focused on application of the information learned in the group to the client's particular circumstances. For example, clients would be taught how to apply proper lifting techniques to the materials and environments encountered in their homes.

Individualized instruction is more appropriate for many clients and caregivers because the personal nature of the tasks that need to be learned does not lend itself to group instruction (eg, bathing). Furthermore, in treatment settings

Compensation		Education	Sample Target Outcomes
Adapt task objects **Assistive devices**	**Adapt the task environment**	**Client/Caregiver Education**	

• Use medication organizer that is acceptable to client
• Use Daytimer™ appointment alarm to signal medication schedule (can set up to 31 alarms per day)
	• Place medications out in a logical place where they will be constantly noticed (eg, kitchen counter) if client is responsible for medication management	• Provide a catalog with relevant assistive devices marked	• Improved adequacy of performance, as indicated by
			  Decreased difficulty
			  Decrease in aberrant task behaviors

• Insert rail on one side of bed so client can use it to pull against when positioning self in bed, lowering self into and raising up from bed
• Use a portable dense foam cushion to place in easy chairs to make it easier to raise self
• Use chair with arms
• Evaluate ability to use walking aids if gait is unsteady
• Install gates by stairs if necessary
	• Add lighting to areas where client is likely to trip
	• Provide a lighted pathway from bedroom to bathroom
	• Repair walking surfaces so they are even
	• Remove tripping hazards
	• Stabilize furniture near natural pathways
	• Make stairways safe
	  Sturdy handrails on both sides
	  Uniform stair height and tread widths
	  Clearly discernable tread widths
	  Top and bottom landings marked with a different color or surface
	• Provide a safe environment for wandering (eg, natural clear pathways)
		• Demonstrate restorative strategies
		• Demonstrate proper use of adapted task objects and assistive devices (eg, walking aid) and have client/caregiver do a return demonstration
		• Provide a catalog with relevant assistive devices marked
		• Provide handouts with drawings or pictures of the strategies or adaptations (eg, stair safety guidelines) and a number to call for assistance
		• Provide a videotape of suggested treatment strategies (eg, indoor safety for wandering pathways), with the client as the subject, if possible, and the practitioner demonstrating the caregiver's role
			• Increased level of independence
			• Improved safety
			• Improved adequacy of performance, as indicated by
			  Decreased difficulty
			  Decrease in aberrant task behaviors

serving a heterogeneous population, the opportunity for group instruction rarely occurs. One-to-one client or caregiver education and training enables the occupational therapy practitioner to obtain immediate feedback from the individual as the session progresses and to alter the amount and focus of learning accordingly.

A vast array of media are available to occupational therapy practitioners to facilitate the learning process. Written materials may be developed specifically for a client or caregiver, or published materials may be used, if appropriate ones are available. Videocassette recorders are widely available, even in clients' homes, and custom or commercially made videotapes can be effective teaching tools. Audiotapes can also be effective, particularly when visual input would be distracting. For example, an audiotape may be used to facilitate visual imagery for relaxation or stress reduction. The Internet is becoming increasingly accessible to the general population, and many occupational therapy clinics now

have Internet access. A wealth of information about various disorders is available through the World Wide Web that is specifically geared toward clients and caregivers. Clients may also find peer support groups through chat rooms or list servers.

Caregiver Training

In addition to evaluating clients' learning capacity, the learning capacity of their caregivers needs to be appraised. Similar to clients, caregivers also have varied learning interests and capacities. In many situations, the caregiver is a family member who is still coping with the emotional effect of having a family member with a disability, whether it is a new mother with a child with cerebral palsy or the spouse of a woman who has had a CVA. Particularly in situations in which the individual is new to the caregiver role, care must be taken to assess the caregiver's capacity to understand and apply the information necessary for safe and effective man-

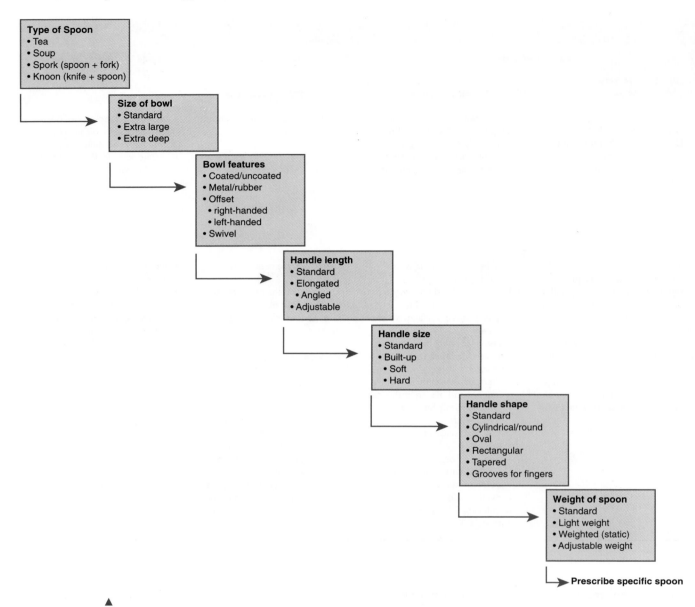

▲
Figure 19-2. Potential decisions for the prescription of one assistive device: An adapted spoon.

agement of the client's needs. Individuals under emotional duress may need more time and repetition to process information accurately. When caregivers are expected to physically assist clients, their physical capacity for providing this assistance also warrants attention.

Caregivers have varied learning styles, and instruction that caters to their preferred style is likely to be the most efficient and effective. Some individuals, for example, are kinesthetic learners. They learn most quickly through "doing." Visual learners may prefer to watch a demonstration of the task several times before attempting it themselves. Others may prefer written instructions. All learners benefit from the opportunity to ask questions to clarify instructions. Me-

dia that support the teaching can be a great asset. Videotapes, for example, provide caregivers with an excellent record of how an exercise or task is to be done. Often, "home or clinic-made" videotapes can be taken of a client's task performance. These productions add little time to the treatment session, because they are recorded as tasks and practiced during treatment. They have the advantage of providing richer and more detailed information than is feasible in oral or written instructions.

When caregivers are helping to carry out a treatment program, the outcome and general treatment strategies should be made clear to them. For remediation programs, clients may need assistance with specific exercises or tasks in

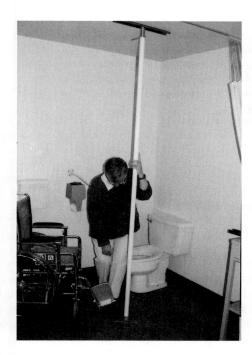

▲
Figure 19-3. A floor-to-ceiling pole that can be used to assist with stability during transfers.

a way that helps restore component skills. Caregivers need to learn specific cuing skills so that "home" programs, whether these are carried out in clients' homes, group homes, or long-term care settings, are carried out accurately. Caregivers are often pivotal in motivating clients. Motivating clients who have disorders that impair motivation, such as depression, can be particularly challenging. Helping caregivers understand that disinterest and lack of motivation are a part of the disorder and providing concrete strategies for managing the "getting going" phase of the home program will foster their success. For clients with behavior problems, such as the catastrophic reactions that often accompany Alzheimer's disease, teaching caregivers behavior management strategies that defuse potentially volatile situations can be invaluable to their success as caregivers.

Caregiver training for assisting clients with functional tasks should focus first on safety for clients and caregivers. The occupational therapy practitioner should emphasize components of the task that promote safety, such as locking the wheelchair brakes or blocking the client's knee to prevent buckling when transferring to and from the wheelchair. As treatment progresses, the occupational therapy practitioner should inform caregivers of the tasks that are safe and unsafe to perform outside of the therapy situation. For example, although a client may be working on bathtub transfers during therapy, skilled facilitation to get in and out safely may be required, making it premature for the client to practice these transfers at home.

When caregivers need to provide physical assistance, they should be trained in using proper body mechanics. Training should include lifting guidelines for transfers or bed mobility, but also more general positioning. Assisting a client in a wheelchair with self-care, such as brushing teeth or feeding, while standing, can cause fatigue of lower back muscles. Taking "care of the caregiver" is frequently overlooked in occupational therapy treatment and is an essential component of the person-task-environment transaction, particularly when it is anticipated that the client will require assistance over a long period.

Grading the Treatment Program

Treatment programs should never be static. It is important to continually progress the client toward the established intervention outcomes. The specific means of grading treatment, when a remediation approach at the performance component level is being implemented, varies depending on the performance component being treated and the treatment medium or procedures being used. Chapter 20 on treatment of performance component deficits provides more specific guidance. If the treatment plan uses both remediation and compensation, the program can be graded by reducing the amount of task and environmental adaptations so that clients use gains made in the performance component areas. Treatment of task disability can be graded by modifying many of the task parameters described earlier in the chapter, including increasing the level of independence, taking more responsibility for safety, enhancing personal satisfaction, reducing the level of difficulty or required exertion, and decreasing the duration or the occurrence of aberrant task behaviors.

GRADE TASK PROGRESSION FROM EASIER TO HARDER

One means of grading a treatment program is to begin with easier tasks and progress to more difficult ones. This progression will be relative to the client's performance deficits. Money management may be relatively easy for a client with quadriplegia to perform once use of a writing tool is mastered, whereas lower extremity dressing would be much more difficult. Conversely, a client with a head injury that resulted in significant cognitive deficits but relatively preserved motor skills, would likely find lower extremity dressing to be relatively easy, but money management extremely difficult.

INCREASE COMPLEXITY WITHIN THE TASK

Rather than progressing from easier to harder tasks, treatment may also be graded by increasing the complexity of a task, that is to say, by progressing from simple to more complex ways of doing it. Cooking skills may extend from very simple preparations, such as cold sandwiches, to more complex, multicourse dinners. Even seemingly simple tasks can often be graded. A sock-donning treatment, for example, might be scaled from using looser, ankle socks, to tighter, knee socks, and finally to panty hose.

SAME TASK IN VARIED PERFORMANCE CONTEXTS

A very critical part of a graded treatment program involves progression from the treatment context to the real-life context in which tasks will actually be performed. This may involve transfer from a clinic to a home setting or the more subtle dynamics associated with the transfer of help from the occupational therapy practitioner to the natural caregiver. The client may be independent in donning a jacket sitting on a mat table in the clinic, while still unable to do it when sitting on a chair with a back, or standing (ie, the way a jacket is typically donned by ambulatory individuals). Providing practice in increasingly demanding performance contexts can facilitate the generalization of skills, thereby enhancing the client's "functional flexibility."

▶TREATMENT OF ADL CONCLUSION

In this section, three broad approaches to occupational therapy treatment for ADL were discussed—namely remediation, compensation, and education. We discussed the necessity of establishing target outcomes for task performance that address (1) value of the task to the client, (2) level of independence in performing the task, (3) safety of task performance, and (4) adequacy of task performance. Adequacy of task performance included the parameters of difficulty, pain, fatigue and dyspnea, duration (efficiency), societal standards, satisfaction, experience, resources, and aberrant task behaviors. Other factors influencing target outcomes and choice of treatment approaches were also presented, including the client's ability to learn, the client's prognosis, the time allocated for treatment, the client's discharge disposition, and the client's ability to follow through with new routines or techniques.

Section 2

Treatment of Activities of Daily Living: Sexuality and Disability

Maureen Freda

Anatomy Knowledge Prerequisites for Sexuality
    Counseling
Physiology Knowledge Prerequisites for Sexuality
    Counseling

Effects of Disability on Sexual Function
    Nervous System Disorders
    Cardiovascular and Pulmonary Disorders
    Musculoskeletal and Orthopedic Disorders
Sexually Transmitted Diseases
Pregnancy and Childbirth
Addressing Sexuality
    Self-Awareness and Interpersonal Communication
    Acknowledgment of Sexuality and Initiation of
        Discussions
    Provision of Information and Counseling Strategies
Sexuality and Disability Conclusion

A dult sexuality is an essential component of our identity and self-image. It is our sense of ourselves as men and women, as people capable of giving and worthy of receiving affection (Neistadt, 1986; Neistadt & Freda, 1987). The ability to express oneself sexually may be altered by functional deficits, feelings of low self-esteem, or other residual effects of disability or illness, but the basic sexual nature of the individual remains (Freda & Rubinsky, 1991). Occupational therapy practitioners can address clients' sexuality needs by providing information about (1) the effects of specific disabilities on sexuality, and (2) adaptive strategies.

▼ ANATOMY KNOWLEDGE PREREQUISITES FOR SEXUALITY COUNSELING

Occupational therapy practitioners involved in sexuality counseling must be knowledgeable about male and female sexual anatomy and hormones. Other areas that should be reviewed before providing sexual counseling are conception, contraception, safe sex practices, and the process of adolescent development of secondary sex characteristics and reproductive capacity. Readers should refer to available biology and physiology texts for this information.

▼ PHYSIOLOGY KNOWLEDGE PREREQUISITES FOR SEXUALITY COUNSELING

Masters and Johnson (1966) have described the physiological changes of the body during the sexual response cycle. This cycle is divided into four progressive phases for both men and women: excitement, plateau, orgasm, and resolution. During the excitement phase, men and women experience initial swelling in breast and genital tissue: the latter results in erection in men and vaginal lubrication for women. These physical changes continue in the plateau phase. During orgasm, or climax, men ejaculate and women experience wavelike contractions down the length of their uterus and vagina. During resolution, all physiological changes gradually return to their normal, preexcitement state. This cycle describes the body's response to sexual stimulation of any kind, that is, intercourse, masturbation, or oral sex.

The physiological process underlying the first three phases is vasocongestion, caused by a combination of arterial dilation and venous constriction. Extra fluid in the congested blood vessels seeps into the surrounding soft tissue, causing the swelling of breast and genital tissues (Masters and Johnson, 1966).

Other physiological changes also occur for both men and women during the sexual response cycle. Beginning in the excitement phase, blood pressure, pulse, breathing rate, and muscle tension rise, reaching a peak at orgasm and gradually returning to normal during resolution. Masters and Johnson (1966), working with subjects aged 21 to 40 years in a laboratory setting, found peak blood pressures of up to 220/130 for men and 200/120 for women, peak heart rates of 110 to 180 beats per minute, and peak breathing rates of 30 to 60 breaths per minute.

Other investigators, working with middle-aged men in their home settings, have found peak heart rates of up to 117.4 beats per minute (Hellerstein & Friedman, 1970). Research has shown peak orgasmic blood pressure in people with hypertension to be as high as 237/138 for men and 216/127 for women (Staff, 1980; *Science News*). Peak metabolic rates last for 10 to 20 seconds during orgasm and return to resting values within about 2 minutes after orgasm. Normal resting values for adults would be 120/80, 72 beats per minute, and 12 breaths per minute for blood pressure, pulse, and breathing rate, respectively (Guyton, 1991).

▼ EFFECTS OF DISABILITY ON SEXUAL FUNCTION

Nervous System Disorders

BRAIN

Diagnoses affecting the brain include **traumatic brain injury** (TBI), cerebral vascular accident (CVA or stroke), cerebral palsy (CP), multiple sclerosis (MS), tumors, epilepsy, **mental retardation**, and Parkinson's disease. Any of these diagnoses can alter a person's sexual functioning. Disorders of the nervous system can affect seminal emission, ejaculation, or both; vaginal lubrication, clitoral engorgement, or orgasm (Zasler, 1991). Frontal lobe lesions can result in disinhibition and sexual acting out, such as public masturbation. However, hyposexuality is more commonly seen following stroke and TBI (Zasler, 1991). Following stroke, men may experience decreased frequency of intercourse and ejaculatory and erectile dysfunction; women may experience decreased vaginal lubrication and orgasmic capacity; libido may decline for both men and women (Sjogren,

Damber, & Liliquist, 1983; Freda & Rubinsky, 1991; Zasler, 1991). These same changes in sexual function have been found in individuals following traumatic brain injury (Kruezter & Zasler, 1989; Zasler, 1991)

Disorders affecting the brain generally do not alter fertility. Some individuals with traumatic brain injury may experience disturbances in gonadal hormone regulation as a result of injury to the hypothalamus, pituitary, or temporal lobes. This could result in impotence in men and infertility in women (Horn & Zasler, 1990).

Some medications prescribed for adults with neurological disorders, such as psychotropic agents and sedating anticonvulsants, can also affect sexual function (Zasler, 1991). It is extremely important for individuals with a disability to understand the possible negative sexuality side effects of certain medications so they can distinguish between disability and medication-related sexual dysfunction. It is equally important for these individuals to consult their physicians relative to possible substitutions or alternatives to troublesome medications. Under no circumstances should individuals take it upon themselves to just stop taking medication.

The following are suggested strategies to deal with the functional sexuality problems often experienced by individuals with brain lesions:

- *Communication deficit*: Use of touch, a communication board, familiar gestures.
- *Sensory deficit*: Use verbal description to replace the sensation; concentrate on sensate areas of the body.
- *Visual deficit*: Emphasize intact senses.
- *Mobility deficit*: Use side-lying and spasticity-reducing positions (utilize neurodevelopmental treatment [NDT] principles).
- *Cognitive deficit*: Use familiar and routinized activities; stay in a nondistracting environment.
- *Tremor*: Use mild restraint or interlock arms with partner for intention **tremors**.
  (Neistadt & Freda, 1987; Freda & Rubinsky, 1991)

SPINAL CORD

Diagnoses that affect spinal cord functioning include amyotrophic lateral sclerosis, MS, **spina bifida**, trauma, and tumors. The degree of sexual dysfunction associated with spinal cord injury is dependent on the level and severity of the lesion. With incomplete lesions, voluntary control of sexual functioning by brain-spinal cord pathways may still be preserved. With complete lesions, cortical input is eliminated. With cervical and thoracic lesions, reflex genital response is still possible through the lumbosacral reflex arcs that control erection and ejaculation in men and vaginal lubrication and orgasm in women. Reflex erection and vaginal lubrication are preserved more often with cervical than with thoracic lesions. The ability to ejaculate is more often preserved in men with lesions in the thoracic area. Lesions in the lumbosacral area can interfere with the genital reflex arcs, resulting in erectile and ejaculatory difficulties in men and lubrication and orgasmic difficulties in women (Smith & Bodner, 1993). Recent studies (Courtois, Charvier, Leriche, & Raymond, 1993) have shown that many men with spinal cord injury underestimate their sexual capability. In a study of individuals with spinal cord injury (SCI) and their partners, Kreuter, Sullivan, and Siosten (1994) found that emotional factors, such as trust and affection along with closeness and appreciation, were essential to maintaining a "positive and satisfying sexual relationship." Fertility is preserved in women with spinal cord injury; although a short period of amenorrhea may occur immediately following injury. Ejaculatory dysfunction in men with spinal cord injury once interfered with their fertility. Now they can pursue electroejaculation followed by insemination of the female partner. However, viability of sperm is still an issue; sperm viability is often affected by temperature regulation problems, urinary tract infections, or medications.

The following are suggested strategies to deal with the functional sexuality problems often experienced by individuals with spinal cord injuries:

- *Erectile dysfunction:* Use vacuum devices, intercorporal injections of papaverine, penile prostheses.
- *Catheter:* Tape tubing along the shaft of the penis after erection for men or onto the abdomen for women
- *Mobility deficits:* Maximize use of unaffected extremities; positions that require less motion on the part of the partner with a spinal cord injury; use of furniture for stability during sexual activity (ie, wheelchair for male seated position, pillows to support side lying, or other such).
- *Sensory loss:* Stimulate sensate parts of the body.
(Neistadt & Freda, 1987)

PERIPHERAL NERVES

Diagnoses that affect peripheral nerve functioning include alcoholism, diabetes, ileostomy, and prostatectomy. Any injury to the peripheral nerves innervating the genitals can affect sexual functioning by blocking the reflex arcs necessary for genital response to sexual stimulation. Men with damage to these nerves can experience difficulties with erection and ejaculation, while women may have difficulties with vaginal lubrication and orgasm. When genital functioning is disrupted, couples need to explore alternatives to coitus and the use of sexual adaptive equipment. The importance of affectionate touch, cuddling, and other expressions of intimacy and sexuality cannot be underestimated in these situations.

Cardiovascular and Pulmonary Disorders

Cardiovascular diagnoses include hypertension and **myocardial infarction**. Clients with these diagnoses often fear that the increases in blood pressure and heart rate that occur during sexual activity will trigger a stroke or heart attack. Research has shown that the risk of sustaining a my-

ocardial infarction during sexual activity is relatively low (Papadopoulos, 1989). Some investigators have suggested that the cardiac cost of sexual activity with a familiar partner is similar to the cardiac cost of activities such as driving a car or climbing two flights of stairs (Hellerstein & Friedman, 1970; Siewicki & Mansfield, 1977). Alternatives to coitus, such as masturbation, generally result in lower peak heart rates and blood pressures during orgasm than does sex with a partner (Wagner & Sivarajan, 1979). Anal sex, however, may lead to irregular heart rhythms secondary to stimulation of the rectal muscle and mucus lining (Cambre, 1978).

If the following signs and symptoms occur related to sexual activity, such activity may not be safe; the client should report these signs and symptoms to his or her physician.

- Heart rate that does not return to normal within 5 to 10 minutes after orgasm
- Chest pain that is new or different and is not relieved by nitroglycerin
- Severe fatigue after sexual activity
- Sleeplessness following sexual activity
- Dizziness
- Palpitations, if you do not usually have them (U.S. Lung Centers, lecture series, 1996)

Some medications prescribed for clients with hypertension or cardiac disease (eg, antihypertensives and digitalis) can interfere with sexual functioning. Additionally, diuretics, or drugs frequently associated with cardiac and pulmonary disorders, can cause erectile dysfunction in some men.

Pulmonary diagnoses include asthma, chronic obstructive pulmonary disease, and emphysema. The increase in breathing rate during the sexual response cycle may cause discomfort for individuals with pulmonary disease.

Two major functional problems that frequently hinder the sexual activity of individuals with cardiac or pulmonary problems are decreased endurance and shortness of breath. Specific suggestions to facilitate comfortable and satisfying sexual activity for these problems include:

- Avoid sexual activity if fatigued or anxious
- Avoid sexual activity in extremely humid, hot, or cold environments
- Wait 3 hours after eating or drinking alcohol before engaging in sexual activity
- Use a well-ventilated room
- Avoid positions that put pressure on the chest wall or diaphragm
- Avoid high-energy positions (try side-lying or spoon positions) (Neistadt & Freda, 1987)
- Relax before, during, and after sexual activity (Papadopoulos, 1989)
- Use energy conservation techniques and planning for sexual activity (ie, do not mow the lawn the same afternoon that you would like to engage in sexual activity)
- Resume sexual activity in familiar surroundings

Musculoskeletal and Orthopedic Disorders

Diagnoses that affect the musculoskeletal and orthopedic system include (1) back and neck sprain or strain, (2) joint replacements, (3) arthritis, (4) **amputation**, (5) trauma, and (6) **scoliosis**. All these diagnostic categories can result in pain, loss of joint ROM, deformity, and fatigue. Because amputation, scoliosis, and arthritis can cause such visible physical effects, individuals with these disorders may suffer emotional as well as mechanical barriers to sexual activity (Buckwalter, Wernimont, & Buckwalter, 1982; Majerovitz & Revenson, 1994). For any chronic conditions, depression, fatigue, or fear of pain may diminish the desire for sexual activity (Neistadt & Freda, 1987). Fear of causing pain or injury to the partner with the disabling condition may also hinder sexual activity; this can often be misinterpreted as a lack of desire (Buckwalter, Wernimont, & Buckwalter, 1982).

The following are suggested strategies to deal with the functional sexuality problems often experienced by individuals with musculoskeletal disorders:

- *Fatigue*: Employ energy conservation techniques
- *Contractures:* Use positions that incorporate contractures
- *Pain:* Use analgesics before sexual activity; avoid positions that use painful body part; for back pain try a seated position; for neck pain avoid positions that encourage head forward droop; for joint pain avoid positions that put prolonged pressure on affected joints.
(Neistadt & Freda, 1987; Buckwalter, et al., 1982)

▼ SEXUALLY TRANSMITTED DISEASES

All people who engage in sexual behavior are at risk for contracting sexually transmitted diseases, including the human immunodeficiency virus (HIV) infection. Therefore, it is important for counseling to include cautions about high-risk behaviors, such as engaging in sexual activity without protective barriers. Protective barriers include latex condoms for coitus or anal sex, and latex squares for oral sex. Vaginal spermicidal foams and gels add an extra measure of protection for women (Kassler, 1993).

▼ PREGNANCY AND CHILDBIRTH

In addition to the normal fears and questions that all women have about pregnancy, women with disabilities must consider the effect the pregnancy will have on the disability and the possible effect the disability will have on the pregnancy. Some disabilities may exacerbate the effects of pregnancy on a woman's body (Freda, Cioschi, & Nilson, 1989). All implications of pregnancy must be considered carefully by women with disabilities. These considerations include medication management, functional changes, access to good obstetrical care, and lifestyle changes. The obstetrician working with a pregnant woman with a disability needs to fully understand the disability or consult with a rehabilitation physician, nurse, or nurse practitioner to identify and appropriately manage disability-specific concerns such as increased spasticity or autonomic dysreflexia.

Occupational therapy practitioners have a role in addressing the functional concerns during pregnancy and childbirth. These concerns include:

- Mobility and balance problems due to increased weight and shift in center of gravity
- Joint instability due to hormonal changes and the softening of ligaments and tendons
- Increased pain due to weight gain and other bodily changes
- Decreased transfer independence due to weight gain and unequal distribution of weight
- Decreased independence in manual wheelchair mobility
- Decreased endurance secondary to diminished respiratory capacity caused by increased uterine size
- Decreased ADL independence (especially lower extremity hygiene and dressing)
- Decreased independence in homemaking due to decreases in mobility
- Positioning difficulties for labor and delivery due to spasticity, contractures, or other deformities.
(Neistadt & Freda, 1987; Freda et al., 1989)

▼ ADDRESSING SEXUALITY

Self-Awareness and Interpersonal Communication

Sexuality is a private and intimate issue. Once the sexuality of another human being is acknowledged the practitioner becomes much closer to the client emotionally and must be careful to maintain the appropriate personal boundaries. This is for the welfare of both the client and the practitioner. It is not good for the client to become too emotionally attached to the practitioner or begin to assign sexual feelings to the existing therapeutic relationship. On the other hand the practitioner cannot be "therapeutic" if the empathy felt toward an individual's situation becomes too personalized.

Practitioners must examine their own beliefs and attitudes before initiation of any sex-counseling sessions with clients. A practitioner who is not comfortable with discussing sex outside of a therapy session should not attempt to do so within the parameters of a therapy session. As a professional dealing with sexual issues, practitioners must be prepared to hear about sexual preferences and activities that may differ greatly from their own; this situation must be met with professionalism, not judgment or disdain (Neistadt & Freda, 1987).

Acknowledgement of Sexuality and Initiation of Discussions

The practitioner can acknowledge the client's sexuality by providing positive feedback about the client's physical appearance and by initiating discussion of sexuality issues. Complimenting a client on a particular blouse or shirt, or noting when a client is well shaved are ways of letting clients know they are still attractive and appealing people.

Initiating discussions about sexuality issues is another way of letting clients know that they are still viewed as sexual beings. Research has shown that most rehabilitation clients have questions about sexuality, but are too hesitant to ask those questions (Neistadt & Baker, 1978). Occupational therapy practitioners do not wait for their clients to initiate discussions about movement or daily-living skills, and they should not wait for clients to initiate discussions about sexuality concerns.

In general, practitioners feel most comfortable initiating discussions about sexuality with clients after they have worked with individuals long enough to develop strong interpersonal rapport and clear pictures of clients' strengths and problems. Additionally, by that time the practitioner will have a better sense of the environment and relationships to which clients will return. The concerns of a long married older man recovering from a stroke will be very different from those of a single, young woman recovering from a spinal cord injury. Both will have very legitimate concerns and issues; the former may have logistic concerns about the resumption of sexual activity with his spouse, whereas the latter may be more concerned with ways to initiate an intimate relationship.

One way for practitioners to initiate these discussions is to start with a general statement, such as: "People who have been in the hospital for a while or who are experiencing difficulties like yours often have questions about sexuality. I have some information about sexuality and disability, so I could try to answer your questions. If I do not have the answers to your questions, I will try and find the answers or refer you to someone on staff who knows more about this area than I do." (Neistadt & Freda, 1987). For clients with limited cognitive abilities, this introduction may have to be modified to, "Do you have any questions about sex?" By introducing the topic in this way the practitioner has given the client permission to ask previously unspoken questions and set the stage for involvement of other professionals if necessary.

Provision of Information and Counseling Strategies

Clients who are younger than 18 years of age or who are not their own legal guardians will need parental or guardian consent for sexuality counseling. Because sexuality is such an emotionally charged issue, the provision of sexuality counseling may not be perceived by parents and guardians as a legitimate part of a general rehabilitation program.

For those clients who are appropriate for counseling there are several different formats in which the information can be shared; how a practitioner provides the information to a particular client will be largely based on the comfort level of that client. Some clients may only be comfortable with reading selected written information in the privacy of their own rooms. For some, that will be a first step, followed by a one-to-one session with the practitioner to ask specific questions not answered by the written material. It is often helpful to include the significant other in these sessions. These private sessions are best suited for clients with very specific concerns about their abilities to engage in certain sexual activities or to procreate.

Group lectures are often used as a way to give general sexual, anatomical, physiological, and disability-specific information. This format gives the added advantage of peer support for sharing sexual difficulties, concerns, and solutions. This type of approach may include clients only, clients and families, or families only. A combination of lecture, written materials, slides, and film are usually effective for this type of session.

Formal sexuality programs are most appropriate for clients who are likely to have both social and physical problems with their sexuality as a result of their disability (eg, clients with head injuries or developmental disabilities). These programs usually involve a series of group meetings to cover all the necessary areas (anatomy, sexual system, contraception, safe sex practices, effects of disability) in detail.

Counseling individuals with a disability about sexuality is a heavy responsibility; the practitioner's response to the client's questions, concerns, and fears may have a lasting effect on the client. The practitioner must employ a nonjudgmental attitude, regardless of the information shared. The main goal for this type of counseling is to be an objective information giver. The practitioner must learn how to really "listen" to what the client is saying and to understand any of the underlying, unspoken fears. Practitioners must maintain eye contact and speak in a very normal tone; a therapeutic, but relaxed atmosphere should be established (Neistadt & Freda, 1987).

▶SEXUALITY AND DISABILITY CONCLUSION

Occupational therapy practitioners have a unique role in sexuality counseling for people with disabilities. The functional perspective that the occupational therapy practitioner can bring to a counseling session is extremely appropriate and helpful in a client's quest to resume sexual activity and once again feel like a sexual being after disabling conditions or accidents interrupt that part of life.

Acknowledgements for Section 2

This section has been adapted from the section appearing in the 8th edition, with the permission of the author, Maureen Neistadt; much of the original work remains and is gratefully acknowledged.

Section 3

Treatment for Work and Productive Activities: Home and Family Management

Kathleen Hilko Culler

Lifestyle Variations
Occupational Therapy Interventions Strategies for
  Home Management and Caregiving
  Remediation
  Compensation
  Environmental Modifications
  Education of Client and Family Members
  Child Care
  Regaining Community Skills
  Training Apartment
  Home Visits
Home and Family Management Conclusion

H ome maintainer is one of the major roles a person may have during a lifetime. A *home maintainer* is a person who has responsibility, at least once a week, for home management tasks (Oakley, 1981). Home management tasks include clothing care, cleaning, meal preparation and cleanup, shopping, money management, household maintenance, and safety procedures (see Appendix F). Successful performance of home management tasks is required for independent community living and requires higher-level organizational and planning skills than performance of self-care tasks (Lawton & Brody, 1969). The role of caregiver is often closely related to that of home maintainer. A *caregiver* is a person who has responsibility, at least once a week, for the care of someone such as a child, spouse, relative, or friend (Oakley, 1981). A major focus of occupational therapy is to help clients return to or assume these two roles.

▼ LIFESTYLE VARIATIONS

Adults have varied responsibilities in the areas of home management and caregiving. Therefore, an occupational therapy practitioner will need to help clients work on tasks and levels of task performance pertinent to their lifestyles. As a way of dealing with this issue, the Rehabilitation Institute of Chicago Instrumental Activities of Daily Living (IADL) protocol (1990) recognizes varying levels of performance for each IADL. For instance, meal preparation and cleanup has five levels of complexity, from easiest to hardest: preparation of (1) self-serve, such as a salad from a grocery store salad bar; (2) cold meals, such as sandwiches; (3) hot beverages, soups, or prepared foods, such as frozen dinners; (4) hot one-dish meals, such as baked macaroni; and (5) hot multicourse meals such as baked chicken with potatoes and vegetables (Rehabilitation Institute of Chicago, 1990). Each successive level requires progressively more sophisticated cognitive, perceptual, and motor performance component skills (see Appendix F for full list of performance component skills). The level of complexity appropriate as a goal for any given client will depend on his or her lifestyle before treatment and the levels of cognitive, perceptual, and motor skills he or she is likely to achieve by the end of treatment. Occupational therapists need to suggest treatment goals and activities for home management and caregiving that are consistent with the client's priorities and anticipated abilities. Therapists can use their activity analysis skills (see Unit V) to determine what levels of task proficiency are a good match for the client's anticipated performance component skill levels.

▼ OCCUPATIONAL THERAPY INTERVENTIONS STRATEGIES FOR HOME MANAGEMENT AND CAREGIVING

There are four types of intervention strategies that can be used with clients demonstrating deficits in home management or caregiving:

1. Remediating performance areas and performance component deficits.
2. Teaching new methods of task performance to compensate for performance area or performance component deficits.
3. Suggesting environmental modifications to make task performance easier.
4. Educating clients and families to support the above approaches or as a means of preventing future problems.

Each of these approaches will be summarized below.

Remediation

The focus of remediation is to improve or restore the client's performance and performance components to pretreatment levels. This approach is appropriate when a client's condition or diagnosis (eg, generalized weakness or deconditioning, acute arthritis) or performance component deficits are likely to improve enough to allow pretreatment levels of task proficiency. For example, a practitioner may teach a client with arthritis exercises to improve the client's shoulder ROM so that he or she could perform meal preparation tasks such as reaching into a cabinet for cooking supplies or dishes. Various parameters need to be considered when grading activities and measuring the effectiveness of treatment using a remediation approach. These parameters include the following:

1. *Physical assistance.* There should be an inverse correlation between the amount of ability demonstrated by the client and the amount of assistance provided by the practitioner or caregiver. That is, as a client displays increased skill in completing a task, the practitioner or caregiver should intervene less frequently.

2. *Supervision and cuing.* Supervision and cuing can include the number of cues given, in addition to the types (written materials, tactile, and verbal) of cues used. Written materials (booklets, handouts, written home programs with illustrations or pictures) can be used to reinforce teaching that has occurred during occupational therapy treatment. Tactile cues can be used effectively to modify or guide client performance (eg, guiding a stroke client's involved arm to reach for a glass in a cabinet). Lastly, the type of verbal cue can affect client performance. While on a community outing to the grocery store, a direct cue provides the client with a specific instruction, such as: "The spaghetti is here," as the practitioner points to the aisle where spaghetti is located. An indirect cue provides assistance to the client in a less directive manner, such as: "Can you find the foods listed on your grocery list?"

3. *Task demands.* Task demands (ie, the amount of cognitive and physical skill required to perform the task) affect quality of client performance. In selecting the type of task, consider the complexity of performance skills demanded by the task. As a general rule, with neurologically involved clients, it is better to select a task with low motor and high cognitive demands or with high motor and low cognitive demands (Chapparo, 1979), and then progress to increasing levels of both. As an example, for a client with stroke, participating in a community outing is an activity that requires high cognitive demand. In addition, the client's mobility may become compromised. Thus, the client may ambulate for a short amount of time, but as the quality of the client's gait decreases, the client may need to complete the community outing in a wheelchair (high cognitive, low motor demand).

4. *Amount of task.* Increasing the number of steps or tasks that a client needs to complete can be indicative of increased proficiency. During a community outing, a client may be able to progress from completing one errand in 1 hour to completing three errands in 1 hour.

5. *Type of task.* Cognitive tasks can be graded from routine and familiar to unfamiliar or new. As an example, it is less demanding for a client to cook a familiar recipe from memory than to follow a new recipe from a cookbook. A task organized by the client without assistance from the practitioner is a high level of performance.

6. *Environment.* Environment plays a role in task performance. A familiar environment (eg, kitchen at home) is less demanding than a new environment (eg, clinic kitchen). In addition, the type of stimulation can vary from a quiet, nondistracting environment, such as a room with no noise or other people, to a distracting, busy environment, such as the community. For clients in wheelchairs, lack of wheelchair accessibility can prohibit the client's ability to access services (banks, restaurant, stores) in the community.

By altering the various parameters in treatment, an activity can be upgraded or downgraded to provide a difficult, but not overwhelming, challenge that results in a successful experience for the client.

Compensation

The compensation approach focuses on using remaining abilities to achieve the highest level of functioning possible in the areas of home and family management. If the client cannot perform these tasks in the usual manner, then adapted techniques or equipment are used to maximize client abilities. This strategy can be used (1) when a client's condition is temporary, such as for hip replacement; (2) when precautions need to be taken; (3) when the condition is not amenable to remediation; or (4) when task speed and proficiency are greatly improved by use of adaptive equipment or adaptive techniques. Use of adaptive techniques is preferable to use of equipment because techniques allow the client more flexibility. Use of adaptive equipment is less preferable because of the cost incurred for equipment purchase and maintenance and the inconvenience of having to transport the equipment for task performance. Table 19–10 outlines specific adaptive equipment and techniques that can be used for various impairments (Hopkins & Smith, 1993; Klinger, 1978; Pedretti, 1996; Trombly, 1989).

Energy conservation and work simplification techniques can help clients perform home management and caregiving tasks in spite of the mobility and endurance problems imposed by many disabilities (American Heart Association, date unknown; Hopkins & Smith, 1993; Pedretti, 1996; Rehabilitation Institute of Chicago (RIC), 1988; Trombly, 1989). These techniques require that the practitioner and client address the following points:

1. Determine what tasks need to be improved; that is, according to the client, what tasks take too long, cause fatigue, or take too much energy.

2. List all the steps of the task, including setup, performance, and cleanup.

3. Analyze the task.
   a. Why is the task necessary?
   b. What is the purpose of the task?

(text continues on page 375)

TABLE 19-10. Adaptive Equipment and Techniques for Home and Family Management Activities

Impairment
One upper-extremity or body side impairment.

Common Diagnoses Resulting in This Impairment
Hemiplegia (cerebrovascular accident (CVA) or head injury), unilateral trauma or amputation, temporary conditions such as burns and peripheral neuropathy.

Rationale for Using Compensatory Strategies
To allow for safe, one-handed performance; to stabilize objects for task completion; with hemiplegia, to compensate for loss of balance and mobility

ADL area	Adaptive equipment	Adaptive techniques
Meal preparation and cleanup	To stabilize objects, consider use of: • Adapted cutting board with stainless steel or aluminum nails for cutting or peeling. Raised corners on the board can stabilize bread to spread ingredients or make a sandwich • Sponge dishes, Dycem™ or suction devices to stabilize bowls or dishes during food preparation. • Pot stabilizer. To allow for safe, one-handed performance: • Adapted jar openers. • Electric appliances such as food processor and hand mixer save time and energy. Note: client safety and judgment need to be considered when electrical appliances are considered. • Rocker knife. • Whisk to mix food. To compensate for decreased standing tolerance and mobility, consider use of: • Utility cart to transport objects. • If cooking is done at wheelchair level or seated, use angled mirror over the stove to watch food on the stove. For cleanup, consider use of: • Handheld spray for rinsing dishes. • Rubber mat at bottom of sink to reduce breakage. • Suction-type brush to clean glassware.	If balance is affected, it is recommended that the task be done in a seated position. • Objects can be stabilized by using the knees. • Pots and pans can be slid across counters, rather than lifted. • To open a jar, place it in a drawer, then lean against it to stabilize it before opening. • Scissors can be used to open plastic bags. • Milk cartons can be opened by using the prolonged portion of a fork. • An egg can be cracked by holding it in the palm of the hand, hitting the egg against the edge of the bowl, and separating the egg shell with the index and middle fingers. For clean-up: • Soak and air-dry dishes for easier clean-up.
Clothing management (laundry, ironing, clothing repair)	• Laundry can be transported to and from and dryer using a wheeled cart.	
Housecleaning	• A tank-type vacuum permits the client to sit and reach areas to be cleaned up. • Long-reach duster. • Long-handled dustpan and brush. • Self-wringing mop.	• Incorporate energy conservation by making bed completely at each corner before progressing to the next corner. • No-wax floors are easier to care for. • If balance and ambulation problems are present, some floor care can be managed from a seated position.
Child care	For feeding use: • High chairs with one-handed tray release mechanism. • Electric baby dish keeps food warm during the meal. • Tongs can be used to remove baby food from heated water. • Use screw top, rather than plastic liner bottles. • If breastfeeding, pillows or commercially available carriers can be used to position the baby.	For feeding: • Prop the infant on pillows, in an infant seat, or against arm or an upholstered chair. If breastfeeding, try various positions to accommodate affected side (sidelying). • Premixed formula can eliminate the need for measuring. • Stabilize the bottle inside a coffee cup and use funnel to pour into bottle.

(continued)

TABLE 19-10. (Continued)

ADL area	Adaptive equipment	Adaptive techniques
	For bathing: • Strap the baby into a suction-based bath seat. For dressing: • Use a Velcro strap on dressing table to reduce squirming. • Use disposable diapers with tab closures/for cloth diapers, use diaper covers with Velcro covers. For transporting child: • Try various child carriers (front, side, and back types available). • Use a bassinet on wheels, a stroller, or a wagon to transport child from room to room.	

Impairment
Reduced upper-extremity range of motion and strength

Common Diagnoses Resulting in This Impairment
Quadriplegia, burns, arthritis, upper-extremity amputation, multiple sclerosis, amyotrophic lateral sclerosis, orthopedic and other traumatic injuries.

Rationale for Using Compensatory Strategies
To compensate for lack of reach or hand grip; to compensate for lack of strength or tolerance for prolonged activity; to allow gravity to assist; to compensate for decreased balance.

ADL area	Adaptive equipment	Adaptive techniques
Meal preparation and cleanup	Consider the use of: • Adapted jar opener. • Foam or built-up handles on utensils. • Universal cuff to hold utensils to compensate for reduced grip. • Long-handled reacher to obtain light-weight objects from overhead or low places. • Wheeled cart to transport objects. • Adapted cutting board. • Loop handles can be added to utensils to substitute for reduced grasp. • If using a walker, a walker basket can help transport objects. For marketing: • Marketing by phone or mail is recommended because many objects may be out of reach in store.	• Joint protective measures for rheumatoid arthritis. • Position electrical appliances within easy reach. This helps to conserve energy. • To conserve energy; work at a seated position. • Use teeth to open containers. • Purchase convenience foods to eliminate food preparation. • Tenodesis action (wrist extension and finger flexion; wrist flexion and finger extension) can be used to pick up lightweight objects. • Use a fork to open milk cartons. • Use lightweight pots, pans, and utensils.
Housecleaning	• Long-handled reacher allows objects be picked up from the floor. • Long-handled sponge to clean bath tub. • Self-wringing mop. • Use lightweight tools such as sponge mops and brooms for floor care.	• Use aerosol cleaners to dissolve dirt before cleaning surfaces. • When making the bed, do not tuck sheets in.
Laundry	• If client is ambulatory, the preference is for a top-loading washer to avoid the need to bend. • Push-button controls on the washer and dryer are easier to use than knobs. If knobs are present, they may need to be adapted. • If client chooses to iron, set iron at a low temperature setting. An asbestos pad can be placed at the end of the ironing board to eliminate the need to stand iron up after each ironing stroke.	• Use premeasured packages of soap or bleach to avoid handling large containers. It may be more economical to buy larger containers and have someone else measure soap or bleach into single packets. Use energy conservation: • Place hangers near dryer to hang permanent press items as they come out of the dryer. Remain seated to do ironing.

(continued)

TABLE 19-10. (Continued)

ADL area	Adaptive equipment	Adaptive techniques
Child care	• If client lacks mobility to get up and down from the floor, then a crib with a swing open side allows the parent in a wheelchair to wheel close to the baby. For feeding: • Feeding can be done with a child in an infant seat or propped up on pillows. • An electric baby dish can be placed in a convenient area to keep food warm throughout the meal. • Formula can be prepared by another family member and placed in bottles for use during the day. For dressing: • Clothing should be large with closures that are easily handled. • Disposable diapers with tabs are easily manipulated.	Use energy conservation: • Have client do the more enjoyable tasks, delegate other tasks to a helper. The safest place to handle an infant is on the floor. All tasks, including sponge bathing, feeding and playing, can be done on the floor. • A method to obtain assistance in an emergency needs to be determined. • Dressing and diapering can be done on a table or desk that allows for wheelchair access.

Impairment
Incoordination of upper extremities

Common Diagnoses Resulting in This Impairment
Head injury, cerebral palsy, CVA, multiple sclerosis, tumors, other neurological conditions

Rationale for Using Compensatory Strategies
To stabilize proximal portion of limbs; to reduce movements distally by using weight; to stabilize objects for task completion; to provide an environment in which client is safe and proficient; to avoid breakage or accidents with sharp utensils or hot food or equipment.

ADL area	Adaptive equipment	Adaptive techniques
Meal preparation and cleanup	• Use heavy cookware, ironstone dishes to aid with distal stabilization. • Use pots and casseroles with double handles to provide greater stability. • Weighted wrist cuffs may reduce tremors. • Use nonslip materials such as Dycem™ to provide stability. • Use adapted cutting board to stabilize food while cutting. • A serrated knife is less likely to slip than a straight-edged knife. • Using a frying basket to cook foods, such as vegetables, makes for safe removal and reduces the chance of burns. • Free-standing appliances, electric skillet, and countertop mixer, are safer than transferring objects out of oven or using handheld mixer. • Use a milk carton holder with handles to pour milk. • A stove with front controls is preferred so the client does not need to reach over hot pots to the back of the stove. • A wheeled cart that is weighted is one alternative for transporting food. • Place a rubber mat or sponge cloth at the bottom of the sink to cushion fall of dishes.	• During food preparation, such as cutting and peeling, stabilize arms proximally to reduce tremors. • Start the stove after the food has been placed on the burner. • Sliding food and dishes over a counter is preferable to lifting to transport food item. • To avoid breakage, soak dishes, rinse with hand sprayer and drip dry—eliminate dish handling.
Housecleaning	• Heavier work tools are useful. A dust mitt is easier to handle than gripping a duster. • Fitted sheets on a bed are recommended.	• Eliminate or store excess household decorations to reduce dusting.

(continued)

TABLE 19-10. (Continued)

ADL area	Adaptive equipment	Adaptive techniques
Laundry	• Premeasured soap and bleach eliminates spills that can occur during measuring. • Eliminate ironing through selection of no-iron clothing and materials.	
Child care	• Use a wide safety strap on dressing table or use a bed. • Use disposable, tape–tab diapers. • Use Velcro closures for infant clothing. • Feeding with a spoon is recommended only if incoordination is mild. • Transporting child: Consider infant carrier or use of bassinet on wheels, stroller, or wagon.	With mild incoordination: • Use stabilizing measure such as holding upper arms close to body and sitting while working. • It is safer to work on the floor while caring for the infant.

Impairment
Mobility impairment without upper-extremity involvement

Common Diagnoses Resulting in This Impairment
Paraplegia, osteoarthritis, lower-extremity amputation, burns, leg and knee fractures and replacement

Rationale for Using Compensatory Strategies
Mobility may be provided by a wheelchair. Wheelchair accessibility includes consideration of work heights, maneuverability, and access to storage, equipment, and supplies.
Other types of mobility devices (walker, crutches) may require increased endurance.

ADL area	Adaptive equipment	Adaptive techniques
Meal preparation and cleanup	• Transport items using a wheelchair laptray. The laptray can be used as a work surface to protect lap from hot pans. • Stove controls should be in the front of the stove. • Use an angled mirror to see the contents of pots.	• Remove cabinet doors to eliminate need to maneuver around them. • Place frequently used items on easy-to-reach shelves, above and below countertop level. Increase height of wheelchair to allow use of standard height countertops.
Laundry Housekeeping Childcare	• Use front-loading washer and dryer. • Use self-propelled lightweight vacuums. For feeding: • Use plastic baby bottles with liners to eliminate the need to sterilize bottles. • Position the baby in an infant seat. The seat can be held or placed on a table. • For highchairs, select a chair with a safety belt and a swing-away tray with one-hand release. For a playpen: • Use an adjustable-height, portable crib with a hinged door for easy access. For lifting, carrying, and transporting: • A converted, lightweight car bed with straps sewn on the side of the bed can be secured to the wheelchair armrests. • With an older child (4 to 5 months old), touch-fastener seat belt can be attached to the wheelchair. • Select stroller with the following features: single handle to allow for one-handed steering, brakes, and opening and closing of stroller should be managed easily. • Attach a safety strap from handle of stroller to waist of parent to prevent stroller from pulling away on an incline.	Safety consideration for all individuals: • Use a phrase or certain voice consistently. • Uses that can be associated with disciplinary action (ie, "touch my chair" if the child is running ahead). • Have children play in rooms that have been child-proofed and where access to the parent is not an issue (ie, child cannot run behind a couch).

c. When and where should it be done?

d. What is the best way for the client to accomplish it?

4. Develop a new method of performing the task. Consider eliminating unnecessary steps, combining motions and activities, rearranging the sequence of the steps, and simplifying the details of the task by taking the following steps:

a. Use correct work height to reduce fatigue and promote good posture. Correct work height in standing should be 2 inches below the bent elbow; in sitting, client should avoid positions that require lifting the shoulders or "winging out" the elbows.

b. Preposition supplies and equipment in work areas. Clear area of unnecessary items. As an example, to pay bills, obtain needed supplies, such as calculator, bills, and stamps, before beginning task.

c. Organize the work center. Having necessary supplies and equipment increases productivity with less effort. In the kitchen, place the can opener near the canned goods. Place the most frequently used items within easy reach on counters or shelves immediately above or below counter height.

d. Use laborsaving devices. This includes using wheels for transport; in the kitchen, using electric appliances, such as an electric mixer and food processor; for outdoors, using an electric garage door opener and motorized lawn mower. Transport heavy objects using wheels.

e. Fatigue can result in poor body mechanics and reduced safety awareness. Regular rest breaks should be incorporated into the client's schedule. The client should alternate light and heavy tasks throughout the day and week. Heavy work tasks, such as cleaning the oven, stripping and waxing floors, or doing yard work, should be delegated to another family member or done by a professional cleaning service.

f. Use proper body mechanics. This includes use of a wide base of support, using both sides of the body and keeping objects close to the body, facing objects when reaching or lifting to avoid twisting, pushing rather than pulling objects, and alternating positions and motions to avoid fatigue.

5. Implement new methods.

Environmental Modifications

Environmental modifications are considered a compensatory strategy. Compared with remediation and compensation, in which the practitioner directly influences client functioning, environmental modification is a means of indirectly maximizing client function. Modifications can range from extensive home modifications to make a home wheelchair accessible, to low-cost strategies, such as removing obstacles to make a household safer for an older person who has impaired vision and mobility.

Education of Client and Family Members

The final type of occupational therapy intervention strategy is client and family education. This is a key component to the occupational therapy treatment plan because the approaches of remediation, compensation, and prevention involve learning new strategies and, more importantly, incorporating these strategies into client and family habits and lifestyles. In some circumstances, the practitioner may provide education to the family in addition to client education or in place of client education. The following issues are central to effective client and family education (Bowling, 1981; Kautzman, 1991):

1. *Have a clear plan about the purpose of the teaching session.* An observable goal for teaching can assist both the practitioner and client regarding expectations and anticipated outcome. Based on client and family motivation, cognitive status, and skill level that need to be achieved, and time availability for the teaching and learning process, the expected outcomes or goals may vary. The three levels of goals include knowledge, application, and problem solving. At the level of knowledge, a client is asked to recall basic facts presented by the practitioner. For example, the practitioner may ask a client to name the five techniques used for good body mechanics. At the application level, the client and family are shown ways of incorporating this information into home management. The practitioner may demonstrate how to use body mechanics when retrieving food from the oven during performance of meal preparation and then ask the client to incorporate the same strategy while performing the task. At the level of problem solving, the client is asked to use information in new situations that have not been demonstrated by the practitioner. For example, the practitioner may ask the client to demonstrate how to use good body mechanics when shoveling snow.

2. *The presentation of information needs to be appropriate to the clients' educational and emotional levels.* The choice of terminology used with a client who has had a few years of formal education should vary from that used with a client who has a college education. Client readiness to receive information will vary. The client may be overwhelmed with life changes caused by the disability and unable to concentrate on issues that the practitioner feels needs to be addressed. Therefore, for a task that a client may not be concerned with, but that will be needed at home, the inpatient practitioner may try to increase client awareness by introducing appropriate adaptive equipment. Once the client has returned home, the motivation to perform in this area may increase. Then the outpatient practitioner can promote client application and problem solving in the outpatient occupational therapy program.

3. *Instructions must be clear.* Clear instructions increase the possibility of client carryover. For example, instead of telling a client to use proper body mechanics for all activ-

ities, it is preferable and more realistic to begin with having the client identify one or two activities that require these techniques. The client may need assistance to do this. Another strategy to increase carryover is to explain the rationale for the therapy recommendations.

4. *Ask open-ended questions to ensure client understanding.* For example: Why is it important for you to incorporate proper body mechanics into your day-to-day activities?

5. *Use client response to determine the amount of information presented during a session.* If the client's attention is waning or if the client's learning ability is decreased, termination of the teaching session is recommended. If the amount of information is extensive, it may be preferable to present it over several sessions. Taking the added time to ensure client competence in performance is time well spent.

6. *Promote the highest level of learning possible, preferably the problem-solving level.* Involve the clients by asking questions about how information presented might affect their lifestyles. For example, a practitioner may ask of an arthritic client: "Which joint protection techniques do you think you would use at home? How could you use these techniques while cooking?" It is preferable to follow this up with client demonstration to ensure that the client has integrated the information into pertinent tasks.

7. *Illustrate or demonstrate the points being taught.* Use of such aids as demonstration, pictures, videotapes, and handouts reinforces teaching and helps the client and family remember the information presented. A study of client-doctor visits found that only half of the information covered was remembered by the client (Ley, 1972). Some of the ways of reinforcing teaching include repeating information throughout the session and allowing adequate time for practice by the client or family members to ensure that they are comfortable with and capable of using the information outside the therapy situation. If the client or family member cannot gain adequate competency or perform the task in a safe manner, then other options such as a paid caregiver or identifying community support (eg, home health aide) need to be considered.

Child Care

For clients who have responsibility for infants, it may be useful to use a life-sized, weighted doll to simulate caregiver tasks. A parent whose ability to perform caregiver tasks safely is questioned should be advised to find help to care for the child.

Regaining Community Skills

Frequently, clients need to access the community for home management tasks, such as grocery shopping and banking. Areas that need to be evaluated include (1) planning, (2) money management, (3) path finding, (4) community safety, (5) use of transportation, (6) mobility, (7) time management, and (8) psychosocial issues, such as exhibiting problem solving to overcome obstacles and interpersonal skills for social interaction. Although a therapist may pursue evaluation and training on an individual basis with a client, community reentry groups are another mechanism that can allow clients discuss and practice community skills. It is helpful if the group is interdisciplinary, with the focus of occupational therapy generally being on tasks and performance components required for successful return to the community. The focus of treatment will vary, based on client diagnosis. For example, for a client who has had a stroke, whose major-limiting factors are in the perceptual and cognitive area, therapy may focus on organization and time management (accomplishing two errands in under 1 hour), ability to attend to a task in a busy environment (finding items on a grocery list in a store), and problem solving (what to do when unable to locate a food item). On the other hand, for a client with a spinal cord injury, whose major limitations are physical, the focus may be on dealing with accessibility and managing personal care tasks in the community (eg, changing a leg bag).

Training Apartment

A training apartment that is available in the health care setting can be used to simulate the experience of returning home and confronting issues that may arise. The time spent in a training apartment may range from 1 hour of individual treatment sessions to 1-to 2-night stays. Given the anticipated circumstances, the client and family members (if appropriate) can attempt personal care and home management tasks required after discharge. This provides an opportunity to identify areas in which the client and family members feel comfortable and to identify issues that need further consideration. The occupational therapy practitioner then can intervene appropriately in preparation for discharge to home.

Home Visits

Often a question arises about whether the client will be safe at home. The purposes of a home visit are to (1) evaluate client level of functional independence and safety at home and (2) provide the client and family with recommendations concerning accessibility, safety, and home modification. A home visit is best done by an occupational and physical therapist together. It is important to explain the purpose of the home visit to family and client. During the home visit, the client should complete activities that typically are performed at home, such as making a bed, transferring in and out of the tub, moving on and off the toilet, and fixing something in the kitchen. The tasks should be relevant to anticipated home responsibilities as well as to client and family experiences.

The results of the home visit should be discussed with the client and family. Recommendations are then written up to reinforce the discussion. Recommendations may vary, based on client circumstances (eg, preferences and financial support). When a home visit is not feasible, obtaining information from the client or family member relative to the discharge environment is a useful option.

►HOME AND FAMILY MANAGEMENT CONCLUSION

The occupational therapy practitioner plays a key role in facilitating a client's return to the roles of homemaker and caregiver. Treatment intervention strategies include remediation, compensation, environmental modification, and education. The therapist selects the treatment strategies on the basis of factors such as client and family goals, client condition, anticipated length of treatment, interdisciplinary goals, and the therapist's professional judgment about skills needed to perform pertinent home management and caregiver tasks.

Section 4

Treatment of Work and Productive Activities: Functional Restoration, An Industrial Rehabilitation Approach

Sherlyn Fenton and Patricia Gagnon

Historical Overview
Work Program Referral Process
Work Program Evaluation
Work Program Treatment
    Frequency and Duration
    Documentation
    Body Mechanics
    Work Conditioning and Work Hardening
    Work-Hardening Team
    Specialized Protocols
    Job Site Analysis
    Vocational Counseling
    Prework Screening
    Prevention Education
Industrial Rehabilitation Conclusion

▼ HISTORICAL OVERVIEW

As early as 1900, work was viewed as an alternative to the custodial care of [individuals with disabilities]. Likewise, industrial therapy was implemented in psychiatric hospitals, where jobs were analyzed according to skill level, physical and mental demands, and potential benefits (Commission on Practice, 1986, p. 841).

Clinical programming related to work has been greatly influenced in the United States by the legislative and political environments of specific eras. Laws, such as the Federal Industrial Rehabilitation Act of 1923, required all American general hospitals dealing with industrial accidents or illnesses to offer occupational therapy. By the 1930s occupational therapists were playing an influential role in the development of the "curative workshops, which were specifically aimed at the injured industrial worker and which utilized work-related activity as the treatment" (Jacobs, 1991, p. 5).

Global politics also played an integral role in the development of occupational therapy in work programs. The late 1940s post-World War II era emphasized retraining and re-education of injured soldiers. Following World War II, the supply of practicing therapists could not meet the demands of the military hospitals. Accredited occupational therapy programs increased from five in 1940s to eighteen in 1945. During this time the industrial economy was also growing. Because of the limited number of able-bodied workers, industries modified work environments to accommodate employees with disabilities. The adoption of the Vocational Rehabilitation Amendments in 1954 further bolstered professional interest in work-related programs. As a result, occupational therapists were instrumental in the development of prevocational exploration. "A priority of therapy was to get soldiers in the best possible shape for their return to a productive civilian life" (Hanson & Walker, 1992, p. 59).

Throughout the next two decades, the economy in the United States shifted from manufacturing industries to service industries. During this period occupational therapy adopted a medical model focusing more on physical, rather than functional modalities. "Occupational therapists were less involved in work programs in the 1950s, 1960s, and early 1970s than ever before in the history of the profession" (Hanson & Walker, 1992, p. 60). However, this low spell was not to last. Workers' compensation legislation and the rising cost of vocational rehabilitation programs created opportunities for occupational therapy practitioners to address the rehabilitation of injured workers.

The 1980s brought unparalleled growth and expansion in rehabilitation for injured workers. Work-hardening programs, which employed occupational therapy practitioners, became an increasingly popular approach to bridging the gap between acute rehabilitation and functional levels of productivity.

Many of the previously described principles of work are apparent in the work-hardening programs of today. Work is still received in the real-world sense and is used "to return the client to gainful employment or homemaking, to improve physical function, to reduce claims and exposure and maintain reserve levels, to provide the clients with independence in the community, and to provide the client with restored earnings." (Hightower-Vandamm, 1981, p. 633)

In 1988, both the Commission on Accreditation of Rehabilitation Facilities (CARF) and the National Advisory Committee on Work Hardening established guidelines for work-hardening programs. The committee presented the following definition:

Work hardening is a highly structured, goal oriented, individualized treatment program designed to maximize the individual's ability to return to work. Work-hardening programs, which are interdisciplinary in nature, use real or simulated work activities in conjunction with conditioning tasks that are graded to progressively improve the biomechanical, neuromuscular, cardiovascular/metabolic and psychosocial functions of the individual. Work hardening provides a transition between acute care and return to work while addressing the issues of productivity, safety, physical tolerances, and worker behaviors. (Ogden-Niemeyer & Jacobs, 1989, p. 1)

Occupational therapy practitioners play a major role in work-hardening programs.

Occupational therapy practitioners of the 1990s find themselves involved with addressing the work-related needs of not only clients, but also of industries and insurance companies. Lost work time, lost dollars, and restricted worker abilities have encouraged employers to become more involved and knowledgeable about the care and management of their injured workers. Injury-prevention programs and worker education are receiving greater emphasis.

In the present atmosphere of change in health care, the guiding principles for a successful industrial rehabilitation program must be quality care, cost containment, and the flexibility to expand services to meet the evolving needs of the marketplace.

Work has been at the core of occupational therapy for the last seven and half decades. The tenets of work, which include providing a way of making a living and giving meaning to one's existence, have remained consistent throughout occupational therapists' use of work in the treatment of physical disabilities during three eras: World War I and II, the era of industrial therapy, and the work-hardening era. Although technological advances and economics have changed the scope of work, it is evident that the work-hardening programs of today have their roots in the work cure of the early 1900s. (Hanson & Walker, 1992; p. 56)

▼ WORK PROGRAM REFERRAL PROCESS

When the return of occupational function is the desired outcome, there are no limits to the scope of diagnoses appropriate for referrals to the work-hardening arena. Whether the injury or illness is acute or chronic, if the ex-

isting condition limits an individual's ability to perform one or more of life's major functions, a functional restoration program may be the appropriate referral. Laborer, homemaker, electrician, computer analyst, or student—all are descriptions of occupations that present with unique characteristics that may require graduated approaches to wellness.

The sources of referrals for work hardening vary as much as the variety of clients. Physicians, occupational medicine nurses, insurance case managers, therapy practitioners, vocational counselors, attorneys, rehabilitation personnel, employers, and self-referrals are some of the many referral sources. Work-hardening programs may be the last stage of a therapeutic process to integrate the individual back into the workforce, or they may be an isolated therapeutic approach to evaluate and determine a worker's functional and physical capabilities. The program outcomes should be behavioral objectives identifying the person's capabilities to perform occupational tasks.

Many programs require a physician's order and a terms of payment agreement before clients begin. Each state and institution must determine policies according to state legislation and professional licensure standards. Once the initial referral is completed, the occupational therapist may be responsible for the initial client screening. Ongoing litigation, or behavioral, psychological, or social factors may delay or prevent initiation of programming.

The advent of managed care has altered the sequence of the admissions process and the programming of work hardening. Instead of having a client in a therapy program, and then measuring the outcome, the managed care approach defines the medical necessity of the program goals and, then, predetermines the services rendered and the duration of treatment.

The sooner the injured worker participates in rehabilitation, the more successful the outcome. Frymoyer found that only 40% of clients with low back pain who had been disabled for 6 months return to work; 1 year later this figure dropped to 20%, and 2 years later, the chances of return to work were nil. These findings suggest that clients who enter a work-hardening program at 6 weeks or less after injury have an estimated 80% to 90% expectation of return to work, whereas the expectation for those who enter a program after 6 months may drop to 20% to 40% (as cited in Niemeyer, Jacobs, Reynolds-Lynch, Bettencourt, & Lang, 1994). Managed care approaches that have determined preferred providers can more easily initiate evaluation and programming to optimize the client's perceived role of worker and facilitate return to work.

The criteria for admission varies, depending on the program and client goals. For example, one program's back school requires a referral from the client's attending physician and accepts clients in four categories: (1) back pain of 1 to 6 months—longer if not a postsurgical client, (2) clients 1 to 3 months postsurgery who are doing well, yet require professional instruction to reach their return to work goals, (3) clients who have returned to work, but experience recurring back problems, and (4) clients who returned to light duty or part-time work following surgery, but who could benefit from the program to reach a higher level of productivity. Client motivation is carefully considered in the selection process as well (Liberty Mutual, 1987).

Other admissions criteria may consider client use or limitation of pain medications, the client's required healing period to assure skin integrity before prosthetic retraining, and any surgical intervention to augment rehabilitative services to allow for the client's increased function (ie, tendon release to increase active ROM after a burn). It is essential that existing programs consider individual circumstances and the client's goals, rather than following a narrow selection process designed to merely support successful program outcomes.

▼ WORK PROGRAM EVALUATION

Tests and programs can vary in length.

For a standard FCE [Functional Capacity Evaluation], the recommended time is four to six hours. The most reliable format is two consecutive days, with the most critical items being presented on the second day. The evaluation time may be longer on the first day than on the second, or it may be allotted equally between the two days. The two-day format allows for retesting for accuracy and evaluating the effect of the first day's work testing on the worker. In some cases, the evaluation on the second day will reveal that the worker has increased physical symptoms (muscle spasm, joint swelling) from work items done on the first day. In other cases, the worker may show increased abilities on the second day (because he or she has worked through the fears and caution) or may show performance on the second day consistent with that of the first day. Therefore, the second test day is highly important to evaluate the effects of work so that recommendations for day-to-day work activity can be made. (Iserhagen, 1988, p. 143).

Although this previous statement is valid, the conservative reimbursement methods of today's managed care typically disallow a second-evaluation day. Therefore, therapists are gathering more initial evaluation information while the client is participating in the actual program.

A referral may be for a Functional Capacity Evaluation (FCE), solely to determine the individual's current physical demand level according to the *Dictionary of Occupational Titles*. The results of this test may define the workers capability to perform a specific job, may investigate effort and present abnormalities, or may be a prescreening to determine a pre-work physical. However, FCE usually defines a baseline for the beginning of a functional restoration or a work-hardening program.

Functional capacity evaluations should be done in a clinic setting, with specific equipment and control of external variables that might influence the test results. Because standardization is an important aspect of the FCE, the equipment and its placement is important. Selection of the items to be tested and arrangement of all testing equipment should be done in advance of an assessment. A

designated space in the department allows smooth transition from one test item to the next and emphasizes the professional aspect of the testing situation. (Iserhagen, 1988, p. 142).

The use of job-specific equipment or tools has become essential with the implementation of the Americans With Disabilities Act (ADA). This policy dissuades the evaluator from using high-technology, generic equipment to determine job specific capabilities (refer to Chapter 15, Section 2 for specific assessment tool descriptions).

▼ WORK PROGRAM TREATMENT

Frequency and Duration

Treatment frequency may vary according to the person's program goals. A client may attend daily and progress from a 2-hour up to a 6-hour, then an 8-hour day. However, if clients are currently at their jobs with restrictions, they may attend in conjunction with work hours. Clients participating in full-time light-duty work may augment their normal work schedule with a program to increase potential to transition into full-time, full-duty work.

Treatment duration is dependent on the person's goals, the client's ability to progress, the opportunity to return to the desired occupational role, and the ability to obtain program reimbursement. Moreover, the severity of injury and the time between injury and program admission may be the most influential factors when considering the treatment duration required to effect a successful discharge outcome (Joe, 1995). Practitioners should keep in mind that program duration should be clearly documented.

Documentation

Thorough documentation systems are an essential part of any successful work-hardening program. From initial evaluation responses to daily documented program reactions, these tools provide the practitioners, clients, and other involved parties with insight and direction for programming and discharge planning. As important as objective measurements are in this type of setting to qualify decision making, subjective perceptions are also influential. However, it is essential for practitioners to document perceptions in measurable terminology. A good example of this practice is the issue of determining the feasibility of clients returning to work. Client attendance, timeliness, ability for transition between program tasks, and the willingness to complete the scheduled day can all be described in the Feasibility Evaluation Checklist (FEC) (Ogden-Niemeyer and Jacobs, 1989, p. 17).

It is critical that practitioners' write reports that are easily understood. Professional terminology should be described in functional terms; jargon, abbreviations, and lengthy narration should be avoided.

The client is also expected to document such items as work task progression, pain levels, and reactions to the therapeutic program on a daily basis. At discharge, a report should include input from both client and therapist and include results from standardized and nonstandardized tests, summary of what goals have been achieved, a comparative analysis of the client's performance from admission to discharge, and any recommendations for accommodations and job modifications (Hertfelder & Gwinn, 1989). The more the practitioner communicates with the involved parties before discharge, the smoother the client's return to work.

Body Mechanics

Many programs include short courses in anatomy for the clients to facilitate their understanding of the mechanical structures and the risk factors they are exposed to while in and out of the workplace. Body mechanics training can minimize, and at times eliminate, the risk of injury. Although there are other factors that help reduce the client's risk of reinjury, knowledge of proper body mechanics in conjunction with a good fitness level is one of the first steps to reaching program objectives.

Work Conditioning and Work Hardening

A functional restoration program is often made up of two components: **work conditioning** and **work hardening**. The work-conditioning portion of the program consists of a fitness program and nonspecific job-simulated work tasks. Strengthening and flexibility through spinal stabilization, lumbar retraining, and cardiovascular exercise all make up a good fitness regimen. Nonspecific job tasks would include lifting at various levels, carrying, pushing, and pulling. These tasks would be part of a progressive schedule to increase strength and endurance, preparing the client for an occupational role to be determined following the functional restoration program.

When the client has occupational goals with well-defined physical and psychological demands, work hardening is appropriate to incorporate job-specific work tasks that progress the client to the physical demand levels of the actual job as listed in the *Dictionary of Occupational Titles* and the actual facility job description. These activities require great collaboration between the practitioner, client, and employer to obtain the actual equipment, tools, materials, and criteria to establish a simulated work environment. The simulated environment should mimic the noise, lighting, timing, and safety issues of the actual workplace as closely as possible.

Job simulations give clients a good opportunity to test their abilities to sustain work-related practices while in a noncompetitive setting. Simulations also give the practitioner and client the chance to consider the need for adapted or modified work practices.

The client generally engages in specific job simulation tasks for 1 to 2 weeks before discharge from the program. To recommend discharge with release to return to a specific job, the rehabilitation team must be able to document the client's ability in relation to the job requirements. For those clients with no specific job to return to, the team must demonstrate either achievement of work-related rehabilitation goals or a plateau in progress (Frantzlett, McCabe, Tramposh, & Tate-Henderson, 1988, p. 216–223).

Since the implementation of the Americans With Disabilities Act (ADA), more workers are able to return to their desired jobs with some type of reasonable accommodation. Just a few years ago such accommodation would not have been considered worth the effort or expense; now employers are realizing that their most valuable asset is their workforce.

Work-Hardening Team

Because the injured client has lost many different roles (worker, parent, spouse, teammate, homemaker), a comprehensive, interdisciplinary team is required. As practitioners, registered occupational and physical therapists provide clients with the following: (1) quality evaluations; (2) treatment planning, implementation, and progression; (3) documentation according to governmental, reimbursement, and licensure standards; and (4) discharge planning.

The role of licensed assistants is well described by the certification boards. Their job is to assist in client assessments, provide treatments, and document services that have been rendered. A certified occupational therapy assistant (1) contributes observations; (2) coordinates program planning; (3) provides direct services relative to instruction and modification of work practices; (4) observes productivity, safety awareness, and behavior; (5) identifies transitional skills that may be applied to other jobs; (6) reports progress; and (7) assists in getting the client ready for discharge (O'Connor & Calabro, 1993).

Exercise physiologists have a general understanding of how the body responds physiologically to the effects of exercise. They play an integral role in the work-conditioning phase of a functional restoration program.

The roles include demonstration and instruction in correct stretching and exercise techniques, flexibility, strength, and conditioning components. These conditioning components may include a home exercise program, education and reinforcement of proper body mechanics, provision of information regarding physiologic responses and treatment of physiologic changes, instruction on nutritional aspects of a healthy lifestyle, provision of continuous motivation and support on a daily basis with constant contact, performance of case management duties, and monitoring progress (Hardway, 1993, p. 73).

From administering an interest checklist, updating a resume, to establishing actual client and employer interviews, the vocational counselor is often the final rehabilitative contact before the client re-enters the workplace. The vocational counselor's role has been as a facilitator, to the point of actually entering the workplace with the employee to complete job coaching. "Vocational rehabilitation is a long-standing feature of workers' compensation systems. By facilitating injured workers' early return to work, rehabilitation both aids the worker and helps to control workers' compensation costs" (Gardner, 1985, p. 1).

The Commission on Accreditation of Rehabilitation Facilities (CARF) has mandated that psychological services be offered in a work-hardening program. On admission, clients complete a battery of psychological screenings to assess attitudes, experiences, motivation, and pain tolerances.

Psychological services can be offered in a group setting, on a one-on-one basis, or as a consult to the rest of the team. Many barriers to recovery include perceptions, attitudes, and emotions that have nothing to do with the actual injury. Direct psychological services are received by only a minority of work-hardening participants. Occasionally, however, a client may posses so many major barriers to recovery that successful outcome is in question. At these times, the psychologist can provide a psychological assessment and individually focused intervention (Young, 1993, p. 2).

Work-hardening clients may have their own attending physicians, but it is helpful to have a program medical director who is a physiatrist to address the immediate medical questions and concerns of clients and to provide a medical sounding board for team members. The incorporation of physiatry in the clinical setting increases the timeliness of client care efficiency in report distribution to the appropriate parties.

Students, facility occupational health nurses, rehabilitation counselors, insurance case managers, social workers, and medical specialists, all are professionals who may play a part in the functional restoration rehabilitation team. "In the true team concept, all members are responsible for developing a comprehensive program for the client, and should be considered equally responsible for treatment outcomes" (Hardway, 1993; p. 73).

Specialized Protocols

Traditionally, musculoskeletal injuries far surpassed all other diagnoses treated in the functional restoration programs. Yet over the past decade, there has been a steady increase in cumulative trauma or repetitive motion injuries. Physical disorders, such as carpal tunnel syndrome and chronic cervical tension, are just a few of the work-related complaints as a result of the increased use of visual display terminals and highly specialized technology that requires awkward and repetitive movements. These clients may share similar conditions and objectives, such that they can be appropriately treated in a group approach.

In contrast, clients with limitations secondary to burns, electrocution, amputation, and systemic disease present with special circumstances that may require the therapist to consider individual programs with less focus on physical demand levels of a specific job and more emphasis on the restoration of ADL. Program goals may initially address self-care and homemaker skills while deferring vocational goals until the client is deemed medically stable and at a physical endpoint for joint ROM, prosthetic fitting, and pain management techniques. The more complicated the diagnosis, the more important is communication with the other involved parties. Family involvement that reinforces therapeutic approaches can facilitate positive outcomes. At the University of Cincinnati Medical Center the team approach for clients who sustained severe burns and are participating in an aggressive rehabilitation program is described as follows:

The care team meets at least once weekly to map out goals, discuss progress, and make modifications to the treatment plans for each patient. It's not uncommon for there to be 20 people gathered around the table for these meetings (Smith, 1995, p. 71).

Job Site Analysis

Job site analysis (JSA) plays a critical role in the success of the functional restoration program and is completed for several different reasons. A JSA may help the therapist understand the exposures of a specific job, which may increase the understanding of the client's disorder. A JSA also allows the therapist to design an accurate environment to simulate the job-specific tasks. Finally, the JSA establishes the job performance criteria on which program goals are based. The client's performance relative to these goals can then be analyzed so that the therapist can make discharge recommendations, which may consist of the following options: return to work (full duty, modified duty, reasonable accommodations), further vocational exploration and retraining, or additional medical investigation for unresolved symptoms.

The JSA is one of the most effective ways to engage the employer in the work-hardening philosophy and process. It is often the opportunity to request the lending and use of actual tools and materials that are appropriate to be transferred and used in the clinic setting. Whether it is approached from a work-methods analysis or an ergonomic perspective, JSA is a valuable tool in providing a comprehensive work-hardening program. For further explanation of the JSA process, refer to the Chapter 15, Section 2.

Vocational Counseling

If a client cannot return to the (1) same employer, same job; (2) same job, but different employer; or (3) same employer, but different job, the client may be an appropriate referral for vocational counseling. Through combined efforts from rehabilitation staff and vocational counseling, clients can improve job-seeking skills, scholastic aptitudes, and interviewing techniques. They can also explore transitional skills and retraining opportunities that will enhance their current vocational potential.

Prework Screening

Employers often ask therapists to perform prework screenings before an employee or a new applicant is offered employment. Since the inception of the ADA, employers are required to recommend postoffer, preemployment screenings. Iserhagen (1990s) has discussed the implications, accuracy, and ethical issues surrounding these types of evaluations. Although the employer concerns of soaring worker compensation costs, lost work days and productivity, and worker protection are all valid, other concerns of discrimination, disclosure, liability in the failure to identify a potential problem, and the questionable predictive validity of these tests are equally important and should be of significant concern to the therapist. Detailed functional job descriptions and adequate-training periods provided to the returning or new worker are alternatives to these screenings that currently remain highly controversial.

Prevention Education

Injury is epidemic in America and most other industrialized nations and, without a doubt, is one of America's greatest health problems. The word "epidemic" is a key concept here. Whereas injuries as "problems" must be "managed" and "solved," only when injuries are seen in the context of an epidemic does it become obvious that preventative measures are imperative if we are to halt the spread of this killer and crippler (Schwartz, 1991; p. 365).

Prevention programs should incorporate a variety of media to address the various learning styles of the workforce. A 2-hour session may include the following: a short video, simple anatomy review, descriptions of common workplace injuries, an explanation of ergonomic controls (worker, engineering, and administrative), and a clinical practice session. Avoidance of the role of "expert" and allowing the audience to have input from their own experiences facilitates program participation, helps participants buy into new knowledge and methods of safe work practices, and ultimately, fosters safe work practice compliance in the workplace. Schwartz (1991) states, "Occupational therapists have skills, attitudes, and methodologies that are ideal for preventive intervention related to work place injuries and accidents" (pp. 367–368).

►INDUSTRIAL REHABILITATION CONCLUSION

To assure successful outcomes in the industrial rehabilitation arena, the occupational therapy practitioner needs to be cognizant of an ever-changing environment. Moreover, the therapy practitioner must be able to consider all aspects of the case management team and adapt effective client treatment approaches according to criteria often set by someone other than an attending physician. Meeting the goals of the worker, employer, and third-party payer can be very challenging, yet with good communication and well-defined program objectives, this area of specialty is a rewarding career path for an occupational therapy practitioner.

Section 5

Treatment Through Play and Leisure

Susan H. Knox

Play and **leisure** activities are an important treatment media in occupational therapy because of their importance to individuals. Play and leisure activities are used in three ways: (1) as treatment goals (improving play or leisure skills), (2) as treatment modalities (to improve specific skills), and (3) to facilitate playfulness. This section addresses play and leisure throughout the life span, constraints to play and leisure, treatment using play, and treatment using leisure activities.

▼ PLAY AND LEISURE THROUGHOUT THE LIFE SPAN

The terms play and leisure are often used interchangeably, and are usually differentiated by age, in that children play and adults engage in leisure activities. But play and leisure are not synonymous. Play has also been linked to work because the child learns skills and develops interests through play that affect later choices in work and leisure. Children's play experiences lay the foundations for work and leisure through (1) exploration; (2) manipulation and investigation; (3) learning; (4) social interaction; (5) competition, cooperation, and the learning of rules; and (6) the development of competence, self-determination, and personality.

Throughout a person's life, the amount of time spent in activities defined as play, work, or leisure varies. In early childhood, most of the time is spent in play. As children mature, time is divided between school and free-time, later work and nonwork. In older adults, leisure time predominates.

Stages of play and leisure have been summarized by Bergen (1988), Neulinger (1981), and others. Infants spend most of their time in sensorimotor and exploratory play.

They develop mastery over their own bodies and learn the effect of their actions on objects and people in the environment. The stages of this early sensorimotor play have been described by Bergen (1988), Piaget (1962), Rubin (1980), Rubin, Fine, & Vanderberg (1983), and others. By the end of the first year, infants actively explore their surroundings, are beginning to understand cause and effect, and are interested in how things work. In the second year, play centers around combining objects and learning their social meaning. Children begin to classify objects and develop purpose in their actions. Also during the end of the first year and through the second, children are beginning to develop symbolic play and pretense. Social play begins very early with interaction between the infant and mother and by age 3, children engage in complex social games.

Major changes in play occur from ages of 3 to 5 as children learn to adjust to the physical and social environment. Practice and exploratory play gradually shift into constructive play, and children become more interested in the outcome of the activity. Constructive play predominates in this period. Symbolic and pretense play are refined into dramatic and sociodramatic play. Children at this stage begin role play and thus learn about social systems. Garvey (1977) describes four types of roles seen in group play: (1) functional roles (eg, doctor), (2) relational roles (eg, mother–baby), (3) character roles (eg, superman), and (4) peripheral roles with no alternative identity. In addition, social play develops into rough-and-tumble play and emergent games with rules (Bergen, 1988).

Play of the school-aged child has not been studied as extensively as other ages because now children have more obligations on their time—namely school, and play is relegated to nonschool time. The major type of play seen at this stage is rule-governed games (Bergen, 1988) through which children learn reciprocity or turn-taking. Social play and games with rules are particularly influenced by the culture. The physical environments available for play, peer groups, and the types of play encouraged by parents have changed as our society has become more urbanized (Neulinger, 1981). The current emphases on organized sports (eg, Little League) and planned after school activities illustrate some of these changes.

In this stage, one can still observe practice and constructive play, but the play appears to be end-related, rather than means-related. In other words, children practice to develop skills or construct to make a project. Symbolic play tends to be integrated into games with rules such as Dungeons and Dragons or transformed into mental games and language play such as riddles or secret codes (Bergen, 1988). Fantasy play persists in secret clubs, daydreaming, or is substituted for by television.

Adolescents are developing autonomy and are becoming socialized into the adult role. This is a period of transition as obligations, time available for leisure, changes and refinements of interests, family and peer pressures, all affect teen activity (Neulinger, 1981). In a study by Csikszentmihalyi and Larson (1984), the largest single activity of adolescents was socializing. Second was television and third, sports, games, hobbies, reading, and music.

The adult's predominant use of time is in work and raising a family. Multiple factors affect leisure patterns in adulthood such as age, gender, marital status, work roles, whether one has children, and the children's ages. Time available for leisure and habits change as one goes through the stages of the adult. For example, single adults take part in a wider variety of activities outside the home than married people and, in particular, physical recreation or social activities vary between men and women of different ages. The influence of such innovations as television and computers has also changed leisure patterns through the years (Neulinger, 1981).

As people reach middle age and children leave home, time available for leisure increases. Neulinger (1981) stated that the "general trend is for leisure interests and activities to become increasingly restricted with age, despite decreased responsibilities" (p. 580). However, a study by Nystrom (1974) showed that the frequency of participation in activity and variety of activity chosen did not decrease with age, which reinforced the concept of maintenance of activity with aging.

Older adults are thought of as having a great deal of leisure. Broderick and Glazer (1983) found correlations between preretirement leisure participation and those of postretirement leisure, but age, health, mobility, and income played important roles in the amount of leisure and the quality of its enjoyment. Nystrom (1974) found that the most common activity for this age group was television. Second was socializing, and then small handicrafts and reading. He found a slightly higher incidence of passive activities than active ones. Gregory (1983) found a relation between activity and meaning and life satisfaction.

Iso-Ahola (1980s) cited research that showed that types of play in childhood affected adult leisure patterns, but he also showed that leisure patterns change continuously over a life span. He felt that this change is due to the individual's need to seek novel and arousing leisure experiences. The acquisition of new leisure skills and replacement of old also showed the influence of socialization on leisure patterns. There tended to be changes in leisure activities, rather than cessation, as people aged.

▼ CONSTRAINTS TO PLAY AND LEISURE

Play and leisure activities are highly influenced by elements in the environment as well as by the abilities and limitations of the individual. All environments offer supports and constraints to an individual's behavior. Knox (1974) and Michelman (1974) described factors in the environment that either promoted or inhibited play. Factors that promoted play included the availability of objects and persons, freedom from stress, provision of novelty, and opportunities to make choices. Factors that might inhibit play included external constraints, self-consciousness, too much novelty or challenge, limited choices, and excessive competition.

Rubin, et al (1983) listed five components felt to promote play: (1) familiar peers, toys, and other materials; (2) freedom of choice; (3) adults who are nonintrusive or directive; (4) safe and comfortable atmosphere; and (5) scheduling that avoids times of fatigue, hunger, or stress.

The effects of the environment on play can be seen in children who have experienced neglect or long hospitalizations. Severe examples have been seen in some of the reports of children in Romanian orphanages (Cermak, 1996). These children showed severe sensory problems, extreme delay in developmental skills, and difficulties in interacting with others. Other characteristics of the play of deprived children included self-stimulation, limited repertoire of activities, decreased social play, and either increased or decreased fantasy play.

There have been various studies of the effects of hospitalization on children's play (Hartley & Goldenson, 1963; Kaplan-Sanoff, Brewster, Stillwell, & Bergen, 1988; Kielhofner, Barris, Bauer, Shoestock, & Walker, 1983). When children were hospitalized, there was the stress of separation, fear of illness, painful procedures, enforced confinement, and disruption of routines (Kaplan-Sanoff et al, 1988). Some of the effects on play behavior include (1) decreased attention span; (2) decreased endurance; (2) decreased initiative, resourcefulness, and creativity; (4) qualitatively less playfulness; (5) decreased affect; (6) decreased movement; (7) increased anxiety; (8) decreased curiosity; (9) decreased imitation; (10) a slower play pace; and (11) regression to earlier stages of development (Hartley & Goldenson, 1963; Kielhofner, et al, 1983).

McGuire (1985) described constraints to leisure that occur across the life span, the effect of which limits the freedom of choice required for leisure. Constraints can result when there are too many choices and not enough time, thus causing a need to eliminate some choices. Here, the individual has some control over the extent of the limits. Second, attitudes held by the individual result in self-imposed limits on leisure choice. Here, the perception of options is reduced. Third, conditions beyond the individual's control such as health or economic factors may limit options.

▼ EFFECTS OF DISABILITY ON PLAY BEHAVIOR

The play of children with varying disabilities has often been described in the literature (Kaplan-Sanoff, et al, 1988; Mogford, 1977; Rubin, et al, 1983). However, there are problems generalizing across or within disabilities. Even children with the same diagnosis are individuals and respond uniquely in different situations. Some of the problems with the research

on children with disabilities are difficulties in conceptualization, theoretical perspectives, and methodology (Kaplan-Sanoff, et al, 1988). Therefore, descriptions of the play of children with disabilities must be interpreted cautiously. Although, heuristically, it is helpful to examine some of the problems that certain conditions may impose on the child, in actual practice, each child must be considered individually. Bundy (1993) stated that although a child's play may not be typical, it was more important for "children to be good at what they want to do" (p. 218).

Some diseases and conditions limit physical interaction with the environment, with toys and other objects, and to some extent with people. The child with a physical disability may display limited movement, strength, and pain when performing daily activities. Social contacts with family and peers may be disrupted by hospitalizations. These problems may lead to feelings of inadequacy and loss of control. The play characteristics of children with physical limitations may include fear of movement, decreased active play, and preferences for sedentary activities. The child may also have problems with manipulating toys and show decreased exploration. There may be decreased opportunities for social play because of hospitalizations or routines that do not allow for social interaction (Knox, 1980; Miller, 1979).

Children with cognitive impairments, such as those with mental retardation, often show delayed or uneven skills, difficulty in structuring their own behavior, or lack of sustained attention. These may be manifested in play by (1) differences in preferred play material (eg, preference for structured play materials); (2) decreased play strategies; (3) decreased curiosity; (4) need for external cues; (5) inflexible methods of exploration; (6) destructive or inappropriate use of objects; (7) decreased imagination; (8) decreased symbolic play; (9) decreased social interaction; (10) decreased language; and (11) increased observer play (Hulme & Lunzer, 1966; Kaplan-Sanoff, et al, 1988; Knox, 1974; Mogford, 1977; Wehman, 1977).

Several studies have examined the effects of sensory impairment on play, particularly blind or deaf children. Kaplan-Sanoff et al (1988) and Mogford (1977) described the blind child as having delays in developing an integrated impression of the world owing to lack of vision, and delayed motor exploration of surroundings and of objects. The play characteristics of the blind child were difficulty in constructive play, delays in developing complex play routines with others, decreased imitative, and role play.

The deaf child was believed to have problems with decreased inner language, decreased social skills, and decreased understanding of abstract concepts. These were manifested in play by imagination becoming more restrictive with age, and increased time being spent in noninteractive construction play; there was decreased symbolic play, organization of play, and social play, and an increase in solitary play (Kaplan-Sanoff, et al, 1988; Mogford, 1977).

Children who have difficulty interpreting and integrating sensory input often have a limited or distorted perception of themselves and of their world, a decreased ability to plan and execute motor and cognitive tasks, and poor orga-nization of behavior. Play characteristics of these children include either excessive movement or avoidance of move-ment, decreased exploration, decreased gross motor or manipulative play, increased observation or solitary play, increased sedentary play, a restricted repertoire of play, resis-tance to change, distractibility, and destructiveness (Ayres, 1972, 1979; Bundy, 1991; Mogford, 1977).

Children with autism have severe sensory integrative problems as well as social and language deficits (Powers, 1989). Their play is characterized by lack of inner and ex-pressive language, stereotyped movements or types of play, decreased imitation and imagination, lack of variety in play repertoires, decreased play organization, decreased manipu-lation of toys, decreased construction and combining of ob-jects, and decreased social play (Kaplan-Sanoff, et al, 1988; Nelson, 1984; Powers, 1989). Nelson (1984) stated that these children appear to have a fundamental deficit in play greater than what would be expected when examining spe-cific skills.

Children with CP show difficulties in many areas. They may show limited and abnormal movement, sometimes have decreased cognitive abilities, may have sensory impairments, and often lack opportunities for social play (Finnie, 1975). In play, cognitive abilities were the most decisive factor in limiting play, but children with good cognitive abilities could make adaptations to their physical limitations. Other problems include decreased physical interaction with the environment and less interactive play time (Finnie, 1975; Mogford, 1977; Wehman, 1977).

Most of the studies of the play of children with disabili-ties stress the obstacles that the disabling condition place on the children. Mogford (1977) summarized the problems that different disabling conditions have on children's play by stat-ing, "all handicapped children have one thing in common—that their ability to explore, interact with, and master the environment is impaired, with a consequent distortion or deprivation of normal childhood experience" (p. 171). However, in occupational therapy, the practitioner also needs to explore supports for play. It is amazing at times, to watch a child overcome great obstacles so that he or she can en-gage in a favorite activity. These supports will be discussed in relation to intervention.

▼ USE OF PLAY IN TREATMENT

What differentiates free play from therapeutic play? Free play is intrinsically motivated, fun, and is performed for its own sake, rather than having a purpose. In therapy, goals and objectives are established by the therapist. Rast (1986) de-scribed this apparent dichotomy and how play serves as the natural arena within which therapy goals can be achieved. She stated:

Play offers a practical vehicle to enlist a child's attention, to prac-tice specific motor and functional skills, and to promote sensory processing, perceptual abilities, and cognitive development. It also serves to support social, emotional, and language development. In the therapeutic setting, play often becomes a tool used to work to-wards a goal, despite the fact that the goal-oriented, externally controlled aspects of the therapy situation conflict with the essence of play itself (p. 30).

For play to be used successfully in treatment, the child should feel that he or she is choosing or directing the play episode. This is particularly important when the goal is to increase competence in play development. Research has shown that when external constraints are placed on play, it is perceived as work and no longer contains playful elements (Mogford, 1977; Wade, 1985; Rast, 1986).

In a study by Couch (1996), pediatric occupational ther-apists were asked if they felt play was important in treatment and how they used play. Ninety-one percent of the thera-pists rated play as very important. In treatment, 95% used play as a modality primarily to elicit motor, sensory, or psy-chosocial outcomes, whereas only 2% used play as an out-come by itself. The therapists also primarily used adult-directed play versus child-directed play.

The way play is used in treatment is influenced by vari-ous factors: (1) the therapist's frame of reference, (2) the in-stitution's emphasis on improving performance components and skills, (3) reimbursement limitations, and (4) the family's values and concerns for the physical aspects of the child's handicap.

Play as a Treatment Goal

Burke (1993) stated, "An occupation-based view of play is built on basic notions concerning the importance of an occu-pation to an individual" (p. 201). The use of play as a treatment goal has been described within the **occupational science** and **sensory integration** frames of reference. In occupational science, play is viewed as an occupation, determined by the in-dividual and his or her interaction with the environment. Reilly and her students (1974) first studied play systematically and studied the treatment effects of play in developing compe-tent behavior. Reilly described play as the child's occupation and saw occupational behavior as the continuum of play and work. She defined play as a multidimensional system for adap-tation to the environment and felt that the exploratory drive of curiosity underlies play behavior. This drive has three hier-archical stages: exploration, competency, and achievement. Ex-ploratory behavior is seen most in early childhood and is fueled by intrinsic motivation. Competency behavior is fueled by effectance motivation and is characterized by experimenta-tion and practice to achieve mastery. The third stage, achieve-ment, is linked to goal expectancies and fueled by a desire to achieve excellence. Within an occupational science frame of reference, a goal of treatment would be the development of play behavior per se and the development of those elements of playfulness that would fuel competent interaction with the world through play.

In sensory integration, play is also valued as the arena through which sensory integration develops (Ayres, 1972,

1979). Successful play experiences are dependent on adequate adaptive responses to environmental demands that, in turn, are dependent on adequate sensory integration. In therapy, the therapist sets up and manipulates the environment (setting, objects, people) so that the child can choose among activities that potentially offer the "just right" challenge (Lindquist, Mack, & Parham, 1982). During treatment, the therapist constantly adjusts the environment, child, or activity to bring about successful adaptation. An excellent description of the role of play within a sensory integrative framework was provided by Bundy (1991). She concluded:

Play is a powerful tool for treatment. For many individuals, the most important byproduct of occupational therapy may be the improved ability to play. If it is carefully planned and conducted, therapy using the principles of sensory integration may be very helpful in facilitating the development of play. Likewise, play as a part of a well orchestrated treatment plan, can result in improvements in sensory integration. (p. 67)

Mack, Lindquist, and Parham (1982) synthesized the commonalities of play from the occupational behavior and sensory integrative viewpoints that relate to use of play in treatment and to the desired outcome. They stated:

In practice, both approaches deem the therapist responsible for structuring adaptive behavior from the child. Thus, the potency of the environment's influence on development is confirmed by both. But from neither perspective does therapy rely solely on environmental manipulation. The child's initiative and active involvement are critical to the therapeutic process. From both perspectives, the intrinsic motivation or self-direction of the child is primary in guiding therapy, for importance is placed on the child's inner drive toward mastery. Play, then, is the process through which therapeutic goals are achieved. The ultimate goal of therapy—competence in daily life activities—is also shared by both perspectives. (p. 367)

Play as Treatment Modality

Two frames of reference that use play as a modality are the developmental and functional approaches. Play is most often used when a specific skill needs to be taught or when a specific goal needs to be met. Goals and objectives are set depending on how the disability is affecting the role performance of the child. Playful activities are used in a more structured or defined sense as a means to achieve the desired goal.

In the developmental frame of reference, play activities are used to develop physical, cognitive, emotional, or social abilities. The play materials are used to entice the child, such as when a toy is used to encourage a child to crawl or when a busy box is used to teach cause-and-effect concepts. Difficulty preserving the qualities of play may arise when therapy goals or techniques require a more structured "hands-on" approach, such as when using a neurodevelopmental technique; therapist skill and imagination is needed to combine approaches successfully and creatively. Anderson, Hino-

josa, and Strauch (1987) provide helpful suggestions for incorporating play into neurophysiological treatment approaches.

In the functional frame of reference, play is also used to meet a therapeutic end by adaptation of the activity, environment, or in therapeutic handling of the child while he or she is engaged in the activity. For example, a child's favorite toy might be positioned in such a way to improve the child's ROM, or adapted to increase the child's strength.

Facilitating Playfulness

The third way play is used therapeutically is in facilitating playfulness in the child. As was stated in the section on evaluation of play and leisure, what an individual plays with and how they play may not be as important as the affective quality of their play. Some children who have tremendous handicapping conditions manage to obtain great joy and benefit out of play. On the other hand, practitioners often see children who are not playful and do not derive pleasure from even the simplest play interaction. Facilitating playfulness in the child can be an important goal of therapy. Morrison, Metzger, and Pratt (1996) stated,

The more playful child may generalize this flexible approach into environmental interaction beyond play and into other aspects of his or her life. For the child with a condition that impedes his or her ability to interact with the social or physical environment, a flexible (playful) approach may enable the child to succeed more frequently in these difficult situations. (p. 519)

Parham (1992) suggested strategies that a practitioner can use to create a playful atmosphere. The practitioner should express a playful attitude through speech, body language, and facial expressions. Also novelty and imaginary play should be used to facilitate playful participation on the part of the child. Bundy (1991) stated that the practitioner must know how to play to be able to model play for the child. And Bundy (1997) and Morrison, et al (1996) stressed the importance of helping the child develop intrinsic motivation, internal control, ability to suspend reality, and ability to give and read cues, all necessary in developing playfulness.

Adaptations

Considering the environment and the objects within it is critical to creating a play atmosphere for children. Environmental spaces, toys, and equipment should have some flexibility in usage to foster play. In addition, toys and play equipment may need to be adapted for the child to access them optimally. Adaptation of toys and the environment is an important role of the occupational therapy practitioner, especially for the severely involved child. The practitioner must know the properties of toys as well as how to adapt them appropriately. Switches, adaptive keyboards, or provisions for sensory impairment may be necessary for the child to benefit from and be more independent in play.

Parent Education and Training

Working with parents in relation to play is vitally important if there is to be carryover of the skills and abilities learned in therapy into the child's everyday life. Parents of children with disabilities often are so concerned with their child's disability that they view their roles as substitute therapists and try to structure therapy into every aspect of the child's day. Mogford (1977) discussed studies dealing with parents perceptions of and feelings toward play. She cited one study that found parents had a preoccupation with physical progress and speech development and failed to appreciate either the child's need for play and exploration on his or her own or their own roles in encouraging play. Missiuna and Pollack (1991) discussed play deprivation in children with physical disabilities. They described four barriers to free play: (1) limitations imposed by caregivers, (2) physical and personal limitations of the child, (3) environmental barriers, and (4) social barriers. They proposed practitioners should provide support for free play, consultation with parents, consultation with teachers and caregivers, and recommendations about playthings.

Often practitioners need to help parents understand the importance of play for their child and to help them interact with their child playfully. Often the parents need help in knowing how to create a balance between doing things *for* their child and allowing the child to form and carry out his or her own intentions. The practitioner may need to model play behavior for the parent, encourage the parent to enter into and contribute to play sequences, without directing or controlling them, and help the parent organize or adapt the play environment to meet the needs of the child. By actively involving the parents or caregivers, the practitioner helps them appreciate their child's strengths, helps them learn the fun of playing with their child, and helps them develop play skills that will serve them well.

▼ LEISURE IN TREATMENT

People are usually referred to occupational therapy when their performance of daily occupations has been altered as a result of injury or illness. However, practitioners are also involved in prevention and wellness programs when there is the potential for disruption of occupation. A major goal of occupational therapy is to help the individual achieve a balance of meaningful activities in daily life. The same activity may provide different meanings for individuals or different activities may provide the same meaning. To plan effective treatment, the therapist needs to examine leisure performance and its meanings. Bundy (1993) stated: "Only when we know what the benefits of particular leisure activities are to the client can we help that person recapture those same benefits in different activities" (p. 220).

The therapist also needs to explore constraints to the successful performance of activities. The therapist's role is to explore these types of constraints to assist the client in making realistic leisure choices.

Occupational therapists often are involved in leisure counseling. McDowell (1981), in discussing leisure counseling, described seven steps in the process by which one makes choices about activities: (1) awareness, (2) knowledge, (3) skills, (4) resourcefulness, (5) strategies, (6) assertion (doing), and (7) reflection. These steps are all used by the occupational therapy practitioner in treatment. Practitioners assist clients in developing awareness of options and limits. They provide information on the options, help develop skills, and provide resources, thus increasing and refining choices and building competencies. Practitioners also help clients devise strategies for goal achievement and provide opportunities for assertion through performance of activities. Reflection involves evaluation of results by the client and the practitioner. Occupational therapy, with its emphasis on purposeful activity is unique in being able to provide all these steps within a treatment program.

McCree (1993) described steps in the leisure counseling process: (1) evaluation to determine past and present leisure interests; (2) expansion and enrichment of interests and skills by exploring leisure opportunities and examining problems; (3) encouragement of engagement in community leisure programs, activities, and groups; (4) guidance in finding leisure outlets in the community; and (5) follow-up assistance to ensure effective functioning in the community.

Activities that are usually ascribed to leisure are also used by occupational therapy practitioners to achieve specific goals. Crafts and recreational activities provide opportunities for active involvement on the part of the client and can be adapted to meet therapeutic goals. With adults, as with children, it is important to use activities that are both meaningful to the person and are therapeutic.

▶ PLAY AND LEISURE CONCLUSION

This section has reviewed play and leisure throughout the life span and addressed constraints to play and leisure. Play in treatment was discussed in three ways: as a treatment goal, as a modality, and in facilitating playfulness. Leisure was discussed in terms of leisure counseling and utilization of leisure activities. Bundy (1993) stated, "We must actively and systematically promote play and leisure in our clients' lives and in our intervention sessions" (p. 218). Only then can we help our clients achieve a meaningful balance of activities in their lives.

▼ REFERENCES

American Heart Association. (Date unknown). *Five step plan for work simplification* (Handout).

Anderson, J., Hinojosa, J., & Strauch, C. (1987). Integrating play in neurodevelopmental treatment, *American Journal of Occupational Therapy, 41* (7), 421–426.

Ayres, A. J. (1972). *Sensory integration and learning disorders.* Los Angeles: Western Psychological Services.

Ayres, A. J. (1979). *Sensory integration and the child*. Los Angeles: Western Psychological Services.

Bergen, D. (1988). *Play as a medium for learning and development*. Portsmouth, NH: Heinemann Educational Books.

Bowling, B. (1981). *Effective patient education techniques for use with aging patients*. Lexington, KY: University of Kentucky.

Broderick, T., & Glazer, B. (1983). Leisure participation and the retirement process, *American Journal of Occupational Therapy, 37*, 15–22.

Buckwalter, K. C., Wernimont, T., & Buckwalter, J. A. (1982). Musculoskeletal conditions and sexuality (Part I). *Sexuality and Disability, 5* (3), 131–142.

Bundy, A. (1991). Play theory and sensory integration. In Fisher, A. G., Murray, E. A., & Bundy, A. C. (Eds.), *Sensory integration: Theory and practice* (pp. 46–68). Philadelphia: F. A. Davis.

Bundy, A. (1993). Assessment of play and leisure: Delineation of the problem, *American Journal of Occupational Therapy, 47*, 217–222.

Bundy, A. (1997). Play and playfulness: What to look for. In Parham, D. & Fazio, L. (Eds.), *Play in occupational therapy for children* (pp. 52–66). St. Louis, MO: Mosby Yearbooks.

Burke, J. (1993). Play: The life role of the infant and young child. In Case-Smith, J. (Ed.), *Pediatric occupational therapy and early intervention* (pp. 198–224). Boston: Andover Medical Publishers.

Cahill, M. (Ed.) (1987). *Patient teaching* (pp. 19–43). Springhouse, PA: Springhouse.

Cambre, S. (1978). *The sensuous heart*. Atlanta: Piedmont Hospital.

Canadian Association of Occupational Therapists. (1991). *Guidelines for the client-centered practice of occupational therapy*. Toronto: CAOT Publications ACE.

Cermak, S. (1966). Ayres Memorial Lecture, presented at the Sensory International Annual Symposium, June 2, 1996, San Diego, CA.

Chapparo, C. (1979). *Sensory integration for adults*. Workshop sponsored by Illinois Occupational Therapy Association, Glen Ellyn, Illinois.

Clark, F. (1993). Occupation embedded in a real life: Interweaving occupational science and occupational therapy, *American Journal of Occupational Therapy, 47*, 1067–1078.

Commission on Practice. (1986). Work hardening guidelines. *American Journal of Occupational Therapy, 40*, 841–843.

Cope, D. N., & Sundance, P. (1995). Conceptualizing clinical outcomes. In P. K. Landrum, N. D. Schmidt, & A. McLean (Eds.) *Outcome-oriented rehabilitation* (pp. 43–56). Gaithersburg, MD: Aspen.

Couch, K. (1996). *The role of play in pediatric occupational therapy*, unpublished master's thesis, University of Washington, Seattle, WA.

Courtois, F. J., Charvier, K. F., Leriche, A., & Raymond, D. P. (1993). Sexual function in spinal cord injury men. I. Assessing sexual capability. *Paraplegia, 31*, 771–784.

Csikszentmihalyi, M. & Larson, R. (1984). *Being adolescent*, New York: Basic Books.

DaCunha, J. P., & Tackenberg, J. (Eds.) (1989). *How to teach patients*. Springhouse, PA: Springhouse.

DeJong, G., & Sutton, J. P. (1995). Rehab 2000: The evolution of medical rehabilitation in American health care. In P. K. Landrum, N. D. Schmidt, & A. McLean (Eds.), *Outcome-oriented rehabilitation* (pp. 3–42). Gaithersburg, MD: Aspen.

Dunn, W. (1993). Measurement of function: Actions for the future. *American Journal of Occupational Therapy, 47*, 357–359.

Dunn, W., Brown, C., & McGuigan, A. (1994). The ecology of human performance: A framework for considering the effect of context. *American Journal of Occupational Therapy, 48*, 595–607.

Evans, R. W., Small, L., & Ling, J. S. (1995). Independence in the home and community. In P. K. Landrum, N. D. Schmidt, & A. McLean (Eds.) *Outcome-oriented rehabilitation* (pp. 95–124). Gaithersburg, MD: Aspen.

Finnie, N. (1975). *Handling the young cerebral palsied child at home* (2nd ed.). New York: E. P. Dutton & Co.

Frantzlett, C., McCabe, N., Tramposh, A., & Tate-Henderson, S. (1988). Components of functional capacity evaluation. In S. J. Iserhagen (Ed.), *Work injury management and prevention* (pp. 216–223). Baltimore, MD: Aspen.

Freda, M., Cioschi, H., & Nilson, C. (1989). Childbearing issues for women with physical disabilities. *Physical Disabilities Special Interest Section Newsletter, 12* (2), 1–4.

Freda, M., & Rubinsky, H. (1991). Sexual function in the stroke survivor. In Goldberg, G. (Ed.). *Physical Medicine and Rehabilitation Clinics of North America, 2*, 634–658.

Fried, L. P., Herdman, S. J., Kuhn, K. E., Rubin, G., & Turano, K. (1991). Preclinical disability: Hypotheses about the bottom of the iceberg. *Journal of Aging and Health, 3*, 285–300.

Gage, M., Noh, S., Polatajko, H. J., & Kaspar, V. (1994). Measuring perceived self-efficacy in occupational therapy. *American Journal of Occupational Therapy, 48*, 783–790.

Gardner, J. (1985). Vocational Rehabilitation in Workers Compensation. *Source Book Issues and Evidence*, June 1–2, p. 1.

Garvey, C. (1977). Play with language. In B. Tizard & D. Harvey, (Eds.). *Biology of play*. Philadelphia: J. B. Lippincott.

Gift, A. G., & Pugh, L. C. (1993). Dyspnea and fatigue. *Nursing Clinics of North American, 28*, 373–384.

Gregory, M. D. (1983). Occupational behavior and life satisfaction among retirees. *American Journal of Occupational Therapy, 37*, 548–553.

Guyton, A. C. (1991). *Textbook of medical physiology* (8th ed.). Philadelphia: W. B. Saunders.

Hagedorn, R. (1995). Environmental analysis and adaptation. In R. Hagedorn (Ed.). *Occupational therapy: Perspectives and processes* (pp. 239–257). Melbourne, Australia: Churchill Livingstone.

Hansen, R. A., & Atchison, B. (1993). *Conditions in occupational therapy: Effect on occupational performance*. Baltimore: Williams & Wilkins.

Hanson, C. S., & Walker, K. (1992). The history of work and physical dysfunction. *American Journal of Occupational Therapy, 46*, 56–61.

Hardway, J. (1993). The exercise physiologist on the work hardening team. *Rehab Management*, August/September, p. 73.

Hartley, R., & Goldenson, R. (1963). *The complete book of children's play*. New York: The Cornwall Press.

Hellerstein, H. K., & Friedman, E. H. (1970). Sexual activity and the post coronary patient. *Archives of Internal Medicine, 125*, 987–999.

Hertfelder, S., & Gwin, C. (1989). Work hardening guidelines. *Occupational therapy in work programs* (pp. 277–280). Rockville, MD: American Occupational Therapy Association.

Hightower–Vandamm, M. (1981). Nationally speaking: The role of occupational therapy in vocational evaluation, part 2. *American Journal of Occupational Therapy, 35*, 631–633.

Hopkins, H., & Smith, H. (Eds.) (1993). *Willard and Spackman's occupational therapy* (8th ed.). Philadelphia: J. B. Lippincott.

Horak, F. (1991). Assumptions underlying motor control for neurologic rehabilitation. In *Foundation for physical therapy, contemporary management of motor problems: Proceedings of the II step conference* (pp. 11–27). Alexandria, VA: Foundation for Physical Therapy.

Horn, L., & Zasler, N. (1990s). Neuroanatomy and neurophysiology of sexual function. *Journal of Head Trauma Rehabilitation, 5*, 1–13.

Hulme I., & Lunzer, E. A. (1966). Play, language and reasoning in subnormal children. *Journal of Child Psychology and Psychiatry, 7*, 107.

Iserhagen, S. (1988). Functional capacity evaluation parameters. *Work injury management and prevention* (pp. 142–143). Baltimore: Aspen Publications.

Iserhagen, S. (1990). Pre-work screening: Is it ethical? Is it legal? Does it work? Should we do it? *Industrial Rehabilitation Quarterly, 3* (1): 7–47.

Iso-Ahola, S. E. (1980s). *The social psychology of leisure and recreation*. Dubuque, IA: William C. Brown.

Jacobs, K. (1991). History of work practice in occupational therapy. In K. Jacobs (Ed.). *Occupational therapy: Work-related programs and assessments* (2nd ed.). Boston: Little, Brown & Company.

Joe, B. (1995). Effective work programs. *OT Week, 9* (48), 12–13.

Johnston, M. V., Keith, R. A., & Hinderer, S. R. (1992). Measurement standards for interdisciplinary medical rehabilitation. *Archives of Physical Medicine & Rehabilitation, 73*, S-3–S-23.

Kaplan-Sanoff, M., Brewster, A., Stillwell, J., & Bergen, D. (1988). The relationship of play to physical/motor development and to children with special needs. In Bergen, D. (Ed.). *Play as a medium for learning and development* (pp. 137–162). Portsmouth, NH: Heinemann.

Kassler, W. (1993). *An introduction to HIV.* Redwood City, CA; Benjamin/Cummings Publishing.

Kautzman, L. (1991). Facilitating adult learning in occupational therapy patient education programs. *Occupational Therapy Practice, 2*, 1–11.

Kielhofner, G., Barris, R., Bauer, D., Shoestock, B. & Walker, L. (1983). A comparison of play behavior in nonhospitalized and hospitalized children, *American Journal of Occupational Therapy, 37*, 305–312.

Klinger, J. (1978). *Mealtime manual for people with disabilities and the aging* (2nd ed.). Camden, NJ: Campbell Soup Company.

Knox, S. (1974). A play scale. In Reilly, M. (Ed.). *Play as exploratory learning* (pp. 247–266). Beverly Hills: Sage Publications.

Knox, S. (1980). Occupational therapy for the child with juvenile rheumatoid arthritis, *Proceedings of model community programs for arthritic children*, Washington, DC.

Krueter, M., Sullivan, M., & Siosten, A. (1994). Sexual adjustment after spinal cord injury (SCI) focusing on partner experiences. *Paraplegia, 32*, 225–235.

Kruetzer, J. S., & Zasler, N. D. (1989). Psychosexual consequences of traumatic brain injury: Methodology and preliminary findings. *Brain Injury, 3*, 177–186.

Law, M., Cooper, B., Strong, S., Stewart, D., Rigby, P., & Letts, L. (1996). The person-environment–occupation model: A transactive approach to occupational performance. *Canadian Journal of Occupational Therapy, 63*, 9–23.

Lawton, M. P., & Brody, E. (1969). Assessment of older people: Self maintaining and instrumental activities of daily living. *Gerontologist, 9*, 179–186.

Ley, P. (1972). Comprehension, memory and the success of communications with the patient. *Journal of Instructional Health Education, 10*, 23–29.

Liberty Medical Center Brochure (1987). *Restoring the promise of the future*, June.

Lindquist, J., Mack, W., & Parham, D. (1982). A synthesis of occupational behavior and sensory integrative concepts in theory and practice, part 2: Clinical applications, *American Journal of Occupational Therapy, 36*, 433–437.

Lorig, K., & Fries, J. F. (1990). *The arthritis helpbook* (3rd ed.). New York: Addison-Wesley.

Mack, W., Lindquist, J., & Parham, D. (1982). A synthesis of occupational behavior and sensory integrative concepts in theory and practice, part 1: theoretical foundations. *American Journal of Occupational Therapy, 36*, 365–374.

Majerovitz, S. D., & Revenson, T. A. (1994). Sexuality and rheumatic disease. The significance of gender. *Arthritis Care and Research, 7*, (1), 28–34.

Masters, W. H., & Johnson, V. E. (1966). *Human sexual response.* Boston: Little, Brown.

Mathiowetz, V., & Bass Haugen, J. (1995). Remediation of motor behavior: Contemporary task oriented approach. In C. A. Trombly (Ed.), *Occupational therapy for physical dysfunction* (4th ed.) (pp. 510–527). Baltimore: Williams & Wilkins.

McCree, S. (1993). *Leisure and play in therapy.* Tucson, AZ: Therapy Skill Builders.

McDowell, F. (1981). Leisure: Consciousness, well-being and counseling. *Counseling Psychologist, 9* (3), 3–31.

McDowell, I., & Newell, C. (1996). *Measuring health: A guide to rating scales and questionnaires* (2nd ed.) New York: Oxford University Press.

McGuire, F. (1985). Constraints in later life. In M. Wade (Ed.). *Constraints on leisure.* Springfield, IL: Charles C. Thomas.

Michelman, S. (1974). Play and the deficit child. In M. Reilly (Ed.).

Play as exploratory learning (pp. 157–208). Beverly Hills, CA: Sage Publications.

Miller, J. (1979). *Juvenile rheumatoid arthritis.* Littleton, MA: PSG Publishing.

Missiuna, C., & Pollock, N. (1991). Play deprivation in children with physical disabilities: The role of the occupational therapist in preventing secondary disability. *American Journal of Occupational Therapy, 45*, 882–888.

Mogford, K. (1977). The play of handicapped children. In B. Tizard & D. Harvey (Eds.). *Biology of play* (pp. 170–184). Philadelphia: J. B. Lippincott.

Morrison, C., Metzger, P. & Pratt, P. (1996). Play. In J. Case-Smith, A. Allen, & P. Pratt (Eds.). *Occupational therapy for children* (3rd ed.) (pp. 504–523). St Louis, MO: C.V. Mosby.

Niemeyer, L., Jacobs, K., Reynolds-Lynch, K., Bettencourt, C., & Lang, S. (1994). Work hardening: Past, present, and future—The Work Programs Special Interest Section National Work Hardening Outcome Study. *American Journal of Occupational Therapy, 48*, 327–329.

Neistadt, M. E. (1986). Sexuality counseling for adults with disabilities: A module for an occupational therapy curriculum. *American Journal Of Occupational Therapy, 40*, 542–545.

Neistadt, M. E., & Freda, M. (1987). *Choices: A guide to sex counseling with physically disabled adults.* Malabar, FL: Robert Krieger.

Neistadt, M. E., & Baker, M. F. (1978). A program for sex counseling the physically disabled. *American Journal of Occupational Therapy, 32*, 646–647.

Nelson, D. (1984). *Children with autism.* Thorofare, NJ: Slack.

Neulinger, J. (1981). *The psychology of leisure* (2nd ed.). Springfield, IL: Charles C. Thomas.

Nystrom, E. P. (1974). Activity patterns and leisure concepts among the elderly. *American Journal of Occupational Therapy, 28*, 337–345.

Oakley, F. (1981). *Role checklist.* Presented at Workshop on Enhancing Clinical Effectiveness: Practical application of the model of human occupation. University of Illinois at Chicago, July 24 and 25, 1989.

O'Connor, K., & Calabro, T. (1993). Roles of the occupational therapist and certified therapy assistant. *Work Programs Special Interest Section, 47* (12), 3–4.

Ogden-Niemeyer, L., & Jacobs, K. (1989). Definition and history of work hardening. *Work hardening: State of the art* (pp. 1–17). Thorofare, NJ: Slack.

Papadopoulos, C. (1989). *Sexual aspects of cardiovascular disease.* New York: Praegar.

Parenté, R., & Herrman, D. (1996). *Retraining cognition: Techniques and applications.* Frederick, MD: Aspen.

Parham, D. (1992). Strategies for maintaining a playful atmosphere during therapy. AOTA *Sensory Integration Special Interest Section Newsletter, 15*, 2–3.

Pedretti, L. (1996). *OT practice skills for physical dysfunction.* St. Louis: C.V. Mosby.

Piaget, J. (1962). *Play, dreams and imitation in childhood.* London: William Heinemann.

Pollock, N., Baptiste, S., Law, M., McColl, M. A., Opzoomer, A., & Polatajko, H. (1990). Occupational performance measures: A review based on the guidelines for the client-centered practice of occupational therapy. *Canadian Journal of Occupational Therapy, 57*, 77–81.

Powers, M. (1989). *Children with autism.* Rockville, MD: Woodbine House.

Quintana, L. A. (1995). Remediating perceptual impairments. In C. A. Trombly (Ed.). *Occupational therapy for physical dysfunction* (4th ed.) (pp. 529–537). Baltimore: Williams & Wilkins.

Rast, M. (1986). Play and therapy, play or therapy. *Play: A skill for life* (pp. 29–42). Rockville, MD: American Occupational Therapy Association.

Rehabilitation Institute of Chicago Occupational Therapy Department (1988). *Work simplification/energy conservation principles* (handout). Chicago: RIC.

Rehabilitation Institute of Chicago Occupational Therapy Department (1990). *Instrumental activities of daily living (I-ADL) protocol.* Chicago: RIC.

Rehabilitation Institute of Chicago Occupational Therapy Department (1991). *RIC Revised functional assessment protocol.* Chicago: RIC.

Reilly, M. (1974). *Play as exploratory learning.* Beverly Hills, CA: Sage Publications.

Rogers, J. C., & Holm, M. B. (1989). The therapist's thinking behind functional assessment, I. In C. Royeen (Ed.). *Assessment of function: An action guide,* Rockville, MD: American Occupational Therapy Association.

Rogers, J. C., & Holm, M. B. (1991). Task performance of older adults and low assistive technology devices. *International Journal of Technology and Aging, 4,* 93–106.

Ross, F. (1992). The use of computers in occupational therapy for visual scanning training. *American Journal of Occupational Therapy, 46,* 314–322.

Rubin, K. H. (1980). *Children's play.* San Francisco: Jossey-Bass.

Rubin, K., Fein, G., & Vandenberg, B. (1983). Play. In P. Mussin (Ed.). *Handbook of child psychology,* Vol IV (pp. 694–774). New York: John Wiley & Sons.

Schwartz, R. (1991). Prevention of work-related injuries. In K. Jacobs (Ed.). *Occupational therapy in work related programs and assessments* (pp. 365–368) (2nd ed.). Boston: Little, Brown & Co.

Shumway-Cook, A., & Woollacott, M. H. (1995). *Motor control: Theory and practical applications.* Baltimore: Williams & Wilkins.

Siewicki, B. J., & Mansfield, L. W. (1977). Determining readiness to resume sexual activity. *American Journal of Nursing, 77,* 604.

Sjogren, K., Damber, J. E., & Liliquist, B. (1983). Sexuality after stroke with hemiplegia. I. Aspects of sexual function. *Scandinavian Journal of Rehabilitation Medicine, 15,* 55–61.

Smith, R. (1995). Burn rehabilitation. *Rehab Management, 4* (8), 67–71.

Smith, E. M., & Bodner, D. R. (1993). Sexual dysfunction after spinal cord injury. *Urologic Clinics of North America, 20,* 535–542.

Staff. (1980s, November 29). Love and hypertension. *Science News,* p. 344.

Tack, B. B. (1991). *Dimensions and correlates of fatigue in older adults with rheumatoid arthritis.* Unpublished doctoral dissertation, University of California at San Francisco.

Taylor, L. P., & McGruder, J. E. (1996). The meaning of sea kayaking for persons with spinal cord injuries. *American Journal of Occupational Therapy, 50,* 39–46.

Trombly, C. (Ed.) (1989). *Occupational therapy for physical dysfunction.* Baltimore: Williams & Wilkins.

Trombly, C. (1993). Anticipating the future: Assessment of occupational function. *American Journal of Occupational Therapy, 47,* 253–257.

Trombly, C. (1995a). Occupation: Purposefulness and meaningfulness as therapeutic mechanisms. 1995 Eleanor Clarke Slagle Lecture. *American Journal of Occupational Therapy, 49,* 960–972.

Trombly, C. (1995b). Planning, guiding, and documenting therapy. In C. A. Trombly (Ed.) *Occupational therapy for physical dysfunction* (pp. 3–40). Baltimore: Williams & Wilkins.

US Lung Centers (1996). *Sex and heart disease lecture series.* US Lung Centers.

Verbrugge, L. M. (1990). The iceberg of disability. In S. M. Stahl (Ed.). *The legacy of longevity: Health and health care in later life* (pp. 55–75). Newbury Park, CA: Sage.

Wade, M. (1985). *Constraints on leisure.* Springfield, IL: Charles C. Thomas.

Wagner, N. N., & Sivarajan, E. S. (1979). Sexual activity and the cardiac patient. In R. Greene (Ed.). *Human sexuality: A health practitioners text* (pp 192–201). Baltimore: Williams & Wilkins.

Watts, N. T. (1990). *Handbook of clinical teaching.* New York: Churchill Livingstone.

Wehman, P. (1977). *Helping the mentally retarded acquire play skills.* Springfield, IL: Charles C. Thomas.

Young, D. (1993). Psychological services. In Work-hardening programs. *Work Programs Special Interest Section Newsletter, 47* (3), 2.

Zasler, N. (1991). Sexuality in neurologic disability: An overview. *Sexuality and Disability, 9* (1), 11–27.

Chapter 20

Treatment of Performance Components

Section 1

Sensory Reeducation

Janet Waylett-Rendall

Goals of Sensory Reeducation
Evaluation Related to Sensory Reeducation
Sensory Reeducation Treatment Techniques
Sensory Reeducation Conclusion

S ensory reeducation is a combination of techniques used to teach those with peripheral nerve injuries how to interpret and make functional use of the abnormal impulses injured nerves relay to the brain (Dellon, 1981). Sensory reeducation is necessary after peripheral nerve injury because peripheral reinnervation is not perfect and return of functional sensation is poor, especially in adults with nerve laceration. Peripheral nerves can regenerate, but the physical structures laid down during regeneration almost never resume fully normal physiological function. That is, regenerated peripheral nerves do not conduct nerve impulses normally. The brain's interpretation of abnormal afferent impulses results in abnormal sensation. Abnormal sensation can put clients at risk for injury. Decreased pain

and temperature sensation, for example, would make a person more likely to be scalded by hot water because the person would not accurately perceive the water's temperature and would not immediately feel pain from scalded skin. Clinical and laboratory studies support the effectiveness of sensory reeducation in improving functional use of altered sensation for clients with nerve injuries.

▼ GOALS OF SENSORY REEDUCATION

The ultimate goal of sensory reeducation is to improve or enhance useful sensation. Corollary goals are to (1) prevent burns or other injuries, and (2) facilitate use of the affected hand in vision-occluded functional activities. As mentioned earlier, people with diminished pain and temperature sensation are at risk for burns. In addition, people with decreased touch and proprioception are at risk for overuse injuries because they use excessive force when manipulating tools and other objects to gain sensory feedback. Over time this excessive force causes overuse injuries to muscles, tendons, and joints. People with peripheral nerve injuries are also more susceptible to skin injuries. Damage to the autonomic nerve fibers of peripheral nerves results in loss of sweating, causing the skin to become dry and cracked. Dry and cracked skin is more easily broken than normal skin, which is kept moist by sweat. The ability to manipulate objects without using vision to compensate for diminished somatic sensation is important for some vocational tasks and for everyday activities such as identifying keys in a pocket or purse by feel.

▼ EVALUATION RELATED TO SENSORY REEDUCATION

Before providing sensory reeducation treatment, occupational therapists need to do a thorough evaluation of skin and muscles innervated by the damaged nerve. Chapter 16, Section 1, provides details about sensory and motor assessments. Two issues specific to sensory reeducation evaluation will be mentioned here: hypersensitivity and stereognosis.

Recovering peripheral nerves cause varying degrees of hypersensitivity during regeneration. Severe hypersensitivity can be a serious detriment to sensory reeducation. Therefore, occupational therapists need to evaluate the degree of hypersensitivity to see if a given client is appropriate for sensory reeducation training. Clients with severe hypersensitivity need to receive desensitization training before beginning a sensory reeducation program. Desensitization involves graded and repetitive application of physical stimuli to the affected body part (Waylett-Rendall, 1995). For example, clients may first be asked to touch soft objects, such as cotton balls or a terry cloth towel. When touching these objects becomes tolerable, the client would be asked to rub the soft objects over the affected skin in a slow, rhythmic fashion. To progress further, the client would follow this same sequence with smooth, hard objects, such as books or the handles of tools or utensils. Finally, the client should be able to touch rough, hard objects, such as a scouring pad, without discomfort.

Stereognosis—the ability to recognize familiar objects by tactile exploration—is the highest level of discriminative sensory function. As such it is an important indicator of the success of a sensory reeducation program.

▼ SENSORY REEDUCATION TREATMENT TECHNIQUES

Clients with good cognitive function and high levels of motivation are the best candidates for sensory reeducation program. The first level of sensory reeducation is to teach the client how to compensate for a lack of **protective sensation** (eg, pain and temperature sensation) by using vision and residual somatic sensation. To wean away from these compensatory techniques, clients need to engage in a program that combines graded sensory stimulation and use of the affected hand in functional activities.

Treatment sessions focusing on sensory stimulation should last about 10 to 15 minutes to allow optimal client concentration. Localization of touch is worked on first. Touch the client's finger or an area on the hand with your fingertip or the eraser end of a pencil, first with the client's eyes open and then in the same place with the client's eyes closed. In the eyes-closed condition, the client concentrates on remembering the sensory and visual images of being touched and tries to point to the area of skin just touched. Discriminatory touch is worked on next to help clients determine the tactile similarities and differences between objects. For this, commercially available training programs exist to teach shape, texture, and object identification. Alternately, a practitioner could assemble grades of cloth (highly textured to finely woven), sandpaper, metal (rough to smooth) or wood for discrimination training. Stereognosis is worked on last by practice in recognizing objects with vision occluded (Callahan, 1995).

Clinicians have noted the most dramatic functional improvement in sensibility in clients who actively use the involved extremity during activities of daily living (ADL) such as self-care. Use of the affected extremity in work simulation and avocational activities is also helpful in promoting the return of more normal sensation.

▶ SENSORY REEDUCATION CONCLUSION

Sensory reeducation after peripheral nerve injuries can prevent disability by helping clients adjust to and use their post-injury sensation during their day-to-day activities. For further details on sensory retraining, readers should refer to specialty texts on this topic, such as the ones cited in this section.

Section 2

Neuromuscular Treatment: Sensorimotor Techniques
Rebecca Dutton

Rood Treatment
 General Inhibition Techniques
 Specific Inhibition Techniques
 Facilitation Techniques
 Treatment Sequence
 Rood Conclusion
Neurodevelopmental Treatment
 Inhibition Techniques
 Facilitation Techniques
 Treatment Stages
 Neurodevelopmental Treatment Conclusion
Proprioceptive Neuromuscular Facilitation Treatment
 Treatment Principles

▼ ROOD TREATMENT

General Inhibition Techniques

Rood's inhibition techniques are based on prolonged sensory stimuli. There are three general inhibition techniques that relax the entire body. Slow, rhythmic rocking, or rolling from side-lying to supine, or from sidelying to prone relax the entire body. Slow, continuous, manual stroking of the spine while the client is prone also relaxes the entire body. Stroking hands alternate, such that as one hand reaches the coccyx, the second hand starts at the occiput to provide continuous, moving, deep finger pad pressure on both sides of the spinous processes. Stroking is repeated for only 3 minutes (Randolph, 1975), because too long may cause sympathetic rebound or even stop the client's breathing (McCormack, 1990). Firm, prolonged manual pressure on the upper lip, the soles of the feet, and palms of the hands also produces general relaxation (McCormack, 1990).

Specific Inhibition Techniques

There are three inhibition techniques that target specific muscles. Neutral warmth consists of covering a body part for 5 to 10 minutes to trap body heat. Firm, prolonged manual pressure applied perpendicular to the longitudinal axis of a tendon with increasing pressure causes that specific muscle to relax. Examples include pressing on the pectoralis major tendon in the armpit, the biceps tendon on the proximal forearm, and the hamstrings tendon at the back of the knee (Randolph, 1975). Prolonged manual pressure activates the Golgi tendon organ (GTO) which rapidly produces a relatively short-lived inhibition of the specific muscle (O'Sullivan, 1988). Prolonged mechanical pressure can also be applied by outside objects such as platform shoes to inhibit plantar flexion, a cone in the hand to inhibit finger flexion, an orthokinetic cuff on the triceps or wrist extensors to inhibit the extensors, and kneeling on all fours to inhibit the quadriceps (Randolph, 1975). These mechanical objects provide continuous pressure on tendinous insertions. They produce a relatively short-lived relaxation of the targeted muscle groups (O'Sullivan, 1988). The Pacinian corpuscle (Umphred & McCormack, 1985) or GTO (McCormack, 1990) may be responsible for the inhibition.

Facilitation Techniques

Rood's facilitation techniques are based on brief sensory stimulation of a specific muscle group. Although stimulation of exteroceptors of the skin, such as fast brushing and icing, were used in the past, these techniques are not used today because they are unpredictable (Umphred & McCormack, 1985). Yet, proprioceptive facilitation techniques are still widely used.

The first facilitation technique is quick stretch. This light, quick stretch helps initiate a muscle contraction. It is administered when the targeted muscle is in a lengthened position, such as quickly stretching the triceps by fully flexing the elbow. The practitioner must give a submaximal stretch because pain will cause withdrawal (Randolph, 1975). Quick stretch produces a very short-lived contraction via the muscle spindle Ia nerve fibers (O'Sullivan, 1988), so it must be done just before the client is asked to contract the muscle. A quick stretch in submaximal range done a moment before an active contraction requires good timing, which comes only with practice.

The second facilitation technique is muscle tapping. It is performed by striking the belly of the targeted muscle with the fingertips as the client is contracting the muscle to produce a movement. Tapping stimulates quick stretch receptors (Randolph, 1975) and produces a relatively short-lived contraction via the muscle spindle Ia fibers (O'Sullivan, 1988). Umphred and McCormack (1985) say muscle tapping is fairly nondiscriminatory and not highly effective at teaching muscle control. Muscle tapping can radiate along the bone to stimulate undesired muscles and make the limb shake so that coordinated movement is difficult. A low-intensity stimulus is better because it is less likely to produce these unwanted effects.

The third facilitation technique is high frequency vibration. A vibrator is applied over a muscle belly to produce a tonic holding contraction that adds strength to an already-contracting muscle (Trombly, 1995c). This activates the Ia afferent of the muscle spindle. Effects peak within 30 to 60 seconds and last only as long as the stimulus is applied (O'Sullivan, 1988; Umphred & McCormack, 1985). If the vibrator is placed over a tendon or a small muscle, vibration may conduct along the bone, producing undesired facilitation of adjacent muscles. The exact frequency is debated. Trombly (1995c) suggests 100 to 300 Hz, whereas Umphred & McCormack (1985) say that a frequency of over 200 can cause skin damage and a frequency of over 150 can cause discomfort or pain. Duration should not exceed 1 to 2 minutes because of heat and friction (McCormack, 1990). Vibration is contraindicated in a very young child with an immature central nervous system (O'Sullivan, 1988). Applying vibration near joints in children may interfere with bone cell production in the growth plate (McCormack, 1990).

The fourth facilitation technique is resistance. Rood used resistance to promote cocontraction (Stockmeyer, 1967). Muscle spindle afferents and GTOs fire in proportion to the amount of resistance applied (Umphred & McCormack, 1985). Resistance is especially important at the end of range. As movement progresses into shortened ranges, a muscle contraction performed without resistance may unload the muscle spindle, which will decrease facilitation from stretch reflexes (O'Sullivan, 1988). Resistance to muscles in shortened range facilitates deeper, tonic postural muscles (McCormack, 1990). Resistance also enhances kinesthetic awareness, which may assist motor learning.

The fifth facilitation technique is joint traction, which activates phasic joint receptors of the flexors as the practitioner gently pulls on the limb (Randolph, 1975). The sixth facilitation technique is joint compression, which facilitates the extensors (Randolph, 1975). Compression is applied along the longitudinal axis of the bone, either manually or with weights, to achieve more compression than body weight alone can provide. For example, the practitioner can apply manual resistance into a client's hand and up the longitudinal axis of the arm while the arm is supported in an extended position. Joint compression during weight bearing activates tonic joint receptors, which facilitates holding postures (O'Sullivan, 1988). Because the body is normally stabilized in mid to shortened ranges, compression is typically applied in functional positions. For example, the practitioner can apply manual compression straight down through the head and spine while the client is sitting. Both joint traction and joint compression improve joint awareness.

Treatment Sequence

Inhibition and facilitation techniques are used in a treatment sequence that Rood divided into four stages (Randolph, 1975). She called the stages reciprocal innervation, coinnervation, heavy work, and skill. Today we use Stockmeyer's terms, which are mobility, cocontraction, mobility superimposed on stability, and skilled movement (Stockmeyer, 1967). Each of these stages will be defined and illustrated through examples.

The first stage, *mobility*, is defined as phasic, reciprocal limb movement through full range while fully supported in supine, rolling over, and prone. For example, in supine, light stroking of the palms or soles of the feet make the arms and legs cross over the anterior surface of body (Randolph, 1975). Rood called this supine withdrawal, because it is a total flexor protective response. She used it to obtain flexion and adduction when a client was dominated by extension (McCormack, 1990).

The second stage, *cocontraction*, is defined as simultaneous tonic contractions of all muscles around a joint to maintain the postures of neck cocontraction, prone on elbows, all fours, and standing. For example, neck cocontraction is achieved by positioning the client prone on a table with his or her head hanging unsupported over the edge with the

eyes focused directly downward to make the chin tuck (Randolph, 1975). Scrubbing with fingertips just above the ears facilitates simultaneous long neck flexion and extension. The practitioner should provide an activity that requires head righting (Trombly, 1995c). As the head bobs into flexion, the extensors are stretched and facilitated to contract; hence, it is important to have well-established neck flexors before asking for cocontraction in this position (McCormack, 1990). However, cocontraction is contraindicated for clients with severe brain damage. It encourages rigid holding to prevent falling at the expense of moving within the posture to interact with the environment.

The third stage, *mobility superimposed on stability*, is defined as movement of proximal limb segments with the distal ends of the limbs fixed on a base of support. This stage includes weight shifts while prone on elbows, on all fours, and standing. For example, weight shifts on all fours takes the form of rocking. While rocking, extensor thrust in the legs is inhibited by weight bearing on the patellar tendon (Randolph, 1975). The practitioner must prevent overstretching of the long finger flexors of the hands by allowing the fingers to partially flex. Weight shifts on all fours enable the client to eventually lift one or two limbs, which permits crawling (Trombly, 1995c). Weight shifts also prepare the client for equilibrium responses (McCormack, 1990).

Mobility superimposed on stability is produced by what Rood called heavy-work muscles. These muscles are medial (neck, trunk, scapula, pelvis), deep, fleshy or fibrous, one-joint, low-energy, red aerobic muscles that perform cocontraction and antigravity work that requires less cortical control (Randolph, 1975). They are primarily the extensors, abductors, and external rotators. Rood's assumption that mobility superimposed on stability must be activated before proceeding to skilled movement is controversial. Trombly (1995c) says that this assumption is wrong because distal and proximal motor systems are controlled separately. McCormack (1990) says this assumption applies primarily to the upper extremity where scapular stability is needed before finger dexterity is possible.

The fourth stage, *skill*, is defined as movement of distal limb segments while proximal segments stabilize. Skill includes hand use and walking. It is produced by what Rood called light-work muscles. These muscles are lateral (eg, arms, thumb), superficial, tendinous, multijoint, high-energy, white anaerobic muscles that perform phasic, skilled movements that require cortical control (Randolph, 1975). They are primarily flexors, adductors, and internal rotators.

Rood Conclusion

Rood identified general inhibition techniques that relax the entire body and specific inhibition and facilitation techniques that target specific muscles. These techniques are applied in four stages called mobility, cocontraction, mobility superimposed on stability, and skill. Rood's exteroceptive facilitation techniques have not stood the test of time. Co-contraction is contraindicated for severely spastic individuals. Her assumption that mobility superimposed on stability must precede skill is still debated. Yet her inhibition and proprioceptive facilitation techniques are so commonly used today that her contribution in this area has faded into anonymity.

▼ NEURODEVELOPMENTAL TREATMENT

Inhibition Techniques

The neurodevelopmental treatment (NDT) frame of reference has six methods that inhibit **spasticity**. They include passive elongation, proximal limb dissociation, reflex-inhibiting patterns (RIPs), inhibitory positioning and **orthotics,** normal weight shifts, and normal limb movements free in space.

The first inhibition technique is passive elongation. Spastic muscles can become shortened and stiff. This shortening elongates the antagonists, which gives these antagonists a poor mechanical advantage because muscles are weakest when stretched out at the end of range (Norkin & Levangie, 1992). To restore the balance between agonist and antagonist, tight, spastic muscles need to be elongated before all muscles around a joint are asked to contract (Adams, 1982). To elongate a muscle, apply slow, even pressure, such that movement is almost imperceptible, to avoid intolerable pain. Hold the limb by grasping bony areas, such as either side of the elbow, or by cupping a nonspastic muscle, such as the triceps, with an open hand. Avoid a circumferential grip that makes the practitioner's fingertips press on a muscle belly.

The second inhibition technique is proximal dissociation, defined as separate movements of adjacent proximal body parts (Adams, 1982). For example, the head rotates while the shoulder girdle remains still, or one hip flexes while the other hip extends. Brain-damaged clients with spasticity often lack proximal dissociation. A client may need to have the scapula dissociated from the neck and rib cage while supine before rolling to sidelying. Once scapular muscles relax, the practitioner can gently protract the scapula, flex the shoulder, and extend the elbow to prevent the hemiplegic arm from becoming trapped under the body as the client rolls to the edge of the bed.

The third inhibition technique is RIPs. Once the spastic muscles are partially elongated, the limb is relaxed enough to be placed in an RIP so the client can perform a movement (Adams, 1982). RIPs ensure that the limb is as far away as possible from pathological **synergy** patterns when the client first tries to move. The practitioner initially wants the flexion synergy bound upper extremity to be as far away from flexion and internal rotation as possible. The practitioner assists shoulder external rotation and elbow extension

with the arm abducted to the side to inhibit upper extremity and trunk flexion (Adams, 1982). Similarly, the practitioner can place the extended arm in front of the body if a client's flexion synergy exhibits especially strong scapular retraction. Then the client moves the sound or involved limb while the practitioner uses key points to maintain the RIP to inhibit synergy and spasticity.

During an RIP, the practitioner can grasp proximal key points of control, such as the head, trunk, pelvis, shoulder, or elbow, or grasp distal key points, such as the forearm, hand, knee, or foot. Regardless of which key point is used, the practitioner must not interfere with the client's movement during a functional activity. RIPs are never used to rigidly hold a position.

The practitioner also wants the extension synergy-bound lower extremity far away from extension and internal rotation. For example, if a client has a stiffly extended lower extremity in sitting, the practitioner can grasp the knee and foot to pull the hip into external rotation and abduction before flexing the hip and knee. This antiextension synergy RIP is a very effective way to put the hemiplegic foot back on the wheelchair footrest.

Clients must be taught to use RIPs during activities of daily living (ADLs) because spasticity escalates as clients exert themselves when they are cognitively and emotionally challenged. A few minutes of therapy is not enough to inhibit spastic muscles and ensure carryover.

Clients can be taught to use distal key points to perform RIPs during ADLs. The client can inhibit the upper extremity flexion synergy by clasping hands together with the hemiplegic thumb on top of the sound thumb and then extending both arms in front of the body. This clasped hands position enables the client to inhibit upper extremity flexion and retraction while rolling over in bed. While standing up, extending the arms in front of the body also shifts the center of gravity forward and pulls the pelvis into anterior tilt. Without this upper extremity RIP, posterior tilt may pull the client's center of gravity backward and facilitate the lower extremity extensor synergy, which thrusts the client backward in the chair.

Clients can be taught to use proximal key points of control to perform RIPs during ADLs. The client can inhibit the lower extremity extension synergy while sitting to dress by flexing and then crossing the hemiplegic leg over the sound leg, or while rolling in bed, by sliding the sound foot underneath the hemiplegic knee to flex it. The client can also inhibit the upper extremity flexion synergy by dangling the shirt sleeve between his or her legs. As the client bends forwards to drop the hemiplegic arm in the sleeve, the weight of the heavy arm pulls the scapula into protraction, which inhibits the upper extremity flexion synergy. This facilitates elbow extension so the arm slides more easily into the open sleeve.

The third inhibition technique is inhibitory positioning devices and orthotics, which keep shortened, spastic muscles in elongated positions (Adams, 1982). While sleeping, a client with hemiplegia can lie on the sound side with the spastic arm in front of the body resting on a pillow at shoulder height. This protracts the scapula and extends the elbow to inhibit the upper extremity flexion synergy. The hemiplegic leg is semiflexed to inhibit the lower extremity extension synergy. Positioning devices can also ensure symmetrical sitting. Excessive anterior or posterior pelvic tilt can be inhibited by inserting a hard seat in the wheelchair. Lateral trunk flexion can be corrected by inserting a hard seat in the wheelchair and resting whichever arm is lower on an arm trough or lapboard. Orthotics that inhibit the upper extremity flexion synergy include the spasticity reduction splint, finger abduction splint, and serial casting (Linden, 1995).

The fourth inhibitory technique is miniature weight shifting to inhibit rigid fixing (Adams, 1982). Axial weight shifts are easiest to achieve while sitting, because this stabilizes the legs so that the trunk has to move in response to the practitioner's handling. Axial weight shifts include shifting the trunk forward, backward, sideways, and with rotation. During limb weight shifts, the distal end of an extremity, such as the elbow or hand, stays in contact with the support surface while the proximal joints move. One example of a high-level limb weight shift is having an ambulatory client lean on a kitchen counter top with the hemiplegic hand to improve balance while reaching for objects in the refrigerator with the sound hand. Initially, the client needs maximal assistance to keep spasticity and pathological patterns under control during active weight shifts. Normal limb movements that are independent of pathological synergies are inhibitory (Adams, 1982). Normal movements include distal dissociation of the forearm, wrist, fingers, and ankle. Distal dissociation requires the client to move distal body parts individually, rather than as a whole unit in a synergy pattern. One example of teaching distal dissociation is helping the client perform supination and wrist radial deviation to keep a spoon level during feeding so that the food does not spill.

Both weight-shifting and normal limb movements can inhibit abnormally high tone, but they can also stimulate spasticity if the client strains. Therefore, both must be used with caution. Early high-quality movements are possible if the practitioner provides maximum support and requires minimum range of motion (ROM).

Facilitation Techniques

Neurodevelopmental treatment uses several facilitation techniques including joint compression, joint traction, and manual resistance (Adams, 1982). These techniques are explained in the foregoing Rood section. NDT also facilitates with active weight shifts that can both inhibit and facilitate because they first make muscles contract and then relax as the limb moves from flexion to extension and back again. One facilitation technique that is unique to NDT is placing and eccentric lowering (Adams, 1982; Bobath, 1978). Placing is the ability to hold a limb suspended in the air and then decrease muscle tone enough for the practitioner to move the limb anywhere in space. Initially the limb is kept perpendicular to the ground so that gravity has less effect. This keeps muscle tone low and gives the client better control. While the client is sitting, the practitioner can place the upper extremity in a flexion RIP and raise the arm overhead. The practitioner then briefly lets go several times to see if the client can hold the RIP position. If the client can hold the position for a few seconds, the practitioner helps the client slowly lower the arm. The practitioner should use key points of control to keep the limb in the RIP pattern during lowering. As the limb becomes parallel to the floor, gravity pulls on the long limb so the client may strain more, experience spasticity, and lose control unless given physical assistance.

Treatment Stages

The NDT inhibition and facilitation techniques must be administered together in three stages (Dutton, 1995). The first stage is to give the sensation of how both normal tone and movement feel. Purposeful activity is not used because the client needs to look at his or her moving body without being distracted by cognitive challenges and emotional stress. The practitioner returns to this first stage whenever abnormal tone or pathological patterns overpower the client's intended movement.

The second stage of facilitation and inhibition is to let the client initiate movement during a purposeful activity, while the practitioner maintains inhibition or facilitation. Research has shown that practicing repetitive motions, such as rocking side to side, does not generalize to open tasks that require the motor system to respond to changing conditions (Sabari, 1991). Purposeful activities are used in this second stage because they provide cognitive and emotional challenges that the client does not always anticipate. Purposeful activities also tell clients why they have to perform specific movements (Dutton, 1995). For example, clients learn that leaning forward with anterior tilt while sitting helps them stand up. Equipment used in an activity also requires the client to use visual input to plan movements and anticipate and correct errors. The client can take responsibility for planning only if the practitioner waits for the client to initiate a purposeful motion.

The second stage usually lasts for several days and requires frequent return to stage 1 when the client exhibits abnormal tone or pathological movements. It is vital to achieve both stages 1 and 2 within a single treatment session. Initially, the sensation of what normal feels like is very fleeting. If you do not ask clients to initiate movement as soon as they recognize how normal feels, you will not see carryover.

The third stage of facilitation and inhibition is to fade control. Initially, this means changing from proximal key points to distal key points. For example, if the hand is still stiffly flexed, the practitioner can move his or her hands from the scapula and humerus down to the forearm and hand to assist supination, wrist extension, and thumb abduction. Eventually, it means removing all physical assistance. If a client cannot move independently with quality movements for even a few seconds, the practitioner should reevaluate his or her long-term goals and discharge plans.

Neurodevelopmental Treatment Conclusion

Neurodevelopmental treatment repeatedly uses facilitatory and inhibitory techniques to achieve high-quality movements during three stages of treatment. These stages are to give the sensation of how normal feels, to let the client initiate, and to fade the practitioner's control.

▼ PROPRIOCEPTIVE NEUROMUSCULAR FACILITATION TREATMENT

Proprioceptive neuromuscular facilitation (PNF) was championed by Knott and Voss (Voss, Ionta, & Myers, 1985). They agreed with their contemporaries that sensory-motor principles guide motor learning, such as cephalocaudal development and establishing a balance between agonist and antagonist by reciprocal innervation. Yet Knott and Voss made a unique contribution by generating a set of seven general principles for approaching the client (Myers, Mukoyama, & Becker, 1985; Voss et al, 1985).

Treatment Principles

The first PNF principle states that normal movement is diagonal: not linear. People do not drink from a glass by moving each joint in a series of linear, anatomical planes; they lift the glass by moving the arm in a graceful, diagonal arc. Diagonal patterns consist of simultaneous flexion and extension, abduction and adduction, external and internal rotation. Pure exercise is usually done in linear planes, which may not prepare clients for normal diagonal movements that require coordination of all the muscles around a joint. This first PNF principle asks practitioners to ask themselves if the kind of movements they are using in treatment are functional, diagonal movements.

The second PNF principle states that distal timing produces smooth movement. During normal movement, distal segments move first, while proximal segments stabilize early in the range. Distal timing is ultimately what practitioners are trying to achieve when they use NDT proximal key points of control to produce proximal stability. However, proximal stability alone is not enough; distal movement is needed to manipulate objects in the environment. This PNF principle asks practitioners to remember that smooth, distal timing is needed to make clients functional.

The third PNF principle states that vision leads movement. When the eyes track a target, the body follows. For example, when clients perform a diagonal limb pattern, they are asked to track one of their own hands. As the eyes follow the hand, the head moves, which causes the limbs and trunk to move through a greater ROM. It is not necessary to use PNF patterns to take advantage of this principle of vision leading movement. Occupational therapy practitioners use purposeful activities that require visual tracking to manipulate objects (Myers et al, 1985). This PNF principle asks practitioners to think about the negative effect on ROM if they always let clients stare straight ahead or look down at one body part while exercising.

The fourth PNF principle states that clients should coordinate movement with breathing to reduce pain, which increases ROM. For example, when clients perform a diagonal limb pattern, they are asked to breath in as they raise their arms and breath out as they lower their arms. This PNF principle asks practitioners to practice what they know about breathing by teaching clients to breathe as they move whenever decreased ROM caused by pain interferes with purposeful activity.

The fifth PNF principle states that the practitioner should use concise verbal commands when teaching the client to move normally. For example, for a diagonal pattern performed while sitting, the practitioner may tell the client to hold his or her arms out to the side at a 45-degree angle to the body and abduct thumbs so they point down at floor. The practitioner then says, "close hands, turn palms up, cross arms." Then, as the client lowers his or her arms, the practitioner says "open hands, turn palms down, uncross arms." Knott and Voss felt that clients who knew what was expected of them would master movements more quickly. Although practitioners do not consistently use verbal commands as precise as these, practitioners find verbal instruction helps when an adult client is trying to second-guess the practitioner by performing an unwanted motion.

The sixth PNF principle states that proprioceptive tracking helps clients relearn movement by mimicking the practitioner's normal movements. To allow the client to track the practitioner's movements, the practitioner must move slowly and maintain firm manual contact with the client's body. To prove to yourself that proprioceptive tracking is effective, stand facing a partner and place your palms an inch away from your partner's palms (Myers et al, 1985). Try to track your partner's arm movements using vision alone. Try again while lightly touch your partner's fingertips as he or she moves. Finally, repeat with your palms firmly pressed against your partner's palms as your partner moves slowly. This PNF principle reminds practitioners that their hands are a powerful teaching tool. Although visual demonstration and light touch are less physically invasive, they are poor substitutes for firm manual contacts and slow movement that permit proprioceptive tracking to enhance motor learning.

The seventh PNF principle states that the practitioner must stand on a diagonal line and rotate his or her whole body to help the client execute normal diagonal movements. For example, to help a client who is lying supine perform an upper extremity diagonal pattern, the practitioner faces away from the client while holding the client's pronated hand with his or her two hands. The practitioner must stand on an imaginary diagonal line to maintain the client's shoulder in 45 degrees of abduction (Myers et al, 1985). The practitioner says "close hand, turn palm up, cross arm." As the client's arm begins to move, the practitioner rotates his or her whole body to encourage the client's arm to supinate and externally rotate. The practitioner then moves towards the client, walking on the diagonal line, as the client's arm crosses the chest.

Having the practitioner walk on the diagonal and rotate his or her entire body accomplishes two things. First, it keeps the practitioner's hands soft and gentle because strength comes from the practitioner's whole body instead of just from the practitioner's hands and arms. Second, as the practitioner's body rotates and moves on the diagonal, the practitioner's hands automatically guide the client's limb in a natural diagonal movement. When practitioners try to consciously think about how to move a client's limb, the resulting movement is often unnatural and lacks smoothness.

The large body movements used in PNF are a stark contrast to the way practitioners usually help clients move during functional activities. Picture a practitioner standing next to a client during assisted feeding. The practitioner moves the client's hand and elbow, but firmly plants his or her feet on the floor and does not move his or her body. It is difficult to consciously teach the small adjustments of forearm, wrist, and hand needed to keep the spoon level while assisting shoulder and elbow movements. This last PNF principle asks practitioners to use their entire body as an instrument to gently teach natural diagonal movement.

Facilitation Techniques

In addition to general principles, Knott and Voss developed specific facilitation and inhibition techniques (Voss et al, 1985). Facilitation is subdivided into direct and indirect techniques. Direct facilitation, such as stretch stimulus, manual resistance, and manual contacts, applies stimulation directly to the weak muscles. Stretch stimulus positions the client in a lengthened position as far away as possible from where the client will end up just before the client moves. For example, the practitioner can stretch a client's hand wide open before asking the client to make a fist. It is easy to learn how to safely administer stretch stimulus because the gentle, nonabrupt stretch is released by the client's movement. Maximal manual resistance is the maximum the client can take and still move through full ROM. Assistance is given at the beginning of range and then resistance gradually builds up as the client moves. This technique is more difficult to learn because the practitioner must take care not to overpower the client.

Brief manual contacts facilitate the muscle directly under your hand. To prove the power of manual contacts to your-self, get a strength baseline. While sitting, hold your arm in 90 degrees of shoulder abduction as someone standing behind you uses one hand to try to make you lower your arm. Let this person scratch your pectoralis major on the arm just tested. Repeat the strength test. Why did you lower your arm the second time? The brief manual contact facilitated an adductor, the pectoralis, which inhibited the abductors by reciprocal innervation. Be careful where you touch your clients because your hands are powerful facilitators. A variety of prescriptive manual contacts is a quintessential characteristic of PNF (Voss et al, 1985).

Indirect facilitation occurs by "irradiation." Muscle activity is facilitated in stronger muscles, which excites weaker adjacent muscles. The diagonal patterns themselves cause irradiation. Having the client move his or her shoulder and elbow excites more distal muscles and vice versa. Bilateral symmetrical patterns cause irradiation as muscle activity in one limb excites the other limb. Finally, developmental patterns, such as using upper extremity diagonals to initiate rolling, cause activity from limb muscles to irradiate to the trunk and vice versa.

Inhibition Techniques

There are many PNF inhibition techniques (Voss et al, 1985). A commonly used one is called hold-relax. For example, ask a client with tight hamstrings to lie supine. The practitioner will grasp the client's leg and slowly perform a straight-leg raise with the knee extended. When resistance is felt, the client is told to "hold" by using an isometric hamstring contraction to press his or her straight leg down against the practitioner's hands. The practitioner resists enough to tire the tight muscle without overpowering the isometric contraction. After a few seconds, the practitioner asks the client to relax and then raises the leg farther into the range. This process is repeated every time resistance is felt.

Proprioceptive Neuromuscular Facilitation Conclusion

Knott and Voss developed seven unique principles for approaching the client. Unlike other theorists, they differentiated between direct and indirect methods of facilitation and emphasized powerful techniques that can be implemented with the practitioner's hands instead of devices such as vibrators and brushes.

▼ SENSORY INTEGRATIVE TREATMENT

Before a sensory integrative (SI) treatment session begins, the practitioner (1) designs a therapeutic physical environment, (2) selects equipment based on general principles, and (3) selects equipment based on diagnosis.

Designing the Physical Environment

Designing a therapeutic physical environment includes ordering SI equipment and finding a large physical space. Suspension equipment is absolutely essential for providing vestibular input. This equipment should include a 500-lb suspension system anchored securely on beams in the ceiling to accommodate nets, hammocks, bolsters, and swings (Clark, Mailloux, & Parham, 1989). Other essential equipment includes scooter boards and ramps, a trapeze, a minitrampoline, mats for falling, large therapy balls, cardboard stacking blocks, small balls and bean bags for tossing, hula hoops and Thera-band for pulling oneself around, and sucking items, such as 4-ft plastic straws (Kimball, 1993). To safely accommodate activities, such as scooter board obstacle courses, swinging equipment that must be placed a safe distance from the walls, and climbing and jumping, the practitioner must have a large room (Kimball, 1993). Yet too large a space may invite hyperactivity, so having moveable partitions to subdivide the space is recommended (Clark et al, 1989).

Accidents can happen with SI equipment (Ayres, 1972). This equipment challenges children who are unskilled at movement and who may lack judgment about what is dangerous. Practitioners can prevent serious accidents by ordering safer materials, such as wood, plastic, and cardboard, instead of metal, removing unnecessary equipment that the child may run into, placing mats wherever the child may fall, and keeping suspension equipment low to the ground and in good repair.

Selecting Equipment Based on Principles

After the practitioner designs the physical environment, he or she is ready to select equipment based on general principles. First, the practitioner should select equipment that requires the desired response, instead of planning for a specific activity (Kimball, 1993). For example, the practitioner can select equipment that requires axial flexion and motor planning. Which game the child plays is negotiated after the child arrives because the practitioner wants the child to be self-directed. Yet, the practitioner should eliminate distractions and provide a variety of enticing equipment that the child can choose among to reach the therapeutic goal (Kimball, 1993). The child is often able to choose exactly the kind of activity that organizes sensory input and produces an **adaptive response** (Ayres, 1979).

Second, the practitioner should select equipment that permits simple activities first and more complex activities later (Kimball, 1993). Start by having equipment that makes use of centrally programmed positions such as sitting and standing. Gradually encourage the use of unusual positions such as being prone on a scooter board or playing on all fours. Start by having equipment that enables the child to bear weight on a stable surface such as a chair. Gradually introduce unstable surfaces such as nets and bolsters. Start by having the child perform the activity alone. In later sessions, introduce extra equipment so the child can do the activity with another child.

Third, the practitioner should select equipment that provides a multisensory experience. Multiple sensory modalities are more powerful because they require intersensory integration (Kimball, 1993). Ayres (1979) described a multisensory game called "net hockey." While prone in nets, the child and his practitioner hit a soft ball back and forth with plastic sticks. Swinging in the net introduced vestibular input. Using strong neck cocontraction to hold up his head and propel himself with his hands on the floor generated proprioceptive input. Watching the moving ball produced visual input and required eye coordination. This is one example of a multisensory activity.

Selecting Equipment Based on Diagnosis

In addition to these three general principles, the practitioner selects equipment based on the treatment sequence for specific SI disorders. The practitioner should always address sensory modulation problems first because threatening sensations cannot be integrated (Ayres, 1972; Kimball, 1993). Meaningful interpretation of sensory input is necessary before an adaptive response can be made. Children with **tactile defensiveness** and gravitational insecurity need lots of tactile and vestibular stimulation, but may avoid it. Therefore, the child who feels threatened by tactile or vestibular sensation should first engage in self-administered stimulation.

Treatment for sensory modulation may start with firm brushing on the back of the arms to decrease arousal. However, sensory stimulation should be experienced as part of an adaptive response during a meaningful activity. Therefore, brushing is often followed by joint compression during an activity, like crawling though a tunnel, and by vestibular activities, like lying prone on a swinging bolster. The bolster swing adds touch pressure where the body touches the swing and proprioception because of the limb cocontraction needed to hold on (Ayres, 1976). To maintain normal modulation of sensory input, some children need a maintenance program called a "sensory diet" (Kimball, 1993). This may include a home stimulation program and activities such as roller skating and gymnastics.

Second in the treatment sequence is remediation of vestibular bilateral integration (Ayres, 1972, 1976; Kimball, 1993). This disorder requires facilitation of flexor and extensor tone, cocontraction, equilibrium, and bilateral coordination. Flexor tone is required to hold onto a trapeze. Extensor tone is needed while going down a ramp on a scooter board. Cocontraction of neck and mouth is needed when sucking juice through a 4-ft plastic straw. Limb cocontraction is needed to hold onto a hoola hoop as the practitioner pushes and pulls the child around while the child sits on a scooter board. Equilibrium is required to kick a small ball while sitting on a large ball. Bilateral coordination is required to jump rope or hit a tether ball with a bat.

Third in the treatment sequence is remediation of end-product abilities (Ayres, 1972, 1976; Clark et al, 1989). For example, to stimulate praxis, use unfamiliar activities and emphasize ideation and sequencing. Have the child set up an obstacle course and figure out how to navigate it. Have the child kick a ball backwards or crawl through a tunnel on two knees and one hand.

Once the practitioner selects and sets up equipment based on general principles and a specific diagnosis and removes distracting equipment, the therapy session begins. The role of the practitioner includes (1) observing precautions, (2) employing a therapeutic use of self, (3) monitoring and assisting adaptive responses, and (4) documenting progress.

Observing Precautions

Despite the best planning, the practitioner must be prepared to observe precautions. Sensory integrative equipment provides very strong sensory input and can produce sensory overload, overinhibition, and strong emotional responses. Sensory overload occurs when vestibular and light tactile stimuli over excite the reticular-activating system (Ayres, 1972). During treatment, watch for subtle signs of withdrawal, such as repeated yawning, and for more obvious signs of withdrawal such as destructive behavior, flushing or blanching of the face, nausea, and unusual perspiration. If these signs of sensory overload do not subside within a few minutes after treatment stops, the child can be calmed with slow rocking on a large therapy ball or deep pressure on the child's body. If the child experiences nightmares or movement after going to bed, the practitioner should consider temporarily reducing the amount of stimulation.

Overinhibition of the brainstem is another precaution (Ayres, 1972; Clark et al, 1989). Watch for signs of cyanosis and decreased respiration by making sure that the child can talk to you. If these signs appear, monitor the child's pulse and respiration for up to 30 minutes after treatment. If needed, apply excitatory stimuli, such as light touch, to the child's feet and face.

Strong emotional responses to therapy can increase the risk of accidents which require precautions (Ayres, 1972). Sensory input has a strong effect on the limbic system, which regulates emotions. After several months of therapy, a child may exhibit profound and pervasive emotional changes such as euphoria (exaggerated elation), depression, or resistance. These emotional changes signal positive neurological changes, but they can be overwhelming. The practitioner should consider temporarily reducing expectations for the few weeks it usually takes for emotional lability (highly changeable emotions) to subside.

Therapeutic Use of Self

The therapeutic use of self includes establishing trust and using a therapeutic style of interaction. First, it is essential for the practitioner to create an atmosphere of safety (Ayres, 1972; Kimball, 1993). The child will tolerate treatment sooner if the practitioner respects the child's fear. Once the practitioner establishes trust by not imposing sensory input, the child is more likely to gain self-confidence through self-directed stimulation and adaptive responses. As a general rule, what is pleasant is integrative and what is unpleasant is disorganizing. The practitioner must also use an appropriate therapeutic style of interaction. The practitioner can be minimally verbal or highly verbal; be subdued or enthusiastic (Clark et al, 1989). Kimball (1993) recommends giving constant verbal feedback or constantly eliciting verbalization so that the child will have a greater understanding of what he or she is doing. When Ayres demonstrated SI treatment in a video (1976), she made sparse, subdued comments and watched the child so she could mimic and assist his interactions with the equipment. She let the playful aspects of the game emerge naturally. Therapeutic styles work best when they match the child's individual needs.

Monitoring and Assisting Adaptive Responses

Once therapy has begun, the practitioner must also monitor the child's adaptive responses and assist, rather than instruct, the child. Ayres said "it takes courage to let a child appear to waste time as he fumbles and resists and explores his own way" (1979; p. 151). The practitioner can help the child get started by asking him what he is about to do. The practitioner can demonstrate or help the child with the movements he or she wants to perform. Only as a last resort, should the practitioner offer specific suggestions. For example, the practitioner can provide the first part of a sequence and let the child verbalize the next step (Kimball, 1993). Clark et al (1989) call this monitoring process "artful vigilance." It involves repeatedly using the child's responses to determine when and how much structure to give and when and how much assistance to give as the session progresses.

Documenting Progress

Finally, because frequent administration of the Sensory Integration and Praxis Tests is not acceptable, the practitioner must document progress by noting increased duration, repetition, or quality of movement during therapeutic activities. The practitioner may record how many seconds the child can roll inside five big inner tubes tied together or count how many times the child can capture a tether ball in an open Clorox bottle. The practitioner may note improved quality of movement. Initially, the child may drag his or her legs and need moderate physical assistance to propel the scooter board forward 3 feet. During later attempts, the child may maintain full leg extension while independently propelling the scooter board around corners.

Sensory Integrative Conclusion

Sensory integrative treatment includes designing a therapeutic physical environment, selecting equipment based on general principles and a specific SI diagnosis, observing precautions, employing a therapeutic use of self, monitoring and assisting adaptive responses, and documenting progress exhibited during therapeutic activities.

Section 3

Neuromuscular Treatment: Strengthening

Debbie Pinet

D eficits in strength can affect a person's ability to complete ADLs, work, and leisure pursuits. Without adequate strength, a person cannot participate in meaningful activities. Strength deficits can be at the levels of impairment, disability, or handicap. Factors such as pain, edema, adhesions and contractures, abnormal tone, and sensory deficits, limit muscle function and result in strength impairment. Decreased strength can also lead to joint deformity owing to imbalances between agonist and antagonist muscles. If the strength impairment is not treated, a disability or dysfunction in occupational performance areas can occur because the person will not have the sufficient strength to complete ADLs, work, or leisure activities such as bathing, carpentry, or tennis (Rogers & Holm, 1994).

Strength impairments can additionally affect the individual's role performance. An individual's successful participation in roles such as parent, worker, student, partner, or athlete depend on sufficient muscle strength. A handicap exists if a person's disability interferes with accomplishing the tasks required of a specific role. (Rogers & Holm, 1994).

▼ DESCRIPTION OF STRENGTH

"Strength is the ability of a muscle or muscle group to produce tension and a resulting force in one maximal effort, either dynamically or statically, in relation to the demands placed upon it" (Kisner & Colby, 1990, p. 10). Skeletal muscles are made up of many individual muscle fibers that act as contracting units. Muscle fiber contraction requires stimulation by a motor neuron. One motor nerve and all the attached muscle fibers form a motor unit. Stimulation of the motor unit occurs via the motor end plate, which is an enlargement at the end of the nerve fiber. At this neuromuscular junction, a neurotransmitter is released that causes the muscle fibers to contract as a motor unit. When the muscle fibers contract, they generate an amount of tension or force that is applied to the muscle, its tendon, and the bone to which the tendons are connected. This force can either promote movement of the attached bones, or provide stability and maintenance of a position. The amount of force produced is related to the number of motor units being stimulated. The greater the number of motor units firing, the stronger the tension, as more muscle fibers are contracting (Kisner & Colby).

▼ TYPES OF MUSCLE CONTRACTIONS

There are two basic categories of muscle contractions: isometric and isotonic. During an isometric muscle contraction, the motor units stimulate the muscle fibers to increase the tension in the muscle, but the muscle does not shorten for joint movement. Stability at the joint occurs as the force generated in the muscle is equal to gravity or any other applied resistance. An example of an isometric contraction would be maintaining a grasp on a blowdryer (finger flexors and thumb opposition).

Isotonic contraction of a muscle involves changes in the muscle fiber's length, resulting in joint movement. Two types of isotonic contractions are possible: concentric or eccentric. During concentric contraction, the muscle shortens to allow motion. The force generated in the muscle is increased to overcome resistance to movement. A concentric contraction of the biceps (elbow flexors) would occur when the blowdryer is raised to dry the wet hair. The tension in the biceps increases to move the forearm up against the resistance of gravity. During eccentric contraction, the muscle fibers of an already shortened muscle, must now lengthen to resist a force and produce a controlled joint motion. A eccentric contraction would occur at the biceps, when slowly lowering the blowdryer after drying the hair. (Pedretti, 1996; Trombly, 1995b). Both isometric and isotonic muscle contractions are needed to perform ADLs, work, and leisure activities.

▼ FACTORS AFFECTING MUSCLE STRENGTH

Edema, adhesions and contractures, abnormal muscle tone, and sensory deficits all influence the muscle's ability to contract. Edema and adhesions are associated with the inflammatory response that occurs whenever there is **trauma** to the body. During inflammation, the blood vessels dilate, thereby sending additional white blood cells to the damaged area. This results in edema or extra fluid in the tissues surrounding the muscles; this edema causes swelling. Fibrin, a sticky substance, is deposited to clot the blood and reduce the edema in the area. Fibrin also causes the development of adhesions, or the holding together of two superficial surfaces. The stronger the adhesions, the greater the chance of muscle atrophy because the adhesions prevent the muscle from lengthening or shortening to generate an adequate contraction. The edema, if left untreated, can place pressure on nerves, blood vessels, and various joint structures, delaying healing and causing pain and stiffness. Expedient prevention and treatment of edema is critical to maintain joint integrity and optimal muscle functioning. Active ROM for fluid absorption and soft tissue mobility, elevation of the edematous extremity, compression of the tissues through retrograde massage, wrapping or pressure garments, and the use of ice for vasoconstriction, are all interventions to address edema (Pedretti, 1996).

Abnormalities in muscle tone, or tightness, can lead to contractures. A contracture occurs when there is permanent shortening of a muscle caused by spasm or **paralysis** (Thomas, 1993). Trombly additionally defines *contracture* as "the inability to move a body part because of soft tissue shortening or bony ankylosis" (1995b, p. 74). The shortened muscle fibers limit joint ROM and can negatively affect completion of occupational performance areas, as well as cause pain and sensory changes due to immobility. Prevention of contractures occurs with stretching, joint positioning, and neurophysiological approaches to facilitate normal muscle tone and motor control. Muscle strengthening is not focused on until normal muscle tone is achieved (Pedretti, 1996). (Please see Section 2 in this chapter for specific neurophysiological treatment approaches).

Accurate sensory processing contributes to coordinated movement. The inclination to move is partly based on sensory feedback. Without adequate sensation, movement can be ineffective despite recovery of motor functioning. A thorough sensory evaluation must be performed in conjunction with an evaluation of active ROM and manual muscle testing. Treatment of sensory deficits can be remedial or compensatory, depending on the cause of the deficits. (Please see Section 1 of this chapter for details on this topic). When sensory deficits are present, a strengthening program should include precautions to prevent injury from lack of sensory feedback to the muscle.

▼ PRINCIPLES AND CHARACTERISTICS OF STRENGTHENING ACTIVITIES

Resistance

Once a strength impairment is identified, the occupational practitioner designs a treatment plan to increase the strength needed for occupational performance tasks. According to the overload principle, to increase strength, the load or force applied to the muscle must exceed the capacity of that muscle, causing recruitment of more motor units. Resistance is often used to stimulate muscle contraction. The greater the intensity or the amount of resistance applied, the more motor units are recruited (Kisner & Colby, 1990). The intensity of the load, rather than the number of completed repetitions, has the most influence on the development of muscle strength. More motor units firing cause a larger force in the muscle tension, which means more muscle strength (Hamill & Knutzen, 1995; Umphred, 1995; Lillegard & Terrio, 1994).

Gravity is one force that places a load on muscles during contraction. The amount of this force is dependent on the plane of movement, either against gravity, or in a gravity-eliminated or lessened plane. Muscles have to work harder to move a body part against gravity than when moving in a horizontal or gravity-eliminated plane. The muscle grade awarded through manual muscle testing determines the plane of movement for muscle strengthening. Muscles should be able the move joints through the full available ROM in a gravity-eliminated and then against gravity plane, before external loads or forces are applied to them.

Types of Contraction

The type of muscle contraction stimulated influences the development of strength. "A muscle produces the most force output when contracting eccentrically (lengthening) against resistance. The muscle produces slightly less force when contracting isometrically (holding) and the least force when contracting concentrically (shortening) against a load" (Kisner & Colby, 1990; p. 11).

Most functional activities require a combination of muscle contractions. Muscle groups respond in different patterns, depending on the demands of specific tasks. These response patterns can be classified as open or closed chains of movement or kinetic links. The chain is considered closed when the distal end of an extremity is bearing weight. When the extremity is free distally, the chain is considered open to a variety of movement possibilities (Goldstein, 1995). A closed-chain movement uses eccentric and concentric muscles contractions and the force of the person's body weight to add a load to the muscle. An example would be a pushup where the hands are bearing weight and the body is raised and lowered slowly over the hands. An example of an open-chain movement would be a biceps curl in which a weight is held in the hand and the elbow is flexed toward the shoulder and then lowered back down. Eccentric and concentric muscle contractions are also used in this example. Closed-chain movement are more representative of the muscle functioning needed in ADL (Hamill & Knutzen, 1995).

Speed of Contraction

The speed of muscle contraction affects strengthening. Greater forces or torques are produced at slower speeds of movement, for there is more time to recruit additional motor units. This results in greater strength (Kisner & Colby, 1990). Factors such as the frequency of the program, the number of repetitions performed, the duration of activities, and the rest periods additionally influence successful muscle strengthening. Specific strengthening programs will be discussed later in this chapter.

Muscle Endurance

Muscle endurance is needed for maximal participation in everyday tasks. Muscle endurance is related to strength because it is "the ability to contract repeatedly or generate tension and sustain that tension over a prolonged period of time."(Kisner & Colby, 1990, p. 12).

Muscle endurance is developed through high-repetitions and low-stress load to the muscle (less than 50% of maximal intensity). As endurance increases, a muscle is able to perform a greater number of contractions or hold against a load over an extended period. This enables longer participation in chosen activities. (Buchner & Coleman, 1994).

▼ DESCRIPTION OF SPECIFIC EXERCISE PROGRAMS

Exercise programs are designed based on a number of factors. The occupational practitioner considers the muscle grade and muscle endurance levels, precautions for movement, prognosis, and the activity demands of the individual's preferred occupational performance areas. Exercise programs used in occupational therapy can be described as passive, isotonic active-assistive, isotonic active, isometric without resistance, isotonic resistive, isometric resistive, and isokinetic (Pedretti, 1996; Trombly, 1995b).

Passive Exercise

This type of exercise involves passive joint ROM and passive stretching of tight soft tissue. No active muscle contraction occurs. Therefore, these activities are not used for strengthening. The purpose is to achieve joint flexibility by maximally stretching the muscle fibers to prevent any loss of active ROM. The stretching is done by the occupational therapy practitioner applying a force to the limited soft tissue while moving the joint through the full ROM. The stretching is done in the direction opposite that of the tightness and is completed slowly to allow the tight structures to lengthen without rupturing. The occupational therapy practitioner holds the joint at the end ROM for 15 to 30 seconds to effectively stretch the tissue (Kisner & Colby, 1990). A twice-daily routine of at least three repetitions of passive ROM exercises and stretching is recommended to maintain joint mobility (Pedretti, 1996). Stretching can also be done by machines which, when attached to joints, continually move the joint through a preset ROM. When only one upper extremity is affected, passive ROM and stretching can be accomplished by using overhead pulleys, where the unaffected upper extremity actively pulls the affected extremity through the available ROM. Passive ROM and stretching should be performed cautiously when there is inflammation, limited sensory feedback for pain detection, and prolonged immobilization, which can lead to osteoporosis or tendon and ligament tears. Positioning of the joints to avoid deformity development should also be done in conjunction with a passive exercise program.

Isotonic Active-Assistive Exercise

This type of exercise requires isotonic muscle contractions. It is used with clients who have muscle grades of trace, poor minus, and fair minus. The person actively moves the joint as far as possible, then some kind of outside force assists with moving the joint the remainder of the ROM. The additional assistance can be provided manually by either the client or the occupational therapy practitioner moving the affected extremity. Another option is the use of equipment, such as a pulley system, mobile arm supports, overhead suspension slings, or a table top upper extremity skate board, to assist in obtaining maximal ROM. Active-assistive exercise in a gravity-eliminated plane is used when the muscle grades are trace to poor minus, whereas active-assistive exercise in an against gravity plane is appropriate for fair minus muscle grades. As the client gains more strength, there is less reliance on the outside assistance. The person participates in an active-assistive exercise program until full active ROM is achieved.

Isotonic Active Exercise

This form of exercise also requires isotonic muscle contractions; however, the client moves fully through the available

ROM without any assistance or additional force applied to the joint (Lillegard & Terrio, 1994). A client who has muscles grades of poor to fair can participate in this type of program. Active exercise in a gravity-eliminated plane is used when muscle grades are poor to fair minus, whereas active exercise in an against gravity plane is appropriate for fair muscles grades. The goal is to increase strength by increasing the frequency, repetitions, and duration of the exercises, or changing the plane in which the exercises are performed.

Isometric Without Resistance Exercise

These exercises are useful when active ROM is not possible or is prohibited following surgery or a flare-up of rheumatoid arthritis. The goal is to maintain muscle strength through isometric muscle contractions. The client contracts the muscle, increasing the tension, and holds the joint in a stable position for approximately 5 seconds. Then the muscle is relaxed and the procedure is repeated. Isometric muscle contraction causes an increased in both systolic and diastolic blood pressure; therefore, it is not recommended for clients who have cardiac conditions (Pedretti, 1996; Lillegard & Terrio, 1994).

Isotonic Resistive Exercise

Once a client is able to move the joint through the full ROM against gravity, the next step to improve muscle strength and endurance is adding an extra load to the muscle. During these strengthening exercises, the load is applied to the muscle contraction by using a number of different items, including weights and dumbbells, springs, pulleys, rubber bands, resistive putty, strengthening machines, or everyday objects (Figs. 20–1 and 20–2). The client should have muscle grades of fair plus to participate in this type of program. Isotonic muscle contractions are used and can be either concentric or eccentric. Proper breathing is necessary to prevent excessive demands on the heart. Exhalation is done when lifting a load and inhalation is initiated during the lowering of the load (Lillegard & Terrio). Precautions for resistive exercise include prolonged fatigue and soreness, muscle contraction imbalance between agonist and antagonist, substitutions by other stronger muscles, and overstretching owing to weakness (Trombly, 1995b).

There are two specialized resistive exercise programs, the DeLorme method of progressive resistive exercise(PRE), and the Oxford technique of regressive resistive exercise (RRE). These exercises should be completed once a day for four or five times per week (Pedretti, 1996). In the DeLorme method, the muscle is allowed a warmup period leading to full muscle contraction. The first step involves determining the maximal load or weight the client can lift through the entire ROM for ten repetitions. Then a program is designed where the client completes ten repetitions with a weight that is 50% of the maximal load, progresses to do ten more repetitions using a weight that is 75% of the

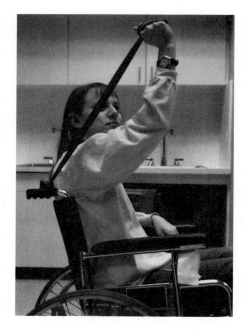

▲
Figure 20-1. Use of an elastic band to provide isotonic, resistive, against gravity exercise for the triceps.

maximal load, and then finishes with ten repetitions using the maximal weight. The client rests for a period of 2 to 4 minutes between progressions with the different weights.

The Oxford technique is basically the reverse approach of the DeLorme method; in the Oxford technique the client begins at maximal weight and lifts a lesser load with

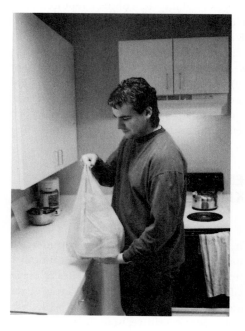

▲
Figure 20-2. Example of applied load to biceps contraction when lifting groceries against gravity.

each set of ten repetitions. The reasoning behind this approach is that the muscle fatigues with more contractions; therefore, the muscle can not effectively contract responding to the increased loads. This approach may be more useful in the beginning of therapy, until the muscle can make more gains in recruiting motor units (Pedretti, 1996).

Isometric Resistive Exercise

During this form of exercise, no joint motion occurs as the muscle is contracting isometrically against some additional force. The outside force can be applied by the occupational therapy practitioner pushing against the held contraction or the client can hold a weight distally while maintaining a stable proximal joint position. These exercises have the same uses and precautions as isometric without resistance exercises.

Isokinetic Exercise

Isokinetic exercise combines the characteristics of both isometric and isotonic resistive exercise. Equipment, such as an isokinetic dynamometer, is used that control the speed of movement, the amount of load on the muscle, and the stimulation of motor units through the full ROM (Lillegard & Terrio, 1994; McArdle, Katch, & Katch, 1991). The use of isokinetic exercise equipment is generally part of a physical therapy treatment program and not a exercise modality typically used by occupational therapy practitioners.

▼ OCCUPATIONAL THERAPY TREATMENT CONTINUUM AND STRENGTHENING

The occupational therapy practitioner identifies strength impairments through formal and informal evaluation. Treatment occurs within the occupational performance framework to address deficits in performance components and performance areas. The occupational therapist chooses activities and methods that fall within a treatment continuum. The treatment continuum has four stages characterized by the types of activities used during the phases of recovery. The stages are in order of progression: adjunctive methods, enabling activities, purposeful activity, and occupational performance and occupational roles. The continuum does not necessarily follow a strict sequential progression. The occupational therapy practitioner may use activities from more than one of the stages to address strength impairments, depending on the severity of the deficit and its effect on the performance areas (Pedretti, 1996).

In the early stages of strength recovery, the occupational therapy practitioner may use adjunctive methods, or procedures preparing the client for participation in meaningful activities. Muscle weakness, pain, edema, or limitations in joint ROM prevent maximal performance of ADL, work, and leisure. The occupational therapy practitioner focuses on treating these performance component deficits using exercise, joint positioning, edema control, and sensory stimulation (Pedretti, 1996).

The use of enabling activities characterizes stage 2 of the treatment continuum. Enabling activities can be thought of as prerequisites or stepping stones to other more difficult or complex tasks (Pedretti, 1996). The client might not have adequate strength to perform previous carpentry activities. Completing a simple woodworking project using sanding blocks of differing weights would increase the strength, enabling future resumption of meaningful work roles.

During stage 3, the occupational therapy practitioner presents activities that the client has identified as meaningful (Fig. 20–3). These tasks are chosen to improve performance areas and roles specific to that client. Studies of effectiveness of goal-directed purposeful activity versus exercise, indicate that purposeful activity is more motivating and shows other benefits to the individual (Trombly, 1995b, p. 240). The activities at this stage may be graded to increase in difficulty, or adaptive equipment can be provided to facilitate successful completion of tasks (Pedretti, 1996). The carpenter now can use lighter-weight tools to construct a bookcase. The weight of the tools, the plane of movement, and the length of time spent working on this project can be increased to achieve the strength required for the worker's role.

The last stage of the treatment continuum is not always reached by clients. During stage 4 the emphasis is on maximum functioning and resumption of roles in the selected environment (Pedretti, 1996). The client with strength impairments may participate in a work-hardening program to improve endurance for return to the carpentry job. If the client has reached a plateau in the strengthening program, the occupational therapy practitioner focuses on educating the client in job modifications. By using the treatment continuum, the occupational therapy practitioner addresses the client's impairment in strength and the resultant effect on occupational performance areas.

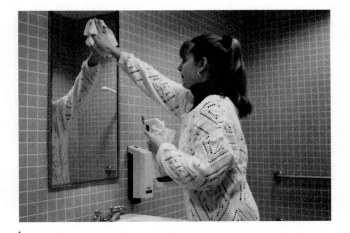

▲

Figure 20-3. Home management activity for upper extremity strengthening and resumption of previous roles.

►**STRENGTHENING CONCLUSION**

Adequate muscle strength is necessary for an individual to participate in selected occupational performance tasks. Through the continuum of occupational therapy, clients can regain or maximize strength to perform activities that give meaning to their lives. The focus of any strengthening program in occupational therapy should be based on the client's identified roles and chosen environments for occupational performance.

Section 4

Neuromuscular Treatment: Upper Extremity Splinting

Elaine Ewing Fess and Judith Hunt Kiel

▼ PURPOSE

Splints are external devices, made from a variety of materials, that are applied to treat upper extremity problems resulting from injury, disease, birth defects, or the aging process. Splints serve one or more of four basic functions: (1) Splints may be used to support, immobilize, or restrict a body part to allow healing after inflammation or injury to tendon, vascular, nerve, joint, or soft tissue structures. (2) Splints may be used to correct or prevent deformity. To achieve the "full potential of active joint motion of the hand, the remodeling of joint and tendon adhesions often requires the prolonged slow, gentle, passive traction that can best be provided by splinting" (Fess & Philips, 1987, p. 72). (3) Splints may be used to artificially provide or assist motion to supple hands (normal passive ROM) that are incapacitated by muscle weakness or paralysis. By placing joints in better positions, or through use of assistive components, splints may allow hands to achieve functional motion more effectively. (4) Splints may serve as bases for attachment of self-help devices. Ranging from simple to complex, splints may be prefabricated or custom-designed and fitted. Because of the complex and multifaceted elements involved in designing splints, it is inappropriate to link a specific splint with a specific diagnosis. Therefore, this section is based on anatomical, kinesiological, biomechanical, and physiological concepts, rather than diagnoses.

▼ CLASSIFICATION, NOMENCLATURE, AND COMPONENTS

Many ways of classifying splints have been used, including external configuration, mechanical characteristics, source of power, materials, and anatomical part, to name a few (Fess, Gettle, & Strickland, 1981; Long & Schutt, 1986; Malick, 1978, 1979). In taking a major step toward eliminating confusion and redundancy in existing nomenclature, the American Society of Hand Therapists (1992) adopted a Splint Classification System (SCS). Created by a specially appointed committee of nationally and internationally recognized splinting experts, this system categorizes splints in an organized, logical, and practical manner, replacing more colloquial terminology that often described properties of splints themselves, without consideration for purpose or intent. Splints in this classification system are *not* categorized according to the presence of dynamic or static components.

The SCS defines splints according to a series of four descriptors: anatomical focus, kinematic direction, primary purpose, and inclusion of secondary joints (Fig. 20–4). Anatomical focus defines the primary joint(s) or segments(s) affected by the splint (eg, metacarpal phalangeal (MP) or interphalangeal (IP) joints; wrist, thumb, or finger segments). Kinematic direction designates which way the primary joints or segments are moved (eg, flexion, extension, rotation). The primary purpose of a splint is described as one of three options: mobilization, immobilization, or restriction. Primary purpose mobilization splints enhance or encourage motion; primary purpose immobilization splints stop motion; and primary purpose restriction splints allow motion only in a partial, predetermined

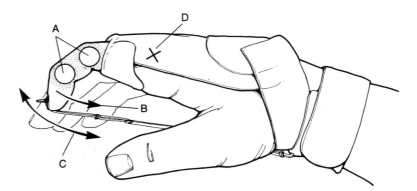

▶

Figure 20-4. Splints are grouped in the following manner: (*A*) anatomic focus (IP joints); (*B*) kinematic direction (flexion); (*C*) primary purpose (mobilization); and (*D*) number of secondary joints (one). According to the SCS, this is an IP flexion mobilization splint, type I.

range. The fourth descriptor indicates the number of joints in a longitudinal pattern that are included in the splint, but are not considered the primary focus joints. These joints are defined as secondary joints. If no secondary joint is included in a splint, it is designated as type 0; one secondary joint is type 1; two secondary joints are type 2, and so forth. The combination of the four descriptors accurately defines a splint without becoming lost in a multitude of specific design options. For example, a "cock-up splint" is considered to be a wrist extension immobilization splint, type 0, and an "MP arthroplasty splint" is categorized as an index through little MP extension-radial deviation mobilization splint, type 1.

The SCS enhances communication between medical personnel by defining the important aspects of splints, while leaving decisions about design options to those who actually fabricate splints. This allows therapists greater flexibility and use of their knowledge bases.

Although a finished splint presents a unified and solid configuration; in reality, it is an assemblage of integrated and interdependent components, each with a specific function and name designation (Bradley, 1968; Fess et al, 1981; Fess & Philips, 1987; Kiel, 1983). Component terminology is usually based on function of the part or on its anatomical location.

While designating a splint, the therapist decides what the splint is to accomplish and what approach will provide optimal results. Experienced therapists often think in terms of components rather than final splint configurations, mentally putting together selected splint parts to build a splint, the final shape of which may be familiar or, as is often the case, completely original. Above all, it is important that a creative flexibility be maintained, allowing the therapist to draw from what is available to design and prepare a splint that best suits the needs of a specific hand problem. Understanding splint components, their potential combinations, and their capabilities provides flexibility.

▼ EVALUATION AND EXERCISE

Evaluation provides the guidelines for treatment. Splinting and exercise programs cannot be established or carried out without careful evaluation and reevaluation of extremity

volume, ROM, sensibility, strength, dexterity, physical daily living skills, and job requirements (see Unit VI for further details). (Sensibility is the "capacity to receive and respond to stimuli" [Thomas, 1993, p.1779], whereas sensation is "a feeling or awareness...resulting from the stimulation of sensory reaceptors" (Thomas, 1993, p. 1778). In testing situations, clients are asked to receive and respond to simuli, not just to receive.].

Treating clients with upper extremity problems requires continual evaluation and problem solving. Splinting must be combined with a carefully supervised exercise program. Although splinting increases passive ROM, active exercise provides critical gliding of musculotendinous units and pericapsular structures.

▼ FUNDAMENTAL CONCEPTS

Anatomy, Kinesiology, Biomechanics

The occupational therapist must first understand the complex and intricate interrelations of normal anatomical structures, their kinesiologic functions, and their biomechanical and physiological ramifications before attempting to interpret, define, and treat the abnormalities that accompany upper extremity problems. Many excellent books and articles are available on upper extremity anatomy, kinesiology, and biomechanics. The reader is encouraged to independently pursue these subjects in greater detail. A careful review will provide a solid foundation from which therapeutic intervention may be directed.

Physiology

Living tissue responds in a predictable manner in its efforts to achieve homeostasis and healing. The normal physiological response to injury results in an alteration and replacement of normal structures with scar tissue. Therefore, it is important to understand the wound-healing process for surgical and therapeutic intervention to be effective (Madden & Arem, 1981; Peacock, 1984; Strickland, 1987). Tissue healing follows a normal sequence that includes inflammation, fibroplasia, and scar maturation. Wound contracture begins at 2 to 3 days and continues until a tension balance is achieved between the healing tissue and surrounding soft tissue. Excessive scar in specialized tissues of the hand, such as tendon, bone, and joint, may lead to sever impairment of function. Scar results not only from accidental injury, but also from surgical intervention and improperly applied therapeutic techniques (Brand & Hollister, 1993; Fess & Philips, 1987; Strickland, 1987). Factors that cause increased scar formation include greater wound size, contamination, additional injury, and persistent edema. Although edema is part of the normal inflammatory response, if it is allowed to persist in the hand with its compact and mobile structures, the result will be marked tissue scarring and fibrosis (Bunnell, 1944; Hunter, Schneider, Mackin, & Callahan, 1990; Strickland, 1987).

Rest or Stress

Scar remodeling is the foundation on which hand therapy treatment is based, and the fundamental question of rest or stress of living tissue is dependent on physiological timing (Brand, 1985; Strickland, 1987). The inflammatory phase is characterized by transient vasoconstriction followed by vasodilation of local small blood vessels and migration of white blood cells. Allowing the removal of dead tissue and foreign bodies by phagocytic cells, the acute inflammatory response generally subsides within several days. During this time, the injured part is usually immobilized to promote healing (Fig. 20–5). In special instances for which control of scar is critical, as with tendon gliding, early motion programs may be initiated (Fig. 20–6) (Duran, Coleman, Nappi, & Klerekoper, 1990; Evans, 1990; Kleinert, Kutz, & Cohn, 1975).

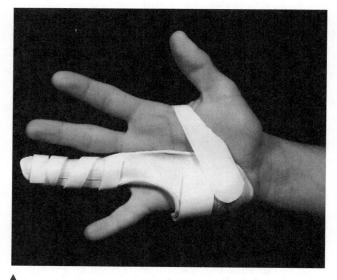

▲
Figure 20-5. To promote healing, this ring-finger immobilization splint, type 0, stops motion at all three joints. (From Fess, E. E., & Philips, C. A. [1987]. *Hand splinting: Principles and methods* [2nd ed.]. St. Louis: C. V. Mosby.

Fibroplasia begins on the fourth or fifth day and continues for 2 to 4 weeks. As collagen fibers increase, the tensile strength (resistance to rupture) of the wound increases. During this stage, active motion may be initiated, and splints may be used to protect healing structures or to control unbalanced forces of uninjured musculature (Fig. 20–7).

Changes in the architecture of the collagen fibers occurs during the scar maturation phase. Collagen becomes more organized, and tensile strength continues to increase (Madden & Arem, 1981). Carefully graded resistive activities may be added to existing active motion exercises, and gentle corrective splinting may be initiated (Fig. 20–8).

As wounds age, their edges contract and the area of scar becomes smaller. Remodeling of scar is a normal process that continues throughout life. Although a scar may not totally disappear, the deposition of new collagen and resorption of old collagen is a constant, ongoing process within the scarred area as well as in normal uninjured tissue. This remodeling process may be altered even in long-standing soft tissue contractures. Application of prolonged gentle traction is the key to influencing the remodeling process, and this is best done through a carefully supervised splinting program (Brand & Hollister, 1993; Fess & Philips, 1987).

Timing for splinting programs must take into consideration all the above information while treating specific abnormalities on an individualized basis. Although diagnoses may be similar, no two clients respond in exactly the same manner to injury and subsequent therapeutic intervention.

Splints may be used to immobilize healing tissues, or they may permit controlled motion to influence adhesion formation and enhance tensile strength of repaired structures. They may be used to correct existing joint deformity by providing constant gentle tension to remodel existent contracted, adherent, or scarred soft tissue structures. In the presence of supple joints and good tendon glide, splints may be used to maintain normal joint motion, and when muscle function is impaired, they may substitute for weak or absent muscle function. The timing is different for each of the foregoing situations. Consequently, it is imperative that the physiological implications be thoroughly understood before embarking on a method of treatment. Too much force applied to healing tissue causes tearing and rupture, whereas too little force directed to stiffened joints or adherent soft tissue structures may result in little to no alteration of offending scar (Brand, 1985, 1990; Fess & Philips, 1987; Strickland, 1987).

Position of Deformity

The presence of dorsal edema encourages a predictable position of deformity with the wrists flexed, MPs in hyperextension, IPs in flexion, and the thumb adducted (Bunnell, 1944; Flatt, 1983; Strickland, 1987; Weeks & Wray, 1978). Acting as a biological "glue", the protein-rich edema fluid fills the interstices of the collateral ligaments and the soft tissues surrounding tendons and joints. An interstice is a "space

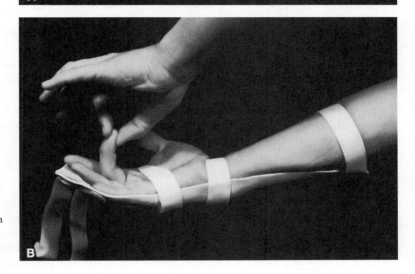

► *Figure 20-6.* Early passive motion of repaired superficialis and profundus tendons of the long finger is permitted in this wrist–finger immobilization splint, type 0. (From Fess, E. E., & Philips, C. A. [1987]. *Hand splinting: Principles and methods* [2nd ed.]. St. Louis: C. V. Mosby.

or gap in a tissue or structure of an organ" (Thomas, 1993, p.1007). Injured tissues, those immediately adjacent to the injury, and those in general proximity may all become involved as the fluid is replaced by collagen, forming scar and limiting both active and passive motion (Bunnell, 1944). Maintaining collateral ligament length by means of antideformity positioning is a fundamental concept to effective hand rehabilitation (Flatt, 1983; Hunter et al, 1990; Strickland, 1987, Weeks & Wray, 1978). It is important to understand the anatomy of each joint and the involvement of surrounding structures because the splinting position of choice differs significantly between the MP and IP joints.

Wrist position is the key to the posture of more distal digital joints (Flatt, 1983). Injury often results in adoption of a protective posture of wrist flexion. Additionally, the presence of dorsal edema places distension pressure on the extrinsic extensor tendons. This edema, coupled with a posture of wrist flexion, pulls the MP joints into extension or hyperextension which, in turn, causes the IP joints to flex in a compensatory manner (Strickland, 1987). This zigzag collapse of the longitudinal arch is both predictable and preventable and may be averted by eliminating the instigating

posture of wrist flexion. Providing there are no extenuating circumstances that would be contraindicated, the antideformity position for the wrist is neutral or dorsal extension. Because of the cam configuration of the metacarpal head, the collateral ligaments are lax with the MP joint in extension (Bunnell, 1944; Flatt, 1983; Strickland, 1987). Injury or chronic edema around the joint can result in deposition of new collagen around the slackened ligaments, allowing

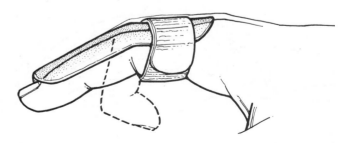

▲ *Figure 20-7.* Full PIP flexion is allowed, but Extension beyond 25° is blocked in this PIP extension-restriction splint, type 0.

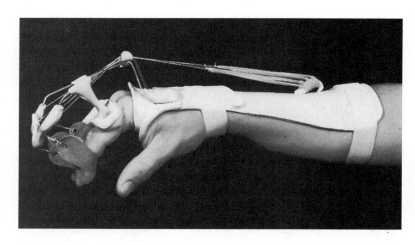

◄ *Figure 20-8.* Gentle tension is applied to remodel extrinsic flexor tendon adhesions and tight PIP pericapsular structures in this PIP extension-mobilization splint, type 2. (From Fess, E. E., & Philips, C. A. [1987]. *Hand splinting: Principles and methods* [2nd ed.]. St. Louis: C. V. Mosby.

them to shorten through tissue remodeling. Flexion is limited according to the degree of ligament shortening.

The IP joints are hinge articulations permitting motion in only one plane. Often the result of poor positioning after injury, IP flexion contractures usually involve shortening of the palmar plate and collateral ligaments (Strickland, 1987). Additionally, adhesion of the palmar skin, flexor tendons, or flexor tendon sheaths may be associated.

Functionally devastating, thumb web space contractures may involve skin, fascia, or musculature of the first web space (Flatt, 1983; Strickland, 1987; Weeks & Wray, 1978). Resulting from direct injury, ischemia, or chronic edema, secondary stiffening of the carpal metacarpal (CMC) joint may occur. Distension pressure on the extensor pollicis longus from dorsal edema also contributes to a posture of thumb adduction.

Functional Position Versus Antideformity Position

For many decades, the functional position (wrist, 20- to 30-degrees extension; MPs 45-degrees flexion; proximal interphalangeal (PIPs), 30-degrees flexion; distal interphalangeal (DIPs), 20-degrees flexion; and thumb abducted) for the hand was considered the posture of choice in hand splinting (Fig. 20–9) (Bunnell, 1944; Malick, 1979; Wynn Parry, 1981).

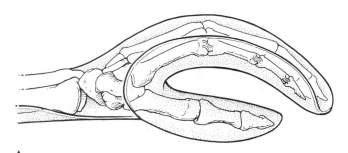

▲ *Figure 20-9.* With the MPs in 45° of flexion and the IPs in 20° to 30° of flexion, in the traditional functional position the collateral ligaments are lax.

When an entire hand required immobilization, it was placed in a functional position unless special circumstances dictated otherwise. In the 1960s, hand specialists began to reevaluate this traditional approach, initially with specific diagnoses such as burns (Evans, Larson, & Yates, 1968; Koepke, Feallock, & Felle, 1963; Von Prince & Yeakel, 1974). This led to better understanding of the anatomical configuration of the joints of the hand and of the role that the wrist and collateral ligaments play in producing a predictable pattern of deformity. "The position desired is not necessarily a functional position, but rather one which will prevent the deformity caused by contracture" (Von Prince & Yeakel, 1974; p. 30). As a result, an antideformity (safe) position was developed that maintained collateral ligament length, considerably diminishing chances of development of MP extension, IP flexion, and thumb CMC adduction contractures with immobilization. It is now thought that this antideformity position should be used as a preventive measure whenever a hand that has a tendency to develop stiffness requires immobilization for an extended time period. This excludes instances when other postures are prescribed to promote healing of specialized tissues, as with flexor or extensor tendon repairs or fractures, or when functional needs dictate alternative measures, as with the development of a tenodesis hand.

In light of better knowledge, the functional position now may be viewed as that hand posture from which function is most easily initiated. To attain a functional position, soft tissue length, especially that of the collateral ligaments of the small joints of the hand, must be present. Maintenance of collateral ligament length requires that the wrist be positioned in neutral to slight extension, the MPs flexed 70 to 90 degrees, the IPs held in full extension, and the thumb CMC joint positioned in full abduction or extension, otherwise known as the antideformity position (Fig. 20–10).

Mobilizing Splints: How Much Force

Splinting, the method of choice for increasing passive ROM, provides prolonged gentle stress that positively influences collagen remodeling and tissue growth. Too much

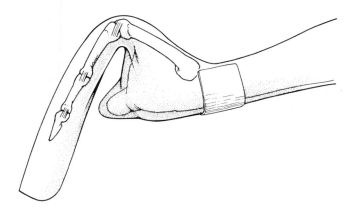

▲
Figure 20-10. In the antideformity position, with MPs flexed 70° to 90° and IPs in extension, the collateral ligaments are at maximal length.

force too quickly causes microscopic tearing of tissue, and the cycle of scar production begins anew (Brand, 1990; Brand & Hollister, 1993; Bell-Krotoski & Fess, 1995; Fess & Philips, 1987; Strickland, 1987).

Force applied to prevent contracture should be just enough to properly position the involved segment. Because the hand is already supple, measurement of the force used is not necessary as long as care is taken not to overcorrect by applying more force than is required to place the hand in the desired position (Fig. 20–11) (Fess & Philips, 1987). Forces used to correct joint deformity must be carefully monitored. Depending on structures involved and physiological timing, experienced therapists use forces between 100 g and 300 g (Brand & Hollister, 1993; Bell-Krotoski & Fess, 1995; Fess et al, 1981; Fess, 1984; Fess & Philips, 1987; Malick, 1978; Pierson, 1978). Caution must be exercised when using commercial splints because certain designs create forces that greatly exceed safe parameters (Bledsoe, 1991; Fess, 1988).

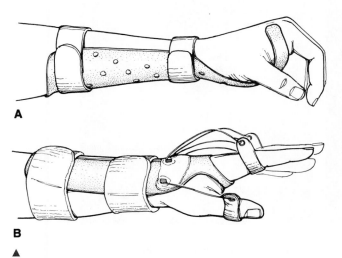

A

B

▲
Figure 20-11. In a hand in which passive motion is normal but active motion is limited, as with a radial nerve palsy, splints may be used to position the wrist (*A*), or to position the wrist and MP joints (*B*).

Elastic or Inelastic Traction

Traditionally, elastic traction has been the method of choice for splinting directed at correction of joint deformity. In addition to rubber bands and elastic thread, springs are now available in differing strengths (Roberson, Breger, Buford, & Freeman, 1988).

As a result of the work of Brand (1952) and Bell (1987; Bell-Krotoski, 1990), the value of inelastic traction for correcting joint deformity is better understood. Minimal force applied by a series of splints that are refitted every 2 to 3 days is an effective method for increasing passive ROM of stiffened joints, especially when chronic.

▼ PRINCIPLES OF SPLINTING

The use of splints in rehabilitation programs is a serious undertaking and should not be regarded lightly. When employed appropriately, splinting is very effective; however, misuse of a splint through ignorance or haste can lead to dire consequences, resulting in needless additional injury to an already debilitated extremity. To provide a splint that meets individual client requirements, fits comfortably, and functions efficiently, certain basic criteria must be achieved. These criteria are relevant to the creation of all splints, regardless of intent of application, final configuration, or material from which they are constructed. Integration of the principles of mechanics, design, construction, and fit will generate splints that are appropriate, wearable, and functional.

Mechanical Principles

Because splinting involves direct application and manipulation of external forces to the extremity, it is important to understand basic principles of mechanics (Brand & Hollister, 1993; Bell-Krotoski & Fess, 1995; Fess et al, 1981; Fess & Philips, 1987). Use of mechanical principles helps make splints comfortable, durable, and effective, and diminishes chances of additional injury secondary to splint application.

Mechanically, splints may be grouped into two categories: those that apply three-point pressure (Brand, 1990; Fess et al, 1981; Fess & Philips, 1987; Malick, 1978) and those that pull adjacent articulated bony segments together through circumferential pressure (P.Van Lede, personal communication, February, 1991). Most splints employ three-point pressure; however, a few frequently used splints fall into the circumferential pressure category. Three-point-pressure splints function through a series of reciprocal forces, with the middle force directed opposite the two end forces (Fig. 20–12). In the circumferential pressure splint, the middle reciprocal force is absent (Fig. 20–13). Those engaged in designing and fitting splints must understand the fundamental differences between these two types of splints to use them correctly and to anticipate potential problems

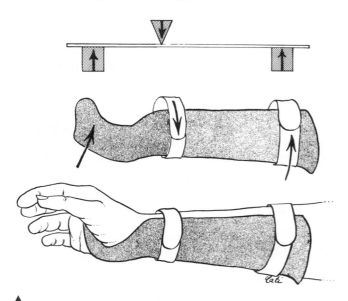

▲
Figure 20-12. Arrows indicate the three points of pressure applied by this writst immobilization splint, type 0. (From Kiel, J. H. [1983]. *Basic hand splinting: A pattern designing approach.* Boston: Little, Brown.)

arising from their application. For example, pressure necrosis is most likely to occur at the point of application of the middle reciprocal force in a three-point-pressure splint, whereas the forces in a circumferential splint are equally dissipated over two or more opposing surfaces. The latter are more likely to precipitate edema problems owing to their inherent circumferential design.

Pressure and shear may be reduced by increasing the surface area of the splint and by ensuring contiguous fit on the extremity. Short, narrow splints or components are often problematic because they apply forces to a small area, creating pressure necrosis of underlying soft tissue. Longer splint designs increase mechanical advantage and make splints less susceptible to causing pressure problems (Fig. 20–14). Rolling or flanging splint edges, especially those at the proximal or distal ends, also diminishes shear and pressure forces (Fig. 20–15). Additionally, dangerous shear forces may be diminished by attaching the splint snug to the extremity and by aligning articulated splint components with their respective anatomical joint axes, eliminating friction between splint and soft tissue surfaces as the extremity is moved. Splint strength and durability is also enhanced through the use of wider and longer components and through providing material contour.

Understanding the effects of proximal or distal joints within the longitudinal ray is another critical concept. Cor-

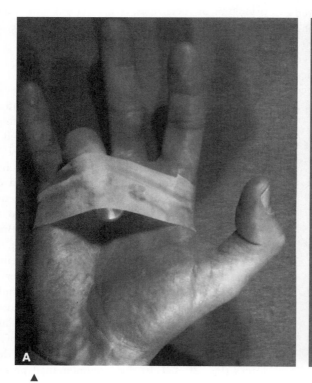

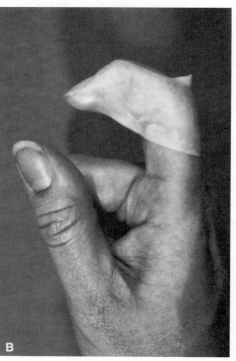

▲
Figure 20-13. The finger flexion-mobilization splint, type 0 (*A*) and IP flexion mobilization splint, type 0 (*B*) are examples of circumferential pressure splints. The middle reciprocal force is absent in both splints. (From Fess, E. E., & Philips, C. A. [1987]. *Hand splinting: Principles and methods* [2nd ed.]. St. Louis: C. V. Mosby.

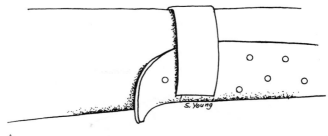

▲
Figure 20-15. To reduce pressure, it is often helpful to flange splint edges. (From Kiel, J. H. [1983]. *Basic hand splinting: A pattern designing approach.* Boston: Little, Brown.)

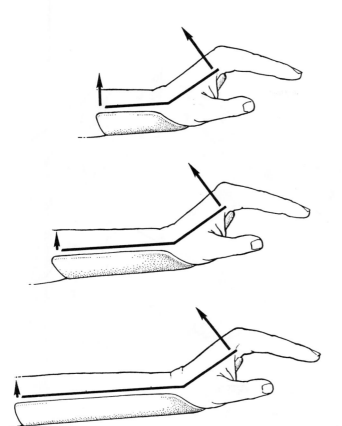

▲
Figure 20-14. The amount of proximal force required to support the weight of the hand in a splint is diminished by increasing the length of the forearm bar. (From Fess, E. E., & Philips, C. A. [1987]. *Hand splinting: Principles and methods* [2nd ed.]. St. Louis: C. V. Mosby.)

rective forces may be abated or rendered ineffective if normal or relatively less stiff joints are not controlled when fabricating splints to mobilize stiff joints (Fig. 20–16).

When splints are used to effect joint motion, a 90-degree angle of approach of the mobilizing force must be used to avoid compression or distraction of articular surfaces. If the splint has been fitted to increase motion of a stiffened joint, a 90-degree angle of approach must be maintained as the joint motion changes through adjustments to the outrigger length. This mobilization force must also be perpendicular to the joint axis of rotation (Fig. 20–17). Additionally, components that provide immobilizing or stabilizing forces, such as straps or dorsal phalangeal bars, should have a 90-degree angle of approach to the joint or segment being immobilized or stabilized.

Design Principles

Principles of design may be divided into two categories: general and specific (Fess et al, 1981; Fess & Philips, 1987). General principles incorporate broad concepts that help generate a splint that is practical for both the client and the therapist, whereas more specific principles focus the splint design on individual client requirements.

General principles include client factors, such as age, intelligence, motivation, body size, activity level, socioeconomic status, proximity to the clinic, length of time the splint will be used, and the exercise program that will be prescribed. Splints should be as simple as possible, allowing optimal function and sensation of the extremity. Generally, they also should provide ease of application and removal. For children or for clients who cannot or will not accept responsibility for their treatment, however, splints may need to be designated to discourage voluntary removal. When one acknowledges that splints are inherently strange-looking devices at best, care should be taken to make them aesthetically pleasing through attention to detail and neatness. The design should also allow efficient construction and fit, thereby controlling time and economic factors. These general principles are taken into consideration by the therapist during the early stages of design. They are approached not in lock-step, one, two, three fashion, but rather, as a simultaneous mental balancing of multiple factors.

Specific principles of design provide substance and detail to the emerging splint configuration. Decisions made at this point are based on specific personal, technical, and medical considerations, leading to substantially different splint configurations for seemingly similar diagnoses or therapeutic needs. Key primary joints are identified, and the purpose of the splint is reviewed. It should be determined whether the splint is intended to immobilize structures, partially restrict motion, increase passive motion, substitute for active motion, or serve as a base of attachment of self-help devices. The surface of the extremity on which the splint will be based is determined, and secondary joints that need to be controlled or positioned are noted. Areas of diminished sensibility are identified, as are anatomical variations, soft tissue defects, suture lines, and the presence of external or internal hardware, such as pins, plates, and screws, or external fixators. Because application of a splint often alters internal and external forces to proximal or distal joints, the kinetic effects of the splint must also be considered, including what will be the forces on unsplinted joints and what will be the ramifications to extrinsic and intrinsic musculotendinous struc-

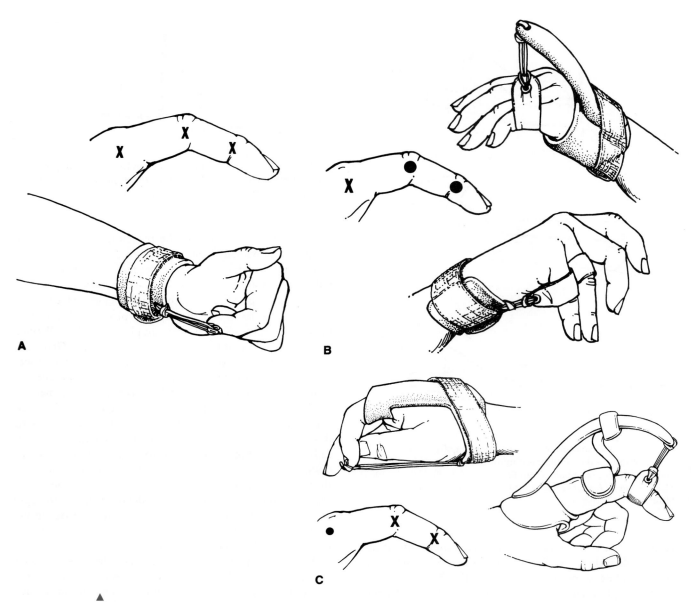

Figure 20-16. (*A*) When all joints within the digit are similarly stiff, a single-mobilizing force may be used to affect all three joints. (*B*) If joints distal to the stiff joint are normal, the mobilizing force should not include the normal joints. (*C*) When proximal joints are less stiff than the joint being mobilized, splints must be designed to control the less stiff joints, allowing the full effect of the mobilizing force to be focused on the more problematic joint.

tures. Mechanical principles directly influence splint structure and shape. Splint designs must also be reflective of the inherent properties of the splinting materials to be used.

All these factors and many more have considerable influence on the final splint configuration. It is easy to understand, in light of the foregoing information, why "cookbook" approaches to splinting are potentially dangerous. With such a plethora of individual variables requiring attention, no single splint design is always appropriate for a given diagnosis or circumstance.

Construction Principles

Principles of construction (Bradley, 1968; Fess et al, 1981; Fess & Philips, 1987; Kiel, 1983) encompass concepts related to splint durability, aesthetics, and comfort. Careful adherence to these principles provides a well-finished, wearable product that will withstand the rigors of daily use. Because splinting materials vary considerably in their respective physical properties, the type of heat, temperature, and the equipment employed to fabricate splints should be matched

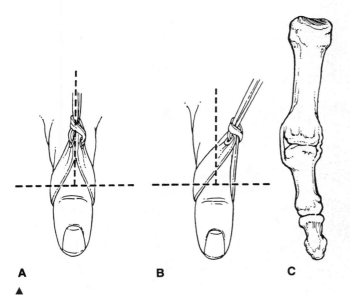

A   B   C

▲

Figure 20-17. The mobilizing force also must be perpendicular to the joint axis of rotation. If it is not, unequal stress is placed on the joint, and attenuation of the greater stressed collateral ligament may occur. (From Fess, E. E., & Philips, C. A. [1987]. *Hand splinting: Principles and methods* [2nd ed.]. St. Louis: C. V. Mosby.

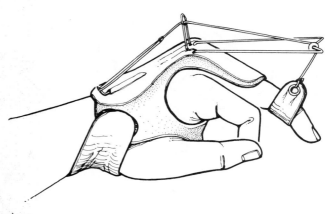

▲

Figure 20-18. Splint corners should be rounded. Internal or external corners that are not rounded create potential for weakness in the splint or pressure for the patient, as well as poor aesthetic quality.

appropriately with the materials used. For the protection of both client and therapist, safety precautions should be observed during all stages of construction. To achieve a good aesthetic effect, splint edges should be carefully smoothed, and both internal and external corners of components, including straps, should be rounded appropriately (Fig. 20–18). The hook portion of hook-and-loop fastening systems should be completely covered; joined components should be secure; and rivets or fastening devices should be finished, eliminating points or surfaces that might inadvertently cause injury or catch on clothing. Ventilation may be provided as necessary, and padding should be secured without surface overlap or wrinkling. Straps also need to be secured on one end to prevent loss or confusion with adjacent straps.

Fit Principles

The best design concepts and fabrication techniques may be rendered useless if a splint is not well fitted. The principles of fit (Bradley, 1968; Fess et al, 1981; Fess & Philips, 1987; Kiel, 1983; Malick, 1978, 1979) serve as guidelines to this technically demanding final phase. It is at this point that the previously discussed principles come together to provide a well-functioning splint.

Mechanical principles play an important role during the fitting of a splint. Contiguous fit of the splint to the extremity reduces pressure on bony prominences as well as soft tissue. Optimal, 90-degree rotational forces prevent migration of the splint and associated components, such as finger cuffs

(Fig. 20–19). Careful alignment of splint articulations with anatomical joint axes eliminates friction, and use of optimal leverage increases comfort and durability.

Anatomical considerations are also critical during fitting. Skin creases serve as anatomical guidelines to articular motion. If motion is desired at a given joint, the splint should be fitted so that it does not impinge on skin creases corresponding to the joint. Because it is frequently impaired by poorly fitted splints or casts that inadvertently limit MP motion, the distal palmar crease should be free of splint material if the MP joints are to be permitted full ROM. The same is true of the thenar crease. If full CMC joint motion of the thumb is required, the splint must not cross to the radial side of the thenar skin crease. Bony prominences should be identified and the splint contoured to provide a smooth, close fit. In some cases, such as the radial styloid process at the wrist, the splint material may be molded to avoid contact, or padding may be employed to reduce forces under a narrow component, such as a dorsal phalangeal bar (Brand, 1990; Brand & Hollister, 1993). Splints that incorporate the second through fifth metacarpals should exhibit the dual oblique angles resulting from the combination of progressive radial to ulnar metacarpal shortening and from the relative mobility of the fourth and fifth metacarpals (Capener, 1956). Both transverse and longitudinal arches should be supported. Careful attention should be directed toward digital joints on which corrective traction is applied. Rotational force applied in a direction that is not perpendicular to the axis of joint rotation results in unequal stress to pericapsular structures, causing irrevocable attenuation or lengthening of one of the two supporting collateral ligaments.

When fitting a splint, it is important to remember that the configuration of the hand and extremity change with movement. For example, as the fingers flex, the relative length of the dorsum of the hand elongates, whereas the

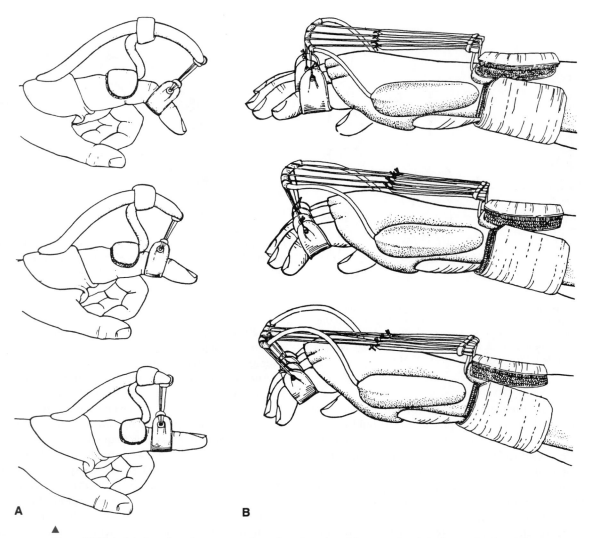

A   B

▲
Figure 20-19. As joint motion changes, outrigger length and position must be altered to maintain a 90° angle of approach of the mobilizing force. (From Fess, E. E., & Philips, C. A. [1987]. *Hand splinting: Principles and methods* [2nd ed.]. St. Louis: C. V. Mosby.)

palmar surface undergoes a relative shortening. The converse is true, but to a lesser extent as the fingers are extended to neutral position. Opposition of the thumb results in similar changes, but it is the relative width of the hand that is altered, with dorsal width increasing and palmar width shortening as the thumb is moved in an ulnar direction. Any splint that allows motion must be fitted to adapt to these kinematic changes.

In addition to assessing component parts as they are constructed and fitted, it is important to mentally evaluate and reevaluate the entire splint as a whole, including those portions already completed. If one aspect of a splint is poorly constructed or fitted, it may cause other components or portions of the splint to be incorrect.

▼ APPLICATION

Pattern Construction

Once a design has been created mentally, it usually progresses through a pattern stage before becoming reality. Many methods have been published for constructing patterns (Fess & Philips, 1987; Kiel, 1983; Malick, 1978, 1979; Tenney & Lisak, 1986; Ziegler, 1984), each with merits and drawbacks. Ultimately, pattern fabrication seems to be dependent on the personal preference and style of the individual therapist. Experienced therapists often use entirely different methods of pattern construction, with end results being very similar. Additionally, it is not uncommon to find experienced therapists who adapt commercially available, precut splint blanks, or who opt to fit a splint without the use of patterns. Newer materials for which inherent physical properties facilitate stretching, draping, and molding are more forgiving. Therapists with limited splinting experience, however, should be cautioned that attempts to make splints without patterns can lead to expensive, frustrating, and time-consuming errors.

An effective method of pattern construction is taping individual paper splint components to form the whole of a splint (Bradley, 1968; Fess et al, 1981; Fess & Philips, 1987; Kiel, 1983). This is particularly useful for novices or in circumstances requiring unusually complicated designs.

Materials

The number of companies that provide material for the construction of splints can be overwhelming. Most of these companies provide several types of materials along with aids to facilitate the splint construction process (AliMed, 1996; North Coast Medical, 1996; Smith & Nephew Roylan, Inc, 1996; Sammons & Preston, 1996). A skilled therapist not only must understand splinting theory and technique, but also is responsible for keeping current with new splinting products—adding, replacing, or rejecting as clinic requirements dictate (Cailliet, 1976). Although not all splinting needs may be purchased commercially, it is important to investigate and identify those that facilitate the fabrication process.

Excluding plaster of Paris and those materials from which specialized components are constructed, most basic splinting materials used today are low-temperature thermoplastics. With heat, these materials become soft and pliable, and when cooled, they retain the shapes to which they were conformed. Although thermoplastic materials differ in chemical content and physical properties, they may be grouped into two categories. The more plastic group has a polycaprolactone base, and the more rubber group has a polyisoprene base (Bell-Krotoski & Fess, 1995; Breger-Lee & Buford, 1991; Shafer, 1989). This provides a wide array of materials that may be matched selectively to individual client problems and therapist preferences.

Qualities that influence the degree of material and moldability include stretchability, drapability, rebound, and elastic memory (J. Hobbs, personal communication, October 1991). These characteristics are present in varying degrees in most thermoplastic materials and directly affect therapist effort required for forming splints.

Highly moldable materials require little therapist effort to conform. Once heated and cut to shape, these materials drape and stretch easily, allowing close, contiguous fit with minimal therapist intervention. These highly drapable materials are often easier to control by using gravity-assisted positions during fitting. This is especially helpful when working with splints designed for large surface areas. It is also possible to roll these materials into balls or tubes with no visible seams. Most highly moldable materials require close monitoring of applied heat levels because too-high temperatures result in excessive material softening and flow.

Rebound and elastic memory refer to the degree to which heated, stretched, or molded materials tend to return to their original sizes and shapes. Materials with large amounts of rebound or elastic memory require more therapist intervention to fabricate splints. Because these materials are inherently less drapable, they must be carefully held in place until cool to prevent inadvertent loss of shape. Although materials possessing rebound properties attempt to return to their original manufactured shape to some degree when heated, they are altered somewhat by stretching and molding and are unable to achieve completely their premolded flat, smooth configurations. On the other hand, high elastic memory materials return to their original flat manufactured shape with little or no alteration when heated and left unattended.

The thermoplastic and memory qualities of splinting materials require constant awareness of the importance of completely cooling finished splints or sections of splints during fabrication. Splints or portions of splints that remain warm are susceptible to loss of shape, conforming to surfaces on which they have been placed, or simply returning to their original flat shape. Without proper caution, it is also possible to accidentally direct heat to completed areas while working on adjacent spots, thereby requiring reforming of previously finished areas. The properties of thermoplasticity and elastic memory also require that clients be cautioned to clean splints in cool water and to store splints away from heat sources when they are not being worn.

Hot air and hot water most frequently are used to heat thermoplastic materials so that they may be cut, assembled, and fitted. Usually, heat guns are chosen for application of dry heat, although dry electric skillets may be employed with specific materials. Hair dryers may be used for materials with relatively low heat thresholds, and occasionally, an electric burner may suffice. With a burner, however, it is difficult to direct the heat to individual splint parts. It is important to note that gas burners should be avoided because some materials are flammable. Wet heat may be obtained by heating water in electric skillets, large cooking pans, hydrocollators, specialized splinting pans, or commercial restaurant steam tables. Hot water has the advantage of heating materials evenly. Although specific portions of splints may be heated in hot water by dipping, there may be areas that cannot be accessed without affecting adjacent finished parts. To avoid accidental burns to the client or therapist when using hot water, it is critical to thoroughly dry materials before fitting.

Care must be used with all materials when tracing patterns to avoid leaving unsightly and undesirable residual marks on completed splints. Finding implements that make marks that are visible during transfer and cutting stages, but dissolve or erase after these stages have been completed, is a continual challenge for therapists. Maintaining clean work areas is also important for fabricating splints because it is easy for dirt or scraps of material to become embedded in warm splint surfaces.

Therapists involved in splinting must thoroughly read information sheets provided with thermoplastic materials to identify the best and most efficient methods for working with each material. Techniques for cutting, heating, smoothing edges, and bonding with or without solvent often differ considerably from material to material.

Plaster of Paris-impregnated bandage, an often overlooked, older splinting material, continues to be used by experiences hand rehabilitation specialists. Although it has a tendency to absorb moisture and wound exudates and is not as durable as plastic, plaster is inexpensive, has superior capacity to conform, and allows skin to breathe. Plaster bandage is especially useful when correcting joint deformity through serial casting (Bell, 1987; Bell-Krotoski, 1990). Because plaster tends to soften when exposed to moisture, clients must be cautioned to keep their plaster splints dry.

▼ TROUBLESHOOTING AND EVALUATION

As therapists make splints, supervise the construction of splints, or examine splints that have been brought to the clinic by clients, there are guidelines that may be followed to ensure that these splints are designed, fabricated, and fitted appropriately. Because therapists often need to evaluate splints extemporaneously, it is helpful to be familiar with these guidelines. A list of splint evaluation criteria (Table 20–1) provides an organized approach to evaluating splints (Fess & Philips, 1987; Kiel, 1983). During this process, it is important to remember to evaluate the splint as a whole as well as its individual components.

Exercise

Splints and exercise must be carefully integrated to allow clients to achieve their full rehabilitation potential (Fess & Philips, 1987; pp. 325-369). Unfortunately, in practice, splinting has sometimes been viewed incorrectly as an isolated treatment technique. Splints are used to improve passive motion, substitute for weakened or lack of active motion, or infrequently, are fabricated to provide resistive exercise. The effect of splinting on active ROM is a secondary benefit that may occur after the attainment of these goals. Involving voluntary use of extrinsic and intrinsic upper extremity musculature with adhesion-free tendinous excursions, active motion is the key factor to establishing and maintaining hand function.

Before active ROM may be realized, corresponding passive joint motion must be present. For this reason, splinting is often used early in rehabilitation programs when exercise alone is insufficient to achieve or maintain motion. There are many instances when exercise alone is appropriate, but there are very few times, if any, when splinting may be used as an isolated entity.

Additionally, the occupational therapist must remember that use of a corrective splint to improve passive motion involves application of forces to effect tissue remodeling. This application of resistance must be appropriate to the level of physiological timing of the problem. If resistive exercises are not appropriate, corrective splinting may also be inappropriate.

Evaluation measurements provide the guidelines from which coordinated splinting and exercise programs are orchestrated (Fess, 1990; Fess & Philips, 1987; pp. 103-121). Without these measurements, treatment intervention is directionless and limited in effectiveness, potentially causing more harm than good. Evaluation, splinting, and exercise are intricately intertwined in hand rehabilitation.

Creation of splint-wearing schedules is dependent on individual client circumstances and physiological timing. When splints are applied to influence tissue healing or remodeling, they must be worn for long periods to affect collagen realignment and tissue growth. Concomitantly, it is important to maintain or improve normal gliding capacity of adjacent structures. This requires delicate balancing between splint and exercise routines. Because clients with identical diagnoses may respond differently to therapeutic intervention, it is insufficient and often detrimental to adhere to rigid, predetermined protocols. Dictated by specific evaluation data and physiological parameters, treatment programs are tailored to individual client needs. Some programs are relatively straightforward and uncomplicated, whereas others require constant alteration to keep pace with changing requirements. For example, a client who needs to improve passive ROM of a PIP joint may be instructed to repeat a splint-wearing and exercise routine every 2 hours throughout the day that involves wearing the PIP extension splint for 1 hour and 45 minutes, then removing the splint and exercising for 15 minutes, and then repeating the routine. Other programs may be more complicated. For example, it is not unusual for clients to have limitation of both flexion and extension, requiring that extension and flexion splints be alternated. Using the previously described splint-wearing and exercise cycle, a client may be instructed to do three cycles with the extension splint, and on the fourth cycle, to substitute the flexion splint. This repetition of a 3:1 splint extension to flexion ratio with exercise is used throughout the day. If a client does not seem to have problems with developing stiffness in adjacent digits or joints, it may be appropriate to decrease the frequency of exercise. Conversely, if stiffness is a problem, exercises may be prescribed more often (e.g., every 45 minutes). The key to effective splint-wearing and exercise regimens is to reevaluate frequently and to alter programs according to these measurements.

Special circumstances may also influence splint-wearing and exercise routines, and the astute therapist realizes that

TABLE 20-1. Splint Evaluation Criteria

Need
1. Is application of splint necessary on initial examination?
2. Does it continue to be necessary on reevaluation?

Design
Given the diagnostic requirements, does the splint meet general design concepts, including adaptation for:
1. Individual client factors (age, motivation, intelligence, clinic proximity)
2. Duration of time splint is to be used (temporarily, semipermanent, permanent)
3. Simplicity (no irrelevant parts; splint is applicable and pertinent to the need)
4. Optimal function (splint allows usage and performance without unnecessary reduction of motion)
5. Optimal sensation (splint permits as much sensory input as possible)
6. Efficient fabrication (no extraneous parts or procedures, such as the use of reinforcement parts instead of curving contour, bonding instead of uninterrupted coalescing of components, straps instead of contiguous fit, inappropriate use of padding)
7. Application and removal (appropriate to individual client factors)
8. Client suggestions (requested adaptation that would not alter or jeopardize splint function)
Given the diagnostic requirements, does the splint meet specific design concepts, including adaptation for:
9. Influencing primary and secondary joints (motion allowed or restricted appropriately; components accomplish intended functions)
10. Attaining purpose (support, immobilize, or restrict motion; prevent or correct deformity; provide or assist motion; or provide attachment base for devices)
11. Effect on joints not included in splint; kinetic effects (avoids application of contraindicated forces to nonsplinted joints)
12. Anatomical variables (surface of application appropriate, healing structures protected as necessary, external hardware considered)
13. Exercise regimen (permits efficient execution of prescribed therapeutic exercises)

Mechanics
Given the diagnostic requirements, does the splint meet mechanical criteria, including adaptation for:
1. Reduction of pressure and shear (length and width of components appropriate; edges flanged as required; contiguous fit of components present)
2. Immobilization or stabilization forces (90-degree angle of approach to involved segment or joint)
3. Mobilization forces (90-degree angle of approach to segments mobilized, perpendicular to joint axes)
4. Magnitude of mobilization forces (supple joint: force sufficient to position segment; stiff joint: force does not exceed safe limits)
5. Difference of passive mobility of successive joints (relative stiffness of joints considered; mobilizing force is not abated at less stiff or normal joints)
6. Material strength (properties of material correlate with strength requirement; curving contour present at potential weak areas)
7. Elimination of friction and shear (joint axes aligned with splint articulations; contiguous fit present)

Construction
Given the diagnostic requirements, does splint fabrication and workmanship provide:
1. Good overall aesthetic appearance
2. Corners rounded, edges and surfaces smooth and flanged appropriately
3. Joined surfaces stable and finished (bonds solid, securing devices of sufficient number and correctly applied; internal edges smoothed, securing devices finished)
4. Ventilation (appropriately placed, splint strength not jeopardized)
5. Padding and straps secured

Fit
Given the diagnostic requirements, has the splint been fitted appropriately to adapt to:
1. Anatomical structure (bony prominences, arches, dual obliquity, skin creases)
2. Ligamentous stress (mobilization, restriction, or immobilization forces correctly applied to avoid damage or attenuation)
3. Joint alignment (anatomical axes aligned with splint articulation; splint does not shift inappropriately on extremity)
4. Kinematic changes (splint does not inappropriately inhibit motion of unrestricted or partially restricted joints)
5. Contiguous fit of components on extremity

Client Education
Given the diagnostic requirements, does the splinting program include consideration of and instructions for:
1. Wearing times and exercise regimen (reflects physiological timing; is adapted to client routine; is understood by client)
2. Donning and doffing (process explained and demonstrated, understood by client)
3. Wearability (client gadget tolerance not exceeded; interfaces such as stockinette or powder used appropriately; acceptable to age and personality characteristics)
4. Precautions (written and verbal instructions provided, understood by client)

Although an attempt has been made to provide a complete listing, these criteria should not be considered all-inclusive.

occasionally more creative approaches may be helpful in re-minding clients to exercise on a regular basis. Television buffs readily adapt to exercising during commercials, whereas people working on an assembly line may be able to exercise only during breaks. Family members must be included when a child is wearing a splint, and school personnel may also need to be informed about wearing and exercise routines. Written instructions for splint-wearing and exercise times should always be used to augment verbal instructions.

Eliminating the excercise portion of a program, night splints may be the same as those used during the day, or they may have an entirely different, often more simple, design. This requires careful monitoring and alteration of both day and night splints as changes occur.

Psychological Effect and Compliance

Because hands are constantly in use and visible, application of a splint often has psychological and socioeconomic rami-fications. Therapists must be aware of the influence these factors may have on client compliance. In reality, no splint may be considered beautiful, no matter how well designed and fabricated. Those clients who have greater physical lim-itations seem to be more accepting of splints, whereas el-derly people often have difficulty adjusting lifetime habits, and teenagers often are unwilling to accept anything that makes them different from their peers (Hopkins, 1966). Other client conditions possibly causing noncompliance (eg, chemical dependence, lack of motivation, mental retar-dation) need to be identified as soon as possible. An unwill-ingness or inability to carry out instructions reliably may re-sult in further damage or injury to the client.

In general, a client's gadget tolerance (Anderson, 1965; Feinberg & Brandt, 1981; Herman, 1984; Hopkins, 1966) may be enhanced if the benefits of wearing the splint are readily apparent. Client education is critical to achieving optimal functional results. It is important that clients be well informed about all aspects of their injury or illness and treatment program so they become integral members of the rehabilitation team. Indeed, the client is the most important member of the team, and should be treated as such.

Precautions

Because splints are foreign bodies applied to living tissue surfaces, clients must be taught to monitor the status of their splinted extremities. The presence of pain, reddened areas, blisters, swelling, rashes, or other problems associated with wearing a splint must be reported to the therapist immedi-ately, and use of the splint should be discontinued until the situation is evaluated (Cannon et al, 1985). Self-examination instructions should be given to clients in writing, including telephone numbers for reporting problems.

Splint care instructions should also be provided in writ-ing. Clients should be cautioned about exposing their splints to warm or hot temperature, such as hot water, heaters, or stoves. Additionally, they need to be reminded not to leave splints in hot car interiors. Thermoplastic splints may lose or alter their configurations in conditions such as these.

▼ MANAGEMENT

Written Documentation

"When writing a note in a client's medical record about a splint, the same rules that apply to all professional writing should be used. In regard to the splint itself, the following. . . must be included" (Kiel, 1983, pp. 136–142): client name, identification number, age, sex, hand dominance, race, and ambulatory status provide basic information. Although the name and number usually appear on every page, the re-maining data may be noted only once. The date, diagnosis, reason for referral, and referring physician are important in confirming the referral and application of the splint and in es-tablishing good communication with the physician. This in-formation is also important for third-party reimbursement procedures.

Initial baseline measurements of volume, ROM, sensibil-ity, strength, and dexterity define extremity condition be-fore splint application. Results from other tests are included as needed. Documentation of passive and active ROM is es-pecially important if a splint is designed to improve joint motion. In the initial note, the splint is described, and the extremity to which it is fitted and the date of fitting are recorded. The purpose of the splint is briefly explained and its effect on the extremity confirmed, verifying that the splint does what it was designed to do. Wearing and exercise instructions are noted, and precautions are defined. Any un-usual splint components or functions should also be in-cluded in the chart at this time. Additionally, documentation of explanations to the client, nursing personnel, and family members should be delineated and, if possible, their level of understanding noted.

Notes from reevaluation sessions should include date and pertinent evaluation measurements, with emphasis on iden-tification of specific changes noted in the splinted extremity. Modifications made in the splint or in the splint-wearing and exercise program should be described in detail. Nota-tion that these modifications were explained to the client and pertinent others and that new instructions were pro-vided in writing also should be recorded.

In practices in which many splints are fabricated, the use of standard forms may simplify and shorten the documenta-tion process. In some cases, these forms are designed to meet the dual needs of client education and medical-legal docu-mentation.

Although clinics may differ slightly in the approaches, the foregoing criteria are fundamental to documentation of splinting endeavors. With litigation procedures on the rise, no splint should be fitted to a client without careful and thorough explanation in the medical record.

Cost and Pricing

Most clinics develop a standard price list for frequently made splints that reflects material cost, therapist time, and overhead expenses per individual splint (Kiel, 1983; pp. 136-137). These prices are based on average-fitting times and average-sized hands or extremities. Although extremes may occur, over time they are incorporated into the general client population and a mean cost of materials and time is attained per splint design.

Material expense includes the cost per inch, or per square inch, of the amount of splint, strap, and padding materials used in each splint. Nonusable scraps are included as part of the cost of the splint. The individual cost of prefabricated components, fasteners, rivets, and so forth is also added to establish a basic price. Use of specialized products such as bonding solution and cooling spray must also be considered and is usually included on a general per application cost.

Therapist time involved in fabrication, fit, and explanation of the splint is added to the material expense. Therapist time is often figured at the same rate per hour used for other clinic treatments. To be representative of an average-experienced therapist, times for novice or highly specialized therapists are not used for determining splint prices. Therapist time involved in reevaluating and altering finished splints on subsequent visits to the clinic may be included in the initial price of the splint or may be assessed on a time per alteration basis. Unfortunately, complicated splints often involve time-consuming alterations that considerably increase the price of the splint. Cost economy to the client is another reason for opting for a simple splint design.

▶SPLINTING CONCLUSION

Many factors must be considered when splinting the upper extremity. The shear number of these variables makes it readily apparent that cookbook approaches must be avoided. Splints should be direct reflections of the individual clients for whom they are made. Factors that must be considered when creating splints include anatomical structures involved; type of surgical repair; physiological timing; individual client variables; kinetic and kinesiological variables involving splinted and unsplinted joints; and the philosophic orientation of the physician and the therapist. When used appropriately, splints are an important and integral aspect of upper extremity rehabilitation.

Section 5

Motor Control Theories and Models: Emerging Occupational Performance Treatment Principles and Assumptions

Clare G. Giuffrida

Motor Control Models
    Central or Peripheral Central Nervous System Control
    Distributed and System Models of Motor Control
Motor Control Approaches Proposed for Therapeutic Intervention
    Task-Oriented Model
    Motor Relearning Program
    Contemporary Task-Oriented Approach
Motor Control Conclusion

The motor control and learning approach is not a singular theory for intervention. Rather, it is a set of concepts, theories, and models that exist and are proposed to explain both the regulation and control of normal move-

---

ETHICS NOTE
DOES ADVANCED CERTIFICATION ENSURE COMPETENCE?
Penny Kyler and Ruth A. Hansen

Jackie is an occupational therapist, with 12 years of practice. She is a certified hand therapist (CHT). She is aware that a new hand therapy clinic is opening in the area. They do not, at present, have any CHTs on staff. One of Jackie's clients tells her that his insurance will no longer cover Jackie's treatment. The insurance will, however, cover treatment at the new hand therapy clinic. Jackie's client asks her opinion of the new clinic, and the caliber of the staff.

1. Is it legally and ethically appropriate to share your personal views about other professionals with a client? If so, under what circumstances?
2. What methods should a practitioner use to determine whether a professional colleague is competent?
3. Does advanced certification or credentialing ensure competence to practice? What are the limits on this interdependence? ■

ments, as well as, the factors and processes involved in normal motor learning.

Understanding motor control implies knowledge about what is controlled and how the controlling processes are organized (Horak, 1991). Normal motor control implies the ability of the central nervous system (CNS) to use current and previous information to coordinate effective and efficient movement strategies. In motor control, the nature and cause of movement is studied. That is, the multiple determinants of movement such as the physiological, biomechanical, neurological, psychological, and environmental factors are investigated (Shumway-Cook & Woollacott, 1995).

Rosenbaum (1991) has proposed that the central issues in motor control revolve around the multiple factors determining movement selection, movement sequencing, and the coordination of perception and action in goal-directed activities. For instance, a fundamental question for motor control theorists is how stability is maintained and controlled while the individual acts in and on the environment. In the context of occupational performance, this question becomes: How is postural stability and movement regulated and controlled for an individual engaged in an occupational performance such as dressing while sitting on a bed?

Motor learning is directed more to understanding how movements are acquired and modified with practice. Schmidt (1988) has defined motor learning as a set of processes associated with practice or experience leading to permanent changes in the capability for skilled acts. Shumway-Cook and Woollacott (1995) have proposed that motor learning develops from a complex set of perceptual, cognitive, and action processes developed in response to individual-task-environment interactions.

The field of motor control and learning is providing occupational therapy with new ideas for understanding the nature, cause, acquisition, and modification of movement subserving optimal occupational performance. The following section provides a synopsis of the prevailing motor control theories and their implications for occupational therapy treatment. Chapter 26, Section 5, contains more detail about motor learning principles.

▼ MOTOR CONTROL MODELS

Central and Peripheral Central Nervous System Control

REFLEX MODEL
Description
The classic experiments of Sir Charles Sherrington provided the basis for the reflex model of motor control (Sherrington, 1947). In these experiments, nervous system processes were inferred by motor outputs in response to sensory inputs given to unconscious anesthetized animals. By stimulating specific sensory receptors, Sherrington in-

duced a variety of distinct stereotyped movements in animal preparations.

Reflexes are the basis for all movements in this model of motor control (Easton, 1972). This model and therapeutic approaches derived from it assumes that sensory input controls motor output. This view of motor control is "peripheralist," for motor control in this model depends on peripheral sensory input controlling the motor response. The nervous system, therefore, is a passive recipient of sensory stimuli that trigger, coordinate, and activate muscles that can excite more sensory systems to activate more muscles (Horak, 1991). This sensory motor input–output relation became incorporated into therapeutic techniques to cause or induce movement with clients demonstrating limited movement patterns.

Clinical Implications
Horak (1991) proposed several clinical implications from this model. The first involves the role of the therapist in identifying reflexes in their clients and predicting from this the client's quality of motor function. This is seen in therapeutic approaches in which therapists identify reflexes in young children and adults with CNS nervous system disorders. Second, this model implies that stereotypical reflex responses can be elicited if appropriate stimulation is provided. In therapy, this occurs when practitioners elicit righting reactions by moving a child or adult on a therapy ball or rocker platform.

Limitations
In this model of motor control, the reflex is the basic building block for coordinated behavior. Considerable evidence now exists that coordinated movement is not controlled by a series of integrated reflexes (Bradley & Bekoff, 1989; Towen, 1984). Deafferentation studies by Polit and Bizzi (1979) support the hypothesis that sensory feedback is not necessary, as originally thought, for accurate movement production. Sensory feedback, however, is necessary for adjusting to environmental demands and learning movements (Horak, 1991). The reflex model also cannot explain or account for sequences of movements occurring so rapidly that sensory feedback from the preceding movement cannot trigger the next. For example, a concert pianist moves from one key to the other so rapidly at times that there is not time for sensory information from one stroke to activate the next. Novel movements, variability in context-dependent responses, and reflexes being controlled consciously are not accounted for in this model (Horak, 1991).

HIERARCHIAL MODEL OF MOTOR CONTROL
Description
Sir Hughlings Jackson in 1932 articulated the hierarchial model of motor control (Foerster, 1977). In this model control of movement is organized hierarchically from the lowest levels in the spinal cord, to intermediate levels in the brainstem, to the highest levels in the cortex. This model provides a central view of motor control in that normal movements

are governed by CNS motor programs that were originally conceived of as specifying muscle-activation patterns. Keele (1968) defined motor programs as a set of muscle commands that is structured before a movement sequence begins and allows the sequence to be carried out uninfluenced by peripheral feedback.

Although there are still considerable controversies about what constitutes motor programming, the hierarchial model clearly separates high-level movement control and low-level reflexive control. This model along with the reflex model became further articulated as the reflex-hierarchial model or programming model of motor control, which also serves as the basis for neurotherapeutic approaches (Mathiowetz & Haugen, 1995).

Clinical Implications

The neurodevelopmental and sensory integration approaches are based on a model of hierarchial organization in the CNS (Montgomery, 1991). Many forms of CNS dysfunction are considered disruptive to higher-level control of movement. Released reflexes are thought to interfere with or block coordinated movement patterns. Therefore, a reasonable goal for therapy is to identify and prevent primitive reflexes from dominating or interfering with higher-level goals. Strategies designed to enhance control are seen in the neurorehabilitation approaches. These strategies can include both sensory-integration procedures and facilitation and inhibition techniques. Both are means of developing more control in the nervous system.

Limitations

In light of classic observations of motor behavior, there are several limitations to this model. For example, low levels of control, such as demonstrated in spinal cord control, dominates motor control when necessary. Lower-level control is seen in cats walking on a treadmill, despite total transections preventing control from higher centers. Also, coordinated reflexive locomotor movement patterns, such as walking, trotting, and galloping, do not appear to require top-down control.

The assumption that motor development and recovery of functions follows a stepwise or hierarchial progression from reflex-driven movements to internally commanded movements is also challenged in light of recent research. Studies are demonstrating that motor development does not always follow a set sequence. For example, learning to reach and kick appears to begin with predictive self-generated movement that become increasingly responsive to ongoing sensory feedback (Thelen, Kelso, & Fogel, 1987; von Hofsten, 1980).

There are other limitations encountered in this model, such as the model's inability to account for the interfacing of reflex and voluntary control seen in a variety of situations. Voluntary movements are accompanied by automatic synergistic activity and ongoing postural adjustments. There is also a reciprocity between reflexive and voluntary control, for sensory feedback can serve to adjust voluntary actions, whereas reflex activity can be influenced by voluntary control. For example, instructions to release or resist a movement modify unexpected perturbations to the limb (Shumway-Cook & Woollacott, 1995).

Distributed and System Models of Motor Control

DISTRIBUTED MODELS OF MOTOR CONTROL

Description

In this model, control of movement is not conceptualized as being located either centrally or peripherally. As scientists looked at different motor behaviors and other characteristics of the movement system, a concept of distributed control of movement emerged [ie, the internal and external forces acting on this system were considered (Keshner, 1991)]. Distributed models of motor control are not unidirectional. Rather, they allow for communication within the nervous system to take place in ascending, descending, and lateral arrangements. The control hierarchy is not perceived as a descending chain of command, but as an overlapping circular network in which each level influences those above and below it. Various sites within and throughout the system are part of the process underlying and controlling movement. Some models of distributed control, however, minimize the relevance of the nervous system. Control of movement is seen as distributed throughout many working systems, including mechanical and environmental factors. There are several different theories about distributed control of movement.

Systems Theory. Bernstein, a Russian scientist, was among the first to look at internal and external forces acting on the body to understand the characteristics of the system being moved. The body was considered to be a mechanical system with mass, and subject to external forces, such as gravity, as well as inertia and movement-dependent forces. Bernstein asked questions related to (1) the function of the system in a continually changing environment, (2) the properties of the initial conditions affecting movement, and (3) the body as a mechanical system influencing the control process (Shumway-Cook & Woollacott, 1995).

Bernstein was also responsible for identifying what is known as "the degrees of freedom problem." In describing the mechanics of the system, Bernstein noted that many degrees of freedom need to be controlled for coordinated movement to occur. For example, there are many joints that can flex, extend, or rotate, and these options complicate the control of movement. Therefore, control involves converting the body into a controllable system (Schmidt, 1988).

Bernstein's solution to this problem was proposing that hierarchial control exists to simplify the body's multiple degrees of freedom. He proposed (1) that groups of muscle were constrained to act together as units, and (2) these units were activated at lower levels in the system.

Dynamical Action Theory (Synergetics). This perspective comes from the study of dynamics or synergetics, the study of how parts of systems work together. Dynamical action theory asks two fundamental questions: (1) How do patterns and organization emerge from orderless parts? and (2) How do systems change over time? A fundamental principle of this theory is self-organization. This principle states that when a system of individual parts comes together, its collective elements behave in an ordered fashion. For motor control, there is no need to have a higher center issuing commands to achieve coordinated output (Rosenbaum, 1991).

Descriptions of these self-organizing systems are expressed mathematically, with the critical features of the system being nonlinear properties. Nonlinear behavior is described as a situation in which the system goes into a different behavioral pattern after one parameter is altered and reaches a critical value. For example, as an animal walks faster and faster, there is a point at which it breaks into a trot and later into a gallop. In this example, the parameter being altered is walking speed and the accompanying behavioral changes are the animal's walking, trotting, and galloping.

Dynamic Pattern Theory. This is an operational approach to the study of coordinated movement (Keshner, 1991). Dynamic pattern theory incorporates aspects of Bernstein's systems theory and dynamic action theory. It is an attempt to define terms and provide behavioral and mathematical predictions for coordinated movement patterns. The basic concepts follow:

1. The human system exhibits self-organizing behavior.
2. The human system is a many-element system that can be described by a few elements, which are referred to as collective variables. Collective variables are the fewest number of variables that completely describe the behavior (Heriza, 1991). For example, Heriza (1991) proposes that for humans, walking is a highly complex behavior characterized by a specific movement pattern. The new walker compresses the many degrees of freedom available from the muscles, bones, joints, tendons, neurons, and motor units to the relatively few degrees of freedom observed in walking. In this example, a complex behavior, walking, becomes characterized by a description of the behavior, the specific movement pattern.
3. Collective variables characterize movement patterns and capture the systems cooperating to produce the movement; movement is more than just muscles and motor neurons. For instance, kicking, stepping, and throwing a ball are examples of coordinated movement patterns. Again, an example by Heriza (1991) helps to clarify this. In intralimb coordination, such as seen within one limb in kicking or stepping, the identified collective variables are (1) the timing of the individual movement phases, such as flexion and extension; (2) phase lags, defined as the time between the onset of movement of one joint relative to another joint; and (3) the relation of individual joints to each other.
4. The identification of phase transitions is basic to understanding behavior. *Control parameters* are variables that shift the movement from one form to another. Control parameters act to reorganize the system. In the example of intralimb coordination as well as in interlimb coordination, behavioral states can drive the system. For instance, when an infant is asleep or drowsy, little kicking is noted. If the infant is aroused, the spatial and temporal pattern of kicking is observed. If the infant is in a crying state, a new pattern emerges that is described as a rigid coactivation of all the muscles into stiff mobility. Therefore, control parameters can be defined as essential components that are nonspecific to the movement behavior. In this example, the control parameters can reside in (1) the individual, such as behavioral state; (2) the environment (eg, gravity); (3) the social environment (eg, the caretaker); or (4) in the goal or in the task. New coordinated patterns emerge because old patterns become unstable and the system is driven to a new state. Changes in the control parameters push the system to a new state. During these shifts in phase or phase transitions, the prevailing movement pattern becomes less stable and more easily perturbed by the control parameter (Heriza, 1991).
5. The study of the stability or instability of behavior during transition periods is essential to understanding pattern change in complex systems. In this approach movement behavior and control can be aptly described by a set of collective variables and control variables associated with phase transition (Haugen & Mathiowetz, 1995).

Clinical Implications

Systems theories take into account factors other than the nervous system in controlling movement (eg, the physical characteristics such as the mass of the system being moved). These theories have enlarged the understanding of the multiple factors responsible for controlled movement. The individual is seen as active in the environment, with movement a product of many systems.

Limitations

The role of the nervous system is minimized in these theories. Transitions in movement patterns are explained in terms of mathematical function and variables. These theories primarily seek physical explanations for movement characteristics.

PARALLEL DISTRIBUTED PROCESSING THEORY
Description

Computer analysis and simulations are also providing models and theories for motor control. These are recent efforts to develop models of higher-level processes based on information from imaging studies about neural processing and patterns of neural activity. These attempts start by asking how the brain might achieve higher-level processing rather than asking how the brain actually achieves such processing. Modeling starts from a basic understanding of how neurons work and asks: How could higher level function be achieved by connecting basic elements like neurons together? (Anderson, 1995).

The parallel distributed processing (PDP) theory of motor control describes how the nervous system processes information for action. It reflects current knowledge in neuroscience about the serial and parallel processing of the nervous system Serial processing is processing of information through a single pathway, whereas parallel processing is processing information through many pathways (Kandel, Schwartz, & Jessell, 1991). Parallel distributed processing is unique in its emphasis on explaining neural mechanisms associated with motor control. Neural modeling, computer simulation of nervous system functioning, has correctly predicted aspects of processing in both the perception and action systems. As neural modeling develops, it may provide further knowledge on how the nervous system solves particular problems.

Clinical Implications

Modeling of function and dysfunction can be integrated into clinical practice. Shumway-Cook and Woollacott (1995) propose that a PDP model could be used to predict how changes within the nervous system affect function. As an example, the theory predicts that parallel redundant pathways exist in the system and a loss of a few elements will not necessarily affect function. The loss of elements beyond a certain threshold, however, may affect the capacity of the system to function. This idea, threshold of dysfunction, is demonstrated in many pathological cases such as in Parkinson's disease.

Limitations

The PDP theory of motor control is a tool to think about the way in which the nervous system works. Some of the proposed functions are not replicated in nervous system processing, and modeling cannot fully account for what is known about nervous system processing.

ECOLOGICAL THEORY
Description

This theory was developed by James Gibson (1966) and explores the interaction between the motor (action) system and goal-directed behavior. Environmental information was seen as relevant to action in the environment. Perception, rather than sensation, is important to the individual acting on the environment. From this perspective, determining how the individual detects information in the environment, the form of this environmental information, and how this information is used to modify and control movement is important. In ecological theory, the organization of movement is dependent on the active exploration of tasks, the environment, and the individual's multiple ways to accomplish a task.

Clinical Implications

A major contribution of this perspective is seeing the individual as active in the environment and the environment as crucial in determining movements. Active exploration of the environment allows the individual to develop multiple ways to accomplish a task.

Limitations

This approach has enlarged the understanding of the interaction between the organism and environment. Research is at the level of the organism-environment interface. This approach has not contributed significantly to knowledge about the organization and function of the nervous system, a primary concern of practitioners intervening in motor control problems based on traditional neurotherapeutic approaches.

TASK-ORIENTED THEORIES
Description

In this theory, motor control is understood by identifying what problems the central nervous system has to solve to accomplish a motor task. By task, Greene (1972) was referring to the fundamental problems, such as the degrees of freedom problem described by Bernstein, that the CNS is required to solve to accomplish a motor task. Peter Greene (1972) proposed that this approach could provide the basis for a more coherent picture of the motor system.

Clinical Implications

This perspective suggests practicing functional tasks for retraining in therapy. It acknowledges the role of perceptual, cognitive, and action systems to accomplish tasks (Greene, 1972). It requires an understanding of motor strategies used to accomplish a task as well as an understanding of the perceptual basis for action and the cognitive contributions to actions.

Limitations

There is a lack of agreement about the fundamental tasks of the CNS. There is also lack of agreement on the essential elements being controlled within a task. For example, in studying postural control, some scientists consider the essential goal of the postural system to be control of head position. Other scientists studying postural control think that controlling the center of mass position to attain body stability is the essential goal of postural control (Shumway-Cook & Woollacott, 1995).

▼ MOTOR CONTROL APPROACHES PROPOSED FOR THERAPEUTIC INTERVENTION

New approaches to intervening with motor performance deficits that affect occupational performances have evolved. These therapeutic approaches are based on traditional motor control models as well as on more contemporaneous models of how movement is controlled.

Task-Oriented Model

The task-oriented approach (Horak, 1991; Gordon, 1987) targets both peripheral and central control systems. In line with system models of motor control, the task-oriented model assumes that control of movement is organized around goal-directed functional tasks. Clients are taught to accomplish goals for functional tasks. By practicing a wide variety of movements, the client solves different types of motor problems. The assumptions seen in Table 20–2 guide treatment.

Along with these assumptions and guidelines, Horak (1991) suggests organizing questions around several areas in treating clients with motor performance deficits. These areas are the client's behavioral goals, movement strategies, musculoskeletal constraints, compensatory strategies, and need for adaptations. An example of questions about these areas follows:

1. Behavioral goals: Are the practitioner's and client's goals the same?
2. Movement strategy: What are the organizing principles of a normal movement strategy?
3. Musculoskeletal constraints: How much of the motor deficit in a neurologically impaired client is due to a deficit in the musculoskeletal system, rather the neural components?
4. Compensatory strategies: Has the client found the most effective strategy?
5. Adaptation: How must a movement strategy be adapted to accomplish a task in a new environmental context?

TABLE 20-3. Assumptions Guiding Motor Relearning Approach

- In regaining motor control, learning is required. This learning follows the same principles and factors as those incurred in normal learning. Therefore, practice, receiving feedback, and understanding the goal are essential for treatment.
- Motor control is exercised in both anticipatory and ongoing modes.
- Sensory input is related to motor output and helps modulate action.
- Control of a specific task can be effectively regained by practice of that specific motor task in various contexts.
- Conscious practice of tasks builds up awareness of the ability to elicit motor control activity.
- Progression of practice is from conscious awareness to practice at a more automatic level to assure that a skill is learned.
- Cognitive function is emphasized. If the client is to learn, then the environment must encourage the learning process.
- When clients can perform a task effectively and efficiently without thinking about it in a variety of contexts, learning is assured to have occurred.
- Contemporary theories of motor control emphasize distributed control rather than a top-down or bottom-up approach. Therefore, in the motor relearning program, recovery is directed to relearning control through many systems.
- The client is defined as an active participant in the treatment process. The major goal in rehabilitation is to relearn effective strategies for performing functional activities.
- The role of the therapist is to prevent the use of inefficient strategies by the client.
- The program addresses seven categories of functional daily activities: upper limb function, orofacial function, sitting up over side of bed, balanced sitting, standing up and sitting down, balanced standing and walking.

(Carr & Shepard, 1987)

TABLE 20-2. Assumptions Guiding Task-Oriented Approach

Assumptions	Treatment Principles
• Movement is controlled by the individual's goals.	• The goal of therapy is to teach clients to accomplish goals for functional tasks.
• A wide variety of movement patterns can be accomplished with a task.	• Therapists do not treat or limit therapy to one normal movement pattern.
• Facilitation of normal movements is not necessary.	• Therapists try to teach the nervous system how to solve different motor problems by practicing in a wide variety of situations.
• The nervous system adapts continually to its environment and musculoskeletal constraints.	• The therapist seeks to manipulate these environmental and musculoskeletal systems to allow for efficient purposeful behavior.
• The nervous system is not a passive recipient of sensory stimuli, but actively seeks to control its own perception and actions.	• Client needs to practice motor behaviors motivated by the goal of task accomplishment.
• Voluntary and automatic control systems are interrelated.	• Clients are encouraged to assist voluntarily in accomplishing a motor behavior with therapist's encouragement.
• Multiple system involvement results in movement.	• The therapist and the environment provide feedback.
• The nervous system is exposed to its own specific environment.	• The therapist must design interventions in which practice of controlled movements is outside structured sessions.
• The nervous system seeks to accomplish goals with remaining systems after injury.	• The therapist helps the client identify and use compensatory strategies.

(From Horak, 1991 & Gordon, 1987)

Motor Relearning Program (Carr & Shepherd, 1987)

The motor relearning program is a synthesis of the prevalent contemporary models of motor control and the motor-learning process (Sabari, 1995). It is specific to the rehabilitation of clients following stroke. The program is based on four factors thought to be essential for the learning of motor skill and assumed to be essential for the relearning of motor control: (1) elimination of unnecessary muscle activity, (2) feedback, (3) practice, and (4) the interrelation between postural adjustment and movement. In this program, treatment is directed to relearning of control, rather than to activities incorporating exercise or to facilitation or inhibition techniques.

Treatment is directed to enhancing motor performance and emphasis is on practice of specific tasks, the training of controllable muscle action and control over the movement components of these tasks. The major assumptions about motor control underlying this approach are listed in Table 20–3.

To provide this program, a four-step sequence is followed for skill acquisition. Step 1 is an analysis of the task, including observation. Step 2 is practice of missing components, including goal identification, instruction, practice, and feedback, with some manual guidance. Step 3 is practice of the task adding reevaluation and encouraging task flexibility. Step 4 targets transfer of training (Carr & Shepherd, 1987).

Contemporary Task-Oriented Approach

Haugen & Mathiowetz (1995) have proposed a task-oriented approach based on a systems model of motor control and influenced by contemporary developmental and motor-learning theories. This model takes into account the interaction between the personal characteristics or systems of the person such as the sensory-motor system and the performance context. Occupational performance emerges from the interaction between personal characteristics and performance contexts as seen in Table 20–4.

In this approach recovery from brain damage is defined as the client's discovery of what skills remain to perform tasks (Haugen & Mathiowetz, 1995). The role of the practitioner in this approach is to take into account all systems as potential variables to explain the behavior of each client at a specific time. For example, the flexor pattern of spasticity seen with cerebrovascular accident (CVA) clients can be the result of more than neural components and, therefore, more than the sensory motor system needs to be evaluated. Each

---

TABLE 20-4. Assumptions Guiding Contemporary Task-Oriented Approach

Assumptions	Treatment Principles
• Functional tasks help organize behavior. Recent research suggests that parameters of motor behavior are not performance components but in fact functional goals (Burton & Davis, 1992; Gentile, 1992; Heriza, 1991; Thelen, 1989). • Occupational performance emerges from the interaction of multiple systems that represent the unique characteristics of the person and the performance context. • After CNS damage or other changes in personal or environmental systems, clients' behavioral changes reflect their attempts to compensate and achieve functional goals. • Personal and environmental systems are hetarchially organized. There is no inherent ordering of the personal and environmental systems in terms of their influence on motor behavior. There is also no inherent ordering within the system, even within the CNS. • A person must practice and experiment with varied strategies to find optimal solutions for motor problems and develop skill in performance.	• As the primary purpose of motor behavior is to achieve functional goals, therapists are to begin and end therapy by focusing on occupational performance. The emphasis on task performance and evaluation is primarily at the disability level using the World Health Organization Model of Disablement (1980). • The therapist assesses all systems that are contributing to problems in functional performance or supporting optimal performance, keeping in mind the tasks the person currently does or would be doing in the future. As the client brings to the situation a unique constellation of characteristics, the therapist makes the client's perspective the focus of assessment. The client determines the important goals and roles necessary for occupational performance. • Movement patterns used for compensation and achievement of functional goals must be understood fully. The evaluation of occupational performance must include an examination of the process (actual movement patterns), the outcome, and the stability or instability of observed motor behavior. • Evaluation strategies consider all personal and environmental systems. Those interfering the most with performance are evaluated first. • As part of treatment, clients are to practice, experiment and problem solve to achieve functional goals. Treatment planning is to develop and implement learning opportunities for clients with problem-solving abilities. When clients are unable to problem solve, the therapist may need to train them to use given routines.

(From Haugen & Mathiowetz, 1995)

client is seen as unique because each individual has a course of recovery that reflects his or her specific problems and environmental demands specific to his or her functions in a unique environment. The assumptions in Table 20–4 are proposed to guide treatment.

►MOTOR CONTROL CONCLUSION

Models of motor control and learning can guide occupational therapy interventions for clients with motor performance deficits. More detail on the models presented here can be found in sources in the reference list. Practitioners need to be aware that as scientific knowledge about movement evolves, new models of practice may emerge. Practitioners have a responsibility to keep up to date on current motor control and learning research, so that they can provide clients with the most effective treatment possible for motor deficits.

Section 6

Cognitive–Perceptual Retraining and Rehabilitation

Joan Pascale Toglia

▼ OVERVIEW OF TREATMENT APPROACHES

Cognitive perceptual difficulties can significantly affect an individual's abilities to perform everyday tasks, fulfill former roles, and maintain personal-social relationships. The aim of occupational therapy intervention for people with cognitive–perceptual dysfunction is to decrease functional limitations and enhance occupational role performance. Although the ultimate goal of intervention with this population is clear, there are different perspectives concerning the means by which this can best be accomplished. For example, as discussed in Chapter 18, occupational therapy intervention can emphasize the underlying performance components as a prerequisite to function or can focus directly on functional tasks and occupational behaviors. The former approach seeks to change or remediate the impaired cognitive–perceptual skills, whereas the latter approach focuses directly on task performance. Within each of these approaches, there are significant differences in the areas targeted for intervention as well as in underlying assumptions concerning individuals' abilities to learn and generalize information. The characteristics of different intervention approaches as well as the underlying assumptions are explored in this section. Factors that are critical in influencing selection of treatment approaches are discussed and methods for systematically integrating treatment approaches are illustrated. Finally, the application of different treatment methods to specific areas of cognitive perceptual dysfunction is described.

▼ CAPITALIZING ON THE ASSETS: THE FUNCTIONAL APPROACHES

The functional approach begins by identifying the tasks or activities that are of most concern to the client and caregiver. It capitalizes on the individual's assets to improve task performance. The functional approach can be subdivided into three different intervention techniques: (1) adaptation of the task or environment, (2) functional skill training, and (3) compensation.

Adaptation of the Task or Environment

Adaptation involves changing, altering, or structuring the task or environment to prevent disruptive behaviors or accidents, minimize cognitive or perceptual demands of a task, minimize caregiver burden, and support or maintain the client's level of functioning (Radomski, Dougherty, Fine, & Baum, 1993). For example, to prevent wandering behavior in a confused and disoriented individual, the environment may be adapted by placing a decoration on a door handle to make it less recognizable as a door handle or by placing wallpaper on a door so that it blends in with the surrounding walls and is less salient or recognizable as a door.

In addition, a caregiver may be trained to alter or structure the task or environment to support the individual's level of function. For instance, the individual may not be able to attend to the task of preparing a meal, but may be able to perform individual components such as mixing the salad and folding napkins in half for the table setting. Engagement in purposeful task components may maintain the client's level of function and prevent disruptive behaviors (Radomski et al, 1993). Allen (1993), in Chapter 26, discusses a cognitive disability approach that provides guidelines for matching the individual's cognitive level with activity demands.

Adaptations seek to change the task or environment, rather than the person. The presence of another person is required to implement the adaptation (Toglia, 1993b). Caregiver burnout and stress can interfere with the caregivers ability to effectively carry out adaptive strategies. Treatment needs to focus on providing support, education, and training to the caregiver instead of direct treatment to the client. The caregiver needs to understand the client's limitations to be an active participant in modifying and adapting tasks or the environment. Adaptations should directly address the problems and needs identified by the caregiver and be designed in collaboration with the caregiver (Campbell, Duffy, & Salloway, 1994). Adaptations can produce rapid changes in function. However, the effects of adaptation are limited to the task or environment adapted and are dependent on reliability and consistency of the caregiver or significant other for success.

Functional Skill Training

Functional skill training or task-specific training involves rote repetition of a specific task with gradually fading cues. Emphasis is on the mastery of a specific task, rather than on the underlying skills needed to perform the task. Behavioral techniques, including positive reinforcement, contingent reinforcement, and backward chaining, are often incorporated into structured and repetitive training of an action sequence. Treatment involves breaking down a specific task into subcomponents and systematically recording the number of prompts required for each subcomponent (Giles, 1992; Glisky, Schacter, & Butters, 1994). Table 20–5 illustrates how the task of brushing teeth is broken down into subcomponents. The practitioner records the number of cues or assistance required for each subcomponent of the task. Gradually the number of cues provided by the practitioner is reduced. Rote repetition of the activity capitalizes on procedural learning or memory for the actual performance of tasks, not memory of a specific set of facts (Glisky, 1995). Structured functional skill training has been effective with individuals with severe memory disorders in a number of different case studies (Giles & Clark-Wilson, 1988; Giles & Shore, 1989; Glisky & Schacter, 1988).

Functional skill training requires learning from the individual, but the learning expected is primitive or associative. In **association learning**, individuals' behaviors are a direct response to environmental stimuli, thus learners are unable to deal with more then minor changes in the task stimuli or environment. Learning is characterized by hyperspecificity (Neistadt, 1994b). Glisky, Schacter, and Butters (1994) found evidence that considerable overlearning of a specific task may increase the ability of severely amnesic individuals to transfer and perform the task with greater variations.

Functional skill training has been demonstrated through case studies to produce significant changes in self-care and

TABLE 20-5. Functional Skill Training: The Method of Vanishing Cues			
Brushing Teeth	**Number of Cues for Each Substep**		
	Day 1	*Day 2*	*Day 3*
Selects toothbrush and toothpaste	3	2	2
Opens toothpaste	2	1	1
Puts toothpaste on toothbrush	3	3	2
Turns on water and wets brush	1	1	0
Brushes teeth—all sides	1	0	0
Fills cup with water	0	0	0
Rinses mouth	0	1	0
Total number of cues	10	8	5

The task is broken down into substeps and the number of cues required for each substep is documented on a daily basis and gradually faded.

work performance in severely impaired individuals (Giles & Shore, 1989; Glisky et al, 1994; Wehman, 1991). However, treatment addresses only one task or routine at a time. Extensive training, time, and effort may be required to achieve success within one task sequence and environment. Proponents of this method have argued that treatment of the cognitively impaired adult should take place in the context in which the individual will function, for persons with brain injury are unable to **generalize** learning (Giles, 1992; Glisky et al, 1994; Mayer, Keating, & Rapp, 1986). However, if the individual is unable to cope with minor unforseen events, or slight changes in routine, even performance within the same context will be compromised. The ability to cope with minor changes, minor disruptions in routines, and unforseen circumstances is a part of daily life even within the same context.

Compensation

Compensation teaches the individual to bypass or minimize the effects of the impairment by using a substitute method to perform a task. The client is expected to initiate and implement use of an external aid or strategy to enhance task performance in a variety of different situations. This requires some awareness and acceptance of one's deficits as well as the ability to generalize use of a learned strategy (Toglia, 1993b). An example is use of a memory notebook to compensate for memory loss. Independent use requires that the individual recognizes that he or she is having difficulty with his or her memory and perceives the need to write things down as a help in remembering. In addition, it requires initiation of use of the book in a variety of different situations.

Summary of the Functional Approaches

The different techniques within the functional approach have different requirements and assumptions concerning learning. For example, adaptation seeks to change the task or environment, rather then the person. Functional skill training requires a primitive level of learning, which is hyperspecific to the task and environment, whereas compensation often requires the individual to apply a learned strategy to a variety of situations. The three techniques can be viewed on a continuum from those that do not expect the individual to change or learn, to those require learning and generalization from the client. The assumptions and requirements of different treatment techniques need to be matched with the abilities of the client.

▼ ADDRESSING THE IMPAIRMENT

In contrast with the functional approach, which minimizes use of the impaired skill, remedial approaches place an emphasis on improving and restoring the underlying cognitive and perceptual performance components. Demands are placed directly on the impaired skill. Learning and generalization are expected to occur. Remedial approaches seek to change the individual's skills, rather the manipulate the task or environment (Neistadt, 1990). The conceptualization of cognition and perception determines what is addressed in treatment. Three different remedial approaches are described: (1) the Affolter approach, (2) cognitive remediation, and (3) the multicontext approach. Each of these approaches reflect different conceptualizations of the underlying cognitive perceptual impairment.

Sensory Motor Deficits: The Affolter Approach

The sensory motor approaches view cognitive–perceptual symptoms as a reflection of inadequate assimilation and integration of vestibular, tactile, proprioceptive, and kinesthetic information. They are based on the assumption that the development of sensory motor skills provides a foundation for the development of complex cognitive and perceptual skills.

The Affolter method views cognitive perceptual problems as a reflection of inadequate tactile-kinesthetic input and environmental interaction. The tactile-kinesthetic perceptual system is considered to be essential for "adaptation and the development of more complex performances" (Davies, 1985, p. 2). It is assumed that clients who fail in complex behaviors receive inadequate tactile-kinesthetic input. Therefore, treatment uses guiding or tactile–kinesthetic stimulation to facilitate interaction between the environment and individual. Therapy focuses on the input of tactile–kinesthetic information, rather than on production or performance. Specific cognitive perceptual skills are not addressed. Instead, there is an emphasis on improving information processing by guiding the individual through problem-solving interactions with tasks and the environment. During guiding, the practitioner places his or her hand over the dorsal aspect of the client's hands and guides movement as the client performs a functional task (Davis, 1992). Examples of tasks that may be used include peeling a banana, cutting an apple, dialing a telephone, and setting a table.

The task and environment are continually varied to promote learning. Effective guiding emphasizes constant contact with surfaces to maximize tactile and kinesthetic input and interaction with the environment, rather than moving in free space. When the practitioner feels that the client is taking over, assistance is gradually reduced. If the practitioner feels that a breakdown in performance is about to occur, additional assistance is provided. Guiding enables the client to experience successful task performance and interaction with the environment. The practitioner does not let the client fail. There is an assumption that learning takes place through repeated successful experiences. During guiding there is no verbal instruction or feedback. The assimulation and organization of cognitive–perceptual processes is stimulated through guided movements during tasks that involve exploration and problem-solving interactions with the environment. Signs of effectiveness of guiding include increased attention span, increased eye contact, changes in facial expressions, improved initiation and problem solving (Davies, 1985, 1992).

The Affolter approach differs from traditional remedial approaches in that it uses functional and meaningful tasks. It is considered remedial because treatment aims to improve the individuals underlying sensory motor abilities and enhance the ability of the person to take in and process information.

The Affolter approach provides an alternative to treatment particularly for globally aphasic or apraxic individuals who do not respond to verbal or visual cues. Although the Affolter approach emphasizes successful experiences, it should be remembered that motor-learning studies have found that motor learning is enhanced when the individual is given the opportunity to make errors and learn from mistakes (Poole, 1991). Motor learning is also enhanced when the client is given the opportunity to initiate the task (Sabari, 1991). At this time, there are no research studies that have systematically investigated effectiveness of the Affolter approach.

Deficits in Specific Skills: Cognitive–Perceptual Remediation

In traditional cognitive–perceptual remedial approaches, cognitive skills are conceptualized in terms of higher cortical skills which are divided into discrete subskills such as attention, discrimination, memory, sequencing, categorization, concept formation, and problem solving. These skills are hierarchically organized from simple to complex. Lower-level skills provide the foundation for more complex skills and behaviors (Toglia, 1992). For example, in treatment, attentional skills are addressed before higher-level skills such as problem solving. Visual perceptual skills are considered to be separate from cognitive skills and include hierarchially organized skills, such as form constancy, figure-ground, position in space, spatial relations, and visual closure. Evaluation, as described in Chapter 16, seeks to identify deficits in specific skill areas. Treatment emphasizes practice of the specific cognitive or perceptual skills that have been identified as being deficient. For example, if the individual has a deficit in attention, treatment may consist of a graded series of attention exercises. If the individual demonstrates impaired performance on a figure-ground task, treatment involves repetitive practice with graded figure-ground tasks.

Drills or exercises involving tabletop or computer tasks are systematically graded in difficulty by either gradually removing cues or by gradually increasing the difficulty level of the task. Ben-Yishay & Diller (1983) and Diller, Ben-Yishay, Gerstman, Gordon, and Weinberg (1974) have pro-

vided guidelines for remedial tasks: (1) define the stimulus parameters of treatment tasks, (2) systematically grade task difficulty from simple to complex, (3) establish a hierarchical sequence of cues with gradual fading of cues, (4) establish criteria for success. This latter guideline requires data about normative performance, which is lacking for many remedial tasks.

Methods and materials used in remedial treatment are often abstract (eg, block designs, shapes) and are closely related to evaluation tasks. There is an assumption that improvement in underlying cognitive or perceptual skills will have a greater influence on behavior than direct functional skill training because learning will spontaneously generalize to a wider range of tasks. For example, if improvement in the ability to construct a block design is observed during treatment, it is assumed that there will also be improvement on all other tasks that require underlying constructional skills, such as making a sandwich. Thus, treatment aims to influence a number of different tasks by improving the underlying cognitive subskills. This has also been referred to as the "transfer training approach" (Toglia, 1992).

Remediation of cognitive–perceptual subskills is based on the assumption that direct practice of the impaired skill promotes recovery or reorganization of that skill. Information on functional reorganization and adult brain plasticity supports this view. For example, it has been postulated that some parts of the brain may take over new functions, or work together in different ways as a result of environmental experiences (Luria, 1973). However, as Neistadt (1994b) observed "because both remedial and adaptive treatment approaches stimulate clients to learn new behaviors, neither approach can claim to take advantage of adult brain plasticity more than the other" (Neistadt, 1994b, p. 426).

Most outcome studies on cognitive remediation have been conducted with the adult brain-injured population. Recently, there has been interest in applying cognitive remediation programs to the schizophrenic population (Green, 1993). Several studies have demonstrated changes in cognitive–perceptual skills as a result of focused cognitive training (Ben-Yishay, Piasetsky, & Rattok, 1987; Ruff et al, 1989; Sohlberg & Mateer, 1989a). However few studies have systematically explored the extent to which these improvements generalize to everyday function. In addition, there are few studies that have actually compared the results of different treatment approaches. One study that compared remedial intervention with a functional approach for adult men with head injures found that task-specific learning occurred in both groups (Neistadt, 1992).

Although it is unclear whether remedial intervention improves function, it may be that awareness and insight improves as a result of remedial intervention. Because remediation emphasizes repetitive practice of the impaired skill, awareness and insight into one's deficits may increase as a secondary effect. This awareness is necessary for sustained participation and motivation in treatment and may eventually allow some individuals to more effectively use compensatory strategies. Several authors have observed a positive relation between awareness and positive outcome in cognitive remediation (Barco, Crosson, Bolesta, Werts, & Stout, 1991; Ben-Yishay & Diller, 1993; Bergquist & Jacket, 1993; Diller, 1994; Lam, McMahon, & Priddy, 1988).

Inefficient Use of Processing Strategy: Strategy Training

Strategy training focuses on training individuals to change their approach, style, or technique for a wide variety of tasks. In dynamic approaches to treatment, cognitive perceptual problems are conceptualized in terms of deficiencies of processing strategy. *Processing strategies* are defined as "organized approaches, routines or tactics which operate to select and guide the processing of information" (Toglia, 1992; p. 108). Deficiencies in processing strategies account for difficulties on several different tasks. For example, a tendency to overfocus on details may interfere with a visual perceptual task, a memory task, or a problem-solving task.

An example of an approach that uses processing strategies is the multicontext approach described in Chapter 26. Treatment targets a processing strategy that interferes with a variety of different tasks and is most responsive to cuing. This strategy is identified with dynamic assessment procedures described in Chapter 16, Section 2. If an individual requires cues more then 25% of the time, then the activity chosen may be too difficult for the client. The exception to this is when the goal is to increase awareness. In this case, the practitioner may design the treatment task to elicit numerous errors so that there are repeated opportunities for clients to experience feedback and gain insight from their mistakes.

Separate cognitive perceptual skills are not addressed in the multicontext approach. For example, the individual may demonstrate a tendency to miss important details in tasks that are unfamiliar and include 15 to 20 pieces of information. The individual may be taught to highlight important information with a color highlighter (external strategy) and to remember to choose important information before making a decision or attempting to solve the problem (internal strategy). The individual then practices the application of the targeted strategies within a variety of tasks and environments using different movement patterns. Task complexity is increased after application of the targeted strategy has been observed in a variety of different situations. Once the individual demonstrates the ability to apply the same processing strategies in a variety of different situations, the complexity or difficulty level of treatment tasks is increased.

The multicontext approach focuses on both impaired skills and areas of strength and thus contains both compensatory and remedial components (Toglia, 1991a). This approach assumes that transfer of learning will occur in some clients only if it is directly addressed during treatment. Al-

though there are several case reports that support the use of strategy training in brain-injured individuals (Cicerone & Wood, 1987; Nelson & Lenhart, 1996; Trexler, Webb, & Zappala, 1994) , the use of a multicontext approach to treatment has not been systematically investigated or compared with other intervention approaches.

▼ AN INTEGRATED MODEL OF TREATMENT: MIXING AND MATCHING TREATMENT TECHNIQUES

Although the different treatment approaches have different requirements and underlying assumptions, they are not mutually exclusive. The different treatment approaches may be used sequentially or concurrently. Gianutsos (1989) proposes that remediation that focuses on improving and restoring skills is often a more successful starting point for a therapeutic relationship: "If exercise does not lead to improved function, the individual will begin to welcome and appreciate compensatory methods..." (Gianutsos, 1989; p.vii). Others propose that treatment should start with remediation as a foundation for developing cognitive subskills. Treatment should then progress to integrating remedial strategies into functional activities. Neistadt (1994a) suggests that different treatment approaches are appropriate at different stages of recovery or severity. In individuals with severe impairments, adaptation or functional skill training may be most effective, for individuals with milder deficits, remediation may be effective. Different treatment approaches may also be used to address different areas of dysfunction in the same individual. For example a practitioner may choose to use a compensatory approach or adaptive approach to address the individual's memory deficits and a remedial approach to address visual scanning and unilateral neglect problems.

The Dynamic Interactional Model of Cognition proposes that a mismatch between the individual's capabilities, the task, and the environment results in the expression of cognitive symptoms (Toglia, 1992). This model provides a framework for simultaneously using and integrating the remedial and functional approaches. In treatment, one needs to begin activities at the information-processing level of the individual. This may require breaking down the components of a task and adapting some features of the environment and task while simultaneously emphasizing practice of a targeted strategy or cognitive subskill. The question of whether occupational therapy intervention should focus on improving or on restoring the impaired cognitive perceptual skills or on capitalizing on the individual's assets should be rephrased to the following set of questions: How much change is expected from the individual? How much is the individual expected to learn and generalize? How much does the task or environment need to be changed or altered to meet the information processing capabilities of the individual? Table 20–6 illustrates how different treatment approaches can be simultaneously used within a functional task by emphasizing the interaction of the individual, the task, and the environment. The factors that influence the selection of treatment are described in the following.

Factors Important in Selecting and Choosing Treatment

As you read the scenarios in Box 20–1, think about the treatment approach that you would emphasize.

The two scenarios describe the same clinical symptoms, but the performance contexts are different. How did the differences in context influence the emphasis in treatment that you would use? What influenced your selection? There is no absolute right or wrong answer.

In scenario 1, the individual is 10 years postinjury, so the potential for change in the underlying cognitive skills is assumed to be minimal. A remedial approach which focuses on improving memory and attention skills would not be warranted unless there was some evidence of potential for further improvement. Compensatory strategies, such as use of a memory notebook or a checklist could be considered; however, the individual denies any difficulty in memory or attention. This lack of insight will present a major obstacle

▼
BOX 20-1

Scenario 1

Mr. X is a 24-year-old with a 10-year history of attention and memory problems related to a head trauma sustained at age 14. He has difficulty recalling conversations and events that occurred just hours before. During performance of a task he easily loses track of the steps and repeats some steps twice, while omitting other steps all together. Mr. X denies any difficulty with his concentration or memory and would like to return to school. He currently lives at home with his parents who care for him.

Scenario 2

Mr. Z is a 64-year-old with attention and memory problems related to a head trauma sustained 3 weeks ago. He has difficulty recalling conversations and events that occurred just hours before. During performance of a task he easily loses track of the steps and repeats some steps twice, while omitting other steps all together. Mr Z is well aware of his difficulties, but is very depressed by them. For example he states "I can't even remember what I ate for breakfast. What good am I? If I have to give up my business, my life is over." Mr. Z was recently widowed and lived alone before his accident.

TABLE 20-6. Integration of Treatment Approaches: The Match Between the Individual, Task, and Environment

Task: Putting on a button down shirt

Task Components that Client has Difficulty With	Improve Underlying Skills of the Person (Remedial)	Person Utilizes a Different Task Method (Compensation)	Adaptation of Task (Other people change the task)	Adaptation of Environment (Other people change the environment)
Difficulty selecting clothes from the closet (requires excessive time and they are often mismatched).			Garments preselected.	Garments removed from busy closet and placed on hanger outside the closet by caregiver.
Put on shirt quickly without properly positioning (eg, puts hand in wrong end of sleeve). Tends to visually focus on parts of objects and fails to appreciate the "whole."	Practice monitoring pacing speed of performance. Scan entire garment. Practice getting an impression of the "whole" before locating the pieces.	Use strategy of finding label to check proper orientation before putting garment on.	Solid garments without distracting patterns selected by caregiver.	
Loses track of sequence of steps (especially when interrupted or distracted).	Practice attending to all steps and monitoring distractions.	Remember to read each step on checklist before execution. Check off each step after completion.	Checklist provided by caregiver.	Quiet environment— telephone, radio turned off.

(Adapted from Toglia, J. [1996]. A multicontext approach to cognitive rehabilitation. Supplemental manual to workshop conducted at Hospital–Cornell Medical Center, New York.)

to independent initiation and use of compensatory strategies. Caregiver training, task and environmental adaptation, as well as the possibility of functional skill training to increase performance on a specified task appear to be the most appropriate areas of treatment emphasis. Treatment techniques to increase awareness (as described later in this section) may be attempted as a prerequisite to use of compensatory aids. External memory aids, such as memory notebook training, may be introduced using task-specific-training methods in combination with maximum prompts and external cues for their use; however, success will likely be dependent on the individual's ability to gain some awareness and acceptance of his disability.

In scenario 2, the individual is only 3 weeks postinjury so that the potential for change in the underlying skills is presumably present. In addition, the individual is very aware of his problems. This would appear to make him a prime candidate for remedial techniques; however, the individual is also very depressed by his deficits. He may not be able to emotionally cope with an approach that focuses on the impairment. An approach that will provide greater opportunities for success and control over his environment may be the initial emphasis in treatment. For example, adaptive techniques in which the caregiver or practitioner presents one-step directions at a time may make it easier for Mr. X to follow task instructions. Training in use of compensatory strategies, such as use of a memory notebook to keep track of daily events and conversations and use of a checklist to assist in keeping track of task steps that have already been completed, may enhance task performance. As Mr. X gains self-confidence and control, remedial tasks that focus on improving attention may be gradually introduced if Mr. X is able to tolerate them.

Some of the factors that influence the selection of treatment include the potential for learning, performance context, personality and emotional characteristics, and awareness. A description of how each of these factors influences the selection of treatment follows.

POTENTIAL FOR LEARNING

The extent to which the practitioner believes that the client has the capacity for change and learning is one major factor that determines the treatment emphasis. As discussed previously, some treatment approaches expect the person to change, whereas others seek to change the task or environment to enhance function. The potential that a person has for learning or further change is evaluated by gathering information from many different sources. As discussed previously, dynamic assessment methods can provide an indication of the person's responsiveness to cues. This information needs to be examined within the context of the length of time since the injury or illness, the stage of recovery, the severity and type of injury, the age of the client, and the prognosis. All of these factors also provide indications for the person's potential for further change. For example, those clients who are younger or have localized lesions may be expected to demonstrate greater recovery than those who

have diffuse injuries or are older. In addition, the length of time in which the practitioner expects to treat the person can influence treatment selection. Suppose for example, that the practitioner only expects to see the client for 1 or 2 weeks. It is unlikely that a remedial approach could make a meaningful change within this time frame. An approach such as adaptation may be more likely to show meaningful changes within a shortened time frame; however, the effects of treatment may be narrow and restricted to the specific task or environment that was adapted.

PERFORMANCE CONTEXT

The expected discharge environment, the individual's premorbid level of functioning, the degree of support from family or friends, the culture and family values, and the skills needed in the discharge environment, all are performance context factors that need to be considered in treatment. A person who lives alone requires a different set of skills than one who is married and has three small children. A person who previously worked as a lawyer requires a different set of cognitive skills to return to work than one who previously worked as a janitor. The cognitive and perceptual skills needed to return to former roles and occupations are individual and vary tremendously. The practitioner needs to analyze the skills, roles, and occupations required for the client to function in his or her environment. This analysis provides the context for goal setting and treatment selection.

EMOTIONAL AND PERSONALITY CHARACTERISTICS: OBSTACLES TO TREATMENT

There are several personality and emotional characteristics that can present obstacles to some of the treatment approaches described in the foregoing. Some of these characteristics may be part of a reaction to the illness and temporary, whereas others may be part of the person's premorbid personality. In either case, these personality blocks need to be identified and the practitioner, along with the team, needs to determine if treatment should assist the client in working through the obstacle or in bypassing it. These characteristics and the effect that they may have on treatment selection are described in the following sections.

Premorbid Personality Characteristics

Some people may have lifelong patterns of personality characteristics that may present obstacles for treatment. For example, consider the person who has always been resistant to change, has always been set in his or her own ways of doing things, and has been unable to modify or change his or her style even when that style has been unsuccessful. It may be particularly difficult for this type of person to adopt compensatory strategies (Gross & Schutz, 1986). Compensation often requires modification of a routine or task. It involves a willingness to change the way one has done something for the past 20 years and adopt a new task method.

Similarly, consider the person who has always been fearful of failure. He or she may have a lifelong pattern of avoidance or withdrawal from difficult situations. Mistakes may have always been accompanied by a defensive position rationalization. This person may not be emotionally capable of dealing with treatment that emphasizes the areas of weakness or impairments. Treatment may need to emphasize opportunities for success and control.

Secondary Psychological Reactions

Secondary psychological reactions following brain injury can cause significant stress, anxiety, and depression, all of which further diminish cognitive functioning. The person with brain injury may experience repeated failures, a loss of hope, a sense of vulnerability and helplessness, a loss of productivity, uncertainty about the future, constant comparison to premorbid functioning by others, a loss of mastery over the environment, a loss of self-esteem, a loss of autonomy, low frustration tolerance, loneliness, and a sense of social isolation. All of these can lead to significant despair and depression (Fine, 1993; Sbordone, 1991). A person who is having difficulty psychologically coping with his or her deficits and is overwhelmed by them may not be able to emotionally deal with tasks that focus on the deficits (eg, remedial approach). Although the person may have the physical and cognitive potential to progress, he or she may not be emotionally ready to participate in an approach that brings out the areas of weakness. Rather then choosing a remedial approach, treatment may initially emphasize a functional approach aimed at providing opportunity for success and control and increasing self esteem and a sense of self-worth.

Helpless Adjustment Style

Some individuals appear to seek dependency, rather than independence. They may not be motivated to learn strategies that would allow them to be independent in self-care skills. For example, a client may state "I am old and I have done everything for everyone else for years. It is time for my family to take care of me." The appearance of helplessness may effectively attract positive attention from family members and friends. A sense of self-esteem may be based on the ability to attract help from others (Gross & Schutz, 1986) . This lack of desire for independence may be either a maladaptive coping style or a value that is shared by the individual's culture or family system. Treatment may need to deemphasize independence in self-care skills and emphasize function in other areas, such as leisure activities. It is essential that the caregiver or family is involved in the goal-setting and treatment-planning process.

Learned Helplessness

Some persons may desire independence but believe that "whatever I do, things won't change. No matter how hard I try, my situation will remain the same." The person who perceives a loss of control over the situation may not persist or actively participate in treatment (Gage & Polatajko, 1994). Treatment for **learned helplessness** may need to emphasize techniques that help the client gain some insight and sense of control over difficulties.

AWARENESS

Lack of awareness is a major obstacle to several of the treatment approaches discussed earlier. It results in poor motivation and compliance, lack of sustained effort and persistence, unrealistic expectations, incongruence between goals of the client and family, impaired judgment and safety, and inability to efficiently use compensatory strategies (Barco et al, 1991; Bergquist & Jacket, 1993). "Clients who lack awareness of their deficits may, if compliant, go through the motions of rehearsing a strategy, but are clearly not engaged in the process. Consequently, the likelihood of the client putting the strategy to functional use is minimal" (Ylvisaker, Szekeres, Sullivan, & Wheeler, 1987, p. 140) . Awareness has been related to positive treatment outcome (Ezrachi, Ben-Yishay, & Kay, 1991; Lam et al, 1988; Melamed, Groswasser, & Stern, 1992).

An inability to choose goals that are realistic and attainable presents a major obstacle to client-centered treatment. The practitioner has to assist the client in focusing on skills needed for the "here and now" and should avoid direct disagreements or confrontations with the client. The caregiver or family should participate in the goal process, and treatment should be aimed toward narrowing any discrepancy between the client's goals and those of the family. The practitioner needs to enthusiastically create a supportive and nonthreatening atmosphere that allows the client to gain insight without accompanying frustration, anxiety, and depression. The way in which treatment sessions are presented sets a tone and atmosphere that can be effective in enhancing active participation in treatment. The following statement is an example of introducing the purpose of cognitive rehabilitation to a client.

"After a brain injury, it is common to have changes in the ability to quickly think and organize information. At times, things may seem like a jumbled jigsaw puzzle. It takes time to sort things out and to recognize the changes that have occurred. The first step in getting better is recognizing and understanding some of the changes that have occurred and getting to know your limits. If you know what type of difficulties you may run into, it will be easier to stay a step ahead. As we do different tasks, I can help you see some of the areas that may give you difficulty so that you can stay a step ahead. This will not be easy, but if you are willing to give this a try, I believe it will make it easier for you to function."

Treatment for clients with decreased awareness of their deficits should emphasize and reinforce the processes of recognizing errors, initiating strategies, and using self-monitoring techniques. Concrete and measurable goals that emphasize the process of error anticipation and recognition should be established for each week and charted or graphed to measure progress (Toglia, 1992). There may be times when a client demonstrates such strong denial and rationalizations of his or her mistakes that they may be unresponsive to therapeutic efforts. For example, a client may say "Yes, I know my memory is not like it used to be, but a lot of people have bad memory—It won't interfere with my ability to work. My memory was never that good... If I forget what I was supposed to do, I'll just ask someone else. What is the big deal?" The type of person who overrationalizes errors is difficult to engage in treatment. As discussed earlier, strong denial may be indicative of a psychological defense reaction, rather than decreased awareness resulting from brain injury. It is important to introduce deficits in a way that promotes self-understanding and control. The entire team, including the family, needs to use a consistent approach to assist the client in gaining awareness. However, the practitioner may need to be prepared to let this client try and fail, but be there when things collapse.

Over the past few years, interest in the area of awareness and awareness training has significantly increased. However, this is still a relatively new area of investigation. Few attempts have been made to systematically address the issues of awareness in treatment, although initial studies indicate that direct intervention may be effective in some groups of clients (Boake, 1991; Cicerone & Giacino, 1992; Soderback, Bengtsson, Ginsburg, & Ekholm, 1992). The following is a description of some of the treatment techniques that can be used to enhance awareness.

Self-Prediction

Self-prediction involves asking the person to anticipate or predict his or her performance on a task. The client may be asked to indicate on a rating scale whether the task will be easy or hard or to predict specific parameters of performance. For example, the accuracy of performance, the time required to complete the task, or the number of verbal cues required, all may be estimated before actually performing a task. The emphasis is on accurately predicting level of performance, rather than on increasing accuracy of performance. Immediately following task performance, the actual performance results are compared with predicted results and any discrepancies are discussed (Toglia, 1991a). Cicerone and Giacino (1992) reported success in the use of self-prediction in two clients with executive dysfunction secondary to head injury.

Feedback

Feedback needs to be direct and consistent. It should be directed at the specific behaviors that are targeted for change. Whenever possible, feedback should be presented in the form of charts or graphs because they are concrete and easily understood. For example, if the goal is to increase use of the memory notebook, every time the client initiates its use, a check mark could be recorded on a chart. This assists the client in recognizing and monitoring the desired behavior.

Videotape Feedback

A videotape of the client that demonstrates the deficit area affecting performance may be used to enhance awareness. Videotape feedback is concrete and it allows the client to see what the difficulty is as it is occurring, rather than discussing it after the fact. Soderback, Bengtsson, Ginsburg, and Ekhom (1992) and Boake (1991) have described the success of videotape feedback in clients with stroke and head injury.

Structured Error Monitoring System

Cicerone and Giacino (1992) describe a procedure during which the client's performance is stopped immediately when an error is made and the client's attention is focused on the error. The client is required to keep a record of his or her own errors and systematically compare responses on subsequent trials.

Self-Evaluation

Immediately following performance of a task, the client may be asked to rate his or herself on targeted behaviors (Toglia, 1991a). Questions may include: "Have I attended to all the necessary information? Did I check over my work?"

Self-Questioning

Questions that are designed to cue the client in monitoring his or her behavior may be written on an index card or memorized by the client. At specific time intervals during the task, the client is expected to stop and answer the same two or three questions such as: "Am I sure that I am looking all the way to the left?; Am I paying attention to the details?; Am I going too quickly?" (Fetherlin & Kurland, 1989).

Role Reversal

The practitioner performs a task and makes cognitive errors. Cognitive symptoms such as distractibility or impulsivity may be exaggerated and role played by the practitioner during the task. The client observes the practitioner's performance and is asked to identify the errors and hypothesize why the errors occurred (eg, the practitioner was distracted by a conversation occurring outside the room). The emphasis of this technique is on increasing error detection skills (Ben-Yishay & Diller, 1983).

▼ WORKING WITH A MULTIDISCIPLINARY TEAM

A strong interdisciplinary approach is needed to address the complexity of issues that arise from cognitive–perceptual problems. In addition to the occupational therapy practitioner, the treatment team may include a neuropsychologist or psychologist, social worker, speech and language pathologist, recreational therapist, and physical therapist. Other disciplines may include nursing, psychiatry, special education, and optometry. Each discipline brings its own perspective and philosophy to the treatment team. It is important that the treatment team discuss their different viewpoints and agree on an overall team philosophy to provide a well-integrated program. Team goals should be identified as well as specific discipline goals. The family and client should be involved in team discussions and provide input into the overall treatment plan.

The multicontext treatment framework can be used to guide an interdisciplinary treatment program. The team should emphasize the same major goals during treatment, rather than working on separate skills. For example, the speech and language pathologist may address attention problems within the context of language material, such as listening to tapes or conversations; the neuropsychologist may use remedial attentional exercises; the physical therapist may reinforce attention through motor tasks; and the occupational therapy practitioner may address attentional strategies within the context of self-care tasks, household tasks, community skills, leisure activities, or work-related tasks. Although the tasks vary, the skills and strategies emphasized may remain similar across the different disciplines, as described in the multicontext approach.

Some treatment teams choose to give the responsibility of training specific cognitive and perceptual skills to specific disciplines. For example, the occupational therapy practitioner addresses visual perceptual problems, whereas the speech and language pathologist addresses language problems, and the psychologist addresses higher-level cognitive problems. Although this clearly delineate roles and prevents duplication of services, it is clearly fragmented and may be more comfortable for the different disciplines than for the client. The client with brain injury is struggling to make sense out of the chaos and confusion in his or her mind. A strong integrated approach that assists the person in seeing patterns of behaviors across different tasks is strongly advocated, rather than one that reinforces only the fragmentation that the client already perceives.

The **certified occupational therapy assistant** works in collaboration and partnership with the registered **occupational therapist** to implement aspects of the occupational therapy intervention plan. Once the targeted behaviors for treatment have been clearly identified, the certified therapy assistant and occupational therapist collaborate to choose a variety of different tasks that can be used to reinforce the desired behaviors. For example, if the use of a checklist to perform multistep tasks has been determined to be an emphasis in the treatment program, the certified therapy assistant may reinforce the use of this strategy during a variety of different activities, such as a trip to the supermarket, planning a meal, or organizing a calendar. The results are discussed with the occupational therapist. Together the occupational therapist and the certified therapy assistant may decide to modify the strategy (decrease the size of the checklist, reduce the number of steps listed to a key outline, or eliminate the need to check off each step as it is completed) or upgrade the complexity of the treatment activities.

▼ ADDRESSING THE COGNITIVE–PERCEPTUAL COMPONENTS

The following section reviews treatment techniques for the cognitive–perceptual components. Each area describes techniques that target change in the person (specific skill training and strategy training), and change in the task and environment (adaptation). Although these techniques are separated for the purpose of discussion, treatment should simultaneously incorporate both areas to meet the information-processing abilities of the client, as discussed earlier in this section. Awareness and self-monitoring techniques should be embedded within treatment approaches that seek to change the person, because the effective use of self-cuing and strategies requires awareness and self-monitoring skills. The Affolter approach and the functional skill training approach are not addressed in this section because they are used in the same way with a wide range of cognitive and perceptual deficits; however, they should be kept in mind as an option for treatment.

Disorientation

Disorientation and confusion are symptoms of severe attention and memory problems and can overshadow performance on all tasks. Treatment can be approached from different perspectives.

SPECIFIC SKILL TRAINING

Reality orientation programs involve reviewing specific information concerning person, place, and time. The key treatment principles are structure and consistency. The same orientation questions or facts should be reviewed several times a day according to an established routine or time schedule. All team members should participate in the program whenever possible. The amount of information reviewed at each session and the expectations for recall should be gradually expanded according to the person's abilities.

Orientation to person is addressed before orientation to place or time. In cases of severe disorientation, the same three or four key personal facts may be reviewed in the form of multiple choice questions, several times a day. If the client has difficulty, additional cues may be provided. For example, if the person does not accurately recall his or her grandchildren's names, pictures of the grandchildren can be shown or the first letter of the names can be provided. Gradually the amount and type of information the individual is asked to recall may be expanded. The individual may be asked to independently retrieve information and may be given additional cues or multiple choices only when necessary.

The daily review of information may be graded by moving from orientation to person and place, toward orientation to time, daily schedule, and current events. The response to each question, as well as the number and type of cues that are needed should be recorded. A fact sheet that includes personal information can be kept in the client's room for use by all team members to verify the correct facts. The emphasis is on increasing the client's ability to retrieve correct orientation facts through repeated questioning. Retrieval of the same information over and over is hypothesized to strengthen the retrieval pathways and increase the likelihood of accurate recall (Harrell, Parente, Bellingrath, & Lisicia, 1992).

A reality orientation program aims to help the individual feel connected to who he or she is. Family members should be asked to bring in a tape of the client's favorite music, a picture album with labels showing family events and holidays, favorite magazines or books, or videotapes of family members or family events. An audiotape or videotape can also be created by a family member to review orientation information and explain what has happened and why the person is in the hospital. These items can be used to assist in cuing the individual to retrieve accurate facts.

Structured orientation review sessions may also be conducted within a group setting. A group setting may enhance attention, motivation, and participation in some clients. Group projects, such as a collage that involves a holiday theme or season, may be used to improve orientation.

Orientation questions can also be incorporated into a bean bag toss game, a board game, or a family feud-style game (Toglia & Golisz, 1990). Each game format places different demands on attention, memory, and orientation. For example, the family feud-style format requires a quick speed of response, whereas the board format requires the ability to keep track on one's turn, playing piece, and position on the board. The cognitive demands of each playing format need to be matched with the abilities of the group.

STRATEGY TRAINING

Strategy training in individuals who demonstrate disorientation consists of training the individual to use external cues to reduce confusion. The individual is trained to look for cues when he or she is feeling confused or is having difficulty recalling orientation information. For example, an information poster that contains orientation facts can be placed on a wall, closet, or eventually inside a drawer or notebook. When the client is asked orientation information, he or she is expected to locate the information poster to verify responses or to find the correct answers. A memory book that includes pictures and names of familiar people, important life events, and such, can also be placed in a key location within the room. An alarm preprogrammed to ring several times a day can be used to cue the individual to read his or her orientation fact book.

A calendar posted on the wall or closet may be helpful in orienting the individual to time. If the individual has poor selective attention, a single piece of paper with the day and date written daily, rather than a monthly calendar, may be needed.

To assist the client in finding his or her room, directional arrows may be placed in the hallway, and tape indicating the route to his or her room can be placed on the floor. Key landmarks can be pointed out and made more salient with arrows or colored tape.

Initiation or use of any of these external cues needs to be immediately reinforced and praised by the practitioner. The practitioner should keep track of each time the individual initiates use of an external cue by recording it on a chart or visual graph. In addition, points can be used to reinforce the desired responses. The frequency of use of external cues should be tracked and gradually faded until the orientation

information is internalized. In addition, the individual should be trained to look for orientation cues (clocks, calendars, or other) in different environments.

ADAPTATION OF TASK OR ENVIRONMENT

An alarm clock or talking watch that automatically announces the date and time on an hourly basis may be used to assist the individual in maintaining orientation to time. An adaptation such as this does not require initiation of the individual. In addition, large brightly colored clocks can be placed in the individual's room, or a large brightly colored sign with the day and date can be placed on the closet door. A large colored sign of the client's name can be placed on the door, to reduce the likelihood of the person entering the wrong room. The saliency of these key items are likely to automatically capture the client's attention without effort. The color and location of the cue signs may need to be changed periodically to prevent habituation (Giles & Wilson, 1993). In addition to the use of external cues, the caregiver may be trained to structure each day with a set routine. Daily repetition of the same schedule may assist in decreasing confusion.

Attention

SPECIFIC SKILL TRAINING

In remedial training, specific components of attention are addressed in a hierarchical manner. Treatment typically begins with simple reaction-time tasks, to address problems in alertness, and progresses to tasks involving attentional flexibility and divided attention. Table 20–7 presents sample treatment activities used to address different attentional components. In general, remedial studies in the area of attention have shown positive results in both brain-injured and schizophrenic populations (Benedict et al, 1994; Ben Yishay et al, 1987; Brown, Harwood, Hays, Heckman, & Short, 1993; Sohlberg & Mateer, 1989a).

In addition to remedial tabletop and computer tasks, gross motor activities such as ball throwing, or hitting a balloon have also been used to increase alertness and reaction time. Shimelman and Hinojosa (1995) found no significant differences on test scores measuring attention following gross motor activity; however, they did note positive changes in attention behaviors, such as scanning and self-checking.

STRATEGY TRAINING

In strategy training, the emphasis is not on training specific attentional skills, but on training use of a strategy to control the emergence of attentional symptoms, such as distractibility, impulsivity, or a tendency to loose track or overfocus on details. Self-instruction is one possible strategy for attentional problems. Self-instruction involves saying each step of a task aloud to focus attention on the task and inhibit distractions and stereotypical behaviors. It may also involve saying self-cues or task instructions out loud. Gradually, the

TABLE 20-7. Attentional Process Training Program (ATP)

Attentional Components	Sample Treatment Tasks
Sustained Attention (Concentration)	• Shape and number cancellation worksheets—Find the target number(s) or shape(s). • Listen for a target number or letter on a tape.
Selective Attention (Focusing attention on selected stimuli)	• A distractor overlay is placed over number and shape cancellation worksheets to make it more difficult to identify the relevant targets. • Listen for target letters or numbers on a tape with the addition of background noise.
Alternating Attention (Switching attention from one stimuli to another)	• Cancellation worksheet—the client is asked to alternate between canceling odd and then even numbers in response to the examiner saying "change." • Worksheet requiring adding or subtracting pairs of numbers in response to the examiner saying "change."
Divided Attention (Paying attention to more than one stimuli at a time)	• Client performs a cancellation worksheet while listening and responding to target numbers or letters on a tape. • Sort cards by suit while turning over any card that contains a target letter in the spelling of its name.

(Sohlberg & Mateer, 1989a)

client is trained to say these cues silently, rather than out loud. Webster and Scott (1983) report the success of using a self-instructional strategy in improving concentration in a 24-year-old male 2 years after a head injury. Other strategies that may be emphasized in treatment include (1) taking "time outs from a task" when concentration begins to fade, (2) remembering to get a sense of the whole situation before attending to the parts, (3) monitoring a tendency to become distracted by either internal thoughts or external stimuli, and (4) remembering to look all over and actively search for additional information before responding.

Strategy training can be integrated within simple or complex tasks, depending on the level of the client. Strategy training begins by identifying a targeted behavior or strategy that influences performance on a wide variety of different tasks and is most responsive to cues, as identified through dynamic assessment procedures. The task parameters under which attentional symptoms emerge are clearly defined. In all cases, the practitioner assists the client in monitoring the use of the targeted strategy or behavior by recording the frequency with which the strategy is initiated and used across different tasks that meet the level of the client.

ADAPTATIONS OF TASK OR ENVIRONMENT

Adaptations designed to minimize attention demands involve reducing or limiting the amount of information presented to the client at any one time. Examples include (1) simplifying task instructions so that only one step is presented at a time, (2) reducing the number of items or choices presented to the client at any one time, (3) preselecting relevant objects needed for tasks, and (4) task segmentation or presenting only one component of a task at a time (Toglia, 1993b). Moulton, Taira, and Grover (1995) found that segmenting the task of feeding and presenting one food item at a time to dementia clients, rather than presenting a cluttered food tray, decreased the amount of assis-

tance required, improved food and fluid intake, and qualitatively improved behavior.

The enhancement or reduction of salient visual cues in the environment can be used to promote desired behaviors. For example, limiting clutter and distraction in the environment, such as taking the telephone off the hook, closing the window, or turning off the radio, can prevent an individual from becoming sidetracked off a task. In the task of brushing teeth, for example, unnecessary items should be removed from the sink, and the items required for use should be made salient with contrasting colors. The contrasting colors of the toothpaste, toothbrush, and cup provide a cue to assist the individual in attending to the different items.

Visual Processing

VISUAL FOUNDATION SKILLS

Treatment of visual foundation skills, such as visual acuity, contrast sensitivity, oculomotor skills, and visual fields, generally involves adaptations and compensation; however, remedial exercises may be recommended for individuals with oculomotor deficits or visual field deficits.

Specific Skill Training

Oculomotor Skills. Range of motion eye exercises to the involved muscle has been advocated for individuals with eye muscle paresis. For example, if the lateral rectus muscle of the right eye is weakened, the individual may be asked to move the eyes as far as possible to the right and "hold it for a few seconds." Optometrists who specialize in vision therapy may recommend specific eye exercises for oculomotor deficits that can be reinforced during occupational therapy sessions and real-life tasks (Efferson, 1995).

Visual Fields. There is some evidence that deficits in visual fields can be decreased with intensive stimulation and training in saccadic eye movements (Warren, 1993; Zihl, 1979, 1981). This can be done by having the individual fixate on a central target on a wall in a dim room while a penlight is used to simultaneously flash a small circle of light within the blind field. The individual is encouraged to guess the location of the light in the blind field.

Adaptations of Task or Environment

Visual Acuity. Deficits in visual acuity are frequently addressed with corrective lenses; however, adaptation of the environment may also be helpful, particularly if eyeglasses are unable to correct acuity. Adaptations that may be beneficial include: (1) large print reading materials, (2) a talking watch or clock, (3) a talking calculator, (4) a telephone with preprogrammed numbers, (5) a telephone with voice recognition, (6) dialing feedback or large numbered buttons, (7) talking books, (8) adaptations to the computer (working with large fonts, using talking word-processing programs, key finders), (9) colored knobs on cabinets or door handles, or (10) magnifiers. In addition, use of halogen and fluorescent light provides high-intensity light with minimal glare. The contrast between objects within a task or the environment should be increased whenever possible. For example, finding a white toothbrush on a white shelf is much more difficult than locating a red toothbrush on a white shelf. Pouring coffee into a white cup may be much safer than pouring coffee into a black cup.

Oculomotor. Patching one eye according to different schedules may be recommended by an optometrist or ophthalmologist to eliminate double vision during task performance. One type of eye-patching regimen is to alternate the patch on each eye on a daily or hourly basis. Time without the patch may be recommended so that the eyes will attempt to gain fusion. Some eye specialists do not advocate eye patching at all because it may contribute to eye weakness and discourage any attempts by the brain to overcome the double vision. Fresnel prisms, applied to the client's eyeglasses, may be recommended as an alternative to eye patching to reduce or eliminate double vision (Efferson, 1995).

Visual Field Deficits. Prisms place a peripheral image to a more central area of the retina. Rossi, Kheyfets, and Reding (1990) found that prisms improved visual perceptual test performance in stroke clients with visual field cuts or unilateral inattention. However, scores on a functional assessment did not improve. The effectiveness of prisms and its carryover to function needs further study. Prisms distort the visual world and clients with visual perceptual problems may have difficulty adjusting to them.

VISUAL SCANNING AND UNILATERAL INATTENTION
Specific Skill Training

Visual Scanning. Training that aims at increasing the speed, scope, and organization of visual scanning has been used to train individuals to compensate for visual field deficits as well as to address problems in unilateral inattention. Kerkhoff, MunBinger, and Meier (1994) found that systematic training of saccadic eye movements in clients with visual field deficits increased visual search field sizes, restored oculomotor functions, and improved performance in functional visual activities. Williams (1995) described an individual with a scotoma in the central field who demonstrated functional gains with a scanning program that aimed at improving the speed and preciseness of saccadic eye movements.

Unilateral Inattention. Visual-scanning training has also been used to remediate **unilateral inattention**. However, the emphasis in this treatment is not on the preciseness and speed of eye movements, but on increasing awareness and attention to the affected side. In unilateral inattention, clients demonstrate a decrease in eye movements to the affected side. This decrease in eye movements reflects a decrease in attention to one side of the environment (Toglia, 1991b). Several authors have reported that visual-scanning training improves performance on specific tasks, but the effects do not generalize to functional performance (Ross, 1992; Wagenaar, Van Wieringen, Netelenbos, Meijer, & Kuik, 1992). However, these studies used only one or two graded scanning tasks during treatment. In contrast, studies that have reported positive functional outcomes have used a wider combination of treatment tasks. Antonucci and colleagues (1995) and Pizzamiglio and colleagues (1992) have reported functional gains following a visual-scanning program that involved practicing visual scanning in four different types of scanning tasks. Training included practice in functional activities. Antonucci and associates (1995) also suggests that differences in the intensity and duration of treatment may account for differences in outcome between different studies. Studies that have 5 to 8 weeks of training at least three times a week have produced more positive results.

Scanning tasks usually involve locating specific letters, numbers, shapes, or objects from an array of stimuli. Remedial exercises include cancellation tasks, such as putting a line through all the letter "As" on a page, or circling all the "thes" in a paragraph. Large-sized scanning boards can be constructed or purchased that require scanning and reaching in larger space. Computerized scanning programs are available that involve quickly locating or matching a shape, letter, or number that appears on the screen in random locations. These programs generally provide information on the time it takes for the individual to locate targets in different quadrants of the visual field. Electronic-scanning devices, such as the Dynavision 2000, have also been used to practice quickly locating and following targets in the visual fields. The Dynavision 2000 is a large electronic-scanning board in which the user has to hit lighted target buttons before they are extinguished. The apparatus can generate a variety of different types of scanning and reaction time tasks. Klavora, et al (1995) found that visual reaction time and scanning training with the Dynavision 2000 improved driving performance in stroke clients with marked visual and attentional difficulties.

The space in which scanning is required needs to be considered when designing treatment. Some individuals have more difficulty searching for items in large spaces, whereas others have more difficulty with tasks involving detailed inspection in smaller spaces. Scanning in large spaces can be easily combined with motor goals. Items such as playing cards or everyday objects can be spread on the floor, wall, or table to encourage reaching, weight shift, or specific motor patterns.

Because unilateral inattention has been hypothesized to be related to a decreased level of arousal on the affected side, gross motor activities that increase general arousal and alertness have been used in combination with scanning activities to increase attention to the affected side. Studies have found that vestibular input with caloric stimulation increases gaze and attention to the affected field (Cappa, Sterzi, Vallar, & Bisiach, 1987). In addition to vestibular input, tactile input may also aid in visual scanning. For example, Warren (1993) suggests that scanning training will be more effective if the client is required to physically manipulate what he or she is scanning.

Weinberg and colleagues (1977) designed systematic training techniques that incorporated a combination of remedial and strategy training techniques during reading and scanning tasks. For example, they used graded anchoring, pacing the speed of scanning, feedback, and decreasing the density of the stimulus. Anchoring involves placing a vertical line in the left hand margin of the page to serve as a cue to attend to the left. The individual is instructed to find the anchor before reading each line. Initially a red line may be used to capture attention to the left side. Gradually the saliency of the cue may be faded and a thin pencil line can be used as an anchor. Each line may also be numbered sequentially on both sides to assist clients in orienting themselves spatially to a page and in moving from one line to another without skipping lines (Diller et al, 1974; Weinberg et al, 1977).

Recently, Robertson, Tegner, Tham, Lo, and Smith (1995) taught clients with chronic unilateral inattention to mentally tell themselves to "pay attention". Although the focus was on the general ability to sustain attention, rather than on directly addressing visual scanning, significant improvements in unilateral inattention as well as sustained attention were found. This suggests that unilateral inattention may be remediated by techniques aimed at general attentional skills, rather than focused visual-scanning training.

Strategy Training

Scanning strategies need to be trained within tasks that meet the information-processing abilities of the client. Table 20–8 describes task parameters that can be used as a guide in grading the difficulty of visual-scanning treatment activities.

During treatment some task parameters are held constant, while others are changed. For example, the number of items, and the horizontal arrangement may be held constant while the task is graded in difficulty by narrowing the spacing between items. This requires strategies aimed at pacing the speed of visual scanning and paying attention to details. On the other hand, changing the arrangement of items from a horizontal predictable pattern to an unpredictable scattered pattern requires a more systematic and organized approach to the task. Different visual search strategies can be emphasized by manipulating the features of the task. In treatment, some task parameters are held constant, while others are varied to emphasize particular skills and strategies.

Internal strategies that may be emphasized in a variety of different situations include teaching the client to consciously employ a systematic and organized scanning method, such as initiating search on the affected side and scanning in an organized pattern (eg, horizontally, vertically, or circular). Treatment should assist the client in identifying task arrangements that require different types of scanning patterns. For example, the client needs to recognize that stimuli arranged in horizontal rows is scanned most efficiently with a left-right horizontal scanning pattern. In addition, clients need practice in recognizing the type of visual situations in which they are most vulnerable to missing information or making errors.

Persons with unilateral inattention do not always know when they are attending to the left side. They frequently think that they are looking to the left when, in fact, they are not. Treatment needs to assist clients in finding external cues that will provide feedback about when they are attending to the left. An emphasis in treatment should include teaching the client to find the edges of a page or the periphery of stimuli, before beginning a task, and marking it with an anchor such as colored tape, a colored highlighter, a bright object, or placement of his or her arm. For example, clients with unilateral inattention may be instructed to "look for your left hand as you are doing the task. When you see your left hand, then you know you are on the left side." Robertson (1991) and Robertson, North, and Geggie (1992) have reported that use of the affected upper extremity for pointing or reaching during search tasks activates or enhances somatosensory spatial representation and decreases unilateral inattention. The use of auditory cuing has also been used successfully to decrease unilateral inattention. In a case report described by Seron, Deloche, and Coyette (1989), a beeper or alarm device was placed in the client's left-sided pocket. The client was required to scan space and attend to the left to turn off the sound.

The visual search strategies described in the foregoing can be integrated within a wide variety of tasks. For example the client can practice scanning or locating specific information in train schedules, spreadsheets, the telephone book, menus, calendars, movie clocks, or maps. He or she may practice (1) finding all the dimes or paper clips in a

TABLE 20-8. Grading Visual Scanning Tasks

Task Parameter	Easy (Less attention and effort)		Difficult (Greater attention and effort)	Demands with Increased Complexity
Discriminability	Target items are easy to discriminate and grossly different from surrounding items	→	Target items are more detailed and similar to the surrounding items	Greater demands on visual acuity, contrast sensitivity, selective visual attention, ability to recognize distinctive cues, pattern recognition
Arrangement	Organize into predictable format such as horizontal rows	→	Randomly scattered and/or overlapping so that some features of objects are partially obscured	Greater demands on saccadic eye movements, strategies to keep track of visual stimuli, ability to change search pattern
Spacing Between Stimuli	Even-spaced distance between each item and each line	→	Items are close together and/or unevenly spaced	Greater demands on saccadic eye movements and focal attention
Amount	Only one or two items are presented at any one time	→	Increased amount of items are presented simultaneously	Greater demands on selective attention, and strategies to keep track of visual stimuli
Predictability	The client knows the exact number of targets that need to be found	→	The number of targets is unknown	Greater initiation of exploration and search in peripheral fields
Timing	Untimed	→	Time limit for search	Greater demands on reaction time, sustained attention and the speed of oculomotor skills
Meaningfulness	Meaningful and familiar stimuli provide a context which cues visual search	→	Unfamiliar or meaningless stimuli (eg, random string of numbers, pictures, words)	Greater demands on initiation and visual search. Fewer cues to direct eye movements and visual search
Number of targets and rules	Find one target item	→	Find two or more different items (eg, "Cross out the letters, A and H, when they are preceded by the letter O")	Greater demands on visual memory and the ability to keep track of visual information
Size of Space	Space for scanning is large (not always easier)	→	Space for scanning is small (This is not necessarily harder)	Greater dependence on peripheral fields and visual search. Requires initiation of active visual exploration
Sample activity	4 objects on the bathroom counter—cup, toothbrush, comb and razor. Find the toothbrush (objects are grossly different)	→	Looking at a large menu. Identify the number of meat items between $8.00 and $11.00	Nearly all task parameters are changed to illustrate simple and complex visual scanning tasks. In treatment, only one or two task parameters should be changed at any one time

draw with scattered and overlapping objects, (2) finding specific items in a draw or shelf or magazine, (3) scanning for a particular type of a greeting card, (4) locating items within a certain price range in a food circular , and (5) scanning a bookshelf or supermarket shelf for a particular item. The movement pattern, context, and content of the tasks should vary while the same strategy is practiced repeatedly in tasks that match the abilities of the client.

Unilateral inattention is frequently accompanied by disturbances in awareness. Any treatment program must incorporate awareness training techniques, such as those described earlier (Diller & Riley, 1993). Videofeedback, self-prediction, self-questioning, and self-instructional techniques all can be integrated into the treatment of unilateral inattention (Toglia, 1991b). Frequently, clients with unilateral inattention demonstrate improvement when they are cued to use a strategy. However, these same clients may not spontaneously carryover use of the strategy independently due to decreased ability to anticipate and recognize errors. Awareness training and self-monitoring strategies need to be deeply embedded within treatment.

Adaptations of Task or Environment for Unilateral Inattention

To minimize the need to attend to the left, it has been suggested the environment be rearranged so that key items such as the telephone, nurse call button, bedside table, and radio or television are on the affected side. However, a study by Kelly and Ostreicher (1985) found no significant difference in functional outcome in clients whose hospital rooms were rearranged in this way.

Lennon (1994) described the successful use of large colored paper markings on the edges of tables, corners, and elsewhere to prevent collision in clients with unilateral inattention. The clients were trained to look for these markers. Markers were gradually faded. Performance improved and was maintained with removal of markers; however, effects did not generalize to other environments. Calvanio, Levine, and Petrone (1993) described use of an adapted plate to increase feeding skills in a client with a severe case of left inattention and a dense left hemianopia. The authors devised a sectioned plate with raised edges that was mounted on a lazy Susan so that it could be rotated. As the client pushed at her food with the fork, the plate rotated so that all the food eventually came into view. This eliminated the need for scanning or head turning to the left.

VISUAL DISCRIMINATION, VISUAL SPATIAL, AND VISUAL CONSTRUCTIONAL SKILLS: SPECIFIC DEFICITS

Specific Skill Training

The deficit-specific approach to visual perception addresses deficits in specific visual perceptual skills through graded tabletop worksheets, exercises, and practice drills (Siev, Freishtat, & Zoltan, 1986). Computer-assisted visual perceptual tasks that simulate tabletop worksheets and exercises are also used in treatment. Such tasks have the advantage of providing a controlled rate of stimulus presentation, an objective record of the client's accuracy and speed of discrimination, and objective feedback (Ross, 1992).

Basic visual perceptual skills, such as difficulty in discriminating objects or shapes, are addressed in treatment by repetitively practicing object or shape matching and identification skills. Real objects are used before line drawings of objects .

Specific deficits in form constancy are addressed by practicing identifying and matching objects that have subtle differences in size, position, or shape. Figure-ground discrimination is practiced by identifying objects or shapes presented within an array of other objects, and visual closure is practiced by identifying objects that are partially hidden.

Complex visual-processing skills are addressed by using tasks that require matching abstract designs or detailed shapes, or identifying subtle differences between complex pictures or designs. The target designs or shapes may be rotated to address spatial skills, fragmented to address visual closure skills, or embedded within another figure or scene to address figure-ground skills.

Tasks that involve copying designs are used to practice visual spatial and constructional skills. For example, copying pegboard designs, dot-to-dot designs, block designs, or parquetry block designs of increasing difficulty require the ability to position and arrange items in their proper spatial relations. Block design tasks may be graded by copying the block designs directly on top of the design card to copying the construction next to the design card. They are also graded by moving from a three-dimensional to a two-dimensional model or design card. Neistadt (1989) suggests that parquetry block designs can be graded from easiest to hardest as follows: (1) colored cards with the outline of each block; (2) black and white cards with the outline of each block; (3) colored cards without the outline of all the blocks; and (4) black and white cards without the outline of all of the blocks. There is currently no evidence that training on visual perceptual worksheets or block designs and parquetry blocks generalizes to function.

Strategy Training

In strategy training, treatment aims to maximize the client's ability to process visual information by providing strategies to enhance his or her ability to take in and assimilate information efficiently. Different task parameters can be manipulated to emphasize different visual-processing strategies. Table 20–9 and Table 20–10 illustrate this and provide guidelines for grading visual discrimination tasks. Treatment involves a careful manipulation of tasks parameters—holding some task parameters constant while systematically changing others to emphasize specific aspects of visual processing. The use of strategies is practiced within tasks that match the visual processing level of the client. Strategy training targets behaviors that have been identified as available to clients and responsive to cuing.

Adaptation of Task or Environment

The key guideline in minimizing the effects of visual perceptual difficulties is to make the distinctive features of objects more salient with color cues. An example is placing color tape on buttons to operate appliances or using salient color cues on objects to make them easier to locate and discriminate (eg, bright pink tape on a medication bottle to make it easier to identify in the medicine cabinet). Cues, such as colored marks or tape at spatial landmarks (tape recorder, wheelchair footrests), reduce spatial demands and makes it easier to orient and align pieces together.

Written material can be perceived with greater ease if there are spaces between lines and a felt tip pen is used to provide greater contrast instead of a pencil. Paper with raised lines makes it easier for clients with spatial difficulties to maintain alignment of lines during writing.

Visual stimuli, such as items on a shelf or sentences on a page, that are large and are arranged in an organized manner, with large spaces between items, are easier to perceive. Consistent locations for objects in the refrigerator, closet, or drawer increase predictability and provide contextual cues for recognition.

The caregiver should be instructed to decrease visual distractions in the room or within a task by limiting designs,

TABLE 20-9. Visual Discrimination: Task Grading

Task Parameters	Simple (Less attention and effort) →	Complex (Greater attention and effort)	Demands with Increased Complexity
Familiarity of stimuli	Familiar stimuli (eg, simple shapes, everyday objects, letters, words) →	Less familiar (eg, unusual objects, abstract unfamiliar shapes)	More difficult to pick up distinctive features
Directions	Structured (eg, matching or point to specific items) →	Unstructured (eg, "Tell me what you see")	Requires initiation and organized visual search strategies
Distinctive features	Readily apparent (eg, regular pen—the pen point is the distinctive feature) →	Obscure or partially hidden features (eg, novelty pen that looks like a candy cane)	Greater visual attention. More difficult to recognize objects—Increased likelihood of misperception
Degree of detail	Little to no detail →	Fine detail	Greater demands on visual attention
Contrast	High contrast (eg, red sock with white socks) →	Low contrast (eg, light beige and white socks)	Harder to determine where one item ends and another begins; greater demands on selective attention
Background	Soft backgrounds, solids, non-patterned → →	Confusing and distracting backgrounds, patterns	Greater visual selective attention
Context	Within environmental context (eg, grooming item in bathroom)	Outside of context (eg, grooming item in therapy area)	Greater visual attention to critical features. Fewer cues for recognition

Task parameters such as the amount and arrangement, which are described in Table 20-8, are also applicable to visual discrimination.

TABLE 20-10. Constructional Task Grading

Task Parameters	Simple	→	Complex	Demands with Increased Complexity
Model	3D model to copy	→	No model: figure out how the pieces fit together	Greater demands on planning and problem-solving strategies
Familiarity	Prior experience	→	Unfamiliar	Greater visual analysis and discrimination
Number of pieces, lines, or details	1–2	→	>12	Greater selective attention and discrimination
Spatial alignment	Nonprecise	→	Precise placement and orientation of angles, pieces	Greater attention to detail
Regularity of pieces	All same size and shape	→	Pieces are different sizes and shapes	Greater discrimination
Color	Different colored pieces	→	Pieces are all the same color	Less contrast, greater spatial analysis
Choose stimuli	Use preselected pieces. Design provides outline for placement of each piece	→	Decide and find pieces from a large array	Greater demands on visual search, discrimination, planning, and decision making
Error feedback	Immediate feedback with errors (eg, pieces do not fit together or construction collapses)	→	Requires close inspection to detect errors	Greater self-monitoring. Harder to recognize and detect errors

(Adapted from Toglia J. [1993]. Treating individuals with constructional apraxia. Handouts from presentation at AOTA—Advanced Apraxia Institute: Assessing and Treating Adults. Denver, CO, Dec. 3–4, 1993.)

patterns, and using solid colors with high contrast. Patterns, designs, and decorations make it harder to select and recognize critical features of an object. For example, Mr. D saw a paper clip with a bright pink decorative heart decal on it. He looked at the object and thought it was something rather peculiar. He did not recognize it as a paper clip. When the therapist covered the decoration, he immediately recognized the object. The brightly colored decoration had captured his visual attention and made it difficult for him to recognize the distinctive features. Although treatment focused on recognizing critical features of objects, the use of patterns and designs were avoided on clothes to enhance his ability to dress.

The caregiver should also be trained to introduce only a small amount of visual information at one time. For example, during grooming, the caregiver may be instructed to have no more than two objects on the sink counter at the same time. When the client is finished with the first two objects needed for the task, the caregiver introduces the next two objects.

Motor Planning

SPECIFIC SKILL TRAINING: LIMB APRAXIA

Treatment of motor-planning deficits may emphasize either the production aspect or the conceptual aspect of motor planning (Roy, 1985). Techniques that address the orientation of an object or limb in space, or the timing, sequence, and organization of the motor elements, aim to enhance the pro-

duction aspect of motor planning. For example, if a movement pattern is performed in an awkward or clumsy manner with unnecessary fixation or movements, the therapist may provide physical contact to limit the inappropriate or extraneous movements while simultaneously using guiding methods to facilitate a smooth motor pattern. Hand over hand assistance or light touch may be used to guide a movement pattern along a specific trajectory pattern or to guide the manipulation of objects (Okkema, 1993). Through repeated practice in different tasks, such as reaching for an object on a shelf or washing one's face, the client begins to learn the movement patterns that feel "right," and the therapist gradually withdraws assistance. For some persons, light touch on the distal components of the extremity may be more effective in guiding motor patterns, whereas for others heavier contact and deep pressure may be more effective. It should be kept in mind that deep proprioceptive input and contact has an inhibitory effect on normal people, whereas light touch tends to have a more facilitatory effect (Farber, 1993).

Familiar tasks that are performed in context are easier for persons with motor-planning disorders because the context provides cues that facilitate the desired action. Treatment can be graded by gradually introducing tasks and environments that have less stability and predictability, such as negotiating around obstacles in a crowded store. Table 20–11 provides guidelines for grading and manipulating tasks parameters in treatment. In grading motor-planning tasks, it is suggested that only one or two task parameters are changed

TABLE 20-11. Task Grading for Motor Planning		
Simple	→	**Complex**
Automatic, overlearned tasks	→	Unfamiliar tasks
Everyday objects	→	Less familiar objects
Single gestures	→	Gestures involving multiple movement elements
Meaningful gestures	→	Meaningless gestures
Transitive gestures (eg, brushing teeth)	→	Intransitive gestures (eg, salute)
1–2 steps	→	Multiple steps
Imitation	→	Movement to command
Small object or target	→	Large object or target
Total body movements	→	Discrete smaller movements
Movement toward body	→	Movement away from body
Bilateral	→	Unilateral
Proximal movements required	→	Distal movements
Symmetrical	→	Asymmetrical
Repetitive actions, movements	→	Nonrepetitive
In context	→	Out of context
Stable, predictable, stationary environment	→	Changing, unpredictable, moving environment
Closed loop	→	Open loop
Fixed posture (stationary)	→	Dynamic posture (in motion)

Note: Transitive gestures involve pretended object use: Intransitive gestures do not involve pretended object use (From Toglia J. [1993]. Treating individuals with limb apraxia. Handouts from presentation at AOTA—Advanced Apraxia Institute: Assessing and Treating Adults. Denver, CO, Dec 3–4, 1993.)

at a time while the other parameters are held constant. However, the context in which the task is performed should vary widely. Clients who uses a lot of extra fixation, cocontraction, or proximal movements may benefit from biofeedback, or sensory feedback, to limit extraneous movements and inhibit unnecessary fixation patterns.

Treatment that addresses the conceptual aspect of motor planning focuses on facilitating the client's understanding of how an object is used or a gesture is performed. Remedial treatment techniques involve practicing the ability to use gestures, objects, or pantomime according to a hierarchical treatment sequence and have been described in the literature (Cubelli, Trentini, & Montagna, 1991; Helm-Estabrooks, 1982).

STRATEGY TRAINING

Clients may be taught to use verbal, visual, or tactile cues to enhance movement. For example, the client may be taught a mental practice strategy. Before performing a task, the client imagines himself or herself performing the task in a smooth, accurate, and coordinated manner. Visual imagery or mental practice may be enhanced by asking the client to arrange a picture or action sequence of the task. In addition, the person may be asked to imagine how an object should look in his or her hand before picking it up—for example, imagine the orientation of the object, the way the fingers should be positioned, and so forth. Incorrect patterns of movement, such as holding an object the wrong way, can also be visualized with an emphasis on having the client mentally practice correcting the movement.

In addition to visual mental practice, the client can be taught to verbally rehearse an action sequence by rehearsing the steps out loud, then gradually whispering the steps, and finally, saying them silently. Self-monitoring strategies can be used to teach a client to monitor unnecessary cocontraction, incomplete actions, or difficulty in switching direction of movements.

Another strategy is to teach a client to associate the movement pattern with a rhyme, rhythm, musical tune, visual image, or word. Initially, the musical tune or rhythm may be provided externally; then gradually, the client should imagine the rhythm or tune silently to himself or herself while performing the task.

ADAPTATION OF TASK OR ENVIRONMENT

Attention to the critical features of a task can facilitate action and motor planning. Techniques that increase the saliency of a task include (1) colored tape on the handle of a draw, utensil, or faucet to assist the client in proper grasp placement; (2) use of a fluorescent color ball to make it easier to catch or hit; and (3) use of a colored nail to make it easier to hit with a hammer. Attention to the wrong cue or less important cues can result in an inappropriate motor response and can interfere with actions. Thus, patterns and designs on utensils, clothing, or other items should be avoided.

Other adaptations include training the caregiver to modify task instructions so that the activity is broken into one command at a time (Lamm-Warburg, 1988). Simple whole commands (eg, "Get up") may put the activity on an automatic level and effectively enhance motor planning .

Adaptive equipment should be selected with caution for the apraxic client. For example, some adaptations such as a button hook, one-handed can opener, reacher, one-handed shoe tying, or one-arm drive wheelchair may be confusing for clients with **apraxia** and place greater demands on motor-planning abilities. Other adaptations such as elastic waist trousers, elastic buttons, Velcro fasteners, wash mitts, slip-on shoes, or elastic shoelaces may simplify the task or motor pattern required to manipulate or hold objects, reduce the number of steps, and facilitate function in the client with apraxia.

Memory

SPECIFIC SKILL TRAINING

Memory exercises and drills have been used in attempts to remediate memory. These repetitive exercises that involve practicing remembering numbers, letters, words, shapes, or locations are commonly seen in computerized memory remediation programs. Although memory has been shown to improve on specific training tasks, there is little to no evidence that such training generalizes to other material. Some investigators have suggested that an indirect approach to the treatment of memory disorders may be most effective.

Memory deficits can be closely related to other cognitive deficits, particularly attention. An indirect approach treats other cognitive skills, such as attention or organization, rather than memory itself. Although memory is not addressed directly in treatment, it is expected to increase as a result of improvement in other cognitive skills (Toglia, 1993a). For example, Sohlberg and Mateer (1989b) reported improvement in memory function following a remedial attentional program. In addition to remedial approaches, functional skill training has been used successfully to teach clients with severe memory disorders rote, but complex tasks.

STRATEGY TRAINING

Another method commonly used to address memory problems is the training of internal strategies. Memory strategies may be directed primarily at encoding operations (getting information in) or the retrieval phase of memory (getting information out). Encoding strategies include (1) chunking or grouping similar items together, (2) the story method or linking a series of facts or events into a story, (3) rehearsal or repeating information over and over to oneself, and (4) rhymes or recalling a fact by changing the fact into a rhyme. Retrieval strategies include (1) alphabetical searching or going through the alphabet letter by letter attempting to find the first letter of a forgotten item, (2) retracing ones steps backward to find a missing object or to recall an event, and

(3) thinking of associated information to cue the recall of a new fact or event. Training in internal strategies is most appropriate for individuals with mild memory deficits or for those who have other areas of cognition intact. The client needs to practice using one or two targeted memory strategies in a variety of different tasks such as remembering a telephone number, news headlines or events, items that need to be bought in a store, stories, or instructions to an activity (Harrell et al, 1992). During practice on different memory tasks, a variety of self-monitoring techniques may also be used (Toglia, 1993a).

Self-Questioning Cards

While studying the items to be remembered, the client is given a cue card with questions such as: "Am I trying to group together related items? Am I repeating each item to myself several times?"

Prediction

The client is asked to predict his or her score before and immediately following a memory task.

Memory External Strategies and Aids

External aids include (1) timers, (2) tape recorders, (3) alarm clocks, (4) electronic devices, (5) computers, (6) pillbox organizers, (7) lists, (8) daily planners, and (9) notebooks. External aids, such as notebooks or tape recorders, store information that the individual may have difficulty remembering. Other aids, such as alarm clocks, serve to remind an individual to perform an action. The successful use of an external memory aid requires training. The client needs to practice initiating and using the aid in a variety of different situations.

The introduction of external aids may need to be graded during treatment. In the initial stages, the client may be expected to use the aid only when its use is initiated by another person. Gradually, the client may be trained to initiate the use of the aid independently. The number of times the person initiates or carries the external aid can be charted, graphed, or awarded points, to provide concrete positive feedback and enhance motivation. The most commonly used external memory strategy is the memory notebook. The memory notebook needs to be designed with the individual's needs and lifestyle in mind. Sample sections in a memory notebook could include (1) personal facts, (2) names of people to remember, (3) calendar and schedule, (4) things to do (daily, within next week), (5) daily log of important events, (6) conversations, (7) important upcoming events, (8) summary of readings (articles, newspaper), (9) medication schedule, and (10) directions to frequently traveled places. Initially, the notebook should begin with one or two sections and gradually increase if the client is able to handle it. Table 20–12 lists some of the common obstacles that need to be addressed during memory notebook training.

Memory notebook training needs to take place within the context of a variety of activities. Therapy sessions may include practicing initiating reading or taking notes in the memory notebook. For example, the client may be asked to (1) summarize simulated or actual conversations, (2) take telephone messages, (3) listen and summarize the news or an interview on the radio or television, (4) summarize an article, or (5) summarize the key steps in a new recipe, game, or task. In addition the client may be asked questions that involve reviewing and rereading the memory notebook. Sohlberg and Mateer (1989c) outline three phases of memory notebook training. In the acquisition phase, the client is taught the purpose and names of different notebook sections through systematic and repetitive questioning. The application phase involves role-playing situations in which the individual is expected to document in the notebook, and the adaptation phase involves training within the context of functional activities.

ADAPTATIONS OF TASK OR ENVIRONMENT

Tasks and environments can be rearranged so that they place fewer requirements on memory. Examples include (1) cue cards or signs in key places (eg, sign on door before leaving—"take keys and. . ."), (2) labeling the outside of drawers or closets to minimize the need to recall the location of items, (3) providing directions one step at a time to reduce memory demands, and (4) providing checklists to assist in keeping track of task steps. The caregiver can also be trained to use methods that increase the likelihood that the client will remember material, such as (1) asking the individual to repeat any instructions or important information in his or her own words, (b) encouraging the person to ask questions, and (3) presenting the material in small groups, clusters, or categories (Wilson, 1995).

Executive Functions, Organization, Problem Solving

SPECIFIC SKILL TRAINING

Executive functions are best addressed with unstructured tasks that require the individual to initiate and plan goals, monitor time, make choices, and establish priorities. Commercial games, such as Mastermind, Sequence, and Othello, can be modified and graded to address planning skills, generating different alternatives, and fully analyzing the situation befor making a move. Typical remedial tasks for organization include (1) associating objects that belong together, (2) identifying the similarities or differences between two words or objects, (3) grouping picture cards into categories, and (4) sequencing a series of action pictures. Logic worksheets, logic grids, and puzzles, such as the Tower of London and Tower of Hanoi, have been used to address problem-solving skills.

STRATEGY TRAINING

Verbal mediation has been reported to be an effective strategy in improving executive function and self-regulation

TABLE 20-12. Obstacles to the Use of a Memory Book and Techniques for Overcoming Them

Obstacles	Sample Techniques
Decreased insight into memory problems	• Use book that looks "normal" or less conspicuous • Write explanation for book and place inside cover of book • Videotape or audiotape of discussion involving importance of book • Highlight forgotten information during rereading • Use of prediction and estimation techniques
Initiate carrying memory book	• Book is kept in a consistent location • Signs in room; on door etc. that say "Take Book" • Book is a distinctive color (eg, yellow, orange) • Positive reinforcement, praise, or points for carrying book
Difficulty initiating writing and rereading memory book	• Preprogrammed message alarms • Posted signs (eg, "Read Book") • Positive reinforcement; scoring system • Use during therapy—not after • Consistent daily time schedule for writing or rereading book • Log in immediately after an event or session—gradually lengthen time of entries
Difficulty finding the correct place to write in the book	• A system for discarding old or useless information • Daily review of notebook sections • Start with only one or two color-coded sections • Bookmark or "Post it" to mark the page and date to write on
Difficulty including the relevant information	• Structured note taking: Each page contains an outline—Gradually reduce the structure • Practice having patient ask others to clarify or summarize conversations to assist journal entry • Increase effectiveness and efficiency of note taking: Practice summarizing; identifying the main point of articles, conversations and so on • Place checkmark or star next to "good" entries • Practice in reducing notes to "key retrieval cues"; single words; phrases

(Adapted from Toglia, J [1996]. A multicontext approach to cognitive rehabilitation. Supplement manual to workshop conducted at New York Hospital–Cornell Medical Center, New York.)

deficits (Cicerone & Wood, 1987; Von Cramon, Matthes-Von Cramon, & Mai, 1991). For example, Cicerone and Wood (1987) report the successful use of a self-instructional procedure in a client with impaired planning ability and poor self-control secondary to head injury. Intervention involved requiring the client to verbalize a plan of action before and during execution of a task. Gradually, the client was instructed to whisper, rather than talk aloud, and eventually, talk silently to himself. Generalization to real-life situations was observed after an extended time period that included training in self-monitoring.

Training in problem-solving strategies frequently involves teaching the person the steps of the problem-solving process. The goal in treatment is to replace an impulsive and disorganized approach with a systematic and controlled approach to planning and solving problems. This approach has been used with individuals with schizophrenia as well as with individuals with brain injury. A problem-solving framework such as IDEAL (Table 20–13) (Bransford & Stein, 1984) can be practiced in a variety of different tasks. The steps of the problem-solving process are reinforced with use of self-questioning techniques. For example, self-questioning cue cards with the following types of questions can be used during problem-solving tasks:

• What do I need to do?
• Do I need more information?
• What do I have to do next?
• Am I getting stuck?
• Have I identified all the critical information?
• Do I understand the problem?
• Am I being sidetracked by irrelevant details?
• Am I becoming stuck in one approach?
• What are all the possible solutions? Did I choose the best one?

The problem-solving strategies described in the foregoing can be practiced in simulated or actual functional problem-solving situations. Table 20–13 provides a description of the features of simple and complex problem-solving tasks.

Broad checklists or task guidance systems are commonly used to assist the individual in initiating, planning, and carrying out a task systematically. Checklists may be specific to a particular task (eg, checklist for making a salad), or they may be designed broadly so that they can be used in a variety of similar tasks (eg, checklist for food preparation or cooking tasks).

Treatment should incorporate practice in identifying the situations or tasks in which use of a checklist may be help-

TABLE 20-13. Task Grading for Problem Solving

	Simple	Complex	Demands with Increased Complexity	Sample Complex Treatment Tasks
Identify the problem	Immediate problem is clear and readily apparent. Examples: Shampoo bottle is empty; toaster is unplugged.	Requires sorting out information to determine where the real problem exists.	Places greater demand on initiation; exploration, attention to the environment and the ability to predict ahead, establish goals.	Emphasis on problem recognition or selection of goals. Recognize that a bill entry is missing in a checkbook activity.
Define the problem precisely	All the necessary information is presented. A small amount of information relevant to the problem is presented.	Requires searching for additional information needed to solve the problem. A large amount of information: both relevant and irrelevant is included.	Greater demands on selective attention strategies, choosing priorities, simultaneously attending to details and keeping the whole situation in mind. Requires processing of multiple information and strategies for keeping track of a large number of factors.	Emphasis on discriminating between relevant and irrelevant information (eg, identifying relevant information in a travel advertisement or "Find the two least expensive restaurants that deliver lunch in the area.")
Explore possible strategies	Limited choices and solutions. The problem may be approached only in one or two ways. Can be solved with trial and error.	Many different possibilities.	Requires ability to generate, plan, test, and reject different hypotheses and formulate alternative solutions. Greater demands on flexibility and abstract thinking.	Generation of ideas and alternatives (eg, "How many different combination of coins can make 65? You are going to visit a friend in another state for 2 weeks. List everything you will need to do before you leave. Now you are going away for 3 months. How would you revise your list?")
Act	One to three steps External time monitor	Multiple steps Internally monitoring time	Greater demands on self-regulation and self-monitoring of behaviors and time.	Set a time goal and ask client to monitor time during an activity.
Look at the effects	Incorrect solution is readily apparent and prevents success.	Incorrect solution is not readily apparent. Requires actively comparing solution with original problem.	Requires greater self-monitoring strategies.	Have client fill out a structured self-evaluation rating form or checklist. Gradually reduce the structure of the rating form.

(Adapted from Toglia, J. [1996]. A multicontext approach to cognitive rehabilitation. Supplement manual to workshop conducted at New York Hospital–Cornell Medical Center, New York.)

ful. The client may be given the opportunity to practice the same task with and without the use of a checklist to enhance awareness. Initially, the goal in treatment may be to have a client follow a checklist established by the therapist or caregiver. Eventually, the client may be given checklists with missing steps and asked to review the lists to identify the missing components. Finally, the client may be required to create a checklist independently. Burke, Zencius, Wesolowski, and Doubleday (1991) described four case studies of individuals with executive dysfunction for whom checklists were used to improve the ability to carry out routine vocational tasks.

Decreased initiation, one of the hallmark features of executive dysfunction, can significantly interfere with the ability to use and apply a learned strategy. For example, a person with deficits in executive functions may use a strategy effectively when cued, but may not use the strategy spontaneously because of a failure to initiate its use. External cues such as alarm signals may be used to prompt the client to initiate a task or to use a particular strategy within an activity. An alarm signal programmed to go off every 10 or 15 minutes can cue the individual to use a checklist or to self-evaluate his or her work before continuing. Preprogrammed alarm messages (on a watch or electronic scheduler) can also cue the client to initiate an errand, make an important telephone call, take medications, or go to an appointment.

ADAPTATIONS OF TASK OR ENVIRONMENT

Adaptations that minimize demands on executive functions and problem-solving skills include training a caregiver to preorganize a task or task materials. For example, all the items needed for grooming can be arranged by the caregiver on the sink in the sequence in which they are used. As an alternative, one task step can be introduced at a time. These adaptations limit the need for planning and organization.

People who have difficulty with initiation, organization, and decision making require structure. Open-ended questions such as "What do you want to eat?" should be avoided. Clients who have difficulty in initiation will have a great deal of difficulty in answering open-ended questions. Questions should provide a limited number of choices whenever feasible.

A predictable and structured daily routine enhances the client's ability to initiate tasks and should be established and monitored by a caregiver. Audiotape instructions that cue the person to initiate a task and perform each task step at a time in its proper sequence have been reported to be successful. Schwartz (1995) describes use of a tape recorder with a personalized message and automatic timer to prompt a client with executive dysfunction to begin his morning routine. The tape included questions that elicited verbal responses such as "When you see the three Ss (shower, shave, and shampoo) what do you do?" To reinforce the tape message, written cues were placed on the bedroom door directing the client to the bathroom. After 3 months, the client completed two to three of the five morning tasks daily. Eventually, the tape-recorded message was discontinued and the client was effectively able to progress to a checklist.

▶ COGNITIVE–PERCEPTUAL CONCLUSION

The different treatment approaches discussed in this section all ultimately aim to enhance the individual's function. Some of the approaches seek to do this by emphasizing change in the task and environment, whereas others seek to change the person's behavior or skills. The extent to which learning and awareness are required for success differs among the varying approaches and needs to be considered in selecting treatment. In clinical practice, a combination of techniques that aim to change the person, task, and environment is recommended. However, at times, it is most appropriate for treatment to emphasize one aspect more than another. The decisions about what to treat and how to treat it constitute a complex clinical reasoning process that is dependent on the therapist's conceptualization of cognitive function and dysfunction as well as the client's level of insight, potential for learning, emotional-psychological characteristics, and the performance context.

The treatment of cognitive–perceptual components is moving away from a traditional deficit-specific approach. Newer treatment approaches such as the Affolter Method (Davies, 1985) and the Multicontext Approach (Toglia, 1991a) have emerged that emphasize information processing rather than separate cognitive–perceptual skills. There are an increased number of case reports that document training in strategies, rather than the repetitive practice of specific skills (Trexler et al, 1994). The role of awareness and strategy training has been increasingly emphasized within cognitive rehabilitation over the past few years (Barco et al, 1991; Ben-Yishay & Diller, 1983; Birnboim, 1995; Bruce, 1994). In addition, recent studies in cognitive rehabilitation reflect a trend toward incorporating a wider variety of treatment tasks, including practice within functional contexts (Antonucci et al, 1995). Finally, there is a growing acknowledgment that the different treatment approaches are not mutually exclusive, but can be integrated and used simultaneously to promote function.

Section 7

Treatment for Psychosocial Components: Intervention for Mental Health

Susan C. Robertson

> **Occupational Therapy's Contribution to Facilitating Mental Health**
> **The Occupational Therapy Process**
>   Goals of Intervention
>   Implementation
> **Intervention for Mental Health Conclusion**

To achieve mental health, one must develop an identity that is based on healthy functioning. Mental health is an attribute everyone needs to function effectively in society. Mentally healthy people (1) have a sense of well-being; (2) have the psychological makeup to realize their goals; (3) think, feel, and act within social boundaries; and (4) achieve goals that are valuable in the person's social context (Waterman, 1992, p. 51). Practitioners need to address the mental health needs of all clients, regardless of diagnosis.

People experiencing impairment, disability, or handicap are confronted with the need to change premorbid personalized images. By doing so, they can re-create their sense of who they are, incorporating both strengths and limitations imposed by the disability. A young woman with an eating disorder must contend with both physical and emotional aspects of her illness. At the same time she forces herself to take nutrition and limit exercise for her physical health, she must change her self-image. She must become reacquainted with herself in a healthy body, doing things that protect and nurture her self.

The concept of the self is a familiar theme throughout occupational therapy literature. The American Occupational Therapy Association's (AOTA) Uniform Terminology (AOTA, 1994) lists self-concept, self-expression, and self-control as key areas we address through occupation. These are important aspects of mental health and provide us with a way to begin to look more closely at the person, as a whole being, in therapeutic interventions.

▼ OCCUPATIONAL THERAPY'S CONTRIBUTION TO FACILITATING MENTAL HEALTH

If our goal is to facilitate adaptation and accommodation, we must help the people we serve learn how to perform occupations in different ways (Schkade & Schultz, 1992; Schultz & Schkade, 1992). During the process of changing their usual occupational routines, clients can discover new things about themselves. The skillful practitioner helps clients integrate this new self-knowledge into a new identity. This newer version of the person is one with a repertoire of adaptive strategies for adjusting to functional losses associated with illness.

Where does the person with a disability start in building a new self-concept that will help him or her navigate through life with different functional skills? Most start by learning how to do familiar tasks. By structuring important experiences that build performance components, in a therapeutic environment, practitioners provide the opportunity for people to learn how to live with a disability and to link their past and future roles.

The role of worker can be an important part of one's identity. Understanding how productive activities fit within the individual's values is often a first step to understanding occupational intervention. What roles does the person have in vocational activities? Observing and talking about how neurobiological disability has affected work performance provides important information about meaningful and appropriate interventions. A person with bipolar disorder may experience difficulties with dressing, grooming, and sleep, which ultimately influence successful performance of productive activities. As an occupational therapy practitioner, you may provide information about dress codes for jobs this client might want and help this person meet those dress codes to assure success on a job interview.

Managing a home and caring for others can be part of a worker role. Proper nutrition is a key factor in maintaining

mental health, and is supported by shopping, meal preparation and cleanup, and household cleaning. A person who becomes unable to perform these activities because of recurring panic attacks, agoraphobia, or suicidal tendencies may begin by focusing on orientation, sequencing, and symptom-specific coping strategies during occupational therapy. These skills could then be used to organize the kitchen work space for safe, efficient meal preparation.

▼ THE OCCUPATIONAL THERAPY PROCESS

Occupational therapy practitioners help the individual select, then engage in, activity that brings meaning to his or her life. We focus on the identity, the being—*the self*—of a person during collaborative therapeutic interventions. The thrust of treatment is threefold. Involvement in occupation is central. Learning through occupation is what enables change. New or different functional capabilities must be integrated within the person's self-concept.

Goals of Intervention

Evaluation precedes treatment planning. Synthesis of evaluation data provides information about clients' valued activities, motivation, and the functional deficits that help or hinder their occupational performance. On the basis of this information, practitioners need to collaborate with clients to form goals for optimal functioning in performance areas of importance to clients. Treatment goals must link performance components and areas. Often, a set of subskills is targeted, such as initiation of activity, social conduct, and self-expression.

Whether occupational therapy intervention is aimed at performance components, performance areas, or identity, communication about therapeutic goals is crucial. Practitioners strengthen the therapeutic relationship by thoughtfully acknowledging the person's strengths, confirming the difficulties losing function poses, and respecting the discipline and commitment it will take to make basic changes in lifestyle.

Implementation

Occupational therapy involves fostering change within the context of dynamic interactions among the occupation (Trombly, 1995a), ways of relating negotiated by client and practitioner (Peloquin, 1993), and the environment in which engagement in occupation occurs. (Dunn, Brown, & McGuigan, 1994). This task–relationship–environment pattern is a complex process requiring attention to the many factors that can influence the person's ability to learn by doing (Fidler & Fidler, 1978), including perceptions of nonverbal behavior (Sviden & Saljo, 1993). Structuring the events of a session is the link between the treatment goal and the potential for learning through experience. Organizing parts of the task opens opportunities to experiment with accommodating to disability.

It is the unique interaction of task, relationship, and environment that helps individuals involved in the change process see themselves differently, to experiment with possible self-attributes, then select those that will be incorporated into the self-concept. The process of self-development must be done with a combination of interaction with others and self-awareness and reflection. The self develops to protect the individual, to ensure survival at the minimum and, ideally, to expand quality of life. The purpose of active relationship with meaningful occupation is to help the person rediscover the self that has survived illness and disability.

FEEDBACK

Involvement in doing is not the full therapeutic process. Doing must be accompanied by examining what happened and how it worked. Discussing each session, then, is a pivotal element in understanding the outcome of the cooperative work. Sometimes, it is useful to communicate observations and suggest modifications as the session is in progress. Other times, it is more useful to complete the task and then reflect on what helped and minimized performance. Most often, though, the most useful approach is to do both—offer pointers during occupation, then summarize and highlight key concepts at the end of the session.

THERAPEUTIC RELATIONSHIP

Chapter 10 discusses therapeutic use of self. As you read it, consider the meaning of *self* in the term. There is an interdependence of self-development between practitioner and client. Your self, your sense of who you are, your professional identity, develops as you interact with others. That is the self you bring to therapeutic relationships.

The very process involved in a therapeutic relationship assumes that your self will be developing, too. You will see yourself as the client sees you. As you address self-development with the person you are helping, you will continually contribute to your own self-development as a person and as an occupational therapy practitioner. Both you and your client offer each other views about the self that can be provided only through interactions with others. Bringing therapeutic use of self to each professional relationship requires one's own ability to regulate the self, maintain a keen sense of self-awareness, and allow the professional self to be influenced by the people being served.

INTERVENTION TO FOSTER SELF-MANAGEMENT

The underlying function of the self is to regulate behavior, to maintain mental health, and maximize each person's productive contribution in valued roles in society. Occupational therapy practitioners would be likely to use various strategies to help the client cope, to appraise stressors to the self in various situations (Gage, 1992). Some of those strategies are listed in the following. The practitioner will help the client to:

1. Define sensorimotor, cognitive, and psychosocial processes that disrupt adaptive function and stability.
2. Set boundaries for behavior and recognize when to set limits.
3. Seek feedback that develops self-awareness.
4. Integrate aspects of psychological values, interests, and self-concept that are demonstrated through involvement in occupations.
5. Organize strategies to respond to negative symptoms.
6. Problem solve by setting goals, monitoring progress, and resolving impediments to healthy functioning.
7. Cope by committing to managing performance for mental health.
8. Separate illness from personality and work to change negative self-expressive behaviors stemming from personality and temperament.
9. Maintain health through medication compliance, monitoring side effects, and seeking guidance as needed.
10. Balance exercise, nutrition, and meaningful occupation in a weekly schedule.
11. Learn to analyze activity and read environmental cues to manage time and occupations.
12. Generate different ways to react to stressors and initiate them in stressful situations.
13. Develop support systems to assist in self-management.

INTERVENTION TO FOSTER HEALTHY SELF-CONCEPT

Self-concept is our definition of the goals, values, and beliefs that "give direction and meaning to life" (Waterman, 1984; p. 331). Knowing who we are unifies our actions, pulls the various parts of ourself into a cohesive whole. Occupational therapy can help a person develop a self-concept that supports the person as a functional being. Some possible approaches are listed in the following. The practitioner will help the client to

1. Describe and demonstrate performance component areas that were particularly skillful before the accident.
2. Describe and demonstrate performance component areas that were challenging before the accident.
3. Discuss how limited ability to perform sequencing, spatial operations, and problem solving, for example, will influence his or her ability to achieve what he or she had hoped for in life.
4. Honestly express reactions to loss of functioning self (fear, anger, sadness).
5. Identify his or her most significant values and interests.
6. Brainstorm to develop adaptive approaches to occupations of interest.
7. Evaluate possible ways of adapting to engage in occupa-

tion, keeping an open mind, and determining what components best support performance areas.

8. Link successful aspects of current function in a picture of a future functioning self who is healthy, despite disability or handicap.

INTERVENTION THAT BUILDS MOTIVATION

Motivation is what links performance with outcome. It is the means people use to initiate, sustain, and direct psychological or physical activities to satisfy needs. Motivation may be conscious or unconscious, biological or cognitive, extrinsic (food, water, sex, social approval) or intrinsic (requiring modification of cognitive structures). But the essence of motivation is that it organizes the self to manage behavior. Occupational therapy can help articulate the motivators that lead to changes in self-functioning and evaluate the intensity and focus of the individual's motivation schema. Some strategies follow. The practitioner will help the client to

1. Gear selection and design of occupational interventions toward expression of self values.

2. Use knowledge of most significant past achievements to structure and monitor occupational interventions.

3. Demonstrate and evaluate achievements in personal action that have been admired by others.

4. Describe impediments to performance and demonstrate approaches to overcoming procrastination or low achievement.

5. Incorporate occupations and relationships that have become more important since onset of disability.

INTERVENTION TO FOSTER SELF-DEVELOPMENT

Occupational therapy can help a person develop a self-concept by providing opportunities for sensorimotor exploration and interactions with others. Some strategies for achieving this follow. The practitioner will help the client to

1. Perform meaningful occupations that require familiar sensorimotor skills.

2. Perform meaningful occupations that require new and challenging sensorimotor skills.

3. Learn how to actively influence his or her environment.

4. Compare and contrast his or her abilities with those of others, building self-control and patterns of social conduct suitable for self-management.

5. Assert greater control over interpersonal skills to foster typical peer relationships.

INTERVENTION RELATED TO PHYSICAL ATTRIBUTES

Physical attributes are linked to self-concept. Changes in physical skills and features that can accompany illness can have a profound effect on how people feel about themselves. Occupational therapy intervention may address physical attributes of illness. Some suggestions follow. The practitioner will help the client to

1. Consistently attend to grooming, bathing, hygiene, dressing, and health maintenance.

2. Develop approaches to social conduct that maximize coping skills.

3. Select clothing for a variety of social situations and dress accordingly.

4. Convey a self-image consistent with self-concept in work and productive activities.

INTERVENTION FOCUSED ON PERSONALITY AND TEMPERAMENT

Personality is our usual style, a typical way of doing things, a predictable emotional reaction to what happens around us. Temperament is a "constitutionally determined behavioral style which is somewhat stable over time" (Bornstein & Lamb, 1988; p. 389). Occupational therapy practitioners consider personality and temperament in treatment. Some strategies follow. The practitioner will help the client to

1. Assess personality characteristics and their effect on self-management.

2. Monitor emotional reactions to life events and seek help when needed to control self-expression.

3. Plan healthy approaches to managing different life situations: pilot test these in role play situations.

INTERVENTION RELATED TO COGNITION AND LEARNING STYLES

Some impairments do not influence premorbid cognitive functioning. But diseases that affect cognitive or psychosocial skills are more likely to have negative effects on information processing and learning. Occupational therapy strategies for adapting to learning and cognitive style are listed in the following. The practitioner will help the client to

1. Define learning styles that help and hinder learning and generalization.

2. Demonstrate use of a variety of learning approaches and evaluate the effectiveness of each.

3. Recognize different approaches to information processing and initiate use of suitable approach in occupational interventions.

INTERVENTION TO PROMOTE SELF-ACCEPTANCE

Self-acceptance is "the ability to be pleased with oneself in the absence of external feedback from others" (Harter, 1983; pp. 364-365). Occupational therapy consistently works to promote self-acceptance through function. Several strategies are listed. The practitioner will help the client to

1. Become aware of strengths and limitations in psychological values, interests, and self-concept.

2. Learn about the self by evaluating performance.

3. Tolerate inability to be perfect in all endeavors as an element of self-management.

4. Adjust to ambiguities and inconsistencies in self in efforts to improve self-control.

5. Accept less desirable characteristics or competencies as part of coping strategy to reduce stress.

►INTERVENTION FOR MENTAL HEALTH CONCLUSION

Occupational therapy's focus has long been on the whole person and his or her ability to live a healthy life. The ultimate outcome of occupational therapy is for clients to be able to create healthy lives for themselves, despite impairments, disabilities, or handicaps. To achieve this outcome, practitioners need to consider and address the psychosocial needs of all clients, using intervention strategies such as the ones suggested in this section.

Section 8

Treatment for Psychosocial Components: Pain Management

Joyce M. Engel

Defining Pain
Occupational Therapy Evaluation of Pain
    Behavioral
    Cultural, Familial, and Spiritual
Occupational Therapy Practitioners' Role in Pain
    Management
      Medication Intake
      Physical Activity
      Communication of Pain
      Relaxation Training
      Biofeedback
      Cognitive Restructuring
      Distraction
      Social Support
      Cutaneous Stimulation Modalities
Pain Management Conclusion

A pproximately 79 billion dollars are spent annually on **pain** care in the United States alone (Supernaw, 1995). The costs of human suffering are inestimable. The presence of pain may affect a person's performance of ADL and may disrupt role performance.

▼ DEFINING PAIN

Pain has typically been conceptualized as a neurophysiological event that involves a complex pattern of emotional and psychological arousal. According to the definition of the International Association of the Study of Pain (1979), "Pain is an unpleasant sensory and emotional experience associated with actual or potential tissue damage or described in terms of such damage" (Mersky, 1986; p. S217). This definition emphasizes the multidimensional nature as well as the inherent subjectivity of pain.

Although definitions of pain are varied, most authors agree that **acute** and **chronic pain** should be differentiated (Fordyce, 1976; McCaffery, 1979). Pain associated with tissue damage, irritation, inflammation, or a disease process that is relatively brief (ie, hours, days, weeks), regardless of intensity, is frequently referred to as *acute pain* (eg, postsurgical pain). Acute pain serves a biological or adaptive purpose by directing attention to injury, irritation, or disease and signaling the necessity for immobilization and protection of an injured area such as a laceration (Katz, Varni, & Jay, 1984). In contrast, pain that persists for extended periods of time (ie, months or years), that accompanies a disease (eg, rheumatoid arthritis), or is associated with an injury that has not resolved within an expected time frame is referred to as *chronic pain* (Turk & Melzack, 1992). Chronic pain complaints can be further differentiated. Chronic, periodic pain is acute, but intermittent (eg, migraine headaches). Chronic, intractable, nonmalignant pain is present most of the time, with intensity varying (eg, low back pain). Chronic, progressive pain is often associated with malignancies (Turk, Meichenbaum, & Genest, 1983). Chronic nonmalignant pain does not appear to serve a biological purpose and is often experienced in the presence of minimal or no apparent tissue damage (Johnson, 1977). The most frequently treated types of recurrent painful conditions seen by occupational therapy practitioners include headache, low back, arthritis, cancer, myofascial, and extremity pain (Engel, 1993). Theories about pain suggest that multidimensional evaluation and intervention are necessary to achieve adequate pain control.

▼ OCCUPATIONAL THERAPY EVALUATION OF PAIN

Effective management of pain depends on accurate and multidimensional pain evaluation. Proper evaluation requires the use of valid and reliable instruments for determining pain effects before and after treatment. Several methods for pain evaluation have been used to measure clinical pain.

Behavioral

Behavioral evaluation may be used to identify behaviors in need of change and to identify environmental or organismic variables that trigger specific pain behaviors (Fordyce, 1976; Keefe, 1982). Practitioners have broadened their view of behavior to include not only overt, but also covert and physiological responses (Sanders, 1979).

OVERT

Overt motor behavior or observable pain responses (eg, medication use, limping) and well behaviors are commonly targeted for evaluation. Persons experiencing pain may rub the pain site, grimace, and demonstrate atypical body posturing. A behavioral interview of the client and a significant other is often used to evaluate these behavioral patterns (Fordyce, 1976; Turk et al, 1983). This interview, coupled with activity diaries, can aid in the analysis of when and in what situations pain interferes with daily activities (Keefe, 1982; Potts & Baptiste, 1989). Clients, however, may be poor or biased self-observers. Indirect evaluation of pain may then be inferred from physical parameters (eg, ROM), job absenteeism, decreased activity levels, and degree of health care utilization. These measures combined with behavioral observations of the client's performance of ADL, including work and leisure performance, may provide a more accurate and complete appraisal of the person's functional status (Caruso & Chan, 1986; Flower, Naxon, Jones, & Mooney, 1981; McCormack & Johnson, 1990).

COVERT

Because pain is a private, internal event that cannot be directly observed, evaluation of the pain experience is frequently through client self-report of pain intensity, pain affect, and pain location. The three most commonly used methods to assess pain intensity are the Verbal Rating Scale (VRS), the Numerical Rating Scale (NRS), and the Visual Analog Scale (VAS) (Jensen & Karoly, 1992). The VRS consists of a list of adjectives ranging from *no pain* to *extreme pain* to describe different levels of pain (Table 20–14). In contrast, the NRS requires clients to rate their pain on a scale from 0 to 10 or 0 to 100, with the understanding that 0 is equal to *no pain* and the 10 or 100 is equal to the *most ex-*

TABLE 20-14. Verbal Rating Scale (VRS)

Mild
Discomforting
Distressing
Horrible
Excruciating

Illustration of the five-point VRS typically used to determine treatment outcome and is part of the McGill Pain Questionnaire.

TABLE 20-15. Numerical Rating Scale (NRS)

Please indicate on the line below the number between 0 and 100 that best describes your pain. A zero (0) would mean "no pain" and a one hundred (100) would mean "pain as bad as it could be." Indicate only one number.

———————

Illustration of the 101-point NRS. The 101-point NRS provides more response categories than the 11-point NRS.

cruciating pain possible (Table 20–15). Finally, the VAS consists of a line, typically 10 cm long, for which the ends are labeled as the extremes of pain (eg, *no pain* to *pain as bad as it could be*) (Fig. 20–20).

These rating scales are easy to administer and score, have good evidence for construct validity, are sensitive to treatment, and are used fairly reliably by clients. **Psychometric** problems, however, exist. For example, the distances between VRS are unknown, but are typically treated statistically as if they were equal (Jensen & Karoly, 1992).

Pain affect refers to the emotional arousal and disruption caused by the pain experience. A commonly used measure of pain affect is the affective subscale of the McGill Pain Questionnaire (MPQ) (Melzack, 1975). Affective qualities of pain include fear, tension, and autonomic properties. Vocabulary, language, or cognitive limitations of the client, however, may limit the usefulness of these instruments. In addition, verbal report of a private stimulus is dependent on the client's cooperation, and may be distorted by the client's motives, attitudes, and self-interests (ie, escape from responsibilities) (Kazdin, 1980; Strong, Ashton, Cramond, & Chant, 1990).

PHYSIOLOGICAL

Physiological pain responses are the third major category used in the behavioral evaluation of pain. Hyperactivity of the sympathetic nervous system is considered one of the major psychophysiological mechanisms of chronic pain (Bonica, 1977). Changes in these physiological indicators may also be seen with other subjective phenomena (anxiety), making it difficult to detect a pattern of responses unique to pain (Stewart, 1977).

In addition, Sternbach (1974) and McCaffery (1979) have suggested that a process of adaptation of physiological pain responses exists, which results in the physiological parameters returning to near normal. Another major problem

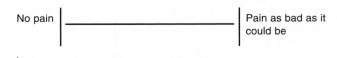

▲
Figure 20-20. Visual analog scale (VAS)

in using physiological responses as measures of pain is that overt, covert, and physiological responses typically do not correlate highly, and research has not yet determined which is the most valid measure (Katz, Varni, & Jay, 1984).

Cultural, Familial, and Spiritual

Cultural, familial, and spiritual influences are other important factors to be considered by the occupational therapy practitioner in pain evaluation and intervention, especially when the pain etiology is unclear (Chapman & Turner, 1990; MacRae & Riley, 1990; Parker & Cinciripini, 1984). Each culture, family, and religion has its own system of values and attitudes about pain (Baptiste, 1988; Niemeyer, 1990). Depending on the culture, the individual may be rewarded, ignored, or punished for emitting pain behaviors.

▼ OCCUPATIONAL THERAPY PRACTITIONERS' ROLE IN PAIN MANAGEMENT

Behavioral methods for chronic pain management are indicated as a treatment for persons with chronic nonmalignant pain who are (1) receiving excessive pain-related medications, (2) not participating in routine ADL (deactivation), (3) engaging in too much postural guarding, (4) demonstrating inappropriate pacing for task completion, and (5) engaging in excessive health care use (Fordyce, 1990). Coordinated, goal-directed, **interdisciplinary** team (physician, clinical psychologist or psychiatrist, occupational therapy practitioner, physical therapist, vocational specialist) services may be offered on an inpatient or outpatient basis with the scope and intensity of medical, psychosocial, and vocational services matched to the client's needs (Commission on Accreditation of Rehabilitation Facilities, 1996).

Medication Intake

To encourage discontinuation of analgesics, muscle relaxants, and tranquilizers, their use is shifted from a pain-contingent to a time-contingent basis. Fordyce (1976) recommended that following baseline, the medications be delivered in a color- and taste-masking liquid medium ("pain cocktail") at fixed time intervals, with the systematic reduction of the proportion of active ingredients over time. By providing adequate medicinal coverage on a time-contingent basis, the learned behavioral chain between overt pain expressions and medication intake is abolished (Grzesiak, 1982). Linking detoxification to a reactivation program (physical retraining, social support) facilitates this process (Fordyce, 1990).

Physical Activity

Increasing the client's activity level is the cornerstone of most chronic pain management treatment programs and is a major area of occupational therapy intervention. Intervention involves positively reinforcing (praising) the client's attempts at physical activity or exercise. Activity increases are done on a gradual basis with the client working to "tolerance" (gradual increase in task completion) as opposed to "pain" before a scheduled rest period. Resting at the time of the pain onset or elevation is avoided because it may reinforce the pain behaviors (Fordyce, 1976; Grzesiak, 1982). Group or individual progressive mobility, strengthening, and endurance exercises or activities are routinely scheduled daily to assist the client in achieving maximal functional status. Modalities (heat or cold) may be applied to prepare the client for exercise.

Proper use of posture, body mechanics, energy conservation, and joint protection techniques are also emphasized as a means of pain reduction (Caruso & Chan, 1986; Giles & Allen, 1986). Adaptive equipment and splinting may be prescribed to enhance independent performance of ADLs (Tyson & Strong, 1990).

Communication of Pain

Discrimination training is directed at enhancing stimulus control so that the client discusses pain with appropriate people (such as health care providers) at appropriate times and places. People interacting with the person experiencing chronic nonmalignant pain are instructed to avoid giving attention and sympathy for either verbal or nonverbal expressions of pain and to praise the client's achievements and efforts to cope with pain. Social skills training may also be used by the occupational therapy practitioner, during which the client is taught and reinforced for using behaviors not revolving around the pain experience in social contacts. Involvement of the partner or significant other in stress or anger management, resolution of sexual dysfunction, and goal-setting skills may make up part of the total treatment package (Fordyce, 1990; Turk, Meichenbaum, & Genest, 1983).

Relaxation Training

Relaxation training may involve teaching the client to systematically contract and relax the major skeletal muscle groups (**progressive muscle relaxation**), the silent repetition of phrases about the ideal psychophysiological state (autogenic training), or the purposeful use of images to achieve a desired goal (guided imagery). The potential benefits of these approaches are the reduction of anxiety, distraction from pain, alleviation of skeletal muscle tension, reduction of fatigue, improved sleep, enhancement of other pain relief measures, and a sense of control over pain (McCaffery, 1979; Turner & Romano, 1990). Research suggests that relaxation rehearsal may be helpful in the reduction of the person's perceived pain frequency, intensity, or duration, and achievement of functional goals (Engel & Rapoff, 1990a; Strong, Cramond, & Mass, 1989d).

Biofeedback

Relaxation training may include the use of biofeedback to help the client learn voluntary control of musculoskeletal and vascular responses that may precipitate a pain episode. Biofeedback has been used effectively for a wide variety of pain complaints, most notably headache; low back, neck, and shoulder pain; and temporomandibular joint syndrome (Blanchard & Ahles, 1990; Engel & Rapoff, 1990b).

Cognitive Restructuring

Cognitive restructuring includes educational and training components. Clients are educated about the role of cognition and emotions in pain and the interrelations among pain, **stress**, and tension. Clients are taught that emotional reactions to and behaviors after an event depend to a large extent on a person's thoughts. Together, the clinician and the client examine whether negative thoughts are realistic. Distorted negative thoughts are then replaced with more realistic positive ones (Tan, 1982).

Distraction

Increased pain awareness may result from a lack of distracting activities. Therefore, it is advantageous for persons experiencing pain to learn how to distract themselves more effectively when exposed to noxious stimuli (painful medical or rehabilitation procedures) and low environmental stimulation, and during periods of minimal activity. Clients cannot attend as much to pain when concentrating on something else. Cognitive distraction techniques, therefore, involve the person actively redirecting attention to something other than pain (doing a puzzle) or focusing inward (reminiscing), but not directly on the pain. Involvement in purposeful activity has been demonstrated to improve pain tolerance (Heck, 1988; McCormack, 1988). A balance of work, recreation, and social activities is of value in distracting attention away from pain (Hanson & Gerber, 1990; Heck, 1988).

Social Support

The importance of social support in facilitating behavior change cannot be underestimated. Support groups may (1) assist persons suffering from pain by helping them realize that others have endured similar circumstances, (2) provide a neutral place to express feelings, and (3) provide opportunities for learning coping strategies. Support groups can ease the transition from terminating treatment to self-management and the maintenance of behavioral change.

Cutaneous Stimulation Modalities

TRANSCUTANEOUS ELECTRICAL NERVE STIMULATION

Transcutaneous electrical nerve stimulation (TENS) is a noninvasive pain relief measure consisting of cutaneous (skin) stimulation. A TENS unit consists of a battery-powered generator that sends a mild electrical current through electrodes placed on the skin at or near the pain site, stimulating A nerve fibers. TENS use has had some success in relieving acute and chronic painful conditions caused by abnormalities in nerve structures, the skeleton, muscles, pain of ischemic origin in the extremities, and angina pectoris. Its use is contraindicated in clients with pacemakers. In addition, the unit should not be placed on the anterior aspect of the neck to avoid stimulation of the carotid nerves and possible **hypotension**. Skin irritation is another possible side effect and, in rare instances, an aggravation of the pain complaint occurs. Individual adjustment of the technique and client status after 3 months is recommended (Sjölund, Eriksson, & Loeser, 1990).

MASSAGE

Massage may be used in preparation for exercise and to improve functional performance. Stimulation of peripheral receptors in the skin is produced by repetitive rhythmic movements of the practitioner's hands (stroking, kneading, rubbing) or devices in a centripetal direction. This stimulation induces muscle relaxation and arteriolar dilation or constriction, increases local blood circulation, improves muscle flexibility, loosens scar tissue, and increases emotional well-being. Conditions that may respond to massage are arthritis, sprain, strain, muscle spasm, bursitis, and contusion. Massage is contraindicated in the presence of an acute inflammatory process, thrombophlebitis, lymphangitis, acute burn, dermatitis, malignancy, advanced arteriosclerosis, nephritis, and severe debilitation (Lee, Itoh, Yang, & Eason, 1990).

THERMOTHERAPY

Heat from hydrocollator packs penetrates the skin superficially. Heat may also be applied with a hot water bottle, an electric heating pad, or a chemical pack. These devices may be useful in reducing muscle spasm, spasticity, bursitis, and tendinitis. Edema, swelling, and tissue damage may be aggravated by heat. Because packs may be heavy and bulky, they may not be suitable for tender regions. Heating pads should not be used by persons with impaired sensation.

Paraffin therapy produces increased skin tissue temperature while decreasing the temperature of subcutaneous tissue. Paraffin may be helpful in relieving arthritis pain of the small joints of the hands and feet. It is contraindicated where there is a skin opening, rash, infection, or dermatitis (Lee et al, 1990).

CRYOTHERAPY

In addition to heat, cold can also improve pain control by elevating the pain threshold (the minimal level of noxious stimulation at which the person first reports pain). Similar to heat, cold can reduce muscle spasm secondary to joint or skeletal injury, and spasticity. Edema, swelling, and tissue damage may be decreased by cold. Joint stiffness, however, may be aggravated. Cold can be applied with packs, sprays, or an ice stick for massage. Contraindications to cryotherapy include vascular insufficiency, an anesthetic area, Raynaud's phenomenon, and intolerance to cold (Lee et al, 1990).

A variety of other physical agents (ultrasound, diathermy, whirlpool therapy) that have the benefits of heat or cold are available. Evaluation by a physical therapist would help determine whether the client is an appropriate candidate for such approaches. The occupational therapy practitioner is cautioned to comply with federal and state laws and American Occupational Therapy Association statements when using physical agent modalities.

VIBRATION

Vibration may mask the discomfort of low-intensity stimulation and reduce the perceived pain intensity. Electric and battery-operated vibrators of varying shapes and sizes may be used with or without heat, cold, or medication (McCormack, 1988). Good relief from this approach has been reported for chronic postherpetic neuralgia (Crue, Todd, & Maline, 1975) and **phantom limb pain** (Russell cited in McCaffery, 1979). Anecdotal reports of low back pain relief have also been noted (McCaffery, 1979).

▶PAIN MANAGEMENT CONCLUSION

Occupational therapy practitioners have a core role in providing therapeutic activities that enable the client with pain to develop the skills and tolerances necessary for the attainment of self-care, vocational, and leisure goals. Because of the complex nature of pain, a "cure" is not readily available. Consequently, treatment efforts cannot simply emphasize the reduction of the pain experience. Ideally, interventions need to focus on improving functional levels and coping strategies, while being sensitive to the client's belief and value systems.

Section 9:

Treatment for Psychosocial Components: Stress Management

Gordon Muir Giles and Maureen E. Neistadt

Physiological Responses to Stress
    The General Adaptation Response
    Psychological Responses to Stress: The Interaction
      of Person and Stressors
Stressors
    Types of Stressors
    Mediating Factors
Stress and Occupational Therapy
    Stress Management Techniques
    General Guidelines for Choice of Technique
Stress Management Conclusion

S tress is the collection of physical and psychological changes that occur in response to a perceived challenge or threat; it is the outcome of an interaction between the person and the environment. People's resources (personality and social supports), their appraisal of situations, and their capacity to handle those situations influence their stress reactions and the effects of stress on their health. This section describes physiological and psychological responses to stress, common causes of stress, stress management techniques, and guidelines for choosing techniques for particular clinical situations.

▼ PHYSIOLOGICAL RESPONSES TO STRESS

The General Adaptation Response

Selye (1978) describes the body's stress reaction as the **general adaptation response**. This response occurs in three stages: the alarm reaction, the adaptive or resistive stage, and the exhaustion phase. Not everyone experiences all three stages. The exhaustion phase is reached only when the person either becomes stuck in the alarm stage or goes through the alarm and adaptive stages too often.

ALARM REACTION

The alarm reaction is the fight-or-flight response that prepares a person to meet a challenge or threat. During this stage, the cerebral cortex activates the reticular activating system to increase general alertness. The cortex also activates the autonomic nervous system and endocrine systems by way of the hypothalamus. The sympathetic branch of the autonomic nervous system increases heart rate, blood pressure, perspiration, muscle tone, and cell metabolism. Blood vessels just under the skin constrict, and digestion is slowed. The endocrine system releases hormones from the adrenal and thyroid glands, which increase the supply of glucose and help cells accelerate their metabolism. In addition, the hypothalamus triggers the release of β-endorphins from the pituitary. β-Endorphins are endogenous opiate proteins that elevate mood and decrease pain perception. They have also been linked to immune system suppression (Shavit et al, 1985). It is the combination of nervous system and endocrine system response that leads to the term neuroendocrine stress reaction.

ADAPTIVE OR RESISTIVE STAGE

In the adaptive or resistive stage, the body returns to its pre-excited state and recovers from the physiological strains of the alarm stage. Stress-prone or overstressed persons, who may interpret even normal events as negative stressors, are often unable to reach this stage. They develop an extended alarm reaction until their bodies enter the exhaustion phase. People who are able to successfully move to the adaptive stage may also reach the exhaustion phase if they experience too many stressors.

EXHAUSTION PHASE

The exhaustion phase is a reaction to the constant high metabolic demands of the alarm stage. During this phase, the neurophysiological ability to respond to stressors is effectively abolished.

CHRONIC STRESS

The physiological demands of chronic stress have been linked to many disorders. Chronic stress can depress immune system functioning, increasing vulnerability to disease and compromising recovery.

Psychological Responses to Stress: The Interaction of Person and Stressors

Stress arises from an imbalance between the demands of a situation and a person's appraisal of his or her ability to cope with those demands. Individual differences in motivation and cognition lead to markedly different reactions to potential stressors. For example, moving to a new apartment might be perceived as exciting by one person and upsetting by another. Lazarus (1993) says personality factors and environmental variables interact to influence persons' perceptions of potential stressors. Aldwin (1994) suggests that seemingly distinct levels of analysis—biological, psychological, and sociological—can further our understanding of stress and coping. For example, the structure of a culture influences a persons well-being both directly through the allocation of resources and indirectly by influencing characteristic levels of stress (Aldwin, 1994).

▼ STRESSORS

Any agent or circumstance capable of triggering stress reactions is called a stressor (Selye, 1978). Knowing the sources of stress can help predict and control the amount of stress a person feels. Clients can be taught to monitor physical and psychological markers of stress and to use these as cues to implement stress reduction techniques. Here we discuss categories of stressors (physical or environmental, major life events, chronic strains, and hassles) and mediating factors [ie, factors that modify the effect of the stressor on the person (personality factors, behaviors, support, and sociocultural factors)].

Types of Stressors

ENVIRONMENTAL STRESSORS

Physical or environmental stressors include noise, crowding, poor lighting, inadequate ventilation, and environmental pollutants. Excessive or continuous noise (90 dB or higher) can cause high blood pressure and hearing loss. Crowding can make people irritable and aggressive. Poor lighting and ventilation have been reported to cause eye irritation, headaches, nausea, and drowsiness in workers. Daily exposure to environmental stressors makes a baseline coping demand on our nervous systems, reducing the reserve capacity required for other forms of stress (Neistadt, 1993).

MAJOR LIFE EVENTS

Major life events can be divided into (1) exposure to extreme or nonnormative events, such as natural or man-made disasters (fires, floods, tornadoes, earthquakes, war); and (2) normative major life changes, such as marriage or bereavement. Reactions to major life events can be acute, chronic, or both. If persons are exposed to events that involve serious threat (actual or threatened death or serious injury to themselves or a loved one) they may later experience posttraumatic stress disorder (PTSD). The symptoms associated with extreme trauma include persistent reexperiencing of the event, avoidance of stimuli associated with the event, a numbing of responsiveness, or a persistent overarousal (American Psychiatric Association, DSM-IV, 1994). The management of individuals with PTSD is a specialized area of practice and is not discussed here. However many of the techniques used in the context of stress management are appropriate for use in an integrated PTSD program.

Major life changes that alter social roles and relationships, such as marriage, divorce, job change, serious illness, or the death of a loved one, can increase susceptibility to stress, especially when several of these changes occur within a brief time period. Multiple major life changes within 1 year correlate with a higher risk of injury or illness (Holmes & Rahe, 1967; Rahe, 1979). Cohen, Tyrrell, and Smith (1991) found a linear relation between an index of stress and the probability of developing a cold following viral challenge. Although both positive and negative life events do seem to have an effect, there is increasing evidence that it is not change per se, but the quality of the change that is potentially damaging to people; specifically events that are undesired, unscheduled, nonnormative, and over which the individual has no control are detrimental.

CHRONIC STRAIN

An area of chronic strain that has received considerable attention is the effect of employment on health. High-stress occupations have been defined as those with high psychological demands and limited decision-making freedom (Karasek, 1979). Psychological strain, increased cardiovascular risk, and decreased general health have been linked to high-stress occupations (Karasek et al, 1988; Lerner, Levine, Malspeis, & D'Agostino, 1994; Siegrist, Peter, Junge, Cremer, & Seidel, 1990; Siegrist, Peter, Motz, & Strauer, 1992). In addition to high strain and low control, low social support at work may contribute to risk of cardiovascular disease (Johnson & Hall, 1988).

Health care workers have been studied extensively relative to the effect of chronic job strain on their physical and psychological well-being. Many health care workers seem to be at risk because of the long hours and frequent changes in shift, leading to disruptions in sleep–wake cycles. Such schedule irregularities have been correlated to a high number of stress-related errors on the job (Neistadt, 1993). Caregiver burden has also been studied (McNaughton, Patterson, Smith, & Grant, 1995).

HASSLES

Minor changes or day-to-day aggravations can also act as stressors. These vexations can have a cumulative effect and are magnified during periods of major life changes. Major life changes, in addition to their immediate effect, can create a "ripple effect" of continuing minor hassles. It is possible to think about this effect as one of primary and secondary stressors. For example, providing care to an impaired loved one may be stressful in and of itself, but may also interfere with employment and produce economic problems as secondary stressors.

Mediating Factors

A number of factors seem to either exacerbate or diminish the effect of stressful events or life circumstances. These "mediating factors" may provide avenues for important interventions to minimize the effect of stress on health.

PERSONALITY FACTORS

Stress-prone people see change as a threat, feel helpless in controlling their environment, and have a sense of alienation about their lives. Personality factors associated with poor responses to stress include anger, cynicism, external locus of control, neuroticism, depression, and irrational beliefs (McNaughton et al, 1995).

Personality traits that appear to be associated with resilience (resistance to stress) include constructive thinking (Epstein & Meier, 1989), hardiness (Hills & Norvell, 1991), dispositional optimism (Scheier & Carver, 1987), hope (Snyder et al, 1991), self-efficacy, mastery and internal locus of control, and possibly, conscientiousness (Friedman et al, 1995).

BEHAVIORS

Behaviors with potential health consequences, such as alcohol use, smoking, and drug abuse, can compromise our capacity to deal with stress and create their own sets of stressors (eg disrupted family relationships, job loss, illness, and injury). Ironically, these negative behaviors are sometimes part of the individual's attempt to manage stress (Bradstock et al, 1988; Budd, Eiser, Morgan, & Gammage, 1985; Gottlieb & Green, 1984; Mehrabian & Straubinger, 1989; Wills, 1986). Stress is not the only determinant of negative health behaviors, however, with both parents and peers having important influences on potentially health-damaging behaviors (Flay et al, 1994).

Health-promoting behaviors increase our capacity to cope effectively with stress. Positive **health behaviors**, such as regular exercise, regular meals, nutritionally balanced diet, and getting enough sleep, are associated with parental modeling of these behaviors (Lau, Quadrel, & Hartman, 1990); also, psychological factors, such as self-efficacy (Grembowski et al, 1993) and positive affect (Griffin, Friend, Eitel, & Lobel, 1993), social support, and the existence of a social network (Gottlieb & Green, 1984), contribute to coping.

SOCIAL SUPPORT

The degree to which a person is connected to others may influence health in a more fundamental way than by reducing negative health practices. Numerous studies now report a relation between social support and health and mortality (Hibbard & Pope, 1993; Reynolds & Kaplan, 1990; Vogt, Mullooly, Ernst, Pope, & Hollis, 1992). Berkman & Syme (1979) found that people who lacked social support were more likely to die than those with social support. The association between social ties and decreased mortality was independent of socioeconomic status, health practices, obesity, physical activity, or the use of preventative health services. Social support has many dimensions, including emotional and material assistance, and information and referral.

SOCIOCULTURAL FACTORS

Larger sociocultural factors, such as overcrowding, may complicate other types of stressors. Little disposable income may force people to live in an unsafe neighborhood, placing them under chronic stress. Unemployment is a risk factor for mortality even when socioeconomic factors are accounted for (Moser, Fox, & Jones, 1984). Interestingly, the risk extends to the wives of the unemployed who also show a raised risk of mortality. Mortality was particularly high from malignant neoplasms, accidents, poisonings, and violence (Moser, et al, 1984). Stressors such as life events, family interaction, and lack of social support appear to play a role in exacerbations of schizophrenia, and increased stressors appear to increase hospital admissions.

TYPES OF COPING

Coping appears to be highly contextual, depending on the type of stressor, the environmental conditions, and the state of the person under stress. Lazarus (1993) suggests that the type of coping likely to be employed depends on the appraisal of whether or not anything can be done to change the situation. He describes two basic types of coping responses: problem-focused coping and emotion-focused coping. If the person believes that something can be done, problem-focused coping predominates. The person is likely to actively interact with the environment and attempt to gain mastery and to change the situation so that it becomes less stressful. If people believe that nothing can be done to change the situation, they are likely to use emotion-focused coping, which involves changes in the way the stress is attended to (denial) or changes in the way the event is understood and integrated into their lives. Both types of coping are useful and help people manage stressors. Problems arise if a particular type of coping is misapplied; what is highly adaptive in one context may be counterproductive in another. For example, emotional-focused coping (such as denial) could be effective in helping people cope with the fear that they were already infected with the human immunodeficiency virus (HIV), but would be disastrous if it prevented them from adopting safe sexual practices or from obtaining needed medical care (Weitz, 1989).

▼ STRESS AND OCCUPATIONAL THERAPY

Occupational therapy clients are particularly prone to some of the stressors just mentioned. Illness and disability themselves are major life changes and can cause social roles changes and generate a host of minor aggravating changes in daily activities. Learning the culture of the hospital can be extremely stressful to some clients (Spencer, Young, Rintala, & Bates, 1995). Changes in appearance or behavior can leave a client constantly fearful of rejection.

On the other side of the therapeutic relationship, practitioners have to deal with job-related stressors that can lead to burnout, chronic fatigue, and irritability. Time pressures are intense in many settings, with demands for direct treatment, documentation, inter- and intradepartmental communication, and staff training being made constantly and simultaneously. With the current changes in the health care system, many clinics are experiencing drastic changes in types of caseload and client or staff ratios.

Stress Management Techniques

Stress management techniques have been developed to help relieve chronic stress and its effects. These techniques are learned behaviors that interrupt the nervous system's stress reactions. A brief description of some techniques and hints about teaching them follow. References for each technique can be consulted for more detail.

COPING SKILLS TRAINING

Coping skills training is a multimodal approach to helping individuals with stress-related problems. It involves both

---

RESEARCH NOTE
RESEARCH CAN DEMONSTRATE WHICH TREATMENT PRODUCES THE MOST IMPROVEMENT

Kenneth J. Ottenbacher

The observation is often made that treatment in occupational therapy involves a mixture of art and science. The art of treatment is reflected in the fact that intervention programs change as the result of clinical creativity and problem solving. The science refers to those components of treatment that are predictable and can be systematically measured, controlled, and evaluated. All occupational therapy intervention programs represent dynamic and evolving systems for interacting with consumers, families, and other professionals. These systems combine elements of clinical creativity and research.

We know that systems of treatment evolve, and we assume that the evolution produces activities and devices that are more effective, efficient, and safer than previous techniques. How do systems of treatment change? And, how do we know that the new methods are more effective, efficient, and safer? Ideally, new treatment activities are based, at least in part, on research findings from the professional literature. For example, an assessment instrument used to identify depression may be revised to include new items or a modified scoring format that previous research has demonstrated is easier to understand and more sensitive. Change is only improvement if we can demonstrate that the changes produce better results. Research can help occupational therapists differentiate between change and improvement when selecting among treatment approaches. ■

cognitive and behavioral techniques and usually occurs in a group format. A typical coping skills-training program might include the management of physiological arousal (relaxation training), time management training (to help the individual develop a daily schedule with both work and leisure time activities), cognitive restructuring (in which individuals identify cognitive distortions associated with stressful events), and social skills or assertiveness training. In coping skills training clients are encouraged to work on specific stressful events and to recognize how they can effect change in their lives (Meichenbaum & Cameron, 1983). Coping skills training has been effective with clients with many types of stress-related problems (Bradshaw, 1993; Ehlers, Stangier, & Gieler, 1995; Starkey, Deleone, & Flannery, 1995; Tallant, Rose, & Tolman, 1989; Taylor, 1995; Wigers, Stiles, & Vogel, 1996).

AEROBIC EXERCISE

Aerobic exercise involves, repetitive, rhythmic contractions of the large muscles of the legs and arms. Examples are walking, running, bicycling, and swimming. Aerobic exercise appears to be an effective mood-regulating behavior (Thayer, Newman, & McClain, 1994). Aerobic exercise has been demonstrated to be effective in the relief of pain and stress-related disorders (Wigers et al, 1996). Anyone planning to start an aerobic exercise program should first be seen by a physician for a complete physical examination; all exercise programs should begin gradually and work slowly toward increased difficulty to avoid injuries. Specific guidelines for setting up individualized aerobic exercise programs are available from other sources (American College of Sports Medicine, 1991).

AUTOGENIC TRAINING

Autogenic training uses autosuggestion or self-hypnosis and mental imagery to achieve relaxation. Autosuggestion typically involve imagining sensations of physical heaviness and warmth to achieve muscle relaxation and vasodilation. Imagining oneself in settings where one would feel warm, comfortable, and heavy can facilitate these autosuggestions. Learning this process requires considerable practice and is not recommended for people who are agitated or actively psychotic (Courtney & Escobedo, 1990). Controlled trials suggest that autogenic training is an effective adjunctive treatment for stress-related conditions (Ehlers et al, 1995).

COMMUNICATION SKILLS

Both psychiatric and medical disorders can be exacerbated by stressful communication with significant others (Bradshaw, 1993; Ehlers, Osen, Wenninger, & Gieler, 1994). Practicing effective communication skills, such as clarifying expectations, defining needs honestly, and providing tactful and constructive feedback, can decrease the number of stressful misunderstandings. Social skills training and assertiveness training programs are an important part of stress

management for certain client populations (eg, persons with chronic pain).

DEEP BREATHING

Deep (diaphragmatic) breathing involves slowly inhaling and exhaling to reduce tension in the shoulders, trunk, and abdomen. The process begins with focusing on normal breathing in a quiet and comfortable place. This is followed by a period of deep inhalation and slow exhalation. During inhalation, the abdominal muscles should be relaxed. During exhalation, the abdominal muscles should be contracted. It is often helpful to rest a hand lightly on the abdomen during this process.

Deep breathing is relatively easy to learn, requires no equipment, and can be done anywhere. Deep abdominal breathing has been demonstrated to reduce physiological responsiveness (Forbes & Pekala, 1993).

LAUGHTER

The healing power of humor has received much attention from health care professionals over the past few years. Some writers have suggested that laughter may stimulate the release of endorphins, the brain's endogenous opiates, thereby helping to alleviate pain and stress (Cousins, 1979). It is important for practitioners to remember that therapy does not have to be solemn to be effective.

MEDITATION

Meditation involves focusing attention on a rhythmic, repetitive word, phrase, or sensation (eg, breathing, heart rate) to achieve relaxation. Benson (1975) has suggested that this mental process blocks the stress response of the sympathetic nervous system by activating the anterior hypothalamus, which controls the parasympathetic nervous system. This technique requires considerable practice and can take many months to learn.

PROGRESSIVE RELAXATION EXERCISES

Progressive relaxation exercises involve tensing and relaxing muscle groups, one group at a time, from head to foot. This technique teaches the difference between muscle tension and muscle relaxation by exaggerating the contrast between the two tone states. The learning sequence for this technique is (1) systematic tensing and relaxing of muscle groups to verbal cues, (2) systematic relaxing of muscle groups to verbal cues, and (3) relaxation of muscle groups by autosuggestion. Progressive relaxation exercises require discipline and practice, and they can take months to learn completely (Jacobsen, 1938). Progressive relaxation is not recommended for clients with upper motor neuron lesions and spasticity. Because these exercises involve isometric muscle contractions, they are not recommended for clients with **hypertension** or cardiac disease (Courtney & Escobedo, 1990; Smith & Lukens, 1983). Progressive relaxation appears to be an effective mood regulatory behavior (Thayer et al, 1994), and it increases skin temperature and decreases pulse rate, suggesting that it can reduce physiological reactivity (Forbes & Pekala, 1993).

TIME MANAGEMENT

Time management techniques include realistically scheduling and organizing time, setting priorities about task accomplishments, making lists, setting limits, and accepting the fact that everything cannot be done at once. An appropriate schedule should include both work and leisure time activities.

VERBALIZATION

Talking to friends and acquaintances about stressors can help reduce stress. Friends can offer different perspectives, new suggestions, and support, all of which are helpful in extricating a person from feeling stuck with a problem situation. Talking problems over with friends and increasing social contact may be an effective mood regulation strategy (Rippere, 1977).

General Guidelines for Choice of Technique

SELF-ASSESSMENT

Guided self-assessment of individual stressors and stress reactions is the first step in designing an appropriate stress management program. The guiding can be done by someone else or by structured forms that the person can fill out independently. The Holmes-Rahe Life Change Index (Holmes & Rahe, 1967) or the Stress Management Questionnaire (Stein & Nikolic, 1989) can help identify stressors. Other forms are available to help people assess their physical, emotional, and behavioral stress responses (Vitaliano, Russo, Carr, Maiuro, & Becker, 1985). Care should be taken to interpret scores on formal stress scales as gross, relative indications of stress levels and behavior patterns only. On the Holmes-Rahe scale, for instance, the statistical correlation between higher scores and the risk of illness or injury, although positive, is relatively weak. A list of the categories of stressors mentioned earlier might be a more useful, less restrictive, and less suggestive way to structure a person's self-assessment.

GENERAL FACTORS

Some stressors can be avoided; others cannot. Some general factors to consider in suggesting stress management techniques for people or deciding on such techniques for oneself are (1) the length of time it take to master the stress reduction technique versus how much time is available, (2) the nature of the persons lifestyle and daily routine, (3) the level of financial and interpersonal support available to the person, and (4) the person's commitment to change.

For example, meditation takes many months to learn properly and could not be taught within a short hospital stay. Deep breathing techniques, on the other hand, are rela-

tively easy to learn, require no outside equipment, and can generally be taught quickly.

▶STRESS MANAGEMENT CONCLUSION

Although not everyone needs formal stress management training, it is important to remember that all clients are in stressful situations by virtue of their illness or disability. Effective stress management programs can be part of individual or group therapy sessions and are particularly helpful for those with stress-related illnesses or with high stress levels that seriously impede their functional progress.

▼ REFERENCES

Adams, M. (1982). Bobath certification eight week course. Memphis, TN.

Aldwin, C.M. (1994). *Stress, coping and development.* New York: Guilford Press.

AliMed (1996). *Orthopedic rehabilitation products catalogue.* Dedham, MA: AliMed, Inc.

Allen, K. C. (1993) Lesson 11: Creating a need-satisfying, safe environment management and maintenance approaches. In C. B. Royeen (Ed.), *AOTA Self-Study Series: Cognitive Rehabilitation.* Rockville, MD: American Occupational Therapy Association.

American College of Sports Medicine (1991). *Guidelines for exercise testing and prescription* (4th ed.). Philadelphia: Lea & Febiger.

American Occupational Therapy Association (AOTA) (1994). Uniform terminology for occupational therapy—third edition. *American Journal of Occupational Therapy, 48,* 1047–1054.

American Psychiatric Association. (1994). *Diagnostic and statistical manual of mental disorders.* (4th ed.) Washington. Author.

American Society of Hand Therapists, Splint Classification System (1992). *Splint classification system.* Chicago, IL: The Society.

Anderson, J. R. (1995). *Cognitive psychology and its implications.* New York: W. H. Freeman & Co.

Anderson, M. H. (1965). Upper extremity orthotics (p. 421). Springfield, IL: Charles C. Thomas.

Antonucci, G., Guariglia, A., Magnotti, l., Paolucci, S., Pizzamiglio, L., & Zoccolotti, P. (1995). Effectiveness of neglect rehabilitation in a randomized group study. *Journal of Clinical and Experimental Neuropsychology, 17,* 383–389.

Ayres, A. J. (1972). *Sensory integration and learning disorders.* Los Angeles: Western Psychological Services.

Ayres, A. J. (1976). *Sensory integration.* Two day workshop presented at the University of Tennessee, Memphis, TN.

Ayres, A. J. (1979). *Sensory integration and the child.* Los Angeles: Western Psychological Services.

Baptiste, S. (1988). Chronic pain, activity and culture. *Canadian Journal of Occupational Therapy, 55,* 179–184.

Barco, P. P., Crosson, B., Bolesta, M. M., Werts, D., & Stout R. (1991). Training awareness and compensation in postacute head injury rehabilitation. In J. S. Kreutzer & P. H. Wehman (Eds.), *Cognitive rehabilitation for persons with traumatic brain injury* (pp. 129–146). Baltimore: Paul Brookes Publishing Co.

Bell, J. A. (1987). Plaster casting for the remodeling of soft tissue. In E. E. Fess & C. A. Philips, *Hand splinting: Principles and methods* (pp. 449–466). St. Louis: C.V. Mosby.

Bell-Krotoski, J. A. (1990). Plaster cylinder casting for contracture of the interphalangeal joints. In J. M. Hunter, L. H. Schneider, E. J. Mackin, & A. D. Callahan (Eds.), *Rehabilitation of the hand* (3rd ed.) (pp. 1128–1133). St. Louis: C.V. Mosby.

Bell-Krotoski, J., & Fess E. E. (1995) (Eds.). Biomechanics (special issue). *Journal of Hand Therapy, 8* (2).

Benedict, R. H. B., Harris, A. E., Markow, T., McCormick, J., Nuechterlein, K. H., N., & Asarnow, R. F. (1994). Effects of attentional training on information processing in schizophrenia. *Schizophrenia Bulletin, 20,* 537–546.

Benson, H. (1975). *The relaxation response.* New York. Avon Books.

Ben-Yishay, Y., & Diller, L. (1983). Cognitive remediation. In M. Rosenthal, E. Griffith, M. Bond, & J. Miller (Eds.), *Rehabilitation of the head injured adult* (pp. 367–391). Philadelphia. F. A. Davis.

Ben-Yishay, Y., & Diller, L. (1993). Cognitive remediation in traumatic brain injury: Update and issues. *Archives of Physical Medicine and Rehabilitation, 74,* 204–212.

Ben-Yishay, Y., Piasetsky, E. B., & Rattok, J. (1987). A systematic method for ameliorating disorders in basic attention. In M. Meir, A. Benton, & L. Diller (Eds.) *Neuropsychological rehabilitation* (pp. 165–181). New York: Guilford Press.

Berkman, L. & Syme, S. L. (1979). Social networks, host resistance, and mortality: A nine-year follow-up study of Alameda County residents. *American Journal of Epidemiology, 109,* 186–204.

Bergquist, T. F., & Jacket, M. P. (1993). Awareness and goal setting with traumatically brain injured. *Brain Injury, 7,* 275–282.

Birnboim, S. (1995). A metacognitive approach to cognitive rehabilitation. *British Journal of Occupational Therapy, 58* (2), 61–64.

Blanchard, E. B., & Ahles, T. A. (1990). Biofeedback therapy. In J. J. Bonica (Ed.), *The management of pain* (2nd ed.) (pp. 1722–1732). Philadelphia: Lea & Febiger.

Bledsoe, S. (1991). Comparison of the force magnitude of PIP flexion and extension commercial spring coil and springy wire splints to a commercial accordion spring configuration. Proceedings of the American Society of Hand Therapists. *Journal of Hand Therapy, 4* (1), 27–28.

Boake, C. (1991). Social skills training following head injury. In J. S. Kreutzer & P. H. Wehman (Eds.), *Cognitive rehabilitation for persons with traumatic brain injury* (pp. 181–190). Baltimore: Paul H. Brookes.

Bobath, B. (1978). *Adult hemiplegia: Evaluation and treatment* (2nd ed.). London: William Heinemann Medical Books.

Bonica, J. J. (1977). Neurophysiological and pathologic aspects of acute and chronic pain. *Archives of Surgery, 112,* 750–761.

Bornstein, M. H., & Lamb, M. E. (Eds.) (1988). *Developmental psychology: An advanced textbook.* Hillsdale, NJ: Lawrence Earlbaum Associates.

Bradley, T. K. (1968). *Basic Splinting Manual.* Indianapolis, IN: Indiana University Medical Center, Occupational Therapy Program.

Bradley, N. S. & Beckoff, A. (1989). Development of locomotion: Animal models. In M. Woollacott and A. Shumway-Cook (Eds.), *The development of posture and gait across the life span* (pp. 48–73). Columbia, SC: University of South Carolina Press.

Bradshaw, W. H. (1993). Coping skills training versus a problem-solving approach with schizophrenic patients. *Hospital and Community Psychiatry, 44,* 1102–1104.

Bradstock, K., Forman, M. R., Binkin, N. J., Gentry, E. M., Hogelin, G. C., Williamson, D. F., & Trowbridge, F. L. (1988). Alcohol use and health behavior lifestyles among U. S. women: The behavioral risk factor survey. *Addictive Behaviors, 13,* 61–71.

Brand, P. W. (1952). Reconstruction of the hand in leprosy. *Annals of the Royal College of Surgeons of England, 11,* 350–356.

Brand, P. W. (1985). *Clinical mechanics of the hand.* St. Louis: C.V. Mosby.

Brand, P. W. (1990). The forces of dynamic splinting: Ten questions before applying a dynamic splint to the hand. In J. M. Hunter, L. H. Schneider, E. J. Mackin, & A. D. Callahan (Eds.), *Rehabilitation of the hand* (3rd ed.) (pp. 1095–1100). St. Louis: C.V. Mosby.

Brand, P. W., & Hollister, A. (1993). *Clinical mechanics of the hand* (2nd ed.). St. Louis: C.V. Mosby.

Bransford, J. D., & Stein, B. S. (1984). *The ideal problem solver.* New York: W. H. Freeman & Co.

Breger-Lee, D. E. & Buford W. L. (1991). Update in splinting materials

and methods. In E. J. Mackin, & A. D. Callahan (Eds.), *Hand clinics* (pp. 569–585). Philadelphia: W. B. Saunders.

Brown, C., Harwood, K., Hays, C., Heckman, J., & Short, J. E. (1993). Effectiveness of cognitive rehabilitation for improving attention in patients with schizophrenia. *The Occupational Therapy Journal of Research, 13,* 71–86.

Bruce, M. A. (1994). Cognitive rehabilitation: Intelligence, insight, and knowledge. In C. Royeen (Ed.), *AOTA self study series: Cognitive rehabilitation.* Baltimore: American Occupational Therapy Association.

Buchner, D. M., & Coleman, E. A. (1994). Exercise considerations in older adults: Intensity, fall prevention and safety. *Physical Medicine and Rehabilitation Clinics of North America, 5,* 357–375.

Budd, R. J., Eiser, J. R., Morgan, M., & Gammage, P. (1985). The personal characteristics and life-style of the young drinker: The results of a survey of British adolescents. *Drug and Alcohol Dependence, 16,* 145–157.

Burke, W. H., Zencius, A. H., Wesolowski, M. D., & Doubleday, F. (1991). Improving executive function disorders in brain injured clients. *Brain Injury, 5,* 241–252.

Bunnell S. (1944). *Surgery of the hand* (pp. 198–203). Philadelphia: J.B. Lippincott.

Cailliet, R. (1976). *Hand pain and impairment* (2nd ed.). Philadelphia: F. A. Davis.

Callahan, A. (1995). Methods of compensation and reeducation for sensory dysfunction. In J. M. Hunter, E. Mackin, & A. Callahan (Eds.). *Rehabilitation of the hand* (4th ed.) (pp. 701–714). Philadelphia: C.V. Mosby.

Calvanio, R., Levine, D., & Petrone, P. (1993). Elements of cognitive rehabilitation after right hemisphere stroke. *Neurologic Clinics, 11,* 25–57.

Campbell, J. J., Duffy, J. D., & Salloway, S. P. (1994). Treatment strategies for patients with dysexecutive syndromes. *The Journal of Neuropsychiatry and Clinical Neurosciences, 6,* 411–418.

Cannon, N. M., Foltz, R. W., Koepfer, J. M, Lauck, M. F., Simpson, D. M., & Bromley, R. S. (1985). *Manual of hand splinting.* New York: Churchill Livingstone.

Capener, N. (1956). The hand in surgery. *Journal of Bone and Joint Surgery, 38B* (1), 132.

Cappa, S., Sterzi, R., Vallar, G., & Bisiach, E. (1987). Remission of hemineglect and anosagnosia during vestibular stimulation. *Neuropsychologia, 25,* 775–782.

Carr, J. H., & Shepherd, R. B. (1987). *A motor re-learning program for stroke* (2nd ed.). Rockville, MD: Aspen System.

Caruso, L. A., & Chan, D. E. (1986). Evaluation and management of the patient with acute back pain. *American Journal of Occupational Therapy, 46,* 347–351.

Chapman, C. R., & Turner, J. A. (1990). Psychologic and psychosocial aspects of acute pain. In J. J. Bonica (Ed.). *The management of pain* (2nd ed.) (pp. 122–132). Philadelphia: Lea & Febiger.

Cicerone, K. D., & Giacino, T. J. (1992). Remediation of executive function deficits after traumatic brain injury. *NeuroRehabilitation, 2* (3), 12–22.

Cicerone, K. D., & Wood, J. C. (1987). Planning disorder after closed head injury: A case study. *Archives of Physical Medicine and Rehabilitation, 68,* 111–115.

Clark, F., Mailloux, Z., & Parham, D. (1989). Sensory integration and children with learning disabilities. In P. N. Pratt & A. S. Allen (Eds.). *Occupational therapy for children* (2nd ed.) (pp. 457–509). St. Louis: C.V. Mosby.

Cohen, S., Tyrrell, D. A. J., & Smith, A. P. (1991). Psychological stress and susceptibility to the common cold. *New England Journal of Medicine, 325,* 606–612.

Commission on Accreditation of Rehabilitation Facilities. (1996). *Standards manual for organizations serving people with disabilities.* Tucson, AZ: Author.

Courtney, C., & Escobedo, B. (1990). A stress management program: Inpatient to outpatient continuity. *American Journal of Occupational Therapy, 44,* 306–311.

Cousins, N. (1979). *Anatomy of an illness as perceived by the patient.* New York: Bantom Books.

Crue, B. L., Jr., Todd, E. M., & Maline, D. B. (1975). Postherpetic neuralgia-conservative treatment regimen. In B. L. Crue, Jr. (Ed.). *Pain: Research and treatment* (pp. 289–292). New York: Academic Press.

Cubelli, R., Trentini, P., & Montagna. C. G. (1991). Re-education of gestural communication in a case of chronic global aphasia and limb apraxia. *Cognitive Neuropsychology, 8,* 369–380.

Davies, P. M. (1985). *Steps to follow.* New York: Springer Verlag.

Davis, J. Z. (1992). The Affolter method: A model for treating perceptual disturbances in the hemiplegic and brain-injured patient. *Occupational Therapy Practice: Is That OT?, 3* (4), 1–88.

Dellon, A. L. (1981). *Evaluation of sensibility and reeducation of sensation in the hand.* Baltimore: Williams & Wilkins.

Diller, L. (1994). Finding the right treatment combinations: Changes in rehabilitation over the past five years. In A. L. Christensen & B. P. Uzzell (Eds.), *Brain injury and neuropsychological rehabilitation: International perspectives* (pp. 1–15). Hillsdale, NJ: Lawrence Erlbaum Associates.

Diller, L., Ben-Yishay, Y., Gerstman, L. J., Goodkin, R., Gordon, W., & Weinberg, J. (1974). *Studies in cognition and rehabilitation in hemiplegia* (Rehabilitation Monograph No. 50): Institute of Rehabilitation Medicine, New York University Medical Center.

Diller, L., & Riley, E. (1993). The behavioral management of neglect. In I. H. Robertson & J. C. Marshall (Eds.). *Unilateral neglect: Clinical and experimental studies* (pp. 293–306). Hillsdale, NJ: Lawrence Erlbaum Associates.

Dunn, W., Brown, C., & McGuigan, A. (1994). The ecology of human performance: A framework for considering the effect of context. *American Journal of Occupational Therapy, 48,* 595–607.

Duran, R. J., Coleman, C. R., Nappi, J. F., & Klerekoper, L. A. (1990). Management of flexor tendon lacerations in zone two using controlled passive motion postoperatively. In J.M. Hunter, L.H. Schneider, E.J. Mackin, & A.D. Callahan (Eds.). *Rehabilitation of the hand* (3rd ed.) (pp. 410–413). St. Louis: C.V. Mosby.

Dutton, R. (1995). *Clinical reasoning in physical disabilities.* Baltimore: Williams & Wilkins.

Easton, T. (1972). On the normal use of reflexes. *American Scientist, 60,* 591–599.

Efferson, L. (1995). Disorders of vision and visual perceptual dysfunction. In D. A. Umphred (Ed.). *Neurological rehabilitation* (3rd ed.) (pp. 769–802). St. Louis: C.V. Mosby.

Ehlers, A., Osen, A., Wenninger, K., & Gieler, U. (1994). Atopic dermatitis and stress: The possible role of negative communication with significant others. *International Journal of Behavioral Medicine, 1,* 107–121.

Ehlers, A., Stangier, U., & Gieler, U. (1995). Treatment of atopic dermatitis: A comparison of psychological and dermatological approaches to relapse prevention. *Journal of Consulting and Clinical Psychology, 63,* 624–635.

Engel, J. M. (1993). Pain management. In H. L. Hopkins and H. D. Smith (Eds.). *Willard and Spackman's occupational therapy* (8th ed.) (pp. 596–604). Philadelphia: J. B. Lippincott.

Engel, J. M., & Rapoff, M. A. (1990a). A component analysis of relaxation training for children with vascular, muscle contraction, and mixed-headache disorders. In D. C. Tyler & E. J. Krane (Eds.). *Advances in pain research therapy* (Vol. 15, pp. 273–290). New York: Raven Press.

Engel, J. M., & Rapoff, M. A. (1990b). Biofeedback-assisted relaxation training for adult and pediatric headache disorders. *Occupational Therapy Journal of Research, 10,* 283–299.

Epstein, S., & Meier, P. (1989). Constructive thinking: A broad coping variable with specific components. *Journal of Personality and Social Psychology, 57,* 332–350.

Evans, R. B. (1990). Therapeutic management of extensor tendon injuries. In J. M. Hunter, L. H. Schneider, E. J. Mackin, & A. D. Callahan (Eds.). *Rehabilitation of the hand* (3rd ed.) (pp. 492–511). St. Louis: C.V. Mosby.

Evans, B. E., Larson, D. L., & Yates, S. (1968). Preservation and restoration of joint function in patients with severe burns. *Journal of the American Medical Association, 204* (10), 91–96.

Ezrachi, O., Ben-Yishay, Y., & Kay, T. (1991). Predicting employment in traumatic brain injury following neuropsychological rehabilitation. *Journal of Head Trauma, 6,* 71–84.

Farber, S. (1993). OT intervention for individuals with limb apraxia, Paper presented at the AOTA Neuroscience Institute: Treating Adults with Apraxia, March 20, 1993, Baltimore, MD.

Feinberg, J., & Brandt, K. D. (1981). Use of resting splints by patients with rheumatoid arthritis. *American Journal of Occupational Therapy, 35,* 173–178.

Fess, E.E. (1984). Rubber band traction: Physical properties, splint design, and identification of force magnitude. *Journal of Hand Surgery, 9A,* 610. (From the Proceedings of the American Society of Hand Therapists.)

Fess, E. E. (1988). Force magnitude of commercial spring-coil and spring-wire splints designed to extend the proximal interphalangeal joint. *Journal of Hand Therapy, 1* (3), 86–90.

Fess, E. E. (1990). Documentation: Essential elements of an upper extremity assessment battery. In J. M. Hunter, L. H. Schneider, E. J. Mackin, & A. D. Callahan (Eds.). *Rehabilitation of the hand* (3rd ed.) (pp. 53–81). St. Louis: C.V. Mosby.

Fess, E. E., Gettle, K. S., & Strickland, J.W. (1981). *Hand splinting: Principles and methods.* St. Louis: C.V. Mosby.

Fess, E. E., & Philips, C. A. (1987). *Hand splinting: Principles and methods* (2nd ed.). St. Louis: C.V. Mosby.

Fetherlin, J. M., & Kurland, L. (1989). Self-Instruction: A compensatory strategy to increase functional independence with brain injured adults. *Occupational Therapy Practice, 1* (1), 75–78.

Fidler, G. S., & Fidler, J. S. (1978). Doing and becoming: Purposeful action and self-actualization. *American Journal of Occupational Therapy, 32,* 305–310.

Fine, S. (1993). Lesson 3: Interaction between psychosocial variables and cognitive function. In C. B. Royeen (Ed.). *AOTA self-study series: Cognitive rehabilitation.* Rockville, MD: American Occupational Therapy Association.

Flatt, A. E. (1983). *Care of the arthritic hand* (4th ed.) (pp. 15–35). St. Louis: C.V. Mosby.

Flay, B. R., Hu, F. B., Siddiqui, O., Day, L. E., Hedeker, D., Petraitis, J., Richardson, J., & Sussman, S. (1994). Differential influence of parental smoking and friends' smoking on adolescent initiation and escalation of smoking. *Journal of Health and Social Behavior, 35,* 248–265.

Flower, A., Naxon, E., Jones, R. E., & Mooney, V. (1981). An occupational therapy program for chronic back pain. *American Journal of Occupational Therapy, 35,* 243–248.

Foerster, O. (1977). The motor cortex in man in light of Hughlings Jackson's doctrines. In: O. D. Payton, S. Hirt, & R. Newman (Eds.). *Scientific basis for neurophysiologic approaches to therapeutic exercise* (pp. 13–18). Philadelphia: F. A. Davis.

Forbes, E. J., & Pekala, R. J. (1993). Psychophysiological effects of several stress management techniques. *Psychological Reports, 72,* 19–27.

Fordyce, W. E. (1976). *Behavioral methods for chronic pain and illness.* St. Louis: C.V. Mosby.

Fordyce, W. E. (1990). Contingency management. In J. J. Bonica (Ed.). *The management of pain* (2nd ed.) (pp. 1702–1710). Philadelphia: Lea & Febiger.

Friedman, H. S., Tucker, J. S., Schwartz, J. E., Martin, L. R., Tomlinson-Keasey, C., Wingard, D. L., & Criqui, M. H. (1995). Childhood conscientiousness and longevity: Health behaviors and cause of death. *Journal of Personality and Social Psychology, 68,* 696–703.

Gage, M. (1992). The appraisal method of coping: An assessment and intervention model for occupational therapy. *American Journal of Occupational Therapy, 46,* 353–362.

Gage, M., & Polatajko, H. J. (1994). Enhancing occupational performance through an understanding of perceived self efficacy. *American Journal of Occupational Therapy, 48,* 783–790.

Gentile, A. (1992). The nature of skill acquisition: Therapeutic implications for children with movement disorders. In H. Forssberg & H. Hirschfield (Eds.). *Movement disorders in children* (pp. 31–41). Basel: S. Karger.

Gianutsos, R. (1989). Forward. In M. M. Sohlberg & C. Mateer (Eds.). *Introduction to cognitive rehabilitation: Theory and practice*, (pp. vii–viii). New York: Guilford Press.

Gibson, J. J. (1966). *The senses considered as perceptual systems*. Boston: Houghton Mifflin.

Giles, G. M. (1992). A neurofunctional approach to rehabilitation following severe brain injury. In N. Katz (Ed.). *Cognitive rehabilitation models for intervention in occupational therapy*, (pp. 195–218). Boston: Andover Medical Publishers.

Giles, G. M., & Allen, M. E. (1986). Occupational therapy in the treatment of the patient with chronic pain. *British Journal of Occupational Therapy, 49*, 4–9.

Giles, G. M., & Clark-Wilson, J. (1988). The use of behavioral techniques in functional skills training after severe brain injury. *American Journal of Occupational Therapy, 42*, 658–669.

Giles, M. G., & Shore, M. (1989). A rapid method for teaching severely brain injured adults how to wash and dress. *Archives of Physical Medicine and Rehabilitation, 70*. 156–158.

Giles, M. G., & Wilson, C. J. (1993). *Brain injury rehabilitation: A neurofunctional approach*. East Sussex UK: Chapman & Hall.

Glisky, E. L. (1995). Computers in memory rehabilitation. In A. D. Baddeley, B. A. Wilson, & F. N. Watts (Eds.). *Handbook of memory disorders* (pp. 557–575). New York: John Wiley & Sons.

Glisky, E. L., & Schacter, D. L. (1988). Acquisition of domain-specific knowledge in patients with organic memory disorders. *Journal of Learning Disabilities, 21*, 333–339.

Glisky, L. E., Schacter, D. L., & Butters, A. M. (1994). Domain-specific learning and remediation of memory disorders. In M. J. Riddoch & G. W. Humphreys (Eds.). *Cognitive neuropsychology and cognitive rehabilitation* (pp. 527–548). East Sussex, UK: Lawrence Erlbaum Associates.

Goldstein, T. S. (1995). *Functional rehabilitation in orthopaedics*. Gaithersburg, MD: Aspen Systems.

Gordon, J. (1987). Assumptions underlying physical therapy intervention: Theoretical and historical perspectives. In. J. H. Carr, R. B. Shepherd, J. Gordon, A. M. Gentile, & J. M. Held (Eds.). *Movement science: Foundation for physical therapy in rehabilitation* (pp. 1–30). Rockville, MD: Aspen Systems.

Gottlieb, N. H., & Green, L. W. (1984). Life events, social network, lifestyle, and health: An analysis of the 1979 national survey of personal health practices and consequences. *Health Education Quarterly, 11*, 91–105.

Green, M. F. (1993). Cognitive remediation In schizophrenia: Is It time yet? *American Journal of Psychiatry, 150*, 178–187.

Greene, P. H. (1972). Problems of organization of motor systems. In R. Rosen & F. M. Snell, (Eds.). *Progress in theoretical biology* (pp. 304–338). San Diego: Academic Press.

Grembowski, D., Patrick, D., Diehr, P., Durham, M., Beresford, S., Kay, E., & Hecht, J. (1993). Self-efficacy and health behavior among older adults. *Journal of Health and Social Behavior, 34*, 89–104.

Griffin, K. W., Friend, R., Eitel, P., & Lobel, M. (1993). Effects of environmental demands, stress, and mood on health practices. *Journal of Behavioral Medicine, 16*, 643–661.

Gross, Y., & Schutz, L. E. (1986). Intervention models in neuropsychology. In B. Uzzell & Y. Gross (Eds.). *Clinical neuropsychology of intervention* (pp. 179–204). Boston: Martinus Nijhoff Publishing.

Grzesiak, R. C. (1982). Cognitive and behavioral approaches to management of chronic pain. *New York State Journal of Medicine, 82* (1), 30–38.

Hamill, J., & Knutzen, K. M. (1995). *Biomechanical basis of human movement*. Baltimore: Williams & Wilkins.

Hanson, R. W., & Gerber, K. E. (1990). *Coping with chronic pain: A guide to patient self-management*. New York: Guilford Press.

Harrell, M., Parente, F., Bellingrath, E., & Lisicia, K. (1992). *Cognitive rehabilitation of memory: A practical guide*. Gaithersberg, MD: Aspen Publication.

Harter, S. (1983). Developmental perspectives on the self-system. In P. H. Mussen (Ed.). *Handbook of child psychology*, (Vol. 4), (pp. 275–386). New York: John Wiley & Sons.

Haugen, J., & Mathiowetz, V. (1995). Contemporary task-oriented approach. In C. Trombly (Ed.). *Occupational therapy for physical dysfunction* (pp. 510–529). Baltimore: Williams & Wilkins.

Heck, S. A. (1988). The effect of purposeful activity on pain tolerance. *American Journal of Occupational Therapy, 42*, 577–581.

Helm-Estabrooks, N. (1982). Visual action therapy for global aphasics. *Journal of Speech and Hearing Disorders, 47*, 385–389.

Heriza, C. (1991). Motor development: Traditional and Contemporary Theories. In M. Lister (Ed.). *Contemporary management of motor control problems* (pp. 99–126). Alexandria, VA: American Physical Therapy Association.

Herman, H. (1984). Compliance with splint wearing schedule on a burn unit. *Journal of Hand Surgery, 9A*, 610. (From the Proceedings of the American Society of Hand Therapists.)

Hibbard, J., & Pope, C. (1993). The quality of social roles as predictors of morbidity and mortality. *Social Science and Medicine, 36*, 217–225.

Hills, H., & Norvell, N. (1991). An examination of hardiness and neuroticism as potential moderators of stress outcomes. *Behavioral Medicine, 17*, 31–38.

Holmes, T. H., & Rahe, R. H. (1967). The social readjustment rating scale. *Journal of Psychosomatic Research, 11*, 213–218.

Hopkins, H. (1966). Self-help aides. In S. Licht (Ed.), *Orthotics etcetera* (9th ed.; p. 647). New Haven, CT: Elizabeth Licht.

Horak, F. (1991). Assumptions underlying motor control for neurologic rehabilitation. In M. Lister (Ed.). *Contemporary management of motor control problems* (pp. 11–28). Alexandria, VA: American Physical Therapy Association.

Hunter, J. M., Schneider, L. H., Mackin, E. J., & Callahan, A. D. (Eds.). (1990). *Rehabilitation of the hand* (3rd ed.). St. Louis: C.V. Mosby.

Jacobsen, E. (1938). *Progressive relaxation*. Chicago. University of Chicago Press.

Jensen, M. P., & Karoly, P. (1992). Self-report scales and procedures for assessing pain in adults. In D. C. Turk & R. Melzack (Eds.). *Handbook of pain assessment* (pp. 135–151). New York: Guilford Press.

Johnson, J. V., & Hall, E. M. (1988). Job strain, work place social support, and cardiovascular disease: A cross-sectional study of a random sample of the Swedish working population. *American Journal of Public Health, 78*, 1336–1342.

Johnson, M. (1977). Assessment of clinical pain. In A. K. Jacox (Ed.). *Pain: A source book for nurses and other health professionals* (pp. 139–166). Boston: Little, Brown & Co.

Kandel, E., Schwartz, J. H., & Jessell, T. M. (Eds.) (1991). *Principles of neural science* (3rd ed.). New York: Appleton & Lange.

Karasek, R. A. (1979). Job demand, job decision latitude and mental strain: Implications for job redesign. *Administrative Science Quarterly, 24*, 285–308.

Karasek, R. A., Theorell, T. T., Schwartz, J., Schall, P., Pieper, C., & Michela, J. L. (1988). Job characteristics in relation to the prevalence of myocardial infarction in the US HES and HANES. *American Journal of Public Health, 78*, 910–918.

Katz, E. R., Varni, J. W., & Jay, S. M. (1984). Behavioral assessment and management of pediatric pain. In M. Hersen, R. M. Eisler, & P. M. Miller (Eds.). *Progress in behavior modification* (Vol. 18, pp. 163–193). New York: Academic Press.

Kazdin, A. E. (1980). *Research design in clinical psychology*. New York: Harper & Row.

Keefe, F. J. (1982). Behavioral assessment and treatment of chronic pain: Current status and future directions. *Journal of Consulting and Clinical Psychology, 50*, 896–911.

Keele, S. (1968). Movement control in skilled motor performance. *Psychological Bulletin, 70*, 387–403.

Kelly, M., & Ostreicher, H. (1985). Environmental factors and outcomes in hemineglect syndromes. *Rehabilitation Psychology, 30,* 35–37.

Kerkhoff, G., MunBinger, U., & Meier, E. K. (1994). Neurovisual rehabilitation in cerebral blindness. *Archives of Neurology, 51,* 474–481.

Keshner, E. (1991). How theoretical framework biases evaluation and treatment. In M. Lister (Ed.), *Contemporary management of motor control problems* (pp. 37–49). Alexandria, VA: American Physical Therapy Association.

Kiel, J. H. (1983). *Basic hand splinting: A pattern designing approach.* Boston: Little, Brown & Co.

Kimball, J. G. (1993). Sensory integrative frame of reference. In P. Kramer & J. Hinojosa (Eds.). *Frames of reference for pediatric occupational therapy* (pp. 87–175). Baltimore: Williams & Wilkins.

Kisner, C., & Colby, L. A. (1990). *Therapeutic exercise: Foundations and techniques.* Philadelphia: F. A. Davis.

Klavora, P., Gaskovski, P., Martin, K., Forsyth, D. R., Heslegrave, J. R., Young, M., & Quinn, P. R. (1995). The effects of dynavision rehabilitation on behind-the-wheel driving ability psychomotor abilities of persons after stroke. *American Journal of Occupational Therapy, 49,* 534–542.

Kleinert, H. E., Kutz, J. E., & Cohn, M. J. (1975). Primary repair of zone two flexor tendon lacerations. In American Academy of Orthopaedic Surgeons, *Symposium on tendon surgery in the hand* (pp. 91–104). St. Louis: C.V. Mosby.

Koepke, G. H., Feallock, B., & Felle, I. (1963). Splinting the severely burned hand. *American Journal of Occupational Therapy, 17* (4), 147–150

Lam, C. S., McMahon, B. T., & Priddy, D. A. (1988). Deficit awareness and treatment performance among traumatic head injury adults. *Brain Injury, 2,* 233–242.

Lamm-Warburg, C. (1988). Assessment and treatment strategies for perceptual deficits. In S. O'Sullivan & T. J. Schmitz (Eds.). *Physical rehabilitation: Assessment and treatment* (2nd ed.) (pp. 93–120). Philadelphia: F. A. Davis.

Lau, R. R., Quadrel, M. J., & Hartman, K. A. (1990). Development and change in young adults' preventive health beliefs and behavior: Influence from parents and peers. *Journal of Health and Social Behavior, 31,* 240–259.

Lazarus, R. S. (1993). From psychological stress to the emotions: A history of a changing outlook. *Annual Review of Psychology, 44,* 1–21.

Lee, M. H. M., Itoh, M., Yang, G. W., & Eason, A. L. (1990). Physical therapy and rehabilitation medicine. In J. J. Bonica (Ed.). *The management of pain* (2nd ed.) (pp. 1769–1788). Philadelphia: Lea & Febiger.

Lennon, S. (1994). Task specific effects in the rehabilitation of unilateral neglect. In M. J. Riddoch & G. W. Humphreys (Eds.). *Cognitive neuropsychology and cognitive rehabilitation* (pp. 187–203). East Sussex UK: Lawrence Erlbaum Associates.

Lerner, D. J., Levine, S., Malspeis, S., & D'Agostino, R. B. (1994). Job strain and health-related quality of life in a national sample. *American Journal of Public Health, 84,* 1580–1585.

Lillegard, W. A., & Terrio, J. D. (1994). Appropriate strength training. *Medical Clinics of North America, 78,* 457–477.

Linden, C. A. (1995). Orthoses: Purposes and types. In C. A. Trombly (Ed.). *Occupational therapy for physical dysfunction* (4th ed.) (pp. 551–582). Baltimore: Williams & Wilkins.

Long, C., & Schutt, A. H. (1986). Upper limb orthotics. In J. B. Redford (Ed.). *Orthotics etcetera* (3rd ed.) (pp. 198–277). Baltimore: Williams & Wilkins.

Luria, A. R. (1973). *The working brain* (Basil Haigh, Trans.). New York: Basic Books.

MacRae, A., & Riley, E. (1990). Home health occupational therapy for the management of chronic pain: An environmental model. *Occupational Therapy Practice, 1* (3), 69–76.

Madden, J. W., & Arem, A. (1981). Wound healing: Biologic and clinical features. In J. Sabiston (Ed.). *Davis-Christopher textbook of surgery* (12th ed.) (pp. 265–286). Philadelphia: W. B. Saunders.

Malick, M. H. (1978). *Manual on dynamic hand splinting with thermoplastic materials* (2nd ed.). Pittsburgh: Harmarville Rehabilitation Center.

Malick, M. H. (1979). *Manual on static hand splinting* (3rd ed.). Pittsburgh: Harmarville Rehabilitation Center.

Mathiowetz, V., & Haugen, J. (1995). Evaluation of motor behavior: Traditional and contemporary views. In. C. Trombly (Ed.). *Occupational therapy for physical dysfunction* (pp. 157–187). Baltimore: Williams & Wilkins.

Mayer, N. H., Keating, D. J., & Rapp, D. (1986). Skills, routines, and activity patterns of daily living: A functional nested approach. In B. P. G. Uzzell (Ed.). *Clinical neuropsychology of intervention* (pp. 205–222). Boston: Martinus-Nijhoff Publishing.

McArdle, W. D., Katch, F. I., & Katch, V. L. (1991). *Exercise physiology: Energy, nutrition and human performance.* (3rd ed.). Malvern, PA: Lea & Feiger.

McCaffery, M. (1979). *Nursing management of the patient with pain.* Philadelphia: J. B. Lippincott.

McCormack, G. L. (1988). Pain management by occupational therapists. *American Journal of Occupational Therapy, 42,* 582–590.

McCormack, G. L. (1990). The Rood approach to the treatment of neuromuscular dysfunction. In L.W. Pedretti & B. Zoltan (Eds.). *Occupational therapy practice skills for physical dysfunction* (3rd ed.) (pp. 311–333). St. Louis: C.V. Mosby.

McCormack, G. L., & Johnson, C. (1990). Systems for objectifying clinical pain. *Occupational Therapy Practice, 1* (3), 21–29.

McNaughton, M. E., Patterson, T. L., Smith, T. L., & Grant, I. (1995). The relationship among stress, depression, locus of control, irrational beliefs, social support and health in Alzheimer's disease caregivers. *Journal of Nervous and Mental Disease, 183,* 78–85.

Mehrabian, A., & Straubinger, T. (1989). Patterns of drug use among young adults. *Addictive Behaviors, 14,* 99–104.

Meichenbaum, D., & Cameron, R. (1983). Stress inoculation training: Towards a general paradigm for training in coping skills. In D. Meichenbaum and M. E. Jaremko (Eds.). *Stress reduction and prevention.* New York: Plenum.

Melamed, S., Groswasser, Z., & Stern, M. S. (1992). Acceptance of disability, work involvement and subjective rehabilitation status of traumatic brain injured patients. *Brain Injury, 6,* 233–243.

Melzack, R. (1975). The McGill Questionnaire: Major properties and scoring methods. *Pain, 1,* 277–299.

Mersky, H. (1986). Classification of chronic pain: Description of chronic pain syndromes and definitions of pain terms. *Pain* (Suppl. 3), S217.

Montgomery P. (1991). Neurodevelopmental treatment and sensory integrative theory. In M. Lister (Ed.). *Contemporary management of motor control problems* (pp. 135–137). Alexandria, VA: American Physical Therapy Association.

Moser, K. A., Fox, A. J., & Jones, D. R. (December 8, 1984). Unemployment and mortality in the OPCS longitudinal study. *Lancet, 2*(84–15), 1324–1329.

Moulton, H. J., Taira, E. D., & Grover, R. (1995). *Utilizing occupational therapy and families at mealtimes with nursing home residents with dementia.* Presentation at Gerontological Society on Aging, Annual Conference, Los Angles, CA, November.

Myers, B., Mukoyama, S., & Becker, P. (1985). *Proprioceptive neuromuscular facilitation.* Two week course presented at the Rehabilitation Institute of Chicago.

Neistadt, M. E. (1989). Normal adult performance on constructional praxis training tasks. *American Journal of Occupational Therapy, 43,* 448–455.

Neistadt, M. E. (1990). A critical analysis of occupational therapy approaches for perceptual deficits in adults with brain injury. *American Journal of Occupational Therapy, 44,* 299–304.

Neistadt, M. E. (1992). Occupational therapy treatments for constructional deficits. *American Journal of Occupational Therapy, 46,* 141–148.

Neistadt, M. E., (1993). Stress management. In H. L. Hopkins and H. D. Smith (Eds.). *Willard and Spackman's occupational therapy* (8th ed.) (pp. 588–596). Philadelphia: J. B. Lippincott.

Neistadt, M. E. (1994a). Perceptual retaining for adults with diffuse brain injury. *American Journal of Occupational Therapy, 48*, 225–233.

Neistadt, M. E. (1994b). The neurobiology of learning: Implications for treatment of adults with brain injury. *American Journal of Occupational Therapy, 48*, 421–430.

Nelson, D. L., & Lenhart, D. A. (1996). Resumption of outpatient occupational therapy for a young woman five years after traumatic brain injury. *American Journal of Occupational Therapy, 50*, 223–228.

Niemeyer, L. O. (1990). Psychologic and sociocultural aspects of responses to pain. *Occupational Therapy Practice, 1*(3), 11–20.

Norkin, C.C., & Levangie, P.K. (1992). *Joint Structure and Function* (2nd ed.). Philadelphia: F. A. Davis, Philadelphia.

North Coast Medical (1996). *Hand therapy catalog, 1996.* San Jose, CA: North Coast Medical.

Okkema, K. (1993). *Cognition and perception in the stroke patient.* Gaithersburg, MD: Aspen Publishers.

O'Sullivan, S. B. (1988). Strategies to improve motor control. In S. B. O'Sullivan, & T. J. Schmitz (Eds.). *Physical rehabilitation: Assessment and treatment* (2nd ed.) (pp. 253–278). Philadelphia: F. A. Davis.

Parker, L. H., & Cinciripini, P. M. (1984). Behavioral medicine with children: Applications in chronic disease. *Progress in Behavior Modification, 17*, 136–165.

Peacock, E. E. (1984). *Wound repair* (3rd ed.). Philadelphia: W. B. Saunders.

Pedretti, L. W. (1996). *Occupational therapy: Practice skills for physical dysfunction.* St. Louis: C.V. Mosby.

Peloquin, S. M. (1993). The patient-therapist relationship: Beliefs that shape care. *American Journal of Occupational Therapy, 47*, 935–942.

Pizzamiglio, L., Antonucci, G., Judica, A., Montenero, P., Razzano, C., & Zoccolotti, P. (1992). Cognitive rehabilitation of the hemineglect disorder in chronic patients with unilateral right brain damage. *Journal of Clinical Experimental Neuropsychology, 14*, 901–923.

Polit, A., & Bizzi, E. (1979). Characteristics of motor programs underlying arm movements in monkeys. *Journal of Neurophysiology, 42*, 183–194.

Poole, J. L. (1991). Application of motor learning principles in occupational therapy. *American Journal of Occupational Therapy, 45*, 531–537.

Potts, H., & Baptiste, S. (1989). An occupational therapy medico-legal programme for chronic pain patients. *Canadian Journal of Occupational Therapy, 56*, 193–197.

Radomski, V. M., Dougherty, P. M., Fine, B. S., & Baum, C. (1993). Lesson 10: Case studies in cognitive rehabilitation. In C. B. Royeen (Ed.). *AOTA self-study series: Cognitive rehabilitation* (pp. 668). Rockville, MD: American Occupational Therapy Association.

Rahe, R. H. (1979). Life change events and mental illness: An overview. *Journal of Human Stress, 5*, 2–9.

Randolph, S. L. (1975). Neurophysiological principles of sensory stimulation. Five day workshop presented at the University of Tennessee in Memphis, TN.

Reynolds, P., & Kaplan, G. A. (1990). Social connections and risk for cancer: Prospective evidence from the Alameda County study. *Behavioral Medicine, 9*, 101–110.

Rippere, V. (1977). "What is the thing to do when you are feeling depressed?" A pilot study. *Behavior Research and Therapy, 15*, 185–191.

Roberson, L., Breger, D., Buford, W. L., & Freeman, M. (1988). Analysis of the physical properties of SCOMAC springs and their potential use in dynamic splinting. *Journal of Hand Therapy, 1* (3), 110–114.

Robertson, I. (1991). Use of left versus right hand in responding to lateralised stimuli in unilateral neglect. *Neuropsychologia, 29*, 1129–1135.

Robertson, H. I., Tegner, R., Tham, K., Lo, A., & Smith, N. I. (1995). Sustained attention training for unilateral neglect: Theoretical and rehabilitation implications. *Journal of Clinical Neuropsychology, 17*, 416–430.

Robertson, I. H., North, N.T., & Geggie, C. (1992). Spatiomotor cuing in unilateral left neglect: Three single case studies of its therapeutic effects. *Journal of Neurology, Neurosurgery, and Psychiatry, 55*, 799–805.

Rogers, J. C., & Holm, M. B. (1994). Accepting the challenge of outcome research: Examining the effectiveness of occupational therapy practice. *American Journal of Occupational Therapy, 48*, 871–876.

Rosenbaum, A. (1991). *Human motor control.* San Diego: Academic Press.

Ross, F. (1992). The use of computers in occupational therapy for visual scanning. *American Journal of Occupational Therapy, 46*, 314–322.

Rossi, W. P., Kheyfets, S., & Reding, J. M. (1990). Fresnel prisms improve visual perception in stroke patients with homonymous hemianopia or unilateral visual neglect. *Neurology, 40*, 1597–1599.

Roy, E. A. (1985). *Neuropsychological studies of apraxia and related disorders.* Amsterdam: Elsevier Science Publishers.

Ruff, R. M., Baser, C. A., Johnston, J. W., Marshall, L. F., Klauber, S. K., Klauber, M. R., & Minteer, M. (1989). Neuropsychological rehabilitation: An experimental study with head injured patients. *Journal of Head Trauma Rehabilitation, 4*, 20–36.

Sabari, J. S. (1991). Motor learning concepts applied to activity based intervention with adults with hemiplegia. *American Journal of Occupational Therapy, 45*, 523–530.

Sabari J. (1995). Carr and Shepherd's motor relearning programme for individual's with stroke. In. C. Trombly (Ed.). *Occupational therapy for physical dysfunction* (pp. 501–510). Baltimore: Williams & Wilkins.

Sammons, F., & Preston, J.A. (1996). *Sammons Preston catalog 1996.* Bolingbrook, IL: Sammons Preston.

Sanders, S. H. (1979). Behavioral assessment and treatment of clinical pain: Appraisal of current status. In M. Hersen, R. M. Eisler, & P. M. Miller (Eds.). *Progress in behavior modification* (pp. 249–291). New York: Academic Press.

Sbordone, R. J. (1991). Overcoming obstacles in cognitive rehabilitation of persons with severe traumatic brain injury. In J. S. Kreutzer & P. H. Wehman (Eds.). *Cognitive rehabilitation for persons with traumatic brain injury* (pp. 105–116). Baltimore: Paul Brookes.

Scheier, M. F., & Carver, C. S. (1987) Dispositional optimism and physical wellbeing: The influence of generalized outcome expectancies on health. *Journal of Personality, 55*, 169–210.

Schkade, J. K., & Schultz, S. (1992). Occupational adaptation: Toward a holistic approach for contemporary practice, part 1. *American Journal of Occupational Therapy, 46*, 829–837.

Schmidt, R. (1988). *Motor control and learning.* Champaign: Human Kinetics Publishers.

Schultz, S., & Schkade, J. K. (1992). Occupational adaptation: Toward a holistic approach for contemporary practice, part 2. *American Journal of Occupational Therapy, 46*, 917–925.

Schwartz, S. M. (1995). Adults with traumatic brain injury: Three case studies of cognitive rehabilitation in the home setting. *American Journal of Occupational Therapy, 49*, 655–667.

Selye, H. (1978). *The stress of life.* New York. McGraw-Hill.

Seron, X., Deloche, G., & Coyette, F. (1989). A retrospective analysis of a single case of neglect therapy: A point of theory. In X. Seron & G. Deloche (Eds.). *Cognitive approaches in neuropsychological rehabilitation.* Hillsdale, NJ: Lawrence Erlbaum Associates.

Shafer, A. (1989). Demystifying splinting materials. In *O. T. product news 1.* Dedham, MA: AliMed.

Shavit, Y., Terman, G. W., Martin, F. C., Lewis, J. W., Liebeskind, J. C., & Gale, R. P. (1985). Stress, opiod peptides, the immune system and cancer. *Journal of Immunology, 135*, 834s–837s.

Sherrington, C. S. (1947). *The integrative action of the nervous system.* New Haven: Yale University Press.

Shimelman, A., & Hinojosa, J. (1995). Gross motor activity and attention in three adults with brain injury. *American Journal of Occupational Therapy, 49*, 973–978.

Shumway-Cook, A., & Woollacott, M. (1995). *Motor control: Theory and practical application.* Baltimore: Williams & Wilkins.

Siegrist, J., Peter, R., Junge, A., Cremer, P., & Seidel, D. (1990). Low status control, high effort at work and ischemic heart disease: Prospective evidence from blue-collar men. *Social Science and Medicine, 31,* 1127–1134.

Siegrist, J., Peter, R., Motz, W., & Strauer, B. E. (1992). The role of hypertension, left ventricular hypertrophy and psychosocial risk in cardiovascular disease: Prospective evidence from blue collar men. *European Heart Journal, 13* (Suppl. D), 89–95.

Siev, E., Freishtat, B., & Zoltan, B. (1986). *Perceptual and cognitive dysfunction in the adult stroke patient: A manual for evaluation and treatment.* Thorofare, NJ: Slack.

Sjölund, B. H., Eriksson, M., & Loeser, J. D. (1990). Transcutaneous and implanted electrical stimulation of peripheral nerves. In J. J. Bonica (Ed.), *The management of pain* (2nd ed.) (pp. 352–357). Philadelphia: Lea & Febiger.

Smith, D. A., & Lukens, S. A. (1983). Stress effects of isometric contraction in occupational therapy. *Occupational Therapy Journal of Research, 3,* 222–242.

Smith & Nephew Rolyan, Inc. (1996). Splinting and rehabilitation products for occupational therapists and physical therapists, 1996 catalog. Germantown, WI: Smith & Nephew Rolyan.

Snyder, C. R., Harris, C., Anderson, J. R., Holleran, S. A., Irving, L. M., Sigmon, S. T., Yoshinobu, L., Gibb, J., Langelle, C., & Harney, P. (1991). The will and the ways: Development and validation of an individual-differences measure of hope. *Journal of Personality and Social Psychology, 60,* 570–585.

Soderback, I., Bengtsson, I., Ginsburg, E., & Ekholm, J. (1992). Video feedback in occupational therapy: It's effect in patients with neglect syndrome. *Archives of Physical Medicine and Rehabilitation, 73,* 1140–1146.

Sohlberg, M. M., & Mateer, C. A. (1989a). *Attention process training.* San Antonio, TX: Psychological Corporation.

Sohlberg, M. M., & Mateer, C. A. (1989b). *Introduction to cognitive rehabilitation: Theory and practice.* New York: Guilford Press.

Sohlberg, M. M., & Mateer, C. A. (1989c). Training use of compensatory memory books: A three stage behavioral approach. *Journal of Clinical Neuropsychology, 11,* 871–891.

Spencer, J., Young, M. E., Rintala, D., & Bates, S. (1995). Socialization to the culture of a rehabilitation Hospital: An ethnographic study. *The American Journal of Occupational Therapy, 49,* 53–62.

Starkey, D., Deleone, H., & Flannery, R. B. (1995). Stress management for psychiatric patients in a state hospital setting. *American Journal of Orthopsychiatry, 65,* 446–450.

Stein, F., & Nikolic, S. (1989). Teaching stress management techniques to a schizophrenic person. *American Journal of Occupational Therapy, 43,* 162–169.

Sternbach, R. A. (1974). *Pain patients: Traits and treatment.* New York: Academic Press.

Stewart, M. (1977). Measurement of clinical pain. In A. K. Jacox (Ed.). *Pain: A source book for nurses and other health professionals* (pp. 107–137). Boston: Little, Brown, & Co.

Stockmeyer, S. (1967). An interpretation of the approach of Rood to the treatment of neuromuscular dysfunction. *American Journal of Physical Medicine, 46,* 900–961.

Strickland, J. W. (1987). Biologic basis for hand splinting. In E. E. Fess & C. A. Philips (Eds.). *Hand splinting: Principles and methods* (2nd ed.) (pp. 43–70). St. Louis: C. V. Mosby.

Strong, J., Ashton, R., Cramond, T., & Chant, D. (1990). Pain intensity, attitude and function in back pain patients. *Australian Occupational Therapy Journal, 34,* 179–183.

Strong, J., Cramond, T., & Maas, F. (1989). The effectiveness of relaxation techniques with patients who have chronic low back pain. *Occupational Therapy Journal of Research, 9,* 184–192.

Supernaw, R. B. (1995). The role of pharmacotherapy in pain management. *Orthopaedic Physical Therapy Clinics of North America, 4,* 519–540.

Sviden, G., & Saljo, R. (1993). Perceiving patients and their nonverbal reactions. *American Journal of Occupational Therapy, 47,* 491–497.

Tallant, S., Rose, S., & Tolman, R. (1989). New evidence for the effectiveness of stress management training in groups. *Behavior Modification, 13,* 431–446.

Tan, S. (1982). Cognitive and cognitive-behavioral methods for pain control: A selective review. *Pain, 12,* 201–228.

Taylor, D. N. (1995). Effects of a behavioral stress-management program on anxiety, mood, self-esteem, and T-cell count in HIV-positive men. *Psychological Reports, 76,* 451–457.

Tenney, C., & Lisak, J. (1986). *Atlas of hand splinting.* Boston: Little, Brown & Co.

Thayer, R. E., Newman, R., & McClain, T. M. (1994). Self-regulation of mood: Strategies for changing a bad mood, raising energy and reducing tension. *Journal of Personality and Social Psychology, 67,* 910–925.

Thelen, E. (1989). Self-organization in developmental processes: Can systems approaches work? In M. R. Gunnar & E. Thelen (Eds.). *Systems and Development* (pp. 77–177). Hillsdale, NJ: Lawrence Erlbaum Associates.

Thelen, E., Kelso, J., Fogel, A. (1987). Self-organizing systems and infant motor development. *Developmental Review, 7,* 39–65.

Thomas, C. L. (Ed.) (1993). *Taber's cyclopedic medical dictionary* (17th ed.). Philadelphia: F. A. Davis.

Toglia, J. P. (1991a). Generalization of treatment: A multicontextual approach to cognitive perceptual impairment in the brain injured adult. *American Journal of Occupational Therapy, 45,* 505–516.

Toglia, J. P. (1991b). Unilateral visual inattention: Multidimensional components. *Occupational Therapy Practice, 3,* 18–34.

Toglia, J. P. (1992). A dynamic interactional approach to cognitive rehabilitation. In N. Katz (Ed.). *Cognitive rehabilitation: Models for intervention in occupational therapy* (pp. 1041–1043). Boston: Andover Medical Publishers.

Toglia, J. P. (1993a). *The contextual memory test manual.* Tucson: Therapy Skill Builders.

Toglia, J. P. (1993b). Lesson 4: Attention and memory. In C. B. Royeen (Ed.). *AOTA Self-Study Series: Cognitive Rehabilitation,* (pp. 4–72). Rockville, MD: American Occupational Therapy Association.

Toglia, J. P., & Golisz, K. M. (1990). *Cognitive rehabilitation: Group games and activities.* Tucson, AZ: Therapy Skill Builders.

Towen, C. L. (1984). Primitive reflexes—conceptual or semantic problems? *Clinics in Development Medicine, 94,* 115–125.

Trexler, L. E., Webb, P. M., & Zappala, G. (1994). Strategic aspects of neuropsychological rehabilitation. In A. L. Christensen & B. P. Uzzell (Eds.). *Brain injury and neuropsychological rehabilitation: International perspectives* (pp. 99–123). Hillsdale, NJ: Lawrence Erlbaum Associates.

Trombly, C. A. (1995a). Occupation: Purposefulness and meaningfulness as therapeutic mechanisms—1995 Eleanor Clarke Slagle Lecture. *American Journal of Occupational Therapy, 49,* 960–972.

Trombly, C. A. (1995b). *Occupational therapy for physical dysfunction.* Baltimore: Williams & Wilkins.

Trombly, C. A. (1995c). Rood approach. In C. A. Trombly (Ed.). *Occupational therapy for physical dysfunction* (4th ed.) (pp. 437–445). Baltimore: Williams & Wilkins.

Turk, D. C., Meichenbaum, D., & Genest, M. (1983). Pain and behavioral medicine. New York: Guilford Press.

Turk, D. C., & Melzack, R. (1992). The measurement of pain and the assessment of people experiencing pain. In D. C. Turk & R. Melzack (Eds.). *Handbook of pain assessment* (pp. 3–12). New York: Guilford Press.

Turner, J. A., & Romano, J. M. (1990). Cognitive-behavioral therapy. In J. J. Bonica (Ed.). *The management of pain* (2nd ed.) (pp. 1711–1721). Philadelphia: Lea & Febiger.

Tyson, R., & Strong, J. (1990). Adaptive equipment: Its effectiveness for people with chronic lower back pain. *Occupational Therapy Journal of Research, 10,* 111–112.

Umphred, D. A. (1995). *Neurological rehabilitation* (3rd ed.). St. Louis,: C. V. Mosby.

Umphred, D. A, & McCormack, G. K. (1985). Classification of common facilitory and inhibitory treatment techniques. In D. A. Umphred (Ed.). *Neurological rehabilitation*. St. Louis: C.V. Mosby.

Vitaliano, R., Russo, J., Carr, J., Maiuro, R., & Becker, J. (1985). The ways of coping checklist: Revisions and psychometric properties. *Multivariate Behavioral Research, 20,* 3–26.

Vogt, T., Mullooly, J., Ernst, D., Pope, C., & Hollis, J. (1992). Social networks as predictors of ischemic heart disease, cancer, stroke and hypertension: Incidence, survival and mortality. *Journal of Clinical Epidemiology, 45,* 659–666.

Von Cramon, D.Y., Matthes-Von Cramon, G., & Mai, N. (1991). Problem solving deficits in brain injured patients: A therapeutic approach. *Neuropsychological Rehabilitation, 1,* 45–64.

von Hofsten, C. (1980). Predictive reaching for moving objects by human infants. *Journal of Experimental Psychology, 30,* 383–388.

Von Prince, K. M., & Yeakel, M. H. (1974). *The splinting of burn patients.* Springfield, IL: Charles C. Thomas.

Voss, D. E., Ionta, M. K., & Myers, B. J. (1985). *Proprioceptive neuromuscular facilitation* (3rd ed.). Philadelphia: Harper & Row.

Wagenaar, R. C., Van Wieringen, P. C. W., Netelenbos, J. B., Meijer, O. G., & Kuik, D. F. (1992). The transfer of scanning training effects in visual inattention after stroke: Five single-case studies. *Disability and Rehabilitation, 14* (1), 51–60.

Warren, M. (1993). Lesson 7: Visuospatial skills: Assessment and intervention strategies. In C. B. Royeen (Ed.), *AOTA self-study series: Cognitive rehabilitation.* Rockville, MD: American Occupational Therapy Association.

Waterman, A. S. (1984). *The psychology of individualism.* New York: Praeger.

Waterman, A. S. (1992). Identity as an aspect of optimal psychological functioning. In G. R. Adams, T. P. Gullotta, & R. Montemayor (Eds.). *Adolescent identity formation: Advances in adolescent development* (Vol.4) (pp. 50–72). Newbury Park, CA: Sage Publications.

Waylett-Rendall, J. (1995). Desensitization of the traumatized hand. In J. M. Hunter, E. Mackin, & A. Callahan (Eds.). *Rehabilitation of the hand* (4th ed.) (pp. 693–700). Philadelphia: C.V. Mosby.

Webster, J. S., & Scott, R. R. (1983). The effects of self-instructional training on attentional deficits following head injury. *Clinical Neuropsychology, 5,* 69–74.

Weeks, P. M. & Wray, R. C. (1978). *Management of acute hand injuries: A biological approach* (2nd ed.). St. Louis: C.V. Mosby.

Wehman, P. H. (1991). Cognitive rehabilitation in the workplace. In J. Kreutzer & P. H. Wehman (Eds.). *Cognitive rehabilitation for persons with traumatic brain injury* (pp. 269–288). Baltimore: Paul H. Brookes.

Weinberg, J., Diller, L., Gordon, W. A., Gerstman, L. J., Lieberman, A., Lakin, P., Plodges, G., & Ezrachi, O. (1977). Visual scanning training effect on reading related tasks in acquired light brain damage. *Archives of Physical Medicine and Rehabilitation, 58,* 479–486.

Weitz, R. (1989). Uncertainty and the lives of persons with AIDS, *Journal of Health and Social behavior, 30,* 270–281.

Wigers, S. H., Stiles, T. C., & Vogel, P. A. (1996). Effects of aerobic exercise versus stress management treatment in fibromyalgia. *Scandinavian Journal of Rheumatology, 25,* 77–86.

Williams, T. A. (1995). Low vision rehabilitation for a patient with a traumatic brain injury. *American Journal of Occupational Therapy, 49,* 923–926.

Wills, T. A. (1986) Stress and coping in early adolescence: Relationship to substance use in urban school samples. *Health Psychology, 5,* 503–529.

Wilson, A. B. (1995). Management and remediation of memory problems in brain-injured adults. In A. D. Baddeley, B. A. Wilson, & F. N. Watts (Eds.). *Handbook of memory disorders* (pp. 451–479). Chichester: John Wiley & Sons.

Wynn Parry, C. B. (1981). *Rehabilitation of the hand* (4th ed.). Boston: Butterworths.

Ylvisaker, M., Szekeres, S. F., Sullivan, D. M., & Wheeler, P. (1987). Topics in cognitive rehabilitation therapy. In M. Ylvisaker & E. M. R. Gobble (Eds.). *Community re-entry for head injured adults* (pp. 137–215). Boston: College-Hill Press.

Ziegler, E. M. (1984). *Current concepts in orthotics.* Menomonee Falls, WI: Rolyan Medical Products.

Zihl, J. (1979). Restitution of visual function in patients with cerebral blindness. *Journal of Neurology, Neurosurgery, and Psychiatry, 42,* 312–322.

Zihl, J. (1981). Recovery of visual functions in patients with cerebral blindness: Effects of specific practice with saccadic localization. *Experimental Brain Research, 44,* 159–169.

Chapter 21

Treatment of Performance Contexts

Section 1: Person–Task–Environment Interventions: A Decision-Making Guide

Section 2: Assistive Technology in Occupational Therapy

Section 1

Person–Task–Environment Interventions: A Decision-Making Guide

Margo B. Holm, Joan C. Rogers, and Ronald G. Stone

Historically, occupational therapy practitioners have been recognized for expertise in the direct observation of clients' performance of the everyday tasks that define and bring meaning to their clients' lives (Fisher & Short-DeGraff, 1993; Guralnik, Branch, Cummings, & Curb, 1989; Trombly, 1993, 1995). The unique contribution of occupational therapy, as a profession, is at the level of functional task performance: namely, the person–task–environment (PTE) transaction. In considering function at this level, we bring cognizance of the influence of the factors *within* the client (sensorimotor, cognitive, and psychosocial abilities and impairments) during the client's *transaction* with specific tasks and task environments.

This section is divided into six major subsections. The first subsection begins with a brief review of occupational therapy frames of reference that highlight PTE relations. The review serves to document the increasing attention that is being given to explaining the way in which humans influence their environments and the way in which environments influence humans. The PTE transaction is then described in terms of its component parts and their synergistic interactions. This discussion provides needed background for understanding the PTE transaction in health and disease, that is function and dysfunction. In the second subsection, the PTE transaction is placed in the context of rehabilitation and occupational therapy theoretical perspectives. This discussion provides core concepts for understanding occupational therapy approaches to managing performance discrepancies. In subsection 3, the two major approaches to managing performance discrepancies—bottom-up and top-down—are defined and described. The top-down approach is selected as the approach of choice for meeting the challenges of the emerging system of managed health care. The subsection concludes with a discussion of the nature of performance discrepancy. Thus, subsection 3 sets the stage for the delineation of decision points for occupational therapy interventions. Subsection 4 presents a clinical decision making guide for determining whether performance discrepancies originate from deficits in skills or habits. This determination aids the occupational therapy practitioner in understanding the nature of a performance discrepancy and, thereby, in planning appropriate interventions. Subsection 5 concentrates on the establishment of target functional outcomes and their management through environmental interventions. In this subsection, five intervention strategies are defined and illustrated through clinical cases. The section concludes with a short summary (subsection 6) and at the end of this book, Appendices H, I, J delineate sources for obtaining resource materials in print, by telephone, and through the Internet or with software.

▼ PERSON—TASK—ENVIRONMENT TRANSACTION MODELS

Safe, efficient, satisfactory, and independent performance of activities of daily living (ADL), work and productive, or play and leisure tasks is dependent on a successful PTE transaction. Ecological models, those concerned with interactions between persons and their environments, address the PTE transaction. Occupational therapists have historically acknowledged the contribution of the environment to task performance, with early leaders Slagle (1922), Meyer (1922), and Haas (1944) suggesting the adaptation of environmental characteristics as one means of improving the function of clients. However, serious attempts to translate this philosophy into practice models are of more recent origin. Since the 1980s, several ecological models have been presented in the occupational therapy literature to assist practitioners' understanding of the PTE transaction.

In 1982, Rogers (1982) borrowed concepts from the behavioral sciences to modernize and enrich the fundamental premises about the link between function and the environment articulated in our early philosophy. Independent behavior was viewed as a function of the competence and autonomy of the person and the behavior-evoking aspects of the physical, social, and temporal environment. Normally, habits of daily living enable humans to respond automatically and appropriately to a variety of environmental demands. The balance between person capabilities and environmental demands may be disrupted by disease-associated or age-related physical, cognitive, and affective impairments. A fundamental therapeutic strategy for raising capability, lowered by impairment, is to lower environmental demands, and raise them gradually as competence improves. Kiernat (1982) further articulated the concept of the environment as a therapeutic modality.

Barris (1982) developed the concept of environment in conjunction with the Model of Human Occupation proposed by Kielhofner and Burke (1980). Accordingly, persons choose environments to become involved with based on such environmental properties as novelty, complexity, or compatibility with interests and values. Environmental demands for performance, which are associated with the peo-ple and objects available in the environment, strongly influence the development of roles, habits, and skills. The development of competence involves the ability to interact successfully with an increasingly broader range of environments. Thus, the model clarifies environmental properties and their influence on persons.

Like Barris, Howe and Briggs (1982) also used **general system theory** to describe the person–environment relationship. In their Ecological Systems Model, humans and their environments shape each other. Persons are at the center of the ecosystem and are surrounded by three interacting environment layers—the immediate setting, social networks and institutions, and ideology. These layers comprise the life space for the performance of life task and roles. Behavior is functional if person—environment interactions enable persons to achieve goals that are consonant with their views of quality of life.

When defining occupation, Nelson (1988) made a distinction between occupational form and occupational performance. He argued that occupational performance or action, can be understood only in the context of occupational form; that is, "an objective set of circumstances, independent of and external to a person" (p. 633). One dimension of occupational form involves the physical stimuli present in the environment, including the materials used, the surrounding environment, the human context, and temporal relationships. A second dimension of occupational form is the sociocultural milieu. The first dimension focuses on the doing aspect of performance while the second dimension emphasizes the symbolic aspect (eg, values and norms). According to Nelson (1988), occupational performance then is the action elicited, guided, or structured by an occupational form.

Holm and Rogers (1989) described the PTE transaction as a relationship between the abilities and behaviors required of a task performer and the inherent properties, procedures, equipment, and materials involved in functional tasks. Emphasis was placed on the natural setting, as opposed to the clinical setting, as a means of eliminating contrived environmental influences. Subsequently, Rogers and Holm (1991a) adapted Lawton's (1982) ecological model of aging to explicate further the PTE transaction. Lawton (1982) described behavior [B] as a function [f] of person capability [P] and environmental demand [E], or $[B = f\ (P, E)]$, and noted that as a person's capabilities become impaired, the influence of the environment (ie, environmental **press**) on behavior increases. By implication then, task performance is dependent on the match between the capabilities of the person and the demands that the environment places on those capabilities. Lawton's formula was revised by Rogers and Holm (1991a) to highlight the role of nonhuman environmental elements in task performance by including assistive technology devices (ATD) for the person, objects in the environment (OE), or the structural environment (SE), into the equation as a method of equalizing the person capability–environmental demand relationship, as follows:

B = f [(P + ATD) × OE × SE] (ATD for the person, such as a listening device)

B = f [P × (OE + ATD) × SE] (ATD for task object, such as a built up spoon)

B = f [P × OE × (SE + ATD)] (ATD for structural environment, such as a ramp)

By incorporating ATD into the equation, task performance becomes a function of a person's capabilities, enhanced by ATD, interacting with environmental demands, reduced by the ATD.

Another ecological model was introduced by Christiansen and Baum (Christiansen, 1991), namely the person–performance–environment (PPE) model. In their model, personal factors (ie, motivation, experience, beliefs, abilities, and skills) are viewed as intrinsic enablers of performance. Performance includes activities, tasks, and roles of occupations, and the environment includes physical, social, and cultural factors. A unique contribution of this model is the emphasis on a person's capabilities as enablers for their activity and task performance.

In the University of Southern California (USC) Model of Human Subsystems That Influence Occupation (Clark et al, 1991), occupational behavior is portrayed as emerging from six internal subsystems—physical, biological, information processing, sociocultural, symbolic–evaluative, and transcendental. These human subsystems interact with the external environment, which is comprised of the sociocultural context and the person's history.

The Occupational Adaptation frame of reference (Schkade & Schultz, 1992; Schultz & Schkade, 1992) includes the person, the occupational environment, and the interaction of these factors during occupation. This frame of reference focuses on the client's experience of self in relevant occupational contexts and the use of meaningful occupations to affect the client's *internal* **adaptation** process rather than *outward* measures of performance. Desired outcomes of the occupational adaptation model are effective, efficient, and satisfying responses to the demands posed by the environment (Brayman, 1996).

The **Ecology of Human Performance (EHP)** framework, proposed by the occupational therapy faculty of the University of Kansas (Dunn, Brown, & McGuigan, 1994) differentiates between a task and the person's performance of the task, thus adding one more dimension to a person capability–environmental demand model. The EHP defines person, task, performance, and context, using the *Uniform Terminology for Occupational Therapy*, 3rd ed. (Uniform Terminology; American Occupational Therapy Association [AOTA], 1994), and describes possible relationships among the four components. In addition, five collaborative approaches to intervention (ie, **establish or restore**, **alter**, **adapt**, **prevent**, and **create**), incorporating all four components of the EHP framework are described.

In a further theoretical development of the Model of Human Occupation, Kielhofner (1995) identified the environment as influencing occupational behavior through affording and pressing. In the former, the environment affords opportunities for performance, whereas in the latter it presses for certain types of behavior. The physical environment was conceptualized as comprised of natural and built environments and objects. The social environment consists of social groups and occupational forms; that is, rule-bound action sequences. The physical and social environments intertwine to create occupational behavior settings; that is, meaningful contexts for occupational performance.

Similar to the EHP framework, the Person–Environment–Occupation Model (Law et al, 1996) also separates the concept of occupation from the performance of the occupation, and emphasizes the consequences to occupational performance when there is any change in the person, the environment, or the occupation. The model is designed to help occupational therapy practitioners take into consideration the temporal aspects of occupational routines, not only on a daily, weekly or monthly basis, but also from a life span development perspective.

Finally, task analysis, which is essential to occupational therapy practice, merits recognition as an ecological conceptual framework. In essence, task analysis defines the relationship between the person and the environment as an action (eg, reaches) oriented toward an object (eg, into the cupboard). As a theoretical approach, task analysis has been highly developed in human factors. A human factors approach to capability–demand models uses task analysis to divide tasks into discrete sequential steps, and then defines the physiological (eg, actions, postures, grasps), sensory (eg, feels, sees), and cognitive (eg, searches, scans) requirements for successful task completion (Faletti, 1984). The occupational therapy practitioner then makes a comparison of the demands of each step of the task, including environmental demands, with the capabilities of the person. When the task–environmental demands are greater than the person's capabilities, the specific area for intervention is targeted (Clark, Czaja, & Weber, 1990; Czaja, Weber, & Nair, 1993).

This brief review of ecological models has ascertained that the PTE transaction has been described from numerous perspectives, and with differential emphases on the various components. A common theme emerging from them is that clients apply their capabilities to accomplish a task, at a given time, using the objects available, in a specific place. The outcomes of task performance in terms of parameters such as independence, safety, and quality depend on the transactions between and among the capabilities of the person, the demands of the task, and the demands of the physical, social, cultural, and temporal context in which the task takes place. Just as our attempts to understand the occupational functioning of clients has led to a refinement of the factors within clients, so too, our attempts to understand the interface between persons with disabilities and their life demands will lead to a refinement of the factors outside clients that are critical for their community integration and reintegration. As used in this section, a performance transaction implies a negotiation or arrangement among three factors—person capabilities, environmental demands at the task level, and environmental demands at the physical and social levels. After defining and describing each of these factors separately, they will be viewed in concert in the discussion of the transaction and of performance discrepancy.

Person (Client) Capabilities

Client capabilities are generic task abilities or task-specific skills. Sensorimotor, cognitive, and psychosocial abilities underlie, support, and enable the performance of multiple tasks. Examples of these abilities are range of motion (ROM), attention span, and coping skills. They are called performance components in the Uniform Terminology (AOTA, 1994). Generic abilities are coalesced into unique combinations to form task-specific skills. Examples of these skills are meal preparation, leisure exploration, and medication management. They are called performance areas in the Uniform Terminology (AOTA, 1994). Task-specific skills are developed through training and practice; that is, through the learning and repetition of the PTE transaction in formal and informal situations.

Environmental Demands

Environmental demands are extrinsic to person capabilities. These demands occur at two levels: the level of the task and the level of the surrounding physical and social environment.

TASK DEMANDS

Client capabilities are challenged by the requirements of tasks, which are usually referred to as task demands. Task demands are identified through task analysis, which is the analytic process of breaking tasks down into discrete, sequential steps (Creighton, 1992; Cynkin, 1979). Task analysis identifies the actions that clients are to perform in relationship to objects. For example, to make a cup of tea, clients must:

Action	Object
Locate	Tea bag and drinking container
Place	Tea bag in drinking container
Obtain	Container for water
Obtain and heat	Water
Pour	Water on tea
Remove	Tea bag

The actions comprising task performance are highly influenced by the objects used to perform them, which include the task materials, tools, and equipment. Task objects have inherent properties that influence the strength or force of the task demand. For instance, pancake batter presents less resistance when stirred than a stiff cookie dough; a plastic garbage bag placed on a car seat provides less resistance than cloth seat covers when transferring into and out of a car; an overhead knit shirt has stretch capabilities whereas an overhead cotton weave shirt does not stretch when it is donned. When calculating the demand properties of a task, the nature of the inherent properties of task objects must be analyzed. For example, one method we can use to analyze the properties of task objects is based on the effect they have on our senses. When touched, lifted, carried, pushed, or pulled, task objects can be slick, sticky, wet, dry, greasy, crumbly, hard, soft, warm, cold, sharp, scratchy, smooth, heavy, and light. When visualized, they can be large, small, colorful, bright, dull, far, near, and have distinct shapes and patterns. When listened to they can produce loud, soft, irritating, soothing, and inaudible sounds. Task objects can taste sweet, sour, salty, and bitter, and emanate odors that are pleasant, noxious, or unnoticeable. In some environments, the inherent properties of objects may also be hazardous to health, such as certain chemicals, solvents, heavy metals, and radiation materials (Brigham, Engelberg, & Richling, 1996). Task materials (eg, bread, shirt, shampoo bottle), tools (eg, fork, drill, ice cream scoop), and equipment (eg, computer, stove, work bench) vary based on their function, design, size, and shape (Cynkin, 1979; Demore-Taber, 1995; Hagedorn, 1995a; Levine & Brayley, 1991; Rogers & Holm, 1991a).

The properties of task objects can be used to increase and decrease task demands. For example, if we consider the actions required and the properties of the foregoing task objects, the task demands for making a cup of tea can vary greatly. Heating water for a cup of tea can be accomplished by heating the water in a teapot or a pan on the stovetop, heating a cup of water in a microwave, using an electric kettle, or placing an electric heating element into the cup. The tea leaves can be loose in a can, contained in a tea bag, or ground into powder for "instant" tea. The tea can be served in a ceramic mug, a plastic mug, a china cup, or the lid on a thermos. Thus, the task steps, and inherent properties and design of specific task objects used to perform a task have a strong influence on the task demands and performance outcomes.

SURROUNDING PHYSICAL AND SOCIAL ENVIRONMENT DEMANDS

In addition to the demands inherent in tasks performed with available objects, task performance is also influenced by the surrounding physical and social environment (Christiansen, 1991; Dunn et al, 1994; Law et al, 1996; Rogers, 1982). The properties of the physical environment usually include space, arrangement, equipment controls, surface heights, lighting, temperature, noise, humidity, vibration, and ventilation (Demore-Taber, 1995; Hagedorn, 1995a; Jacobs & Bettencourt, 1995; Raschko, 1991). Each of these properties has been further delineated in architectural (Raschko, 1991), anthropometric (Diffrient, Tilley, & Bardagjy, 1974), **ergonomic** (Jacobs & Bettencourt, 1995), and occupational health and safety literature (Brigham et al, 1996; Carson, 1994; Moore & Garg, 1995). Not only are there static aspects of the physical environment to be considered, but there are also the dynamic aspects: machines that have moving parts, temperatures that fluctuate, noise levels that rise and fall, humidity that rises and falls, and ventilation that fluctuates. Moreover, some environments, including new office buildings and homes, are referred to as "sick" environments because of how they affect the performance of those who work or live in them. These environments are deemed sick because of inadequate ventilation systems, asbestos insulation, radon, improperly functioning cooling systems, or old plumbing systems that deliver water tainted with lead (Brigham et al, 1996).

The demands of the physical environment may compound those of the task. If a toilet is on the second floor of a two-story house and a client cannot climb stairs, the client will not be able to get to the toilet to use it. A portable toilet may need to be purchased or rented and installed in a first floor bedroom or closet to reduce the demands of physical structures. Furthermore, if space in the bedroom is restricted, or if there is no lighting in the closet, the safety of toilet transfers may be compromised, and adaptations may need to occur to reduce the negative effect of environmental demand.

Often environmental demand is viewed solely in terms of the physical environment. However, the social environment also influences role and task performance. The social environment includes more than the mere number of persons in the home, school, or workplace. The knowledge, skills, habits, expectations, values, attitudes, and motivations of these persons create a social climate that fosters or hinders task performance. Cultural beliefs, norms, customs, and practices also influence the social environment (Hagedorn, 1995a). Moreover, persons arrange the physical, social, and temporal environments. They select and place task objects, organize and govern social groups, and establish daily schedules and the pacing of tasks. In so doing, they set the overall level of stimulation (eg, too much, just right, too little) surrounding persons during task performance (Christiansen, 1991; Gerdner, Hall, & Buckwalter, 1996; Hall & Buckwalter, 1987). At any given time a person can have numerous roles (eg, worker, parent, husband, grandparent, coworker, volunteer, client, or social activist), each of which has task demands that occur in separate or overlapping social environments.

The Transaction

Clients are not passive recipients of the effects of their environments. Rather, they act on, as well as are acted on, by task and physical and social environmental forces, thereby creating a transactional relationship that is characterized as an interdependence between person capabilities and the demands of the task and surrounding environment (Dunn et al, 1994; Law et al, 1996; Lawton, 1982; Rogers, 1982). For example, a client, who is unable to get up the stairs to the

bathtub, may install a shower on the first floor of the home, provide a stair lift to the second level, or resist dependency-reinforcing bed bath caregiving actions and bathe at the kitchen sink. Each of these decisions would change the task objects and the surrounding environment and, in turn, these environmental changes would alter the PTE transaction.

When Demands Exceed Capabilities: Performance Discrepancy

When the capabilities of a client are sufficient to manage the demands of the task and surrounding environment, the client's performance and the level of performance that is expected, required, or desired are congruent. However, when demands exceed capabilities, task performance is compromised, and there is a discrepancy between actual performance and what is expected, required, or desired (Lawton, 1982; Mager & Pipe, 1984). The performance discrepancy can be reduced, eliminated, or prevented by establishing or restoring capabilities, reducing task or environmental demands, or a combination of these two methods (Dunn et al, 1994; Law et al, 1996; Rogers, 1982). With the diminishment of client capabilities through disease, trauma, age-related changes, developmental disorders, psychological maladaptation, or environmental deprivation, clients become more susceptible to environmental influences. They have fewer internal resources and less energy to resist environmental forces or to devise adaptive strategies to counteract them (Lawton, 1982). By manipulating the environment therapeutically to accommodate diminished capability it may be possible to improve task performance.

▼ THE PTE TRANSACTION AND MODELS OF FUNCTION AND DYSFUNCTION

The PTE transaction is a composite of person capabilities influencing and being influenced by the demands of objects and of the ambient physical and social environment. Now that we have a better understanding of the PTE transaction, and before we examine further the nature of performance discrepancies, we will view the PTE transaction from the overall perspective of rehabilitation and occupational therapy science. This perspective will assist us in understanding occupational therapy approaches to fostering competent PTE transactions.

Clients are referred for occupational therapy services primarily because there is a discrepancy in current role or task performance compared with the performance that is expected or required of them, or desired by them. These performance discrepancies are usually the result of a specific pathology and its consequences for daily living. The World Health Organization (WHO) (WHO, 1980; Wood, 1980) defined the consequences of pathology in terms of a hierar-

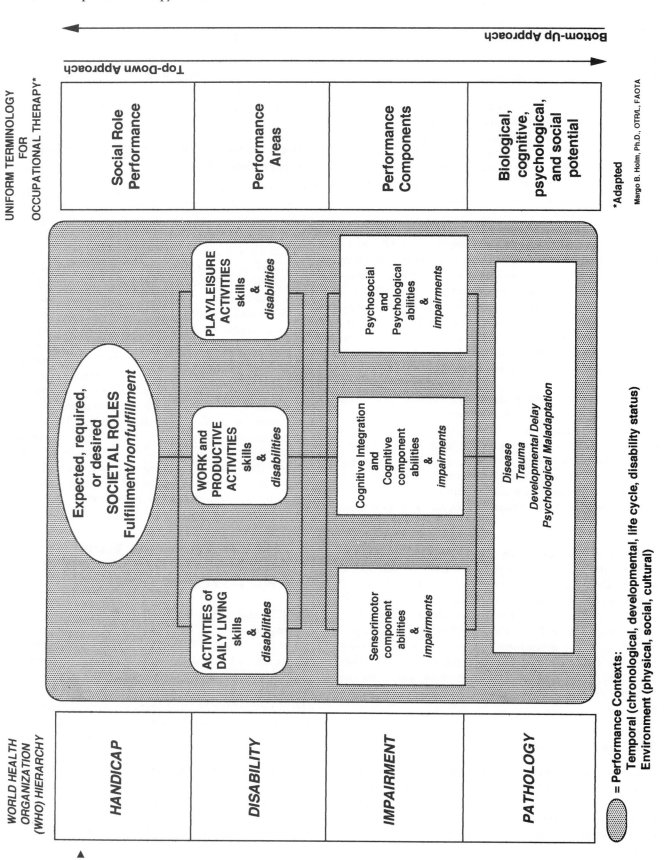

Figure 21-1. The relationship of concepts. (From the World Health Organization [WHO] Model and the Uniform Terminology for Occupational Therapy, 3rd ed.)

chy of impairment, disability, and handicap. The term disablement encompasses the experience of pathology at all three levels. In occupational therapy, disablement is conceptualized along a continuum of dysfunction to function in a three dimensional hierarchy consisting of performance components, occupational areas, and role performance. The term occupational functioning encompasses all dimensions of the hierarchy. There are similarities and differences between the hierarchy proposed by the WHO and that implicit in the Uniform Terminology (AOTA, 1994). Figure 21–1 depicts the relationship between the WHO model of pathology, impairment, disability, and handicap (WHO, 1980; Wood, 1980) and the Uniform Terminology (AOTA, 1994) scheme of the performance components, occupational areas, and role performance.

Pathology, according to the WHO model, is a disruption of normal body systems or processes, and clients referred for occupational therapy services present with various diseases, traumas, developmental delays, and psychological maladaptations. Because the Uniform Terminology contains no concept paralleling pathology, we have added biopsychosocial potential as the lowest level on this hierarchical scheme. If a pathology has no cure, or goes untreated, clients may experience impairment, or dysfunction at the level of an organ or organ system (eg, restrictions in ROM or short-term memory loss). The Uniform Terminology concept that corresponds to impairment is the performance components—the client's sensorimotor abilities, cognitive integration and cognitive abilities, and psychosocial and psychological abilities. If impairments cannot be reduced, eliminated, or prevented, they may be severe enough to cause disability. Clients experience disability as dysfunction in the performance of ADL, work and productive tasks, and play or leisure tasks. Task performance in the occupational areas of ADL, work and productive activities, and play and leisure is the Uniform Terminology equivalent of disability. When disability is substantive, or chronic, and a client is unable to fulfill expected, required, or desired societal roles, the experience of pathology is known as handicap. Occupational role performance, the corresponding level for handicap in the Uniform Terminology, is the adequate fulfillment of one's societal roles.

Thus, the WHO and Uniform Terminology perspectives of disablement are similar in using a trilevel hierarchy for the consequences of pathology—biopsychosocial potential—at progressively higher levels of organization of the human system. However, they differ insofar as the WHO model emphasizes dysfunction, whereas the Uniform Terminology emphasizes function. Thus, the WHO model accents the dysfunction associated with disablement while the Uniform Terminology can be applied to a function-to-dysfunction continuum. In both perspectives, the PTE transaction becomes particularly salient at the second level of the hierarchy (ie, disability and occupational areas), and it maintains significance at the third level of the hierarchy (eg, handicap and occupational role). Hence, factors that are essentials to the PTE transaction, although external to clients, must be taken into account when intervening for disability (ie, dysfunction in occupational areas) or handicap (ie, occupational role dysfunction). It should also be noted in Figure 21–1 that both models are embedded within temporal, physical, social, and cultural environments.

▼ OCCUPATIONAL THERAPY APPROACHES TO PERFORMANCE DISCREPANCY

The hierarchy of occupational functioning provides a useful perspective for delineating the two major evaluation and intervention approaches for performance discrepancies used in occupational therapy. Trombly (1993, 1995) labeled these the bottom-up and top-down approaches.

Bottom-Up Approach to Performance Discrepancy

Occupational therapy practitioners, when using a bottom-up approach, focus evaluation and intervention on the client's generic task abilities, specifically, on impairments according to the WHO model and performance components in the Uniform Terminology scheme (see Fig. 21–1). For Mrs. Fisher, a 63-year-old client, who sustained a right cerebrovascular accident (CVA), the practitioner might focus the evaluation on muscle tone, reflexes, postural control, visual–motor integration, and short-term memory. Interventions are remedial in nature, with the intent of restoring abilities lost secondary to stroke. The rationale underlying the bottom-up approach is that generic task abilities support tasks in all occupational areas and that by restoring these abilities to their normal state, task performance, which was previously dysfunctional, automatically becomes functional, because the abilities needed to perform these tasks are once again intact. Once generic abilities are restored, some remedial interventions may be devised for task and role performance to reintegrate newly restored generic abilities into everyday task performance in the client's self-care, work and productive, or play and leisure roles. This intervention would not need to be extensive, however, because the "cure" of impairments reestablishes clients' capabilities, and task reactivation occurs rapidly, particularly for well-learned and well-practiced everyday skills. Hence, the bottom-up approach to performance discrepancy is efficient because the restoration of task abilities returns clients to their premorbid (ie, preinjury, preillness) condition, and task and role performance are resumed at their prior level.

The bottom-up approach permits the occupational therapy practitioner to focus the evaluation and intervention on discrete components of performance without initially having to consider the demands of tasks or the surrounding physical and social environment. Mrs. Fisher's muscle tone, reflexes, and postural control can be evaluated on a mat table and her visual–motor integration and short-term memory can be evaluated through tests as she sits in her wheelchair. Neurodevelopmental interventions to normalize tone, inhibit abnormal reflex patterns, and improve postural control can also be implemented with Mrs. Fisher on the mat table. Interventions to resolve problems in form constancy, visual closure, figure-ground perception, and short-term memory can be implemented through paper and pencil exercises done on a lapboard. For the most part, environmental interactions are limited to test and intervention objects and instructions. The demands of real-life situations are introduced into the intervention plan once generic abilities have been restored, or their improvement has plateaued. For example, because Mrs. Fisher has not yet achieved full voluntary control of her hemiplegic extremities and cannot perform transfers in a normal manner, her occupational therapy practitioner practiced bed and toilet transfers with her to help her integrate postural control techniques and inhibition of abnormal tone and reflexes into these procedures.

Top-Down Approach to Performance Discrepancy

The second major approach to occupational therapy evaluation and intervention—the top-down approach—begins by establishing performance discrepancies at the highest level, that is, the WHO level of handicap or the Uniform Terminology level of role performance (see Fig. 21–1). It then moves to the tasks necessary to sustain valued roles; that is, to the WHO level of disability, or to the Uniform Terminology level of performance in occupational areas (Holm & Rogers, 1989). Finally, the focus is transferred to generic abilities that support task and role performance, or to the WHO level of impairment, or to the Uniform Terminology level of performance components. The fundamental rationale underlying the top-down approach is that even though impairments cannot always be cured, performance in valued roles can be improved through adaptive task performance associated with these roles. The following logic undergirds this rationale: (1) evaluation and intervention begin with tasks that are of value to clients (ie, necessary for carrying out valued roles); (2) factors external to clients that contribute to performance discrepancies can be identified during task performance; (3) inferences about probable external causes of performance discrepancies can be verified by changing task or surrounding environmental demands during task performance, thereby reducing or resolving the performance discrepancy; (4) abilities and impairments can be observed as they interact synergistically in the performance of real-life tasks; and (5) a more focused evaluation of impairments can occur in the context of task performance, to formulate appropriate intervention strategies to restore, establish, or prevent loss of generic abilities (Mathiowetz, 1993; Trombly, 1993, 1995).

For our client, Mrs. Fisher, who sustained a right CVA, the occupational therapy practitioner would begin by evaluating Mrs. Fisher's roles that are most likely to be affected following a stroke. Mrs. Fisher values most her roles as a wife and homemaker. She enjoys cooking for her husband and baking for her grandchildren, who visit her every Tuesday. She is also concerned about her role as a self-carer. In addition to walking, feeding, bathing, toileting, dressing, and hygiene, Mrs. Fisher mentions medication management and emergency communication in conjunction with self-care. Once the most salient tasks comprising each role have been identified, performance-based evaluation is initiated to identify task abilities and disabilities. In-depth task evaluations are needed to identify the specific point in a task sequence where breakdown occurs and to develop clinical hypotheses about the impairments responsible for this breakdown. Intervention strategies to reduce environmental demands involving compensatory methods of task performance, the use of adaptive equipment, and modification of the ambient physical and social environments may be implemented. These compensatory strategies may resolve performance discrepancies relatively quickly. They may be permanent or temporary solutions to performance discrepancies. If temporary, they enable successful task performance, while impairment-oriented interventions are instituted to restore task performance.

The top-down approach to performance discrepancies permits the occupational therapy practitioner to initially focus evaluation and intervention on the roles and responsibilities that define a client's life in the community. The demands of tasks and the surrounding physical and social environment are integral to the occupational therapy process from the beginning. Mrs. Fisher, for example, indicated that her present concerns center on her roles as self-carer, wife, grandparent, and homemaker. She is anxious about her ability to carry out these roles following her stroke. Ideally, evaluation of the critical tasks that constitute her homemaker role (eg, meal preparation, household maintenance, clothing care, and such) and her self-carer role (eg, bathing, toileting, dressing, and so forth) is carried out in her home so that information obtained about the PTE transaction is accurate and valid. Under less than ideal conditions, these tasks are evaluated in an occupational therapy clinic. Accuracy and validity of information is increased under clinical conditions by simulating as much as possible the environmental demands that Mrs. Fisher will face in her own home at discharge. For example, because the bathroom in the Fisher home is too narrow to allow Mrs. Fisher to turn her wheelchair around in the bathroom while she is sitting in it, the occupational therapy practitioner trained Mrs. Fisher to back her wheelchair into the clinic bathroom, thus simulating how she would have to perform this maneuver at home. This procedure enables Mrs. Fisher to transfer to a tub bench, as well as the toilet, toward the stronger, unaffected side of her body. She can then collapse the wheelchair and reposition it in the opposite direction before transferring out of the bathtub. Turning the chair allows her to again transfer toward her stronger, unaffected side. The space needed to turn the chair is less when she is not in the chair because her thigh length does not need to be taken into account. Neurodevelopmental interventions to improve postural control, by normalizing muscle tone and inhibiting abnormal reflex patterns, would be incorporated into transfer practice exercises.

Advantages and Disadvantages of the Two Approaches to PTE Transaction Discrepancies

THE BOTTOM-UP APPROACH

An advantage of the bottom-up approach to PTE discrepancies is that intervention aimed at establishing or restoring generic abilities may benefit many tasks. For example, increasing muscle strength or ROM in the upper extremities will facilitate all tasks for which these abilities were deficient. Similarly, reducing apathy will foster reengagement in previously neglected occupational areas. Likewise, correcting visual-sequencing deficits will enhance the performance of all tasks negatively affected by this impairment. Thus, potentially, by remediating physical, cognitive, or affective impairments, multiple task disabilities can be treated simultaneously.

Because the bottom-up approach emphasizes performance factors that are internal to clients, the role of external, environmental factors is extremely limited. Therefore, this approach is economical to administer because occupational therapy practitioners do not need to assess or manage the demands of tasks and the surrounding physical and social environment as they impinge on these abilities.

Nonetheless, an inherent disadvantage of the bottom-up approach is that improvements in generic abilities may not generalize to tasks. Generalization may not occur for several reasons: First, abilities-oriented interventions concentrate on the components of task performance that are common to many tasks. However, task performance requires the application of these common abilities to the specific demands of individual tasks. Improvements in visual figure-ground perception demonstrated on paper and pencil tests, using black and white stimulus materials, may not enable clients to identify hazards, such as water spills, on a multicolored and patterned vinyl floor surface. Second, when abilities are exercised in isolation from tasks, they are not integrated with the other abilities that are also needed to perform these tasks. In other words, discrete abilities-oriented interventions do not acknowledge either the interaction between task-related abilities or their coalescence in the PTE transaction in which the discrete abilities will be used. Perceiving a water spill on the floor must be accompanied by the decisional capacity to motor plan to avoid the spill and the neuromuscular strength and endurance to execute walking around it. Finally, generalization may not occur because, although abilities may be improved, they may not be improved sufficiently to meet task demands. An increase in ROM of 10 degrees at the shoulder joint will still be inadequate for grooming if 25 degrees more motion is needed to comb hair on the back of one's head.

The bottom-up approach may also result in the identification and treatment of impairments that may not actually be causing performance dysfunctions. A deficit score on a test of visual figure-ground perception may not translate into performance deficits in well-learned daily-living skills. Without assessing the PTE transaction during tasks, the meaning of impairments for performance is vague.

The bottom-up approach is generally initiated with the intention of switching to the top-down approach if full recovery does not occur, or once maximum benefit is obtained from remedial interventions. The danger in this tactic is that too much intervention time may be spent on remediating impairments. At the outset of intervention, it is difficult to predict if full recovery will be achieved, and occupational therapy practitioners are prone to persist in remedial interventions as long as gains are being made. Unfortunately, if full recovery is not achieved, there may be little intervention time left for addressing task disabilities. Clients may then be deprived of independent, safe, and adequate task performance that could have been achieved—or achieved more readily—through compensatory interventions. The risk of clients being discharged from therapy before maximum improvement in task performance has been achieved has been intensified by managed care and reduced time allocations for rehabilitation.

Another disadvantage of the bottom-up approach, is that clients may not see the connection between interventions aimed at discrete impairments (eg, motor control exercises, visual scanning programs on a computer, stacking cones) and improvement of their daily life task performance. Hence, they may be less motivated to participate in occupational therapy. However, by educating clients and their families about the connection between impairment reduction and task improvement, this disadvantage may be overcome.

THE TOP-DOWN APPROACH

A primary advantage of the top-down approach (Trombly, 1993) is that evaluation and intervention center on role and task performances that are meaningful to clients, yet discrepant with the performance that is expected, required, or desired. Contingent to this advantage are two additional benefits. First, because the occupational therapy process focuses on role and task performances that are meaningful to clients, the relevance of therapy for improving daily life is readily apparent to clients (Trombly, 1993). Thus, motivation to participate in therapy is heightened. Second, role and task performance are influenced directly by the intervention. Real-life performance is both the medium and the outcome of therapy.

The top-down approach also has the advantage of reinforcing and expediting an approach that people often implement naturally when problems are experienced in task performance (Fried, Herdman, Kuhn, Rubin, & Turano, 1991). When difficulties are encountered in doing tasks, we tend to seek the assistance of others, use a tool to help us, or try a different way of performing the task. These compensatory procedures foster task completion. Because the top-down approach enhances procedures that humans turn to naturally when problems are encountered, it is familiar to clients; hence, it is likely to be well-accepted by them.

The top-down approach provides a further advantage at the point when intervention switches from a role or task focus to an impairment orientation. The top-down approach facilitates the identification of impairments in the context of tasks and roles; consequently, the relevance of impairments for role and task performance is known. In contrast, in the bottom-up approach, where impairments are evaluated in isolation, their relevance for role and task performance can only be inferred. The visual–perceptual impairments tests identified through a paper or pencil test may or may not impair task performance. The identification of role and task-related impairments, in turn, enables a more targeted evaluation of impairments, as well as more precisely directed remedial interventions.

The disadvantage of the top-down approach is that evaluation and intervention are task-specific, with no or minimal transfer from one task to another. Moreover, for intervention to be maximally effective, it must occur in the occupational context in which the client lives, works, or plays. Thus, the approach requires the occupational therapy practitioner to take into account the complexity of environmental factors that impinge on performance.

INTERVENTION APPROACH FOR THE 21ST CENTURY

The predominant approach to the occupational therapy process over the past several decades has been the bottom-up approach and restorative interventions. Nonetheless, even with its disadvantages, the top-down approach, and its concomitant compensatory interventions, is the best fit for the emerging system of health care delivery. Leaders within occupational therapy, health care financing and administration, and consumers themselves have called for this reversal of emphasis.

Within occupational therapy, Dunn (1993) in an article entitled *Measurement of Function: Actions for the Future*, proposed the following:

We need to consider the fact that a contextual approach to assessment provides an opportunity to identify what the person needs or wants to do. It is essential for occupational therapy to begin assessment at this level and to create goals for services from this list of expressed needs. This strategy has the advantage of engaging the person's motivational system, providing another mechanism to facilitate a successful outcome (p. 357).

Rogers and Holm (1989; Holm & Rogers, 1989, 1991; Rogers, Holm, & Stone, 1997) have stressed the pivotal position of task performance and compensatory interventions for

maximizing performance gains. Mathiowetz (1993) in a discussion of physical performance component evaluation and intervention for function noted that it is possible for some clients to have grip or pinch strength within normal limits, but not be able to accomplish necessary functional tasks, and for others to have grip or pinch strength below normal limits, yet be able to accomplish all their functional tasks. He further points out that the kinesiology literature suggests that motor learning is task-specific, with little carryover to other tasks; thus, the best way to improve motor function is to practice the task for which it is required. According to Trombly (1993), "we have no definitive study in occupational therapy that indicates that a person's occupational functioning is better as a result of restorative therapy rather than adaptive therapy" (p. 255), and Wood (1996) summarized concerns about a singular use of the bottom-up approach to PTE transaction discrepancies (Humphrey, Jewell, & Rosenberger, 1995; Neistadt, 1994a, 1994b; Trombly, 1995) by noting that there "has been increasing evidence that improvements in performance components do not necessarily translate into competent functioning in everyday life" (p. 631).

More compelling arguments for the top-down approach have come from health insurance companies, because they can define acceptable outcomes of therapy through their reimbursement practices. For example, Blue Cross of California defined a meaningful outcome of therapy as "one in which the activity level achieved by the patient. . . is that level necessary for the patient to function most effectively at home or at work" (Stewart & Abeln, 1993, p. 213). Another parameter of acceptability, a utilitarian outcome of therapy, is defined as a functional outcome that is economically and efficiently achieved (Stewart & Abeln, 1993).

Finally, the disability rights movement has also promoted compensatory approaches that focus on environmental adaptation, because the compensatory approach does not assume that there is something wrong with the person with a disability that needs to be "fixed" or "changed." Instead, the compensatory approach concentrates on the environment and its demands, probing to identify how it affects performance, and then seeking to work around it, or to capitalize on it (Dunn, 1993; Verbrugge, 1990). As Verbrugge notes, the request of advocacy groups for individuals with lifelong impairments is: "Change the milieu, not me" (p. 68).

Performance Discrepancy: Person Capability Versus Environmental Demand

This subsection focuses on pathology experienced at the level of disability; that is, task performance in the three occupational areas. This is a pivotal level that stands at the interface between role performance and the components of performance. The fulfillment of societal roles is dependent on a client's ability to perform a unique combination of tasks in ADL, work and productive tasks, and play and leisure tasks. The ability to safely, efficiently, satisfactorily, and independently carry out everyday tasks is, in turn, dependent on the sensorimotor, cognitive, psychosocial, and psychological abilities of the client.

The role of the environment in task performance becomes more salient as one moves up the hierarchy from abilities to tasks to roles. At the level of tasks and roles, the environment, in terms of objects, structures, and people, is inextricably linked to client capabilities. Numerous methods of adapting the client's performance environment to achieve, restore, or improve function, and prevent dysfunction are available. Rather than devising an approach to environmental modifications for each pathology, impairment, or disability experienced by clients, we chose to develop a clinical decision-making guide to help occupational therapy practitioners systematically determine the nature of the performance discrepancy. This evaluation provides the basis for determining the most appropriate type of environmental modification. The guide, consisting of a series of questions, is used to determine the nature of a client's performance discrepancy, specifically, if it is a skill or habit deficit, and to formulate intervention strategies that will meet target outcomes within the constraints of the health care service delivery system (Fig. 21–2). In this subsection, emphasis is on the *decision-making process* leading to environmental adaptations for enhancing the PTE transaction, rather than on presentation of a compendium of adaptive environmental solutions, which are prone to change rapidly as technologies improve. Case examples are used to illustrate the guide. To serve more practical needs for information about the availability of specific technologies and services, three appendices for accessing information via printed materials, telephone, and computer are included at the end of this book. Concepts included in the guide are based on the *Uniform Terminology for Occupational Therapy*, 3rd ed (AOTA, 1994), human factors methodologies (Czaja et al, 1993; Faletti, 1984), the Ecology of Human Performance framework (Dunn et al, 1994), a Model for Skill and Habit Acquisition (Rogers & Holm, 1991b), and a Model of Occupational Functioning (Trombly, 1995).

Two approaches to managing performance discrepancies have been described: bottom-up and top-down (Trombly, 1993). Employing the top-down approach to clinical problem-solving suggested by Trombly (1993), the clinical decision-making guide presented in Figure 21–2 begins with the identification of the discrepancy between a client's current role and task performance and that which is expected, required, or desired (Mager & Pipe, 1984; Rogers & Holm, 1991b). For example, parents may indicate that their son does not interact with toys, children, or adults in the same manner that their other children did at age 3 1/2, and the preschool that they wish their son to attend requires age-appropriate dexterity and social skills. A worker who sustained a rotator cuff injury wishes to return to work, but finds that he cannot sustain the motions required for operating the surge machine for 2 consecutive hours, the minimum standard required by the Occupational Health and Safety Office. A middle-aged adult with **developmental delay**, who

was moved into a group home 1 week ago after the death of his surviving parent, refuses to come out of his room and is aggressive with staff. The group home's admission criteria stipulate that residents must participate in daily activities and chores, and must not exhibit aggressive or self-destructive behaviors. An older adult wishes to return to her senior apartment following her stroke, but she is unable to meet two of the residency criteria: managing her medications and preparing two light meals per day. In each of these situations, there is a discrepancy between the client's current capabilities and the demands of the physical or social environment. The specific nature of the discrepancy helps to focus the evaluation and guide effective intervention.

Nature of the Performance Discrepancy

Two broad categorizations of the nature of a performance discrepancy are skill deficit (Fleishman, 1966; Fleishman & Quaintance, 1984; Gentile, 1987) and habit deficit (Cubie & Kaplan, 1982; Florey & Michelman, 1982; Kielhofner & Burke, 1985; Rogers, 1986; Rogers & Holm, 1991b). When the PTE transaction is unsafe, inefficient, unsatisfactory, or dependent on others, the decision-making guide is designed to help clinicians ascertain if the performance discrepancy is due to a skill or habit deficit. Once this determination is made, environmental adaptations can be incorporated to reduce the environmental demand to match the client's performance level. If the probable cause of the performance discrepancy is a skill deficit, environmental adaptations can be incorporated that reduce environmental demand, thereby potentiating the client's level of skill. Likewise, if the probable cause is a habit deficit, short-term environmental adaptations can be incorporated, which substitute for habit acquisition and reduce the performance discrepancy, until enough time has passed to develop or restore routines and habits. For intervention approaches that focus on development and restoration of person capabilities see Chapter 20, and Units VIII, IX, and X.

SKILL AND SKILL DEFICIT

Skill is a task-specific ability to perform proficiently the requirements of a task (Fleishman, 1966). The standards for proficiency are determined both internally and externally. Internally, individuals determine a level of skill proficiency that is acceptable to them, and externally family members, teachers, friends, employers, and coworkers establish skill proficiency levels for tasks that are adequate to meet societal standards. Skill is acquired by practicing tasks under the supervision of an expert, who monitors performance and provides corrective guidance for errors. Skill deficit is a lack of ability to meet the proficiency standards set by oneself or others for performing a task. Because skill is task-specific, failure to meet the standards for one task does not necessarily mean that the standards for other tasks are not being met. Additionally, skill proficiency can be influenced by the task, or by physical and social environments.

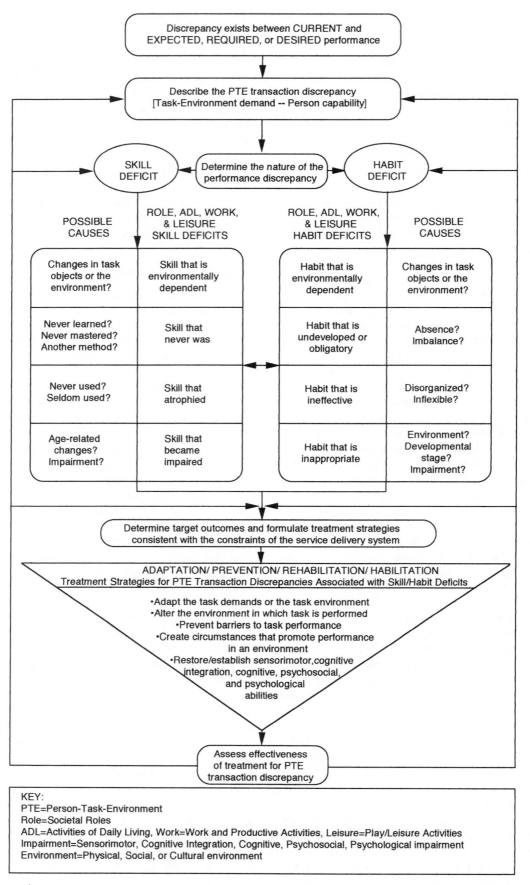

Figure 21-2. A clinical decision-making guide for person–task–environment transaction interventions.

HABIT AND HABIT DEFICIT

Several skills linked together into a sequence constitute a routine; routines linked together constitute a habit. Habits are usually developed over time as a means of making performance more efficient (Kielhofner & Burke, 1985; Rogers 1986; Rogers & Holm, 1991b). Habits are patterns of daily living that are unique to each person and are laborsaving mechanisms that enable humans to accomplish expected, required, or desired everyday tasks in an efficient manner. The acquisition of habits is more difficult than the acquisition of skills because habits involve more complex units of behavior and are dependent on the existence of at least a minimal level of proficiency. Habits, for example, involve morning care routines versus grooming skills. While skills are individualized by the style in which they are performed, habits are individualized by the sequence in which tasks are linked into routines. After arising in the morning, some individuals proceed by toileting, taking a bath, eating, brushing teeth, and dressing, whereas others begin with brushing teeth and then move to toileting, bathing, dressing, and eating. Habits are also embedded within each morning care task. For example, some individuals perform upper extremity dressing first and then lower extremity dressing, while others dress in the reverse order or in a more random fashion. Habit deficit is the cessation or disruption of daily living routines. The individuality of habits makes them more difficult to assess and treat than skill deficits. Similar to skills, habits are acquired over time, but unlike skills, which can be demonstrated within a single session, evaluation and intervention for habit discrepancies must occur over time to validate their existence, consistency, and effectiveness. As with skills, the task and the physical and social environment can also affect habits.

RELATIONSHIP BETWEEN SKILLS AND HABITS

Skills and habits are interdependent and inextricably linked (Rogers & Holm, 1991b). For a skill to be included in a routine or habit, it must be present. For example, unless an individual possesses skill in dressing, grooming, preparing meals, changing oil in the car, or mowing a lawn, routines and habits cannot be developed in association with these tasks. If skills are absent, inadequate, or impaired, routines and habits may not be developed, or may be disrupted. Likewise, skills must be used frequently to be adequately maintained, and refined (Mager & Pipe, 1984; Rogers & Holm, 1991b).

▼ A CLINICAL DECISION-MAKING GUIDE FOR PTE TRANSACTION INTERVENTIONS

The decision-making guide displayed in Figure 21–2 is designed to lead the occupational therapy practitioner step by step through a decision-making process to rule out probable causes of performance discrepancy during a PTE transaction. The top-down approach was chosen because it enables the occupational therapy practitioner to begin with the roles and tasks that are meaningful to the client, and also because observation of the PTE transaction at the role or task level incorporates both person capabilities and environmental demands. The decision-making guide prompts examination of discrepancies in performance from the perspective of skill deficits or habit deficits. Skill and habit were chosen because clients with physical impairments most often exhibit problems with skills, whereas clients with cognitive and psychological impairments may also exhibit problems with habits. Skill deficits will be examined first, because skills are requisite for habit development and maintenance. Skills that may be environmentally dependent are discussed first, because unfamiliar task objects or surrounding environments can negatively influence a client's performance even if no impairments are present. Subsequently, the guide helps you explore whether the skill was ever learned, never used, or seldom used. Finally, the guide prompts you to examine age-related changes in the client or impairments as probable causes of skill deficits.

If skill deficits are ruled out or resolved and a performance discrepancy remains, the guide begins with consideration of whether the habit is environmentally dependent. If task objects or physical and social environments change, habits and routines can be disrupted and can explain performance discrepancies. The guide goes on to encourage examination of whether habits were ever developed, are obligatory in nature, are ineffective, or are socially inappropriate. Once the nature of the performance discrepancy is established, the guide continues, by prompting the establishment of target outcomes and consideration of appropriate intervention strategies to reduce environmental demand.

Is it a Skill Deficit?

There are several types of skill deficits (Fig. 21–3) and, as indicated in the decision guide, they can be grouped into four general categories: skills that may be environmentally dependent, skills that were never learned or mastered, skills that are never or seldom used, and skills that are impaired.

CHANGES IN TASK OBJECTS OR ENVIRONMENT?

Is performance discrepant because of changes in task objects or because of the surrounding environment? When occupational therapy practitioners evaluate task performance, they establish the conditions under which this takes place. They select the task objects to be used during the evaluation, establish the interpersonal climate, and determine the level and kind of help that will be offered during the evaluation. Except when the evaluation takes place in the naturalistic setting— that is, in the client's home, school, or workplace—they also select the physical environment; for example, the occupational therapy clinic or the client's room in a hospital or re-

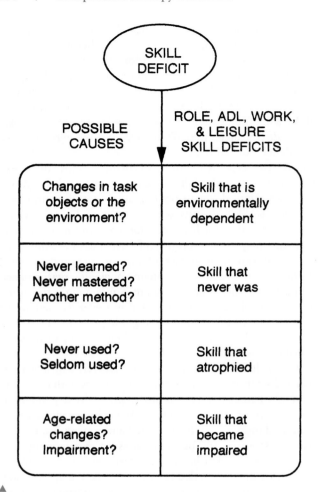

▲

Figure 21-3. **Skill deficits influencing the person–task–environment transaction and their possible causes.**

habilitation center. The evaluation conditions may facilitate or hinder task performance, or may be neutral to it, depending on a client's capabilities. Hence, these conditions are one possible cause of a performance deficit. During an occupational therapy evaluation, for example, Ms. Chu, a 67-year-old single woman with macular degeneration, who was recovering from a below-the-knee amputation of her right leg secondary to diabetic neuropathy, was unable to interpret a utility bill or write out a check. The amputation was healing well, and she was alert and oriented immediately postoperatively and thereafter. Ms. Chu reported that she had always taken care of her own finances and had balanced her checkbook before coming into the hospital. At home, however, Ms. Chu used enlarged checks and a template to locate the lines on the check. After completing the check, she used a high intensity halogen lamp and a magnifying glass to check her work. Without her usual task objects, as much as she tried to please the occupational therapy practitioner, she was unable to complete the checking tasks. She

was rated as having a skill deficit by the occupational therapy practitioner, who did not explore the implications of the evaluation materials on her task performance, and was concerned about the possible emergence of cognitive impairment.

Skill deficits similar to those induced by occupational therapy evaluation objects may occur when clients change their living, learning, working, or playing environments. Mrs. Booker, for example, called the Geriatric In-Home Assessment Program because she noted that her mother, who had recently moved to a senior apartment, was burning food quite frequently and seemed to be storing "garbage" in the refrigerator. The evaluation revealed that the client was having difficulty learning to use the electric range, because she had cooked on a gas one for the past 64 years. Furthermore, she was storing left-over food temporarily in the refrigerator because the garbage container was located in the basement, ten floors down, and this was too far to go everyday.

Skill deficits may be induced by social as well as physical environments and objects. The mere presence of the occupational therapy practitioner overseeing task performance during an occupational therapy evaluation may be sufficient to disrupt performance because the feeling of being observed and evaluated may make clients nervous or anxious. Persons in the environment may also be remiss in their responsibility for arranging task objects. For example, clients with moderate dementia can often perform tasks when they are reminded to do so by being given task objects by their caregivers. Without this reminder from caregivers, however, task performance may not occur.

A change of environment, either temporarily or permanently, challenges clients' adaptive capacities. Skill deficits may occur in a new environment because task performance was environmentally dependent on specific task objects or physical or human environments in the usual performance setting. Occupational therapy practitioners need to be sensitive to skill deficits that may be environmentally induced so that ratings of performance are not artificially lowered because clients are not using their usual task objects or performing in their usual environments. Ascertaining the degree of difference between usual and the clinic's task objects and arrangements will help in discerning if the skill deficit is due to environmental dependence. If performance does not seem to be affected by environmental factors, perhaps the skill was never learned or mastered, is not used frequently, or has not been required recently.

NEVER LEARNED OR MASTERED?

Is Performance Discrepant Because a Skill Was Never Learned or Mastered?

Before a determination can be made that the performance discrepancy is caused by the pathologies or impairments, it is necessary to ascertain if the skill was ever learned or mastered (Mager & Pipe, 1984; Rogers & Holm, 1991b). For instance, if Mrs. James, a 68-year-old widow who sustained a right CVA, has difficulty writing out a check and balancing a checkbook ledger, it is important to ascertain if she knew how to do these tasks before she had her stroke. Mrs. James reports that she always used cash and money orders before she was married. Mr. James handled all the family finances until his death 2 years ago and Mrs. James' daughter has taken over her finances since then. Thus, her inability to do these tasks is most likely due to a skill deficit caused by lack of learning. A skill that was never learned or never mastered requires habilitation, not rehabilitation. More important, however, is the need to determine if the skill is even needed, and if it is needed, the proficiency level that will be required. Following a traumatic injury, or the onset of a deteriorating neurological condition, for example, a move to a new apartment, assisted-living center, or group home may require skills that are deficient due to lack of learning or mastery. Such lifestyle changes may also require the use of previously learned, but never or seldom used skills.

Is Performance Discrepant Because Another Method Was Learned or Mastered?

Another factor to consider at this point is whether the client uses a method different from the one required in the evaluation to accomplish the same task. As part of an evaluation protocol, an occupational therapy practitioner may ask a client to review a utility bill, write a check for the amount on the bill, and balance the checkbook ledger. The client, however, may always use money orders to pay bills, and thus have adequate money management skills, even though check-writing skills are deficient. If it is determined that the *relevant* skill (ie, ability to pay bills) was learned and mastered, and that another method of task performance is familiar to the client, then changes in task objects or the task environment are logical factors to consider as precipitating a skill deficit.

NEVER OR SELDOM USED?

Is performance discrepant because the skill is never or seldom used? Skills may not be demonstrated or may be inadequate or unsafe because they have been dormant for months or years. Meal preparation and laundry skills have often atrophied in married men of the Second World War generation because their wives have been doing these tasks for them since they were discharged from the armed forces some 40 years ago. Widows of the same generation frequently report that they have not managed finances since their marriage because their husbands did this. Thus, data about clients' task performance history is required to determine the frequency and recency of skill use. Again, if a skill has not been adequately practiced, perhaps habilitation is needed, not rehabilitation. If you can rule out, however, that the performance discrepancy is not due to lack of opportunity to use it frequently or recently, then age-related sensorimotor, cognitive, psychosocial, or psychological changes or recent impairments may impede skill performance.

AGE-RELATED CHANGES OR IMPAIRMENTS?

Is Performance Discrepant Because of Age-Related Changes?

In older adults, normal age-related changes in motor, cognitive, psychosocial, or psychological abilities may interfere with task performance. The effects of these age-related changes may be compounded by new and preexisting pathology-associated impairments. Identifying the contribution of aging and pathology to skill deficits requires good observation skills against a background of knowledge of normal aging and the classical manifestations of pathologies. Mr. Carl, a 67-year-old farmer, who required a left above-elbow amputation following a World War II injury in 1945, was seen in the outpatient clinic following surgery for a herniated lumbar disc. He reports that many of the problems he currently experiences with bending, lifting, pulling, and pushing were not apparent even 10 years ago when he was younger and stronger. At 67 years, however, Mr. Carl reports that he does not have the strength he had previously, and he can no longer use brute force and one-handed lifting as he used to do. With decrements in functioning associated with the normal-aging process, persons usually make gradual accommodations in how they carry out tasks. If these accommodations no longer enable safe or adequate performance, however, it may be necessary to reduce the environmental demands to match current client capabilities.

Is Performance Discrepant Because of Impairments?

Impairments reflect the expression of pathology on organs and organ systems. Mr. Ken, a 46-year-old self-employed electronics sales representative, who sustained a left CVA, has difficulty writing out checks and balancing a checkbook ledger. Before his stroke, however, Mr. Ken managed the family's finances, as well as the financial aspects of his business. Hence, the most likely causes of his skill deficits are the residual impairments from his stroke. Although he is left-hand dominant, and can manipulate a pen adequately, his aphasia and impulsivity impair the quality of his financial skills. Although the classic impairments and disabilities associated with pathologies, such as CVAs and multiple sclerosis, are enumerated in medical textbooks, the classic pattern is rarely exhibited in individual clients, and the occupational therapy practitioner must be sensitive to unique manifestations. Moreover, skill deficits may arise from a combination of new and preexisting impairments.

Is it a Habit Deficit?

After it has been ascertained that a performance discrepancy may not be attributable to a skill deficit, evaluation of habit deficits is begun. As indicated on the decision guide (Fig. 21–4), habit deficits generally fall into four categories: those that are environmentally dependent, those that are undeveloped or obligatory, those that are ineffective, and those that are inappropriate.

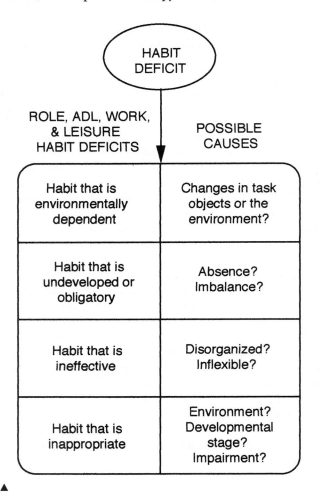

HABIT DEFICIT

ROLE, ADL, WORK, & LEISURE HABIT DEFICITS	POSSIBLE CAUSES
Habit that is environmentally dependent	Changes in task objects or the environment?
Habit that is undeveloped or obligatory	Absence? Imbalance?
Habit that is ineffective	Disorganized? Inflexible?
Habit that is inappropriate	Environment? Developmental stage? Impairment?

▲

Figure 21-4. Habit deficits influencing the person–task–environment transaction and their possible causes.

CHANGES IN TASK OBJECTS OR THE ENVIRONMENT?

Is performance discrepant because of changes in task objects or because of the surrounding environment? Habits that are environmentally dependent can be triggered by task objects (eg, toothbrush, zipper, blouse with buttons down the front), physical environments (eg, bathroom, lunchroom, assembly work station), and social environments (eg, baseball practice, religious services). When PTE transactions do not reveal any obvious routines or habits, before concluding that these have not been developed, it is appropriate to determine if the environment precludes a client from maintaining usual routines and habits. Hospitals and long-term care facilities (LTCF) are often unsupportive of habit acquisition and maintenance because they are organized around the routines established by staff. The schedules of hospital clients and LTCF residents revolve around nursing shifts and dietary schedules. Hospitalized clients are not allowed to self-medicate, thus eliminating the opportunity to demonstrate the habits that support their medication management skills.

Residents of LTCF who toileted independently at home, but are considered mobility impaired by LTCF criteria, may become incontinent frequently while waiting for assistance to ambulate to the bathroom. Mental health settings provide disincentives to habit maintenance and encourage dependency on staff with policies that require the removal of razors, fingernail polish, and manicure scissors for safety reasons, and lock up watches, money, and denture tablets for security purposes.

Because habits can be environmentally dependent (eg, which drawer a person automatically reaches for to obtain toothpaste), a move to a new room within a hospital or LTCF, and certainly a move to a new home, can cause a temporary disruption or cessation of intact habits and routines. For example, during an evaluation of meal preparation, Mrs. Dodd seemed confused. Even though she had been oriented to the kitchen in the occupational therapy apartment, she opened and closed doors and drawers trying to located items and repeatedly turned appliances on and off. However, an alternative explanation to confusion is that her cooking habits are somewhat attached to the kitchen in which she has cooked for 52 years, including the location of utensils and food supplies and the equipment controls. Clarification of the usual task environment, as well as the usual patterns and routines the client engages in, can help the occupational therapy practitioner arrange the task environment and provide the relevant task objects necessary for efficient and adequate task performance. If such accommodations are made, and performance is still discrepant, perhaps the habits are undeveloped.

ABSENCE OR IMBALANCE?

Is Performance Discrepant Because of an Absence of Habits?

The absence of habits and routines reflects a lifestyle that lacks sufficient structure and is relatively unpredictable. In young children, there may be an absence of self-initiated habits, but even toddlers quickly accommodate to routines and habits established by family members and daycare staff. When habits and routines are absent in their environments, children may not develop age-appropriate skills and may experience difficulty adjusting to preschool or school environments (Kramer & Hinojosa, 1993). Furthermore, if regular attendance at school is not in a child's repertoire, skill development is likely to be negatively influenced. For adolescents and adults in the work environment, the absence of habit patterns that support on-time arrival at the workplace, follow-through with assigned tasks, or adherence to safety procedures can negatively affect the ability to obtain or retain a job, even when the worker is highly skilled (Barris et al, 1985). If habits have been in place, but are suddenly disrupted because of a major illness in the family, relocation, or the apathy associated with depression, a performance discrepancy may also become evident (Kramer & Hinojosa, 1993). With the reduced time for rehabilitation in managed care, it is difficult to help clients develop routines that may become habits over time. Furthermore, in the inpatient setting, the usual physical or social environment that trigger and support a habit is not found. This affords the opportunity to creatively use educational techniques to help clients develop routines and habits to organize their lives and make tasks more efficient. If habits and routines are present, but performance is still discrepant, then habit imbalance is possible.

Is Performance Discrepant Because of an Imbalance of Habits?

Habit imbalance can take the form of routines lacking in number, diversity, type, and pacing of activities (Cubie & Kaplan, 1982; Florey & Michelman, 1982; Kielhofner & Burke, 1985; Rogers, 1986; Rogers & Holm, 1991b) as well as an obligatory adherence to habits and routines (Barris et al, 1985). Physical, cognitive, and psychological impairments can cause clients to severely restrict the type of activities they pursue, and the frequency with which they pursue them. For example, before an automobile accident that resulted in central cord syndrome and paresis in all four extremities, Mr. Jotel, a 48-year-old divorced man, jogged every morning and lifted weights 5 nights a week. Although he recently returned to his position as a tax auditor for the Internal Revenue Service, he is dissatisfied with his present lifestyle. During a recent on-site job analysis, he reported that he spends all his waking hours performing either self-care or work tasks, and further, that "if this is all that my life is going to be from now on, it isn't worth it."

Imbalance can also take the form of habits or routines that clients treat as obligatory. Impairments associated with dementia and obsessive–compulsive disorders can result in this type of imbalance. Mrs. Craven, who is 84 and has moderate cognitive impairment from dementia of the Alzheimer's type, spends many hours each day watching Lawrence Welk videotapes. Some days she will watch the same tape eight to ten times. Whereas she used to be quite social, Mr. Craven is unable to coax her to go out to visit with relatives or accompany him to the store. Mr. Craven has difficulty scheduling meals so that they coincide with the ending of the videotapes, and his wife gets upset if he turns them off to have her come into the kitchen to eat. In obsessive–compulsive disorders, habit imbalance usually takes the form of rituals, such as hand-washing (Bonder, 1991). Because these rituals are repeated often, such as hand-washing every 15 minutes, they tend to disrupt the normal rhythm of task performance. Changes in either the physical or social environment may serve to trigger new routines, serve as distracters from obligatory habits, or prevent the carrying out of routines due to lack of trigger stimuli, or presence of new stimuli. If discrepant performance cannot be attributed to an imbalance in habits and routines, perhaps disorganization or inflexibility of response is affecting performance.

DISORGANIZATION OR INFLEXIBILITY?

Is Performance Discrepant Because of Habit Disorganization?

When a smooth rhythm of daily routines is not evident in the client's PTE transactions, habit disorganization may be the reason. Pathologies such as **traumatic brain injury**, **stroke**, **depression**, **attention deficit disorder**, and **bipolar affective disorder** can result in impaired attention span, decreased ability to concentrate, impulsiveness, indecisiveness, and apathy, all of which can contribute to habit disorganization. Clients with habit disorganization tend to focus on the here-and-now and fail to plan for upcoming events, making them absent, unprepared, or late for appointments or tasks. For example, during the evaluation of personal care tasks, the occupational therapy practitioner observed that although Mr. Takada prepared for bathing and shaving by collecting his soap, towel, and razor, he left them on his dresser when he went into the bathroom. When he returned to his side of the room, presumably to get bathing and shaving materials, he noticed his clothes, which had been stacked on the bed by the nursing aide. He then proceeded to dress and when finished dressing, he put his razor, soap, and towel in his dresser. For habits to become automatic as well as purposeful, practice in planning, organizing, and implementing efficient routines is needed (Bransford & Stein, 1984). Habits that are only partially in place or disorganized, yield ineffective performance, as do inflexible habit patterns.

Is Performance Discrepant Because of Inflexible Habit Patterns?

Inflexibility of response can also disrupt habits and routines (Kielhofner & Burke, 1985). Characteristics of inflexibility are the inability to change routines to accommodate unanticipated or changing circumstances, as well as an inability to adjust emotionally when routines are changed. For clients who cannot vary routines or habits when necessary, or who become upset, agitated, angry, or confused when habits are disrupted, task and role performance may be discrepant because of inflexible habit patterns (Rogers & Holm, 1991b). A widow who still "cooks for two," even though this means extra cost and effort, is an example of how inflexible habit patterns influence everyday task performance. A client who has recently undergone a coronary artery bypass graft after years of high fat and cholesterol intake, and complies with his severe dietary restrictions while complaining through every meal, is an example of someone who becomes upset when habits are changed. Social support for changes in habits can aid adjustment when changes need to occur that are difficult for clients to accept. Inflexible habit patterns can also serve as an adaptive response for skill deficits, by conserving the response repertoire. Some inflexible habits are adaptive, rather than maladaptive, and it is critical for the occupational therapy practitioner to gather sufficient information about clients to be able to make this distinction. A client who checks every electrical outlet and touches each burner on an electric range before leaving the house, may have developed this routine because of short-term memory deficits. It may be an adaptive strategy designed to prevent fires that was developed after having left a burner or an iron on when out of the house. If the client's habits or routines seem ineffective, but not due to disorganization or inflexibility, then perhaps they are just inappropriate for the time or situation in which they occur.

INAPPROPRIATE ENVIRONMENT?

Is performance discrepant because the habit is enacted in the wrong environment? Many everyday tasks are linked to specific environments, such as bathrooms, kitchens, and bedrooms. Clients with cognitive or psychological impairments may carry out acceptable habits in an inappropriate environment, thereby making them unacceptable. Julian, an ambulatory 18-year-old male with severe developmental delay recently began to masturbate during mealtimes when in the dining room of the group home. Although this habit would be appropriate in the privacy of his bedroom or in the bathroom, Julian enacted his habit in the wrong environment; therefore, his performance is discrepant with social norms. Cues from significant members of the client's social environment may be needed to clarify behaviors that are acceptable and unacceptable in a specific environment. If a discrepancy is not due to performance in the wrong environment, it may be developmentally inappropriate.

DEVELOPMENTAL STAGE?

Is performance discrepant because the habit pattern is inconsistent with the client's developmental stage? Although exceptions are made based on pathology and impairment, society has certain expectations of "appropriate" behavior based on a person's age and stage of development (Eisenberg, Sutkin, & Jansen, 1984). A 12-year-old girl who sucks her thumb when stressed or tired runs the risk of ridicule by peers, because this performance is age-inappropriate. Similarly, adults who have the habit of "pouting" or "sulking" in the workplace also display a performance discrepancy. Whereas such behavior is frequently observed in children and teenagers, it is inappropriate for adults and is usually not tolerated by coworkers in the work environment. Again, cues from peers or supervisors in the social environment are helpful for eliminating developmentally inappropriate habits and supporting those that are consistent with a person's age and stage. If routines and habits are still discrepant, but not because they are inconsistent with a client's age or developmental stage, then impairment must be considered as a probably cause.

IMPAIRMENT?

Is performance discrepant because of impairment? Many pathologies can result in impaired judgment, leading to occasional or chronic socially inappropriate behavior (Bonder, 1991; Eisenberg, Sutkin, & Jansen, 1984; Hansen & Atchison, 1993; Reed, 1991). Since she sustained a left CVA, 71-year-old Sister Mary Joseph has had expressive aphasia. When she does speak she repeats a phrase, consisting of several four-letter words, that would have brought her ruler down on the knuckles of any child she taught who uttered even one of them. In the room next to Sister Mary Joseph is Mr. Graves, a 57-year-old longshoreman. Mr. Graves has also sustained a left CVA, and every time he has visitors he cries. Mrs. Graves had never seen her husband cry, and she was particularly concerned about his crying because some of their friends had mentioned that they had stopped visiting because they were embarrassed by his outbursts and did not know how to respond to them. The nursing staff had to explain to Mrs. Graves about emotional lability (rapidly changing emotions) and its relationship to stroke. Another client, 43-year-old Mr. Jackson, sustained a traumatic brain injury in a car accident 2 months ago, and insists on touching and grabbing the female hospital personnel he encounters. His family indicated that although he always liked to "kid around" with friends and coworkers, he never acted on his teasing and would certainly not have touched or grabbed anyone before his accident. In each of these instances, impairments have resulted in habits that are inconsistent with the clients' premorbid personalities and are viewed by friends and family in the social environment as "inappropriate."

▼ TARGET OUTCOMES

We have focused on one systematic clinical decision-making guide for identifying the nature of performance discrepancies and their probable causes. Once the client or the client's advocates have identified the level of task performance that is required, desired, or expected for each discrepant PTE transaction, target functional outcomes can be established (Fig. 21–5). The client and the occupational therapy practitioner then need to collaboratively establish the rank order in which target outcomes will be addressed and performance discrepancies resolved, taking into account the severity of the client's impairments and the constraints of the service delivery system (Evans, Small, & Ling, 1995; Hagedorn, 1995b). As some performance discrepancies are resolved, others may be identified, and further evaluation may be needed to assess sensorimotor, cognitive, and psychosocial impairments and develop long-term outcomes aimed at establishing or restoring generic abilities (Rogers, Holm, & Stone, in press; Trombly, 1993, 1995).

The Ecology of Human Performance Model (EHP) (Dunn et al, 1994) identifies five intervention strategies that incorporate the environment. By using the utilitarian parameters of economy and efficiency to guide intervention, we organized the intervention strategies into the top-down approach shown in Figure 21–5. Therefore, we begin discussion at the top with the adapt strategy, because of its potential for an immediate resolution of the performance

Determine target outcomes and formulate treatment strategies
consistent with the constraints of the service delivery system

ADAPTATION/ PREVENTION/ REHABILITATION/ HABILITATION
Treatment Strategies for PTE Transaction Discrepancies Associated with Skill/Habit Deficits

•Adapt the task demands or the task environment
•Alter the environment in which task is performed
•Prevent barriers to task performance
•Create circumstances that promote performance
in an environment
•Restore/establish sensorimotor,cognitive
integration, cognitive, psychosocial,
and psychological
abilities

Assess effectiveness
of treatment for PTE
transaction discrepancy

Figure 21-5. The top-down approach to intervention for person–task–environment performance discrepancies.

discrepancy and end with the establish or restore strategy, which may delay resolving the performance discrepancy until generic abilities are developed or redeveloped. After each intervention strategy is defined, it is illustrated with case scenarios involving skill and habit deficits.

Adapt

Adapt contextual features and task demands so they support performance in context. Therapeutic interventions can adapt contextual features and task demands so they are more supportive to the person's performance. In this intervention, the therapist changes aspects of context and/or tasks so performance is more possible. This can include enhancing some features to provide cues, or reducing other features to reduce distractibility (Dunn et al., 1994, p. 606).

ADAPT ENVIRONMENT FOR SKILL DEFICIT

Mrs. Hill is a 63-year-old woman with a 20-year history of multiple sclerosis, resulting in bilateral numbness and weak-

HISTORICAL NOTE
SUSAN TRACY'S VISION: THE NEED TO FOCUS ON MEANING

Suzanne M. Peloquin

Susan E. Tracy started a program of manual arts at the Adams Nevine Asylum in Boston, the first course designed to train nurses as crafts instructors. She left a legacy of her views in a book published years before the founding of the Society for the Promotion of Occupational Therapy.

Tracy thought that the crafts teacher had to be "thoughtful of the deeper needs of her patient" (1913, p. 10). She believed that an instructor who met those needs realized larger gains:

If a nurse can prove to the patient who chafes against his limitations that there is really a broad highway of usefulness opening before him of which he knew not, the mental friction is diminished and satisfaction steals in, while the whole physical organism prepares to respond by improved conditions. (1913, p. 171)

Tracy's vision of broad pathways to usefulness is an inspiring one. It reminds therapists today to explore those treatments that press past impaired sensation or limited motion to reach their clients' more basic needs for satisfaction and meaning. ■

Tracy, S. E. (1913). *Studies in invalid occupation: A manual for nurses and attendants.* Boston: Whitcomb and Barrows.

ness below the hips, decreased sensation in the hands, and low back pain with prolonged sitting. Because of several recent falls from her wheelchair when transferring, her family wants her to have an attendant while her husband is at work. She adamantly rejected their suggestion. Because Mrs. Hill had used a ladder successfully in the physical therapy clinic to get back into her chair, the occupational therapy practitioner recommended that a similar ladder be installed in the home. A suitable site was located, and recently, when she slipped to the floor during a transfer from bed to wheelchair, she crawled to the ladder, pushing her wheelchair ahead of her and used the ladder successfully to get back in her chair (Fig. 21–6).

Mrs. Charles is an 83-year-old woman with a 5-year history of macular degeneration, resulting in loss of central vision and fluctuating acuity in her peripheral vision. She has always enjoyed sewing items for craft fairs, but she can no longer see to thread the needle on her sewing machine, even when she uses a wire needle threader. She also cannot see the tension and stitch settings on the machine. The occupational therapy practitioner suggested a lighted magni-

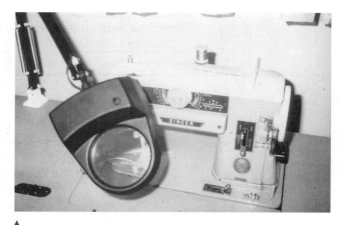

▲

Figure 21-7. A lighted magnifier used to adapt a sewing task.

fier, which has enabled her to continue a meaningful pastime (Fig. 21–7).

Jason is a 5-year-old boy with cerebral palsy (spastic quadriplegia). His parents signed him up to play T-ball in the summer league. The occupational therapy practitioner made a T-ball platform (Fig. 21–8) for Jason that provided him with adequate hip and trunk support so that he could stand without his walker and swing the bat. After Jason and his par-

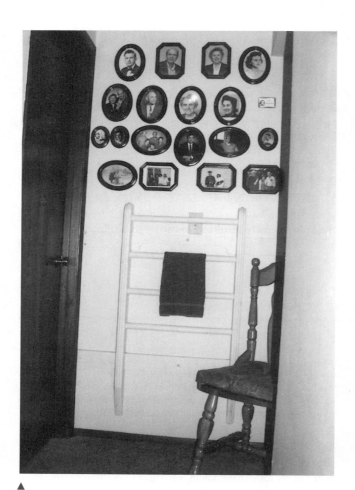

▲

Figure 21-6. A wall ladder designed to blend in with the decor of the home environment.

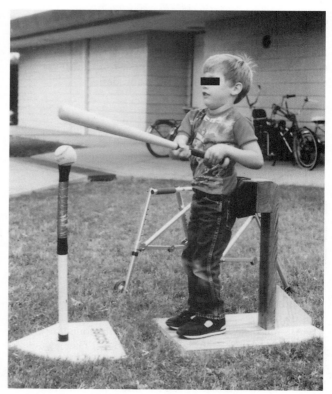

▲

Figure 21-8. A pelvic stabilizer—enabling both hands to hold the bat! (Stabilizer built by Steve Shores, MOT, OTR/L; Good Samaritan Hospital, Puyallup, WA.)

ents met with the T-ball coach, and he saw the platform, he adapted the game so that all batters positioned themselves on Jason's T-ball platform, and made the rule that if a child was at bat, then another child would run bases. These adaptations of the physical environment and the social environment (game rules) enabled Jason to play summer league T-ball.

Keenan is a 3 year-old-boy with a closed head injury. His occupational therapy practitioner adapted Bigfoot (a motorized ride-on vehicle) with hand controls so he could have functional mobility in his yard and neighborhood (Fig. 21–9). Two other modified ride-on-toy vehicles are shown in Figures 21–10 and 21–11. The vehicle in Figure 21–10 has been adapted by adding a positioning chair and a lever switch to move the vehicle forward. The vehicle in Figure 21–11 has been adapted with the addition of a car seat for postural stability, and has been fitted with a joystick for vehicle control. The ride-on-toy vehicles are battery-operated, can be purchased in any major toy store, and enable children with mobility impairments to explore their environments, and enjoy functional mobility with their peers. The vehicles were adapted by an occupational therapy practitioner, and are fitted with a safety control so that the practitioner or parent can override the system and stop the car.

ADAPT ENVIRONMENT FOR HABIT DEFICIT

Mrs. Hansen is a 52-year-old woman, who is confined to bed and has an organic brain disorder secondary to a brain tumor. Unable to communicate her wants and needs, she screams to get assistance from the LTCF staff. Eventually, she began to scream all the time when left alone. Because of her screaming, other residents avoided her and the staff placed her in her room with the door shut to reduce the distur-

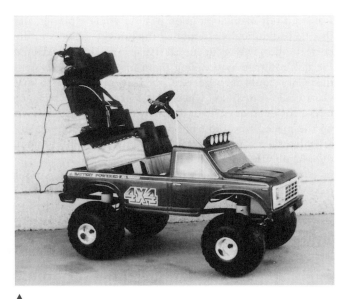

▲
Figure 21-10. Adapted motorized vehicle with a positioning chair added. (Motorized vehicle adapted by Steve Shores, MOT, OTR/L; Good Samaritan Hospital, Puyallup, WA.)

bance to others. The occupational therapy practitioner suggested using an audiocassette tape player and headset with tapes of music that she liked in the past. The family brought in the tapes, and within 1 week, Mrs. Hansen's screaming was reduced to only one or two cycles a day.

Gary is a 17-year-old boy with cerebral palsy (hemiplegia) and moderate mental retardation. As part of his Individualized Vocational Plan, he spends 3 hours each day in a work program. He was assigned to the lawn decorations assembly crew to develop work habits. The special education teacher notified the occupational therapy practitioner that

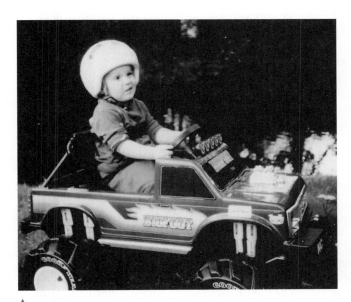

▲
Figure 21-9. Adapted motorized vehicles such as this Bigfoot™ enable functional mobility and exploration capabilities for children with motor impairments. (Motorized vehicle adapted by Steve Shores, MOT, OTR/L; Good Samaritan Hospital, Puyallup, WA.)

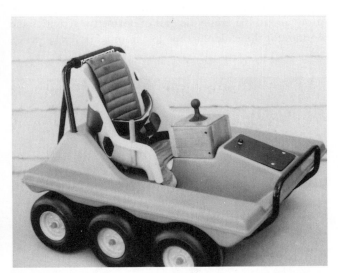

▲
Figure 21-11. Motorized vehicle adapted with a car seat and joystick. (Motorized vehicle adapted by Steve Shores, MOT, OTR/L; Good Samaritan Hospital, Puyallup, WA.)

Gary did not maintain a good posture while working, and that he had difficulty assembling the pinwheel pieces in the correct order. The occupational therapy practitioner adapted the task routines by breaking them into several extra steps that Gary could manage. She put nails in a board so that Gary could sort the pinwheel pieces in the basket by color in the correct sequence for assembly (Fig. 21–12), then pick up the pieces from the nail board in correct sequence, and assemble them onto a jig for the next student to continue the assembly. In regard to posture, the occupational therapy practitioner observed that once Gary became engaged in his tasks, he forgot about his posture. To solve this problem, a tape player with one of Gary's favorite tapes was attached to a switch plate. To trigger the switch plate, Gary had to have most of his hand on the switch, and to accomplish this, he had to develop the habit of sitting upright instead of listing to left with his shoulder protracted, elbow flexed, and wrist flexed.

Mr. Jakke is a 48-year-old man with a 10-year history of multiple sclerosis, resulting in bilateral lower extremity weakness and numbness, decreased balance, and decreased sensation in his hands. Following the last exacerbation of symptoms, Mr. Jakke has been unable to transfer independently into his car, and the family decided to invest in a car that would suit his needs. The occupational therapy practitioner referred them to a company that specialized in adapting vehicles to meet the needs of the user. Mr. Jakke's van (Fig. 21–13) has a remote control for opening the door, closing the door, and positioning the driver's seat, thus enabling him to transfer easily in and out of the van. The van also features hand controls. Although these adaptations do not seem "economical," they enable Mr. Jakke to take his children to school and transport and pick them up from social activities. He can also take himself to therapy and support groups, while his wife is at work. If Mr. Jakke could not drive, the cost to him (ie, loss of therapy, loss of support, isolation) and to the family (ie, loss of normative activities and routines for the children; time lost from work for his wife),

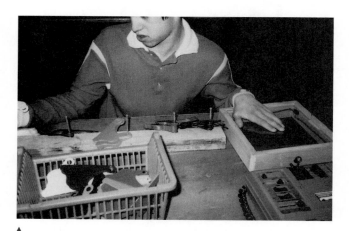

▲
Figure 21-12. Switch plate adapted to trigger the tape player if the student's hand is placed firmly on the switch.

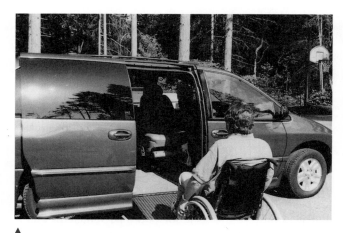

▲
Figure 21-13. This adapted van allows the driver to open the door with a remote control and then enter the van on a ramp. The ramp folds into the door when it closes, and the driver transfers into the bucket seat and engages the hand controls.

could easily cost more in the long term, than did the adaptations to the van.

Mark is a 18-year-old young man whose diagnosis is undifferentiated schizophrenia. As an outpatient he has been seen by an occupational therapy practitioner as part of a supported employment program. Mark is being placed in a fast-food restaurant and is assigned to work in the supply room and on the grill. To develop appropriate work habits, Mark has been supplied with a Neuropage System (Hersh & Treadgold, 1994) that is programmed to get him up in the morning, cue him about items to bring to work, and cue him about which medications are to be taken when the pager activates. The target outcome is to decrease the reliance on the paging system, with Mark being on time for work and having his medication blood levels remain within the therapeutic window.

Alter

Alter actual context in which people perform. Therapeutic interventions can alter the context within which the person performs. This intervention emphasizes selecting a context that enables the person to perform with current skills and abilities. This can include placing the person in a different setting that more closely matches current skills and abilities, rather than changing the present setting to accommodate needs. (Dunn et al, 1994, p. 606)

ALTER ENVIRONMENT FOR SKILL DEFICIT

Before Mr. Jakke and his family moved into their new home, several alterations were made to enable successful PTE transactions using a wheelchair. After the occupational therapy practitioner and the contractor reviewed relevant dimensions (Fig. 21–14), several alterations were made in the physical environment. The plumbing was recessed under the bathroom sink, thereby allowing Mr. Jakke to roll under the sink without worrying about burning his insensate lower extrem-

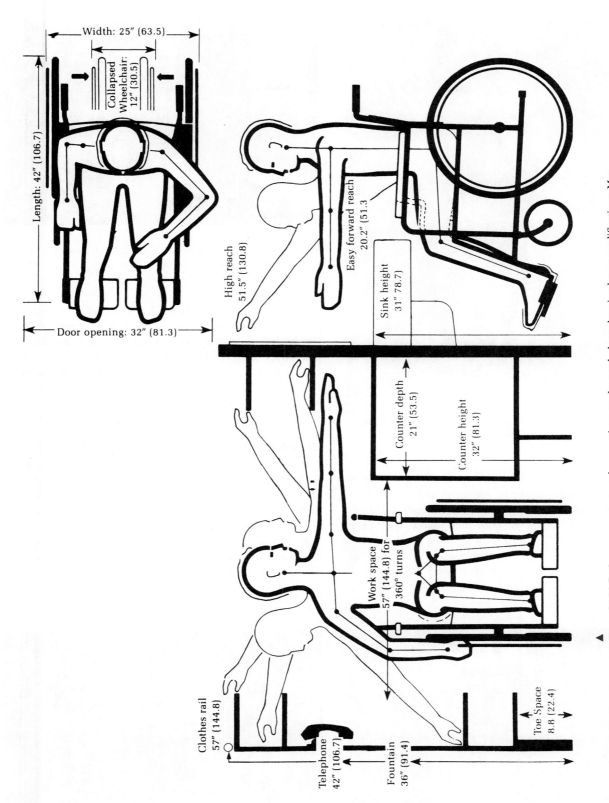

▲ *Figure 21-14.* Basic measurements and proportions can be used when planning home modifications. Measurements are given in inches and centimeters. (Adapted from Diffrient, N., Tilley, A. R., & Bardagey, J. (1974). *Humanscale 1/2/3.* Cambridge, MA: MIT Press, Designer, Henry Dreyfuss Associates.)

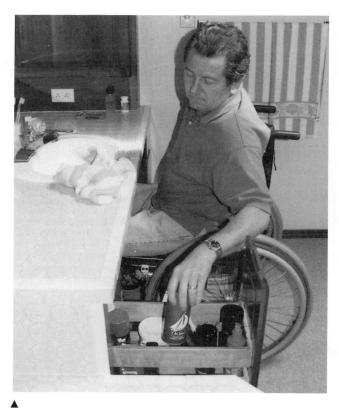

▲
Figure 21-15. Recessed plumbing and double deep drawers allow easy access to the sink area from a seated position.

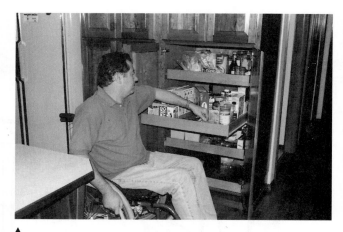

▲
Figure 21-17. Shallow drawers on gliders make all goods accessible from a seated position.

ities on the pipes, and two drawers were made into one deep drawer so that items could be obtained and stored easily from a seated position (Fig. 21–15). The standard 15-inch high toilet was replaced with an 18-inch high toilet for easier transfers. The oak "grab bars" for standing pivot transfers, which are next to the toilet, double as towel racks (Fig. 21–16). In the kitchen, static shelves were replaced with pull-out drawers for easier access to items (Fig. 21–17). The

microwave oven was placed by the cutting board (Fig. 21–18). With weakness and some loss of sensation in his hands, this allows Mr. Jakke to remove a hot dish from the microwave oven to the counter, reposition it, move it from the counter to the cutting board, reposition it; and, then move it from the cutting board to the table. Finally, a counter was built into the laundry room that enabled Mr. Jakke to fold laundry while seated in his wheelchair (Fig. 21–19).

ALTER ENVIRONMENT FOR HABIT DEFICIT

Mr. Bitner is a 68-year-old man with dementia of the Alzheimer type (DAT). He is a retired pharmaceutical company executive, and he and his wife Anne enjoy entertaining family and friends in their home. Mr. Bitner's current stage of DAT includes increased memory loss, resulting in continuous repetitive questioning of Mrs. Bitner, difficulty concentrating, loss of interest in previous activities secondary to memory loss and depression, withdrawal from social activities, and constant pacing. Mrs. Bitner has tried to rearrange

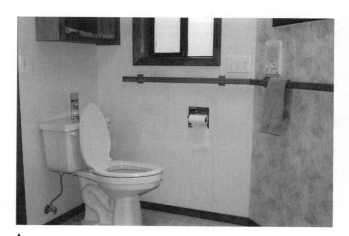

▲
Figure 21-16. The oak grab bars also serve as a towel rack, and the "extra-high" toilet enables an easy side-to-side transfer from a wheelchair.

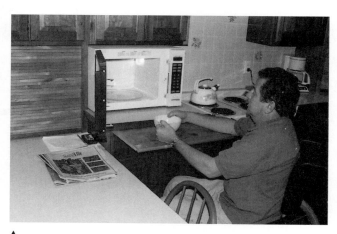

▲
Figure 21-18. The placement of the microwave oven enables hot items to be "stepped-down" to the cutting board and then transferred to the table with ease.

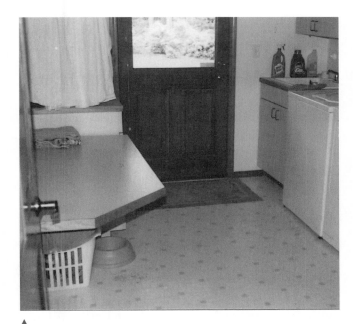

▲
Figure 21-19. The laundry table is angled to allow a clear pathway for the wheelchair, and the counter height is 32 in. for ease of use when seated, with clear access underneath.

their home to accommodate the pacing, but his habit of constantly asking questions or repeating phrases has taken its toll on her patience. She is no longer able to leave her husband unattended, and he is unable to function without her assistance. Two weeks ago Mr. Bitner sustained bilateral Colles' fractures when he tripped over a coffee table in the family room. After assisting Mrs. Bitner with suggestions for her husband's personal care, the occupational therapy practitioner also provided her with information about an **adult day care** program for individuals with dementia, that would provide him with a low-stimulus environment designed for his current level of functioning, and provide Mrs. Bitner, his caregiver, with some respite.

Prevent

Prevent the occurrence or evolution of malpractice [*sic*] performance in context. Therapeutic interventions can prevent the occurrence or evolution of barriers to performance in context. Sometimes, therapists can predict that certain negative outcomes are likely without intervention to change the course of events. Therapists can create intervention to change the course of events. Therapists can create interventions that address person, context, and task variables to change the course, thus enabling functional performance to emerge. (Dunn et al, 1994, p. 606)

PREVENT SKILL DEFICIT BY CHANGING ENVIRONMENTAL DEMAND

Mr. Alder is a 72-year-old man with a 30-year history of rheumatoid arthritis, and a 10-year history of type II diabetes. Following a mild right CVA, his wife was concerned about how she would manage him during bathtub transfers.

Mr. Alder liked to soak twice a day in the bathtub because this relieved his arthritis pain. The home health occupational therapy practitioner recommended a spring-loaded mechanical bathtub seat (Fig. 21–20) that allowed him to safely transfer into the bathtub, move down to and up from the bottom of the bathtub, and transfer out of the bathtub, thus preventing falls.

Mrs. Prescott is a 51-year-old woman with a fast-progressing dementing illness of unknown origin. She was hospitalized in a psychiatric unit after she lost 30 lb in 2 months, exhibited **apraxia** during everyday tasks, and became extremely labile. At discharge, she is unable to dress herself, remember how to use silverware, and is incontinent. Her family wishes to care for her at home, and has hired a live-in attendant. The occupational therapy practitioner met with the family and the attendant to demonstrate a hierarchy of assists that are available to them to maintain the skills Mrs. Prescott still retains, and to provide the necessary support as her capabilities decrease. The occupational therapy practitioner showed them a videotape he made while assisting Mrs. Prescott during a meal. As he showed the caregivers the videotape, he identified lower-level verbal cues as they were given, middle-level gestural cues, and higher-level physical assists (physical guidance and total assistance). He then discussed using lower-level assists before higher-level assists, the need to vary the type of assists from day to day as her performance fluctuates, and the increased use of higher-

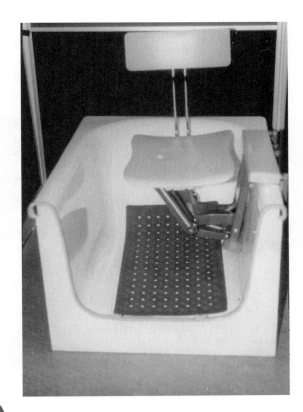

▲
Figure 21-20. The mechanical tub seat is spring-loaded and raises from the tub bottom with a weight shift and a simultaneous pushing up on the tub edges.

level assists as her dementia progresses. The practitioner gave each caregiver a list of the types of assists that Mrs. Prescott has required with personal care tasks, explaining each one, and then responding to questions. Although Mrs. Prescott's progressive deterioration of skill deficits cannot be prevented, the appropriate level of cues from the social environment can prevent a faster rate of skill deterioration.

PREVENT HABIT DEFICIT BY CHANGING ENVIRONMENTAL DEMAND

Mrs. Sandwick is a 94-year-old woman with **congestive heart failure**, **osteoarthritis**, and profound deafness, which is corrected slightly with bilateral hearing aids. Following the death of her sister, Mrs. Sandwick began to withdraw from social activities. Staff in the LTCF noticed that she no longer responded to their conversations, and they had difficulty communicating with her about medications, schedule changes, or her needs. She also stopped going to the activity room, which she had previously frequented twice daily. Following a hip fracture, Mrs. Sandwick was seen by the occupational therapy practitioner, who also had difficulty communicating with her, and thus tried using a Pocket Talker with a magnetic loop to enhance her hearing aids, and an attached microphone (Fig. 21–21). Mrs. Sandwick's eyes lit up at hearing the practitioner's words. She began asking questions about the device and how she could obtain one "so she could hear again and go back to the activity room." The family obtained the listening device for Mrs. Sandwick, which reversed her social withdrawal, and prevented miscommunication as well as possible depression.

Create

Create circumstances that promote more adaptable/complex performance in context. Therapeutic interventions can create circumstances which promote more adaptable performance in context. This therapeutic intervention does not assume a disability is present or has the potential to interfere with performance. This therapeutic choice focuses on providing enriched contextual and task experiences that will enhance performance. (Dunn et al, 1994, p. 606)

CREATE ENVIRONMENTS THAT ENHANCE SKILL

Ms. Yi-Sun is the occupational therapy practitioner at Vintage LTCF, and was asked by the administration to create an environment that would be safe for residents with dementia to wander and pace when they became anxious. With the assistance of students from the nearby educational program for occupational therapy assistants, she designed stations in the hallway where residents could stop and wind pocket watches, fold towels, sort and stack heavy plastic dishes, watch fish in an eye-level aquarium, and pick up finger foods. Outside, in the fenced in patio area they built raised plant boxes that could be tended without bending, and placed fencing around areas where the ground was uneven or there were tripping hazards that could place residents at risk for falls (Fig. 21–22).

CREATE ENVIRONMENTS THAT ENHANCE HABIT

Mr. Jakke had always liked being outdoors. Several years ago he had taken up gardening and was accustomed to spending about 2 hours each morning tending his vegetables, flowers, and bonsai trees. He had previously used a portable kneeler–bench that provided support for kneeling or sitting. However, he was no longer able to use this because of increased lower extremity spasticity. Hence, his morning gardening routine came to a halt. The occupational therapy

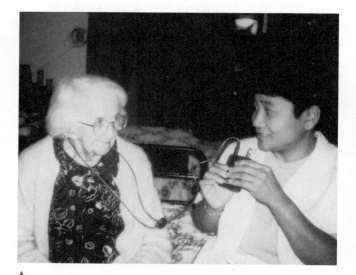

▲
Figure 21-21. The Pocket Talker magnetic loop around the nursing home resident's neck enhances the magnification of sound in her bilateral hearing aids, thus allowing easier communication with those in her social environment.

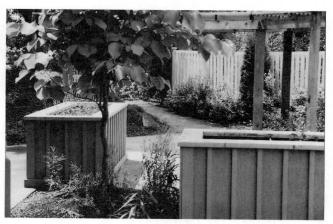

▲
Figure 21-22. The wandering paths and built-up planter enable nursing home residents to pace and wander in a safe and attractive environment.

practitioner suggested raised gardens for his vegetables and flowers (Fig. 21–23), and a fence with shelves to tend and display his bonsai trees.

Establish or Restore

Establish/restore a person's abilities to perform in context. Therapeutic intervention can establish or restore person's [*sic*] abilities to perform in context. This emphasis is on identifying a person's skills and barriers to performance, and designing interventions that improve the person's skills and experiences. (Dunn et al, 1994, p. 606)

ESTABLISH OR RESTORE SKILL FOR PERFORMANCE IN A SPECIFIC ENVIRONMENT

Mrs. Kochinski is an 86-year-old woman with multi-infarct dementia, who currently resides in an assisted-living center. Because she was having difficulty locating her room after meals and other activities, the occupational therapy practitioner helped her put some "favorite" pictures of herself and her husband (circa 1940) on her door, and then cued her to find the door with her pictures after each meal and activity session (Fig. 21–24). In 3 days, her "wayfinding" skills were established for her new environment.

ESTABLISH OR RESTORE HABIT FOR PERFORMANCE IN A SPECIFIC ENVIRONMENT

Andrew is a 13-year-old boy who has a recent diagnosis of attention deficit disorder. He has his own room, and a desk for studying, but he becomes easily distracted and rarely completes his homework. Andrew's psychologist works with an occupational therapy practitioner consultant, whom he asked to evaluate Andrew and make recommendations. Her recommendations were: "After removing all items from Andrew's desk except the desk lamp, and all posters from the walls surrounding his desk, have Andrew study in a dark room with only the desk lamp on and the items necessary for a particular assignment on his desk. In addition, have Andrew wear a Walkman that plays a tape of 'white noise.' This

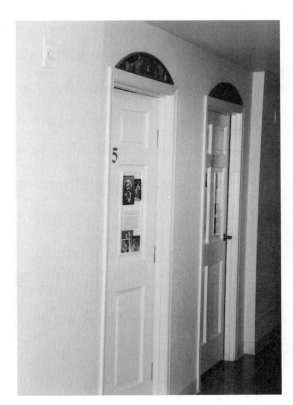

▲
Figure 21-24. Familiar cues in a new environment help nursing home residents "find their way home."

will help to reduce environmental stimulation. Have Andrew study at the same time every evening, and go through the same routines to set up his study area until habit patterns are established and maintained." The intervention was successful.

►PERSON—TASK—ENVIRONMENT INTERVENTIONS CONCLUSION

Occupational therapy practitioners have expertise in the analysis of performance discrepancies in the PTE transaction that occurs when our clients engage in meaningful tasks in relevant environments. Our knowledge base, derived from the biological, physical, behavioral, and occupational sciences, also prepares us to identify and implement efficient and economical interventions that will enable our clients to perform meaningful tasks in a safe, independent, satisfactory, and efficient manner. The clinical decision-making guide presented in this section was designed to prompt clinicians to consider a top-down approach to the evaluation of skill and habit performance discrepancies. Moreover, given the need to achieve functional outcomes in limited time frames (Christiansen, 1993, 1996; Cope & Sundance, 1995) we recommended several of the compensatory environmental intervention strategies delineated by Dunn et al (1994) as the initial

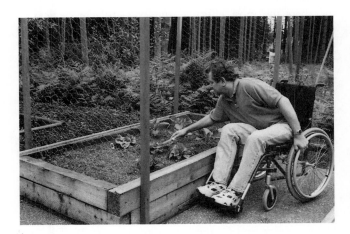

▲
Figure 21-23. The raised gardens enable the tending of plants from a seated position.

approach to performance discrepancy, followed by restorative strategies.

Appendices H, I, and J at the end of this book are provided as resource compendiums to this section. They are not meant to be exhaustive listings of resources, but rather to provide examples of resources that are available to occupational therapy practitioners and their clients. They are meant to stimulate further research for resources by providing sample categories and examples of what is available in the private and public sectors. Consistent with the decision-making guide, within each Appendix for this chapter there are resources for person support, task–environment adaptation, as well as resources for family members, advocates, caregivers, employers, coworkers or friends in the client's environment. In summary, the guide presented in this section is meant to provide a pathway through the decision-making processes required to enhance person capabilities and reduce or change environmental demands to enable clients to achieve successful PTE transactions. The following section discusses assistive technology options that might be considered during those decision-making processes.

Section 2

Assistive Technology In Occupational Therapy

Beverly K. Bain

Therapeutic Foundation
Evaluation Of Clients, Tasks, Devices, And Environments
Switches and Control Interfaces And Input Devices
Augmentative and Alternative Communication
Powered Mobility
Environmental Controls
> Telephones
> Monitoring Systems
Assistive Technology Conclusion

F or most people technology makes things easier. For people with disabilities, however, technology makes things possible. Mary Pat Radabough (1990)

Historically, occupational therapy has used adaptive equipment to enhance the functional abilities of clients in self-care, work, and leisure. With advances in technology have come new assistive devices that can increase functional abilities and offer independence for clients of all ages at various functional levels. Technological devices, such as powered wheelchairs and remote environmental control systems (ECUs), are used by physically and sensory impaired clients to perform ADLs not possible a decade ago; specially adapted computers and augmentative communication aids now make it possible for severely disabled, nonverbal children to participate in classrooms, for adults with impaired hand functions to become gainfully employed, and for individuals with physical, sensory, or psychosocial disabilities to enjoy leisure time activities in the community.

The Technology-Related Assistance for Individuals with Disabilities Act (1988) defines an *assistive technology* device (ATD) as "any item, piece of equipment, or product system, whether acquired commercially off-the-shelf, modified, or customized, that is used to increase, maintain, or improve the functional capabilities of individuals with disabilities" (29 USC 2202 [2] 1988). This broad definition includes "low-technology" devices that can be purchased from electronic or specialty stores, such as a simple attachment to a standard lamp that allows a person to turn on a lamp with the touch of a hand, rather than fumbling with a hard to find small switch. The definition also includes complex "high-technology" devices, such as a powered computerized wheelchair that enables a person to control the chair, turn on and off lights and appliances, use the telephone, and operate an augmentative communication aid and a computer through one integrated system. The ATDs addressed here are switches, powered wheelchairs, powered scooters, adapted vehicles, verbal communication aids, and ECUs.

The knowledgeable occupational therapy practitioner can use these advanced devices to increase, maintain, and improve the functional capabilities of many clients. Assistive technology services are also mandated by the Technology-Related Assistance Act and include "any service that directly assists an individual with a disability in the selection, acquisition, or use of assistive technology services" (29 USC 2202 (3) 1988). The competent therapist must be able to (1) assess the client; the tasks, needs, and goals of the client; the technological device; and the environments in which the device will be used; (2) select with other interdisciplinary team members the most effective and cost-efficient devices to meet the client's needs and abilities; (3) train the client and caregiver in the use and maintenance of the device; (4) document the client's abilities and needs, the selected devices, and all the environments where the devices will be used; (5) reevaluate the client, the tasks, all devices, and environments periodically; (6) contribute to the development, research, and field testing of new devices; and (7) serve as consultants to other professionals and caregivers. For more detail see AOTA's *Assistive Technology Competencies for Occupational Therapy Practice* (Hammel, 1995).

Assistive technology can be viewed as a system of four integrated and interdependent components: (1) the client; (2) the tasks and goals that the client needs to accomplish; (3) the device; and (4) the environments (Fig. 21–25). Each component must be evaluated in the context of the others, selected on the basis of how it interfaces with the others,

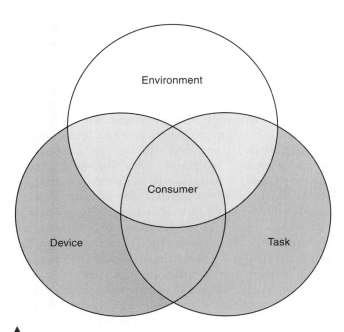

▲

Figure 21-25. Consumer, task, environment, and device model.

and applied as it interacts with the others. Devices are being developed very rapidly, some are extremely expensive, many are purchased only once, and too frequently they are underused or abandoned (Batavia & Hammer, 1990; Phillips, 1992). The occupational therapist can no longer think of each new device on the market as best for all clients. Each client must be evaluated and trained from a holistic perspective, each device must be evaluated and selected by an interdisciplinary team, and both the immediate and the future environments must be considered, if the client is to accomplish the desired tasks and achieve his or her goals. Given the rapid pace of development, occupational therapists need to know the therapeutic concepts and principles related to technology that are built on the profession's body of knowledge because these remain constant.

▼ THERAPEUTIC FOUNDATION

In the area of occupational therapy rehabilitation technology practice, the therapeutic foundation is based mainly on the following frames of reference: *biomechanical*, specifically, **work simplification** and energy conservation; *acquisitional*, the learning and maturation theories; and *rehabilitation*, for adaptations of devices and environmental modifications (see Unit VIII).

Biomechanical work simplification and energy conservation principles are the basis for prescribing battery-powered wheelchairs for persons with high-level spinal cord injuries to reduce the physical energy needed for wheelchair movement and to increase the energy available for ADL, work, play, and leisure activities. ECUs are used to control lights

and appliances, simplify work, and conserve energy for persons with low physical tolerance, including individuals with multiple sclerosis (MS), muscular dystrophy (MD), amyotrophic lateral sclerosis (ALS), arthritis, cardiac disease, or burns. In the future, as *robots* become less expensive, they can be used to conserve the energy of both the user and caregiver in the home and workplace.

The acquisitional frame of reference relates to learning the "specific skills needed for successful interaction in the environment" (Mosey, 1986; p. 433). For example, clients with lower-extremity impairments can learn to interact successfully in their environments by learning to use powered wheelchairs and adapted vans to solve their mobility problems. Children with severe, multiple disabilities can learn to participate in activities and games by using a switch to control appliances or toys.

The major learning theories relevant to the occupational therapy process include classical conditioning, operant conditioning, and social or imitational conditioning. When teaching a client to use an ATD, the therapist may use one learning theory or a combination. For example, an augmentative communication aid is prescribed for a nonverbal person who might randomly press various keys on the aid. If that person accidentally strikes a certain key and hears the communication aid speak the word *food* and the person strikes the key again and the response is repeated, the person has learned through conditioning that pressing a designated key gives a definite response. That person can further learn, through operant conditioning, that striking a series of keys (receiving positive reinforcement each time) expresses the desire to have lunch because the synthesized voice says, "I want to eat lunch now." Furthermore, this person may learn through social imitation that the preferred way to ask for lunch is to use the augmentative communication device, rather than pounding on the table or making grunting noises.

The rehabilitation frame of reference includes the therapeutic application of adaptive equipment and modification of the environment to compensate for physical and sensory impairments or deficits. Assistive technology devices are a new dimension of adaptive equipment, and through the application of devices, such as power scooters and ECUs, many environments require fewer adaptations. Environmental modifications have also been enhanced by the technological and ergonomic advances in tool and work environment designs. Technology is congruent with the philosophical assumption that "rehabilitation must be dynamic and keep in step with both scientific advances and changes in society" (Hopkins & Smith, 1983, p. 135). Based on rehabilitation assumptions, an occupational therapy treatment program for a severely involved client with a C4 quadriplegia, for example, would be to teach the person to use an ECU to compensate for the lack of hand manipulative skills; a powered wheelchair to foster independent mobility; and a computer to increase possible education, avocational, and vocational activities, enabling the client to be involved in a community. In addition, the treatment process may include technological adaptations of the home, school, and workplace environments to help the client live a more purposeful and satisfying life.

The domain of concern for the profession—the occupational performances of ADLs, school, work, play, leisure, and recreational activities—can be enhanced through the application of assistive technology (AT). ECUs, powered wheelchairs, computers, and augmentative communication devices can increase a client's function in each area. However, the client's motor, sensory, cognitive, psychological, and social abilities must be carefully evaluated before the selection or application of any technological device. For example, each ATD must be activated, which requires some form of motor function (this can be in the form of pressing a switch, blinking an eye, or saying a command); each device has some form of feedback, which is usually visual or auditory, requiring sensory integration; and each device requires a certain amount of cognitive ability, such as learning sequencing to control an ECU or computer. In addition, psychologically the client must be motivated to use the equipment for any device to be effective.

Occupational therapy's fundamental concern is ensuring the client's capability throughout the life span to perform with satisfaction those tasks and roles essential to productive living and to the mastery of self and environment. Technology can be used throughout the life span; for example, infants at risk can operate toys that allow them to interact and learn from the environment, and the elderly can use powered scooters and ECUs to increase their independence in performing tasks safely. Technology, however, should not be considered the only solution. Rather, technology provides an extension of the abilities of selected clients treated by a reflective therapist who has thoroughly assessed each component, the various ATDs, and the environments in which the individuals will use them.

▼ EVALUATION OF CLIENTS, TASKS, DEVICES, AND ENVIRONMENTS

A primary responsibility of the occupational therapist is to undertake a holistic evaluation of the client; the needs, tasks, and goals of the clients; various ATDs; and possible environments in which the devices will be used. A structured evaluation is necessary in view of the available devices, the increasing number of clients being referred to occupational therapy for aids, the price range of different devices, and, as more architectural barriers are removed, the greater level of participation in community life by people with disabilities. Professionals should not randomly match the latest device on the market with every client but must systemically evaluate each client's functional need for each device and all possible environments in which the client will use the device.

A valid technological evaluation should be a collaborative team effort that includes the client, physician, occupational therapist, physical therapist, social worker, teacher, vendor, and caregiver. The trained occupational therapist contributes valuable and unique professional skills to the evaluation team, including the ability to assess clients with disabilities in all performance components, the ability to analyze skills required to successfully use an ATD, and the ability to position clients. Most devices are activated by switches; therefore, the optimal control sites, the anatomical parts of the body that are used to activate the switches, can best be determined by a therapist who evaluates a client's motor abilities. For example, a client who has a deficit in motor control in the upper and lower extremities may use head or neck or eye movements to activate the switches that propel the powered wheelchair. In addition, the therapist must evaluate the client's spatial and depth perception abilities as well as cognitive ability. Furthermore, an experienced therapist is cognizant of the psychological implications of adaptive equipment for a client and can determine the best time to introduce ATDs into the treatment program.

For severely involved clients who require complex technology systems, the primary occupational therapist (1) gathers data about the client's background and needs, (2) evaluates the client's abilities, and (3) relates this information to an occupational therapy technology specialist. The specialist should (1) have knowledge of and experience with various devices, (2) evaluate the client with several devices before recommending the appropriate ATD, (3) continue to evaluate both the client and AT system during the training process, (4) teach the client all applications and maintenance of the ATD, and (5) coordinate the integration of all technological and standard equipment that the client requires. In settings in which off-the-shelf technological devices are used, a certified occupational therapy assistant, consulting with a specialist, is able to follow through with the application of the ATD and report when reevaluation of the client or ATD or maintenance of the ATD is required.

A structured assessment instrument has been developed and field tested with various populations, including adults and children with severe physical disabilities, adults with sensory impairments, and clients with developmental disabilities (for a complete description and a copy of the form, see Bain, 1989). The primary areas to consider in the problem-solving approach to the evaluation of clients for ATDs by the entry-level therapist are presented in this section, with specific guidelines for switches, powered wheelchairs, augmentative communication aids, ECUs, and adapted computers.

Each part of the technology system must be evaluated to ensure that the most appropriate device is selected and used effectively by the client. The four major areas of evaluation for ATDs are (1) data collection of the client's background and needs; (2) evaluation of client's abilities, including positioning; (3) planning with the client, caregivers, and rehabilitation team members; and (4) selection of appropriate ATD that will enhance the client's functional abilities throughout the day and in a variety of environments. As with all evaluations for any assistive or adaptive equipment, a problem-solving approach is essential. The following guidelines have proved to be effective:

- What are the client's needs and goals?
- What are the client's abilities?
- What ATD would be appropriate based on the client's needs, goals, and abilities, considering: (1) the input, throughput, output, and display characteristics; (2) the commercial availability of an ATD or the adaptability of a commercial ATD; (3) safety and reliability; (4) practicality; and (5) affordability.
- Where will the ATD be used? (Consider all present and possible future environments.)
- Based on the evaluation of the client, the ATD, and the environments in which the ATDs will be used, various ATDs should be tried with the client. (Most vendors and manufacturers of ATDs will lend therapists equipment on a trial basis).
- Where can the ATD be ordered, and will it need to be adapted?
- Who will train the client to use the device, and how many treatment sessions will be required?
- Who will document the evaluation, and where?
- When should the client, ATD, and environment be reevaluated and by whom? (Table 21–1)

These guidelines may be modified to meet the clinical setting and the qualifications of the rehabilitation technology team members. Many sites will not have all members of the desired team, and frequently, the occupational therapist will be responsible for the coordination of the team evaluation.

TABLE 21-1. Steps in a Problem-Solving Approach to the Evaluation of Consumers for Assistive Technology Devices (ATDs)

Steps	Part of System	Problem	Action

1.	Task	Identify the tasks the consumer needs to accomplish with the ATD
		   Communication
		   Mobility
		   Environmental controls
		   Computer adaptation
		   Switch interface
			Review records
			
			Interview consumers, caretakers, and family
			
			Observation

2.	Consumer or user	Identify the consumer's abilities in lying, sitting, and standing positions	Formal testing:
			   Motor
			   MMT, reflexes, ROM
			   Coordination
			   Endurance
			   Sensory
			   Psychosocial
			   Cognitive
			   Social
			Interview
			Observation

3.	ATD	Based on 1 and 2, identify possible devices	Characteristics: Input, processing, output, display Commercial availability Safety and reliability Practicality Affordability

4.	Environment	Present and future:
		   Bed or chair
		   Home
		   School or work
		   Community
			Interview
			Observation
			On-site visits

5.	All	Trial period	Try various devices in a variety of environments
6.	ATD	Selection	Order, adapt, or fabricate
7.	Consumer or user	Application	Train in use and maintenance
8.	All	Documentation	Record in all intra- and interdepartmental files
9.	All	Reevaluation	Periodically consumer, ATD, environment, and task(s)

A few words of caution should be noted: Technological devices are usually ordered only once, some are expensive, and many times they are discarded or underused. Therefore, a precise, structured evaluation of each part of the system is worthy of professional time and effort, often requiring two or more sessions. Also, the clinical judgment of the therapist and members of the rehabilitation team should take precedence over the salesmanship of vendors or manufacturers, who may try to influence the selection of devices. The best assistive device is the one that best facilitates the client's functional abilities. It may be an expensive, high-technology, integrated system; or it may be an affordable, low-technology, single piece of equipment. In either case, the decision must be based on clinical knowledge of the entire team, which includes the client and caregiver. For details, see the AOTA *Technology Competencies for Occupational Therapy Practice* (Hammel, 1995) and for assessments of acute and rehabilitation centers see the *AOTA Technology Special Interest Section Newsletters* for March and June 1995.

Currently, there is not one comprehensive interdisciplinary evaluation especially designed for AT. There are separate evaluations for powered wheelchairs, augmentative communication devices (Fishman, 1987), ECUs (Bain, DiSalvi, Gold, Kollodge, & Schein, 1993), and computers (Anson, 1994). O.T. FACT, a software assessment tool developed by Roger Smith (1990), has two sections that are relevant to AT: (1) the use of environment-free scoring behavior, and (2) the use of environmental-adjusted behavior (Smith, personal communication, October 1994). Other AT assessments that should be reviewed are Lee and Thomas (1990), Scherer (1991), and Williams, Stemach, Wolfe, and Stanger (1993).

▼ SWITCHES AND CONTROL INTERFACES AND INPUT DEVICES

Each AT system has four parts: (1) the input, known as the switch or control interface that activates the device; (2) the throughput, which is the processing unit of the device; (3) the output, which is the result of a successful operation; and (4) a display, which is the visual, auditory, or tactile feedback that informs the operator that the system was activated. When one turns on a light by pushing or twisting a switch (input), the electrical current in the building is the throughput and a light turning on, is the output and also the visual display.

Switches enable people with disabilities to interact with their environments, to increase functional activities, and to extend their capabilities. The purpose of switches is to control devices; therefore, in the technology literature, they are usually referred to as control interfaces. It has often been said that the most magnificent technological device or the simplest toy is underused or useless if the person cannot ef-

ficiently operate it; it can also be the most frustrating experience for the client, caregiver, and therapist. Thus the therapist must be certain that the client can readily and efficiently activate the switch or control interface (Box 21–1).

Because switch selection and mounting for ATDs are usually the responsibility of the occupational therapist, the therapist should first evaluate several *control sites* to determine the most accurate, reliable, and efficient movement that the client can make (Wright & Nomura, 1990). Next, the therapist determines the proper mounting system for the switch, which depends both on *where* the switch will be used and with *which* devices it will interface. For example, an ECU or augmentative communication aid needs to be controlled when the user is in bed as well as when the user is in a wheelchair. The trend toward integrated technology warrants the use of one switch to control many ATDs in different modes.

▼ **BOX 21-1**

Guidelines for Switch or Control Interface Selection

1. Establish the optimal position for the client, noting all other functions, especially ADL.
2. Determine what assistive technology devices the client needs to switch to interface (toy, wheelchair, ECU, communication aid, computer, or others).
3. Evaluate the client's physical abilities, considering the sensorimotor, cognitive, and psychosocial components (voluntary control, action, ROM, endurance, speed of response, vision, and so on).
4. Note all precautions (seizures, respiration, fatigue, other).
5. Discuss with the client, or significant others, or both, their thoughts, opinions, and desires.
6. Test the client for two or three possible control sites by observing, formal testing, interviewing, and reviewing the initial evaluation (if the client cannot communicate, be sure to observe all voluntary motions that are accurate, reliable, and efficient). Interview the caregiver.
7. Evaluate the operational features of the switch: activation, force requirements, distance the switch must travel, size of the control surface, durability, feedback, connector type, momentary or latching mode.
8. Analyze the selection technique required by the assistive technology device (direct selection, scanning, or encoding).
9. Determine where the switch will be used (in bed, on wheelchair, at a workstation, or other).
10. Mount the switch temporarily. *Do not hold the switch.*
11. Try the switch with a temporary mounting. If this is not successful, try another switch or change the mounting; if successful, mount the switch permanently and note the position in writing (draw a picture) so all caregivers will be informed.
12. Re-evaluate periodically.

The technology specialist should be able to select several possible control sites at which the client demonstrates purposeful movement by reviewing the physical abilities evaluation, by interviewing the client, and by observing the client's voluntary motion in various environments. Almost any part of the body can be used as an optimal control site; for severely involved individuals that might be the head, eyes, tongue, chin, breath, or voice, as well as the leg or foot.

A wide variety of switches and control interfaces are available commercially, and some can readily be fabricated by the therapist, other clients, family members, or caregivers. The most commonly used switches include the following: (1) mechanical switches, such as joysticks, cushions, treadles, rockers, and pneumatic switches, such as sip and puff switches; (2) electromagnetic switches, such as light beam infrared switches, light-emitting diode (LED) detectors, and optical headpointers; (3) electromyographic switches such as those used to control myoelectric prosthesis; and (4) sonic switches, such as ultrasound and voice switches that convert sound levels to switch closure (Webster, Cook, Tompkins, & Venderheiden, 1985). Different disabilities require different types of switches. A client with a spinal cord injury who has limited motion and muscle power requires a sensitive switch (sip and puff), whereas a client with poor gross motor control may require a strong pressure switch with individual slots, to restrict inadvertent selection.

Single, dual, and multiple switches are used to operate technical aids: for a simple on or off toy, a single cushion switch may be used; for an ECU that requires scanning and then selection, a dual pneumatic switch may be needed; for a powered wheelchair that moves in many directions, a multiple joystick may be required. Switches operate in momentary or latching modes. A momentary switch activates the device only as long as pressure or contact is being applied—for example, a car horn, an electric bed, or a powered wheelchair switch. A latching switch requires one motion to turn on the device, which remains on until the switch is reactivated, disengaging the latch to the off position—for example, a wall light switch or the on and off switch of a computer. Most powered wheelchairs and scooters use switches that allow a smooth gradual acceleration, known as proportional switches.

Switches act as the interface between the person and the device; they activate or deactivate the device and also control the device by direct selection, scanning, or certain encoding techniques. *Direct selection* is the most frequently used and efficient selection technique. It can require more motor control than scanning, which requires higher cognitive and visual-tracking skills. The two types of *scanning* are linear scanning and row-column scanning. In linear scanning, each element is sequentially pointed to, and in row-column scanning, first the row or column is selected, followed by the linear scanning of each element in the selected row or column. The later technique reduces time and effort. *Encoding* can be used with both direct selection and scan-

ning techniques, and it usually requires multiple selections such as Morse code. Encoding is an abbreviation or acceleration selection technique. When recommending a switch or control interface, the therapist should take into consideration which selection technique will be used for each device to integrate the total AT system. For example, many ECUs and augmentative communication aids require scanning techniques, but some powered wheelchairs do not; therefore, whenever possible, all devices should be integrated to use the same switches or control interface with a compatible selection technique.

In communication, for instance, a client using a picture communication board who wishes to convey the desire for a glass of water can indicate that desire by pointing directly to the appropriate picture on the board. If the client is using a more complex communication device that has letters of the alphabet in rows of eight letters per row, however, the client may point first to the third row, where the letter *w* appears, then to each letter in that row until *w* is selected. Speed is an important factor and should be taken into account when choosing the appropriate technical aid. When the message sender can reduce the effort and time it takes to make a selection, the communication becomes more effective. An example of the increased communication speed of high technology might be a computerized communication aid that has been programmed so that when a nonverbal client points at two or three icons, the computerized voice says, "I want a drink of water, please." This communication aid has switch-encoded selection ability, whereby one or more symbols, letters, or words can be coded to convey a complete phrase or sentence.

Most switches require some form of mounting to keep the switch within reach and to permit effective operation. Some switches can be kept in place on table tops, wheelchair trays, or bed rails using Velcro™ with adhesive backing or clamps, a single or multiple joint mounting arm, and a mounting clamp. There are rigid stainless steel tubular mounting arms or flexible gooseneck or caterpillar arms. Switches can also be mounted directly on the client, including the head, chin, or over any muscle on the client's chest or on the roof of the mouth. A rehabilitation engineer may assist the therapist if a customized-mounting system is necessary.

The variety of available interface systems and the range in prices warrant that a therapist check various suppliers' catalogs, carefully evaluate the client's abilities and all the environments where the switch will be used, and integrate the switch and mounting system with the other ADL and hospital equipment the client may use. A primary consideration when selecting a control interface should always be the client's position in lying or sitting, so that reflexes or poor postures are not elicited. If a complex system is used, the occupational therapist should draw a diagram or take pictures so all caregivers mount the switch correctly.

In summary, it should be noted that (1) the selection of the switch or control interface is crucial to the operation of all assistive devices, (2) the occupational therapist is primarily responsible for selecting the switch and mounting system, but collaboration with other team members is essential, and (3) when possible, one switch or control interface system should be selected to integrate all the client's assistive devices.

▼ AUGMENTATIVE AND ALTERNATIVE COMMUNICATION

The basic areas of communication are verbal, conversational, written, and gesturing. Historically, the occupational therapist and the classroom teacher have screened, evaluated, and trained children in the area of written communication. Today, there is an increasing use of computers as writing and drawing aids for the all students, as well as those with disabilities. This section focuses on verbal communication and the vital role of the occupational therpist in collaborating with the speech pathologist, who is usually the technology coordinator of augmentative and alternative communication aids.

Communication aids are defined by the American–Speech–Language–Hearing Association (ASHA) as "physical objects or devices used to transmit or receive messages (e.g. a communication book, board, chart, mechanical, or electrical device or computer)" (ASHA, 1991, p. 10). Augmentative and alternative communication (AAC) systems "attempt to compensate (either temporarily or permanently) for the impairment and disability pattern of individuals with severe expressive communication disorders" (ASHA, 1989, p. 107).

The term augmentative communication is defined as some way of communicating that does not require speech. If someone has a severe physical disability this may be through gesturing, facial expressions, body or sign language, or through the use of picture-letter-word boards, commonly known as communication boards. When a client with physical impairments lacks the motor ability to convey a message, an alternative or augmentative communication system is required. When a communication aid is used, the speed at which the user can locate and select a key, the number of required selections before the aid offers an output, and the quality of the output must be considered. The most frequently used nonelectronic communication system requires the user or communication partner to point to choices to convey messages. Pointing by the user may be done with the hand, with a headpointer, a lightbeam pointer, or with the eyes.

An electronic augmentative communication system uses an electronic device as throughput. The input can be a single pressure switch, a dual rocker-level switch, a joystick, an optical pointer, a keyboard, an eye-blinking switch, or any other control interface that is properly mounted and readily accessible to the user. The output can be by spelling; abbre-

viation; pictures; coding of words, phrases, and sentences by synthesized speech; visual display; printed copy; or a combination of these.

A communication evaluation should begin by identifying all the tasks, needs, and goals of the client and communication partners. The client's cognitive, motor, and hearing abilities that should be assessed for the elements of communication are sender–receiver–feedback. In addition, the client's language and educational skills need to be considered. The environment where the aid is used should be assessed for the mounting of the aid, whether in bed or in a wheelchair.

The key characteristics of any communication system are (1) rate or speed that a message can be conveyed, (2) portability of the aid, (3) its accessibility to the user in various positions, (4) dependability of both manual and electronic power sources, (5) quality of the output, (6) durability, (7) independence of the user, (8) vocabulary flexibility (programmable or fixed), and (9) time required for repairs and maintenance of the aid (Church & Glennen, 1992; Fishman, 1987; Flippo, Inge, & Barcus, 1995; Mann & Lane, 1995).

Team cooperation is required to deliver the appropriate augmentative communication services to a client. In the service delivery of electronic communication, the four substantial contributions of the occupational therapist are (1) holistically evaluating of the client, including physical abilities (eg, seating and positioning, range of motion, coordination, reflexes) and cognitive and perceptual abilities; (2) evaluating and recommending the most effective control interface and selection technique; (3) training the client to access the aid; and (4) collaborating with other team members (Angelo & Smith, 1989; Church & Glennen, 1992; Fishman, 1987). The speech therapist usually determines the client's communication needs, assesses the client's language ability, collaborates in the selection of an aid, and trains the client and his or her major communication partners. Other professional members of the team may include a physician, who is required to sign orders for equipment; a social worker, who may counsel the client and family; a rehabilitation engineer, who may modify the control interface and mounting system; the vendor or manufacturer, who designs and produces the electronic aid; and the special education teacher, who will be responsible for language development and implementation of the aid in the school setting. To be effective, this professional team must work closely with the nonverbal client and the client's communication partners.

As with all assistive devices, the optimum approach to augmentative communication aids includes the following: (1) the aid meets the client's needs; (2) the client, various aids, and all environments in which the aids will be used are carefully evaluated; (3) the selection is the result of collaboration between the client and the rehabilitation technology team members; (4) a backup, standard, nonelectric aid is also available to the client; (5) the augmentative communication aid can be integrated with all other assistive devices; and (6) the aid does not interfere with ADL. The occupational therapy technology specialist needs to be aware of various aids from simple, small, battery-operated aids that can be used bedside for nonspeaking persons (MS, MD, ALS, CVA, and laryngectomy), to complex, programmable, wheelchair-mounted systems that integrate with computers and ECUs. For additional information, speech pathologists, manufacturers, and vendors are available for in-services, workshops, and training institutes. Three variable comprehensive resources are the ASHA booklet *Augmentative Communication*, the International Society for Augmentative and Alternative Communication's (ISAAC) journal which includes proceedings of its biennial conference, and the *Trace Resource Book: 1996–97 Edition* (Borden, Lubich, & Vanderheiden, 1996). The occupational therapist needs to know what equipment is available and the most appropriate control interface. The speech pathologist is responsible for evaluating the client's language communication abilities.

▼ POWERED MOBILITY

Powered mobility is the assistive device that liberates individuals with physical impairments to move about home environments and into the community. Various powered mobility aids are available; those most frequently used are three-wheeled battery-powered scooters, adapted vehicles, powered wheelchairs, and adapted farm vehicles. Powered mobility is a system that begins with proper positioning of the client in an appropriate powered wheelchair or scooter that is maneuverable in accessible environments and is transportable in a car, van, train, plane, and bus. Each part of the mobility system is dependent on the other for functional mobility. The salient characteristics that are desirable for a powered mobility device include safety, comfort, dependability, portability for long-range transportation, ease of maintenance, ease in operation for user and caregivers, and compatibility with other ATDs (ventilators, ECUs).

The occupational therapist is a valuable member of the technology rehabilitation team that selects and then trains clients who need powered mobility. The clients most frequently referred for powered mobility are clients with high-level spinal cord injury—C4 and above; clients with advanced muscle weakness, caused by such diseases as ALS, MS, or MD; and clients with poor coordination in all extremities, such as those with cerebral palsy. Clients of all ages who have to travel long distances and have low levels of endurance usually need powered wheelchairs or scooters. However, they will also need a standard wheelchair as backup when their powered chair is being repaired and for those times when a powered chair cannot be transported. Since 1980, an increasing number of young children have been referred for powered mobility, but always with two main concerns: safety for the user and others, and the potential adverse effects on the child's physical development. There is limited research on the effects of powered mobility of the child, but specialists agree that a comprehensive evaluation of each child's proper positioning, cognitive and perceptual development, and all possible environments where the chair will be used is crucial (Barnes, 1991; Jaffe, 1987; Warren, 1990).

Members of the technology rehabilitation team most responsible for the optimum powered wheelchair system are occupational therapists, physical therapists, rehabilitation engineers, manufacturers or vendors, family members or caregivers, and social service professionals. The occupational therapist has a vital role in evaluating the client holistically; collaborating on the selection of a powered wheelchair system; verifying the chair prescription with the user; training the user and caregivers; and following-up periodically, especially as children grow and adults' physical conditions change. The user's primary therapist and the occupational therapy technology specialist can collaborate on a holistic evaluation of the client's positioning, physical abilities to access the control interface, cognitive ability to follow instructions and use judgment, perceptual skills especially spatial relationships and figure-ground perception, and motivation. Proper positioning is the key to successful use of ATDs. Therefore, it is necessary for the occupational therapist to collaborate with the physical therapist, seating specialist, and caregivers to determine the best seating position before selecting any mobility device. In addition to evaluating the user and his or her environments, the occupational therapy technology specialist should carefully assess the numerous powered wheelchairs that are now available. Some have power that allows the user to stand or recline, some allow the user to stand and move about, and some standard wheelchairs can be converted to motorized by adding a power pack to the back of the chair. The power base is the first portion of the chair that is selected, with special consideration given to types of batteries (lead or gel), safety brakes, any additional powered equipment, such as powered recliners, ventilation or phrenic nerve stimulater platforms.

The technology specialist must also assess the user's optimum control site because power mobility, in particular, requires accurate, reliable, and efficient user control. In addition, the technology specialist is usually responsible for evaluating and recommending the switch control method and mounting system. The most frequently used power wheelchair controlled method is the hand-controlled proportional joystick. A proportional joystick allows for graduation in speed and for smooth acceleration. For persons with limited motion, a proportional joystick can be adjusted with a *short throw* feature which requires approximately 50% less movement than the standard proportional device setting. For persons who have short, jerky, uncoordinated movements, the proportional joystick can be adjusted with a tremor damping feature. Other control methods include (1) pneumatic switches (sip-and-puff breath controls for persons with no functional movements); (2) multiple single switches (mounted on laptrays or head rests for on-off, forward, backward, right and left movements); and (3) microswitches that can be programmed to integrate with

ECUs and augmentative devices as well as program the speed.

Another responsibility of the technology specialist is to collaborate on a detailed wheelchair prescription with other team members. Most wheelchair vendors have worksheets or prescription forms; however, it is recommended that each wheelchair clinic develop its own forms that should be completed by the clinic coordinator and the vendor. It is imperative that the rehabilitation technology team work with a reliable, reputable, dependable vendor who will service the powered chair after it is purchased. Once the chair has been delivered, the therapist should carefully check each part against the prescription and test drive the chair before training the user.

Powered wheelchairs are usually delivered 4 to 6 months after they are ordered; clients need to receive training in powered wheelchair use before this chair arrives. Begin training in a large space by having the client go forward, stop, backward, stop, right, left, make circles. Then practice going around an obstacle course. Training sessions may vary depending on the age, cognitive ability, and physical function of the user. Powered wheelchairs that are equipped with augmentative communication aids, ECUs, computer interfaces, and ventilators require the client to be trained in the entire integrated control system by the therapist or other team members. An integrated control system uses a single input device to operate other ATDs. For example, a joystick on a wheelchair can be programmed through the controller to operate an AAC device, a computer, a power recliner, and an ECU. In addition to training the user with controls, the therapist should train the user in various environments, including on rough and smooth surfaces, indoors and outdoors, on inclines and declines, in large and small spaces (most powered wheelchairs have a turning radius of 30 inches), and in different climatic conditions.

With the passage of the Americans with Disabilities Act (ADA) (1990), there should be an increase in public accommodations, public transportation, and employment opportunities for individuals with disabilities. The primary occupational therapist or certified occupational therapy assistant is qualified to assess the architectural barriers in the user's home, school, work, and community. For example, consider a farmer with no function in his or her lower extremities. He or she may use a standard wheelchair around a barrier-free home with smooth surfaces. Then the farmer goes outside to work where the ground may have sand, gravel, mud, loose soil, and climatic conditions that vary. The farmer will have to transfer from a wheelchair to a hand control truck or tractor or an "all-terrain vehicle." (Freeman, Brusnighan, & Field, 1992). Consider a child who has limited functioning of all extremities and must travel to school in a wheelchair on a bus that allows only dry-cell batteries. The child may need a standard chair with tie-downs on the bus, but to keep pace with other children in the school building and on the playground, the child will need a powered chair.

Other means of power mobility are powered scooters. A powered scooter requires the user to have good sitting balance, good eye–hand coordination, adequate spatial and figure-ground perception, and good judgment (Warren, 1990). Scooters can be used in conjunction with walkers, canes, or standard wheelchairs in the home, workplace, or when traveling in the community by people who have limited stamina. Some can be transported on car racks and some can be broken down into parts for ease in transporting.

Adapted cars and vans are another source of powered mobility for those with limited function of both lower and upper extremities, one arm and one leg, restricted joint motion, or the absence of lower extremities. Scrupulous evaluation must be done by the occupational therapist and the driving specialist before the client is trained and issued a license. In most clinics the primary occupational therapist evaluates the client's perceptual ability; the driving specialist performs both simulated and on-the-road training. Driving standards for individuals with disabilities have been established by the Veterans Administration and most state motor vehicle agencies. Driver training is a specialty area that requires additional training, certification, and experience and is beyond the scope of this section.

The entry-level therapist should be aware of various vehicle adaptations, including proportional steering and hand controls, braking systems and safety backup systems, auxiliary control boxes, and hydraulic lifts. Vans with lifts are the preferred means of transportation for powered wheelchairs with batteries that weigh between 25 and 50 lb and can carry people who weigh 250 lb. Lifts can conserve energy and the time required to transfer a person into a car and push or disassemble the powered wheelchair before placing it into a car. The independence and opportunities gained by a person who is able to drive to attend school, work, and recreational activities must be considered in perspective with the safety of the client and others on the road. Wheelchair and powered wheelchair standards have been developed by the Americans National Standards Institute (ASNI) and Rehabilitation Engineering and Assistive Technology Society of North America (RESNA) committee, which provide the user and professional with information on how the product measures in durability and performance. Powered wheelchair evaluation criteria have also been developed by the National Rehabilitation Hospital. For additional information on powered mobility see *Selected Readings on Powered Mobility* by Trefler, Kozole, & Snell (1986) available from RESNA. Other excellent resources are Jaffe (1987), and Warren (1990).

▼ ENVIRONMENTAL CONTROLS

The ECU is the ATD for which the occupational therapist is mainly responsible; the occupational therapist undertakes the evaluation, selection, client training, and application of the ECU in collaboration with the client, caregiver, and other rehabilitation specialists. An ECU is defined as:

...a means to purposefully manipulate and interact with the environment by alternately accessing one or more electrical devices via switches, voice activation, remote control, computer interface and other technologic adaptations. The purpose of an ECU is to maximize functional ability and independence in the home, school, work, and leisure environment. (Bain, DiSalvi, Gold, Kollodge, & Schein, 1991; p. 55)

In the past 10 years, there has been a technology explosion in commercially available, convenient remote controls for television, lights, telephones, emergency calls, door locks and openers, temperature regulators, and other appliances in the home and workplace. Some are simple systems that control two or three appliances; others are more complex and control over 200 appliances; some can be integrated with augmentative communication aids, wheelchairs, computers, and telephones.

For the person with poor hand skills, ECUs can be operated by switches; for the person with low physical stamina,

tasks can be completed with greater speed and less energy; for the person with pulmonary and cardiac complications who needs constant monitoring, an ECU can be a safety device; and for the caregiver, an ECU saves time and energy by increasing the client's self-reliance, self-confidence, and independence. ECUs can be used by clients of all ages with various levels of function. Some require limited cognitive ability, whereas others require problem-solving, sequencing, memory, and concept formation abilities. Most ECUs have auditory, visual, or tactile feedback and, therefore, can be used by clients with sensory or motor impairment.

Each ECU consists of the four standard AT parts; input, which can include buttons on the device, various switches, computer command, or voice activation; throughput, which can be operated by means of batteries, household current, or household current plus a module, radio waves, ultrasound, or infrared; feedback, which can include the response of the device; and output, which is referred to as the action on or off of the appliances (Fig. 21–26).

The evaluation of a client for an ECU begins with an evaluation of the client's needs and functional abilities; next,

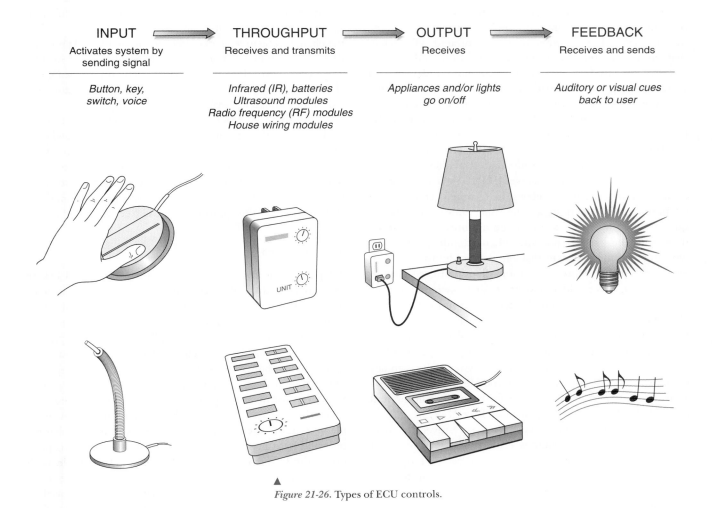

Figure 21-26. Types of ECU controls.

all environments where the ECU will be used must be considered, especially to determine if a portable system is required. Evaluation of the ECU should include the access method, feedback requirements, integration with other equipment; expandability for future use; flexibility (eg, adjustable rate and method of scanning); installation; and cost (Figs. 21–27 and 21–28; Box 21–2).

The selection of an ECU begins with off-the-shelf devices that can readily be purchased from a local electronic store for approximately 200 dollars. Some of these ECU remote controls have small input buttons that can be adapted with dime-size felt pads or grids made of plastic strips. Mouthsticks, universal cuffs, or splints can be used for access if a person has limited hand manipulation skills (see level I, Box 21–2). If a person needs a switch, then levels II, III, and IV ECU are recommended (see Box 21–2). Switch-activated ECUs are available from special AT rehabilitation suppliers. Most use infrared or ultrasound transmissions; some can operate telephones; and some can scan televison channels, operate a VCR, and turn appliances on and off, in and outside a building. Note that ultrasound waves are not transmitted through walls, radio waves have a greater transmission distance, and household AC current has the greatest transmission distance. Infrared signals transmit in direct-line of sight; however, one infrared device can teach other infrared devices. For example, there are infrared AT devices that can teach a television remote-control infrared receiver to accept signals. In addition, some infrared AT devices can send signals to an infrared receiver that converts the signal to house current to operate other appliances. There are also "POWERMIDS" and "LEAP FROGS" that can extend the length of infrared signals from one room to another.

Planning is a crucial step in the selection process for present and future ECUs. To illustrate, a person with a C4 spinal cord injury will need a level III ECU when in bed for calling a nurse, scanning television channels, and making telephone calls; when in a wheelchair, portability is required; when at home or in the community, the environment must be barrier free; and when attending school or working a compact system that can control lights, electrical appliances (tape recorder, rotating file system, computer, mail opener, letter folder, and other such) is required. Because ECUs are not usually funded and if funded are purchased only once, the therapist must evaluate all present and future environments where the ECU will be needed and also how much support will be provided by caregivers. Currently, there are few level II, III, or IV systems that can accomplish all of the foregoing tasks; therefore, it may be necessary to purchase a level III or IV for hospital or home, and a level II for school or workplace (see Box 21–2).

In the future, as robots become less expensive, they may be the ECU of choice. There is available today a robot that is mounted on a powered wheelchair that can pick up a pill from the floor, put it in a person's mouth, reach up to get a glass out of the cupboard, fill it with water, and deliver the water to the person.

After the ECU system has been evaluated and the selection has been completed, the next step is training the client and all caregivers, usually by the occupational therapist. It is important that both the user and caregivers know how to assemble the system, all its capabilities, the routine maintenance, and where repairs can be made. When a user is in the hospital, it is advisable for the therapist to place drawings or pictures of all connections near the user's bed and to give inservice training to the staff. When the user leaves the hospital or rehabilitation center, the user or caregiver should demonstrate to the therapist how to assemble, operate, and maintain the system. Most AT rehabilitation suppliers have catalogs on the ECU application and some will supply videos to the user.

Because the cost of an ECU is rarely reimbursed by insurance carriers, another responsibility for the occupational therapist working in conjunction with the social worker and family is to find funding for the ECU system that best meets the client's needs. Sometimes this may mean beginning with an affordable ($50 to $100), off-the-shelf unit purchased by the family or friends and then progressing to a more comprehensive system as funding becomes available.

When requesting funding for ECUs, rehabilitation technology team members need to include in their calculations the hours and cost of attendant care that will be saved when the client can be independent because of the ECU. At present, there is not sufficient research data to validate these savings. The occupational therapist can wisely spend time by searching electrical specialty shops and trade magazines and by attending workshops to find affordable off-the-shelf ECUs.

Other important factors to consider when prescribing an ECU are its *safety* features, its *durability*, and the *reliability* of the manufacturer. It is frustrating to the client, caregivers, and therapist when the system needs constant repairs or when the manufacturer is not reliable. A classification system has been developed to help the occupational therapist and client select the appropriate ECU (see Box 21–2).

Telephones

Telephones mean safety as well as convenience and leisure for people with disabilities. Numerous technological telephone advances have been made that benefit people with hearing, speaking, visual, and motor impairments. These include the following: for the visually impaired, telephones with enlarged numbers as well as enlarged stick-on numbers that can be applied to any phone. In addition, telephone bills can be printed in braille. Another useful aid for people with visual or motor impairments is to dial the operator (0), who will then assist by dialing the desired number. For people who need assistance dialing 0, there is an overlay that fits over the buttons and requires only a gross motion to push down the 0 button. Other telephone aids for people with motor impairment include telephones that can be controlled by switches or interfaced with an ECU; portable,

(text continues on page 512)

Name _____ Date _____ Age _____ Sex _____
Date of Onset _____ Diagnosis _____
Reason for Referral _____
Major Functional Problem Areas: Communication _____ Manipulation _____
                                Motor _____ Other _____

I. Devices to be Controlled:

Devices	Quantity	Comments
		Location (Bed, wheelchair, school, workplace, other)
		Remote Transmission: IR, Ultrasound, RF
Call Bell		
Emergency Call System		
Telephone		
Intercom		
Lights:		
Lamps		
Overhead		
Bed Control		
Television		
VCR		
Stereo		
Radio		
Tape Recorder		
Fan		
Temperature		
Computer		
Page Turner		
Door Opener		
Door Lock		
OTHER		

II. Possible Access Methods

Direct Selection _____ Scanning _____ Encoding _____

Switch(s) _____ Mounting Hardware _____

Comments:

▲
Figure 21-27. Environmental control systems needs assessment *(continued).*

III. Feedback?   [ ] YES   [ ] NO

Auditory _____ Visual _____ Tactile _____

Comments:

_____

_____

IV. Integration With Other Equipment (check all that apply)

Equipment	Manufacturer/Model
Wheelchair	
Computer	
Communication Aid	
OTHER:	

Comments:

_____

_____

V. Expendability for Future Use

A.   What are the user's goals?

Vocationally:

_____

_____

Avocationally:

_____

_____

Educationally:

_____

_____

B.   Medical Status (Prognosis/Potential for Improvement)

_____

_____

_____

VI. Funding

_____

_____

Additional Comments:

Revised Bain, 1995, from Bain, DiSalvi, Gold, Kollodge, Schein   AOTA Institute 6/1/91   Page 2
BBsa506.107

▲

Figure 21-27. (Continued)

Name of Environmental Control System

Manufacturer (Address & Phone)

Operational Features:

Numbers of Inputs	Methods of Inputs:	Switch		
Type of Access:	Direct Selection	Scanning	Encoding	Voice Activation
Feedback:	Visual	Auditory		

Functional Capabilities:

Momentary	Latching	Both:	
Appliance Control:	Low V	(Check all that are possible)	
Nurse call		Intercom	
Electric bed		TV channel selector	
Radio channel changer		Page turner	
Other			
Telephone Control:			
Direct dial		Operator assist	
Redial		No. of Memory locations	
Battery back-up		Speaker	Head set
Other			

Flexibility:

Adjustable rate of scanning	Adjustable method of scanning		
Interface with various switches			
Access by careproviders			
User programmable			
Integrate with:			
Wheelchair	Computer	Augmentative/Alternative Communication Aids	
Remote control transmission:	Infrared	Ultrasound	Radio

Installation Requires a Specialist: Hard Wiring Requires an Electrician

Mounting Hardware Available

User's Goals:

User's Opinions:

Cost:

Other Possible Systems:

Comments

Revised, Bain 1995, from © Bain, DiSalvi, Gold, Kollodge, Schein AOTA Institute 6/1/91.

▲

Figure 21-28. Environmental control systems evaluation.

BOX 21-2

Classification of ECUs

Level I
- Devices are available off-the-shelf
- Devices do not require an adaptive switch
- Devices use direct selection and may be used with adaptations, such as mouthstick, typing pegs, hand splints, and so forth
- Devices offer primarily latching control; but very limited momentary control
- Devices allow control of on or off functions of appliances and lights (which can also be brightened and dimmed); includes telephones, multiple stand-alone devices, or small units that will control more than one appliance
- Devices may use infrared and radio frequency remote controls

Level II
- Devices are available through specialty equipment manufacturers
- Devices are controlled by an adaptive switch
- Devices use direct selection or scanning
- Devices offer primarily latching control
- Devices allow control of on or off functions of appliances, lights (including brightening and dimming), television, VCR, and so forth, and adapted access to telephone functions
- Devices may use remote control through infrared, radio frequency and ultra sound transmissions

Level III
- Devices are available through specialty equipment manufacturers
- Devices are controlled by an adaptive switch
- Devices use scanning, with the exception of voice activation
- Devices offer both latching and momentary control
- One system allows control of all functions of multiple devices, including full telephone and bed control
- Devices may use remote control through infrared, radio frequency, and ultrasound transmissions

Level IV
- Devices are available through specialty equipment manufacturers
- Devices are controlled by adaptive switch
- Devices use scanning
- Devices offer both latching and momentary control
- One system allows control of all functions of multiple devices, including full telephone and bed control
- Devices incorporate integration with other electrical devices, such as augmentative and alternative communication aids, power wheelchair electronics, and computers using the same switch to access all functions

Level V
- Future developments integrating technology into the community

© Bain, DiSalvi, Gold, Kollodge, Schein. AOTA Annual Conference, Cincinnati, June 1, 1991.

---

lightweight headset telephones; telephones with four-button emergency attachments, memory storage, battery backup, conference call, and redial capabilities. For people with weak voice quality, there are telephones that amplify the voice, and for those with poor voice volume, there are electronic artificial larynxes.

Great advances have been made in technology to increase the telephone capabilities of people with hearing impairments and those who are deaf, including fax and e-mail. The hearing impaired can attach small amplifiers to any handset or purchase a handset with adjustable amplification built-in. Deaf or speech-impaired people can call person-to-person to another deaf person or to anyone, any time of the day, any day of the year, through the use of a telecom-munications device for the deaf and the telephone company dual relay system (check your local telephone directory for details). Section IV of the ADA ensures that interstate and intrastate telecommunications relay services are available to people with hearing and speech impairments.

Monitoring Systems

Personal response systems are technological devices that are worn or carried by people who wish to live alone or who are left alone, such as the frail elderly, people with physical disabilities, or children who are old enough to care for themselves after school, but who need help if there is an emergency. These devices can be activated by various switches; for severely impaired people, sip and puff, light pressure, or eyebrow switches are usually used. The switch sends a signal to a monitoring center, which then puts the user in touch with a relative, friend, neighbor, or an emergency service. Most cardiac users are linked directly to hospital monitoring centers. This device can be cost-effective in reducing nursing home or hospital stays while granting safe independence to the user and comfort to relatives who are unable to offer constant care (Joe, 1990). There are several systems throughout the United States and in many European countries; the client, therapist, and family need to evaluate each system in view of the user's needs. Another means of monitoring people in the same house is an inexpensive (less than 50 dollars) baby monitor, which is sensitive enough to hear breathing anywhere in the house.

The therapist must be cognizant of the client's tolerance to equipment and the psychological factor of being dependent on aids. Every effort should be made to prescribe only the ECU that will enhance the client's functional abilities and improve or maintain the client's independence. Often, the most efficient solution is for the therapist to suggest architectural changes in the environment.

For additional ECU information see the *AOTA Assistive Technology Self Study* (1996) chapter 7, Church and Glennen (1992) for excellent drawings and clear descriptions of ECUs; Mann and Lane (1995) for several pictures and a list; Lange (1995) for a comprehensive selection chart; Dickey, Loeser, and Specht (1995) for concise descriptions; Cook and Hussey (1994) for charts, drawings, and use of robots.

▶ ASSISTIVE TECHNOLOGY CONCLUSION

In the past 10 years, occupational therapist have learned to use AT to extend the abilities of clients of all ages and with varying degrees of function. It is the intent of this section to encourage the entry-level occupational therapist and certified occupational therapy assistant to seek additional information, knowledge, skills, and competency by attending workshops, enrolling in technology courses, and networking with other professional groups.

In 1991, the AOTA formed a special interest group in technology, and additional information can be obtained by contacting the AOTA Division on Practice. Another informative interdisciplinary professional group is RESNA, which publishes a journal, newsletter, proceedings of conferences, special topic booklets, and an excellent resources in the book *Assistive Technology Sourcebook* (Enders & Hall, 1990). RESNA holds national, international, and regional meetings each year; in addition, some states have local groups that meet bimonthly.

As with any specialty area, AT builds on the body of professional occupational therapy knowledge. It is advisable to first learn about switches and control interfaces and then to progress to an area for which your occupa-

tional therapy department or clinical site is responsible, such as toys, wheelchairs, ECUs, or computers. At first, it may seem impossible to keep up-to-date on the rapid advances in technology, but networking with occupational therapists, other professionals, and consumers is beneficial. Remember that AT is one of many tools of the occupational therapy profession and attempts should be made to avoid inappropriate application of high technologies when they are not needed and to use them only when their application is beneficial to the client. Assistive technology can make many tasks possible for many clients when it is based on sound therapeutic foundations, an on-going comprehensive evaluation of all parts of the system, an interdisciplinary team, including the client and caregiver, making decisions on the selection of ATDs, and a focus on the individual client's needs and goals.

Assistive Technology Acknowledgments

I gratefully acknowledge the professional contributions of Margy DiSalvi-Wolf, Judy Gold, Barbara Kollodge, and Ronnie Schein, the editing and reviewing of Dawn Leger, the graphics of Cristina Burwell, and the critiquing by the New York University (NYU) technology students.

▼ REFERENCES

American Occupational Therapy Association (AOTA). (1994). Uniform terminology for occupational therapy—third edition. *American Journal of Occupational Therapy, 48*, 1047–1059.

American Occupational Therapy Association (AOTA). (1995). Assessment of assistive technology. *Technology Special Interest Section Newsletter, 5*, 1&2.

American Occupational Therapy Association (AOTA). (1996). *Assistive technology self-study.* Rockville, MD: AOTA.

American Speech–Language–Hearing Association (ASHA). (1991). Report: Augmentative and alternative communication. *ASHA, 33*(4), (Suppl. 5), 9–12.

American Speech–Language–Hearing Association (ASHA). (1989). Report: Competencies for speech–language pathologists providing services in augmentative communication. *ASHA, 31*, 107–110.

Americans with Disabilities Act. (1988). (Public Law 100–366), 42, USC 12101.

Angelo, J. & Smith, R. O. (1989). The critical role of occupational therapy in augmentative communication services. In American Occupational Therapy Association (AOTA), *Technology Review 89: Perspectives on occupational therapy practice* (pp. 49–54). Rockville, MD: AOTA.

Anson, D. (1994). Finding your way in the maze of computer access technology. *American Journal of Occupational Therapy, 48*, 121–129.

Bain, B. K. (1989). Assessment of clients for technological assistive devices. In American Occupational Therapy Association, *Technology review '89: Perspectives on occupational therapy practice* (pp. 55–59). Rockville, MD: AOTA.

Bain, B., DiSalvi, M., Gold, J., Kollodge, B., Schein, R. (1991, June 1). Environmental control systems: Assessment, selection, and training. Paper presented at the 1991 AOTA Annual Conference, Cincinnati.

Bain, B., DiSalvi, M., Gold, J., Kollodge, B., & Schein, R. (1993). Technology. In H. Hopkins & H. Smith (Eds.), *Willard and Spackman's Occupational Therapy* (8th ed.) (pp. 333–337). Philadelphia: J. B. Lippincott.

Barnes, K. H. (1991). Training young children for powered mobility. *Developmental Disabilities Special Interest Section Newsletter, 14,* 1–2.

Barris, R. (1982). Environmental interactions: An extension of the model of human occupation. *American Journal of Occupational Therapy, 36,* 637–644.

Barris, R., Kielhofner, G., Neville, A. M., Oakley, F. M., Salz, C., & Watts, J. H. (1985). Psychosocial dysfunction. In G. Kielhofner (Ed.). *A model of human occupation* (pp. 248–305). Baltimore: Williams & Wilkins.

Batavia, A. & Hammer, G. (1990). Toward the development of consumer-based criteria for the evaluation of assistive devices. *Journal of Rehabilitation Research and Development, 27,* 425–435.

Bonder, B. (1991). *Psychopathology and function.* Thorofare, NJ: Slack.

Borden, P., Lubich, J., & Vanderheiden, G. (1996) *Trace resource book: 1996–97 edition.* Madison, WI: Trace Research and Development Center.

Bransford, J. D. & Stein, B. S. (1984). *The ideal problem solver.* New York: W. H. Freeman.

Brayman, S. J. (1996). Managing the occupational environment of managed care. *American Journal of Occupational Therapy, 50,* 442–446.

Brigham, C., Engelberg, A. L., & Richling, D. E. (1996). The changing role of rehab: Focus on function. *Patient Care, February 16,* 144–184.

Carson, R. (1994). Reducing cumulative trauma disorders: Use of proper workplace design. *AAOHN Journal, 42,* 270–276.

Christiansen, C. (1991). Occupational therapy intervention for life performance. In C. Christiansen & C. Baum (Eds.). *Occupational therapy: Overcoming human performance deficits* (pp. 3–43). Thorofare, NJ: Slack.

Christiansen, C. (1993). Continuing challenges of functional assessment in rehabilitation: Recommended changes. *American Journal of Occupational Therapy, 47,* 258–259.

Christiansen, C. (1996). Managed care: Opportunities and challenges for occupational therapy in the emerging systems of the 21st century. *American Journal of Occupational Therapy, 50,* 409–412.

Church, C. & Glennen, S. (1992). *The handbook of assistive technology.* San Diego: Singular Publishing Group.

Clark, F. A., Parham, D., Carlson, M. E., Frank, G., Jackson, J., Pierce, D., Wolfe, R. J., & Zemke, R. (1991). Occupational science: Academic innovation in the service of occupational therapy's future. *American Journal of Occupational Therapy, 45,* 300–310.

Clark, M. C., Czaja, S. J., & Weber, R. A. (1990). Older adults and daily living task profiles. *Human Factors, 32,* 537–549.

Cook, A. & Hussey, S. (1994). *Assistive technologies: Principles and practice.* New York: C.V. Mosby.

Cope, D. N. & Sundance, P. (1995). Conceptualizing clinical outcomes. In P. K. Landrum, N. D. Schmidt, & A. McLean (Eds.), *Outcome-oriented rehabilitation* (pp. 43–56). Gaithersburg, MD: Aspen.

Creighton, C. (1992). The origin and evolution of activity analysis. *American Journal of Occupational Therapy, 46,* 45–48.

Cubie, S., & Kaplan, K. (1982). A case analysis method for the model of human occupation. *American Journal of Occupational Therapy, 36,* 645–656.

Cynkin, S. (1979). *Occupational therapy: Toward health through activities.* Boston: Little, Brown & Co.

Czaja, S., Weber, R. A., & Nair, S. N. (1993). A human factors analysis of ADL activities: A capability–demand approach. *Journal of Gerontology, 48,* 44–48.

Demore-Taber, M. (1995). Americans with Disabilities Act work site assessment. In K. Jacobs & C. Bettencourt (Eds.), *Ergonomics for therapists* (pp. 229–244). Boston: Butterworth-Heinemann.

Dickey, R., Loeser, A., & Specht, E. (1995). Environmental control for persons with disabilities. In J. Bedford, J. Basmajian, & P. Trautman (Eds.), *Orthotics: Clinical practice and rehabilitation technology* (pp. 257–286). New York: Churchill Livingstone.

Diffrient, N., Tilley, A., & Bardagjy, F. (1974). *Humanscale 1/2/3.* Cambridge, MA: MIT Press.

Dunn, W. (1993). Measurement of function: Actions for the future. *American Journal of Occupational Therapy, 47,* 357–359.

Dunn, W., Brown, C., & McGuigan, M. (1994). The ecology of human performance: A framework for considering the effect of context. *American Journal of Occupational Therapy, 48,* 595–607.

Eisenberg, M. G., Sutkin, L. C., & Jansen, M. A. (1984). *Chronic illness and disability through the life span: Effects on self and family.* New York: Springer.

Enders, A. & Hall, M. (1990). *Assistive technology sourcebook.* Washington, DC: RESNA Press.

Evans, R. W., Small, L., & Ling, J. S. (1995). Independence in the home and community. In P. K. Landrum, N. D. Schmidt, & A. McLean (Eds.), *Outcome-oriented rehabilitation* (pp. 95–124). Gaithersburg, MD: Aspen.

Faletti, M. V. (1984). Human factors research and functional environments for the aged. In I. Altman, M. P. Lawton, & J. F. Wohlwill (Eds.), *Elderly people and the environment* (pp. 191–237). New York: Plenum.

Fisher, A. G. & Short-DeGraff, M. (1993). Improving functional assessment in occupational therapy: Recommendations and philosophy for change. *American Journal of Occupational Therapy, 47,* 199–201.

Fishman, I. (1987). *Electronic communication aids.* Boston, MA: College-Hill Press.

Flippo, K., Inge, K., & Barcus, J. (1995). *Assistive technology: A resource for school, work, and community.* Baltimore, MD: Paul H. J. Brookes Publishing Co.

Fleishman, E. A. (1966). Human abilities and the acquisition of skill. In E. A. Bilodeau (Ed.). *Acquisition of skill.* New York: Academic Press.

Fleishman, E. A. & Quaintance, M. K. (1984). *Taxonomies of human performance.* Orlando, FL: Academic Press.

Florey, L. L. & Michelman, S. M. (1982). Occupational role history: A screening tool for occupational therapy. *American Journal of Occupational Therapy, 36,* 301–308.

Freeman, S., Brusnighan, D., & Field, W. (1992). Selecting mobility aids for farmers and ranchers with physical disabilities. *Technology and Disability, 4,* 63–67.

Fried, L. P., Herdman, S. J., Duhn, K. E., Rubin, G., & Turano, K. (1991). Preclinical disability. *Journal of Aging and Health, 3,* 285–300.

Gentile, A. M. (1987). Skill acquisition: Action, movement, and neuromotor processes. In J. H. Carr & R. B. Shepherd (Eds.), *Movement science foundations for physical therapy in rehabilitation* (pp. 93–154). Rockville, MD: Aspen.

Gerdner, L. A., Hall, G. R., & Buckwalter, K. C. (1996). Caregiver training for people with Alzheimer's based on a stress threshold model. *Image: Journal of Nursing Scholarship, 28,* 241–246.

Guralnik, J. M., Branch, L. G., Cummings, S. R., & Curb, J. D. (1989). Physical performance measures in aging research. *Journal of Gerontology, 44,* 141–146.

Haas, L. (1944). *Practical occupational therapy.* Milwaukee: Bruce.

Hagedorn, R. (1995a). Environmental analysis and adaptation. In R. Hagedorn (Ed.), *Occupational therapy: Perspectives and processes* (pp. 239–257). Melbourne, Australia: Churchill Livingstone.

Hagedorn, R. (1995b). Intervention. In R. Hagedorn (Ed.), *Occupational therapy: Perspectives and processes* (pp. 175–195). Melbourne, Australia: Churchill Livingstone.

Hall, G. R. & Buckwalter, K. C. (1987). Progressively lowered stress threshold: A conceptual model for care of adults with Alzheimer's disease. *Archives of Psychiatric Nursing, 1,* 399–406.

Hammel, J. (Ed.). (1995). *Assistive technology competencies for occupational therapy practice.* Rockville, MD: AOTA.

Hansen, R. A. & Atchison, B. (1993). *Conditions in occupational therapy.* Baltimore: Williams & Wilkins.

Hersh, N. & Treadgold, L. (1994). Neuropage: The rehabilitation of memory dysfunction by prosthetic memory and cuing. *NeuroRehabilitation, 4,* 187–197.

Holm, M. B. & Rogers, J. C. (1989). The therapist's thinking behind functional assessment, II. In C. Royeen (Ed.), *Assessment of function: An action guide*. Rockville, MD: AOTA.

Holm, M. B. & Rogers, J. C. (1991). High, low, or no assistive technology devices for older adults undergoing rehabilitation. *International Journal of Technology and Aging, 4*, 153–162.

Hopkins, H. L. & Smith, H.D. (Eds.). (1983). *Willard and Spackman's occupational therapy* (6th ed.). Philadelphia: J. B. Lippincott.

Howe, M. C. & Briggs, A. K. (1982). Ecological systems model for occupational therapy. *American Journal of Occupational Therapy, 36*, 322–327.

Humphrey, R., Jewell, K., & Rosenberger, R. C. (1995). Development of in-hand manipulation and relationship with activities. *American Journal of Occupational Therapy, 49*, 763–771.

Jacobs, K. & Bettencourt, C. (Eds.). (1995). *Ergonomics for therapists*. Boston: Butterworth-Heinemann.

Jaffe, K. (Ed.). (1987). *Childhood powered mobility: Developmental technical, and clinical perspectives*. Washington, DC: RESNA.

Joe, B. E. (1990). International symposium focuses on emergency response devices. *Occupational Therapy Week, 4*, 4–5.

Kielhofner, G. (1995). Environmental influences on occupational behavior. In G. Kielhofner (Ed.). *A model of human occupation: Theory and application* (2nd ed.). Baltimore: Williams & Wilkins.

Kielhofner, G. & Burke, J. P. (1980). A model of human occupation, Part I. Conceptual framework and content. *American Journal of Occupational Therapy, 34*, 572–581.

Kielhofner, G. & Burke, J. P. (1985). Components and determinants of human occupation. In G. Kielhofner (Ed.), *A model of human occupation* (pp. 12–36). Baltimore: Williams & Wilkins.

Kiernat, J. M. (1982). Environment: The hidden modality. *Physical and Occupational Therapy in Geriatrics, 2* (1), 3–12.

Kramer, P. & Hinojosa, J. (1993). *Frames of reference for pediatric occupational therapy*. Baltimore: Williams & Wilkins.

Lange, M. (1995). Selecting environmental controls. *Team-Rehab, 6* (11), 43–45.

Law, M., Cooper, B., Strong, S., Stewart, D., Rigby, P., & Letts, L. (1996). The person–environment–occupational model: A transactive approach to occupational performance. *Canadian Journal of Occupational Therapy, 63*, 9–23.

Lawton, M. P. (1982). Competence, environmental press, and the adaptation of older people. In M. P. Lawton, P. G. Windley, & T. O. Byerts (Eds.), *Aging and the environment: Theoretical approaches* (pp.33–59). New York: Springer.

Lee, K. & Thomas, D. (1990). *Control of computer-based technology for people with physical disabilities*. Toronto, Canada: Toronto Press.

Levine, R. E. & Brayley, C. R. (1991). Occupation as a therapeutic medium. In C. Christiansen & C. Baum (Eds.), *Occupational therapy: Overcoming human performance deficits* (pp. 591–631). Thorofare, NJ: Slack.

Mager, R. F. & Pipe, P. (1984). *Analyzing performance problems* (2nd ed.). Belmont, CA: Lake.

Mann, W.C. & Lane, J.P. (1991; 1995). *Assistive technology for persons with disabilities*. Bethesda, MD: AOTA.

Mathiowetz, V. (1993). Role of physical performance component evaluations in occupational therapy functional assessment. *American Journal of Occupational Therapy, 47*, 225–230.

Meyer, A. (1922). The philosophy of occupational therapy. *Archives of Occupational Therapy, 1*, 1–10.

Moore, J. S. & Garg, A. (1995). The strain index: A proposed method to analyze jobs for risk of distal upper extremity disorder. *American Industrial Hygiene Journal, 56*, 443–456.

Mosey, A. C. (1986). *Psychosocial components of occupational therapy*. New York: Raven Press.

Neistadt, M. E. (1994a). Perceptual retraining for adults with diffuse brain injury. *American Journal of Occupational Therapy, 48*, 225–233.

Neistadt, M. E. (1994b). The effects of different treatment activities on functional fine motor coordination in adults with brain injury. *American Journal of Occupational Therapy, 48*, 877–882.

Nelson, D. L. (1988). Occupation: Form and performance. *American Journal of Occupational Therapy, 42*, 633–641.

Phillips, B. (1992). Technology abandonment from the consumer point of view. *NARIC Quarterly, 3*, 2–3.

Radabough, M.P. (1990). Speech given at the RESNA Conference, Washington, D.C., June 1990.

Raschko, B. B. (1991). *Housing interiors for the disabled and elderly*. New York: Von Nostrand Reinhold.

Reed, K. L. (1991). *Quick reference to occupational therapy*. Gaithersburg, MD: Aspen.

Rogers, J. C. (1982). The spirit of independence: The evolution of a philosophy. *American Journal of Occupational Therapy, 36*, 709–715.

Rogers, J. C. (1986). Occupational therapy assessment for older adults with depression: Asking the right questions. *Physical and Occupational Therapy in Geriatrics, 5*, 13–33.

Rogers, J. C. & Holm, M. B. (1989). The therapist's thinking behind functional assessment, I. In C. Royeen (Ed.), *Assessment of function: An action guide*, Rockville, MD: AOTA.

Rogers, J. C. & Holm, M. B. (1991a). Task performance of older adults and low assistive technology devices. *International Journal of Technology and Aging, 4*, 93–106.

Rogers, J. C. & Holm, M. B. (1991b). Teaching older adults with depression. *Topics in Geriatric Rehabilitation, 6*(3), 27–44.

Rogers, J. C., Holm, M. B., & Stone, R. G. (1997). Assessment of daily living activities: The home care advantage. *American Journal of Occupational Therapy, 51*, 410–422.

Scherer, M.J. (1991). The Scherer MPT model: Matching people with technologies. In M. J. Scherer, *Assistive technology device predisposition assessment* (pp. 10–18). Rochester, NY: Scherer Associates.

Schkade, J. K. & Schultz, S. (1992). Occupational adaptation: Toward a holistic approach for contemporary practice, part 1. *American Journal of Occupational Therapy, 46*, 829–837.

Schultz, S. & Schkade, J. K. (1992). Occupational adaptation: Toward a holistic approach for contemporary practice, part 2. *American Journal of Occupational Therapy, 46*, 917–925.

Slagle, E. C. (1922). Training aides for mental patients. *Archives of Occupational Therapy, 1*, 11–17.

Smith, R. (1990). *Administration and scoring manual: OT FACT*. Rockville, MD: AOTA.

Stewart, D. L. & Abeln, S. H. (1993). *Documenting functional outcomes in physical therapy*. St. Louis, MO: C.V. Mosby.

Technology-Related Assistance for Individuals with Disabilities Act. (1988). 29 USC 2202 (2) and (3).

Trefler, E., Kozole, K., and Snell, E. (Eds.). (1986). *Selected readings on powered mobility for children and adults with severe physical disabilities*. Washington, DC: RESNA Press.

Trombly, C. (1993). Anticipating the future: Assessment of occupational function. *American Journal of Occupational Therapy, 47*, 253–257.

Trombly, C. (1995). Occupation: Purposefulness and meaningfulness as therapeutic mechanisms. 1995 Eleanor Clarke Slagle lecture. *American Journal of Occupational Therapy, 49*, 960–972.

Verbrugge, L. M. (1990). The iceberg of disability. In S. M. Stahl (Ed.), *The legacy of longevity: Health and health care in later life* (pp. 55–75). Newbury Park, CA: Sage.

Warren, C. G. (1990). Powered mobility and its implications. In S. P. Todd (Ed.), *Choosing a wheelchair system* (pp. 74–85). Washington DC: Veterans Health Services and Research Administration.

Webster, J. G., Cook, A. M., Tompkins, W. J., & Vanderheiden, G. C. (Eds). (1985). *Electronic devices for rehabilitation*. New York: John Wiley & Sons.

Williams, B. W., Stemach, G., Wolfe, S., & Stanger, C. (1993). *Lifespace access profile: Assistive technology planning for individuals with severe or multiple disabilities*. Sebastopol, CA: Author.

Wood, P. H. N. (1980). Appreciating the consequences of disease: The

International Classification of Impairments, Disabilities, and Handicaps. *WHO Chronicle, 34,* 376–380.

Wood, W. (1996). Legitimizing occupational therapy's knowledge. *American Journal of Occupational Therapy, 50,* 626–634.

World Health Organization (WHO). (1980). *International classification of impairments, disabilities, and handicaps: A manual of classification relating to the consequences of disease.* Geneva: Author.

Wright, C. & Nomura, M. (1990). *From toys to computers: Access for the physically disabled child* (2nd ed.). San Jose, CA: Wright.

▼ RELATED READINGS

Baker, A. C. (1993). The spouse's positive effect on the stroke patient's recovery. *Rehabilitation Nursing, 18*(1), 30–33.

Baum, C. M. (1991). The environment: Providing opportunities for the future. *American Journal of Occupational Therapy, 45,* 487–490.

Carson, R. (1994). Reducing cumulative trauma disorders: Use of proper workplace design. *AAOHN Journal, 42,* 270–276.

Dunn, P. A. (1990). The impact of the housing environment upon the ability of disabled people to live independently. *Disability, Handicap, & Society, 5*(1), 37–52.

Galvin, J. C. & Scherer, M. J. (Eds.). (1996). *Evaluating, selecting, and using appropriate assistive technology.* Gaithersburg, MD: Aspen.

[The book includes a CD that is IBM and Macintosh campatible (Cooperative Database Distribution Network for Assistive Technology) with ABLEDATA, TraceBase, 16 Cooperative Service Directories, 7 Databases including REHABDATA, and a Text Document Library].

Giloth, B. E. (1990). Promoting patient involvement: Educational, organizational, and environmental strategies. *Patient Education and Counseling, 15*(1), 29–38.

Hahn, H. (1993). Equality and the environment: The interpretation of "reasonable accommodations" in the Americans with Disabilities Act. *Journal of Rehabilitation Administration, 17*(3), 101–108.

Hall, G. R., Buckwalter, K. C., Stolley, J. M., Gerdner, L. A., Garand, L.,

Ridgeway, S., & Crump, S. (1995). Standardized care plan. Managing Alzheimer's patients at home. *Journal of Gerontological Nursing, 21,* (1), 37–47.

Heller, K. W., Dangel, H., & Sweatman, L. (1995). Systematic selection of adaptations for student with muscular dystrophy. *Journal of Developmental and Physical Disabilities, 7,* 253–265.

Jackson, J. (1989). En route to adulthood: A high school transition program for adolescents with disabilities. *Occupational Therapy in Health Care, 6*(4), 33–51.

Landry, C. & Knox, J. (1996). Managed care fundamentals: Implications for health care organizations and health care professionals. *American Journal of Occupational Therapy, 50,* 413–416.

Mace, R. L., Hardie, G. J., & Place, J. P. *Accessible environments: Toward universal design.* Raleigh, NC: North Carolina State University.

Marrelli, T. M. (1994). *Handbook of home health standards and documentation guidelines for reimbursement* (2nd ed.). St. Louis, MO: C.V. Mosby.

May, B. J. (1993). *Home health and rehabilitation: Concepts of Care.* Philadelphia: F. A. Davis.

McCunney, R. J. (Ed.). (1994). *A practical approach to occupational and environmental medicine* (2nd ed.). Boston: Little, Brown & Co.

Pynoos, J. (1995). Supportive services? Fine. But how about supportive surroundings? *Perspectives on Aging, 24* (4), 20–23.

Raphael, C. (1987). An architect's viewpoint. *Topics in Geriatric Rehabilitation, 3*(1), 19–25.

Rosenstock, L. & Cullen, M. R. (Eds.). (1994). *Textbook of clinical, occupational and environmental medicine.* Philadelphia: W. B. Saunders.

Ruffing-Rahal, M. A. (1989). Ecological well-being: A study of community-dwelling older adults. *Health Values, 13* (1), 10–19.

Sherrill, C. (1994). Least restrictive environment and total inclusion philosophies: Critical analysis. *Palaestra, 10*(3), 25–54.

Steinfield, E. & Angelo, J. (1992). Adaptive work placement: A "horizontal" model. *Technology and Disability, 1*(4), 1–10.

Tideiksaar, R. (1990). Environment adaptations to preserve balance and prevent falls. *Topics in Geriatric Rehabilitation, 5*(2), 78–84.

York, J. (1989). Mobility methods selected for use in home and community environments. *Physical Therapy, 69,* 736–748.

UNIT VII
CLIENT APPLICATIONS
Maureen E. Neistadt

In Chapter 3, you met Mary Weber and her occupational therapist, Anna Deane Scott. Anna Deane's treatment was extremely effective in helping Mary become more independent in her valued day-to-day activities. Mary said, "In the year that I worked with her I could see small changes in my life and as I got greater control over the details of my life again, the person who I had been started to reemerge." (see Chap. 3; p. 29) Let us look at why this intervention program was so effective in light of what you have read in this treatment unit.

First of all, Anna Deane directed treatment toward activity goals that Mary thought important. Mary said, "...Anna Deane felt her role was not to tell me what to do, but to work with me, to empower me. She asked me constantly what was important to me. What did I

think of something. What did I want to do. And she LISTENED to me." (see Chap. 3; p. 28). Because she felt empowered, Mary was able to engage fully in this treatment process and persist with it despite the fact that, "For every victory,...There were dozens of defeats" (see Chap. 3; p. 29). Empowerment gave Mary hope.

Anna Deane chose to work directly on the occupational performance activities Mary identified as priorities. Though Mary had significant cognitive problems, Anna Deane did not offer Mary remedial drills for her deficits. One reason for this was that Mary was experiencing such serious memory problems, it was unlikely she would be able to transfer learning from remedial drills to functional activities. Second, remedial drills, such as practicing recalling lists of words to improve memory, would have reminded Mary of her deficits and accentuated her sense of loss. Third, and most importantly, Mary was already at home, and often unsafe because of her occupational performance problems. Focusing directly on Mary's occupational performance activities was the quickest way to improve her safety. Anna Deane was concerned about Mary's safety with: (1) personal care, especially in the bathroom, (2) kitchen activities and medication management, (3) telephone use and setting of temperature controls in the house, and (4) community activities such as grocery shopping.

For Mary's most dangerous activities Anna Deane adapted the tasks and environments. For example, Mary reports, "I was afraid of falling in the shower when I was getting spacey from a seizure, so we got a shower chair and a metal bar on the wall and rubber rugs inside the tub and outside the tub. . . . I was also afraid of burning myself on the flames of my gas stove if I was feeling confused, so we got a large electric hot plate and I could heat something up without being afraid of lighting myself or my clothes on fire" (see Chap. 3; p. 28). In both of these examples, the environment was changed to compensate for Mary's deficits and increase her safety.

Other times, Anna Deane taught Mary a strategy for particular tasks, such as unlocking her front doors.

> Anna Deane watched me try to get into the house and said she understood what the problem was. She said when I couldn't get in the outside door with one key, that I should *try the other key*. It had not occurred to me to try the other key. I would stand endlessly with the wrong key doing it over and over again, but when I had this new strategy, it freed me to get into my own house, and each time I opened the door myself it was such a victory. And I began to feel hope for myself. (see Chap. 3; p. 28)

In this case, Mary learned a new approach to the task of unlocking her front doors. Sometimes, for extremely difficult tasks, such as grocery shopping, the strategy was for Mary to have someone do the task for her. In working with Mary, Anna Deane used the processes of listening, observing, and activity analysis. In the front door example, Mary says, "Anna Deane watched me try to get into the house..." (see Chap. 3; p. 28). Anna Deane was able to hypothesize what Mary's difficulty with this task was by watching how she did the task. By Mary's account, she "would stand endlessly with the wrong key doing it over and over again..." (see Chap. 3; p. 28). This behavior of repeating the same thing over and over is called perseveration. Anna Deane noted this behavior and suggested a strategy to get around it—"She said when I couldn't get in the outside door with one key, that I should *try the other key*" (see Chap. 3; p. 28). This strategy worked; therefore, it was not necessary to try to modify the front door system of Mary's apartment.

By studying the neuropsychology test results and keeping careful track of which strategies and adaptations worked and which did not, Anna Deane discerned the kind of cuing Mary needed in order to learn. Mary says, "Anna Deane and I discovered that while it was impossible for me to just follow or understand verbal directions, if I could also watch someone do a task, listen to the directions, even place my hands on the things at the same time, I could after a number of tries, do it again myself" (see Chap. 3; p. 28). Once Anna Deane knew that this combination of demonstration with verbal explanation and hand over hand practice worked for Mary, she was able to use it for all of the activities Mary wanted to master. Throughout the treatment process, Mary and Anna Deane worked together to discover and build on Mary's strengths.

The empowerment and careful trial and error experimentation of this treatment process are central components of all effective treatment. Practitioners need to understand that treatment is not a series of unending successes, but a series of successes and failures that collectively move the client and therapist toward the client's goals.

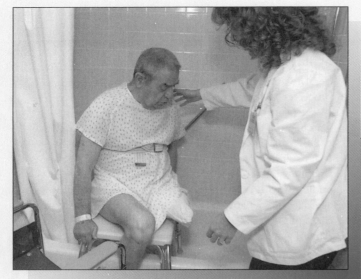

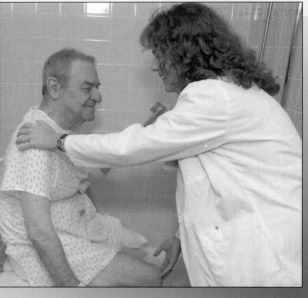

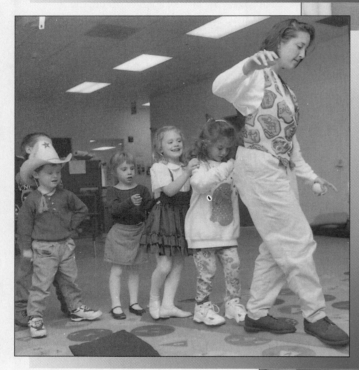

These treatment segments illustrate occupational, rehabilitative, developmental, and learning approaches to occupational therapy intervention. (Photographs courtesy of Gary Samson [top] and Ron Bergeron [bottom], Instructional Services, Dimond Library, University of New Hampshire.)

Unit VIII

Theories That Guide Practice

LEARNING OBJECTIVES

After completing this unit, readers will be able to:

▶ Define the terms theory and frame of reference.

▶ Identify major concepts developed in the occupational behavior tradition.

▶ Identify why systems thinking is important to the Model of Human Occupation.

▶ Identify the general principles of the occupational adaptation frame of reference.

▶ Explain how the Ecology of Performance Theory can be used in practice.

▶ Define rehabilitation.

▶ Identify the use of the rehabilitative frame of reference in practice.

▶ Describe the strengths and limitations of the biomechanical frame of reference.

▶ Explain the evolution of developmental theory from a hierarchical, biologically based linear model, to one that emphasizes the variability in normal development.

▶ Summarize the principles of theory and practice of Sensory Integration.

▶ Describe the strengths and limitations of the Neurodevelopmental Treatment frame of reference.

▶ Define association, representational, and association levels of learning.

▶ Explain the differences between behavioral and cognitive behavioral theories.

▶ Define the levels of functioning in the Cognitive Disability Model.

▶ Discuss the strengths and limitations of using the Multicontextual Approach to treat cognitive perceptual problems.

▶ Identify the strengths and limitations of approaches based on motor-learning foundations.

This unit provides readers with yet another tool for occupational therapy practice—theory. Theories relevant to occupational therapy intervention are organized ways of thinking about client problems, evaluation, and treatment. All occupational therapists think about client problems in terms of occupation. However, sometimes, looking at occupational problems from another theoretical perspective helps a practitioner understand a client's problems more fully and generate better treatment ideas. For example, from an occupational perspective we could say that Mary Weber (see Chap. 3) has difficulty performing activities of daily living (ADLs), work and productive activities, and play and leisure activities primarily because of her performance component deficits in cognition. We could think about working with her on her occupational performance areas or her performance component deficits. But how exactly would we work with her? How would we organize our evaluation and treatment sessions? This is where theory helps. Because Mary is having primarily cognitive difficulties, we could use a treatment approach that has been developed for those types of problems. Joan Toglia's Multicontext Approach, for instance, is a practice approach grounded in learning theory that would provide a practitioner with very specific ideas about how to proceed with Mary's intervention. If Mary's problems were primarily physical, then practice theories derived from rehabilitation perspectives would be helpful. This unit provides an overview of the different theories most frequently used by occupational therapy practitioners. (*Note*: Words in **bold** type are defined in the Glossary.)

Chapter 22

Theory and Frame of Reference

Kathlyn L. Reed

▼ WHAT THEORY DOES FOR A PROFESSION

Theory serves a profession such as occupational therapy by providing answers to eight major issues related to distinctness and viability of the profession. One, theory helps establish that a profession, such as occupational therapy, has a unique body of knowledge that can be articulated. In other words, theory shows what occupational therapy practitioners think occupational therapy is. Two, theory demonstrates the presence of a distinctive occupational therapy approach to health and health care that permits it to be compared and contrasted with other professions for similarities and differences. The distinctive approach relates intervention to improved occupational performance. Three, theory facilitates the growth of the profession as a vital force in the arena the profession is supposed to influence. For occupational therapy the arena to be influenced is health care delivery, including health promotion and illness or injury prevention. Four, theory helps describe and define the domain of concern the profession such as occupational therapy selects as its area of excellence and expertise, such as the relationship of occupation to person, environment, and health. Five, theory enriches practice by providing ways to improve the effectiveness of the profession's work. For example, theories help with professional decision making, problem solving, clinical reasoning, instruction, and economy of thought. (Johnson, 1978). Six, theory can be updated periodically to keep the knowledge base current with (1) new knowledge and skills gained from working with other disciplines, and (2) changes in the political, social, and cultural perspectives. Occupational therapy is especially sensitive to changes in health care delivery patterns and politicosociocultural trends. Seven, theory facilitates communication within the profession between practitioners. For example **Sensory Integra-**tion theory has been the catalyst for many conferences, seminars, writings, and a special interest section of the professional organization. Finally, theory translates intuitive ideas and hunches (conceptual models) into **concepts** and variables that can be organized systematically and studied. Occupational therapy has many ideas and hunches and needs more testable concepts and variables.

▼ DEFINING THEORY

Theory is an organized way of thinking about given phenomena. In occupational therapy, the phenomenon of concern is occupational endeavor. Theory attempts to (1) define and explain the relationships between concepts or ideas related to the phenomenon of interest, (2) explain how these relationships can predict behavior or events, and (3) suggest ways that the phenomenon can be changed or controlled. Occupational therapy theory is concerned with four major concepts related to occupational endeavor: person, environment, health, and occupation. Each of these concepts can be described in several ways. For example, a person can be described by age, gender, interests, educational level, social roles, occupational skills, economic resources, and other attributes. Environment can be described as physical, physiological, psychological, social, or political. Health may be described as good, poor, the opposite of illness, or total well-being. Occupation may be described by tasks, skills, knowledge, years of experience, social recognition, income received, employment status, or socially sanctioned roles. Because the four major concepts in occupational therapy can be viewed from several vantage points, the profession has developed a variety of theories about occupational endeavor. These theories can be categorized into different levels and stages.

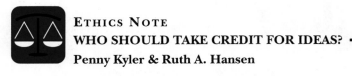

WHO SHOULD TAKE CREDIT FOR IDEAS?
Penny Kyler & Ruth A. Hansen

Sarah is an entry-level masters student and is a graduate assistant in the occupational therapy department. One of her professors asks her to fax the professor's latest article for publication to a journal in another country. Sarah scans the article and notices that the professor has taken full credit for the majority of the theoretical and conceptual constructs in the article. Sarah knows that most of these ideas are from the collaborative work of several professors in the department.

1. What are the limits and constraints on the use of other's ideas?
2. What are the legal and ethical requirements for acknowledgment of sources?
3. Did Sarah violate any ethical or moral standards when she scanned the article?
4. What are the options that Sarah has in this situation? What are the implications for each option? ■

▼ LEVELS OF THEORIES

There are four levels of theory: meta theory, grand theory, middle range theory, and "practice theory." Meta theory focuses on the broader spectrum of a profession. Theories at the meta level tend to be abstract and relate to the profession's viability more than to direct client care (Walker & Avant, 1995). In occupational therapy meta theory centers on the meaning of occupation, on occupational therapy as a "practice discipline" and on occupational therapy as both science and profession. Specific examples would include the idea of an Integrated Theory of Occupational Therapy ("Toward an integrated theory," 1968) and Occupational Science (Yerxa et al, 1989).

Grand theory deals with broad goals and concepts representing the total range of phenomena of concern within a discipline (Chinn & Kramer, 1995). Grand theories tend to be fairly general and may be quite abstract. Examples include Philosophy of Occupation Therapy (Meyer, 1922); Facilitating Growth and Development (Llorens, 1970), and **Model of Human Occupation** (Kielhofner, 1980).

Middle range theories deal with a relatively broad scope of phenomena, but do not cover the full range of phenomena that concern a disciple (Chinn & Kramer, 1995). Sensory Integration (Ayres, 1968); Sensorimotor Therapy (Rood, 1956); and **Cognitive Disability** (Allen, 1985) are examples of middle range theory.

Practice theory gives occupational therapy goals (direction of desired change) and actions occupational therapy practitioners must take to meet the goals (produce the change). For example, using a **biomechanical** practice theory, if the goal is to prevent contractures, the action is to maintain movement in the joint range of motion (ROM).

The four levels of theory are linked together. The meta-theory level clarifies the grand theory level which, in turn, guides middle-range level theory, which directs practice level theory. In reverse, testing of middle-range and practice theory provides input for refining grand theory which, in turn, provides material for changes in meta-theory. All levels of theory pass through different stages of development.

▼ STAGES OF THEORY DEVELOPMENT

There are four stages of theory development in a practice oriented profession: description, explanation, prediction, and control (Dickoff, James, & Wiedenback, 1968; Walker & Avant, 1995). The first stage, descriptive theory, classifies or describes specific dimensions, factors, or characteristics of individuals, groups, situations, or events by summarizing the commonalities found in discrete observations of those individuals, groups, situations, or events. When these descriptions are named or labeled they become concepts (Fawcett & Downs, 1992). Types of descriptive theory include naming theories and classification theories such as topologies and taxonomies. Descriptive theory is the most basic level of theory construction and is used most often when little is known or understood about a phenomenon or phenomena. An example of descriptive theory might be the description of a child who (1) strikes out at another child if touched or brushed lightly while standing in a line at school, (2) hates to have his hair brushed, and (3) refuses to wear wool because it "scratches." This collection of behaviors, plus others, becomes a concept labeled tactile defensiveness.

The second stage of theory development is explanation. Once the concept is labeled, defined, and described, it can be examined in relationship to another or to several other concepts. The purpose of the explanation theories, then, is to propose or suggest reasons for relationships between identified concepts. To continue the example of tactile defensiveness, one might observe that such a child may be labeled as having a behavior problem because the child does not seem to stop the striking out behavior when corrected by teacher or parent. One explanatory theory could be that the relationship between tactile defensiveness and "bad" behavior is the result of neurological factors, rather than failure or refusal to learn better self-control.

The third stage of theory development is prediction. Prediction is based on an understanding of the relationships between concepts. Prediction theories hypothesize that if a particular situation occurs it will likely result in some specific outcome. In the example of tactile defensiveness, it is possible to predict that if a child is tactile defensive, he is then likely to strike out at another child if touched lightly or brushed against while standing in the school lunch line.

The fourth stage of theory development is control. Control theory is based on understanding how prediction works. Knowing that situation A results in situation B we can intervene to stop an undesirable outcome or facilitate a desired outcome. Control theory thus is the most useful stage of theory construction to therapy management. Control theory allows the therapist to make recommendations for better managing the tactilely defensive child in the school and at home. Control theory also provides the rationale for therapeutic interventions that attempt to reduce the tactile defensive reactions by improving the neurological functioning of the tactile system. However, control theory depends on the development of the other three stages of theory construction. Control theory is improved as we improve the description, explanation, and prediction aspects of theory development.

▼ THEORY CONSTRUCTION

Although a detailed description of theory construction is not within the scope of this section, it is important to know the basic construction units of a theory. Each theory is based on a philosophical view of how the world and the objects, human and nonhuman, in the world operate and function. The philosophical views most associated with occupational therapy are humanitarianism, humanism, and holism. A specific philosophical view is expressed in assumptions or board general statements, which may also be called axioms, maxims, and suppositions. Assumptions act as the foundation of a theory. Concepts (constructs or ideas) are built from the basic assumptions. The concepts and their definitions form the basic units of theory construction. The concepts are related to each other through rules of organization that state how the concepts logically fit together. Thus, a theory is organized by putting together philosophical views, assumptions, concepts, and rules of organization.

▼ THEORETICAL FRAME OF REFERENCE IN OCCUPATIONAL THERAPY

Frame of reference is a theory-related term that is used frequently in occupational therapy. According to Mosey (1981, p. 5) "a theoretical frame of reference is a set of interrelated internally consistent concepts, definitions, postulates, and principles that provide a systematic description of and prescription for a practitioner's interaction with his domain of concern. It delineates the nature of the human and nonhuman objects with which the practitioner interacts and in

turn serves as a guide for his actions relative to these objects." Mosey's description is similar to the fourth stage of theory development labeled change or practice theory.

▶ CONCLUSION

A profession must have a theoretical base of knowledge. In a practice or applied profession such as occupational therapy the theoretical base must be translated and developed into specific guidelines for practice that can be continually examined for their effectiveness.

The following chapters describe occupational therapy theories that have been developed from different perspectives on the four major concepts important to occupational endeavor: person, environment, health, and occupation. Although all of the theories presented look at all four concepts, there are distinctive perspectives on some concepts that distinguish different groups of theories from each other. The occupational behavior chapter deals with theories that focus on occupation as an organizing force in peoples' lives. The rehabilitation chapter looks at theories that focus on health as a process of adaptation. The developmental chapter presents theories that focus on the person in terms of neurological and developmental stages. The learning chapter focuses on the person and environment in terms of their relative contributions to learning capacity. Most of the theory discussions include suggestions about how to apply these theories to practice. The case study analyses at the end of the pediatric and adult diagnostic units also demonstrate ways that different theories can be applied to practice to make therapy more systematic and effective.

▼ REFERENCES

Allen, C. K. (1985). *Occupational therapy for psychiatry disease: Measurement and management of cognitive disabilities.* Boston: Little, Brown & Co.

Ayres, A. J. (1968). Sensory integrative processes and neuropsychological learning disability. In *Learning Disorders Vol. 3.* (pp. 41–58). Seattle, WA: Special Child Publications.

Chinn, P. O. & Kramer, M. K. (1995). *Theory and nursing: A systematic approach*, (4th ed). St. Louis: Mosby-Year Book.

Dickoff, J., James, P., & Widenbach, E. (1968) Theory in a practice discipline, Part I. *Nursing Research, 17*, 415–435.

Fawcett, J. & Downs, F. S. (1992). *The relationship of theory and research* (2nd ed). Philadelphia: F. A. Davis.

Johnson, D. E. (1978) State of the art of theory development in nursing. In National League for Nursing, *Theory development: What, why, how?* (pp. 1–10). New York: Author.

Kielhofner, G. & Burke, J. (1980). A model of human occupation. Part one. Conceptual framework and content. *American Journal of Occupational Therapy, 34*, 572–582.

Llorens, L. (1970). Facilitating growth and development: The promise of occupational therapy. *American Journal of Occupational Therapy, 24*, 93–101.

Meyer, A. (1922). Theory of occupation therapy. *Archives of Occupational Therapy, 1*, 1–10.

Mosey, A. C. (1981). *Three frames of reference for mental health.* New York: Raven Press.

Rood, M. (1956). Neurophysiological mechanisms utilized in the treatment of neuromuscular dysfunction. *American Journal of Occupational Therapy, 10,* 220–225.

Toward an integrated theory of occupational therapy (1968). *American Journal of Occupational Therapy, 22,* 451–456.

Walker, L. O. & Avant, K. C. (1995) *Strategies for theory construction in nursing,* (3rd ed). Norwalk: Appleton & Lange.

Yerxa, E. J., Clark, F., Frank, G., Jackson, J., Parham, D., Pierce, D., Stein, C., & Zemke, R. (1989). An introduction to occupational science, a foundation for occupational therapy in the 21st century. *Occupational Therapy in Health Care, 6* (4), 1–17.

Chapter 23

Theories Derived from Occupational Behavior Perspectives

Section 1

An Overview of Occupational Behavior

Laura Barrett and Gary Kielhofner

Historical Context of Occupational Behavior
Occupational Behavior Defined
Occupational Behavior Themes
    Work and Play Adaptation
    The Motivation for Occupation
    Temporal Adaptation
    Occupational Roles
The Influence of Occupational Behavior on the Field

During the 1960s and 1970s, Dr. Mary Reilly, with her colleagues and graduate students at the University of Southern California, developed the occupational behavior perspective to explain why **occupation** was the media and method of the field (Reilly, 1969). The central premise of occupational behavior is "...that man through the use of his hands as they are energized by his mind and will, can influence the state of his own health" (Reilly, 1962, p.2).

▼ HISTORICAL CONTEXT OF OCCUPATIONAL BEHAVIOR

Reilly's effort to develop occupational behavior came at a time when the field had built a strong alliance with medicine (Shannon, 1972; Kielhofner & Burke, 1977). Reilly argued that medicine's influence had resulted in occupational therapy failing to follow the vision of its founders concerning the potential of occupation as a force in the health of humans. Following medicine's lead, occupational therapy defined the effect of client engagement in activity in narrow terms based on **biomedical** and psychoanalytical knowledge. Reilly (1969, p. 300) argued that it was important to distinguish occupational therapy from medicine, noting: "It is the task of medicine to prevent and reduce illness; while the task of occupational therapy is to prevent and reduce the incapacities resulting from illness." From the recognition that occupational therapy had a purpose different from medicine, Reilly stressed building a base of knowledge about occupation and its influence on human welfare from the point of view of the social sciences. Hence, the concepts of occupational behavior are mainly based on ideas from philosophy, psychology, social psychology, sociology, and anthropology.

▼ OCCUPATIONAL BEHAVIOR DEFINED

Occupational behavior includes those activities that occupy a person's time, involve achievement, and address the economic realities of life (Reilly, 1962, 1966). Longitudinally, occupational behavior constitutes the complete developmental continuum from childhood play to adult work (Reilly, 1962; Shannon, 1972; Black, 1976; Moorhead, 1969). In the cross-sectional sense, occupational behavior involves the daily round of work, play, and rest within a physical, temporal, and social environment (Matsutsuyu, 1971; Shannon, 1972). Moreover, occupational behavior involves interaction with the environment and is shaped by the complex, interrelated environments in which one functions (Dunning, 1972; Gray, 1972; Parent 1978; Reilly, 1966).

▼ OCCUPATIONAL BEHAVIOR THEMES

The wide range of topics in occupational behavior can be viewed as comprising four major conceptual themes: work and play adaptation, the motivation for occupation, temporal adaptation, and occupational roles.

Work and Play Adaptation

The concepts of occupation and **adaptation** are closely linked. To begin with, occupation is seen as a landscape on which the person has to adapt. From birth on, the human being is challenged to deal with the necessary tasks of everyday living—occupations. This process begins with the infant's struggle to overcome gravity, proceeds through learning the necessary tasks of self-care and cultural competency, and culminates in the challenge of taking on adult responsibility for productivity (Black, 1976; Matsutsuyu, 1971; Reilly, 1962).

Adaptation in occupation requires that persons have and exercise basic occupational skills that include motor, social decision making, time use, self-care, and specific work and play abilities (Black, 1976; Kielhofner, 1977; Shannon, 1972). When these occupational skills are intact, the person is able to adapt; when illness or disability compromises these skills, adaptation is threatened. Hence, occupational behavior calls attention to how disease and disability affect occupational skills and how these skills can be optimized in the face of chronic impairments.

Occupation is also viewed as a fundamental means through which people cope and adapt in life. One's ability to fill time, to find meaning, and to productively contribute to society are all important elements of how humans adapt through occupation (Florey, 1969; Kielhofner, 1977; Matsutsuyu, 1971; Reilly, 1962). Occupation is also a means of

generating the capacity for adaptations. For example, in play the child learns and integrates the rules and skills that will be required later in life (Robinson, 1977). Through play children experience, explore, and test the world, and in doing so, learn about their own capacities, how the world responds to their efforts, and what expectations others have for their behavior (Hurff, 1980; Michelman, 1971; Robinson, 1977). Finally, people adapt by using occupation to respond to the expectations of society and to validate themselves as social members (Matsutsuyu, 1971).

The Motivation for Occupation

Occupation is founded on the human need to exercise capacity and to achieve a degree of personal mastery over oneself and one's environment (Reilly, 1962). This idea that occupation serves a special human motive was particularly important when Reilly first defined occupational behavior, because thinking at that time was dominated by the psychoanalytical and behavioral tradition that emphasized sexual and physiological needs. Reilly believed it was critically important that occupational therapy identify itself as being in the service of addressing an equally important human need, that of the need to fill one's life with occupation (Reilly, 1962).

Occupation is intrinsically motivating; persons engage in occupation for its own sake—that is, for the rewards of learning, control, and mastery that occur in the midst of performance (Florey, 1969). The intrinsic motive of occupation changes over the life span; it begins with the early motive of curiosity, which fuels exploration, and proceeds to a competency motive for learning and the adult motive for achievement (Reilly, 1966; Florey, 1969).

Experiencing oneself as an agent able to achieve desired outcomes is the product of healthy occupation; it is also the foundation for being motivated to engage in occupation (Burke, 1977). When occupation is prevented or disturbed,

---

HISTORICAL NOTE
SLAGLE'S USE OF HABIT TRAINING: PRACTICE BASED ON REASON

Suzanne M. Peloquin

Eleanor Clarke Slagle, one of the founders of the Society for the Promotion of Occupational Therapy, taught habit training to patients with mental illness. Believing that occupations could be useful and even curative when done habitually, she selected patients who were regressed and chronically ill.

Each patient in habit training was encouraged to get into a routine and to then assume responsibility for it. Excerpts from one patient's case convey a sense of the practice:

May 3, 1926—Admitted to habit training. Will not dress or undress self. Clothing untidy and unbuttoned. Wets and soils the bed. Eats excessively. Masturbation frequent.

June 1 to June 30—Washes and dresses self. Wets and soils less frequently. Polishes floor when continuously supervised. Does low-grade occupation.

July 10 to September 22, 1926—Speaks occasionally. Told superintendent he was "slightly improved." Works on braid-weave rug. Helps attendant with cleaning and clears dishes from table at meals. Appetite more normal. (Wilson, 1929; pp. 196–197)

The belief that treatment needed to be directed by reason and purpose predated more current discussion of theory or frames of reference. Since the profession's inception, hypotheses about the nature of a client's problems and the effects of a therapist's actions have helped guide treatment. ■

Wilson, S. C. (1929). Habit training for mental cases. *Occupational Therapy and Rehabilitaion, 8,* 189–197.

this sense of competence is threatened. Interest also contributes to the motive for occupation. Knowing a person's interests is the key to knowing how he or she is individually motivated (Borys, 1974; Matsutsuyu, 1969).

Temporal Adaptation

Temporality is important to occupational behavior because occupation is the main way that persons occupy time. The theme of temporality can be traced back to the founders of the field who had emphasized that health could be measured by how effectively persons filled time with activity (Shannon, 1972; Kielhofner, 1977). The two most important ideas to emerge in this area were balance and habits.

The achievement of an appropriate balance between the demanding activities of work and the restorative activities of play and rest is seen as essential to health (Shannon, 1972; Kielhofner, 1977). Health requires a rhythm of alternating forms of activity and rest and is realized in the quality of those behaviors that fill time. A lack of balance can, in itself, constitute unhealthy living. Therefore, when an impairment disrupts the balance of occupational life, it is important to restore that balance.

Habits are the basic structures that give temporal order to daily behavior (Kielhofner, 1977). Habits account for those behaviors that become automatic when repeated over time. Furthermore, habits integrate skills into routines of action organized to meet the daily demands of one's life. Consequently, it is not sufficient to have the basic occupational skills. Those skills have to be organized into patterns of behavior that allow one to fulfill environmental expectations and achieve balance.

Occupational Roles

Roles mediate between the requirements of the social environment and the contributions of the individual. When defined as the behavioral expectations that accompany one's occupied position or status in a social system, roles are the primary means through which persons express occupational behavior (Heard, 1977). Occupational roles begin with the child's role of play, proceed through the familial, friendship, and student roles, continue in the adult work role, and culminate in the role of retiree. This sequence of occupational roles is referred to as the occupational career (Black, 1976; Shannon, 1972; Heard, 1977; Kielhofner, 1977; Moorhead, 1969; Reilly, 1966; Matsutsuyu, 1971).

Two important concepts related to roles are socialization and occupational choice. Socialization refers to the series of environmentally based learning experiences by which persons acquire necessary role attitudes and behaviors (eg, learn work skills from role models, and through homework and chores). Occupational choice is the ongoing process through which persons select and commit themselves to occupational roles (eg, student, worker, homemaker, volunteer) (Matsutsuyu, 1971; Moorhead, 1969).

▼ THE INFLUENCE OF OCCUPATIONAL BEHAVIOR ON THE FIELD

The influence of occupational behavior on occupational therapy is probably not best measured by its direct application in practice. Rather, its importance lies in its overall influence on the directions of the field and its richness in generating new traditions. Three effects are probably most notable. The first is that occupational behavior was successful in calling occupational therapist's attention to the need to emancipate itself from medicine and define its practice around the construct of occupation. Second, the occupational behavior tradition is the basis for the occupational science movement currently based at the University of Southern California. Proponents of occupational science are attempting to build a scientific discipline around the study of occupation. Their efforts echo the occupational behavior emphasis on the importance of understanding occupation. Finally, the occupational behavior tradition is the foundation out of which the Model of Human Occupation (MOHO) (Kielhofner, 1995) developed. To a large extent, the aim of the model has been to synthesize many of the themes of occupational behavior into a framework suitable to guide practice. Section 2 discusses MOHO. Sections 3 and 4 present other theories derived from occupational behavior: occupational adaptation and ecology of human performance.

Section 2

The Model of Human Occupation

Gary Kielhofner and Laura Barrett

Subsystems Contributing To Occupational Behavior
Volition
Habituation
Mind–Brain–Body Performance
The Cooperation of Subsystems
The Environment
Application to Practice

The MOHO provides a way of thinking about persons' occupational behavior and occupational dysfunction. Its concepts address motivation for occupation, the routine patterning of occupational behavior, the nature of skilled performance, and the influence of environment on occupation. The model provides a broad framework for gathering data about a client's circumstance, for generating an understanding of the client's strengths and weaknesses, and for selecting and implementing a course of therapy.

The MOHO incorporates a systems view of the human being and emphasizes two main points. The first point is that behavior is dynamic and context-dependent. How one is motivated, what one does, and how one performs, all are dependent on environmental conditions. Underlying motives or capacity interact dynamically with the environment and behavior emerges out of this dynamic interaction.

The second point is that occupation is essential to human self-organization. Human beings are living systems who are unfolding and changing in time. Through their occupations, persons exercise their capacities and generate ongoing experiences that affirm and shape their psyches. Therefore, the order or organization of humans depends on occupational behavior.

Consequently, the MOHO emphasizes that the human system is carried along and shaped by the nature of its occupational behavior. Humans become, to an extent, what they do. In the context of occupations, people create their abilities, self-concepts, and identities. Occupational therapy engages persons in occupational behavior that helps maintain, restore, reorganize, or develop their capacities, motives, and lifestyles.

▼ SUBSYSTEMS CONTRIBUTING TO OCCUPATIONAL BEHAVIOR

The model conceptualizes the human as a system made up of three subsystems: volition, habituation, and mind—brain—body performance. Volition motivates occupational behavior. Habituation organizes occupational behavior into patterns or routines. Mind—brain—body performance provides the performance capacities for occupation.

Volition

Volition is a set of inner dispositions and self-knowledge built through experience. Dispositions are cognitive and emotional orientations toward occupations, such as enjoying, valuing, and feeling competent to perform them. Self-knowledge is common sense awareness of self as an actor in the world. Volitional dispositions and self-knowledge pertain to (1) how effective one is in acting on the world, (2) what one holds as important, and (3) what one finds enjoyable and satisfying. These three areas are referred to as personal causation, values, and interests, respectively. Together they influence and enable one to anticipate, choose, experience, and interpret occupational behavior.

PERSONAL CAUSATION

Personal causation refers to people's capacities and effectiveness. People learn about their capacities and dispositions from experience. They also learn how effective they are in using their capacities to achieve desired outcomes of behavior.

VALUES

Values are beliefs and commitments that define what is good, right, and important. Values influence one's view of what is worth doing or aiming for and what is the proper way to act. Values belong to a common sense, cultural view of life, and are usually associated with strong emotions (eg, feelings of importance, security, worthiness, belonging, and purpose). Hence, values are felt as obligations, and one cannot behave contrary to values without feeling guilty or inadequate.

INTERESTS

The experience of pleasure and satisfaction in occupational behavior generates interests. Interests begin with natural dispositions (eg, the tendency to enjoy physical or intellectual activity) and develop through the acquisition of tastes. People feel their interests as an attraction to participating in certain occupations. This attraction may come from positive feelings associated with either the exercise of capacity, intellectual or physical challenge, fellowship with others, aesthetic stimulation, or other factors. Each person has a unique preference for certain occupations or for particular ways of performing.

VOLITIONAL CHOICE AND NARRATIVE

Personal causation, values, and interests are interrelated in volition and together provide a framework for making sense of experience, for anticipating possibilities for action, and for making choices. Persons make both activity and occupational choices. The former are everyday choices for action, and the latter are choices concerning occupations that will become an extended or permanent part of their lives.

Volition reflects present circumstances, past memories, and anticipation of the future. People integrate their personal causation, values, and interests across time by locating themselves in an unfolding life story, referred to as the volitional narrative (Helfrich & Kielhofner, 1994; Helfrich, Kielhofner, & Mattingly, 1994). Therefore, people experience and make sense of their own volition as an unfolding life story. Moreover, each person chooses occupations as a means of continuing his or her life story.

Habituation

The habituation subsystem organizes occupational behavior into recurrent patterns that are integrated into the rhythms and customs of our physical, social, and temporal worlds. This subsystem includes habits and roles.

HABITS

Habits involve learned ways of doing things that unfold automatically. Through repeated experience a person acquires a kind of map for appreciating and behaving in familiar environments. Because of one's habits one intuitively knows, for example, when it is time to leave for work, what turns to take in driving there, and what step comes next in performing a familiar work task. Habits locate people in the unfolding events and places of everyday life and steer their behavior in the right direction. Habits influence how one performs routine activities, how one typically uses time, and what one's style of behavior is like.

ROLES

Internalized roles give people a social identity and a sense of the obligations that go with that identity. People see themselves as students, workers, parents, and recognize that they should behave in certain ways to fulfill these roles. Roles give people scripts for appreciating their status in social situations and for enacting that role status. Roles influence the manner and content of persons' interactions with others, the tasks they routinely do, and when they do them. Roles place expectations on persons for task performance and for time use, thereby providing structure and regularity to life and channeling people's actions into necessary patterns and tasks.

Together habits and roles allow one to automatically recognize features and situations in the environment and to construct behavior accordingly. Because of one's roles and habits, most routines of daily life unfold automatically and predictably.

Mind–Brain–Body Performance

The mind–brain–body performance subsystem includes the musculoskeletal, neurological, perceptual, and cognitive capacities needed for occupational performance. Effective occupational performance is the result of the unified action of all constituents of the mind–brain–body performance subsystem as they work in collaboration with unfolding circumstances and environmental conditions.

The Cooperation of Subsystems

Occupational behavior always reflects a complex interplay of our motives, habits and roles, and capacities. Hence, the three subsystems must operate in concert with each other, making simultaneous contributions to behavior. We cannot fully understand occupational behavior without reference to all three internal contributing factors.

▼ THE ENVIRONMENT

Our interwoven physical and social environments afford opportunities and press (ie, expectations or demands) for performance. The physical environment consists of the natural and human-made spaces and the objects within them. The social environment includes the gatherings or groups of persons that one joins, and the occupational forms (Nelson,

1988) that persons perform. Occupational behavior settings are composites of spaces, objects, occupational forms, social groups, or combinations thereof, that cohere and constitute a meaningful context. Homes, schools, workplaces, and stores are examples of occupational behavior settings. Occupational life involves rounds of occupational performance in a number of occupational behavior settings.

▼ APPLICATION TO PRACTICE

The volition, habituation, and mind–brain–body performance subsystems, and the environment may all contribute to maladaptive function. When this occurs, the occupational therapist uses the MOHO as a framework for understanding the interrelated factors that contribute to dysfunction. The therapist evaluating a particular client will discover the unique way in which these factors are involved in that person's function and dysfunction. In evaluation, therapists seek out data to answer questions they generate from the theoretical perspective of the model. For example, therapists might ask how a person's habit pattern or personal causation is influencing a problem. They then use the data they collect to make theoretically informed judgments about the answers to such questions and to create a theoretically based explanation of the client's circumstances. This explanation allows the therapist to engage in the process of deciding on and implementing strategies of intervention.

Therapists using the MOHO have various resources on which to draw. Several structured assessments have been developed to collect data when one is using this model (Kielhofner, 1985, 1995). There are also many published articles that discuss the MOHO's application for practice. Additionally, many therapists have developed programs that are systematic approaches to applying this model. These applications represent the breadth of occupational therapy practice from pediatrics to gerontology, in both psychosocial and physical dysfunction and in a wide range of settings. See the Unit Summaries for Units IX and X for applications of this model to specific case studies.

Section 3

Occupational Adaptation: An Integrative Frame of Reference

Janette K. Schkade and Sally Schultz

Intellectual Heritage
Definitions or Assumptions

▼ INTELLECTUAL HERITAGE

Occupational Adaptation is a frame of reference that describes the integration of two concepts long present in occupational therapy thinking: occupation and adaptation. The intellectual heritage dates back to the writings of Adolph Meyer (1922) and continues through contemporary theorists. (See Schkade and Schultz, 1992a, 1992b, for a more extensive discussion of the theoretical underpinnings.) Occupational Adaptation offers a description of an internal adaptation process that occurs through occupation and for occupation. According to this frame of reference, occupations are activities that consist of three properties: active involvement of the individual; personal meaning to the individual; and a process that ends in a product, whether that product is tangible (such as a piece of pottery) or intangible (such as personal satisfaction from helping a friend). Occupational Adaptation was first articulated as a frame of reference in two articles by Schkade and Schultz (1992a,b). A model of the therapeutic intervention approach first appeared in Schkade and Schultz (1993).

▼ DEFINITIONS AND ASSUMPTIONS

The following assumptions undergird the frame of reference: (1) competence in occupational performance is a lifelong process of adaptation to internal and external performance demands; (2) these demands occur naturally within occupational roles and within the context of person–occupational environment interactions; (3) the Occupational Adaptation frame of reference describes this process; (4) dysfunction occurs when there is disruption in the adaptation process; (5) the adaptation process can be disrupted by impairment, disability, or handicapping conditions as well as by stressful life events; (6) the focus of intervention is to maximize the individual's internal adaptation process; (7) improvement in occupational performance is dependent on improvement in the adaptation process.

Occupational Adaptation presents the adaptation process as emerging from an interaction between the person (consisting of idiosyncratic sensorimotor, cognitive, and psychosocial systems) and occupational environments (consisting of work, play and leisure, and self-maintenance functions) in response to occupational challenges. Person systems are what they are because of genetic, environmental, and experiential (phenomenological) subsystems that feed into the person systems and create the idiosyncratic nature of individuals. Likewise, in the occupational environments, physical, social, and cultural subsystems feed into and create the nature of specific occupational environments, or con-

texts in which occupation occurs. Occupational challenges occur within the context of performing occupational roles. Performance expectations from the occupational environment and from the person's own internal expectations influence the challenge experienced.

There are three adaptation subprocesses the individual uses when facing an occupational challenge: the adaptive response generation subprocess, the adaptive response evaluation subprocess, and the adaptive response integration subprocess. These subprocesses function to plan the occupational response, evaluate it, and integrate its outcome into the person as adaptation.

The adaptive response generation subprocess is the anticipatory portion of the adaptation process. It consists of two components: the adaptive response mechanism and the adaptation gestalt. The "mechanism" creates a plan of action for the occupational response by selecting the energy form, the pattern of responding, and the behavior type. The plan calls for the individual to program the three person systems (the "gestalt") to execute the plan of action. The occupational response is the outcome of the interplay between the mechanism and the gestalt. It is assumed that the individual attempts to generate responses that result in some degree of relative mastery. In the adaptive response evaluation subprocess, the extent to which the individual has experienced relative mastery is assessed by the individual. Relative mastery consists of the properties of efficiency (use of time, energy, and resources); effectiveness (extent to which the desired goal was achieved); and satisfaction to self and society (the extent to which the individual was personally satisfied with the response and the extent to which societal influences assessed the response as congruent with performance expectations). If the evaluation subprocess indicates that change in the way the individual interacts with the environment in similar circumstances is needed, the necessary adaptation occurs as a result of action of the adaptive response integration subprocess. The occupational environment also evaluates the outcome of the occupational response. The potential for change in the occupational environment is also present as a consequence.

▼ EVALUATION, TREATMENT, CLIENT–PRACTITIONER INTERACTIONS

Occupational adaptation is not a collection of techniques, but a way of thinking that guides and organizes the intervention process. The essential task of the practitioner is to acknowledge and facilitate the client as the agent of therapeutic change. The practitioner sets the stage for the client to progressively assume the agency role. This is critical in influencing the client's internal adaptation process. To reiterate, it is the internal adaptation process that is the focus for intervention with this frame of reference.

In all phases of the intervention process, collaboration between the client and the practitioner is essential. Articles by Schultz and Schkade (1994) and Ford (1995) describing the use of Occupational Adaptation in home health are recommended as a good place to begin learning about the fundamentals of intervention guided by this perspective. The goal of intervention is to facilitate the client's ability to make his or her own adaptations to engage in occupational activities that are personally meaningful to the client. This is accomplished by enhancing the function of the client's internal adaptation process through using a client-selected occupational role to guide intervention. The therapist evaluates the client's ability to carry out the activities within that role and determines what is helping or hindering the client to experience relative mastery in those activities. A plan is then developed to enhance the capabilities and minimize the negative effect of disabling conditions. The plan consists of two types of intervention: occupational readiness and occupational activity. Occupational readiness addresses deficits in the sensorimotor, cognitive, and psychosocial systems to prepare them (or make ready) for occupational activity. Occupational readiness might include a splint to support the hand in a more functional position, exercise to strengthen weak muscles, training in social skills, or other interventions. Occupational activity engages the client in tasks that are a part of the occupational role selected by the client. For example, if the role is work related, occupational activity will consist of tasks related to that role within the client's expectations and those of his or her occupational environment. An important intervention principle is that all three person systems are always present in every occupational response. This principle requires that therapists always think holistically when planning and carrying out intervention.

▼ STRENGTHS, LIMITATIONS, AND RESEARCH

The strengths of the Occupational Adaptation frame of reference lie in its holistic perspective and its adherence to fundamental ideas of occupation and adaptation inherent in the profession's life and history. It provides a way to think and communicate about occupational therapy intervention that is organized, process oriented, and client-focused. It offers a mechanism (relative mastery) for engaging the client in the evaluation of intervention outcomes, thereby providing a greater potential for the results of intervention to generalize to settings outside the clinic. The results of future use by practitioners and investigation into its essential properties by researchers will identify the limitations present in the frame of reference and shape its continued evolution. Its limitations will only be known as its use becomes more prevalent.

Research on adaptive response behaviors can be found in Garrett and Schkade (1995) and on relative mastery in Pasek

and Schkade (1996). Gibson and Schkade (1997) reported that a group of clients with cerebrovascular accidents demonstrated significantly different functional independence when treated with an Occupational Adaptation approach. Case studies as reported by Ross (1994) add to the knowledge about the effectiveness of intervention with Occupational Adaptation. Other studies are in progress in persons with a range of physical and mental health dysfunction, from school children to the elderly.

Section 4

The Ecology of Human Performance

Winnie Dunn, Linda Haney McClain, Catana Brown, and Mary Jane Youngstrom

Intellectual Heritage
Assumptions Underlying the Ecology of Human Performance: Persons and Their Contexts Are Unique and Dynamic
Definitions
  Person
  Task
  Performance
  Context
  Person-Context-Task Transaction
  Therapeutic Intervention
Application to Practice
Editors' Conclusions

The purpose of this section is to introduce the Ecology of Human Performance (EHP) framework as a model for considering context in occupational therapy practice. The fundamental theoretical postulate of the EHP framework is that ecology, or the interaction between a person and the context, affects human behavior and task performance. Human performance is a transactional process through which the person, the context, and task performance affect each other. Each transaction affects a person's future performance range and options, because the person, the context, or the available performance range may be modified by the experience. In some cases, the most salient variable will be the context, whereas in others, it may be a particular person variable. Frequently, the person–context match is the conspicuous performance issue. Therapeutic intervention from an EHP perspective occurs as a collaboration between the person and family and the occupational therapy practitioner. It is designed to improve performance. Occupational therapy intervention is designed to enhance the person's performance range by changing the following variables: the person, the context, the task, or the transaction among them.

▼ INTELLECTUAL HERITAGE

Scholars from many disciplines have explored the interaction between organisms and their environments. Environmental psychologists have emphasized the relationships between persons and their physical environments (eg, Holahan, 1986; Wicker, 1979). Hart (1979) considered the environment as a medium for social interactions and pointed out that the environment could support social competence. Bronfenbrenner (1979) also discussed the social aspects of context as part of an ecological model for human development. Auerswald (1971) argued that a holistic ecological perspective enabled the practitioner to be concerned with the performance environment as well as the performance demands the person must face.

The construct of context (ie, environment in much of the occupational therapy literature) is elucidated by two primary perspectives within the occupational therapy framework. In the first perspective, context is addressed as part of the intervention process. Llorens (1970) employed the construct of context by explaining occupational therapy intervention as a process of providing environments that assist persons when their developmental evolution has been disrupted. Fidler and Fidler (1978) conceived of context as important as persons develop mastery through their interactions with aspects of the environment. King (1978) characterized interventions as the use of the environment to elicit an adaptive response.

In the second perspective, the relationship between person and environment is conceptualized within general systems theory, in which the person and environment are interdependent as they interact in the system of input, throughput, and output (Reilly 1962). The MOHO (Kielhofner & Burke, 1980), occupational science (Clark et al., 1991), and Nelson's (1988) description of the dynamics of occupational form (ie, context) and occupational performance draw on general systems theory. Others have included environmental factors in their models of occupational therapy (eg, Allen,1992; Howe and Briggs, 1982; Kiernat, 1992; Law et al, 1996; Mosey, 1992; Schkade & Schultz, 1992a; Spencer, 1991).

▼ ASSUMPTIONS UNDERLYING THE ECOLOGY OF HUMAN PERFORMANCE: PERSONS AND THEIR CONTEXTS ARE UNIQUE AND DYNAMIC

1. Persons and their contexts are unique and dynamic.
2. Contrived contexts are different from natural contexts.
3. Occupational therapy practice involves promoting self-

determination and inclusion of persons with disabilities in all contexts.
4. Independence includes using contextual supports to meet your wants and needs.

▼ DEFINITIONS

Person

A *person* is an individual with a unique configuration of abilities, experiences, and sensorimotor, cognitive, and psychosocial needs. Persons are unique and complex and therefore precise predictability about their performance is impossible. The meaning a person attaches to task and contextual variables strongly influences performance (Dunn, Brown, McClain, and Westman, 1994; p.15).

Task

A *task* may be considered an objective set of behaviors necessary to accomplish a goal. An infinite variety of tasks exists for every person. Roles shape a person's tasks.

Performance

Performance is comprised of both the process and the result of the person interacting with context to engage in tasks. The performance range is determined by the transaction between the person and the context.

Context

Context has two aspects: temporal and environmental. Although temporal aspects are determined by the person, temporal features become contextual because of the social and cultural meaning attached to them.

TEMPORAL ASPECTS
1. Chronological: individual's age
2. Developmental: stage or phase of maturation
3. **Life cycle**: place in important life phases, such as career cycle, parenting cycle, or educational process
4. Disability status: place in continuum of disability, such as acuteness of injury, chronicity of disability, or terminal nature of illness (AOTA, 1994).

ENVIRONMENT
1. Physical: nonhuman aspects of contexts; includes the accessibility to and performance within environments having natural terrain, plants, animals, buildings, furniture, objects, tools, or devices
2. Social: availability and expectations of significant individuals, such as spouse, friends, and caregivers; also includes larger social groups that are influential in establishing norms, role expectations, and social routines
3. Cultural: customs, beliefs, activity patterns, behavior stan-

dards, and expectations accepted by the society of which the individual is a member; includes political aspects, such as laws that affect access to resources and affirm personal rights; also, opportunities for education, employment, and economic support (AOTA, 1994; p. 1054).

Person–Context–Task Transaction

The person–context transaction in task performance is the major variable that ultimately governs the performance range. Ecology, or the transaction between a person and the context, affects task performance; task performance, in turn, affects the person, the context, and the person–context transaction.

Therapeutic Intervention

Therapeutic intervention, as illustrated in Figure 23–1, is a collaboration between the person, the family, and the occupational practitioner directed at meeting performance needs utilizing the following strategies:

ESTABLISH OR RESTORE A PERSON'S ABILITIES TO PERFORM IN CONTEXT

One intervention option is to establish or restore a person's skills or abilities. The establish intervention leads toward the attainment of a new skill or ability. The restore option leads toward the reestablishment of a lost skill or ability. Establish and restore interventions target the person; the outcome is a new or renewed skill or ability. This intervention fixes or improves the person, so that performance is improved.

ALTER ACTUAL CONTEXT OR TASK IN WHICH PEOPLE PERFORM

Therapeutic interventions can alter the context or task within which the person performs. This intervention emphasizes selecting a context or task that enables the person to perform with current skills and abilities. This can include placing the person in a different setting or task that more closely matches current skills and abilities, rather than changing the present setting or task to accommodate needs.

MODIFY (ADAPT) CONTEXTUAL FEATURES AND TASK DEMANDS SO THEY SUPPORT PERFORMANCE IN CONTEXT

When employing modify (adapt) intervention strategies, the occupational therapy practitioner finds ways to revise the current context or task demands to support performance in the natural setting. Modify (adapt) approaches encompass compensatory techniques, including enhancing some features to provide cues, or reducing other features to reduce distractibility.

PREVENT THE OCCURRENCE OR EVOLUTION OF MALPRACTICE PERFORMANCE IN CONTEXT

Therapeutic interventions can prevent the occurrence or evolution of barriers to performance in context. Sometimes, practitioners can predict that certain negative outcomes are

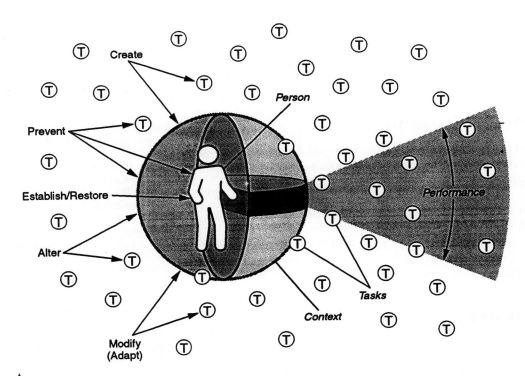

▲

Figure 23-1. Illustration of therapeutic interventions within the *Ecology of Human Performance* framework. The arrows indicate the variables that are affected by each intervention.

likely, without intervention, to change the course of events. Practitioners can create interventions to change the course of events. These interventions may address person, context, task, or a combination of these variables to change the course, thereby enabling functional performance to emerge.

CREATE CIRCUMSTANCES THAT PROMOTE MORE ADAPTABLE OR COMPLEX PERFORMANCE IN CONTEXT

Providers can also design interventions that promote performance in context. The create intervention does not assume a disability is present, or that any factors would interfere with performance. The create intervention focuses on providing enriched contextual and task experiences that will enhance performance for all persons in the natural contexts of life (Dunn, Brown, & McGuigan, 1994; Dunn, Brown, McClain, & Westman, 1994).

▼ APPLICATION TO PRACTICE

Occupational therapy practitioners intervene when people have difficulty with the tasks that make up their occupations. The EHP framework not only considers performance, but also consistently considers the unique nature of performance in context. As review, the primary theoretical postulate fundamental to the EHP framework is that ecology, or the transaction between the person and the context, affects human behavior and task performance, and that performance can be understood only in context. Likewise, task performance affects the person, the context, and the person–context transaction. Therefore, occupational therapy evaluation and intervention options are not constricted to the person variables that affect human performance, but also consider the effects of the context and the person–context match and the effect of the tasks themselves on human performance.

► EDITORS' CONCLUSION

The Model of Human Occupation, Occupational Adaptation, and the Ecology of Human Performance all focus on occupational behavior—the central domain of concern for occupational therapy. All of these theories see occupational behavior as the outcome of interactions between persons and their environments. However, each theory has a different image of the processes behind that interaction. Practitioners can use these different images to gain insight into clients' occupational dysfunctions.

▼ REFERENCES

Allen, C. K. (1992). Models of performance within the cognitive levels. In C. K. Allen, C. A. Earhart, & T. Blue (Eds.), *Occupational therapy treatment goals for the physically and cognitively disabled* (pp. 85–102). Rockville, MD: American Occupational Therapy Association.

American Occupational Therapy Association (AOTA). (1994). Uniform terminology for occupational therapy—third edition. *American Journal of Occupational Therapy, 48*, 1047–1054.

Auerswold, E. H. (1971). Families, change, and the ecological perspective. *Family Process, 10*, 263–280.

Ayres, A. J. (1979). *Sensory integration and the child*. Los Angeles: Western Psychological Services.

Black, M. M. (1976). The occupational career. *American Journal of Occupational Therapy, 30*, 225–228.

Borys, S. S. (1974). Implications of interest theory. *American Journal of Occupational Therapy, 28*, 35–38.

Brofenbrenner, U. (1979). *The ecology of human development*. Cambridge, MA: Harvard University Press.

Burke, J. P. (1977). A clinical perspective on motivation: Pawn versus origin. *American Journal of Occupational Therapy, 31*, 254–258.

Clark, F. A., Parham, D., Carlson, M. E., Frank, G., Jackson, J., Pierce, D., Wolfe, R. J., & Zemke, R. (1991). Occupational science: Academic innovation in the service of occupational therapy's future. *American Journal of Occupational Therapy, 45*, 300–310.

Dunn, W., Brown, C., McClain, L., & Westman, K. (1994). The ecology of human performance: A contextual perspective on human occupation. In C. B. Royeen (Ed.), *AOTA self-study series: The practice of the future: Putting occupation back into therapy*. Rockville, MD: American Occupational Therapy Association.

Dunning, H. (1972). Environmental occupational therapy. *American Journal of Occupational Therapy, 26*, 292–298.

Fidler, G. S. & Fidler, F. W. (1978). Doing and becoming: Purposeful action and self actualization. *American Journal of Occupational Therapy, 32*, 305–310.

Florey, L. L. (1969) Intrinsic motivation: The dynamics of occupational therapy theory. *American Journal of Occupational Therapy, 23*, 319–322.

Ford, K. (1995, March). Occupational adaptation in home health: an occupational therapist's viewpoint. *Home and Community Health Special Interest Section Newsletter*, pp. 3–4.

Garrett, S. & Schkade, J. K. (1995). Occupational adaptation model of professional development as applied to level II fieldwork. *American Journal of Occupational Therapy, 49*, 119–126.

Gibson, J. & Schkade, J. K. (1997). Occupational adaptation with CVA: A clinical study. *American Journal of Occupational Therapy, 51*. 523–529.

Gray, M. (1972). Effects of hospitalization on work–play behavior. *American Journal of Occupational Therapy, 26*, 180–185.

Hall, E. T. (1983). *The dance of life*. New York: Doubleday.

Hart, R. (1979). *Children's experience of place*. New York: Irvington.

Heard, C. (1977). Occupational role acquisition: A perspective on the chronically disabled. *American Journal of Occupational Therapy, 31*, 243–247.

Helfrich, C. & Kielhofner, G. (1994). Volitional narratives and the meaning of therapy. *American Journal of Occupational Therapy, 48*, 318–326.

Helfrich, C., Kielhofner, G., & Mattingly. C. (1994). Volition as narrative: Understanding motivation in chronic illness. *The American Journal of Occupational Therapy, 48*, 311–317.

Holahan, C. J. (1986). Environmental psychology. *Annual Review of Psychology, 37*, 381–307.

Howe, M. C. & Briggs, A. K. (1982). Ecological systems model for occupational therapy. *American Journal of Occupational Therapy, 36*, 322–327.

Hurff, J. M. (1980). A play skills inventory: A competency monitoring tool for the 10 year old. *American Journal of Occupational Therapy, 34*, 651–656.

Kielhofner, G. (1977). Temporal adaptation: A conceptual framework for occupational therapy. *American Journal of Occupational Therapy, 31*, 235–242 .

Kielhofner, G. (1985). *A model of human occupation: Theory and application*. Baltimore, MD: Williams & Wilkins.

Kielhofner, G. (1995). *A model of human occupation: Theory and application* (2nd ed.). Baltimore: Williams & Wilkins.

Kielhofner, G. & Burke, J. P. (1977). Occupational therapy after 60 years: An account of changing identity and knowledge. *American Journal of Occupational Therapy, 31,* 675–689.

Kielhofner, G. & Burke, J. P. (1980). A model of human occupation, Part 1. Conceptual framework and content. *American Journal of Occupational Therapy, 34,* 572–581.

Kiernat, J. M. (1992). Environment: The hidden modality. *Journal of Physical and Occupational Therapy in Geriatrics, 21,* 3–12.

King, L. J. (1978). Toward a science of adaptive responses. *American Journal of Occupational Therapy, 32,* 429–437.

Law, M., Cooper., B., Strong, S., Stewart, D., Rigby, P., & Letts, L. (1996). The person–environment–occupation model: A transactive approach to occupational perfection. *Canadian Journal of Occupational Therapy, 3* (1), 9–23.

Llorens, L. A. (1970). Facilitating growth and development: The promise of occupational therapy. *American Journal of Occupational Therapy, 24,* 93–101.

Matsutsuyu, J. (1969). The interest check list. *American Journal of Occupational Therapy 23,* 323–328.

Matsutsuyu, J. (1971). Occupational behavior–a perspective on work and play. *American Journal of Occupational Therapy, 25,* 291–294.

Meyer, A. (1922). The philosophy of occupational therapy. *Archives of Occupational Therapy, 1,* 1.

Michelman, S. (1971). The importance of creative play. *American Journal of Occupational Therapy, 25,* 285–290.

Moorhead, L. (1969). The occupational history. *American Journal of Occupational Therapy, 23,* 329–334.

Mosey, A. C. (1981). *Occupational therapy: Configuration of a profession.* New York: Raven.

Nelson, D. (1988). Occupation: Form and performance. *American Journal of Occupational Therapy, 42,* 633–641.

Parent, L. H. (1978). Effects of a low-stimulus environment on behavior. *American Journal of Occupational Therapy, 32,* 19–25.

Pasek, P. B. & Schkade, J. K. (1996). Effects of a skiing experience on adolescents with limb deficiencies: An occupational adaptation perspective. *American Journal of Occupational Therapy, 50,* 24–31.

Reilly, M. (1962). Occupational therapy can be one of the great ideas of 20th century medicine. *American Journal of Occupational Therapy, 16,* 1–9.

Reilly, M. (1966). A psychiatric occupational program as a teaching model. *American Journal of Occupational Therapy, 20,* 61–67.

Reilly, M. (1969) The educational process. *American Journal of Occupational Therapy, 23,* 299–307.

Robinson, A. L. (1977). Play the arena for acquisition of rules for competent behavior. *American Journal of Occupational Therapy, 31,* 248–253.

Ross, M. M. (1994, August 11). Applying theory to practice. *O. T. Week,* pp. 16–17.

Schkade, J. K. & Schultz, S. (1992a). Occupational adaptation: Toward a holistic approach to contemporary practice. Part 1. *American Journal of Occupational Therapy, 46,* 829–837.

Schultz, S. & Schkade, J. K. (1992b). Occupational adaptation: Toward a holistic approach to contemporary practice. Part 2. *American Journal of Occupational Therapy, 46,* 917–925.

Schkade, J. K. & Schultz, S. (1993). Occupational adaptation: An integrative frame of reference. In Hopkins, H. & Smith, H. (Eds.), *Willard and Spackman's Occupational Therapy* (8th ed.). Philadelphia: J. B. Lippincott.

Schultz, S. & Schkade, J. K. (1994, September). Home health care: A window of opportunity to synthesize practice. *Home & Community Health Special Interest Section Newsletter,* pp. 1–4.

Shannon, P. (1972). Work–play theory and the occupational therapy process. *American Journal of Occupational Therapy, 26,* 169–172.

Spencer, J. C. (1991). The physical environment and performance. In C. Christiansen & C. Baum (Eds.), *Occupational therapy: Overcoming human performance deficits* (pp. 125–140). New York: Slack.

Wicker, A. W. (1979). *An introduction to ecological psychology.* Cambridge, England: Cambridge University Press.

Chapter 24

Theories Derived from Rehabilitation Perspectives

Section 1: Rehabilitaion Perspectives

Section 2: Rehabilitative Frame of Reference

Section 3: Biomechanical Frame of Reference

Section 1

Rehabilitation Perspectives

Alice C. Seidel

Defining Rehabilitation
Historical Roots of Rehabilitation
Effect of Legislation on Rehabilitation
Occupational Therapy and the Rehabilitation
   Movement

▼ DEFINING REHABILITATION

Rehabilitation is the process of restoring an individual's capacity to participate in functional activities when the capacity has been altered or limited by a physical or mental impairment. The World Health Organization (WHO) defines *rehabilitation* as "the combined and coordinated use of medical, social, educational and vocational measures for training and retraining the individual to the highest levels of functional ability" (cited in Hagedorn, 1992, p. 42). Rehabilitation does not cure the illness or replace lost organ function, but it does enable performance of self-care, work, and leisure activities. Rehabilitation teaches clients compensatory methods for performing activities, provides assistive devices, and adapts environments so that people may function in their social roles and life-worlds (Dutton, 1995; Guillickson & Licht, 1968; Mattingly & Fleming, 1993).

The WHO's model of disablement defines terminology associated with rehabilitation: impairment, disability, and handicap. *Impairment* is the "loss or abnormality of psychological, physiological or anatomical structure or function" (WHO, 1980, p. 47). For example, a person with an amputa-

tion of his or her right forearm, has an impairment of the right upper extremity. When an impairment is severe enough to limit function of a task, the individual has a disability. A *disability* is "any restriction or lack of ability to perform an activity in a manner or within the range considered normal" (WHO, 1980, p. 143). The person with an impaired right upper extremity is unable to tie his or her shoes and, therefore, he or she has a disability. When a person with a persistent disability is unable to complete activities that fulfill the essential responsibilities and duties of a social role, he or she is handicapped. WHO defines *handicap* as a "disadvantage for a given individual resulting from an impairment or disability that limits or prevents the fulfillment of a role that is normal for that individual" (WHO, 1980, p. 183). These definitions provide a framework for describing levels of function among clients who participate in rehabilitation.

▼ HISTORICAL ROOTS OF REHABILITATION

Before the early 19th century, persons with disabilities were cared for by family members within the home. Outside of the immediate family unit, few people knew about the needs of individuals with physical or mental disabilities. Persons with disabilities were isolated and sheltered from societal attitudes about disabilities. In an effort to educate others about the needs of their impaired members, caregiving families formed groups. These groups, formed around families' experiences, became the first formal organizations that advocated for the needs of persons with impairments. They represented the earliest efforts to shift the issues of disability from the family to society. Contemporary consumer advocacy groups and governmental programs that fund rehabilitation programs and services continue this long tradition of societal participation in meeting the needs of persons with disabilities (Groce, 1992; Gullickson & Licht, 1968).

The shift of care from the family unit to the community led to the development of rehabilitation institutions and programs. Rehabilitation facilities were created through the education and advocacy efforts of family organizations. As industrialization forced women, the primary caregivers, to work outside the home, the idea of placing a family member with a disability in a residential rehabilitation center gained societal acceptance. Early facilities did not attempt to teach residents how to achieve independence or functional competency in caring for themselves; instead they provided shelter and basic care (Groce, 1992). This concept of rehabilitation as care giving remained unchanged until World War II (WW II). After WW II, rehabilitation facilities started teaching residents how to function as independently as possible in their daily living activities (ADL).

The change in the philosophy of rehabilitation was created by the large number of WW II veterans who returned from the battlefields with disabilities. Medical advances in the treatment of war injuries enabled large numbers of soldiers to survive, despite permanent physical impairments. These soldiers returned to their hometowns as wounded, disabled veterans who wanted to resume their former social, family, and worker roles. Society could not ignore the needs of men and women who had lost their ability to function normally while serving the country. (Groce, 1992; Gullickson & Licht, 1968).

To meet the needs of these soldiers, veterans hospitals, built in the United States during WW I to provide residential care for veterans, expanded to include restorative services. Funded by the government, veteran hospitals became national leaders in advancing the philosophy of rehabilitation. They provided the most up-to-date medical, social, and vocational services to return veterans to their social roles. Rehabilitation personnel trained to provide occupational therapy, physical therapy, and vocational counseling were prepared in academic programs funded by the government. The mid-1940s, post-WW II, marked the beginning of long-term government funding of rehabilitation programs, facilities, and personnel (Groce, 1992).

Rehabilitation became a medical specialty during the post-WW II era. Chronic illness and diseases became more prevalent and medical advances enabled people to survive accidents and traumatic injuries with permanent disabilities. These changes in health and illness patterns, led to the development of a medical specialty called rehabilitation medicine or physical medicine. Specialists in rehabilitation medicine or physical medicine are called physiatrists; they specialize in serving the medical needs of persons with physical impairments. Initial efforts to organize rehabilitation medicine as a specialty occurred in veterans hospitals which provided a service-delivery model for the development of civilian rehabilitation centers (Licht, 1968).

Rehabilitation medicine highlighted the importance of enabling people with chronic illness and diseases to live productive lives. It also introduced the concept of a treatment team composed of professionals trained in the area of rehabilitation. The rehabilitation team usually includes a physiatrist, physical therapist, occupational therapy practitioner, vocational counselor, and a rehabilitation nurse. Additional members may include a prosthetist, orthotist, speech pathologist, recreational therapist, and psychologist.

Much of the early writing about rehabilitation as a medical specialty suggests that the restoration of physical function dominated the philosophy and goals of programs and professionals. Rehabilitation services for persons with mental illness is given minimal attention and when mentioned, focuses on community reentry (Fidler, 1993).

▼ EFFECT OF LEGISLATION ON REHABILITATION

Federal legislation that funded rehabilitation programs, facilities, services, and training for personnel helped advance rehabilitation in the United States. Vocational rehabilitation received its initial funding in 1918 and 1920 from legislation enacted to support rehabilitation services for individuals with physical impairments. Medical and psychiatric rehabilitation services remained unfunded until the passage of 1943 amendments to the earlier vocational rehabilitation legislation. These amendments strengthened the ability of rehabilitation programs to serve the vocational needs of persons with mental impairments. Subsequent amendments in 1954 and 1963 expanded the concept of rehabilitation from a biorehabilitation to a social rehabilitation model. The shift to a social rehabilitation model emphasized the restoration of an individual "to maximum usefulness to himself, his family and his community" (cited in Reed, 1984, p. 77). The concept of social rehabilitation resulted in federal funds for research and the training of rehabilitation personnel, such as occupational therapy practitioners, who would provide services that enabled persons with disabilities to function in social, family, and community activities (Reed, 1984).

American rehabilitation services and programs during the 1960s and 1970s were affected by the social movements of Civil Rights and deinstitutionalization of persons with chronic mental impairments. The philosophical underpinnings of these movements stimulated the Independent Living Movement which advocated for community reintegration of persons with physical impairments. The Independent Living Movement, funded by vocational rehabilitation amendments, created community-based programs, such as wheelchair repair shops and transportation services, for persons confined to wheelchairs, that enabled persons with disabilities to live in groups homes or assisted-living apartments. Most important, the Independent Living Movement advocated persistently and loudly for the inclusion of persons with disabilities in the mainstream of community life. Rehabilitation professionals and consumers involved in the Independent Living Movement laid the foundation that would eventually become The American Disabilities Act (ADA) of 1993—landmark legislation that ensures the rights of persons with disabilities to fully participate in society.

▼ OCCUPATIONAL THERAPY AND THE REHABILITATION MOVEMENT

Concern for the preservation and restoration of an individual's functional abilities made occupational therapy practitioners early advocates for rehabilitation services. In WW I, "reconstruction aides" provided restorative services at battlefield sites to soldiers suffering from battle fatigue and mental trauma. Reconstruction aides, who later would become trainers of future generations of occupational therapy practitioners, used vocational-based crafts, such as woodworking, to teach soldiers trades they could use in civilian work roles. Reconstruction aides would return from the battlefields to veterans hospitals to continue their restorative work with soldiers. They would eventually establish similar programs in civilian hospitals and train nurses and social workers in the use of activity to rehabilitate individuals institutionalized with mental impairments.

The growth of rehabilitation services after WW II led to an increased demand for trained occupational therapy practitioners. Because of the large number of soldiers returning from WW II battle sites with permanent physical injuries, occupational therapy practitioners began to specialize in the rehabilitation of individuals with physical impairments. The specialty of "physical disabilities" gained popularity among therapists. The areas of prosthetics, orthotics, and the application of assistive devices expanded and became integral parts of the rehabilitation process.

When rehabilitation moved toward a community model, occupational therapy practitioners often spearheaded the development and implementation of programs that occurred in independent-living centers or transitional housing settings.

Occupational therapy practitioners frequently use two practice theories or frames of reference derived from rehabilitation principles: the rehabilitation and biomechanical frames of reference. The following sections describe these frames of reference.

Section 2

Rehabilitative Frame of Reference

Alice C. Seidel

> Philosophy
> Intellectual Heritage
> Definitions and Assumptions
> Effects on Evaluation
> Mechanisms for Change
> Strengths and Limitations
> Future Research

▼ PHILOSOPHY

The rehabilitative frame of reference embraces the philosophy of rehabilitation: to enable a person with a physical or mental disability or chronic illness to achieve maximum function in the performance of his or her daily activities. Rehabilitation is used when medical or surgical remediation of an impairment is not possible or completed (Hagedorn, 1992; Trombly, 1995). Rehabilitation emphasizes an individual's abilities; therefore, the rehabilitative frame of reference focuses on compensatory methods, assistive devices, and environmental adaptations the individual needs to function in spite of his or her impairment.

▼ INTELLECTUAL HERITAGE

Knowledge bases that contribute to the rehabilitative frame of reference include the medical sciences, and the physical and social sciences. The medical sciences help practitioners understand the influence of pathological processes on an individual's abilities to function in ADLs. Physical sciences help practitioners understand the biomechanics of human movement, design or select assistive devices that promote function, and modify an environment to help an individual with a disability function more effectively. The social sciences contribute important knowledge about how individuals and societies respond to chronic illness and disability.

▼ DEFINITIONS AND ASSUMPTIONS

Rehabilitation is the process of helping a person with a disability perform competently in his or her social roles and daily activities. The rehabilitative frame of reference emphasizes the teaching of compensatory techniques; the use of adaptive and assistive equipment; and the modification of environments to eliminate barriers to function. Dutton (1995) identifies five assumptions of the rehabilitative frame of reference:

1. Through the use of compensation strategies and techniques an individual can restore independence when the underlying impairment can not be remediated.
2. A person's level of motivation affects the extent to which an individual regains independence.
3. Environments in which daily activities are performed influence a person's motivation for independence.
4. Rehabilitation involves the teaching–learning process. Therefore, cognitive skills are needed to learn and apply compensatory methods. Motivation enables the individual to participate fully in the teaching–learning process.
5. Clinical reasoning, used by the practitioner, begins with the individual's functional capabilities, then moves to the environments in which the person will function, and then to the types of compensatory strategies the person needs to use his or her capabilities.

▼ EFFECTS ON EVALUATION

In the rehabilitative frame of reference, an evaluation is used to assess a client's function in self-care, work, and leisure activities. The results of this evaluation provides a picture of the person's capabilities and competencies in daily activities. The occupational therapist uses several types of assessment methods: observations of client performance in selected activities, interviews about a client's daily living priorities, and client self-reports about his or her level of competency in daily activities (Dutton, 1995). Most commonly the therapist uses all three assessment methods to evaluate a client's function in daily activities.

Throughout an evaluation, the occupational therapist pays attention to several factors associated with an individual's functional status: (1) characteristics of environments in which the client functions; (2) equipment and economic resources used by the client; (3) levels of supervision and assistance available to the client; (4) developmental expectations for the client's performance; and (5) performance components that are absent or limiting a client's function. The therapist's analysis of evaluation data provides a picture of the client's capabilities and areas that need intervention (Dutton, 1995; Trombly, 1995).

▼ MECHANISMS FOR CHANGE

Occupational therapy practitioners using the rehabilitative frame of reference assume that the client's impairment is stabilized and can not be altered by therapeutic interventions. The client's capacity to function in daily activities, however, can be changed through his or her use of compensatory methods and adaptive equipment. Therefore, the teaching–learning process is a major part of occupational therapy treatment. The practitioner teaches the client compensatory methods to perform ADLs and ways to apply these new techniques to his or her self-care, work, and play or leisure routines (Trombly, 1995).

Change in a client's functional abilities depends on several client-centered factors. The client must demonstrate sufficient motivation to participate in the teaching–learning process and use new compensation methods or assistive devices. The client's cognitive and perceptual performance component skills will influence his or her ability to learn and apply new compensatory methods. The environment in which therapy occurs is essential to a client's learning. This environment needs to include the necessary equipment, objects, and support and feedback systems that contribute to the client's motivation for change and to his or her learning style (Trombly, 1995).

The rehabilitative frame of reference uses daily-living, work, and leisure activities as the purposeful activities of occupational therapy treatment. Treatment programs occur in the environment that is natural for the performance of the daily activities. For example, a practitioner would teach a client compensatory methods for bathing in a fully equipped bathroom that contains the assistive devices and equipment the client needs to achieve competent performance. Opportunities to practice and apply the newly learned compensatory methods are important elements of the treatment process.

Practitioner–client collaboration is important in the rehabilitative frame of reference (Dutton, 1995; Trombly, 1989). The client is expected to cooperate in learning and practicing new compensatory strategies (Hagedorn, 1992). By participating in the problem-solving process of treatment, clients learn skills they will use outside the therapeutic milieu. Practitioners use reinforcers and demonstration to create environments that support client learning. Another important factor in the therapeutic relationship is the occupational therapy practitioner's creativity in devising compensatory methods, adaptive equipment, and learning environments that fit with the client's capabilities and limitations (Trombly, 1995).

▼ STRENGTHS AND LIMITATIONS

The rehabilitative frame of reference has enjoyed a long and successful history in occupational therapy because it includes the core values of occupational therapy. It focuses on a client's capabilities and daily activities that are important to him or her (Hagedorn, 1992). The therapeutic relationship is client-centered and requires collaboration to problem solve and create compensatory methods for the client's performance of everyday activities. The evaluation process addresses a client's interests, roles, resources, environments, and support systems, thereby providing the occupational therapy practitioner a holistic perspective of a client's function in daily activities.

There are limitations to the rehabilitative frame of reference that can not be overlooked. Some ADL instruments lack reliability and validity data and are designed specifically and exclusively for a particular setting (Dutton, 1995). This absence of reliability and validity data limits the use of some ADL evaluations in outcome research.

Successful outcomes in the rehabilitative frame of reference depend heavily on client motivation and participation in the teaching–learning process. The unmotivated client is not addressed in this frame of reference. When compensatory methods do not work or a client is unable to learn new approaches, this frame of reference provides no alternative ones. Also, this frame of reference does not address the psychosocial needs of clients, which reflects its historical linkages to physical medicine.

The rehabilitative frame of reference is linked closely to the medical model and, particularly, to physical rehabilitation, which emphasizes the individual with a physical impairment. Therefore, the rehabilitative frame of reference is most closely associated with the physical disabilities area of occupational therapy practice. The rehabilitative frame of reference is seldom presented as a model for designing occupational therapy programs for clients with mental impairments.

▼ FUTURE RESEARCH

An important area for research in the rehabilitative frame of reference is the establishment of reliability and validity for ADL evaluation instruments so therapists can use these assessment tools to conduct functional outcome studies using the rehabilitative frame of reference. Another area of research is the use of the rehabilitative frame of reference in occupational therapy programs for individuals with mental impairments. Because client motivation is a requisite for successful outcomes under the rehabilitative frame of reference, the contribution and importance of this client characteristic is also an appropriate area for occupational therapy research.

Section 3

Biomechanical Frame of Reference

Rebecca Dutton

▼ INTELLECTUAL HERITAGE

Baldwin was the first health care professional to analyze joint and muscle function during purposeful activity. Before WW I, purposeful activities were used strictly for diversion with psychiatric clients. Baldwin also developed tests to see if clients were achieving their goals of increased range and strength. Dr. Licht added the concern of work tolerance, which we call now refer to as endurance training (Reed, 1984).

▼ DEFINITIONS

The six domains of concern for the biomechanical frame of reference are (1) structural stability, (2) low-level endurance, (3) edema control, (4) passive range of motion (ROM), (5) strength, and (6) high-level endurance (Dutton, 1995).

Increasing passive ROM, strength, and high-level endurance have been biomechanical concerns since the 1940s. Therapists used to be able to assume that structural stability was present before stressing peripheral structures. Changes in the length of hospital stays require therapists to treat clients very early while they still have partially healed bones and soft tissue. It is dangerous to separate structural stability from biomechanical issues in today's health care system.

Endurance used to be placed at the end of the biomechanical treatment sequence because therapists used to get well-rested clients with the ability to tolerate sedentary activity. Today, treatment can begin immediately at bedside in intensive care so that low level endurance, such as the ability to perform morning care while sitting unsupported, may be absent. Endurance now needs to be divided into early low-level and later high-level training. Edema control has been separated from passive ROM because so many techniques have been developed specifically for this problem. Therapists are very aggressive about treating edema because the effects of uncontrolled long-term edema can be devastating.

▼ ASSUMPTIONS

The biomechanical frame of reference has four assumptions (Dutton, 1995):

1. Purposeful activities can be used to treat loss of ROM, strength, and endurance.
2. After ROM, strength, and endurance are regained, the client will automatically regain function.
3. The principle of rest and stress: first, the body must rest to heal itself; then structures must be stressed to regain range, strength, and endurance.
4. The biomechanical frame of reference is best suited for clients with an intact central nervous system (Pedretti & Pasquinelli, 1990) because clients must be able to perform smooth, isolated movements.

▼ EFFECTS ON EVALUATION

Evaluation is restricted to the six domains of concern listed in the foregoing. Only the physician is licensed to evaluate the status of structural stability, by reading x-ray films (Dutton, 1995). Tests for low-level endurance include using cardiac step charts and recording the duration that a client can tolerate a sedentary activity. Therapists have formal evaluations for edema such as volumetry, for ROM such as goniometry, and for strength such as manual muscle testing. Formal tests are supplemented by clinical observations, such as end feels during ROM (Clarkson & Gilewich, 1989), and by specialty tests, such as muscle palpation. Tests for high-level endurance include recording the number of repetitions or duration that a client can perform an activity and using metabolic equivalents (MET) levels (see Table 16–22 in Chap. 16).

▼ EFFECTS ON CLIENT–PRACTITIONER INTERACTIONS

To empower the client, the practitioner must clearly explain the connection between the general deficit, the biomechanical goal, and the functional outcome (Dutton, 1995). For example:

General deficit: loss of ROM of the burned left hand because of hypertrophic scarring.
Measurable biomechanical goal: increasing MP flexion to 70 degrees, PIP flexion to 50 degrees, and DIP flexion to 15 degrees will permit.
Functional outcome: hand closure on gardening tools.

It is vital to link the biomechanical goal, such as increased finger flexion, to a functional outcome, such as gardening. Third-party payers use this link to justify the need for therapy (Allen & Foto, 1991; Dahl, 1990; Pinson, 1991). Clients need to know why they are participating in stressful and sometimes painful treatment. In the foregoing example, the practitioner wants to document an increase in finger flexion. The client wants to know if he can take care of his lovely garden again. The client–practitioner relationship must integrate both agendas.

▼ STRENGTHS AND LIMITATIONS

It is easy to write measurable biomechanical goals because this frame of reference uses quantitative evaluation data, such as degrees of ROM. However, because this frame of reference is one of the oldest treatment approaches, some biomechanical goals may still be written as service goals, which was the standard years ago. Service goals describe what the practitioner will do (Denton, 1987) such as provide heat, manual stretch, splinting, and patient education. Service goals are no longer acceptable for the purposes of reimbursement and research. As shown by the foregoing example, biomechanical goals must be written as outcome goals that describe what new performance components, such as increased ROM, and functional gains the client will exhibit.

The debate about whether both exercise and purposeful activity are legitimate tools of occupational therapy has divided the profession for a long time (Dutton, 1989). Yet, changes caused by managed health care have made time management very valuable. Although exercises can be used to increase strength and endurance, purposeful activities can save time because they tell clients how and when to move. For example, even though free weights could be used to simultaneously perform isometric left arm extension and concentric right arm flexion, why not gradually raise the torque on a compound bow to strengthen the exact muscle groups and types of muscle contractions needed for archery? Many self-care activities, such as eating, dressing, and bathing, are not suited to frequent daily repetitions, but many games, crafts, and work-related tasks inherently require endurance, so why not use them?

Treatment concerns ignored by the biomechanical frame of reference include pain, loss of sensation, and incoordination. Yet many clients with medical conditions, such as burns, spinal cord injuries, rheumatoid arthritis, and traumatic hand injuries, have pain and a loss of sensation that interferes with coordinated movement. These problems cannot be remediated with biomechanical techniques such as resistance and repetitions. Sensory motor treatment approaches are needed to supplement the biomechanical frame of reference for many clients.

▼ FUTURE RESEARCH

Research on functional gains is sparse because practitioners have assumed that functional gains will happen automatically if biomechanical goals are achieved. Yet, practitioners cannot assume that clients will generalize biomechanical gains, even when the clients are cognitively intact and well-educated. Clients may believe that doing home exercises twice a day will maintain gains achieved in the hospital despite constant disuse (Dutton, 1989). A client with a frozen shoulder may not notice that he or she has developed the clever strategy of using lateral trunk flexion to reach for clothes in the closet, despite regaining full shoulder motion. A brief evaluation of a few functional activities may be needed to detect and eliminate unnecessary compensatory habits.

Recent studies on functional gains have been looking for a global connection between biomechanical gains and a composite score for ADL. Glynn and Morgan (1990) found a low correlation between a composite ADL score and the Jebsen Hand Function Test. This finding is logical, because a client needs refined hand function for only a few ADLs, such as buttoning a shirt. Safaee-Rad and colleagues (1990) found that feeding requires no more than 45 degrees of shoulder ROM, so all gains in shoulder ROM are not related to all ADL tasks. What is needed are studies of the relationship between specific biomechanical gains and specific functional outcomes.

▶ EDITORS' CONCLUSION

The rehabilitation and biomechanical frames of reference are both derived from rehabilitation perspectives that have emerged during the history of rehabilitation. Both frames of reference focus on clients' physical impairments. Practitioners using the rehabilitative frame of reference would teach clients to compensate for their physical problems; practitioners using the biomechnical frame of reference would try to remediate specific client impairments. A practitioner might use both frames of reference simultaneously with any given client, teaching adaptations for those performance components that are not likely to improve, and offering remedial treatments for deficits that might improve. Before using either of these practice theories practitioners need to consider the strengths and weaknesses of each in relation to clients' particular situations and priorities.

▼ REFERENCES

Allen, K. A. & Foto, M. (1991). Reporting occupational therapy outcomes with the ICIDH codes. *Physical Disabilities Special Interest Section Newsletter, 14* (2), 2–3.

Clarkson, H. M. & Gilewich, G. B. (1989). *Musculoskeletal assessment.* Baltimore: Williams & Wilkins.

Dahl, M. (1990). *Money and reimbursement versus OT practice.* Pennsylvania Occupational Therapy Association workshop. Philadelphia, PA.

Denton, P. L. (1987). *Psychiatric occupational therapy: A workbook of practical skills.* Boston: Little, Brown & Co.

Dutton, R. (1989). Guidelines for using both activity and exercise. *American Journal of Occupational Therapy, 43,* 573–580.

Dutton, R. (1995). *Clinical reasoning in physical disabilities.* Baltimore: Williams & Wilkins.

Fidler, G. S. (1993). The challenge of change to occupational therapy pratice. In R. P. F. Contrell (Ed.), *Psychosocial occupational therapy.* Bethesda, MD: American Occupational Therapy Association.

Glynn, J. W. & Morgan, V. R. (1990). You can do research in the clinic. *Advance for Occupational Therapy, 6,* 1–3.

Groce, N. (1992). *The U. S. role in international disability activities: A history and a look towards the future.* (Grant # G0087C2013). Oakland, CA: World Institute on Disability.

Gullickson, G. & Licht, S. (1968). Definition and philosophy of rehabilitation medicine. In S. Licht (Ed.), *Rehabilitation and medicine* (pp. 1–13). Baltimore: Waverly Press.

Hagedorn, R. (1992). *Occupational therapy: Foundations for practice. Models, frames of references and core skills.* New York: Churchill Livingstone.

Mattingly, C. & Fleming, M. H. (1993). *Clinical reasoning: Forms of inquiry in a therapeutic process.* Philadelphia: F. A. Davis.

Pedretti, L. W. & Pasquinelli, S. (1990). A frame of reference for occupational therapy in physical dysfunction. In L. W. Pedretti, & B. Zoltan (Eds.), *Occupational therapy practice skills for physical dysfunction* (3rd ed.). Philadelphia: C. V. Mosby.

Pinson, C. C. (1991). Work programs reimbursement: What is happening across the nation? *Physical Disabilities Special Interest Section Newsletter, 14* (2), 4–5.

Reed, K. L. (1984). *Models of practice in occupational therapy.* Baltimore: Williams & Wilkins.

Safaee-Rad, R., Shwedyk, E., Quanbury, A. O., & Cooper, J. E. (1990). Normal functional range motion of upper limb joints during performance of three feeding activities. *Archives of Physical Medicine and Rehabilitation, 71,* 505–509.

Trombly, C. A. (1995). Theoretical foundations for practice. In C. A. Trombly, (Ed.), *Occupational therapy for physical dysfunction.* (4th ed., pp 15–27). Baltimore: Williams & Wilkins.

World Health Organization. (1980). *International classification of impairments, disabilities and handicaps* (ICIDH). Geneva, Switzerland: Author.

Chapter 25

Theories Derived from Infant and Child Developmental Perspectives

Section 1: Overview of Infant and Child Developmental Models

Section 2: Neurodevelopmental Theory

Section 3: Sensory Integration

Section I

Overview of Infant and Child Developmental Models

Rosemarie Bigsby

Historical Perspective on Developmental Models

The Hierarchical Model: Continuity and Predictability in Normal Development

Contextual Models: The Influence of Experience and Features of the Environment

Broadening Frames of Reference for Intervention to Incorporate Changing Views

▼ HISTORICAL PERSPECTIVE ON DEVELOPMENTAL MODELS

The scientific view on infant and child development as a process has changed dramatically during the 20th century. Until the last two decades, developmental theorists viewed development as a predictable, stepwise sequence dependent on maturation of the central nervous system (CNS). Now they see development as a variable process dependent on a complex interaction between a child's biological endowment, the immediate caregiving environment, the community and the society, or culture within which the child is being raised (Freel, 1996; Wachs, 1992).

▼ THE HIERARCHICAL MODEL: CONTINUITY AND PREDICTABILITY IN NORMAL DEVELOPMENT

Early views on development were dominated by observational studies of motor and cognitive development (Gesell, 1928; Piaget, 1952) that presumed a hierarchical model (ie, one in which normal development occurs in a predictable sequence of steps). The process underlying this linear progression in development was thought to be biologically predetermined, and directly related to hierarchical changes in CNS development. Although increasingly complex functions are known to emerge as the CNS develops, brain–behavior relationships are not necessarily as direct as was previously thought. The hierarchical model does not explain the variability and flexibility seen in motor and cognitive behavior among normally developing children, or the profound influence of CNS plasticity and the environment on development.

▼ CONTEXTUAL MODELS: THE INFLUENCE OF EXPERIENCE AND FEATURES OF THE ENVIRONMENT

Periods of variability in performance were recognized by early theorists, who described them as a time of "interweaving" of new, unrefined behaviors with old, established ones (Gesell, 1928); an adaptation sequence involving assimilation of new with previous experiences, accommodation to changing circumstances, and eventual progression to a new, higher level of functioning (Piaget, 1952). This theory of adaptation has held a dominant role in occupational therapy as it incorporates adjustment to disruption or change, as well as the roles of purposeful activity, self-direction, and motivation in coping with stress and challenge (Gilfoyle, Grady, & Moore 1981; King, 1978; Llorens, 1969). Still, this model failed to address those periods in normal development, often just before a shift to a higher level of performance, when infants and young children not only exhibit variability in their behavior, but actually appear to lose previously acquired skills. Using motor develpments as an example, McGraw's longitudinal study during the 1930s was one of the first to suggest that such periods of disorganization may actually perform a function (ie, to fuel development) (Dalton, 1996). Decades later, theorists are returning their attention to these processes, recognizing that motor development is dynamic and variable, "a product of not only the central nervous system but also of the biomechanical and energetic properties of the body, the environmental support, and the specific (and sometimes changing) demands of the particular task" (Thelen, 1995, p. 81).

Dynamical explanations for development of motor control were first put forth by Bernstein (1967), who questioned the feasibility of a motor system that relies on a centrally programmed one-to-one relationship between CNS connections and action. Bernstein proposed that movements are the product of coordinated action by groups of muscles, and they are subject to the biomechanical constraints imposed by the weight and size of the limbs, as well as the demands and opportunities for flexibility inherent in the environment. Dynamical theory posits that the disequilibrium seen before a change in development is the response of a stable system to perturbations imposed by one or several of the foregoing influences. A characteristic of the coordinative structures that support movement is that they are self-regulating (ie, they are "attracted" to their previous stable state after a perturbation, for example, introduction of a new task or challenge). However, in a dynamic system a temporary loss of stability provides the opportunity for change to a new movement strategy. As development proceeds, changes in the body and new task-related challenges within the environment combine to disrupt an otherwise stable pattern of movement, permitting flexibility of response and eventual change. If there is sufficient flexibility within postural components, new movement strategies will be attempted under varying conditions and constraints, and reinforced through use (Sporns & Edelman, 1993). The broader the range of "affordances" (ie, facilitators for action) available within the environment, the greater the possibilities for change (Gibson, 1979). Thus, action, in and of itself, provides an influence on perceptual and motor experience that is unique to the individual.

Dynamical theory does not specifically address the varying degrees of purposefulness and motivation inherent in a task, although the potential influence of such psychosocial factors on development is significant (Thelen, 1995). Sameroff and Chandler (1975) emphasized the need to focus beyond biological risk and genetic endowment, to examine not only environment, but more specifically, the combined contributions of child and caregiver to early development. Thus, the child, the caregiver and the social and physical environment *each* may contribute substantially and interdependently to developmental outcome. This transactional model acknowledges potential effects of socioeconomic status, social support, infant–caregiver reciprocity, and individual behavioral characteristics of infants and caregivers on development. Rather than focusing on single factors, such as medical risk, therapists who wish to assist families in optimizing child outcomes are now encouraged to consider the family within their environment as a contextual unit, thereby involving family members in evaluating needs and identifying priorities for intervention. This approach to service provision, termed family-centered care (Dunst, Trivette, & Deal, 1988; Simeonsson & Bailey, 1990) brings health care professionals closer to understanding the complex interplay of factors that influence a growing child's health and development.

▼ BROADENING FRAMES OF REFERENCE FOR INTERVENTION TO INCORPORATE CHANGING VIEWS

Occupational therapy practitioners need to draw from various developmental models to construct principles for effective pediatric occupational therapy intervention. As research continues to identify factors that influence development to a greater or lesser extent, developmental models, and the treatment principles that are based on them, need to be continually modified. In the interim, it may be useful to approach developmental intervention from two broad perspectives: elements of developmental risk and protection, and "goodness of fit" (Lester et al, 1994). Occupational therapy practitioners might ask: What are the elements of risk and of protection inherent in this child and family system that can influence development? How can occupational therapy intervention be used to reduce risk and strengthen protective factors within the child, the family, and the environment? In this approach, individual needs of the child and caregivers (elements of risk) and capacities of each (elements of protection) are evaluated within the context of the environment. The focus of interventions is to achieve a fit between the needs and capacities of the child, and those of each member of the family system, while considering environmental affordances and influences.

The following sections of this chapter discuss two occupational therapy frames of reference that were derived from hierarchical theory. In light of more current theories, each frame of reference has undergone its own developmental process, emerging in a modified form that takes into account some of the converging influences on development. Successful occupational therapy practitioners will avoid basing their interventions on a single frame of reference which could be grounded in out-dated theory, remaining conscious of the need to continually assess the validity of those theories that underly their approaches to developmental intervention.

Section 2

Neurodevelopmental Theory
Rebecca Dutton

> Definitions
> Intellectual Heritage
> Assumptions
> Effects on Evaluation
> Effects on Client—Practitioner Interactions
> Strengths, Limitations, and Research

▼ DEFINITIONS

The three domains of concern for the **Neurodevelopmental Treatment** (NDT) frame of reference are axial control, automatic reactions, and limb dissociation (Dutton, 1995). Axial control was ignored by other frames of reference until the founders of NDT—the Bobaths—pointed out that postural adjustments of the neck and trunk create an important foundation for all limb movements (Bobath, 1978). **Automatic reactions**, which include righting and equilibrium reactions, were part of evaluations before the NDT frame of reference, but it took the Bobaths to explain their importance in treatment. Automatic reactions enable us to risk movement without the fear of falling (Adams, 1982). Without them, safety exists only in rigidly held postures. Finally, the Bobaths made us understand the importance of proximal limb structures, such as the shoulder and pelvic girdles, to distal limb function (Adams, 1982). These proximal limb structures provide essential proximal stability during the early part of limb motion. The scapula and pelvis also contribute a significant number of degrees of range of motion (ROM) when the arm and leg are moving in midranges (Norkin and Levangie, 1992).

▼ INTELLECTUAL HERITAGE

Berta and Karel Bobath created the NDT frame of reference as a part of their work in the 1940s and 1950s with clients who had cerebral palsy and cerebral vascular acci-dents (CVAs). These were exciting decades when several sensorimotor theories were emerging. As the title implies, the theoretical base for NDT comes both from normal development and neurophysiology. Yet, it is not a pure developmental frame of reference as one example under gross motor trends makes clear.

▼ ASSUMPTIONS

The NDT frame of reference has five assumptions:

1. Teaching normal motor milestones is *not* the proper focus for treatment (Adams, 1982). Normal development is important because it identifies the underlying foundation skills that make motor milestones possible. For example, if midline symmetry is achieved, then a minimum of practice is needed to achieve the motor milestone of independent sitting.
2. You cannot impose normal movement on abnormal muscle tone (Bobath, 1978). Spasticity and hypotonia both produce abnormal movements that become more pronounced with repeated use.
3. Damage to higher centers in the brain produces a release phenomenon (Adams, 1982). Lower centers generate mass, obligatory, stereotyped movements in the form of hyperactive phasic and tonic reflexes and pathological limb synergies.
4. Normal movement is learned by experiencing how normal feels (Adams, 1982).
5. The brain is very plastic and capable of remarkable recovery. Research has substantiated and explained CNS plasticity (Moore, 1986).

▼ EFFECTS ON EVALUATION

Evaluation is limited to axial control, automatic reactions, and limb dissociation. Formal evaluations exist for reflex development and automatic reactions (Fiorentino, 1973), pathological limb synergy (Sawner & Lavigne, 1992), and muscle tone (Dutton, 1995). Clinical observations are needed to evaluate impairments ignored by formal tests, such as symmetrical sitting and placing and eccentric control (Bobath, 1978). Clinical observation is needed to evaluate automatic reactions (Dutton, 1995). Before NDT, automatic reactions test results had poor sensitivity because they were scored only as present or absent.

Normal gross- and fine-motor trends are a valuable source of information about the primitive, transitional, and mature stages of development that identify underlying motor strategies (Dutton, 1995). For example, a gross-motor trend called "flexor to extensor tone," tells us that mature extension is preceded by a transition stage called "extension with retraction" (Dutton, 1995). Extension with retraction is characterized by neck and trunk hyperextension that is yoked to limb extension (Bly, 1991), along with scapular and pelvic retraction and shoulder and hip abduction. This transitional movement strategy is safe for normal infants, but it is very dangerous for brain-damaged individuals who often do not progress to mature extension.

▼ EFFECTS ON CLIENT–PRACTITIONER INTERACTIONS

To empower the client, the therapist must clearly explain the link that connect the general deficit and NDT goal to the functional outcome (Dutton, 1995). For example:

General deficit: poor axial weight shifts are due to
Stage specific cause: spastic lateral trunk flexors.
Measurable NDT goal: active weight shift onto the weight-
   bearing hemiplegic hip with trunk elongation will permit
Functional outcome: hiking the hemiplegic hip to bath with
   minimal assistance while sitting on a tub-seat.

It is vital to link the NDT goal, such as axial weight shifts, with a specific functional outcome, such as bathing. Third-party payers require it (Allen and Foto, 1991; Dahl, 1990) and the client needs to know why shifting onto the hemiplegic side is important. It is difficult for cognitively impaired clients to understand the value of mat exercises. It is even difficult for family and other team members to understand how rocking onto the hemiplegic side makes it possible for the client to go home instead of going to a nursing home. Although other frames of reference use intervention that is obvious to the client, such as using weights to strengthen, the therapist must explain the link between NDT goals and functional outcomes before the client and therapist can become partners.

▼ STRENGTHS, LIMITATIONS, AND RESEARCH

Teaching normal movement strategies is the strength of the NDT frame of reference. You can see from the foregoing example that normal strategies are often made measurable with a qualitative approach. It is important for NDT goals to include qualitative descriptions, because they often show what we are trying to change with our NDT treatment. Practitioners do not want clients to sit for longer periods of time with poor posture. We want clients to sit symmetrically with both shoulders level, equal weight on both hips, hips symmetrically abducted, and feet flat. It is easier to count duration and repetitions, but using only quantitative measurements limits our ability to document the NDT gains that third-party payers and researchers are looking for.

The old debate about using handling exercises versus purposeful activity is fading. Changes have occurred in NDT owing to new research in motor control (Carr & Shephard, 1987; Craik, 1991; Sabari, 1991). For example, practitioners know they will not see carryover if they use only handling exercises to inhibit abnormal muscle tone. Students can be taught to make clients use normal tone by immediately initiating their own movement during purposeful activity (Dutton, 1995). Bly (1991), an NDT certified instructor, recommends using purposeful activities because they are open tasks, in which the environment is constantly changing its demands, instead of having clients practice predictable, repetitive movements on mat tables.

One issue ignored by NDT is the use of visual input during purposeful activities to teach clients to predict and correct movement errors before they occur (Carr & Shephard, 1987; Sabari, 1991). Normal individuals do not use proprioceptive feedback to tell them that they might slip on ice; they see the ice, lower their center of gravity, and take shorter steps to prevent a fall. Clients should learn to use visual input for feed-forward problem solving.

Recent studies on functional gains have been looking for a global connection between NDT gains and a composite score for activities of daily living (ADL). Spaulding and colleagues (1989) found no correlation between wrist spasticity and a composite ADL score. However, there are confounding factors that conceal the relationship between NDT and ADL gains. First, other factors, such as cognitive deficits, contribute to a composite ADL score. Second, a client can gain independence by doing things one-handed; therefore, regaining limb motion to permit two-handed independence will not change the ADL score. What is needed is a study of the relationship between specific NDT goals and specific ADL gains, such as studying wrist spasticity and ADLs that require wrist dissociation, such as cutting with a knife and fork.

Section 3

Sensory Integration
Olga Baloueff

Definition
Intellectual Heritage of the Frame of Reference
   Jean Ayres: The Person and Her Work
   Basic Premises
Assumptions and Neurobehavioral Concepts
Evaluation of Sensory Integration Dysfunction
   Standardized Testing
   Clinical Observations
   Interviews and Questionnaires

▼ DEFINITION

Sensory integration (SI) refers to both a neurological process and a theory of the relationship between the neural organization of sensory processing and behavior (Ayres, 1972a,b,c, 1989; Fisher & Murray, 1991; Parham & Mailloux, 1995). Ayres (1989), an occupational therapist, who developed this theory, defined SI as:

. . . the neurological process that organizes sensation from one's own body and from the environment and makes it possible to use the body effectively within the environment. The spatial and temporal aspects of inputs from different sensory modalities are interpreted, associated, and unified. Sensory integration is information processing. (p.11)

▼ INTELLECTUAL HERITAGE OF THE FRAME OF REFERENCE

Jean Ayres: The Person and Her Work

A. Jean Ayres (1920–1988), began developing the theory of sensory integration in the 1960s and continued to redefine it until her death in 1988 (Clark, 1988). Ayres' early work was influenced by Rood and the Bobaths, who addressed the relationship of sensory stimuli to motor responses in the treatment of neuromuscular dysfunction, and by Piaget who stressed the early sensorimotor experiences as foundation for cognitive development (Fisher & Murray, 1991; McCormack, 1996). Ayres' clinical work with adults and children with neurological and learning problems sparked her interest in the study and evaluation of neurobehavioral functioning and in exploring perceptual and motor contributions to learning (Fisher & Murray, 1991).

Basic Premises

Sensory integration has three basic postulates (Ayres, 1972a, 1979; Fisher & Murray, 1991; Kimball, 1993):

1. The integration of sensory information, especially, vestibular, tactile, and proprioceptive input is fundamental to a person's ability to interact efficiently with the environment.
2. Sensory integration provides a foundation for learning and emotional regulation. Deficits in sensory processing and organization can lead to certain types of conceptual and motor learning.
3. Sensory experiences provided within the context of meaningful activities and resulting in adaptive responses will enhance sensory integration, and in turn enhance learning.

▼ ASSUMPTIONS AND NEUROBEHAVIORAL CONCEPTS

Several assumptions are central to SI theoretical construction (Ayres 1972a, 1979; Fisher & Murray, 1991; Kimball, 1993; Parham & Mailloux, 1995; Stallings-Sahler, 1993).

1. *Sensory nourishment:* Sensory input is critical for brain function. The individual must actively use sensory input to interact with the environment.
2. *Plasticity within the central nervous system:* Through adaptive responses to environmental demands (ie, purposeful activities), changes occur at the neuronal synaptic level.
3. *Developmental sequence:* Sensory integrative processes occur in a developmental sequence as the CNS organizes adaptive responses to sensory information with increasing levels of complexity.
4. *Central nervous system organization:* The brain functions as both an integrated whole and as hierarchically organized interactive systems. Cortical centers are dependent on the brainstem's and the thalamus' functioning for the organization and interpretation of incoming sensory information.
5. *Sensory modalities convergence:* Convergence (integration) of sensory input from all sensory modalities occurs in the reticular formation (brainstem and thalamus), which has a widespread influence over the rest of the brain.
6. *Adaptive response:* An adaptive response contributes to the development of sensory integration. When a person experiences a challenging, but not overwhelming, type of sensory stimulation to his or her CNS, and successfully responds to it, an adaptive response takes place.
7. *Inner drive:* People have an inner impetus to develop sensory integration through their participation in sensorimotor activities and activity preference. The more innerdirected a person's activities, the greater the potential for improving neural organization.

▼ EVALUATION OF SENSORY INTEGRATION DYSFUNCTION

Evaluation of sensory integrative functioning is a multifaceted process. It includes standardized testing and clinical observations. These tests are supplemented by child and parent interviews and teacher questionnaires. Contextual considerations are always taken into account.

Standardized Testing

The primary instrument for identification of sensory integration dysfunction is the Sensory Integration and Praxis

Tests (SIPT; Ayres, 1989). The SIPT evolved from earlier test batteries developed by Ayres (1972b, 1975, 1980): the Southern California Sensory Integration Test (SCSIT) and the Southern California Postrotary Nystagmus Test (SCPNT).

The SIPT is composed of 17 subtests measuring four SI domains: (1) tactile, vestibular, and proprioceptive processing; (2) form and space perception, visual–motor coordination; (3) praxis; (4) bilateral integration and sequencing (Ayres, 1989).

Testing is administered individually, and takes about 2 hours. The SIPT's age range is 4 years through 8 years, 11 months. Scoring is computerized by the publisher, Western Psychological Services (WPS). Administration and interpretation of the SIPT requires specialized examiner training, which is administered through Sensory Integration International (1602 Cabrillo Avenue, Torrance, CA 90501–2819).

As needed, additional testing of specific performance areas or components are administered, such as play, ADL, psychosocial, sensorimotor, and cognitive skills (see Unit IX). Neuropsychological testing may also be part of a comprehensive evaluation.

Clinical Observations

Informal and formal observations of an individual's occupational performance are part of the evaluation process. For children, informal and unstructured observations in natural settings may include, but are not limited to, a child's sitting posture and handling of writing tools, as well as frustration tolerance with the complexity of a task. On the playground, a child's level of participation in games and enjoyment of the activity will also be observed. Formal clinical observations of muscle tone and cocontraction, reflex integration, symmetry, oculomotor, and postural reactions supplement the SIPT (Parham & Mailloux, 1995).

Interviews and Questionnaires

Interviews and questionnaires are given to gather pertinent information, such as (1) referral background and reason for referral, and (2) detailed developmental history, including developmental milestones and sensory history. Teacher's and parents' perceptions of the child's temperament, coping styles, performance in ADL, feeding, play, and school work are also explored. The interviewer should also include children's own perception of their problems, their strengths, and reason for referral.

▼ SENSORY INTEGRATIVE DYSFUNCTION

Sensory integrative dysfunction is a developmental disorder characterized by problems in CNS processing of sensory input (Fisher & Murray, 1991). Three major categories of SI

dysfunction are most often addressed by practitioners: sensory modulation problems, dyspraxia, vestibular and **bilateral integration** deficits (Fisher & Murray, 1991; Kimball, 1993; Parham & Mailloux, 1995).

- *Sensory modulation disorders* are characterized by overresponsivity (hyper) or underresponsivity (hypo) to incoming sensory input. Dysfunction occurs when these fluctuations are extreme and render people inefficient in their interaction with the environment. Such disorders are most common in the tactile (eg, tactile defensiveness) and vestibular systems (eg, gravitational insecurity).
- *Dyspraxia* is a difficulty with the planning and execution of movement patterns of a skilled or nonhabitual nature, originating in childhood.
- *Vestibular and bilateral integration disorders* reflect problems in central vestibular processing. Deficits in coordinating the two sides of the body, poor equilibrium reactions, low muscle tone, and difficulties in communication, organization of behavior, and modulation of arousal are common manifestations of this type of disorder.

▼ SENSORY INTEGRATIVE THERAPY

The specific objectives of SI intervention vary according to the person's individual characteristics and the type of dysfunction. However, several general outcomes of therapy are expected, based on SI theory (Ayres, 1972a, 1979; Koomar & Bundy, 1991; Parham & Mailloux, 1995). These outcomes are:

- Enhancement of the nervous system's processing and organization of sensory input, thereby providing a foundation for improvement in occupational performance as manifested by motor skills, academic learning, language, daily living, and personal–social skills.
- Development of increasingly more complex adaptive responses to controlled sensory input, especially vestibular, tactile, and proprioceptive input.
- Increase in the duration and frequency of adaptive responses.

▼ RESEARCHING THE EFFECTIVENESS OF SENSORY INTEGRATION

Although many clinicians working with children with a wide range of sensory-processing disorders use SI as a frame of reference, conflicting reports exist concerning its effectiveness (Cermak & Henderson, 1990; Cool, 1995; Daems, 1994, Hoehn & Baumeister, 1994).

Relative to future research, Cermak & Henderson (1990) have proposed the development of models to examine the immediate effect of sensory integration procedures as well as models for examining change over time. Coster, Tickle-Degnen, and Armenta (1995) have started to develop a coding system designed to examine therapist–child interaction during sensory integration treatment. Perceptions of individuals receiving SI therapy about its effect on their occupational performance also need to be studied in the future. In summary, sensory integration is still an evolving theory and "critical analysis of SI theory and practice should remain an ongoing process" (Fisher & Murray, 1991; p. 24).

►Editors' Conclusion

The NDT practice theory or frame of reference and sensory integration theory are both derived from hierarchical models of infant and child development that assume predictable, sequential development: of movement in NDT and of sensory processing in SI. Practitioners applying these theories to adults have assumed that adult neural recovery after brain injury recapitulates this hierarchical process. Hierarchical models of development were the only ones available when these theories were initially developed. However, research performed since the development of NDT and SI suggests that hierarchical models provide inadequate and incomplete descriptions of normal development. That is, NDT and SI are based on outdated theories of development. Some techniques from these intervention approaches may work for some clients, but for reasons other than those suggested by the approaches' founders. Practitioners using NDT or SI for intervention need to be mindful that development is more complex than either of these approaches suggests.

▼ REFERENCES

Adams, M. (1982). *Eight week NDT certification course*. Memphis, TN.

Allen, K. A. & Foto, M. (1991). Reporting occupational therapy outcomes with the ICIDH codes. *Physical Disabilities Special Interest Section Newsletter, 14*(2), 2–3.

Ayres, A. J. (1972a). *Sensory integration and learning disorders*. Los Angeles: Western Psychological Services.

Ayres, A. J. (1972b). *Southern California Sensory Integration Tests manual*. Los Angeles: Western Psychological Services.

Ayres, A. J. (1972c). Types of sensory integrative dysfunction among disabled learners. *American Journal of Occupational Therapy, 26*, 13–18.

Ayres, A. J. (1975). *Southern California Postrotary Nystagmus Test manual*. Los Angeles: Western Psychological Services.

Ayres, A. J. (1979). *Sensory integration and the child*. Los Angeles: Western Psychological Services.

Ayres, A. J. (1980). *Southern California Sensory Integration Tests manual: Revised 1980*. Los Angeles: Western Psychological Services.

Ayres, A. J. (1989). *Sensory Integration and Praxis Tests*. Los Angeles: Western Psychological Services.

Bernstein, N. (1967). *The coordination and regulation of movements*. London: Pergamon.

Bly, L. (1991). A historical and current view of the basis of NDT. *Pediatric Physical Therapy, 3*, 131–135.

Bobath, B. (1978). *Adult hemiplegia: Evaluation and treatment* (2nd ed). London: William Heinemann.

Carr, J. K. & Shephard, R. B. (1987). *Movement science: Foundations for physical therapy in rehabilitation*. Rockville, MD: Aspen Publications.

Cermak, S. A. & Henderson, A. (1990). The efficacy of sensory integration procedures, Part II. *Sensory Integration Quarterly, 28*(1), 1–5.

Clark, F. (1988). Lessons we have learned: A history of sensory integration research. *Sensory Integration Quarterly, 26*(3), 3–9.

Cool, S. (1995). Does sensory integration work? *Sensory Integration Quarterly, 23*(1), 1–9.

Coster, W., Tickle-Degnen, L., & Armenta, L. (1995). Therapist–child interaction during sensory integration treatment: Development and testing of a research tool. *Occupational Therapy Journal of Research, 15*(1), 17–35.

Craik, R. L. (1991). Recovery process: Maximizing function. In *Contempory management of motor control problems* (pp. 175–184). Proceedings of the II Step Conference of the American Physical Therapy Association.

Daems, J. (Ed.). (1994). *Reviews of research in sensory integration*. Torrance, CA: Sensory Integration International.

Dahl, M. (1990). *Money and reimbursement versus OT practice*. Pennsylvania Occupational Therapy Association Workshop. Philadelphia, PA.

Dalton, T. C. (1996). Reconstructing John Dewey's unusual collaboration with Myrtle McGraw in the 1930s. *Newsletter of the Society for Research in Child Development, Winter*, 1–3; 8–10.

Dunst, C. J., Trivette, C. M., & Deal, A. G. (1988). *Enabling and empowering families: Principles and guidelines for practice*. Cambridge, MA: Brookline Books.

Dutton, R. (1995). *Clinical reasoning in physical disabilities*. Baltimore: Williams & Wilkins.

Fiorentino, M. R. (1973). *Reflex testing methods for evaluating CNS development* (2nd ed). Springfield, IL: Charles C. Thomas.

Fisher, A. G. & Murray, E. A. (1991). Introduction to sensory integration theory. In Fisher, A. G., Murray, E. A., & Bundy, A. C. (Eds.), *Sensory integration theory and practice* (pp. 3–26). Philadelphia: F. A. Davis.

Freel, K. S. (1996). Finding complexities and balancing perspectives: Using an ethnographic viewpoint to understand children and their families. *Zero to Three, 16*, 1–7.

Gesell, A. (1928). *Infancy and human growth*. New York: Macmillan.

Gibson, J. J. (1979). *The ecological approach to visual perception*. Boston: Houghton Mifflin.

Gilfoyle, E. M., Grady, A. P., & Moore, J. C. (1981). *Children adapt*. New Jersey: Charles B. Slack.

Hoehn, T. P. & Baumeister, A. A. (1994). A critique of the application of sensory integration therapy to children with learning disabilities. *Journal of Learning Disabilities, 27*(6), 338–350.

Kimball, J. C. (1993). Sensory integrative frame of reference. In Kramer, P. & Hinojosa, J. (Eds.), *Frames of reference for pediatric occupational therapy* (pp. 87–175). Baltimore: Williams & Wilkins.

King, L. J. (1978). Toward a science of adaptive responses. *American Journal of Occupational Therapy, 32*, 429.

Koomar, J. A. & Bundy, A. C. (1991). The art and science of creating direct intervention from theory. In Fisher, A. G., Murray, E. A., & Bundy, A. C. (Eds.), *Sensory integration theory and practice* (pp. 234–250). Philadelphia: F. A. Davis.

Lester, B. M., McGrath, M. M., Garcia-Coll, C. T., Brem, F. S., Sullivan, M. C., & Mattis, S. B. (1994). Relationship between risk and protective factors, developmental outcome and the home environment at 4-years-of-age in term and preterm infants. In H. Fitzgerald, B. M., Lester, & B. Zuckerman (Eds.), *Children in poverty: Research, health care, and policy issues* (pp. 197–227). New York: Garland Press.

Llorens, L. (1969). Facilitating growth and development: The promise of occupational therapy. *American Journal of Occupational Therapy, 24*, 93–101.

McCormack, G. L. (1996). The Rood approach to treatment of neuromuscular dysfunction. In Pedretti, L. W. (Ed.). *Occupational therapy: practice skills for physical dysfunction* (pp. 377–399). St. Louis: C.V. Mosby.

Moore, J. C. (1986). Recovery potentials following CNS lesions: A brief historical perspective in relation to modern research data on neuroplasticity. *American Journal of Occupational Therapy, 40,* 459–463.

Norkin, C. C. & Levangie, P. K. (1992). *Joint structure and function* (2nd ed.). Philadelphia: F. A. Davis.

Parham, D. L. & Mailloux, Z. (1995). Sensory integration. In Case-Smith, J., Allen, A. S., & Pratt, P. N. (Eds.). *Occupational therapy for children* (pp. 307–356). St. Louis: C.V. Mosby.

Piaget, J. (1952). *The origins of intelligence in children.* New York: International Universities Press.

Sabari, J. S. (1991). Motor learning concepts applied to activity based intervention with adults with hemiplegia. *American Journal of Occupational Therapy, 45,* 523–530.

Sameroff, A. J. & Chandler, M. J. (1975). Reproductive risk and the continuum of caretaking casualty. In F. D. Horowitz, M. Hetherington, S. Scarr-Salapatek, & G. Siegel (Eds.). *Review of child development research,* Vol. 4, (pp. 187–244). Chicago: University of Chicago Press.

Sawner, K. A. & Lavigne, J. (1992). *Brunnstrom's movement therapy in hemiplegia* (2nd ed.). Philadelphia: J. B. Lippincott.

Simeonsson, R. J. & Bailey, D. B. (1990). Family dimensions in early intervention. In S. J. Meisels & J. P. Shonkoff (Eds.), *Handbook of early childhood intervention* (pp. 428–444). New York: Cambridge University Press.

Spaulding, S. J., Strachota, E., McPherson, J. J., Kuphal, M., & Ramponi, M. (1989). Wrist muscle tone and self-care skill in persons with hemiparesis. *American Journal of Occupational Therapy, 43,* 11–18.

Sporns, O. & Edelman, G. M. (1993). Solving Bernstein's problem: A proposal for the development of coordinated movement by selection. *Child Development, 64,* 960–981.

Stallings-Sahler, S. (1993). Sensory integration: Assessment and intervention with infants. In Case-Smith, J. (Ed.), *Pediatric occupational therapy* (pp. 309–341). Baltimore: Williams & Wilkins.

Thelen, E. (1995). Motor development: A new synthesis. *American Psychologist, 50,* 79–95.

Wachs, T. D. (1992). *The nature of nurture.* Newbury Park: Sage Publications.

Chapter 26

Theories Derived from Learning Perspectives

Section 1: Overview of Learning Theory

Section 2: Behaviorism

Section 3: Cognitive Disability Frame of Reference

Section 4: The Multicontext Treatment Approach

Section 5: Motor Learning: An Emerging Frame of Reference for
Occupational Performance

Section I

Overview of Learning Theory

Maureen E. Neistadt

> **Learning as Information Processing**
>   Levels of Information Processing and Learning
>   Transfer of Learning
> **Evaluation of Clients' Learning Capacities**
> **Treatment Recommendations Related to Learning**
>   **Capacities**

Occupational therapy clients spend most of their treatment time learning. Consequently, occupational therapy practitioners need to know something about learning theory. Learning can be defined as "a relatively permanent change in behavior or in behavior potentiality that results from experience and cannot be attributed to temporary body states induced by illness, fatigue, or drugs" (Hergenhahn, 1976, p. 9). Philosophers since Plato (427 to 347 BC) and Aristotle (384 to 322 BC) have debated over whether the nature of knowledge is primarily determined by the mind (rationalism) or by sensory experience (empiricism). Beginning in the mid-19th century, this debate about the nature of learning evolved into a psychology debate about the best way to explain learning. Some theorists, such as Pavlov (1849 to 1936), Watson (1878 to 1958), and Skinner (1904 to 1990) felt that learning was best explained by observing and describing relationships between behaviors and observable events (associationism, behaviorism). Others,

such as the Gestalt psychologists (late 19th to mid-20th century) or Piaget (1896 to 1980) felt that learning was best explained by making inferences about the mental activities underlying observed behaviors (cognitive theorists). Since the late 1950s, the dominant perspective in learning theory has been information processing (Hergenhahn, 1976; Hintzman, 1978; Ormrod, 1990).

Occupational therapy practitioners use behavioral, cognitive behavioral, and information-processing theories of learning in their practice. Behavioral and cognitive behavioral theories are discussed in Section 2. Sections 3, 4, and 5 discuss three treatment theories derived from an information-processing perspective on learning. This section provides an overview of the information-processing perspective and shows how that perspective can be applied to occupational therapy evaluation and treatment.

▼ LEARNING AS INFORMATION PROCESSING

The information-processing perspective suggests that learning is a process mediated by the brain, with the brain interpreting and relating external sensory impressions and internally stored concepts with each other, much as a computer relates keyboard inputs with internally stored programs (Kantowitz & Roediger, 1980). This information-processing system works best when the information or task to be learned is meaningful to the learner (Jarus, 1994; Mathiowetz & Haugen, 1994).

From an information-processing perspective learning requires effective (1) sensory reception, (2) brain processing, and (3) motor behavior for either movement or communication. Errors in this information-processing system can lead to errors in occupational performance. For example, a person who has difficulty with visual acuity may frequently spill things in the kitchen because he or she can not see objects clearly. A person with slowed brain processing may have difficulty driving on high-speed, heavily trafficked roads because he or she can not process the multiple, rapid inputs in this situation fast enough to make safe-driving decisions. A person with impaired motor responses may have difficulty carrying out a wide range of functional activities. Research has indicated that the brain processing part of this information system operates at different levels of capacity, yielding different types of learning.

Levels of Information Processing and Learning

All healthy adults have the capacity to engage in three types of learning that require differing degrees of information processing: association, representational, and abstract learning (Goldstein & Oakley, 1985). **Association learning**, which happens when an individual makes an association between two events, is mediated by subcortical, or, in some cases, cerebellar structures in the brain. This type of learning is illustrated by a cigarette smoker who learns to associate smoking with drinking a cup of coffee at the end of a meal in a restaurant. For that person, the arrival of the coffee triggers an automatic response to light up a cigarette.

Representational learning involves the "formation of durable internal (including linguistic) representations or images of events, and the creation of a spatio-temporal framework into which events are organized and from which they are retrieved" (Goldstein & Oakley, 1985; p. 14). This type of learning is mediated by the hippocampus and neocortex. Representational learning is illustrated by becoming familiar with cooking a new recipe. Initially, a person might follow the recipe step by step. However, with practice, he or she will begin to rely less and less on the cookbook, and more and more on his or her memory of the recipe and the action sequences needed to complete it. That is, the person will have developed an internal image of how to make this particular dish.

Abstract learning is the "acquisition and storage of rules, knowledge and facts abstracted from unrelated events, independently of a spatio-temporal context" (p. 14). This type of learning is mediated by the neocortex. Abstract learning is illustrated by a client with a stroke who derives the principle of always starting with the affected extremity from one session of upper extremity dressing training, and then applies that principle to lower extremity dressing without being cued to do so.

Abstract learning requires more complex information processing than representational and association learning and representational learning requires more complex information processing than association learning. The neurological capacity for abstract learning develops gradually throughout childhood and adolescence. Children may rely more heavily on association and representation learning than on abstract learning because they have not yet fully developed the ability to think abstractly. Healthy adolescents and adults have access to all three types of learning, but those with brain dysfunction may not. Adolescents and adults with severe brain dysfunction may rely exclusively on association learning, while those with lesser dysfunction may still have access to representational or even abstract learning.

Transfer of Learning

Association, representational, and abstract learners all have different capacities for transferring learning from one activity to another. Toglia (1991) has identified degrees of transfer along a continuum from transfer to very similar to transfer to very different activities. Spontaneous **transfer of learning** across very different activities is also known as generalization.

People relying on association learning can, at best, accomplish near transfer of learning [tasks different in one or two characteristics (Toglia, 1991)]. These individuals would have difficulty transferring learning across different situations, with different sets of stimuli. For instance, a teenager with congenital brain dysfunction who was using association learning might be able to learn to make a cup of instant coffee if the necessary supplies (mug, instant coffee, and other necessities) were set out on the kitchen counter in exactly the same way and the exact same cues were given by the exact same person each time that task was practiced. If any aspect of the activity presentation changed, the association learner might not be able to make the cup of coffee. An association learner would be able to transfer this learning only to very similar situations (eg, to a setup in the same kitchen where the mug or the brand of instant coffee had been changed). The best learning environment for an association learner, then, would be the home setting where he or she will be doing self-care and home management activities.

People engaged in representational learning would be able to tolerate changes in activity setup because they would have an internal image of activity performance against which to compare the immediate environmental stimuli. For instance, representational learners would know to look for missing ingredients in the setup for an instant coffee preparation activity. They would most likely be able to show near and intermediate [tasks different in three to six characteristics (Toglia, 1991)] transfer of learning. That is, after learning to make instant coffee with a given set of supplies in a given kitchen, this learner might be able to make a cup of instant coffee in a different kitchen, with different supplies (different mug, kettle, brand of coffee, and such). These learners might be able to transfer some task strategies learned in therapy clinics to their home settings.

The conceptual framework of representational learners, however, is limited and would be insufficient to deal with major changes in activity presentation. Therefore, home settings are the better learning environments for these learners also. A representational learner, for example, would not be able to problem-solve past a broken stove while making a cup of instant coffee because he or she would be working with only one image of how the activity could be done. An abstract learner, by contrast, would be able to create alternative images for activity completion based on past experiences. When faced with a broken stove, the abstract learner would look for an alternative way to heat the water, based on the abstract knowledge that to heat water, one has to apply some form of energy to it (eg, microwaves). Abstract learners would be able to show far and very far transfer of learning [tasks conceptually similar, but different in all but one or two characteristics (Toglia, 1991)]. For example, after learning to make instant coffee in a kitchen, abstract learners would be able to figure out how to make a cup of instant coffee at a campsite, with supplies that were totally different in appearance from the ones used during training. Abstract learners, then, would be able to transfer activity strategies learned in hospital or outpatient settings to their homes.

▼ EVALUATION OF CLIENTS' LEARNING CAPACITIES

Because learning capacities (association, representational, abstract) are associated with specific abilities to transfer learning, occupational therapist can evaluate clients' learning capabilities by assessing their abilities to transfer learning across different activities. To evaluate transfer of learning, a therapist can change a functional task from one session to the next and see how the client responds. For example, a bathing activity using a basin on the bedside table could be done with soap and toiletries laid out in a line on the table next to the basin one day, and with soap and toiletries laid out in a cluster the next. The client who is unable to perform the activity with this change may not be capable of new learning at all. A client who is confused by this change in task presentation is showing difficulty with near transfer (one characteristic changed) and may be using primarily association learning. A client who can bathe even with changes in position (sitting in a bedside chair instead of lying in bed with the head of the bed raised), arrangement of toiletries, and environment (television or radio on instead of off, or in the bathroom rather than at bedside) is showing capacity for intermediate transfer (three to six characteristics changed) and is demonstrating a capacity for representational learning. A client who can bath successfully in the shower, with their soap and toiletries jumbled together in a plastic basket is showing both far transfer from the bed bath situation and a capacity for abstract learning.

Clients' abilities to transfer learning can change through the course of treatment owing to (1) spontaneous neurological recovery from medical conditions, such as stroke and head injury, and (2) the neurobiological effects of learning (Bach-y-Rita, 1981; Kertesz, 1985; Neistadt, 1994). Clients' transfer of learning capacities, then, should not be considered a static characteristic and need to be reevaluated on an ongoing basis.

▼ TREATMENT RECOMMENDATIONS RELATED TO LEARNING CAPACITIES

General guidelines for treatment can be recommended based on clients' assessed learning capabilities. For clients showing no learning capacity on evaluation, therapists need to recommend adapting the environment and providing clients with whatever assistance they need to perform their daily activities safely.

Clients showing association learning would need a focus on functional activity training, with consistent task setups and treatment schedules. Once an association learner had mastered a particular functional activity, using consistent task setups, then it would be appropriate to vary the activity setup by one characteristic (eg, changing from pullover to button down the front cotton shirts for dressing). Association learners need tremendous amounts of repetition to learn, so something like activities of daily living (ADL) training would have to be done at least five times a week.

For clients showing representational learning, an occupational therapy practitioner would be able to vary three to six characteristics from one treatment session to the next (eg, changing the style and texture of clothing and moving from bedside to a bathroom, for dressing). These clients may need less repetition for learning and so may need only three or four treatment sessions per week for ADL training. Abstract learners can be taught the principles behind adapted functional activity performance during an initial treatment session and may need only a few sessions of practice with the practitioner after that. For example, an abstract learner with a **total hip replacement (THR)** may need only a few sessions to learn THR precautions and the techniques for using long-handled equipment for dressing. Once the abstract learner has the principles of long-handled equipment use down, he or she might be able to practice on his or her own to become proficient with the devices.

Application of learning theory perspectives to practice, then, can help practitioners continually think of more effective ways to teach clients skills and activity adaptations. The following sections provide background on other approaches to practice derived from learning theory.

Section 2

Behaviorism

Gordon Muir Giles

> Intellectual Heritage
> Definitions
>   Basic Principles of Behavior Theory and Therapy
>   Basic Principles of Cognitive Behavioral Therapy
> Research and Relevance of Behavioral Approaches to
>   Occupational Therapy

For the behaviorist, observable behavior is the fundamental subject of study. Behaviorism is best viewed as a general orientation to experimental and clinical work. This section provides a brief overview of some of the basic concepts of behavioral theory.

▼ INTELLECTUAL HERITAGE

J. B. Watson (1913) is considered by some to be the father of American behaviorism. He thought only observable behavior should be the subject of scientific study and that speculations about the thought processes associated with behaviors were irrelevant. To justify this rejection of "mental" explanations, behaviorists pointed out that people have little insight into why they do what they do (Nisbett & Wilson, 1977). Later behaviorists retained this focus on observable behavior, but also started to consider the associated cognitive processes.

During the 1950s, behavioral principles began to be applied to the treatment of psychological problems in humans. Wolpe (1958) developed the principles of systematic desensitization, while Eysenk (1960) and others in England began to define behavioral treatment of psychological problems. Behavioral principles derived from the work of Skinner (1938) began to be applied in mental hospitals in an attempt to ameliorate some of the handicapping behaviors associated with chronic psychosis or mental retardation. For example, token systems were used to help clients develop self-care and social skills required for community living. (In a token system clients are given tokens for positive behaviors—tokens that can be used use to purchase items in a facility store.) During the late 1960s and early 1970s cognitive behavioral therapies were developed. These new therapies considered both observable behavior and the thought processes that went with them. So there are currently two major branches of behavior therapy: behavioral and cognitive behavioral.

Behaviorists focus on observable behavior without reference to the cognitive processes associated with behavior.

Cognitive behaviorists differ from behaviorists in that they regard cognition and behavior as influencing one another. The development of cognitive behavioral therapy was probably the result of two factors. First, the behavioral model, which ignored cognitive appraisal of events, simply did not account for all classes of human behavior. For example, Bandura's (1977) accounts of **vicarious learning** defied traditional behavioral explanations. In vicarious learning, people learn new behaviors by simply watching others perform those behaviors. Second, the cognitive revolution in psychology led to a reevaluation of the role of mental processes in psychiatric disorders. Key theorists, such as Ellis (1962) and Beck (1963), began to emphasis that the cognitive appraisal of events can affect an individual's mood and response to those events.

▼ DEFINITIONS

Basic Principles of Behavior Theory and Therapy

Fundamental to behaviorists' understanding of behavior is the law of effect. The law of effect, first formulated by Thorndike in 1932, states that if an organism's response to a given stimulus is followed by a pleasant event, the association formed between the stimulus and response is further strengthened. If the response is followed by an aversive event, the association is weakened.

In behavioral theory, classes of behavior are identified with reference to the circumstances of their performance. In classical (Pavlovian) conditioning, responses originate with the stimuli that elicit them and are called respondents. Through conditioning, respondents developed in a species through natural selection can come under the influence of new stimuli (conditioned stimuli). This type of learning underlies important human phenomena such as anxiety and anger and is implicated in new areas of research in behavioral medicine (eg, psychopharmacology) (Ader & Cohen, 1993).

In operant (Skinnerian) conditioning, behaviors develop as a result of their effect on the environment. These behaviors (operants) or responses are said to be emitted. The consequence of a response may either raise or lower the rate of similar subsequent emitted behaviors. Events following a response that increase the frequency of that behavior are called reinforcers, and subsequent events that lower the frequency of a particular response are called punishers. Mapping the relationships between responses and their consequences establishes the contingencies of reinforcement. Once a behavior has been established, it is possible to influence the likelihood that it will continue with little or no reinforcement. The tendency for a behavior to cease if it is no longer reinforced is called extinction. Behaviors that occur after an individual observes another person model the behavior are termed vicarious learning behaviors.

Basic Principles of Cognitive Behavioral Therapy

In cognitive behavioral therapy (CBT), the therapist addresses the client's habitual ways of construing the world. CBT suggests that all people have **automatic thoughts**—things they tell themselves about themselves and the world around them. Automatic thoughts are usually highly abbreviated forms of internal speech that reflect habitual and erroneous forms of thinking (cognitive distortions).

Core schemas are the fundamental thoughts people use to construe themselves, others, and the world around them. These core schemas affect people's perceptions of their environments and inform their actions. Core schemas are inferred from a person's actions and words and can be altered by helping people change the ways they think and behave. Core schemas are described by a series of statements about the self, people, and the world, and as a series of if–then statements. For example, "I am (competent, no good).";"People are (friendly, mean).";"The world is (exciting, threatening).";"If (someone ignores me), then (he or she doesn't like me)."

The repetition of automatic thoughts over months or years can change a person. CBT uses a wide range of intervention techniques, such as problem-solving training, to help people make changes in their behavior and thought patterns to improve their mental health. Clients are asked to examine the advantages and disadvantages of certain beliefs, to logically challenge their cognitive distortions, and to change some of their thoughts about the world.

CBT continues to use behavioral interventions such as reinforcement of positive behaviors. The use of behavioral interventions in CBT varies with the type of disorder, the stage of therapy, and the client's individual needs. For example, the treatment of eating disorders requires a strong behavioral focus because behaviors (eg, binging and vomiting) are central to the client's problems.

▼ RESEARCH AND RELEVANCE OF BEHAVIORAL APPROACHES TO OCCUPATIONAL THERAPY

Behavior therapy is a natural fit with the practical, functional focus of occupational therapy. In many instances, occupational therapy practitioners use such behavioral interventions as social skill, assertiveness, relaxation, or problem-solving training, without appreciating that these interventions are grounded in behavioral theory.

Behavioral intervention assists in the acquisition of behavior appropriate to the environment. Much of behavioral treatment can be thought of as an attempt to rectify a person's failure to adapt to a novel environment. Behavior therapy has had a place in medical rehabilitation since the early

1970s (Ince, 1976). For example, research has shown behavioral intervention to be effective in assisting people with developmental disabilities develop self-care and community-living skills (Azrin & Armstrong, 1973; Azrin, Schaeffer, & Wesolowski, 1976). More recently, behavioral therapies have been applied in an increasing number of conditions (Epstein, 1992). For example, behavioral therapy is effective in improving the self-care skills of adults with brain damage (Giles & Clark-Wilson, 1988,1993). Other research has shown the usefulness of behavioral techniques in the treatment of substance abuse and eating disorders (Epstein, 1992; Vuchinich & Tucker, 1988).

Ongoing experiment and theory development have the potential to provide occupational therapy practitioners and others with new practical and effective behavioral treatment strategies. The combination of CBT and occupational therapy allows therapists to examine meanings associated with functional activities: meanings that can interfere with independent functioning (Giles, 1985). CBT's emphasis on behaviors fits into occupational therapy's emphasis on activity analysis and adaptation. Behavior therapy's emphasis on empirical validation of interventions and its emphasis on the validity of single case study research designs are also relevant to occupational therapy.

Section 3

Cognitive Disability Frame of Reference

Claudia Kay Allen

> **Intellectual Heritage**
> **Definitions**
> **Assumptions**
> **Evaluation and Treatment**
> **Strengths and Limitations**

The Cognitive Disability frame of reference provides environmental compensations for people with severe mental disorders. With acute conditions, the Allen Cognitive Levels (ACL) that are part of this frame of reference can be used as a sensitive measure of changes in ability to function (Table 26–1). Acute changes in the ability to function may be explained by medication and the process of natural healing. While ACL changes are occurring, skilled occupational therapy services consist of explaining the functional meaning of changes. The skill is in the interpretation of the change, not in producing the change. When the ACL score remains constant for a period of

TABLE 26-1. Summary of Cognitive Disability Levels

Cognitive Disability Level	Overview of Functional Capabilities
Level 1: Automatic Actions	The person is conscious and responds to internal stimuli. He or she is dependent for all self-care tasks, and requires 24-hour supervision.
Level 2: Postural Actions	The person initiates gross body movements, and may maintain unusual postures. The person may be able to assist in his or her care, but may become distressed or resistive. He or she requires 24-hour supervision.
Level 3: Manual Actions	The person responds to tactile cues, and uses hands to manipulate objects. He or she may engage in repetitive or seemingly pointless actions. Long-term repetitive training may enable the person to perform simple, routine tasks. The person needs cues to stay on-task, and requires 24-hour supervision.
Level 4: Goal-Directed Actions	The person engages in purposeful activity to achieve a short-term goal. Training should be situation specific, because the person thinks concretely and has difficulty generalizing. The person relies on structure in the environment. He or she can complete routine tasks such as dressing, but requires assistance to solve problems or deal with unexpected situations.
Level 5: Exploratory Actions	The person can problem-solve by trial and error, but has difficulty anticipating the results of actions. The person can learn new activities, but needs assistance with activities requiring him or her to plan ahead.
Level 6: Planned Actions	The person can anticipate the effects of future actions and can think abstractly. This makes it possible for him or her to problem-solve and plan future actions in advance. He or she can follow verbal or written instructions without a demonstration.

weeks, no more immediate improvement in ability to function may be expected with stable conditions. Skilled services are required to set up a home program that can be sustained over time. Lists of activities are organized according to the cognitively disabled person's best ability to function. These lists are used to select activities that are realistic and relevant to the individual and possible in the person's social circumstances. Caregiver education is done so that people can use their best ability to function in the least restrictive environment.

This frame of reference attempts to deal with three problems often ignored by other frames of reference: (1) changes in ability to function that would happen anyway, (2) difficulties in capacity to learn, and (3) chronic mental disorders. A hierarchical sequence (ACL) is used to measure the capacity to learn and analyze the learning difficulties in treatment methods. The individual's learning capacity is matched to the demands of the activity (Allen, Earhart, & Blue, 1992, 1993, 1996).

Diagnostic categories that are associated with a global loss of cognitive ability include Alzheimer's disease and other dementias, traumatic brain injury, delirium, multiple sclerosis, Parkinson's disease, schizophrenia, affective disorders, mental retardation, and cerebral palsy. People with any of these mental disorders may live with severe and persistent limitations in their ability to function that can have a devastating affect on their quality of life. Environmental compensations suggest realistic options that people may not realize are possible. By identifying actions and activities that can be done successfully, practitioners are in a position to have a practical influence on the quality of life.

▼ INTELLECTUAL HERITAGE

Most of the credit for the intellectual heritage of this frame of reference must go to the clients who have tried to share their world view with us. While we can assume that we see and think about the world in ways that are similar to those with cognitive disabilities, we also must assume that there are differences. Occupational therapy values that are considered to be important considerations for this frame of reference include (1) treating the whole person as a conscious organism; (2) improving the quality of life; (3) producing a functional outcome that is practical, realistic, relevant, meaningful, and sustainable; (4) helping people with disabilities, their family, and other caregivers feel good about themselves and what they are doing; and (5) objectively helping people adjust to the sorrows of living with a disability.

During the 20th century, persons in other disciplines have not been particularly interested in a holistic view of the preferred actions, activities, and roles of individuals. Related fields of study, such as psychiatry, psychology, and neurology, tend to produce lists of limitations or impairments. The result has been an impairment-driven practice, with countless reminders of what the person can not do. Impairments need to be balanced by abilities.

▼ DEFINITIONS

Six cognitive levels were originally taken from Piaget's description of the sensorimotor period and translated to conform with observations of psychiatric clients (Allen, 1985) (see Table 26–1). Within a few years, a more sensitive scale was needed and created by adding subcategories denoted by a decimal system to the original scale. These subcategories are called the modes of performance. The ADLs common to all areas of practice were analyzed according to 52 modes of performance to determine their levels of cognitive difficulty (Allen, Earhart, & Blue, 1993a).

▼ ASSUMPTIONS

The following assumptions guide the evaluation and treatment of a cognitive disability using this frame of reference:

1. The severity of a mental disorder can be judged by the consequences it has on a person's capacity to think, do, and learn.
2. Mild mental disorders can be compensated for by learning psychological substitutes for normal mental processes.
3. Severe mental disorders can be associated with limited mental abilities that can not be corrected by what the person says or does.
4. Severe mental disorders can be compensated for by providing environmental substitutes for normal mental processes and identifying normal processes that can still be used.
5. The remaining mental abilities can be engaged to do realistic activities that are meaningful to the client, practical for caregivers, and sustainable over time.
6. When people are unable to learn to use psychological compensations effectively, environmental compensations can improve the quality of life of person with cognitive disabilities and their long-term caregivers.

▼ EVALUATION AND TREATMENT

In practice, evaluation and treatment occur continuously and simultaneously. The Allen Battery has been developed to facilitate the continuum of care. The Allen Cognitive Level Screen (ACLS) uses leather lacing to obtain an initial estimate of the person's ability to function. A larger version (Larger Allen Cognitive Level Screen) is available for those with visual impairments. Begin with the smaller one and use the larger one when a visual impairment is confirmed (Allen, Earhart, & Blue, 1992). The Allen Diagnostic Module contains a Sensory Motor Simulation Kit for lower-level clients, and 30 craft projects for moderate- to higher-functioning clients. Crafts are used to evaluate new learning, which is necessary to estimate the person's capacity to adapt to a constantly changing environment (Allen, Earhart, & Blue, 1993). ADL are overlearned and may give an inflated estimate of ability, or can be very difficult to unlearn and change with a physical disability. The Routine Task Inventory (RTI) is an analysis of ADL (Allen, Earhart, & Blue,

1993a). The modes of performance are used to organize the description of abilities, treatment goals and methods, ADLs, and safety precautions for caregivers' education (Allen, Earhart, & Blue, 1996; Allen, Earhart, Blue, & Therasoft, 1996).

▼ STRENGTHS AND LIMITATIONS

Environmental compensations do not aim at teaching skills that can generalize to a wide range of activities. Environmental compensations are designed for people who cannot learn to generalize. The ACL evaluation is used to guide the selection of adaptive equipment, make changes in the home, work, or clinical environment, and modify the type of instructions and cues given. These adjustments are based on an empathetic understanding of how a cognitively disabled person thinks and feels.

Section 4

The Multicontext Treatment Approach

Joan Pascale Toglia

> **Components of the Multicontext Approach**
> Specifying a Processing Strategy for Transfer
> Task Analysis, Establishment of Criteria for Transfer and Practice in Multiple Tasks and Environments
> Metacognitive Training
> Individual Characteristics
> **Strengths, Limitations, and Research**

The Multicontext Treatment Approach addresses the issue of generalization in cognitive rehabilitation. Although it was designed for clients with brain injury, it has also been applied to clients with psychiatric disabilities. The Multicontext Approach is based on the dynamic interactional model of cognition (Toglia, 1992) that was adapted from the cognitive psychology and educational psychology literature on learning and generalization (Bransford, 1979; Brown, 1983, 1988).

The Multicontext Treatment Approach, views learning as an interaction between internal (person) and external (task and environment) variables. Person variables include (1) characteristics of the learner, such as previous experience, skills and knowledge, motivation, attitude, and emotions; (2)

metacognition or the knowledge and regulation of one's own cognitive processes; and (3) processing strategies or the strategies that learners use when presented with information. External variables include (1) task parameters, such as the number of items, arrangement, familiarity, or movement demands; and (2) environmental factors, such as the social, physical, and cultural context. Problems in processing information and learning are understood by analyzing the dynamic interaction between person variables, task variables, and environmental factors (Toglia, 1992) . In some persons, one component may affect learning more than the others. For example, the individual may have difficulty learning the task because of an unfamiliar environmental and cultural context.

In the Multicontext Approach, treatment systematically changes task and environmental variables to enhance the person's ability to process, monitor, and use information across new tasks and situations. The strategies and self-monitoring techniques remain constant in treatment, whereas the environment gradually changes (Toglia, 1991).

▼ COMPONENTS OF THE MULTICONTEXT APPROACH

The components of the multicontext approach are summarized in Table 26–2 and described in the following.

Specifying a Processing Strategy for Transfer

The first step in treatment is identifying a behavior that is targeted for change. A dynamic approach to evaluation (see Chap. 16; Sec. 2) identifies the symptoms or behaviors that

TABLE 26-2. Components of the Multicontext Treatment Approach

Treatment Components	Description
1. Specify a Processing Strategy for Transfer *(The behavior that should be observed in a variety of different tasks).*	**Strategies: 2 types** **Internal:** Use of self-cues, self-reminders, self-instructions, mental rehearsal or visualization (eg, remembering to begin searching on the left side, or remembering to plan ahead). **External:** Use of aids, or interactions with environmental stimuli, such as checklists; anchor for scanning; highlighting most critical points, memory notebook. Strategies (internal or external) may also be characterized by their range of application: **Situational Strategies:** Effective in selected tasks and environments (eg, grouping, rehearsal, visual imagery, scanning left or right). **Nonsituational Strategies:** Nonspecific strategies that are effective in a wide variety of tasks and environments. "context free." For example: planning ahead, stimuli reduction, self-monitoring strategies, pacing speed).
2. Task Analysis and Establishment of Criteria for Transfer *Transfer of learning can occur at different levels.*	Gradually vary the physical or surface features of the task while keeping the underlying conceptual characteristics consistent. **Near Transfer:** Alternate form of the same task. Only 1–2 task parameters are changed. Task is easily recognizable. **Intermediate Transfer:** 3–6 task parameters are changed. The task shares some physical features with the original task, but the similarities are less obvious. **Far Transfer:** All task parameters are changed except for 1 or 2. The task is conceptually the same but physically different. **Very Far Transfer:** Transfer of what has been learned in treatment to everyday functioning.
3. Practice Application of the Strategy in Multiple Environments and Tasks	• Transfer increases with the number of examples and situations provided. • Include practice in identifying situations in which the strategy does not apply. • Difficulty level is not increased until evidence of far transfer is observed.
4. Metacognitive Training *Self monitoring and self regulatory skills are needed to move the patient beyond the cued condition.*	**Metacognitive skills include the ability to:** • Evaluate task difficulty in relation to one's own abilities (awareness). • Predict or anticipate consequences. • Recognize errors or obstacles during task performance. • Monitor and adjust responses according to feedback from the task.
5. Individual Characteristics *Information is better learned and retained when the patient can relate to previously learned material.*	**Motivation and active participation are enhanced when:** • Treatment tasks are chosen with the individual's personality, interests, experiences in mind (tailor treatment to the individual). • The task introduction defines the purpose and enthusiastically creates an atmosphere of challenge. • The goals are defined concretely (eg, measurable scores, ratings for each task). • Each new treatment task is connected with previous treatment tasks and experiences. • The client is assisted in gaining a sense of "control" over their symptoms.

From: Toglia, J. (1996). A multicontext approach to cognitive rehabilitation. Supplemental manual to workshop conducted at New York Hospital–Cornell Medical Center, New York, NY.

are most responsive to cues. Responsiveness to cues indicates that the weakened skill lies right beneath the surface, but shows the potential for function (Toglia, 1992). Thus, the behavior that is targeted for change is not the client's most severe problem, but rather, a behavior or skill that is either inconsistently observed or observed with guidance.

Once the behavior targeted for change is determined, the client is taught to use a particular approach or strategy that is effective in controlling the emergence of the cognitive perceptual symptoms in a variety of different situations (see Table 26–2).

Task Analysis, Establishment of Criteria for Transfer, and Practice in Multiple Tasks and Environments

Task parameters are analyzed and manipulated to place increasing demands on the ability to transfer learning. Trans-

▼
BOX 26-1

Sample Guidelines for Analysis of Surface Task Parameters

Task Parameters That Are Most Likely to Increase Task Difficulty
Degree of detail
Degree of discriminability of task stimuli. Number of background distracters
Number of possible decisions, solutions or choices
Number of task steps, rules or facts to keep track of

Task Parameters That Are Least Likely to Significantly Increase Task Difficulty
Type of stimuli, such as objects, shapes, letters
Attributes of the stimuli, such as the color, texture, size, shape
Task category—kitchen task, grooming task
Environmental context, such as the physical surroundings, number of people
Type of task (craft, gross motor, computer)

Task Parameters That May or May Not Increase Task Difficulty (Depending on the Client's Problem Areas)
Stimuli arrangement, such as scattered, horizontal, overlapping
Movement requirements, such as body alignment, positioning, and active movement patterns
Presentation mode, such as auditory, visual, written
Location of objects or task items; size of space in which task is performed
Initiate or generate plans, ideas or hypotheses

Adapted from: Toglia, J. (1996). *A multicontext approach to cognitive rehabilitation.* Supplemental manual to workshop conducted at New York Hospital–Cornell Medical Center, New York, NY.

fer of learning is not all or none. There are different degrees of transfer, as defined in Table 26–2. Treatment involves analyzing a task to identify its surface characteristics and to determine which task parameters will stay constant in treatment and which task parameters will change. Surface characteristics of a task are its observable or physical features. Examples of task parameters that are likely to increase the difficulty of a task as well as those that may be varied without significantly increasing task difficulty are included in Box 26–1.

Metacognitive Training

Training in self-monitoring skills and awareness needs to be embedded throughout treatment. Specific self-monitoring- and awareness-training techniques were described in Chapter 20; Section 6. To function across situations and environments, the client needs to be able to monitor his or her performance and know when a particular strategy should be applied. Several authors have found that metacognitive training increases the probability of transfer of cognitive skills (Belmont, Butterfield, & Ferretti, 1982; Brown, 1988; Roberts & Erdos, 1993).

Individual Characteristics

The individual needs to be an active participant in treatment. Table 26–2 lists some ways to enhance client motivation and active participation. In addition, the use of charts, graphs, or point systems to reinforce the extent to which the targeted strategy and self-monitoring techniques are used can assist the client in understanding the goals of the individual treatment session (Toglia, 1992).

▼ STRENGTHS, LIMITATIONS, AND RESEARCH

Limitations of the multicontext treatment approach include the time required for treatment planning and the individualized nature of treatment. Because treatment is tailored to the clients previous interests and experiences, clients with the same deficit may be treated with different treatment tasks. This makes it difficult to study this approach empirically.

Although there is no research that compares or contrasts use of the multicontext approach with other treatment approaches, recent case reports and studies support individual components of the multicontext approach, such as strategy training (Nelson, Fogel, & Faust, 1986; Trexler, Webb, & Zappala, 1994), metacognitive training (Birnboim, 1995; Cicerone & Giacino, 1992; Fertherlin, 1989), and use of a wide range of tasks and situations in treatment (Llyod & Curvo, 1994; Sohlberg & Raskin, 1996).

Section 5

Motor Learning: An Emerging Frame of Reference for Occupational Performance

Clare G. Giuffrida

M otor-learning theory is a set or collection of ideas used to explain the acquisition and modification of motor behavior. It is not a singular theory, but several different concepts and theories current in the field of motor learning and control (Shumway-Cook & Woollacott, 1995). This "theory" is increasingly influencing occupational therapy knowledge and treatment.

▼ INTELLECTUAL HERITAGE

Several occupational therapists have introduced ideas, concepts, and principles derived from the field of motor behavior into occupational therapy (Jarus, 1994, 1995; Mathiowetz & Haugen, 1994; Haugen & Mathiowetz, 1995; Poole, 1991; Sabari, 1991). The motor behavior field is focused on investigating the nature, etiology, acquisition, and modification of movements. From these inquiries, theories, models, and principles to explain motor learning and con-

trol have emerged (Schmidt, 1988). These theories, models, and principles reflect the changing focus of the motor behavior field as it has developed.

In the late 1970s the motor behavior field shifted from a strict behavioral stimulus–response orientation to an information-processing orientation, focusing on underlying mental and neural events supporting and producing movement. At this time, a synthesis between neural control and motor behavior research also occurred. Scientists in neural control shifted from examining only neural mechanisms to investigating neural mechanisms during complex movements. This work was characterized by an attempt to find an association between motor behavior and neurological processes, to understand the control of movement (Adams, 1987).

As an increased interest in motor control emerged, the primary focus of motor learning on information processing gradually declined. In the motor control area there was a shift from studying the primacy of the nervous system in controlling movements to investigating other factors and systems regulating movement. The understanding of the physical principles of action became the concern of movement scientists. A reluctance to continue using cognitive–psychological styles of inquiry accompanied this emphasis on studying the physical principles of action that determined movement (Schmidt, 1988). However, counterintuitive findings about the effects of practice schedules (Shea & Morgan, 1979) and contemporary explanations of the role of feedback in learning (Salmoni, Schmidt, & Walter, 1984) have contributed to an increased interest and resumed study of motor learning.

▼ COMMONALITIES BETWEEN MOTOR LEARNING AND OCCUPATIONAL THERAPY

Motor behavior scientists have traditionally focused on motor-learning investigations with "normal" individuals, whereas occupational therapy has focused on restoring or rehabilitating occupational performances in clients (Schmidt, 1991). Many neurorehabilitation treatment approaches within occupational therapy are based on implicit and explicit assumptions about motor control and learning in the normal individual (Mathiowetz & Haugen, 1994). Within the last two decades, those assumptions have been challenged by motor control and learning research. This research has led to a shift away from reflex and hierarchical models for motor learning toward more complex conceptualizations of motor learning and programming (Schmidt, 1988; Schmidt & Bjork, 1992). This shift in knowledge has implications for how occupational therapy practitioners teach clients new movement sequences, such as how to get out of bed after a stroke or how to use a long-handled reacher.

▼ MOTOR LEARNING

Motor learning is described by Schmidt (1988) as a set of processes associated with practice and experience, leading to permanent changes in the capacity for responding and producing skilled action. This definition highlights four aspects essential to learning:

1. Motor learning is the process of acquiring the capability for skilled action.
2. Motor learning results from experience or practice.
3. Motor learning is inferred, based on behavior, and is not measured directly.
4. Motor learning produces permanent changes in behavior.

Learning is distinguished from temporary improvements in performance by relatively permanent changes in behavior. In line with this principle, it is necessary to evaluate performance by testing learning after practice has occurred. If the behavior is learned, it is evident on a test after practice. In the case of a client, this is demonstrated in the following way: the practitioner has the client practice putting on a shirt. The next day at the beginning of the session, the practitioner gives the shirt to the client and says "please put it on." If the client is successful, then the practitioner assumes that the client has retained the skill.

The effectiveness of training or rehabilitation programs are most clearly evaluated by the learner's posttraining performance and the ability to generalize to variations of the skill. Thus, the most effective practice conditions are those leading to the highest performance on either a novel version of the task or on the task performed under novel or variable conditions. For the occupational therapy practitioner planning treatment sessions, this means incorporating more task novelty and variability into sessions to evaluate learning.

The goals of practice, training, and therapy, therefore, become long-term retention, generalizability, and task learning that is resistant to altered contexts. This goal is highly congruent with occupational therapy's emphasis on function and intervention to restore or enhance independence in functional tasks necessary to fulfill occupational roles. Next, the two most important learning variables, feedback and practice conditions (Schmidt, 1988), are discussed.

▼ LEARNING VARIABLES AND FEEDBACK

Feedback is information that the learner receives about performance while learning a skill or a new occupational performance area. This information is frequently under the control of the teacher, experimenter, or practitioner. Feedback serves to inform the learner about the proficiency of his or her response during or after a response and appears critical for learning. Information produced during and after the movement, and the results of the movement on the environment, are received as feedback by the learner. In occupational therapy, as individuals practice putting on items of clothing, they receive feedback from their sensory receptors and the environment as to their success with that activity. This response produced feedback is further divided into intrinsic and extrinsic forms.

Intrinsic Feedback

This form of feedback includes information that is gathered through the individual's available sensory avenues, such as proprioception and vision. It is the inherent information from the sensory receptors during or after movement production. The learner compares this information to a learned reference of correct movement. If there is no reference of correctness, the learner is unable to use feedback to detect errors. Feedback is used in early learning to generate or modify each successive movement pattern. Later, feedback helps compare the movement executed with the reference of correctness that was developed during early learning (Poole, 1991). Clients who have sensory impairments or diminished sensory acuity would have difficulty perceiving the feel of a movement based solely on feedback from the intrinsic mechanisms.

Extrinsic Feedback

Extrinsic feedback is augmented information from an external source and supplements intrinsic feedback (Schmidt, 1988). Extrinsic feedback can be provided as knowledge of results (KR) or as knowledge of performance (KP). These forms of feedback are provided verbally about task success and the learner's performance, respectively.

KNOWLEDGE OF RESULTS

This is verbal, terminal, postresponse feedback about movement outcome in terms of the environmental goal (Schmidt, 1988). Knowledge of results provides information about errors, thus giving the learner information on whether or not to modify the movement on the next attempt. Examples used by practitioners with clients are, "You reached for the plate, not the cup," or "Your shirt is on backwards."

KNOWLEDGE OF PERFORMANCE

This is verbal postresponse augmented feedback about the correctness of the movement pattern that the learner makes (Schmidt, 1988). It is directed toward improving the movement pattern, rather than on providing information about the outcome of the movement in the environment. Examples of knowledge of performance are, "You need to lean forward in your chair to reach for the cup," or "You need to push with both arms to make the scooter go faster." There is more research evidence on the effects of KR on learning than there is on KP. Winstein and Schmidt (1990) suggest that more research is needed on KP, because practitioners seem to use it more often with clients than they use KR.

RESEARCH NOTE
THEORIES ALLOW CLINICIANS TO PREDICT WHAT SHOULD OCCUR IN THERAPY

Kenneth J. Ottenbacher

Research on theory and frames of reference can serve several purposes in occupational therapy. Theories summarize existing knowledge and give meaning to isolated empirical findings. Theories provide a conceptual scaffolding for the interpretation of observations. Theories are also used to explain observations by showing how variables and events are related. For instance, a theory of motor learning might explain the relationship between feedback and feedforward mechanisms in the learning, performance, and retention of a sensorimotor skill, such as buttoning a shirt.

Theories allow clinicians to predict what should occur in therapy, given a set of specific circumstances. A theory of motivation and compliance might assist a therapist in predicting which clients are most likely to engage in specific intervention activities and which clients are likely to resist those same activities.

One important goal of research is to generate and confirm theories. Ideas or clinical hunches that are systematically examined by research may lead to theory (induction), or research may be used to test existing theory (deduction). This circular process of integrating research and theory helps provide a dynamic, clinical environment where clients receive the most effective treatments. ■

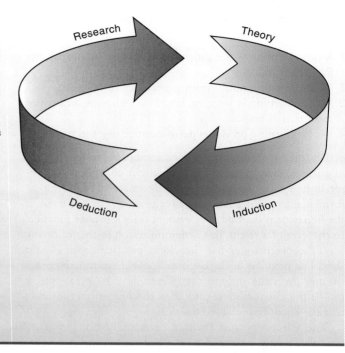

Salmoni, Schmidt, and Walter (1984) have described KR as providing an energizing, guiding, and informational function for the learner. Knowledge of results seems to guide the learner away from error toward the correct response. It tells the learner what went wrong and indicates how to correct it on the next trial. As in the previous example, if the practitioner tells the client that he or she has reached for the plate and not the cup; then, the next time the client will reach for the cup. Thus, KR has a prescriptive role and provides guidance for the learner. Knowledge of results can also keep the subject alert and motivated, particularly on mundane tasks or in long practice periods. This is important in therapy because KR can make extended, difficult treatment sessions more interesting and keep the client engaged.

Knowledge of results, however, can also detract from the learning process. Research by Winstein and Schmidt (1990) has shown that schedules of frequent feedback enhance learning, whereas schedules of continuous feedback interfere with learning. This finding runs counter to traditional viewpoints that less frequent KR degrades learning (Thorndike, 1927; Adams, 1971).

Several explanations have been proposed to explain this finding. The first is that when augmented verbal feedback is provided frequently, the learner's information-processing activities are diverted from the analysis of intrinsic response-produced feedback. This failure to process intrinsic feedback is thought to prevent the learner from being sensitive to the signals and patterns of performance errors. This results in

only effective practice; the frequent KR holds the behavior on task, but results in poor retention and learning because subjects do not develop a sufficient error detection capability (Salmoni, Schmidt & Walter, 1984).

Too much KR, then, can be counterproductive to the learner's processing of intrinsic information and developing of error detection capabilities. Therefore, only intermittent KR should be given during treatment sessions to enhance learning. As to providing KP, research on the learning principles of this form of intrinsic feedback is limited. Evidence by Schmidt and Young (1991), however, suggests that KP may follow the same learning principle as KR.

▼ LEARNING VARIABLES AND PRACTICE CONDITIONS

Massed and Distributed Practice

Massed practice is defined as a continuous practice with no rest periods or practice sessions in which practice time is more than the time for rest between practices. In massed practice, if you have a client practicing transfers, the practice time for the transfer is greater than the rest time between the first and second practice of the transfer. On the other hand, *distributed practice* is defined as practice interspersed with more time between practice for rest. In the example of practicing transfers, the time for rest equals or is more than the time spent practicing the transfer. For tasks having an arbitrary beginning and end, such as running, massed practice decreases performance but enhances learning. For discrete tasks, having a specific beginning and end, research evidence is not as clear on the effects of massed versus distributed practice (Schmidt, 1988).

Whole Versus Part Practice

This involves practicing the entire activity or its component parts. Use of a work simulator, such as a Baltimore Therapeutic Equipment (BTE), is an example of part practice, whereas practicing a complete transfer is an example of whole practice (Poole, 1991). Research evidence indicates that unless the component parts are subskills of each other or natural components of the task, part practice is not as beneficial as whole practice (Winstein, Gardner, McNeal, Barto, & Nicholason, 1989).

Mental Practice

This form of practice involves performing or running through the activity in one's mind without accompanying physical practice. Research indicates that mental practice cannot replace physical practice, but it can produce large effects on the performance of a task. It is hypothesized that mental practice triggers neural circuits underlying physical movement sequences. For clients temporarily unable to practice physically, mental practice of occupational performance tasks may provide a reasonable alternative and supplement to treatment (Shumway-Cook & Woollacott, 1995).

Variable Practice

Variable practice involves varying the conditions of the task across practice trials. In constant practice there are no variations in task conditions. Buttoning different-sized buttons, putting on different blouses, and using different spoons are examples of variable practice. Buttoning the same-sized buttons, putting on the same blouse, and using the same plastic spoon is constant practice. Variable practice appears to be more effective than constant practice, although this finding is more evident in children than adults (Shumway-Cook & Woollacott, 1995).

Schedule of Practice

This form of practice takes into account how different practiced tasks are grouped or ordered in a practice session. Blocked or rote practice is repetitive practice of one task before the next task is introduced in the treatment session (eg, practicing bed to wheelchair transfers before practicing transfers from a wheelchair to a chair). This form of practice leads to enhanced practice performance, but reduced retention when compared with random practice, nonsystematic practice, of the same tasks. Random practice leads to depressed practice performance, but enhanced retention and transfer of learning for the tasks practiced (Shea & Morgan, 1979).

Contextual Interference

The contextual interference effect refers to the finding that practice of multiple tasks in a random or nonsystematic, but repetitive, way results in depressed performance, but greater retention and transfer, when compared with tasks being practiced in a blocked or systematic manner. There are several cognitive explanations for this phenomenon. Lee and Magill (1983) have suggested that practicing different tasks on each trial forces the subject to reconstruct an action plan on each trial, which impairs speed of processing and actions during practice, but enhances retention of the task. Second, Shea and Morgan (1979) have suggested that more intertask and intratask comparisons occur during random practice, leading to more elaborate and distinct memory representations of the tasks and better retention. More recently, Schmidt and Bjork (1992) have suggested that retention is enhanced because more memory retrieval occurs during practice with random practice schedules, and this results in better retention.

The implications of this phenomenon for client intervention and treatment sessions are significant. This phenomenon implies that methods of practice, such as drill or rote practice, are not necessarily the most effective for learning. On the contrary, practicing a variety of tasks in a nonsystematic way is more successful for learning. Therefore, the practitioner may not need to make task practice simple or easy, but rather, demanding and effortful for the client. By varying the order of tasks practiced, the client becomes cognitively engaged and more effective learning can occur.

Guidance

In this practice condition, the learner is physically guided through the practice. Generally, research in this area indicates that physically guiding a learner through the task is no more effective than unguided practice (Shumway-Cook & Woollacott 1995).

▼ MOTOR LEARNING THEORIES

Theories of motor learning are groups of distinct ideas about the nature and cause of the acquisition or modification of movement. Different theories include Adams' (1971) Closed Loop Theory of Learning, Schmidt's (1975) Schema Theory, information-processing-based theories (Glass & Holyoak, 1986), Fitts and Posner's (1967) Stages of Learning, and Newell's (1991) Theory of Learning as Exploration. Each of these motor-learning theories provide different explanations of the processes and external factors significant in motor learning. They all, however, stress that the learner is actively involved in the process and that there is an interaction between the learner and the environment. A detailed exploration of these theories is beyond the scope of this book.

▼ MOTOR-LEARNING POSTULATES FOR OCCUPATIONAL THERAPY EVALUATION AND TREATMENT

Learning variables, practice conditions, and theories derived from motor learning provide a framework for evaluating and treating clients in occupational therapy. The following principles can guide occupational therapy:

1. Motor learning is the individual's active process of acquiring the capability for skilled action through practice and experience and results in permanent changes in behavior.
2. Learning is best evaluated by performance after, not during, practice.
3. Practice and feedback are the two most important variables affecting motor learning.
4. Creating practice conditions that are difficult, such as providing reduced KR and varying the practice schedule, creates an optimal motor-learning environment for the client as intense cognitive effort has to occur.
5. Contemporaneous motor-learning theories are based on a systems model of the individual and the environment and on a distributed model of motor control.

▼ THE INFLUENCE OF MOTOR-LEARNING PRINCIPLES ON OCCUPATIONAL THERAPY EVALUATION AND TREATMENT

Motor-learning principles provide a guide for evaluating and treating the client. These principles encourage active involvement of the learner in the process. However, this also means providing or altering the practice context so that the client receives reduced KR and KP and encounters difficulty in the practice context. Providing therapy in this way may be difficult for practitioners wanting to encourage and support the client while also simplifying task demands.

▼ STRENGTHS AND WEAKNESSES OF THE FRAMEWORK

The motor-learning approach is based primarily on research evidence for normal motor learning. It assumes that this evidence applies to clients engaged in normal motor learning or relearning of activities. Even though this approach is being supported by recent investigations with atypical populations (Hanlon, 1996), it needs to be systematically explored with a variety of clients having different learning needs and different movement problems. For clients having difficulty learning, it may not be the approach to use.

▶ EDITORS' CONCLUSION

Behaviorism, Allen's Cognitive Disability Model, the Multicontext Approach, and Motor Learning are all derived from learning perspectives. Not all of these approaches to intervention will be appropriate for all clients. Behavioral techniques are most appropriate for clients at the association level of learning. Allen's Cognitive Disability Model is most useful for clients who are either unable to learn or able to learn only at the association and representational levels of learning. The Multicontext Approach is appropriate for clients who are able to learn at either the association, representational, or abstract levels. Motor-learning approaches are best used with clients who can learn at the representation and abstract levels. To choose one of these intervention approaches, practitioners need to consider the relative merits of each in relation to a client's particular learning capacities and priorities.

▼ REFERENCES

Adams, J. A. (1971). A closed-loop theory of motor learning. *Journal of Motor Behavior, 3*, 111–150.

Adams, J. A. (1987). Historical review and appraisal of research on the learning, retention, and transfer of human motor skills. *Psychology Bulletin, 101*, 41–74.

Ader, R. & Cohen, N. (1993). Psychoneuroimmunology: Conditioning and stress. *Annual Review of Psychology, 44*, 53–85.

Allen, C. K (1985). *Occupational therapy for psychiatric diseases: Measurement and management of cognitive disabilities.* Boston: Little Brown & Co.

Allen, C. K., Earhart, C. A., & Blue, T. (1992). *Occupational therapy treatment goals for the physically and cognitively disabled.* Rockville, MD: American Occupational Therapy Association.

Allen, C. K., Earhart, C. A., & Blue, T. (1993). *Allen diagnostic manual.* Colchester, CT: S & S/ Worldwide.

Allen, C. K, Earhart, C. A., & Blue, T. (1996). *Understanding cognitive performance modes.* Ormond Beach, FL: Allen Conferences.

Allen, C. K, Earhart, C. A., Blue, T., & Therasoft (1996) . *Allen cognitive levels documentation.* Colchester, CT: S & S/Worldwide.

Azrin, N. H. & Armstrong, P. M. (1973). The "mini-meal"—a method for teaching eating skills to the profoundly retarded. *Mental Retardation, 11*, 9–13.

Azrin, N. H., Schaeffer, R. M., & Wesolowski, M. D. (1976). A rapid method of teaching profoundly retarded persons to dress by a reinforcement–guidance method. *Mental Retardation, 14*, 29–33.

Bach-y-Rita, P. (1981). Brain plasticity as a basis of the development of rehabilitation procedures for hemiplegia. *Scandinavian Journal of Rehabilitation Medicine, 13*, 73–83.

Bandura, A. (1977). *Social learning theory.* Englewood Cliffs, NJ: Prentice-Hall.

Beck, A. T. (1963). Thinking and depression: I. Idiosyncratic content and cognitive distortions. *Archives of General Psychiatry, 9*, 324–444.

Belmont, J. M., Butterfield, E. C., & Ferretti, R. P. (1982). To secure transfer of learning: Instruct self management skills. In D. K. Detterman & R. J. Sternberg (Eds.), *How and how much can intelligence be increased* (pp. 147–154). Norwood, NJ: Ablex.

Birnboim, S. (1995). A metacognitive approach to cognitive rehabilitation. *British Journal of Occupational Therapy, 58*(2), 61–64.

Bransford, J. (1979). *Human cognition: Learning, understanding and remembering.* Belmont, CA: Wadsworth Publishing Co.

Brown, A. (1983). Learning, remembering and understanding. In J.

Flavell & E. Markamn (Eds.), *Handbook of child psychology*, (Vol. 3, pp. 77–158). New York: John Wiley & Sons.

Brown, A. (1988). Motivation to learn and understand: On taking charge of one's own learning. *Cognition and Instruction, 5*, 311–321.

Cicerone, D. K., & Giacino, T. J. (1992). Remediation of executive function deficits after traumatic brain injury. *NeuroRehabilitation, 2* (3), 12–22.

Ellis (1962). *Reason and emotion in psychotherapy*. New York: Lyle Stuart.

Epstein, L. H. (1992). Role of behavior theory in behavioral medicine. *Journal of Consulting and Clinical Psychology, 60*, 493–498.

Fertherlin, J. M. (1989). Self-instruction: A compensatory strategy to increase functional independence with brain injured adults. *Occupational Therapy Practice, 1*(1), 75–78.

Fitts, P. M. & Posner, M. I. (1967). *Human Performance*. Belmont, CA: Brooks/Cole.

Giles, G. M. (1985). Anorexia nervosa and bulimia: An activity oriented approach. *American Journal of Occupational Therapy, 39*, 510–517.

Giles, G. M. & Clark-Wilson, J. (1988). The use of behavioral techniques in functional skills training after severe brain injury. *American Journal of Occupational Therapy, 42*, 658–665.

Giles, G. M. & Clark-Wilson, J. (1993). *Brain injury rehabilitation: A neurofunctional approach*. San Diego: Singular Publishing Group.

Glass A. J. & Holyoak, K. J. (1986). *Cognition*. New York: Random House.

Goldstein, L. H. & Oakley, D. A. (1985). Expected and actual behavioural capacity after diffuse reduction in cerebral cortex: A review and suggestions for rehabilitative techniques with the mentally handicapped and head injured. *British Journal of Clinical Psychology, 24*, 13–24.

Hanlon, R. E. (1996). Motor learning following unilateral stroke. *Archives of Physical Medicine and Rehabilitation, 77*, 811–815.

Haugen, J. & Mathiowetz, V. (1995). Contemporary task-oriented approach In C. Trombly (Ed.), *Occupational therapy for physical dysfunction* (pp. 510–529). Baltimore: Williams & Wilkins.

Hergenhahn, B. R. (1976). *An introduction to theories of learning*. Englewood Cliffs, NJ: Prentice-Hall.

Hintzman, D. L. (1978). *The psychology of learning and memory*. San Francisco: W.H. Freeman & Co.

Ince, L. P. (1976). *Behavior modification in rehabilitation medicine*. Springfield, IL: Charles C. Thomas.

Jarus, T. (1994). Motor learning and occupational therapy: The organization of practice. *American Journal of Occupational Therapy, 48*, 810–816.

Jarus, T. (1995). Is more always better? Optimal amounts of feedback in learning to calibrate sensory awareness. *The Occupational Therapy Journal of Research, 15*, 181–197.

Kantowitz, B. H., & Roediger, H. L. III (1980). Memory and information processing. In G. M. Gazda & R. J. Corsini (Eds.), *Theories of learning* (pp. 332–369). Itasca, IL: F. E. Peacock Publishers.

Kertesz, A. (1985). Recovery and treatment. In K. M. Heilman & E. Valenstein (Eds.), *Clinical Neuropsychology* (2nd ed.; pp. 481–505). New York: Oxford University Press.

Lee, T. D. & Magill, R. A. (1983). The focus of contextual interference in motor-skill acquisition. *Journal of Experimental Psychology: Learning, Memory and Cognition, 9*, 730–746.

Llyod, L. & Curvo, A. (1994). Maintenance and generalization of behaviors after treatment of persons with traumatic brain injury. *Brain Injury, 8*, 529–540.

Mathiowetz, V. & Haugen, J. B. (1994). Motor behavior research: Implications for therapeutic approaches to central nervous system dysfunction. *American Journal of Occupational Therapy, 48*, 733–745.

Neistadt, M. E. (1994). The neurobiology of learning: Implications for treatment of adults with brain injury. *American Journal of Occupational Therapy, 48*, 421–430.

Nelson, A., Fogel, B. S., & Faust, D. (1986). Bedside cognitive screening instruments: A critical assessment. *Journal of Nervous and Mental Disease, 174*, 73–83.

Newell, K. M (1991). Motor skill acquisition. *Annual Review of Psychology, 42*, 213–237.

Nisbett, R. E. & Wilson, T. D. (1977). Telling more than we can know: Verbal reports on mental processes. *Psychology Review, 84*, 231–259.

Ormrod, J. E. (1990). *Human learning. Principles, theories, and educational applications*. New York: Maxwell Macmillan International Publishing Group.

Poole, J. (1991). Application of motor learning principles in occupational therapy. *The American Journal of Occupational Therapy, 45*, 531–537.

Roberts, M. J. & Erdos, G. (1993). Strategy selection and metacognition. Special Issue: Thinking. *Educational Psychology, 13*, 259–266.

Sabari, J. S. (1991). Motor learning concepts applied to activity based intervention with adults with hemiplegia. *American Journal of Occupational Therapy, 45*, 523–536.

Salmoni, A. W., Schmidt, R. A., & Walter, C. B. (1984). Knowledge of results and motor learning: A review of critical appraisal. *Psychological Bulletin, 95*, 355–386.

Schmidt, R. A. (1975). A schema theory of discrete motor skill learning. *Psychological Review, 82*, 225–260.

Schmidt, R. A. (1988). *Motor control and learning*. Champaign: Human Kinetics Publishers.

Schmidt, R. A. (1991) Motor learning principles for physical therapy. In M. Lister (Ed.). *Contemporary management of motor control problems* (pp. 49–64). Alexandria, VA: American Physical Therapy Association.

Schmidt, R. A. & Bjork, R. A. (1992). New conceptualizations of practice: Common principles in three paradigms suggest new concepts for training. *Psychological Science, 3*, 207–217.

Schmidt, R. A. & Young, D. E (1991). Methodology for motor learning: A paradigm for kinematic feedback. *Journal of Motor Behavior, 23*, 13–24.

Shea, J. & Morgan, R. (1979). Contextual interference effects on the acquisition, retention and transfer of a motor skill. *Journal of Experimental Psychology: Human Learning and Memory, 5*, 179–187.

Shumway-Cook, M. & Woollacott, M. (1995). *Motor control: Theory and practical applications*. Baltimore: Williams & Wilkins.

Skinner, B. F. (1938). *The behavior of organisms*. New York: Appleton-Century-Crofts.

Sohlberg, M. M. & Raskin, S. A. (1996). Principles of generalization applied to attention and memory interventions. *Journal of Head Trauma Rehabilitation, 11*(2), 65–78.

Thorndike, E. L. (1927). The law of effect. *American Journal of Psychology, 39*, 212–222.

Toglia, J. P. (1991). Generalization of treatment: A multicontextual approach to cognitive perceptual impairment in the brain injured adult. *American Journal of Occupational Therapy, 45*, 505–516.

Toglia, J. P. (1992). A dynamic interactional approach to cognitive rehabilitation. In N. Katz (Ed.), *Cognitive rehabilitation: Models for intervention in occupational therapy* (pp. 1041–1043). Boston: Andover Medical Publishers.

Trexler, L. E., Webb, P. M., & Zappala, G. (1994). Strategic aspects of neuropsychological rehabilitation. In A. L. Christensen & B. P. Uzzell (Eds.), *Brain injury and neuropsychological rehabilitation: International perspectives* (pp. 99–123). Hillsdale, NJ: Lawrence Erbaum Assoc.

Vuchinich, R. E. & Tucker, J. A. (1988). Contributions from behavioral theories of choice to an analysis of alcohol abuse. *Journal of Abnormal Psychology, 97*, 181–195.

Watson, J. B. (1913). Psychology as a behaviorist views it. *Psychological Review, 20*, 158–177.

Winstein, C. J., Gardner, E. R., McNeal, D. R., Barto, P. S. & Nicholason, D. (1989). Standing balance training: Effect on balance and locomotion in hemiparetic adults. *Archives of Physical Medicine Rehabilitation, 70*, 755–762.

Winstein, C. J. & Schmidt, R. (1990). Reduced frequency of knowledge of results enhances motor skill learning. *Journal of Experimental Psychology: Learning, Memory and Cognition, 16*, 677–691.

Wolpe, J. (1958). *Psychotherapy by reciprocal inhibition*. Stanford CA: Stanford University Press.

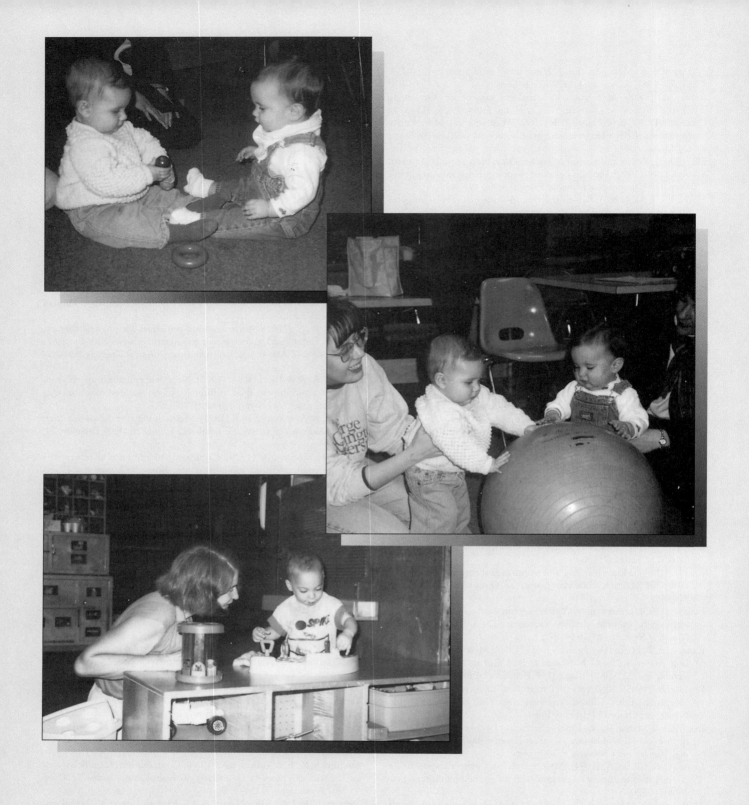

Occupational therapy practitioners encourage the development of occupational performance skills in young children.

UNIT IX

Occupational Therapy: Diagnostic Considerations in Pediatric Practice

LEARNING OBJECTIVES:

After completing this unit, readers will be able to:

▶ Describe the population served by pediatric occupational therapy practitioners.

▶ Define the diagnoses of children receiving occupational therapy and the effect of these diagnoses on occupational performance:

- Developmental delay and mental retardation

- Neurological dysfunction: cerebral palsy, neural tube defects, learning disabilities

- Orthopedic and musculoskeletal dysfunction, including congenital deformities and conditions such as osteogenesis imperfecta, muscular dystrophy, and juvenile rheumatoid arthritis

- Cardiopulmonary dysfunction

- Pediatric acquired immunodeficiency syndrome (AIDS)

- Pediatric psychosocial dysfunction: attention-deficit hyperactivity disorder, conduct disorder, mood disorders, and autism

- Child abuse and neglect

▶ Define and explain evaluation and intervention strategies for children receiving occupational therapy.

Occupational therapy services in pediatrics spans the full spectrum of care from medically focused acute care for children with AIDS, cystic fibrosis, or other conditions, to community-based services in schools and the homes of children. Legislation has stimulated the expansion of services for children from **early intervention programs** to inclusion models in public school settings. Family-centered care has emerged as an important philosophy in providing services. **Family-centered care** recognizes the importance of families in all aspects of intervention and the necessity of tailoring this intervention to the particular needs of the family unit. Unit IX builds on previous units in the book that provided information about the people who seek occupational therapy, occupational therapy practitioners, the principles of occupational therapy evaluation and treatment, and the theories that guide practice. It addresses the specific diagnostic conditions commonly encountered by occupational therapy practitioners working with children. Each chapter describes the specific evaluation and intervention strategies appropriate for these conditions. The unit opens with a chapter that defines developmental disabilities and tells the first part of the story of Patrice, a grade schooler who sustained a closed head injury and just returned to school. The unit closes with the next part of Patrice's story, the plan developed by the interdisciplinary team at his school. This plan demonstrates the use of occupational therapy services in a public school setting. Following Patrice's story are four tables that summarize the major occupational therapy assessment tools. These are organized by performance areas, performance components, and performance contexts. (*Note* Words in **bold** type are defined in the Glossary.)

Chapter 27

Introduction to the Pediatric Population

Olga Baloueff

Developmental Disabilities Defined
   Legislation
   Role of the Family in Services for
   Children

Patrice's Story: A Client and Family
   Narrative
Conclusion

Pediatrics is defined broadly as the period between birth and 21 years of age. During the past two decades, services in pediatric occupational therapy have grown in size and complexity. Over one-third of occupational therapy practitioners today work with children (American Occupational Therapy Association [AOTA], 1995). They practice in contexts such as hospitals, rehabilitation centers, mental health clinics, home health care, school systems, early intervention programs, residential centers, extended care facilities, and community-based centers. This chapter defines developmental disabilities and describes the issues important for occupational therapy practitioners working in this area of practice. The chapter closes by introducing Patrice, a schoolboy, who sustained a closed head injury, and the issues he, his parents, and school personnel encountered when he returned to school after the acute rehabilitative phase of his recovery.

▼ DEVELOPMENTAL DISABILITIES DEFINED

The term **developmental disability** encompasses a group of chronic conditions with either a prenatal, perinatal, or childhood origin. Diverse groups of diagnostic entities are included under this umbrella: mental retardation, cerebral palsy, genetic and chromosomal anomalies, autism, learning disabilities, severe orthopedic impairments, visual and hearing impairments, serious emotional disturbances, and traumatic brain injury (Liptak, 1995). The common characteristic of these disabilities is that they generally affect multiple areas of the child's development and result in dysfunction of several functional areas and components. The disability extends beyond 21 years of age into adulthood and old age.

For each child, outcome in occupational performance areas can be viewed as the result of an interactive triad among the characteristics of the environment, the child, and his or her specific diagnosed condition (Schaaf & Davis, 1992). The relation among these three factors is dynamic and ongoing throughout the individual's life cycle (Fig. 27–1).

Legislation

In the United States, key federal laws mandate and influence the provision of health care, education, and social services for children and youth with developmental disabilities. The first of such laws, the Sheppard–Towner Act, a plan for the "Public Protection of Maternity and Infancy," was enacted in 1921 (Fischer, 1994). Since then, many more legislative mandates have been produced to support the provision and delivery of services for children with disabilities. Occupational therapy is an important component of the range of services mandated by many of these laws. A summary of legislation since 1975 that affect the civil rights and education of children with disabilities is presented in Table 27–1, along with their key issues.

These laws require not only the provision of services for children with, or at risk for, developmental deviations, beginning at birth, but also, that these services be provided in the least restrictive environment. Services are geared to maximize children's individual functional performance in their natural environment. Most importantly, the role of families is central to the decision-making process and to the service delivery.

Role of the Family in Services for Children

Families are the primary social unit in which children live and receive care and nurturing; consequently, they provide the central influence in the lives of their children. The family-focused nature of pediatric practice is linked to the philosophy of occupational therapy that recognizes the impor-

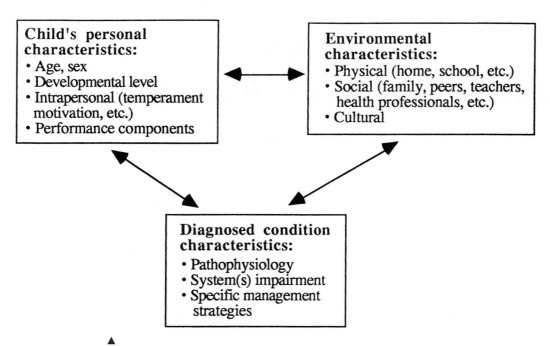

▲

Figure 27-1. Occupational performance is determined by an interactive triad.

TABLE 27-1. Federal Legislation Since 1975 Affecting Health Care and Education for Children with Disabilities

Year Enacted	Public Law Number	Title	Key Issues
1975	PL 94-142	The Education for All Handicapped Children (EHA)	Free appropriate education in the least restrictive environment for all children with "handicaps," ages 5 through 21 years; occupational therapy as a related service to support special education; established IEP; child-centered and educational.
1986	PL 99-457	Amendments to EHA	Part B: programs for preschoolers (3–5 years) with handicaps, with occupational therapy as a related service to special education. Part H: statewide systems of early intervention for infants and toddlers (birth to 2 years); established IFSP, provision of services in natural environment; family-focused; occupational therapy included in direct and primary services.
1990	PL 101-392	Carl D. Perkins Vocational and Applied Technology Education Act	Full vocational educational opportunity for youths with disabilities.
1990	PL 101-476	Individuals with Disabilities Education Act (IDEA)	Reauthorization of EHA Amendments for part H; Part B: educational services for children 3–21 years is permanently reauthorized; autism and traumatic brain injury added to definition of children with disabilities; wording change from "handicapped" to "individuals with disabilities"; transition and assistive technology services to be included in IEP.
1990	PL 101-336	The Americans with Disability Act (ADA)	Mandate making all facets of the public and private sector accessible to persons with disabilities.
1991	PL 102-119	IDEA Amendments	Reauthorized early intervention; established Federal Interagency Coordinating Council.
1992	PL 102-569	Rehabilitation Act Amendments	Transition planning at high-school graduation includes coordination of assistive technology services and rehabilitation system.
1997	PL 105-17	IDEA Amendments of 1997	Restructuring of IDEA into four parts; part C (formerly Part H—early intervention) takes effect in July 1998.

Adapted from Fischer, 1994; Gilkerson, Hilliard, Schrag, & Shonkoff, 1987; Hanft, 1991; Hauser-Cram, Upschor, Krauss, & Shonkoff, 1988; McEwen, 1994; Noonan & McCormick, 1993; Obert, Bryant, & Bach, 1994. IEP, Individualized Education Program; IFSP, Individualized Family Service Plan

RESEARCH NOTE
LEGISLATIVE INFLUENCE ON RESEARCH PRIORITIES IN PEDIATRIC PRACTICE

Kenneth J. Ottenbacher

Intervention programs for children at risk for developmental problems and for those with documented handicaps are now prominent features of the occupational therapy service delivery system. Our ability to provide effective intervention programs for infants and children reflects our understanding of the developmental processes and how events in the life of the child and family are influenced by physical, sensory, or emotional dysfunction.

Research in pediatric occupational therapy has changed dramatically in the past two decades, due largely to mandates generated by federal and state legislation. This legislation has influenced who provides services, where they are provided, what services are delivered, and how they are evaluated. The most significant recent change has been the focus on family-centered intervention programs. These changes have generated new areas of research interest and opportunities for occupational therapists. These research areas are inherently collaborative and interdisciplinary. Evaluation and research questions regarding the most effective and efficient method of service delivery in school systems and related environments will define the future roles of occupational therapists working with children with disabilities and their families. ■

tance of including the family in planning intervention. Specific roles of the family are also addressed in **PL 102–119** and **PL 105–17** concerning the formulation of services, including assessment, intervention, and transitions in and out of school settings, according to the child's chronological age (Table 27–2).

To better understand the importance of the family's influence on a child's development, occupational therapy practitioners must become familiar with the concepts of family system and parent–professional interactions. Families are seen as a dynamic, interacting system of interdependent individuals, called family members (Zeitlin & Williamson, 1994). Each family has its own characteristics, determined by its own patterns of relationships, culture, structure, life cycle, and socioeconomic background (Humphry & Case-Smith, 1995; Zeitlin & Williamson, 1994).

PATTERNS OF RELATIONSHIP

Children's development is largely dependent on their caretaking experiences and social environment (Kochanek, Kabacoff, & Lipsitt, 1990). It is a transactional process, a product of continuous dynamic reciprocal interactions between the child and the experience provided by the family (Sameroff & Fiese, 1990). Contributions from the child and caregiver influence the course of development (Figs. 27–2 and 27–3).

Caregiver's responses influence, but are also determined by, the infant's behavior (Seligman, 1988). For example, infants with severe disabilities, poor sensory modulation, or cognitive impairment challenge parents and their caregiving skills. The behavioral cues of the infant are often intense or difficult to read, and making daily activities, play, and interactions problematic. This often leads to a mutually reinforcing style of ineffectuality, with profound negative consequences for both infant and parent (Greenspan, 1988; Seligman, 1988; Williamson, 1988). Prevention and remediation of such a disastrous chain of behaviors are crucial to the child's development and family functioning.

The quality of the family environment influences children's psychological, social, and cognitive functioning (Garrison & McQuiston, 1989). Family structure, cultural factors, and socioeconomic status are important elements of the family environment. Unit II addresses these topics in greater detail. Family relationships that encourage support of its family members and expression of feelings appear to be the most significant predictors of psychosocial adjustment in children with chronic illness (Daniels, Moos, Billings, & Miller, 1987; Hamlett, Pelligrini, & Katz, 1992; Pelligrini, 1990; Sinnema, 1991; Wallander, Varni, Babani, DeHaan, Wilcox, & Banis, 1989). Conversely, psychosocial dysfunction in children with **chronic illness** is associated with maternal depression, poor coping mechanisms, and less supportive families (Daniels et al, 1987; Hamlett et al, 1992).

EFFECT OF A CHILD WITH DISABILITY ON THE FAMILY

Families of children with disabilities are faced not only with the same pressures and tensions as are all families, but also with a unique set of problems in raising children with special needs. Among the problems frequently encountered by these parents are greater physical and time demands, long-term uncertainty about a child's condition and self-sufficiency in adult years, a feeling of stigma for one's child and the family, and a lack of information and resources on how to meet the needs of the child and the family (Gallimore et al, 1990; Leyser, 1994; Seideman & Kleine, 1995; Shonkoff, Hauser-Cram, Krauss, & Upshur, 1992).

A higher degree of severity of the child's disability or medical condition, or even a lack of diagnosis, are generally most stressful for families (Shonkoff et al, 1992). Additionally, various children's characteristics have been linked to higher levels of parental stress, particularly more difficult temperament, less social responsiveness, more stereotypical behavior patterns, the presence of additional or unusual

TABLE 27-2. IDEA Legislative Provisions for Services by Age Group

Child's Age and Legislation	Program	Setting	OT Role	Basis for Eligibility	Intervention and Documentation	Service Focus	Family Role
0–3 yr	Early intervention program (EIP)	Natural setting	Primary service	Family and child's needs (criteria established by each state)	Individualized Family Service Plan (IFSP)	Family-focused	Central to all facets of IFSP, including assessment
3–5 yr	Early childhood special education program	Natural setting (school, home, center)	Related service as support to special education	Child's developmental disability or delay in specific areas	Individualized Education Program (IEP)	Family-focused but child-centered intervention	Collaborative goal-setting for IEP
5–21 yr	Special education	School setting	Related service	Child's disability support to special education	Individualized Education Program (IEP)	Child-focused affecting the ability to progress effectively in regular education	Collaborative goal-setting for IEP

Adapted from: H. R. 5, The IDEA Amendments of 1997.

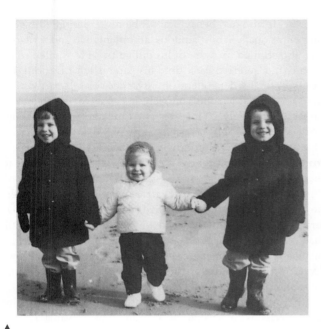

▲
Figure 27-2. Three siblings on a family outing.

caregiving demands, and a slower rate of progress (Shonkoff et al, 1992; Zeitlin & Williamson, 1994).

PARENT–PROFESSIONAL INTERACTIONS

All parents in modern societies have to depend, to some degree, on the expertise and help from professionals for the care and education of their children. But for parents of children with disabilities this dependence is much stronger. The shape and quality of this interaction can influence the way

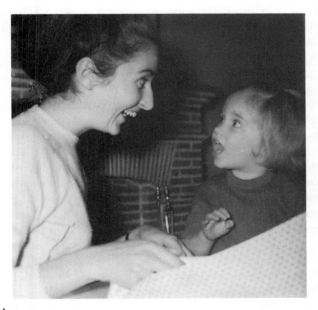

▲
Figure 27-3. Mother and daughter sharing a joyful moment.

parents adapt to meet the needs of their child, other members of their family, and their own.

For occupational therapy practitioners working in pediatrics, the challenge is how best to contribute their expertise and services in ways that will respect the family's integrity and promote competence and independence in children and their parents. Sensitivity, acceptance, and open communication are the essence of this interaction (Briskin & Liptak, 1995; Provence, 1990; Seligman, 1991). Unit IV of this book delineates this process in greater detail.

▼ PATRICE'S STORY: A CLIENT AND FAMILY NARRATIVE

Today, 1 month after the start of school, Susan, a registered occupational therapist and Mary, a certified occupational therapy assistant, are coming to the Pierce Public School. They are meeting with the director of special education, the classroom resources teacher, the physical therapist, the speech therapist, the school psychologist, and Mr. and Mrs. Douce, the parents of a third-grade student named Patrice. As a team, they will discuss Patrice's **individualized education program (IEP)**.

Patrice is a 9-year-old boy, the middle child in a family of three children. He has an 11-year-old sister Marie, and a 7-year-old brother Justin. Patrice and his family immigrated to the United States from Haiti 3 years ago. They left Haiti as political refugees, and came to the Boston area where they knew a few people, including the father's brother and his family.

The children have integrated well into their community and school, but it has been much harder for the parents who had to learn English, find new resources and support, and secure employment. Both parents work, Mrs. Douce as a nurse's aide on the afternoon shift in a nursing home, and Mr. Douce at the Haitian Resources Center. Much of the after-school care is left on the shoulders of young Marie, Patrice's sister.

Patrice is described by his parents and teacher as a handsome, vivacious, energetic boy with an interest in sports, particularly basketball. He is a good student, a quick learner who enjoys reading, art projects, and who excels in spelling and arithmetic skills. But, this was before an accident that changed the family's life.

On a sunny afternoon in early May, after school, Patrice took his bike, but not his bicycle helmet, and went to his friend Bruce's house. Both boys biked to the local playground to play basketball with their friends. The boys had a good time, but suddenly, in the middle of the game, the players began to argue about the rules of the game and about the fact that Patrice had been pushed by another boy and forced to drop the ball. In the middle of the argument, Patrice became angry, kicked the ball into the bushes, jumped on his bike, and pedaled furiously home. At a road intersection, he ignored the traffic signal and did not see a car coming in his direction. The driver of the car tried to avoid the child. Unfortunately, it was too late, and Patrice was hit by the car and thrown from his bike. He lay unconscious on the pavement as the driver of the car and passers-by anxiously waited for the ambulance and the police to arrive.

Emergency medical technicians arrived within minutes of the accident and attended to Patrice right at the scene and in the ambulance. He was transported to a local pediatric trauma center. On arrival at the hospital, he was immediately attended by the trauma team. Patrice was diagnosed as suffering from a closed head trauma, multiple fractures, and contusions. His family was notified of the accident. When the parents arrived at the emergency room, they were immediately taken to the crisis room where they were informed of their son's condition by the doctor, and were assisted by a nurse and a social worker. They saw Patrice lying unconscious, pale, and hooked up to life support units as he was wheeled into the operating room.

Patrice survived the surgery to relieve the intracranial pressure, but his prognosis remained extremely guarded for the following 5 days. He lay in a coma, showing at first only a generalized response to sensory stimuli and pain and facial grimaces in response to light touch and loud sounds. The first 10 days were most stressful for Patrice's family. Their feelings ranged from shock to fear initially, and to hope, guilt, and confusion, as they saw their son hooked up to a respirator and other life support units monitoring every facet of his body. Patrice's mother recalled: "All I could do in the beginning was cry."

The family received enormous support from friends, their church, the parent–teacher organization (PTO) at their children's school, and from the hospital pediatric staff. Through the PTO, meals were brought to the family. The other two children stayed at friends' homes after school until the parents came home after visiting Patrice at the hospital. Members of the church offered their prayers and rides to the hospital.

Patrice's primary nurse, the doctor, his occupational therapist, and physical therapist encouraged the parents to talk to him about his life, about who he was, what he liked to do, to touch him, hug and kiss him. His parents were told that a person in a coma absorbs familiar sounds and people's voices. They encouraged them to tape voices of his sister, brother, and classmates and to play them back to him at different times during the day. The medical team actively involved the family in the care of their son, as well as giving them emotional support .

After 12 days, Patrice came out of the coma, was taken off of the respirator, and 3 weeks after the accident, he was finally medically stable. A family conference with his pediatric team was scheduled to discuss his progress and to plan his discharge to a pediatric rehabilitation center. At that time, he had language problems, such as being slow to respond, speaking unclearly, and difficulty in finding the right words. He also had behavioral problems, exemplified by being emotionally labile, anxious, argumentative and irritable. He also seemed unaware of his difficulties. He wanted to go home, and he cried each time his parents left his room. He was still totally dependent on assistance for self-care activities, and his left leg and arm were in casts. He was able to sit in a chair for only 20 minutes at a time and was on phenytoin (Dilantin) for seizures.

Patrice spent 2½ months in a rehabilitation hospital. A **multidisciplinary team** of clinicians worked with him to help him regain function and go back home and to school. Finally, at the end of August, Patrice went home, to his overjoyed family and friends. He had made an excellent recovery, but his therapists warned his parents that Patrice still had some lingering problems that would affect his performance in daily living, educational, and play activities. However, over time, and with the support of his family and the school team, he would be expected to do well.

In early September, Patrice entered Ms. Fowler's third grade class with several of his previous classmates. This teacher knew well the Douce family because Patrice's sister, Marie, had been in her class when the family first arrived at the school. She is a warm, well-organized teacher, who keeps regular contact with her pupils' parents and who values the services of the special educational team. The classroom is on the first floor, with direct access to the playground.

Physically, Patrice walks independently, with a slight limp on the left side. His balance is fairly good, unless he is tired or runs. Because of poor stamina and difficulty in anticipating the position of the ball or players on the field, participation in the recreational activities with his peers is still limited. This is very frustrating for him. He dresses himself independently and takes care of his toileting needs and grooming, but is somewhat slow. His speech is somewhat laborious at times. He seems to stumble on words, forgets them, and stutters when he is tired. Once this made his classmates laugh, and he became very upset.

In class, at midday he often becomes withdrawn, apathetic, and distracted, especially when the classroom atmosphere is noisy and the children are moving about. He has difficulty with arithmetic and spelling, frequently forgetting a letter or the place of a number. When his teacher corrects him, he often reacts with a temper outburst. Once he threw his papers on the floor and accused her of picking on him unfairly. Mr. and Mrs. Douce remarked that their son has similar tantrums at home, especially if they would give him verbal instructions for various tasks. This is very upsetting to the whole family because they expect their children to be well-behaved and to be polite with them and their teachers.

Finally, Patrice's written work, which always had been well-organized and neatly done, is now sloppy. He often forgets to do his homework for the next day. At this point, Mr. and Mrs. Douce are becoming very worried about their son's behavior at school and at home. Their other two children are resentful at the long disruption in the family's routine. They also do not understand why their brother has changed so much, although he looks well and is able to walk. After speaking with his teacher, it is clear to Mr. and Mrs. Douce that their son needs help with his behavior at home and to keep up with school work.

▶CONCLUSION

To provide quality care in pediatrics, occupational therapy practitioners must recognize issues affecting each family and become familiar with federal regulations shaping the delivery of health and educational services. Parent–professionals interactions are key to the quality of interventions given to children. Patrice's story reflects the complexity of the issues surrounding children who need occupational therapy intervention and their families. The following chapters in this unit will provide an introduction to pediatric practice. The unit closes with a section entitled *Client Applications*, which presents Patrice's evaluation findings and the occupational therapy interventions developed by the occupational therapy practitioners at his school.

▼ REFERENCES

American Occupational Therapy Association (AOTA). (1995). *Membership information.* Bethesda, MD: AOTA.

Briskin, H. & Liptak, G. S. (1995). Helping families with children with developmental disabilities. *Pediatric Annals, 24,* 262–266.

Daniels, D. Moos, R. H., Billings, A. G., & Miller, J. J. (1987). Psychosocial risk and resistance factors among children with chronic illness, healthy siblings, and healthy controls. *Journal of Abnormal Child Psychology, 15,* 295–308.

Fischer, J. L. (1994). Physical therapy in educational environment: Moving through time with reflections and visions. *Pediatric Physical Therapy, 6,* 144–147.

Gallimore, R., Weisner, T. S., Bernheimer, L. P., Guthrie, D., & Nihara, K. (1993). Family responses to young children with developmental delays: Accommodation activity in ecological and cultural context. *American Journal of Mental Retardation, 98,* 185–206.

Garrison, W. T. & McQuiston, S. (1989). *Chronic illness during childhood and adolescence.* Newbury Park, CA: Sage Publications.

Gilkerson, L., Hilliard, A. G., Schrag, E., & Shonkoff, J. P. (1987). *Report accompanying the Education of the Handicapped Act Amendments of 1986 and commenting on P. L. 99–457.* Washington, DC: National Center for Clinical Infant Programs.

Greenspan, S. (1988). Fostering emotional and social development in infants with disabilities. *Zero to Three, 9,* 8–18.

Hamlett, K. W., Pelligrini, D. S., & Katz, K. S. (1992). Childhood chronic illness as a family stressor. *Journal of Pediatric Psychology, 17,* 33–47.

Hanft, B. E. (1991). Impact of federal policy on pediatric health and education programs. In W. Dunn (Ed.), *Pediatric occupational therapy, facilitating effective service provision* (pp. 273–284). Thorofare, N J: Slack.

Hanson, M. J. & Hanline, M. F. (1990). Parenting a child with a disability: A longitudinal study of parental stress and adaptation. *Journal of Early Intervention, 14,* 234–248.

Hauser-Cram, P., Upshur, C. C., Krauss, M. W., & Shonkoff, J. P. (1988). Implications of Public Law 99–457 for early intervention services for infants and toddlers with disabilities. *Social Policy Report, 3*(3), 1–16.

Humphry, R. & Case-Smith, J. (1995). Working with families. In J. Case-Smith, A. S. Allen, & P. N. Pratt (Eds.), *Occupational therapy for children* (pp. 67–98). St. Louis: C.V. Mosby.

Kochanek, T. T., Kabacoff, R. I., & Lipsitt, L. P. (1990). Early identification of developmentally disabled and at-risk preschool children. *Exceptional Children, 56,* 528–538.

Leyser, Y. (1994). Stress and adaptation in orthodox Jewish families with a disabled child. *American Journal of Orthopsychiatry, 64,* 376–385.

Liptak, G. (1995). The role of the pediatrician in caring for children with developmental disabilities: Overview. *Pediatric Annals, 24,* 232–237.

McEwen, I. R. (1994). Perspective, special education legislation and pediatric physical therapy: Past and future influences. *Pediatric Physical Therapy, 6,* 152–153.

Noonan, M. J. & McCormick, L. (1993). *Early intervention in natural environments: Methods and procedures.* Pacific Grove, CA: Brooks/Cole Publishing.

Obert, C. N., Bryant, N. A., & Bach, M. L. (1994). On the road to ADA: The development of health care and education services for children with disabilities. *Children's Health Issues, 2*(2), 8–10.

Pelligrini, D. S. (1990). Psychosocial risk and protective factors in childhood. *Journal of Developmental and Behavioral Pediatrics, 11,* 201–208.

Provence, S. (1990). Interactional issues: Infants, parents, professionals. *Infants and Young Children, 3*(1), 1–7.

Sameroff, A. J. & Fiese, B. H. (1990). Transactional regulation and early intervention. In S. J. Meisels & J. P. Shonkoff (Eds.), *Handbook of early childhood intervention* (pp. 119–149). New York: Cambridge University Press.

Schaaf, R. C. & Davis, W. S. (1992). Promoting health and wellness in the pediatric disabled and at risk population. In J. Rothman & R. Levine (Eds.), *Prevention practice: Strategies for physical therapy and occupational therapy* (pp. 270–283). Philadelphia: W. B. Saunders.

Seideman, R. Y. & Kleine, P. F. (1995). A theory of transformed parenting: Parenting a child with developmental delay/mental retardation. *Nursing Research, 44*(1), 38–44.

Seligman, M. (1991). *The family with a handicapped child* (2nd ed.). Boston, MA: Allyn and Bacon.

Seligman, S. (1988). Concepts in infant mental health: Implications for work with developmentally disabled infants. *Infants and Young Children, 1*(1), 41–51.

Shonkoff, J. P., Hauser-Cram, P., Krauss, M. W., & Upshur, C. C. (1992). Development of infants with disabilities and their families: Implications for theory and service delivery. *Monographs of the Society for Research in Child Development,* No. 230, 57(6).

Sinnema, G. (1991). Resilience among children with special health-care needs and among their families. *Pediatric Annals, 20,* 483–486.

Wallander, J. L., Varni, J. W., Babani, L., DeHaan, C. B., Wilcox, K. T., & Banis, H. T. (1989). The social environment and the adaptation of mothers of physically handicapped children. *Journal of Pediatric Psychology, 14,* 371–387.

Williamson, G. G. (1988). Motor control as a resource for adaptive coping. *Zero to Three, 9*(1), 1–7.

Zeitlin, S. & Williamson, G. G. (1994). *Coping in young children, early intervention practices to enhance adaptive behavior and resilience.* Baltimore: Paul H. Brookes.

Chapter 28

Developmental Delay and Mental Retardation

Olga Baloueff

▼ DEVELOPMENTAL DELAY

Children are considered to have a developmental delay when they are unable to accomplish tasks typical of their chronological age (Clancy & Clark, 1990). The term developmental delay generally refers to a deficit in one or more of the following areas of development: (1) cognitive, (2) physical, (3) communication, (4) social or emotional, and (5) adaptive or self-help skills, as measured by appropriate diagnostic instruments and procedures (Noonan & McCormick, 1993).

Under **Public Law (PL) 105–17** regulations, it is the responsibility of each state to determine the criteria and procedures for establishing developmental delay, and thus the eligibility for services. The law mandates that two groups of infants and toddlers with disability (birth to 3 years) are eligible to receive early intervention (EI) services: those who are developmentally delayed; and those with a diagnosed physical or mental condition that has a high probability of resulting in developmental delays. Additionally, children aged 3 to 5 with developmental delay may, at the state's discretion, be included under the term of children with disabilities and become eligible for special education and related services.

Types and Causes for Developmental Delays

Children may be at risk for developmental deviations for a variety of reasons. Tjossem (1976) identified three groups of infants and young children with or at risk for developmental

delays. These groups, still in use today, identify children with the following issues: (1) established risk, (2) biological risk, and (3) environmental risk. Each of these will be discussed in turn.

Children with established risk are those manifesting early-appearing atypical development related to diagnosed developmental disabilities of known etiology, such as chromosomal, structural, or metabolic defects. Examples are children with Down syndrome, spinal bifida, or visual impairment. Those with biological risk have an increased probability for delayed or atypical development caused by early health factors affecting the developing brain and known to potentially affect the developmental course. Prematurity, low birth weight, malnutrition, and fetal alcohol syndrome are examples of these risk factors. Children with environmental risk are those who, although biologically sound, may experience developmental deviations secondary to depriving social and familial life experiences. Examples are children who live in conditions of poverty, homelessness, or with parents who have a mental illness or mental retardation.

These three categories of risk are not mutually exclusive, and many infants have a combination of risks for developmental deviations. Often it is the number, rather than the nature, of risk factors that determines outcome in children's development and functional performance (Sameroff & Fiese, 1990). For example, a child born prematurely with low birthweight to a mother who has an addiction to drugs and a chaotic lifestyle that limits her ability to properly care for her infant is at greater risk for developmental delays than a child born early in a stable and nurturing family with resources.

Occupational Performance Deficits

Developmental delays manifest themselves in many ways. They can be transient, as in some children born prematurely, or last a lifetime, as in mental retardation. Some other children will develop normally for a period and then regress, such as those with Rett syndrome or Tay-Sachs disease (McEwen, 1994).

In infancy, regardless of the cause of the disability, developmental delays are most apparent in the sensorimotor performance components. Acquisition of motor skills, particularly proximal stability and trunk control, are considered to be essential for the development of mobility, oral-motor, fine-motor, and perceptual-motor skills (Bly, 1994; Vergara, 1993). Children with cardiopulmonary or musculoskeletal problems, mental retardation, or those born very prematurely, typically show developmental delays in the achievement of motor milestones.

During the toddler years and early childhood, additional delays may become evident in language and cognitive development, particularly for children with mental retardation or in children raised in suboptimal environmental conditions (Greenspan & Meisels, 1994). Such delays will have an influence on all performance areas, ranging from activities of daily living (ADL) to play, and early participation in educational activities.

▼ MENTAL RETARDATION

Definition and Prevalence

Mental retardation is a general term used to describe a lifelong developmental disability marked by intellectual and functional skills deficits. According to the American Association on Mental Retardation (AAMR), **mental retardation** is defined by:

. . . substantial limitations in present functioning. It is characterized by significantly subaverage intellectual functioning, existing concurrently with related limitations in two or more of the following applicable skill areas: communication, self-care, home living, social skills, community use, self-direction, health and safety, functional academics, leisure, and work. (1992, p. 1)

It is estimated that about 3% of the general population has mental retardation, and that 12% of children with disabilities (ages 6 to 21) in US public schools are given that diagnosis (Drew, Hardman, & Logan, 1996, p. 14).

Etiology

Mental retardation is a functional deficit associated with a wide range of disabilities. It may be caused by prenatal, perinatal, or postnatal factors, all of them affecting the central nervous system (CNS). There are several categories of causes: chromosomal abnormalities, disorders of metabolism or nutrition, maternal infections and intoxications, disorders of

gestation, CNS malformations, severe environmental deprivation, postnatal brain disease and injury, and frequently, of unknown origin (AAMR, 1992; Bertoti, 1994). The lower the children's IQ, the more neurological and associated problems are generally present with the mental retardation (Drew et al, 1996). Chronic problems range from visual and hearing impairments to heart diseases, seizures, and endocrine disorders.

Diagnosis of Mental Retardation

Three criteria are used in the process of determining a diagnosis of mental retardation (AAMR, 1992; Drew et al, 1996). The first criterion addresses an intellectual functioning level for an IQ of 70 to 75 or below, as measured by appropriate standardized intelligence tests, with consideration of the child's cultural, social, and linguistic background. In the second criterion, the intellectual functioning must coexist with significant disabilities in at least two of the ten adaptive skill areas outlined by the AAMR, such as self-care, communication, and functional readiness. The last criterion specifies that mental retardation must be evident before the age of 18 (Drew et al, 1996).

Although, over the years, the definition of mental retardation has evolved from primary emphasis on subaverage intellectual functioning, the American Psychiatric Association *Diagnostic and Statistical Manual of Mental Disorders,* 4th ed. (DSM-IV) classification system still rates individuals according to their level of intelligence quotient (IQ). These ratings follow: mild (IQ levels of 50 to 55 up to 70); moderate (IQ levels of 35 to 40 up to 50 to 55); severe (IQ levels of 20 to 25 up to 35 to 40); profound (IQ below 20 to 25); severity unspecified, owing to lack of appropriate testing (American Psychiatric Association, 1994).

The final step in the diagnosis and classification process of individuals with mental retardation is a profile of the level of support needed for enabling them to function in society (Drew et al, 1996). The AAMR (1992) suggests four degrees of support: episodic (as needed); limited (for a limited time); extensive (regularly in some environments); and pervasive (constant and intense).

The diagnosis of mental retardation is a multidisciplinary process that views the individual within a life cycle context. This developmental disability is diagnosed most frequently between 5 and 18 years, during the child's school years, with much lower numbers both at preschool and postschool levels (Drew et al, 1996). This distribution relates to the tasks presented to children during their school years, when an ever increasing emphasis is placed on abstract learning, social skills, and independence, as well as the availability of more age-appropriate psychometric measurements for diagnosis.

Prevention

Some forms of mental retardation and associated problems can be prevented through early prenatal care, monitoring of at-risk pregnancies, proper nutrition of infant and mother, and monitoring in infancy for developmental milestones and general health. Family-focused early intervention services are mandated by PL 102–119 to prevent and minimize developmental disabilities by enhancing the capacity of families to meet the needs of their infants and toddlers.

Occupational Performance Deficits

Occupational performance in children with mental retardation is characterized by the following: (1) a much slower rate of learning, (2) **developmental delays**, and (3) impaired functional skills. The impairment level varies according to the severity of the mental retardation, the environmental factors, and the associated problems. Although it is a lifelong chronic disability, there are typical performance deficits and issues at various developmental stages.

Delays in the achievement of developmental motor milestones and atypical sensory processing are often the first performance deficits to be noticed in the first 3 years of life. This is particularly so, for children with Down syndrome or for children with greater than mild mental retardation (Drew et al, 1996; McEwen, 1994). Children with Rett syndrome or Tay-Sachs disease develop normally at first, and then regress later in early childhood. These motor regressions are often the first indication of a more global developmental problem (McEwen). In the preschool years, mental retardation is likely to become evident in delayed language development, perceptual processing, and cognitive integration (Drew et al, 1996; Ramey & Ramey, 1992). As the child prepares for kindergarten and elementary school, delays in cognitive, psychological, social, and self-management skills become increasingly apparent and may have a serious influence on the child's ability to adapt and chances to succeed in a classroom environment (Drew et al; Hardman, Drew, Egan, & Wolf, 1996).

The cognitive and the psychosocial deficits are generally the major issues for the adolescent and young adult with mental retardation. These deficits manifest themselves in dysfunction in all three major performance areas: ADL, work and productive activities, and leisure activities. For individuals with mental retardation, performance contexts can have a major effect on their occupational performance and their ability to adapt and chances to succeed.

▼ EVALUATION OF DEVELOPMENTAL DELAYS AND MENTAL RETARDATION

Evaluation of infants and young children is fundamentally different from older children. In infants and toddlers, all areas of the development are not only interdependent, but are shaped by the quality of the home environment and interaction with the caregiver (Greenspan & Meisels, 1994). Thus, in the evaluation process, the therapist must consider

both the child's biological status and the influence of the environmental factors on the performance areas or components (Bagnato, Neisworth, & Munson, 1993; Benn, 1993; Greenspan & Meisels, 1994).

Part C of PL 105–17 delineates the type of assessment to be administered to young children with developmental delays.

Assessment Guidelines for Infants and Toddlers at Risk for Developmental Delay

1. A multidisciplinary assessment of the unique strengths and needs of the infant or toddler and the identification of services for meeting such needs;
2. A family-directed assessment of the resources, priorities, and concerns of the family and the identification of the supports and services necessary to enhance the family's capacity to meet the developmental needs of their infant or toddler with a disability.

With their emphasis on occupational performance, occupational therapists have a major role in the evaluation of children with developmental delays and with mental retardation. Occupational therapists generally evaluate children's performance areas, sensorimotor components, coping skills, and overall developmental skills, always taking into account the performance contexts (Case-Smith, 1993; Cook, 1991).

Assessments generally comprise **standardized tests** (criterion- or norm-referenced), such as, for example, the Bayley Scales of Infant Development, the Early Intervention Developmental Profile, and the Miller Assessment for Preschoolers. Behavioral observations and family interviews are included in the evaluation process. At the end of this unit, more extensive lists of assessment tools frequently used by occupational therapists to evaluate and screen for developmental and functional deviations are presented (see Tables IX-A, IX-B, and IX-C).

The evaluation process of adolescents and young adults with mental retardation focuses on the major performance areas of self-maintenance tasks, work and productive activities, and leisure activities. Assessment tools also need to be ecologically and functionally relevant (Hardman et al, 1996). Furthermore, it is important to determine the individuals's profile of strengths and needs within the context of his or her cognitive abilities; also, to determine the individual's preferred learning style (Humphry & Jewell, 1993).

▼ TREATMENT OF CHILDREN WITH DEVELOPMENTAL DELAYS AND MENTAL RETARDATION: THE INDIVIDUALIZED FAMILY SERVICE PLAN AND INDIVIDUALIZED EDUCATION PROGRAM

Guidelines for service provision to children with developmental delays and mental retardation are written in **PL**

▼ BOX 28-1

Components of the Individualized Family Service Plan (IFSP)

1. The child's level of function in all developmental areas;
2. The family's strengths and needs related to the support of their child's development;
3. The major outcome to be achieved for the child and the family; the criteria, procedures, and timeline used to determine the degree to which progress toward achieving the outcomes is being made; whether modification or revisions of the outcome are necessary;
4. The specific services needed to meet the unique needs of the child and the family, including the frequency, intensity, and the method of delivery of services;
5. The dates of services (initiation and anticipated duration);
6. The name of the family service coordinator;
7. The transition plan to services from early intervention to preschool services.

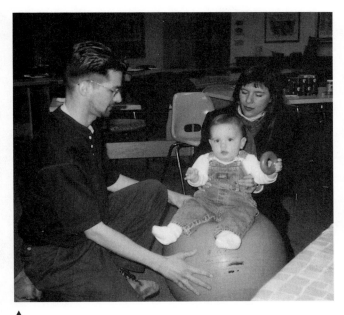

▲
Figure 28-1. Facilitation of equilibrium reactions on therapeutic ball.

105–17. For children younger than 3 years of age, services are spelled out in a family-centered service plan, called the Individualized Family Service Plan (IFSP; Box 28–1). Occupational therapy is included as a direct service in this plan. For children 3 to 21 years of age the Individualized Education Program (IEP; Box 28–2) delineates the plan to facilitate and support the education of the child. Occupational therapy services are included to the extent that they support the child's education. Both the IFSP and IEP provide multidisciplinary services delivered in the child's natural environment and in the least restrictive settings (McEwen, 1994) (Figs. 28–1 and 28–2).

The IFSP is an individualized plan of intervention containing specific information concerning the delivery of services for the child and the family (Slentz & Bricker, 1992). This plan is written in language the parents can understand (ie, lay rather than professional terminology).

An occupational therapy practitioner may use several frames of reference or theories, often simultaneously, in

▼ BOX 28-2

Components of the Individualized Education Program (IEP)

1. The child's present levels of educational performance;
2. The strengths of the child and parents' concern for enhancing their child's education;
3. Annual goals and short-term instructional objectives in all areas where the child needs specially designed instruction;
4. A statement of the specific educational services needed;
5. Extent of regular classroom participation;
6. Projected date for initiation of services and anticipated duration of services;
7. Criteria, evaluation procedures, and schedules for determining (at least once a year) whether instructional objectives are being met.
8. Consideration whether the child requires assistive technology devices and services.

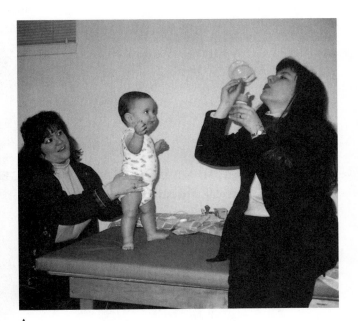

▲
Figure 28-2. Therapist supports the infant's standing balance with his mother's participation.

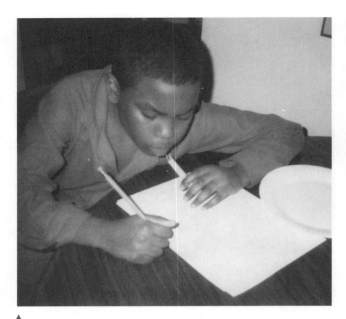

▲
Figure 28-3. In children with handwriting problems, occupational therapists evaluate sitting posture, visual-motor, and fine-motor skills.

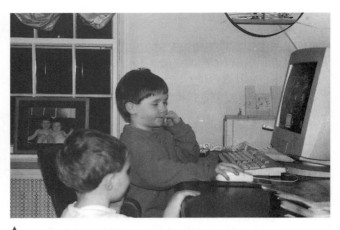

▲
Figure 28-4. Children can be taught to use computers in their preschool years.

treating children's performance deficits. Developmental, sensorimotor, and sensory integration approaches are commonly used to address developmental delays, motor issues, and sensory and perceptual processing. Behavioral approaches, using principles of learning and behavior management, are used to teach functional skills, such as ADL, work skills, and psychosocial skills (Humphry & Jewell, 1993). Environmental adaptations, such as computers, assistive devices, and other adaptations for work and living (Figs. 28–3 and 28–4) are also often used to assist individuals with mental retardation and developmental disability to function at their optimum level (Humphry & Jewell, 1993; McEwen, 1994). These approaches are delineated in the evaluation, treatment, and theory units of this book.

Programs for adolescents with mental retardation must include the development of vocational interests and skills, focusing on employment preparation. Adaptive skills training in such areas as interpersonal relationships, personal appearance, sex education, community mobility, and leisure activities is considered essential for enhancing independence in the community (Drew et al, 1996). After 21 years of age, young adults with mental retardation move from the educational environment to programs for adults. The occupational therapy practitioner has an important role in this passage, ensuring that the functional needs of the individual will continue to be matched for productive living.

►Conclusion

Occupational therapy services to children with mental retardation and developmental disabilities support and enhance development of the children's functional capabilities. This enables them to gain skills in self-care, education and work, and play or leisure to participate as fully as possible in society as they enter adulthood—whether they live at home or in more independent settings in the community.

ETHICS NOTE
IS TREATMENT A RIGHT OR A PRIVILEGE?
Penny Kyler and Ruth A. Hansen

The Lopes family lives in a rural area. Their 3-year-old daughter, Maria, has severe athetosis with quadriplegic involvement. The parents want her to receive occupational, physical, and speech therapy in their home. The local school administrator says that the school cannot afford to provide early intervention in the home. The best that the school district can offer is to provide therapy in a school that is 70 miles from the Lopes' home.

1. Do the parents have the right to expect or demand these services?
2. Does the school have any legal or ethical obligation to provide these services?
3. Are there other possible service delivery options that might work?
4. Is treatment for Maria a right or a privilege?   ■

▼ REFERENCES

American Association on Mental Retardation (AAMR). (1992). *Mental retardation: Definition, classification, and systems of supports* (9th ed.). Washington, DC: Author.

American Psychiatric Association (APA). (1994). *Diagnostic and statistical manual of mental disorders (DSM-IV)* (4th ed.). Washington, DC: Author.

Bagnato, S. J., Neisworth, J. T., & Munson, S. M. (1993). Sensible strategies for assessment in early intervention. In D. M. Bryant & M. A. Graham (Eds.), *Implementing early intervention: From research to effective practice* (pp. 148–156). New York: Guilford Press.

Benn, R. (1993). Conceptualizing eligibility for early intervention services. In D. M. Bryant & M. A. Graham (Eds.), *Implementing early intervention: From research to effective practice* (pp. 18–45). New York: Guilford Press.

Bertoti, D. B. (1994). Physical therapy for the child with mental retardation. In J. S. Tecklin (Ed.), *Pediatric physical therapy* (pp. 363–389). Philadelphia: J. B. Lippincott.

Bly, L. (1994). *Motor skills acquisition in the first year: An illustrated guide to normal development.* San Antonio, TX: Therapy Skill Builders.

Case-Smith, J. (1993). *Pediatric occupational therapy and early intervention.* Stoneham, MA: Butterworth-Heinemann.

Clancy, H. & Clark, M. J. (1990). *Occupational therapy with children.* Melbourne, Australia: Churchill Livingstone.

Cook, D. G. (1991). The assessment process. In W. Dunn (Ed.), *Pediatric occupational therapy: Facilitating effective service provision* (pp. 35–72). Thorofare, NJ: Slack.

Drew, C. J., Hardman, M. L., & Logan, D. R. (1996). *Mental retardation, a life cycle approach.* Englewood Cliffs, NJ: Merrill, Prentice Hall.

Greenspan, S. I. & Meisels, S. (1994). Toward a new vision for the developmental assessment of infants and young children. Zero to Three, 14(6), 1–8.

Hardman, M. L., Drew, C. J., Egan, M. W., & Wolf, B. (1996). *Human exceptionality: Society, school, and family* (5th ed.). Needham Heights, MA: Allyn & Bacon.

Humphry, R. & Jewell, K. (1993). Mental retardation. In H. Hopkins & H. Smith (Eds.), *Willard and Spackman's occupational therapy* (8th ed., pp. 419–430). Philadelphia: J. B. Lippincott.

McEwen, I. (1994). Mental retardation. In S. K. Campbell (Ed.), *Physical therapy for children* (pp. 459–488). Philadelphia: W. B. Saunders.

Noonan, M. J. & McCormick, L. (1993). *Early intervention in natural environments: Methods and procedures.* Pacific Grove, CA: Brooks/Cole Publishing.

Ramey, C. T. & Ramey, S. L. (1992). Effective early intervention. *Mental Retardation, 30,* 337–345.

Sameroff, A. J. & Fiese, B. H. (1990). Transactional regulation and early intervention. In S. J. Meisels & J. P. Shonkoff (Eds.), *Handbook of early childhood intervention* (pp. 119–149). New York: Cambridge University Press.

Slentz, K. L. & Bricker, D. (1992). Family-guided assessment for IFSP development: Jumping off the family assessment bandwagon. *Journal of Early Intervention, 16,* 11–19.

Tjossem, T. D. (1976). *Intervention strategies for high risk infants and young children.* Baltimore: University Park Press.

Vergara, E. (1993). *Foundations for practice in the neonatal intensive care unit and early intervention:* Vols. 1 and 2 Bethesda, MD: The American Occupational Therapy Association.

Chapter 29

Neurological Dysfunction in Children

Rhoda P. Erhardt and Susan Cook Merrill

The scope of pediatric neurological dysfunction includes conditions that are acquired and conditions that are congenital or hereditary. This chapter will focus on three conditions that fall into the latter, developmental category: **cerebral palsy**, **learning disability**, and **neural tube defect**. Acquired conditions, such as **traumatic brain injury** and spinal cord injury, which are also neurological dysfunctions, are discussed in Chapter 36.

Occupational therapy practitioners view all children as constantly developing and modifying the skills necessary to participate in activities that fulfill the varied roles of childhood (Neville, Kielhofner, & Royeen, 1985). For children with developmental disabilities, the process of skill development is altered. Evaluation focuses on analysis not only of the child's abilities and limitations, but also on a thorough analysis of the physical, social, and cultural environments in which performance takes place. Intervention is based on goals created in collaboration with the child, family, and other members of the child's team (Logigian & Ward, 1989). Intervention aims at reducing deficits, thereby maximizing the child's skill development and active participation (Kalscheur, 1992).

▼ TYPICAL DEFICITS IN PERFORMANCE COMPONENTS AND PERFORMANCE AREAS FOR CHILDREN WITH NEUROLOGICAL DYSFUNCTION

Understanding performance deficits in children with developmental or neurological problems requires knowledge of central nervous system (CNS) function, sensory processing and adaptation, development of motor control, and an appreciation for the complexity of development in children. Development is a process in which neurological maturation (including motivation, arousal, and autonomic integrity) interact with external, environmental conditions (Gilfoyle, Grady, & Moore, 1990). These interactions between neurological systems and the environment create feedback loops that modify both the neurological systems and the environment. Development, therefore, proceeds based on previous experiences and genetic programming. Movement puts the child in a relationship with the environment, providing feedback to the nervous system, which promotes more mature movement patterns, and cognitive and social development (Alexander, Boehme, & Cupps, 1993). For most children, maturation occurs through participation in the typical daily activities of play, self-care, and school (Mathiowetz & Haugen, 1994).

Performance Components

Children with neurological dysfunction experience a variety of deficits in sensorimotor, neuromusculoskeletal, and motor control. These deficits, in turn, influence cognitive and psychosocial development, thereby leading to difficulty in the developmental acquisition of skills necessary for the performance areas of self-care, school, and play activities.

SENSORY DEFICITS AND ORGANIZATION

Congenital or hereditary neurological problems in children may result in a wide range of sensory problems. One area of dysfunction often experienced by children with the diagnoses described in this chapter is generalized problems processing sensory information, whether in the presence or absence of specific sensory system deficits. The general ability to process sensations in an organized way is a perceptual skill that directly affects the child's ability to make adaptive responses to the environment. For example, sensory defensiveness can result from poor registration and processing of sensory stimuli and may result in the child withdrawing from, or responding aggressively to, normal touch during bathing, normal sounds of children in a classroom, or the visual stimuli in a typical classroom (Royeen & Lane, 1991).

Additionally, children may have specific sensory systems deficits that impair their ability to make sense of the world around them. For example, a young child with hearing impairment may have difficulty making sense of the social environment because he or she misses parts of conversations or misses nonverbal communication because he or she is concentrating so hard on listening. Often, more than one sensory system is impaired, which complicates the child's ability to understand and participate in meaningful activities at school and home.

Visual Problems

Visual impairment results from problems with any part of the visual system, including eyes, eye muscles, optic nerve, or areas of the cerebral cortex that process visual information (Gersh, 1991b). Optic nerve damage, visual field losses, and cataracts are common in premature infants with retinopathy of prematurity (ROP). These infants may also be partially or totally blind due to injury to visual pathways or visual cortex of the brain. Children with neurological dysfunction may have problems with acuity and focusing, ocular motor performance, or visual perception. For example, almost 75% of children with cerebral palsy are nearsighted, farsighted, have astigmatism, or some combination thereof (Duckman, 1984; Erhardt, 1990; Gersh, 1991a). Such deficits have a tremendous influence on school performance.

Parents of children with developmental disabilities are often aware, even during the first year, that "something is wrong" with their child's eyes. Some of the comments parents tell therapists later are: "His eyes weren't always straight, especially when he was tired"; "She didn't always notice me when I was across the room"; "He wasn't interested in books and pictures"; "She seemed to ignore everything on one side of her body"; "He never watched his hands." New techniques have improved the precision of visual testing for infants and young children, but this still continues to be a difficult area for physicians to make diagnoses.

Vision includes motor as well as sensory components. By 6 months, oculomotor performance in a normal infant is almost identical with that of an adult. Visual reflexes are integrated; that is, they do not interfere with voluntary eye movements. Localization, fixation, ocular pursuit, and gaze shift are accurate and effortless. Coordination of eye muscles is usually related to neuromuscular function of the entire body. Thus, children with delayed integration of general primitive reflexes, such as the **asymmetrical tonic neck reflex**, often show delayed integration of visual reflexes, and those with gross and fine motor developmental delays show inadequate control of voluntary eye muscles (Erhardt, 1990). These oculomotor skills are essential to school-related activities, such as finding a place on a page and scanning a computer screen during computer activities.

Visual perception is defined as the process of obtaining and interpreting information from the environment. It is a cognitive process that involves attaching meaning to sensory stimuli. Visual perception includes discrimination, memory, spatial relationships, form constancy, sequential memory, figure-ground, and closure. This is a key area of occupational therapy evaluation and intervention. Interestingly, children whose movement is limited by neurological dysfunction, but who have normal intelligence, score significantly lower than normal children on motor-free tests of visual–perceptual skills (Menken, Cermak, & Fisher, 1987). Visual–perceptual deficits are also common among children with cerebral palsy and neural tube defects who have hydrocephalus. Visual–perceptual deficits contribute to difficulty in school-related activities, especially reading and writing.

Auditory Problems

Auditory problems, ranging from mild to profound, can involve two types of hearing impairments: sensorineural and conductive. Sensorineural loss is due to damage in the inner ear, the auditory nerve, or both. It may be hereditary, congenital (present at birth), or acquired later in childhood from meningitis, high fever, or medications. Conductive loss is due to anatomical malformation or frequent infections of the middle ear. Middle ear fluid, accompanying colds or allergies, can cause temporary hearing loss, which can be critical during early speech and language development in the first 3 years of life, affecting the performance area of functional communication (Gersh, 1991b). Consequently, physiological auditory deficits not only influence functional communication, but also the ability of the child to process auditory input and respond with appropriate actions.

NEUROMUSCULOSKELETAL DEVELOPMENT

Primitive reflex activity, abnormal muscle tone, and inadequate postural control are the primary deficits in performance that impede the overall development of children with neurological dysfunction, affecting performance in play, activities of daily living (ADLs), and school.

Primitive Reflex Activity

Primitive reflex patterns provide the foundation for the infant's first sensorimotor experiences. However, the child must develop voluntary control of movement, which helps integrate these reflex patterns so that they are available when needed, but are not obligatory. For example, the asymmetrical tonic neck reflex (ATNR) provides opportunities for the infant's first visual awareness of his own hand because head rotation causes extension of the face-side arm in a very stable pattern with neck and arm joints at end ranges. If the child cannot achieve voluntary midrange control, however, the ATNR pattern may become necessary for stability, and symmetry and bilateral eye and hand function will not develop. Many voluntary skills can similarly be traced to certain primitive reflexes. Specific reflexes affecting prehension, for example, prepare the infant for complex voluntary hand skills. Continuation of these primitive reflexes will interfere with development of more refined movement. For example, the grasp reflex sustains early grasp so toys can be brought to the mouth for exploration during play. Persistence of this reflex after 3 to 4 months of age, however, will interfere with the development of skilled voluntary prehension (Erhardt, 1994). Motor maturation proceeds in a cephalo to caudal as well as proximal to distal direction (Scherzer & Tscharnuter, 1990).

Abnormal Muscle Tone

Hypertonia, or high muscle tone, results in slow, difficult movements, requiring excessive effort. Hypotonia, or low muscle tone, interferes with the balance between stability and mobility required for almost all movement, especially antigravity motor control. Many infants with low tone develop hypertonia later as they recruit excessive tone in distal parts, such as hands, when they attempt to move or maintain difficult postures. Fluctuating tone also prevents the development of controlled mobility based on appropriate points of stability. Many children with neurological dysfunction have combinations of muscle tone and movement disorders, distributed in different parts of the body.

Postural Control and Upper Extremity Function

Skilled movement requires complex patterns of muscular coordination, which depend on a foundation of basic motor patterns acquired during early life. All movement requires constant change of posture and adjustment in the center of gravity. Upper extremity function, such as reaching, grasping, and manipulating objects, requires dynamic stability of the shoulder girdle on a stable trunk, and independent movement of the head and arms from the shoulders. This stability develops out of weight-bearing activities of the infant, such as crawling during play (Scherzer & Tscharnuter, 1990). Skilled arm and hand functions also require a dynamically stable sitting base, which allows weight shift during reaching. Thus, all parts of the body are connected, with the pelvis as the central point, and significantly affect upper extremity function (Hypes, 1988). Poor spinal stability can result in excessive flexion or extension of trunk or legs and asymmetry. Without good sitting balance, the hands are not free for manipulation in self-care skills, such as eating and dressing, and school-related activities, such as writing.

Components of voluntary fine motor function include visual regard or inspection, approach or reach, grasp, manipulation, release, and eye–hand interaction or coordination (Erhardt, 1994). In-hand manipulation typically develops during the ages of 1 through 7 years. It refers to movement of an object within a person's hand, such as retrieving coins from a purse or pocket, moving them from fingers to palm, then from palm to fingers to insert into a machine slot one at a time (Exner, 1989). Buttons, zippers, shoelaces, scissors, and other tools are examples for which mastery is expected by the school-aged child and that require the most complex distal movement patterns. The use of eating utensils is one of the first functional tasks in self-care and represents the first purposeful use of tools for most children and, as such, is an important precursor for manipulation of tools used in school, including writing tools and scissors. Use of these fine motor tools is a combination of simple patterns, performed sequentially and concurrently to complete a functional task (Boehme, 1988; Connolly & Dalgleish, 1989).

Visual–Motor Integration

Visual–motor integration is the ability of the eyes and hands to work together in smooth, efficient patterns. Controlled eye movements precede controlled hand movements. At the same time, coordinated hand movements influence the eyes, as both systems exchange information needed for adaptation to rapidly changing environmental conditions (Erhardt, 1992). The coordination of hand and eye depends first on the control of the head, enabling the eyes to monitor the task of the hands. A stable shoulder girdle then dictates the effectiveness of the arm in transporting the hand to its task and maintaining it during manipulation (Penso, 1990). The role of the hand, accomplished through combined movements of the forearm, wrist, and the dynamic palmar arches, is to shape itself around the viewed object (Boehme, 1988).

Cognition

The ability to reason, think, and solve problems in ways that are adaptive develops out of the child's early sensorimotor experiences. Cognitive abilities reflect the highest organization of the nervous system, but they depend on the organization and integrity of lower levels of neurological function. It is often difficult for psychologists to determine intelligence in children with moderate to severe neurological disabilities because current standardized tests are inappropriate for children with physical handicaps who cannot talk or control their hands to respond correctly. In general, however, these children demonstrate a wide range of intelligence, which means that the ability to learn varies greatly. Children with mental retardation usually learn new skills more slowly than other children, may not be as motivated, and do not generalize new skills to similar situations (Gersh, 1991a).

The Medically Fragile Child

More school children are medically fragile and have multiple, severe disabilities. These children require medically related procedures during the school day. Federal legislation dating as long ago as 1978 initiated mainstreaming and inclusion policies that have increased the likelihood that children who are medically fragile and multiply disabled live at home, instead of in institutions, and attend neighborhood schools. School personnel are dealing with issues that had been relegated exclusively to nurses and physicians in the past, such as management of seizure problems. Other health-related procedures, which usually involve school nurses, include postural drainage, shunt care, nasogastric tube and gastrostomy feeding, prosthesis care, catheterization, machine and syringe suctioning, and tracheostomy care. As policies defining the roles of professionals in these situations continue to evolve, occupational therapists and certified occupational therapy assistants must remain knowledgeable about these serious medical conditions and aware of their effects on function (Mulligan-Ault, Guess, Struth, & Thompson, 1988).

Medical treatments, such as medication or surgery, influence the ability of the child who is medically fragile to participate in the environment. The use of drugs for problems associated with neurological dysfunction has a relatively recent, and not always successful, history. Muscle relaxants and tranquilizers—oral, rectal, or injected—have shown limited benefit in reducing muscle tone and involuntary movement in children with cerebral palsy, but they also show unwanted side effects, such as drowsiness, disorientation, weakness, nausea, headaches, or increased drooling (Albright, Cervi, & Singletary, 1991; Armstrong et al, 1991). Medication has always played a significant and essential role in the control of seizure activity. Drugs for attentional deficits and hyperactivity have been useful in some children with learning disabilities, especially to enable the child to participate and benefit from therapy and education (Batshaw & Perret, 1986; Scherzer & Tscharnuter, 1990;). Team members need to be aware of drug side effects that influence behavior and function (Fraunfelder, 1976).

Summary

Children in our society are expected to perform a wide range of activities, which can be categorized as ADLs, play, and productive school participation. Neurological deficits impede the child's ability to explore the environment and engage in typical activities that provide opportunities for the development of necessary skills. Neurological deficits may influence the ways in which a child obtains and processes sensory information and develops motor control, skilled distal movement, visual–motor integration, and cognitive skills. Furthermore, children who are medically fragile are more often remaining at home and attending community schools than in the past. The medical interventions these children receive influence their ability to participate in the typical routines of self-care, play, and school.

▼ OCCUPATIONAL THERAPY EVALUATION AND INTERVENTION OF PEDIATRIC NEUROLOGICAL DYSFUNCTION

Evaluation

The goal of evaluation is to understand the strengths of the child and areas of concern within the context of the environments in which the child participates. Family members and other team members, such as teachers, are integral to this process. They contribute important information about the child's functional vision, hearing, speech, social and emotional development, and cognition. Evaluation is ecological, meaning the child and environment are evaluated as a unit. Evaluation places equal importance on information gathered from formal tests as well as interviews, checklists, and observations of the child's interactions with people and objects (Huber & King-Thomas, 1987).

Pediatric evaluations by occupational therapists should include motor and sensory components of developmental milestones in the areas of movement, play, and self-care skills. Evaluation must describe not only the neurological deficits, but also the functional consequences of those deficits because meaningful intervention is created from evaluation findings (Scherzer & Tscharnuter, 1990). Evaluation of the young child, in particular, should include handling, positioning, bathing, dressing, and feeding. Information about the child's social interaction in all of these contexts should be gathered. The therapist then has a broad perspective of the child's function. As the child matures, evaluation expands to include school and community.

Standardized assessments, such as the Bayley Scales of Infant Development (Bayley, 1993) and the Peabody Developmental Motor Scales (Folio & Fewell, 1983), provide objective measurements for comparing the child's development with established developmental norms. Newer assessments of interest include the Infant–Toddler Developmental Assessment (IDA) (Provence, Erikson, Vater, & Parmeri, 1995) and the Pediatric Evaluation of Disability Index (PEDI) (Haley et al, 1992).

Assessments measuring visual perception are used by occupational therapists, as well as by learning specialists, speech and language pathologists, psychologists, and optometrists. The Motor-Free Visual Perception Test-Revised (MVPT-R) assesses visual–perceptual processing without motor components required (Colarusso & Hammill, 1995). The Developmental Test of Visual Perception (DTVP-2) distinguishes between visual perception and visual motor problems (Hammill, Pearson, & Voress, 1993). The Test of Visual Motor Integration distinguishes among children with a range of ability (Hammill, Pearson, & Voress, 1996).

Although the use of **standardized tests** increases the reliability of the evaluator's judgment, they are not always appropriate for children with moderate to severe developmental disabilities. Standardized tests do not always assess quality of movement, identify improvement in children who change slowly, or measure functional skills (Campbell, 1990; Harris, 1988). Also, most of these tests rely on the child's ability to execute verbal or motor responses, and cannot be used with children who are nonverbal, physically handicapped, or both. Modification of standardized tests to make them more appropriate renders the standardization meaningless (Hacker & Porter, 1987).

Thus, many therapists rely upon a variety of structured, nonstandardized assessments of muscle tone, reflex patterns, motor development, and sensory status, as well as observations of spontaneous behavior (Cook, 1991; Fiorentino, 1973; Knobloch, Stevens, & Malone, 1980; Uzgiris & Hunt, 1975;). For example, the Erhardt Developmental Prehension Assessment (EDPA) measures (1) involuntary (positional-reflexive) arm–hand patterns; (2) voluntary movements of approach (supine, prone, and sitting), grasp and release (dowel, cube, and pellet), and manipulation; and (3) prewriting skills of crayon or pencil grasp and drawings of children (Erhardt, 1994). The motor components of vision can be evaluated with the Erhardt Developmental Vision Assessment (EDVA), which measures (1) involuntary (reflexive) visual patterns, and (2) voluntary (cognitively-directed) movements of localization, fixation, ocular pursuit, and gaze shift (Erhardt, 1990).

Oral-motor function and prefeeding skills can be evaluated within the framework of therapeutic eating programs developed by professionals such as occupational therapists, physical therapists, nurses, physicians, dietitians, and nutritionists (Fee, Charney, & Robertson, 1988; Jelm, 1990; Morris, 1982; Morris & Klein, 1987; Smith et al, 1982). Age-appropriate skills related to eating and oral-motor abilities, such as self-care, mobility, social function, play, and handwriting also need to be evaluated (Coley, 1978; Haley et al, 1992; Knox, 1974; Amundson, 1995).

Comprehensive assessments are necessary when equipment needs to be prescribed. For example, positioning for adaptive-seating devices requires evaluation of the child's medical and surgical history, muscle tone, alignment, and postural control, sensory organization and processing, upper extremity function, cognition, behavior, and communication abilities. The goals of the child and primary caregivers, and the expectations of the child's environmental context are also important (Bergen, Presperin, & Tallman, 1990; Scherzer & Tscharnuter, 1990).

Intervention

Effective intervention for children with neurological deficits depends on the ability of the team to analyze and synthesize all the information gathered during evaluation. The child must be considered within the social context of family, school, and community, as a unique, goal-oriented person who influences the world and is influenced by it, and who is intrinsically motivated to seek stimulation and interaction (McEwen, 1990). Occupational therapy programs for children with neurological deficits are designed to promote adaptation and prevent secondary complications that would occur during development. Adaptation is facilitated through purposeful participation in meaningful and natural activities. By discussing evaluation and intervention in terms of daily life experiences and occupational performance, the team can move away from a focus on pathology toward a focus on finding solutions that promote the child's participation in everyday activities (Gilfoyle et al, 1990). Many therapists combine several intervention approaches, choosing a variety of strategies from established theoretical bases, and individualizing each program according to the child's changing needs as well as their own professional strengths. (Scherzer & Tscharnuter, 1990). Occupational therapy intervention will be described using three domains: developmental, motor control, and positioning and adaptive equipment.

DEVELOPMENTAL APPROACHES

The most widely used developmental approach for children with neurological deficits is **neurodevelopmental treatment (NDT)**. This approach offers specific handling techniques to inhibit abnormal patterns, normalize muscle tone, and facilitate normal movement, which leads to improved ability to carry out ADLs, such as sitting at a table to eat or write, or being able to dress more independently. Please also refer Chapter 25 for a more detailed discussion of the neurodevelopmental frame of reference.

The concept that movement ranges from "least automatic" to "most automatic" is useful in explaining the NDT emphasis on therapeutic handling. Therapeutic handling attempts to obtain active, automatic movement from the child, leading to controlled, purposeful movement. The child responds actively and automatically to specific positioning and handling techniques that facilitate more typical patterns of movement while inhibiting atypical patterns.

Occupational therapy using NDT techniques emphasizes head, trunk, and upper body control toward the acquisition of hand skills for independent self-care, play, school, and community activities. Handling and positioning techniques are designed to normalize muscle tone and obtain postural alignment throughout the entire body, and to prepare both the upper and lower extremities for weight-bearing, weight-shifting, and function (Foltz et al, 1991).

Many therapists who use NDT also incorporate myofascial release techniques into their handling methods. The purpose of myofascial release is to decrease movement restrictions that result from tonal dysfunction. The lengthening of superficial and deep soft tissue is accomplished by changing the viscosity of the fascial ground substance and through gentle and sustained stretch of the muscular elastic components of fascia. The improved structural alignment is then integrated into active postural and movement patterns (Barnes, 1991; Boehme, 1991). These techniques are used by expert therapists who have years of experience and who have had intensive training.

Use of NDT has also been combined with **sensory integration (SI)** intervention, because both developmental approaches address adaptive responses of the individual and use sensory input to produce a motor response. The main difference between the two approaches is that NDT focuses on motor output and the production of motor control, whereas SI focuses on sensory registration, organization, and processing that underlie purposeful responses to the environment (Blanche & Burke, 1991).

Sensory integration evaluation and intervention were developed by occupational therapist A. Jean Ayres for children with learning disabilities and sensory integrative dysfunction (Ayres, 1973, 1979). This frame of reference is also addressed in Chapter 25. Sensory integration is concerned with how the nervous system takes in, organizes, and processes sensory information from the different sensory channels, and the ability to relate input from one channel to that of another to produce an adaptive response (Dunn, 1987; Fisher, Murray, & Bundy, 1991). Information from three basic senses (touch, movement, and position) is used to (1) plan and sequence movements, (2) coordinate both sides of the body, (3) develop balance, (4) coordinate eye and hand movements, and (5) develop body awareness. Many children with neurological dysfunction have problems receiving and processing sensory input, resulting in (1) hyperresponsivity or hyporesponsivity to sensory stimuli, (2) gravitational insecurity, and (3) motor-planning problems (Foltz et al, 1991).

Occupational therapy practitioners who intervene with children who have sensory integration deficits are guided by a number of principles derived from Ayres' theory. Intervention (1) provides controlled, specific sensory input, (2) focuses on the nervous system's ability to organize sensory information for purposeful interaction with the environment, and (3) provides an environment in which the child can direct therapy. Intervention is effective when the child makes adaptive responses (Ayres, 1979; Dunn, 1991).

Intervention using a sensory integrative approach aims to improve registration and integration of sensory input (especially tactile, vestibular, and proprioceptive), develop mature postural and bilateral movement, improve motor planning, and improve body scheme. Practitioners using sensory integration techniques use a wide range of equipment for the child to work on these goals so that the environment can change to meet the child's needs (Richter & Oetter, 1990; Slavik & Chew, 1990).

MOTOR APPROACHES

The motor development, motor learning, and motor control approaches explain and provide intervention strategies for motor dysfunction (Kielhofner, 1992). For motor development, the question is: " How does motor behavior change during age-related growth?" For motor learning, the question is: "How are skills acquired through experience and practice?" For motor control, the question is: "How is the control organized?" (VanSant, 1991). Intervention provides activities organized to create increasing demands for motor development, motor learning, and motor control. This approach views children with neurological dysfunction as unable to perform, and thereby learn, purposeful motor patterns independently owing to the cycle of inadequate or distorted feedback, causing abnormal motor output, resulting in unsuccessful completion of tasks.

Tenets of the motor learning approach support intervention that emphasizes practice of movement patterns in relation to functional tasks. Skill acquisition depends on both the type of task and the subject's stage of learning. Feedback (internal as well as external), facilitation, and practice are important instructional variables.

Stages of motor learning include (1) cognitive (inconsistent performance, must be thought out); (2) associative (more refinement, errors are used to correct performance during practice); and (3) automatic (little cognitive processing, less susceptible to distractions) (Poole, 1991). Most children with disabilities remain in the cognitive and associative stages, with few skills becoming smooth and automatic. Adaptations that promote the child's performance and, therefore, learning of new skills are integral components of this approach. Facilitation includes verbal instruction, demonstration, and manual guidance, always within the context of the whole task (Poole 1991). Refer to Chapter 26, Section 5 for more information about motor learning.

ROLE OF POSITIONING AND ADAPTIVE EQUIPMENT

The development of a positioning program and the use of adaptive equipment involve the integration of both developmental and motor control approaches. Proper positioning not only minimizes the influence of pathological forces on body posture, but provides a stable base of support for performance of developmentally meaningful activities. The principles delineated here apply to children with cerebral palsy, learning disability, and neural tube defects. The more severe the child's neurological dysfunction, the more complex the positioning program. Children with learning disabilities may require modified desks, chairs, and writing tools to enhance writing abilities. Children with cerebral palsy or neural tube defects may require much more extensive positioning program to minimize tonal abnormalities and maximize function.

The positioning program is developed by members of the team, with the caregivers' participation, to ensure that recommended techniques are compatible with established home routines and schedules. Even when optimal seating is achieved using a specific adaptive-seating system, children should experience other positions each day, to provide a variety of sensory experiences (Fraser et al, 1990). Positions may include reclined supine, sidelying, prone, sitting, and standing. A position is appropriate for a child when it meets the following criteria: (1) head midline with slight chin tuck; (2) symmetrical body alignment (eg, in sidelying, head on pillow to align head and spine); (3) independent sitting position which prevents lordosis and stress on hip joints in adduction and internal rotation (eg, long, half-long, and side-sitting); (4) trunk is supported in sitting when using both hands for manipulation (eg, against a wall, in a corner, or in an adapted chair); and (5) child is at eye level to adults during activities to prevent neck hyperextension.

Additional principles specific to an optimum-seated position also consider the child's head, trunk, and extremity positions in relation to each other. For maximal efficiency in sitting the child's (1) head is maintained in the vertical plane; (2) hips, knees, and ankles are maintained at 90 degrees of flexion, unless pelvic thrust or posterior tilt require more hip flexion; and (3) feet are supported. Most equipment for moderately to severely involved children is designed to be extremely adaptable, but continual monitoring is necessary as the child grows, or as changes in performance occur (Bergen & Colangelo, 1985; Taylor & Trefler, 1984). Although commercial equipment may be available for a specific type of problem, many therapists invent or adapt devices.

Strategies for improving handwriting and keyboard use for written communication are based on an understanding of the child's ability to maintain head, trunk, and extremities appropriately. For writing, the hand typically maintains a static grasp of the pencil while the wrist is held in slight extension and the forearm is supinated to about 45 degrees. This position provides the base for dynamic movement of the arm. For using a keyboard, hands are usually held in a pronated position with wrists in slight extension. In addition to appropriate positioning, adaptations for handwriting include (1) adjustment of the work surface with inclines or easels to facilitate postural alignment, and (2) the use of adaptations for crayons, pencils, pens, or markers, such as grips of plastic, foam rubber, or thermoplastic material in triangular, cylindrical, ball, or customized shapes. These grips are also useful for other utensils and tools.

A major challenge for the team and family members is to identify strategies to facilitate communication skills in a child with limited or unintelligible speech. Alternative communication methods are often necessary for them to communicate adequately with others. Augmentative and alternative communication (AAC) systems have dramatically increased these opportunities with a variety of commercial communication boards, voice output communication aides (VOCA), and accessibility switches.

ROLE OF ORAL–MOTOR INTERVENTION

In our society, mealtime is a social occasion; a time to enjoy food and conversation. Motor control problems, such as atypical muscle tone, primitive reflexes, and delayed oral–motor development can make feeding difficult, time-consuming, and often unpleasant for many children and their families. Similarly, children with sensory integrative problems are often unable to tolerate specific textures, flavors, or odors, which can make meal planning and mealtime very difficult.

Without early intervention, eating problems may lead to long-term eating disorders, including rejection of some or all foods or textures, failure to thrive, and disturbed parent–child interaction. In addition, some medical conditions affect feeding, such as respiratory insufficiency and frequent respiratory infections that lead to chronic gagging, coughing, and possible aspiration of food. Nutritional inadequacy is a common problem for children with moderate to severe neurological dysfunction. Oral–motor dysfunction, dental problems, or food refusal, vomiting or gastroesophageal reflux (GER) can result in malnutrition.

The role of occupational therapy in eating problems varies according to the child's problems and environment. The therapist may be part of a team in the **neonatal intensive care unit (NICU)**, or of an outpatient support group program for parents of NICU graduates (Chamberlain et al. 1991). In the home, the occupational therapist provides consultation to family and respite caregivers who help the child eat, to facilitate appropriate methods as well as positive social interaction during the process (Erhardt, 1985, 1986, 1995). In school, the occupational therapy practitioner may provide direct service at lunchtime or consultation to para-professional classroom staff.

Occupational therapy intervention for oral–motor deficits combines developmental and motor control principles and may include (1) overall sensory program that provides organized sensory input, (2) general tactile desensitization techniques beginning with less sensitive body parts, (3) encouragement of mouthing of hands and toys, (4) activities that encourage head and trunk control for proper positioning for eating, (5) oral–motor prefeeding stimulation, and (6) developmental progression in tolerance of food textures.

Summary

Occupational therapy evaluation and intervention consider the child's abilities in the context of environments in which the child functions. Practitioners use intervention strategies appropriate to the child, and most practitioners mingle strategies from developmental and motor learning approaches. By combining strategies, practitioners are able to address the specific needs of a child through direct intervention (such as sensory integration, NDT, or motor learning activities) and through environmental adaptation to enhance the child's performance (such as adaptive equipment for positioning for specific activities or teaching caregivers and teachers specific positioning and handling techniques).

▼ CEREBRAL PALSY

Cerebral palsy is a condition caused by damage to the brain, usually occurring before, during, or shortly after birth (National Information Center for Children and Youth with Handicaps, 1991). It is a static motor impairment, with associated handicaps that may include visual and auditory deficits, seizures, mental retardation, learning disabilities, and oral–motor and behavioral problems. It is not a disease, is neither progressive nor communicable, and is also not "curable" in the accepted sense. Education, therapy, and assistive technology can help persons with cerebral palsy lead productive lives (Batshaw & Perret, 1986).

Cerebral palsy occurs in about 1 of every 500 live births (Schleichkorn, 1993, p. 3). Of these births 10% are estimated to have a hereditary origin, whereas the remainder is attributed to prenatal, perinatal, or postnatal factors (Schleichkorn, 1993, p. 5). For example, during the first trimester, the fetus may be exposed to teratogenic drugs or intrauterine infection. In later pregnancy, placental insufficiency may place the child at risk. Complications during labor, delivery, and the neonatal period include asphyxia, sepsis, and prematurity (noted in at least one-third of all cases). Early childhood disorders affecting the developing brain are meningitis, toxins, and head injury (Batshaw & Perret, 1986; Scherzer & Tscharnuter, 1990; Torfs, Van den Berg, Oechsli, & Cummins, 1990).

A diagnosis of cerebral palsy in the very young child is formulated on the basis of developmental history, abnormal tone, and reflex behavior. In the child who is older than 1 year, the diagnosis can indicate a specific motor type, which is emerging, but is also changing. As the child grows, the extent and degree of involvement can be specified (Scherzer & Tscharnuter, 1990). The younger child demonstrates developmental delay with fairly normal patterns that become more atypical as he or she grows older.

The occupational therapy practitioner working with young children with cerebral palsy recognizes the importance of encouraging them at an early age to take responsibility, be self-reliant, and eventually become assertive in directing their own lives (Magill-Evans & Restall, 1991; Neistadt, 1987). This prepares them for the developmental tasks of adolescence, expected in the dominant American culture, such as achieving emotional independence from parents, establishing close relationships with peers, becoming socially responsible, and exploring vocational options. These tasks are difficult to accomplish from a social position of passivity and helplessness, which is common in young adults with cerebral palsy because of limited mobility, few opportunities to make decisions, and dependence on others for many ADLs.

Consequences of Cerebral Palsy on Development

Because cerebral palsy influences the process of development in children, it is a developmental disability. Cerebral palsy is distinguished primarily by its motor nature from other types of developmental disabilities, such as organic brain deficits, autism, emotional disorders, or mental retardation syndromes (Gersh, 1991a; Scherzer & Tscharnuter, 1990).

ABNORMAL MUSCLE TONE
All movement requires constant change of posture and adjustment in the center of gravity. These automatic, unconscious shifts of postural tone are dynamic and variable, preceding movement as well as accompanying it (Bobath & Bobath, 1972). Typically, children find appropriate points of stability, from which to achieve smooth and comfortable mobility. Without these automatic postural adjustments, the child "fixes" in various parts of the body and cannot perform skilled, efficient movement.

The existence of abnormal muscle tone dramatically affects the development of the child's dynamic movement. Tonal abnormalities in children with cerebral palsy are distributed in patterns of extremity involvement, which depend on which parts of the CNS are involved. These are called (1) monoplegia or involvement of one arm or leg, (2) hemiplegia or involvement of the upper and lower extremities on one side of the body, (3) paraplegia or involvement of both lower extremities, (4) diplegia or involvement of both upper and lower extremities with less involvement in the upper extremities, and (5) quadriplegia or fairly equal involvement of both upper and lower extremities (Gersh, 1991a; Scherzer & Tscharnuter, 1990).

In spasticity, or hypertonia, increased tone creates an imbalance between muscle groups. More than half of all children with cerebral palsy have spasticity caused by damage to the motor cortex, which controls voluntary movement, or to the corticospinal tracts, which link the cortex with nerves in the spinal cord that relay signals to the muscles. Hypertonia (high muscle tone) is often accompanied by persistent primitive reflexes, an exaggerated stretch reflex, and clonus (rapid and rhythmical involuntary muscle contractions, usually in the ankles).

The child with spasticity has difficulty moving from one position to another. Gross and fine motor movements are slow and require excessive effort. Restricted ROM and limited manipulation delays the development of skills necessary for play and self-care. Many children born with low tone develop spasticity later as they recruit excessive tone in their attempt to maintain posture and to move. Flaccidity, or hypotonia, prevents the child from developing cocontraction, the balance of stability and movement needed for purposeful movement.

In athetosis, fluctuating tone leads to poor midrange control. Inadequate fixation of head, shoulders, and trunk owing to lack of cocontraction in proximal joints means that distal control is difficult for activities requiring eye–hand coordination. Nearly 25% of children with cerebral palsy have these involuntary movements caused by damage to the cerebellum or basal ganglia, which process signals from the motor cortex to achieve smooth, coordinated movement and to maintain posture.

Another quarter of children with cerebral palsy demonstrate both spasticity and athetoid movements. These children have lesions in both pyramidal and extrapyramidal areas of the brain (Batshaw & Perret, 1986; Gersh, 1991a). Different types of involuntary extrapyramidal movements have been further subclassified as (1) chorea (abrupt, jerky), (2) athetosis (slow, writhing), (3) dystonia (slow, rhythmic), (4) ataxia (incoordination, imbalance), (5) rigidity ("lead-pipe").

SENSORY DEFICITS

Interpreting and using information from the senses is often impaired in the child with cerebral palsy. Sensory deficits are caused not only by lesions in the sensory areas of the brain that affect any of the sensory systems previously discussed, but also by inadequate or distorted feedback caused by lack of sensory stimulation that results from decreased motor control. Hyperresponsivity or hyporesponsivity can lead to a variety of social and emotional problems. (Foltz et al, 1991; Fraser et al, 1990).

MOTOR DEFICITS

Skilled movement requires complex patterns of motor coordination, which depend on a foundation of basic motor patterns acquired during early life. For children with cerebral palsy, quality of development is as important or even more important than the rate of development. Children with cerebral palsy develop habitual patterns of flexion or extension that limit isolated, selective movements. Instead of being gradually integrated into voluntary movement as the infant matures, these primitive patterns are strong and long-lasting. They cause stereotypic, obligatory postures and movements that are a result of an imbalance between flexion and extension. These movements and postures are incompatible with higher level, automatic balance reactions and complex motor skills (Batshaw & Perret, 1986).

Sustained postural abnormalities lead to soft tissue imbalances, eventually resulting in contractures and skeletal deformities. For example, "tailbone sitting," a common pattern in spastic diplegia, originates from poor balance reactions and postural control in this higher-gravity position. Limited range of hip abduction and flexion also interferes with upright sitting. Compensatory kyphosis (rounding of the back)

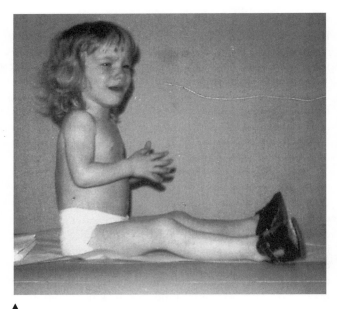

▲
Figure 29-1. A typical sitting position in a child without disability. (Photo courtesy of Joanne Ulven.)

and increased tightness in anterior flexors (neck, trunk, and extremities) become secondary problems, with significant influence on upper extremity function. Figures 29–1 and 29–2 compare the sitting positions of a typical 3-year-old and her twin sister who has spastic diplegia.

Without postural stability for independent sitting, the child's competence in play, self-care, and school activities will be compromised.

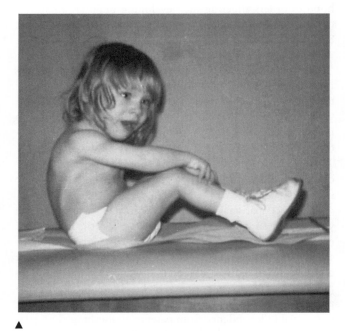

▲
Figure 29-2. The "tailbone" sitting position, common in spastic diplegia. (Photo courtesy of Joanne Ulven.)

Table 29–1 compares developmental postures in prone and sitting of a typical 3-month-old and a 10-month-old child with cerebral palsy, whose postural patterns are delayed, but are fairly typical. By 3 years, atypical patterns emerge and reflect the effects of primitive reflexes and poorly regulated muscle tone. By 11 years of age, his compensatory patterns are well established, as can be seen while he uses electronic equipment for school and communication.

Table 29–2 illustrates the effects of different types of cerebral palsy on muscle tone and movement, as well as general needs of these children.

SEIZURE DISORDERS

Nearly half of all children with cerebral palsy have seizures, involuntary movements or changes in consciousness or behavior caused by abnormal electrical activity in the brain.

Seizures may be partial or generalized, and can affect the motor, sensory, and autonomic systems. Motor symptoms include jerking of muscle groups or an extremity. Sensory seizures cause visual or auditory hallucinations or disturbances of taste or smell. The autonomic system reacts with rapid heart beat, sweating, paleness, flushing, or anxiety. Table 29–3 includes current terminology for generalized seizures, previous terms, and descriptive behaviors.

ORAL–MOTOR DISORDERS

The motor control issues that have been discussed for children with cerebral palsy often affect the facial and oral muscles as well. Eating and communication are two major areas of difficulty for these children. Primitive reflexes interfere with movement patterns such as maintaining stable head and trunk positions, bringing hand to mouth, chewing, and swal-

TABLE 29-1. Typical, Delayed, and Atypical Development and Compensatory Functional Patterns

Position	Typical (3 mo)	Delayed (10 mo)	Atypical (3 y)	Function (11 y)
Prone	Beginning head control and symmetry, elevated shoulders, arms internally rotated, hands fisted or partly open, eyes straight	Incomplete head control and symmetry, elevated shoulders, arms internally rotated, hands fisted, eyes not straight	Inadequate head control asymmetry, elevated shoulders, wrists and hands fisted, eyes not straight (strabismus)	Independent use of electronic keyboard
Sitting	Beginning head control, sitting with trunk support, hands partly open, arms and legs abducted, general low muscle tone	Incomplete head control, sitting with trunk support, hands fisted, arms and legs adducted, low proximal muscle tone, high distal tone	Inadequate head control, sitting with trunk support, athetoid hand posturing, low proximal muscle tone, high distal tone (feet)	External head support needed for control of lighted head pointer with communication system

(Photos courtesy of Carolyn and Grant Hensrud, Mary Rutten, and David Foerster)

TABLE 29-2. Effects of Cerebral Palsy

Type	Muscle Tone	Movement	Needs
Spastic (hypertonic)	Ranging from normal to very high, depending on stimulation	Small, labored, limited, in midrange only, not selective, abnormally learned	Assistance to achieve movement; strong but graded stimulation, time to adjust; avoid excessive effort
Flaccid (hypotonic)	Very low tone with intermittent extensor tone, sinks into gravity in all positions	No cocontraction, full range, but not used, hypermobile joints	Head control, stimulate to increase muscle tone and initiate effort, slow and steady handling, wait for reaction, developmental sequences
Athetoid	Fluctuating from low to normal or low to high	Extreme ranges, no midrange grading, no fixation, large jerky movements, uses asymmetry for stability	Stability, control of entire body, symmetry; reduce movement, avoid overstimulation
Athetoid with spasticity	Moderately high, ranging from normal to high	Poor control in midrange; poor selective movements	Balance, symmetry, midrange control of head, shoulders, and arms
Ataxic	Low or ranging from low to normal	No sustained postural control or fixation, normal but primitive coordination	Sustained posture

(From Bobath, B. (1997, Oct–Nov) NDT 8 week training course. London, England. Unpublished material)

lowing. Other problems may be poor lip closure, jaw or tongue thrust, tonic bite, ineffective swallowing, and hypersensitivity to touch. Lack of automatic swallowing contributes to excessive drooling, with associated problems of hygiene, skin irritation, social concerns, and in severe cases, risk of aspiration (Fraser et al, 1990). Children who are unable to achieve adequate nutrition orally or who are in danger of aspiration may need a temporary nasogastric (NG) tube, or a gastrostomy (G-tube) for longer periods or permanently. The NG tube is inserted into the stomach through the nose, and can be irritating and invasive. The G-tube is a surgical opening between the stomach and outside surface of the abdominal wall, and can be used to supplement eating, or it can be the sole source of nutrition (Fraser et al, 1990).

SURGICAL INTERVENTION

At one time, surgery aimed to eliminate all deformities, but changing priorities have led to a different approach to sur-

gical intervention. Generally, surgery is used to enhance function: (1) to achieve better postural alignment and joint flexibility; (2) to correct deformities so that adapted equipment can be used; and (3) to improve hygiene, such as to open fisted hands for skin care. Upper extremity surgical procedures for children with cerebral palsy involve tendon transfers, small joint arthrodeses, and muscle releases or lengthenings. They have been most beneficial when deformities are mild, and neuromuscular reeducation is provided in follow-up therapy.

Recently, procedures have been developed in which nerves in the spine are cut to reduce muscle tone in the extremities or trunk. The most common of these surgeries, the selective posterior dorsal rhizotomy, has improved some children's sitting, thereby promoting improved upper limb function and facilitation of the child's participation in ADLs, play, and school. Despite its apparent success for some children, some controversy about the procedure exists

TABLE 29-3. Terminology and Descriptions of Seizures

Current Terminology	Previous Terms	Descriptive Behaviors
Absence	Petit mal	Brief, abrupt loss of consciousness for a few seconds, associated with staring or eye blinking, followed by rapid, complete recovery
Infantile myoclonic	Infantile	Sudden, brief, involuntary muscle contractions, producing head drops and flexion of extremities (jackknife)
Tonic–clonic	Grand mal	Muscle stiffening and falling into unconsciousness (tonic phase), followed by rhythmic jerking (clonic phase), breathing problems, drooling, and loss of bladder control, and finally confusion and sleepiness. A seizure brought on by fever is termed a febrile seizure, common in young children.

(Stern, 1994). Because this surgery unmasks substantial weakness when spasticity and tone are reduced, therapists who are part of rhizotomy teams have developed postsurgical protocols to improve upper as well as lower extremity function (Berman, Vaughan, & Peacock, 1990; Bretas & Dias, 1991; Gersh, 1991b; Peacock & Stridt, 1990; Stern, 1994).

Occupational Therapy Evaluation of Children with Cerebral Palsy

Children with cerebral palsy benefit from a comprehensive evaluation, which includes the use of standardized pediatric assessments, observation instruments, and interview protocols. In addition, observations of the child engaged in play, school, and self-care activities can yield important information. Figure 29–3 illustrates observations of a 3-year-old child with athetosis and spasticity. Asymmetry (poor postural alignment) is demonstrated during reaching, with retraction of the opposite arm and shoulder. During bilateral manipulation (Fig. 29–4), the same child's flexor **synergies** are expressed in elevated shoulders, rounded spine, internal rotation of arms and legs, and flexion of elbow and wrist joints, compromising soft-tissue integrity. Because his flexed wrist prevents him from resting his right arm and hand on the table surface, he finds stability instead with his fingers, hyperextended at the metacarpophalangeal (MCP) joints. The subluxed proximal joint of his right thumb is further evidence of this instability and underlying low muscle tone. Figure 29–5 shows the use of a commercial corner seat to provide postural alignment and control (trunk support and a

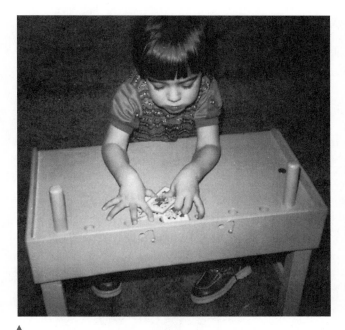

▲
Figure 29-4. Atypical patterns during manipulation. (Photo courtesy of Sallie and John Mooneyham.)

low bench to keep legs apart), and dowels to normalize hand patterns during grasp for stabilization (right hand) and release (left hand). These adaptive strategies, developed through collaborative task analysis between therapist, parent, and child are problem-solving skills that can be learned by the child, who then knowing what adaptations work can

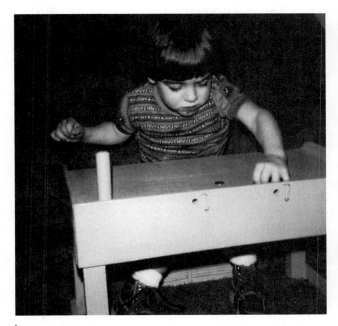

▲
Figure 29-3. Retraction of opposite arm and shoulder during reaching. (Photo courtesy of Sallie and John Mooneyham.)

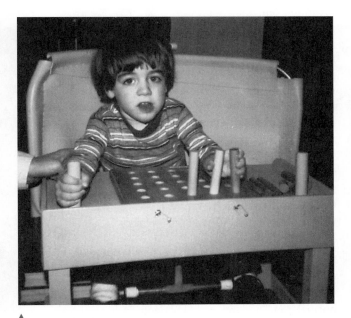

▲
Figure 29-5. External supports to normalize patterns during grasp and release (age 3 years). (Photo courtesy of Sallie and John Mooneyham.)

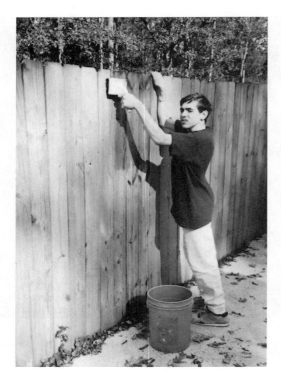

▲
Figure 29-6. External supports to normalize hand patterns during functional activity (age 16). (Photo courtesy of Sallie and John Mooneyham.)

continue to use these throughout life. Figure 29–6 shows the same individual at age 16 years, using appropriate external supports with improved postural alignment and control during the functional household maintenance activity of painting a fence.

Evaluation for an eating program is done by an experienced occupational therapist and includes (1) review of background information (medical considerations, gross and fine motor function, sensory impairments); (2) examination of the mouth and oral structures (lips, teeth, gums, palate, tongue); and (3) observation of the present eating process to assess positioning, developmental components, and responses to food textures, utensils, and presentation methods (Bergen & Colangelo, 1985; Fraser et al, 1990; Morris & Klein, 1987).

Occupational Therapy Intervention with Children with Cerebral Palsy

Neurodevelopmental treatment, an interdisciplinary, developmental approach, is used to enhance the quality of motor performance, teach new movement patterns, and prevent disability resulting from movement that is dominated by abnormal tone and reflexes. This approach requires specific handling techniques that provide clear sensory messages to muscles and joints. Physical, occupational, and speech therapists all use these techniques with children to increase head and trunk control. The occupational therapist uses NDT to develop the motor control necessary for performance of specific daily activities. One goal of NDT, for example, is to provide opportunities for the child to develop patterns for learning self-care skills, such as feeding, dressing, and hygiene (Lilly & Powell, 1990).

Intervention techniques are implemented once the therapist has determined the quality of the movements the child performs independently and where the child needs assistance. The therapist can facilitate all or part of the normal movement pattern by (1) helping the child maintain proper alignment and relationship to the body's center of gravity, (2) guiding the speed and excursion of the movement, (3) inhibiting inefficient patterns, and (4) reinforcing the child's improved movement verbally and by reducing support (Boehme, 1988; Hypes, 1991).

Most children with cerebral palsy need assistance to learn the skills necessary for motor performance because of inadequate upper extremity function and postural deficiencies. With the motor learning approach, the occupational therapy practitioner uses activities from the child's typical routines to provide learning opportunities that are meaningful to the child and caregivers. The practitioner adapts the environment to enhance performance, using a wide variety of positioning and adapted equipment.

Most occupational therapy practitioners combine NDT and motor control approaches in the treatment of the child with cerebral palsy. It is important to use appropriate handling techniques to help the child regulate muscle tone (NDT) while the child practices controlled motor skills (motor control).

SELF-CARE

Parents have many opportunities for therapeutic handling during self-care activities. Therapists can help them understand atypical movement patterns and develop spontaneous and natural handling skills as part of their daily interaction with their child (Stern & Gorga, 1988). Because self-care activities can be especially difficult for families to manage, therapists set up routines that are feasible for the family and that incorporate NDT and motor control approaches. Although some children remain dependent on caregivers for basic needs (Fraser et al, 1990), others gain varying degrees of independence, which can be evaluated by functional assessments such as the Pediatric Evaluation of Disability Index (PEDI) (Haley et al, 1992).

Eating

As mentioned earlier, eating is laden with social and emotional importance in our society. The motor control problems of the child with cerebral palsy often make eating difficult, time-consuming, and unpleasant for both children and their families. Early intervention can reduce the risk of long-term eating disorders, including rejection of some or all foods or textures, failure to thrive, and disturbed parent–child interaction.

The general principles discussed earlier are relevant to oral–motor intervention with children who have cerebral palsy. In addition, a variety of adaptive equipment is available for those whose oral–motor dysfunction does not allow them to put food in their mouths and those who have upper extremity control and oral–motor skills allowing them a degree of active participation in the eating process (Fraser et al. 1990). These devices include a wide variety of dishes, bottles, cups, and spoons, as well as more sophisticated feeding systems.

Figures 29–7 and 29–8 show a child with hypotonia learning to use a ball-bearing feeder to provide the necessary control for using a utensil. Intervention provided manual support and adaptive equipment within the context of feeding. The ball-bearing feeder eventually will become unnecessary as strength and coordination improve through repetitive practice (Fig. 29–9).

Special needs products catalogs are excellent resources for new products. Often, everyday eating equipment can be adapted for the child. For example, if a child with low muscle tone has difficulty lifting a cup to use a straw, a tall sport cup with an added saucer base for stability promotes more normalized postures of head and trunk, as well as independence.

Hygiene

Hygiene includes toileting, bathing, and grooming. Many children with cerebral palsy are incontinent and remain so throughout their lives. Others either can participate in a scheduled toileting program or be independently trained. Occupational therapists and certified occupational therapy assistants often help create toileting programs and recommend equipment. Adapted seats and chairs that provide motor control and comfort can make this process easier and

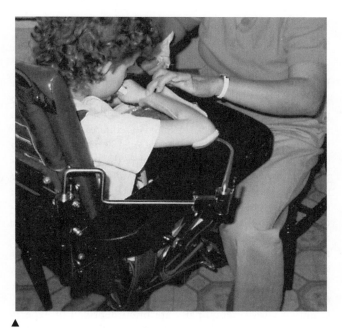

▲
Figure 29-8. An adapted ball-bearing feeder, leading to independent feeding. (Photo courtesy of Carmon and Mike Cymbal.)

more effective. Bathing aids that promote motor control range from portable devices to bathtub or shower seats, chairs, or hydraulic lifts (Fraser et al, 1990). A lightweight portable bath chair that provides head and trunk support has suction cups on the legs for stability in the tub or shower. Practical materials with suggestions for bathing children

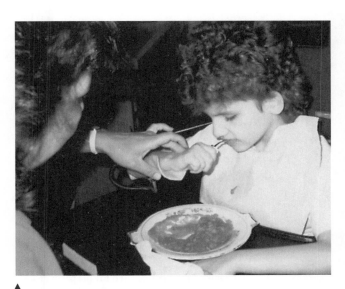

▲
Figure 29-7. An adapted ball-bearing feeder, leading to independent feeding. (Photo courtesy of Carmon and Mike Cymbal.)

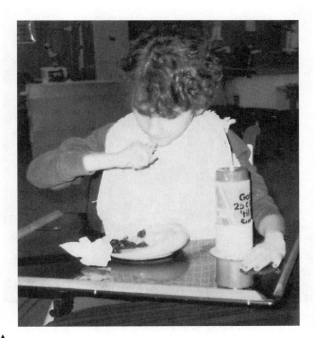

▲
Figure 29-9. Independent feeding. (Photo courtesy of Carmon and Mike Cymbal.)

with cerebral palsy can be individualized and taught to caregivers by therapists (Dunaway & Klein, 1988).

Dressing

Dressing activities provide a perfect opportunity for motor learning. NDT techniques, which emphasize handling to provide proximal stability to foster distal mobility, are useful. For example, support of the pelvis facilitates reaching upward to place an arm into a sleeve or downward to pull on socks. Occupational therapists identify the movement components required (task analysis), and evaluate which of those the child possesses and which compensatory patterns are substituted. Occupational therapists and certified occupational therapy assistants also make recommendations for adapted clothing that can make dressing easier, such as elastic shoe laces, using pants with elastic waists, and pull-over shirts (Boehme, 1985; Fraser et al. 1990).

PLAY

Children with cerebral palsy are often deprived of experiences essential to the development of motor control through play. Barriers to adequate play include (1) limitations imposed by caregivers, who fear injury; (2) physical limitations of the child, whose lack of mobility has prevented exploratory play; (3) environmental barriers in homes, schools, and community; and (4) social barriers. Occupational therapy practitioners can influence these last two barriers by evaluating school playgrounds and making recommendations that allow children with cerebral palsy access to recess activities at school (Stout, 1988).

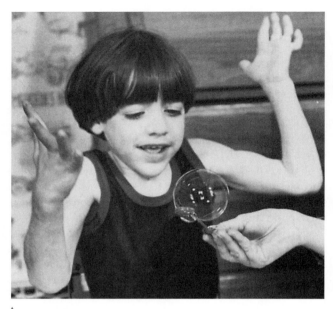

▲
Figure 29-11. Bilateral hand use and eye–hand coordination. (Photo courtesy of Sallie and John Mooneyham.)

Practitioners can help parents establish safe, enjoyable play routines (Missiuna & Pollack, 1991). Parents of children with cerebral palsy often ask practitioners to recommend appropriate toys for birthday or holiday presents. The practitioner can demonstrate specific play procedures for individualized goals, such as head control in prone for downward gaze into a mirror (Fig. 29–10), and eye–hand coordination and bilateral hand use in popping soap bubbles (Fig. 29–11). Figures 29–12 and 29–13 show how the motor skills learned from playing with a switch-adapted, battery-operated toy can serve as preliminary training for operation of a power wheel chair, as well

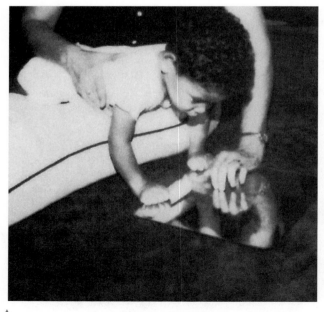

▲
Figure 29-10. Developing head control during mirror play. (From Erhardt, R. P. [1987]. *American Journal of Occupational Therapy, 41,* p. 46. Reprinted with permission of the American Occupational Therapy Association.) (Photo courtesy of Mary Rutten and David Foerster.)

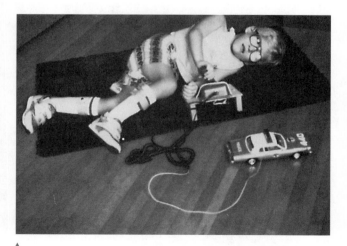

▲
Figure 29-12. A switch-adapted battery-operated toy preparing for power wheelchair operation. (From Erhardt, R. P. [1992]. *Development of hand skills in the child.* Bethesda, MD: American Occupational Therapy Association, p. 28. Reprinted with permission.) (Photo courtesy of Valerie and James Sand.)

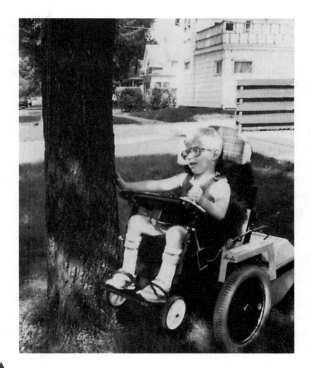

▲

Figure 29-13. Operation of a power wheelchair. (From Erhardt, R. P. [1992]. *Development of hand skills in the child.* Bethesda, MD: American Occupational Therapy Association, p. 28. Reprinted with permission.) (Photo courtesy of Valerie and James Sand.)

as computers, augmentative communication devices, and environmental control systems (Williams & Matesi, 1988).

By integrating NDT and motor control approaches with play into therapy sessions, therapists promote interaction with the environment and mastery of new skills, and develop risk-taking, problem-solving, and decision-making abilities (Reilly, 1974). A child absorbed in play is not focused on the specific motor demands of the activity, and can

be stimulated to use appropriate movement to improve head, trunk, and extremity control during play. The occupational therapist's task analysis skills are used to continually adapt (1) size, shape, or consistency of materials; (2) rules and procedures; (3) position of child or materials; and (4) nature and degree of personal interaction (Anderson, Hinojosa, and Strauch, 1987).

POSITIONING AND ADAPTIVE EQUIPMENT

Application of the principles of positioning mentioned earlier in this chapter is a very important component of occupational therapy intervention with the child who has cerebral palsy. Finding a variety of positions that promote participation in activities while supporting the child in positions that minimize the influences of pathological forces on the body is essential. The positioning program should be developed by members of the team, including caregivers, to ensure that recommended techniques are compatible with established home routines and schedules.

ORTHOTICS

Once the therapist has determined the extent of neuromusculoskeletal deficits, such as ROM limitation (soft tissue integrity), orthotics can be considered to maintain postsurgical correction as one part of the occupational therapy program. The variety of thermoplastic materials used to fabricate customized orthotics provide many options for upper and lower extremities, as well as the trunk (Fraser et al. 1990; Scherzer & Tscharnuter, 1990).

Soft splints, the least restrictive devices, can be constructed from webbing, neoprene, and hook-and-loop fastener material. They do not limit mobility and sensory input as much as thermoplastics. For children with moderate degrees of spasticity, stronger molded thermoplastic materials are necessary to prevent contractures. Ankle foot orthoses (AFO) and shoe inserts provide stability during standing and walking. Spinal orthoses and seating orthoses can be

HISTORICAL NOTE
RUGGLES' WORK WITH A CHILD: THE CARE REQUIRED BY CHILDREN

Suzanne M. Peloquin

Ora Ruggles' work with an 11-year-old boy named Ramon, exemplifies her practice among children. Ramon had little voluntary control, and he twitched and jerked constantly. Painfully shy, he hid himself in dark corners so that he would not be noticed. One day, when the rest of her charges complained that their clay was so lumpy that they were wasting time pressing it through a screen, Ruggles walked Ramon from a corner into the workroom.

As soon as he saw the other children making clay figures, he reproached Ruggles. She countered by showing him

how to press clay through the screen. His uncontrolled shaking worked to his advantage, and the other children soon thanked him for producing clay with such a fine texture. Ramon felt useful and appreciated. The task gave him a chance to connect with others in a venture that highlighted his capacity for fellowship, rather than his disability.

Although in her biography Ruggles never used the word *diagnosis*, her practice took the patient's symptoms and needs into deep consideration. ■

Carlova, J. & Ruggles, O. (1946). *The healing heart.* New York: Julian Messner.

used to support spinal curvatures such as scoliosis, kyphosis, and lordosis (Fraser et al, 1990).

Occupational therapists have also found upper extremity casting, which provides prolonged, gentle stretch to spastic or contracted muscles, to be an effective adjunct to therapeutic techniques. Casts are made with plaster or fiberglass casting tape. Significant results have been reported: increased strength, control, and spontaneous use of the impaired arm, as well as more bilateral hand use during play and transitional movements (Yasukawa & Hill, 1988; Yasukawa, 1990). Use of upper extremity inhibitive weight-bearing mitts during transitional movements such as crawling, can also be used to reduce muscle tone in children (Smelt, 1989). Results with older, more severely impaired children with fixed contractures may be less effective or inconsistent (Cruikshank & O'Neill, 1990). Casting and splinting programs are always integrated into the overall therapy program (Yasukawa & Hill, 1988).

▼ LEARNING DISABILITIES

There are many definitions of learning disabilities (Ayres, 1979; ACLD, 1985; Bashir, 1993; Kavanagh & Truss, 1988; National Advisory Committee on Handicapped Children, 1968; US Department of Education, 1987), all of which include the following elements: (1) that it is a chronic condition of neurological origin that interferes with the development, integration, and use of verbal or nonverbal abilities; (2) that it may occur concomitantly with other handicapping conditions (eg, sensory impairment, mental retardation, serious emotional disturbance), or with extrinsic influences (eg, cultural differences, insufficient or inappropriate instruction), but is not the result of those conditions; and (3) that it affects education, vocation, ADLs, self-esteem, and socialization. Learning disabilities are recognized under ADA regulations, which define an individual with a disability as someone who has a physical or mental impairment that substantially limits one or more major life activities such a learning or working (Latham, 1995).

In the past, learning disability was diagnosed only in children of school age. Now, early identification is the goal (Batshaw & Perret, 1986). Ellenberg and Nelson (1981) found a relationship between transient motor dysfunction in infancy, hyperactivity at 3 years, and learning disabilities at 7 years. Infants and young children who have sensory, emotional, and attentional problems are at risk for learning disabilities and are now being served in early intervention programs that recognize the basis of these regulatory disorders (DeGangi, Berk, & Greenspan, 1988). It is estimated that about 5% of all school-aged children receive special education for learning disabilities (US Dept. of Education, 1987).

Although the exact cause of learning disabilities is unknown, its etiology is considered to be an interaction of environmental influences and genetic inheritance. Sometimes family history reveals parents who had similar problems. Also contributing to the increased risk of learning disabilities is a history of minimal brain damage, caused by prematurity, prolonged labor, or inability to breathe spontaneously after delivery.

Because the primary handicapping condition is assumed to reflect subtle brain damage, some children may benefit from medical intervention, including psychotropic drugs, such as stimulants, which have proved useful for improving attention span and impulse control (Brown, Aylward, & Keogh, 1992). Speech therapists, learning specialists, physical therapists, psychologists, and occupational therapists, all have expertise that can help the child with learning disabilities.

Sensory Integration in Children with Learning Disabilities

The sensory systems provide the mechanism by which individuals learn about and interact with the environment. Information from all sensory systems enables the child to creates maps of the internal as well as external environment. As Ayres (1979) stated:

Sensory integration is the organization of sensation for use. Our senses give us information about the physical conditions of our body and the environment around us. Sensations flow into the brain like streams flowing into a lake. Countless bits of sensory information enter our brain at every moment, not only from our eyes and ears, but also from every place in our bodies . . .

The brain must organize all of these sensations if a person is to move and learn and behave normally. The brain locates, sorts and orders sensations. . . . When sensations flow in a well-organized or integrated manner, the brain can use those sensations to form perceptions, behaviors and learning. When the flow of sensations is disorganized, life can be like a rush-hour traffic jam. (p. 5)

For most children, sensory integration develops out of typical interactions with the environment. Adequate sensory integration allows the child to concentrate, organize information, develop self-esteem and self-confidence, anticipate and solve problems, and develop efficient use of the body and brain (Fisher & Murray, 1991). All of these abilities are essential to academic learning. Although there are many reasons why a child may have a learning disability, if the disability is a result of inefficient sensory integration, several problems may become evident.

One such problem is poorly modulated responses to sensations including touch, movement, visual, or auditory stimuli. This child may be withdrawn, irritable, fearful, unable to concentrate, disorganized, or overly active. For example, deficits in the regulation and interpretation of proprioceptive sensations may be reflected in a child's inability to sit still, write with a pencil using adequate pressure, and work in a small group.

Children with learning disabilities often have poor muscle tone regulation and coordination as a result of poorly integrated vestibular and proprioceptive sensations. Children with low tone will seek positional stability by excessive dependence on school furniture (eg, resting head and arms on desktop while writing, or hooking feet around chair legs). Another common compensation for poorly regulated muscle tone is seen in the child who grasps a pencil too tightly and exerts too much pressure on the paper. These children often rush through tasks, reducing the length of time required to maintain control.

Poor registration or interpretation of sensation makes it difficult for the child to develop a reliable body image or scheme that provides a point of reference for all external spatial relationships. Knowing right from left, up from down, and directionality, all develop from a reliable body image. Reading, writing, organization of self, and of self to the environment, all develop based on an understanding of the body in space. For example, letter or word reversals and irregularities in letter and word size and spacing can be traced to inadequate concepts of directionality. Figures 29–14 and 29–15 show examples of a child's handwriting before (at age 10) and after (at age 11) occupational therapy intervention.

As academic and social demands become more complex, children with learning disabilities often find themselves working increasingly harder to learn "splinter skills," which they cannot generalize to similar tasks. Their efforts to cope with environmental demands without the necessary sensory integrative prerequisites become unsuccessful and frustrating.

Consequences of Learning Disabilities on Development

Performance areas for children include school work, play and leisure, and ADLs. Deficits in performance components are the underlying factors that interfere with successful function. For example, the child who has difficulty completing written assignments in the classroom, may have letter and word reversals contributing to poor spelling, irregularities in letter and word size and spacing, and disorganized sequencing in compositions. Examples of problems with sequencing include disorganized stories, extra letters inserted into words when reading, and inadequate concepts of time. Outside of the classroom, these deficits have the potential to decrease the speed in which the child can complete routine activities such as bathing, dressing, and household tasks.

Knowing that the demands of tasks may be too great, a child may avoid many age-appropriate leisure activities at school or at home, despite the desire to participate with peers. As a result, the child may have difficulty establishing and maintaining friendships. The adolescent may have difficulty developing intimate relationships.

The effects of poor sensory integrative development can influence the child's performance in other areas as well. Self-care activities, such as eating and dressing, are relevant in the child's school environment as well as at home. For example, the child who is much slower and somewhat clumsy will have difficulty in the school cafeteria, and in physical education owing to deficits in coordination or dexterity, motor planning, and organization (Brown, Aylward, & Keogh, 1992; Penso, 1993).

Occupational Therapy Evaluation of Children with Learning Disabilities

The goal of evaluation is to identify problems in sensory integration and the manifestations of those problems. It is critical to identify the child's strengths and adaptive capacities as well. Data from evaluation are used to guide individualized intervention. Strategies for evaluation include record review, medical history, observations, and formal tests that measure specific performance components. Interviews with the

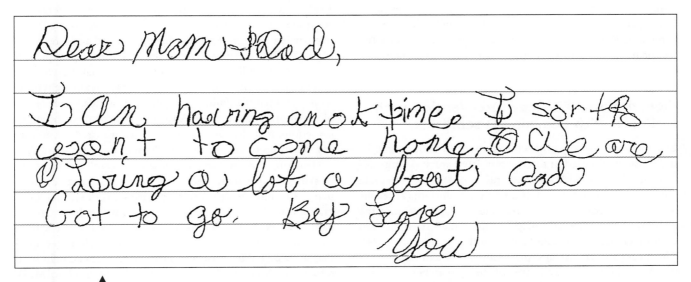

▲
Figure 29-14. Sample of handwriting, age 10, before intervention. (Courtesy of Laurine and David Braukman.)

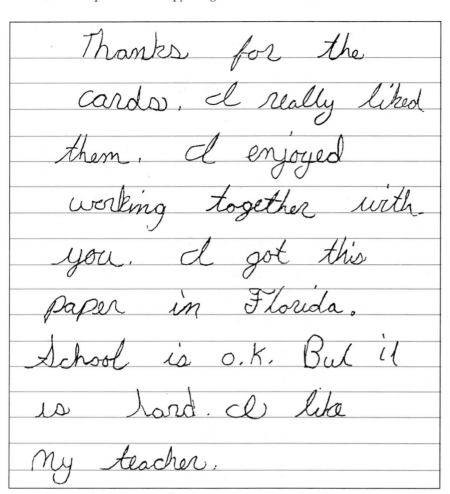

Thanks for the cards, I really liked them. I enjoyed working together with you. I got this paper in Florida. School is o.k. But it is hard. I like my teacher.

◄ *Figure 29-15.* Sample of handwriting, age 11, after intervention. (Courtesy of Laurine and David Braukman.)

child's family or teachers, or both, are essential to identify specific problems. Examples of interviews that are used include the Play Skills History and Sensory History. The Bruininks-Oseretsky Test of Motor Proficiency, the DeGangi-Berk Test of Sensory Integration, the Quick Neurological Screening Test and the Sensory Integration and Praxis Test are formal tests used frequently by occupational therapists.

Occupational Therapy Intervention with Children with Learning Disabilities

Occupational therapy with children with learning disabilities is usually focused in three interrelated areas: (1) improving the child's capacity to register, process, and integrate sensory information through direct intervention; (2) teaching the child compensatory strategies; and (3) adapting the environment to take advantage of the child's strengths and to compensate for the child's areas of deficit (Mason, 1994). The occupational therapy practitioner works closely with parents and teachers in all three of these areas, because consistency of approach and expectations is essential to the child's success.

Direct intervention is aimed at enhancing the function of the child's nervous system to lay the groundwork for improved motor and academic learning (Koomar & Bundy, 1991). The child is provided with opportunities to take in controlled, but enhanced, sensory information through active participation in activities that elicit an adaptive response (Ayres, 1979). The practitioner decides where therapy will start, but the child directs the process by making choices. Sensory integrative intervention requires a flexible environment in which the child can experiment with a wide variety of sensations in a safe place. A variety of suspended and moving equipment, textures, and activities are used in infinite combinations to engage the child's inner drive for mastery.

Teaching the child to compensate for specific deficits can be part of direct intervention or can be a separate component. The child can learn to recognize signs of sensory integration problems and can intervene on his or her own behalf. For example, the middle-school-aged child whose attention starts to wander can use a squeeze ball or get up to sharpen a pencil for proprioceptive input that can help with refocusing. A child who has difficulty keeping school work organized can use a color-coded system which will provide the necessary structure.

Adapting the environment to promote the child's best performance takes into account both human and nonhuman factors. Desk heights and proper writing tools are essential for the child who has low muscle tone and poor fine motor control. A teacher who provides clear expectations for work can help the child who has difficulty staying organized. A classroom structure that allows controlled movement around the room can help the child who needs vestibular and proprioceptive input to control behavior and maintain attention. Helping parents understand their child's sensory needs can provide environments in which the child can experience the kinds of sensations that are most organizing to that child's nervous system.

▼ NEURAL TUBE DEFECTS

Spina bifida is a term used to describe children and adults with a wide variety of neural tube defects. The spine is cleft or split because the vertebrae (bones of the spinal column) do not enclose the spinal cord during the first trimester of pregnancy. This results in abnormal development of the meninges, nerves, and vertebrae (Williamson, 1987).

The prevalence of neural tube defects varies in geographic location and ethnic groups, leading researchers to believe that environmental as well as genetic factors are responsible. In the United States the incidence in 1989 was 0.6 per 1000 births (Yen, Knoury, & Erickson, 1992, p. 1). It is the second most common specific birth defect after Down syndrome. Specific causes are not known, although there is evidence that folic acid deficiency may be related (Williamson, 1987).

Of the three types of spina bifida, the most common and least severe is **spina bifida occulta**. Although there is an opening in the spine, the spinal cord and nerves are not damaged and neurological function is usually intact, or manifested in slight bowel or bladder problems. A dimple, tuft of hair, or nothing may be visible at the site of the defect. Next in severity is **meningocele**. The meninges are pushed out through an opening in the vertebrae, forming a sac, but the spinal cord is intact, and after corrective surgery to remove the sac and reposition the meninges, neurological function is often normal, slight sensory or motor deficits sometimes occur. **Myelomeningocele** is the most severe type of spina bifida, accompanied by significant impairment. The meninges and spinal cord protrude from the vertebral opening to form a sac, with the spinal cord injured below and sometimes above the lesion, resulting in damaged spinal nerves (Williamson, 1987).

Although the lesion can occur at any point on the spinal cord, the most common sites are in the lumbosacral region. Different levels result in specific patterns of motor weakness or paralysis and loss of sensation below the level of the lesion, but these deficits vary widely in terms of asymmetries and clinical pictures of flaccidity and spasticity. Any brain damage will also affect motor, sensory, and perceptual functions. Associated brain anomalies can and do occur. The Arnold-Chiari malformation, for example, is the herniation of the brainstem and cerebellum into the foramen magnum (Gabriel & McComb, 1985). Hydrocephalus can be caused by any number of problems that interfere with production and flow of spinal fluid, resulting in enlarged ventricles and resultant brain damage. Ventriculoperitoneal shunts are usually inserted within the first 2 weeks to relieve pressure on the brain caused by ventricular enlargement.

Consequences of Neural Tube Defects on Development

Although lower extremity impairment is expected in children with spina bifida, reduced control of upper limbs is also common. Cerebellar ataxia that is due to the Arnold-Chiari malformation causes problems regulating the force, rate, and range of voluntary movement. Hydrocephalus may cause damage in the motor cortex, affecting perceptual function as well. Deprivation or distortion of movement experiences interferes with efficiency of motor planning, which depends on the feedback and integration of sensory information from successful motor experiences. Thus, these children have difficulty with cognitive performance components, such as the complex sequences required for eating, dressing, and handwriting.

The neural damage caused by neural tube defects usually results in some sensory-processing problems that affect the development of motor planning, visual–perceptual skills, and bilateral coordination. Other sensory deficits are specific to sensory systems. For example, the visual system may be impaired with refractive errors (farsightedness or nearsightedness), strabismus (owing to muscle imbalance), or nystagmus (rhythmic jerking eye movements). These deficits must be evaluated and treated by an ophthalmologist or optometrist. Children with myelomeningocele and hydrocephalus score lower than normal children on tests of visual perception (Williamson, 1987). Exaggerated, emotional responses to specific sensory stimuli are caused by hyperresponsivity to sensory input eliciting primitive, protective responses. In this guarded state, the child explores the tactile environment less, and tactile discrimination and stereognosis may not develop normally. Auditory defensiveness has also been reported frequently in children with hydrocephalus. Some children talk constantly, which may be protection against excessive auditory input (Knickerbocker, 1980).

Bowel and bladder control presents a special problem for the child with spina bifida. Practitioners should be aware that a child may have internal or external collecting devices, or need intermittent catheterization. Bowel management programs usually include special diets, stool softeners, and regular use of suppositories. As they grow older, most children can gradually become independent in bowel and bladder care (Williamson, 1987).

Medical precautions are related to specific deficits. For example, diminished sensation in the lower extremities puts children at risk for injuries such as burns, abrasions, or even pressure sores on weight-bearing areas. Water temperature for bathing must be carefully monitored, and the child must learn to test the temperature with the hands first.

Lower extremity orthotics and body casts are used extensively for children with myelomeningocele to prevent misalignment, especially after surgery for partial spinal fusion. Adaptive equipment such as crutches and wheelchairs are needed for almost all individuals with neural tube defects. Approximately half of all children with myelomeningocele use a wheelchair, either as their primary means of mobility or for distance mobility. Power wheelchairs or scooters may be necessary, depending on the child's strength, endurance, and lifestyle.

Figure 29–16 shows a 2-year-old child with myelomeningocele who demonstrates a common clinical picture. Observations show low muscle tone proximally (neck, trunk, shoulder, and hips), but fisted hands show how tone is increased distally with the effort to gain stability while using her hands. She compensates for poor sitting balance by using one arm for support, thus bilateral tasks such as opening packages can only be done with one hand. Figure 29–17 shows her at 8 years, compensating for motor and sensory deficits. Weak spinal muscles have resulted in general asymmetry, scoliosis, lordosis, with compensatory head righting. She demonstrates a left exotropic strabismus (left eye deviating outward). Her legs are adducted with the effort to achieve stability during standing and walking. Constant use of the arms for weight-bearing (essential for independent ambulation with forearm crutches) impedes the use of her hands for refined manipulation skills. For this child, stability has been gained at the expense of mobility. According to her

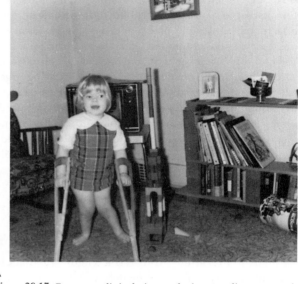

▲
Figure 29-17. Common clinical picture during standing posture in a child with myelomeningocele, age 8. (Photo courtesy of Jean and Paul Anderson.)

mother, after crutch-walking at an amusement park, the child exclaimed "My arms are so tired." Judicious use of a wheelchair could contribute to a balanced use of her arms for manipulation and ambulation. Figure 29–18 shows improved hand use at age 10 after intervention for deficits in postural control and alignment, as well as adaptation of external supports using a chair for trunk support and resting the forearms on the table edge.

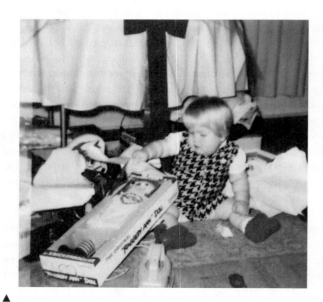

▲
Figure 29-16. Common clinical picture of sitting posture in a child with myelomeningocele, age 2. (Photo courtesy of Jean and Paul Anderson.)

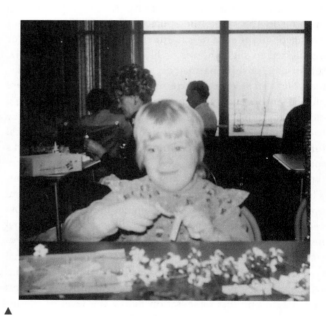

▲
Figure 29-18. Improved hand use in a child with myelomeningocele, age 10, after intervention for deficits in postural control and alignment. (Photo courtesy of Jean and Paul Anderson.)

Occupational Therapy Evaluation of Children with Neural Tube Defects

The sensory and motor problems experienced by children with neural tube defects require occupational therapy evaluation of muscle tone, strength, postural control, visual–perception, and bilateral and fine motor coordination. The occupational therapist evaluates the child within the context of the child's various environments.

Specific pediatric assessments used by occupational therapists include standardized instruments such as the Bayley Scales of Infant Development, the Peabody Developmental Motor Scales, the Motor-Free Visual Perception Test-Revised, and the Developmental Test of Visual Perception. Therapists also use nonstandardized assessments of muscle tone, sensory status, motor skills, and social and self-care skills.

Occupational Therapy Intervention with Children with Neural Tube Defects

Occupational therapy's role should start in early intervention for the child with neural tube defects. A simple NDT program, begun in the first few months, can activate muscles with low innervation and, through repetitive play activities using proper handling techniques, bring them to a functional level, first with gravity eliminated, then against gravity (Stern, 1994).

Occupational therapy practitioners are also involved in the child's preparation for academic learning, which takes place at home and in preschool experiences. Occupational therapists and certified occupational therapy assistants work closely with teachers and parents to design programs to meet the child's needs for individual and group activities in cognitive, communication, motor, and psychosocial skills.

TABLE 29-4. Adaptive Equipment to Facilitate Participation in Developmental Activities*

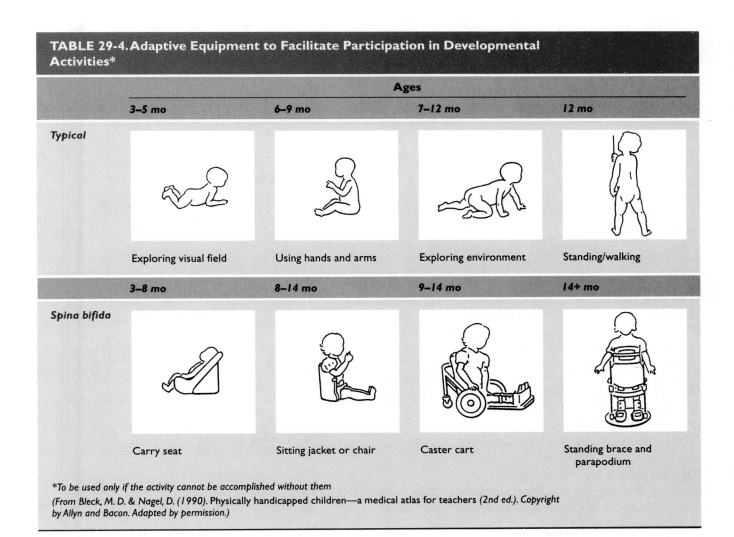

	Ages			
Typical	3–5 mo	6–9 mo	7–12 mo	12 mo
	Exploring visual field	Using hands and arms	Exploring environment	Standing/walking
Spina bifida	3–8 mo	8–14 mo	9–14 mo	14+ mo
	Carry seat	Sitting jacket or chair	Caster cart	Standing brace and parapodium

*To be used only if the activity cannot be accomplished without them

(From Bleck, M. D. & Nagel, D. (1990). Physically handicapped children—a medical atlas for teachers (2nd ed.). Copyright by Allyn and Bacon. Adapted by permission.)

The child's self-esteem develops out of successful early experiences that promote purposeful interaction with the environment. Developmental activities that promote creative play and material exploration include block play and construction, filling and emptying containers, finger painting, clay activities, tearing and crumpling paper, and scribbling or drawing with chalk, crayons, and pencils. Practitioners also facilitate fine motor development during these activities with techniques that promote stability and mobility. The child's learning of motor skills begins with proper positioning and handling, which will promote learning of eating, dressing, hygiene and grooming, and play skills. Repetition is essential to learn these activities. Environmental modifications are important to successful learning for children with spina bifida.

POSITIONING AND ADAPTIVE EQUIPMENT

Careful positioning at home and school is important to prevent orthopedic deformities (contractures and spinal curvatures), maintain skin condition, avoid accidents, promote independence, and achieve optimal use of the upper extremities (Williamson, 1987). A variety of positions should be available for each task, because the child may not be able to move independently into different positions.

EATING

Eating problems in children with spina bifida are similar to those in children with other developmental disabilities and can make eating a difficult, time-consuming, and unpleasant time for children and their families. For children with spina bifida, the problems may include oral hypersensitivity, motor control, and dietary concerns, such as obesity and bowel function. These dietary concerns may place restrictions on the types and textures of foods available to a particular child, limiting the child's sensory and motor experiences. Principles that guide occupational therapy for oral–motor deficits were discussed earlier in this chapter.

FINE MOTOR

Fine motor performance components may also be deficient, because of postural insecurity, sensory processing, and poor eye–hand coordination. Occupational therapy intervention for fine motor delays should consider (1) secure positioning to allow mobility of arms and hands; (2) strengthening of upper as well as lower extremities (Stern, 1994); (3) development of hand skills; and (4) adapted equipment (eg, built-up spoons and writing tools, nonslip mats under dishes or school work).

ENVIRONMENTAL MODIFICATIONS

To foster learning and independence for the child with spina bifida, the environment should have child-sized furniture and smooth carpeting to encourage mobility, and be organized to limit visual and auditory distractions, with well-defined areas for activities. Vertical or inclined work surfaces promote erect posture, increased shoulder and arm strength, and eye–hand coordination. Table 29–4 illustrates the correlation of adapted equipment with appropriate motor experiences during development.

►CONCLUSION

Children with neurological dysfunction offer exciting challenges and opportunities for occupational therapy practitioners. Both occupational therapists and certified occupational therapy assistants are involved with children with neurological deficits in many different settings. Early intervention may begin in the high-risk nursery or in screening programs for infants and toddlers. Preschool programs may be home or center based. Occupational therapy practitioners may provide related services in schools, or be hired by families to supplement school programs. As part of the professional team assisting adolescents with neurological dysfunction make transitions from high school into different levels of domestic and employment situations, the occupational therapy perspective on purposeful engagement in activity is invaluable.

Acknowledgments

Appreciation is extended to the children, parents, and therapists who have graciously given permission for use of their photographs.

▼ REFERENCES

ACLD Newsbriefs. (1985). Pittsburgh, PA: ACLD, Jan/Feb.

Albright, A. L., Cervi, A., & Singletary, J. (1991). Intrathecal baclofen for spasticity in cerebral palsy. *Journal of the American Medical Association, 265,* 1418–1422.

Alexander, R., Boehme, R., & Cupps, B. (1993). *Normal development of functional motor skills.* San Antonio, TX: Therapy Skill Builders.

Amundson, S. J. (1995). *The Evaluation Tool of Children's Handwriting* (ETCH). Homer, AK: OT KIDS.

Anderson, J., Hinojosa, J., Strauch, C. (1987). Integrating play in neurodevelopmental treatment. *American Journal of Occupational Therapy, 41,* 421–426.

Armstrong, R., Steinbok, P., Farrell, K., Cochrane, D., Kube, S., & Fife, S. (1991). Intrathecal baclofen for treatment of spasticity in children. *Developmental Medicine and Child Neurology, 33, Supplement 64 (Abstracts of Annual Meeting),* 27.

Ayres, A. J. (1973). *Sensory integration and learning disorders.* Los Angeles, CA: Western Psychological Services.

Ayres, A. J. (1979). *Sensory integration and the child.* Los Angeles, CA: Western Psychological Services.

Barnes, J. F. (1991, July 19). Pediatric myofascial release. *Occupational Therapy Forum,* 18–19.

Bashir, A. S. (September 22, 1993). Treatment of language disorders in middle school children. *Syllabus of the proceedings of advances in developmental disabilities, learning disabilities, and ADHD.* Philadelphia: Children's Seashore House.

Batshaw, M. L. & Perret, Y. M. (1986). *Children with handicaps* (2nd ed.). Baltimore: Paul H. Brookes.

Bayley, N. (1993). *Bayley Scales of Infant Development.* (2nd ed) San Antonio, TX: Psychological Corporation.

Bergen, A. F. & Colangelo, C. (1985). *Positioning the client with central nervous system deficits: The wheelchair and other adapted equipment* (2nd ed.). Valhalla, NY: Valhalla Rehabilitation Publications.

Bergen, A. F., Presperin, J., & Tallman, T. (1990). *Positioning for function: Wheelchairs and other assistive technologies.* Valhalla, NY: Valhalla Rehabilitation Publications.

Berman, B., Vaughan, C. L., & Peacock, W. J. (1990). The effect of rhizotomy on movements in patients with cerebral palsy. *American Journal of Occupational Therapy, 44,* 511–516.

Blanche, E. J. & Burke, J. P. (1991). Combining neurodevelopmental and sensory integration approaches in the treatment of the neurologically impaired child, Part I, *Sensory Integration Quarterly, 19,* 1–5.

Bobath K. & Bobath, B. (1972). Cerebral palsy. In P.H. Pearson & C. E. Williams (Eds.), *Physical therapy services in the developmental disabilities* (pp. 31–185). Springfield, IL: Charles C. Thomas.

Boehme, R. (1985, November). Self-care assessment and treatment from an NDT perspective. *NDT Newsletter* 1, 5.

Boehme, R. (1988). *Improving upper body control.* San Antonio, TX: Therapy Skill Builders.

Boehme, R. (1991). *Myofascial release and its application to neuro-developmental treatment.* Milwaukee: Boehme Workshops.

Bretas, C. & Dias, L. (1991). Selective posterior rhizotomy. *Developmental Medicine and Child Neurology, 33, Supplement 64 (Abstracts of Annual Meeting),* 26.

Brown, F. R., Aylward, E. H., & Keogh, B. K. (1992). *Diagnosis and management of learning disabilities* (2nd ed.). San Diego: Singular Publishing Group.

Campbell, S. K. (1990). Using standardized tests in clinical practice. In S. K. Campbell (Ed.), *Topics in pediatrics, Lesson 11* (pp. 1–13). Alexandria, VA: American Physical Therapy Association.

Chamberlain, J. L., Henry, M. M., Roberts, J. D., Sapsford, A. L., & Courtney, S. E. (1991). An infant and toddler feeding group program. *American Journal of Occupational Therapy, 45,* 907–911.

Coley, I. L. (1978). *Pediatric assessment of self-care activities.* St. Louis: C.V. Mosby.

Colarusso, D. & Hammill, D. (1995). *Motor-free Visual Perception Test–Revised (MVPT-R).* Novato, CA: Academic Therapy Publications.

Connolly, K. & Dalgleish, M. (1989). The emergence of tool-using skill in infancy. *Developmental Psychology, 25,* 894–912.

Cook, D. G. (1991). The assessment process. In W. Dunn (Ed.). *Pediatric occupational therapy: Facilitating effective service provision* (pp. 34–73). Thorofare, NJ: Slack.

Cruikshank, D. A. & O'Neill, D. L. (1990). Upper extremity inhibitive casting in a boy with spastic quadriplegia. *American Journal of Occupational Therapy, 44,* 552–555.

DeGangi, G. A., Berk, R. A., & Greenspan, S. I. (1988). The clinical measurement of sensory functioning in infants: A preliminary study. *Physical and Occupational Therapy in Pediatrics, 8,* 10–23.

Duckman, R. H. (1984). Effectiveness of optometric visual training in a population of severely involved cerebral palsied children utilizing professional, non-optometric therapists. *Physical and Occupational Therapy in Pediatrics, 4,* 75–86.

Dunaway, A. & Klein, M. D. (1988). *Bathing techniques for children who have cerebral palsy.* San Antonio, TX: Therapy Skill Builders.

Dunn, W. (1987, May). Sensory integration. In *NDT OT Instructor Course,* Akron, Ohio.

Dunn, W. (Ed.). (1991). *Pediatric occupational therapy: Facilitating effective service provision.* Thorofare, NJ: Slack.

Ellenberg, J. H. & Nelson, K. B. (1981). Early recognition of infants at high risk for cerebral palsy: Examination at age four months. *Developmental Medicine and Child Neurology, 23,* 705–716.

Erhardt, R. P. (1995). *Self-feeding in the child with special needs* (video). Maplewood, MN: Erhardt Developmental Products.

Erhardt, R. P. (1994). *Developmental hand dysfunction: Theory, assessment, and treatment* (2nd ed.). San Antonio, TX: Therapy Skill Builders.

Erhardt, R. P. (1992). Eye–hand coordination. In J. Case-Smith & C. Pehoski (Eds.), *Development of hand skills in the child* (pp. 13–33). Bethesda, MD: American Occupational Therapy Association.

Erhardt, R. P. (1990). *Developmental visual dysfunction: Models for assessment, and management.* San Antonio, TX: Therapy Skill Builders.

Erhardt, R. P. (1986). *The consultant's role in evaluation and treatment of eating dysfunction* (video). Maplewood, MN: Erhardt Developmental Products.

Erhardt, R. P. (1985). *Developmental prehension components of independent feeding* (video). Maplewood, MN: Erhardt Developmental Products.

Exner, C. (1989). Development of hand functions. In P. N. Pratt & A. S. Allen (Eds.), *Occupational therapy for children* (pp. 235–259). St. Louis: C.V. Mosby.

Fee, M. A., Charney, E. B., & Robertson, W. W. (1988). Nutritional assessment of the young child with cerebral palsy. *Infants and Young Children, 1,* 33–40.

Fiorentino, M. R. (1973). *Reflex testing methods for evaluating C. N. S. development.* (2nd ed.). Springfield, IL: Charles C. Thomas.

Fisher, A. G. & Murray, E. A. (1991). Introduction to sensory integration theory. In A. C. Fisher, E. A. Murray, , & A. C. Bundy (Eds.), *Sensory integration: Theory and practice.* Philadelphia: F. A. Davis.

Fisher, A. G., Murray, E. A., & Bundy A. C. (Eds.). (1991). *Sensory integration: Theory and practice.* Philadelphia: F. A. Davis.

Folio, R. & Fewell, R. R. (1983). *Peabody Developmental Motor Scales.* Allen, TX: DLM Teaching Resources.

Foltz, L. C., DeGangi, G., & Lewis, D. (1991). Physical therapy, occupational therapy, and speech and language therapy. In E. Geralis (Ed.), *Children with cerebral palsy: A parents' guide* (pp. 209–260). Rockville, MD: Woodbine House.

Fraser, B. A., Hensinger, R. N., & Phelps, J. A. (1990). *Physical management of multiple handicaps.* Baltimore: Paul H. Brookes.

Fraunfelder, F. T. (1976). *Drug-induced ocular side effects and drug interactions.* Philadelphia: Lea & Fabiger.

Gabriel, R.S. & McComb, J. G. (1985). Malformations of the central nervous system. In J. H. Menkes (Ed.), *Textbook of child neurology.* Philadelphia: Lea & Febiger

Gersh, E. S. (1991a). What is cerebral palsy? In E. Geralis (Ed.), *Children with cerebral palsy: A parents' guide* (pp. 1–32). Rockville, MD: Woodbine House.

Gersh, E. S. (1991b). Medical concerns and treatment. In E. Geralis (Ed.), *Children with cerebral palsy: A parents' guide* (pp. 57–90). Rockville, MD: Woodbine House.

Gilfoyle, E. M., Grady, A. P., & Moore, J. C. (1990). *Children adapt: A theory of sensorimotor-sensory development* (2nd ed.). Thorofare, NJ: Slack.

Hacker, B. J. & Porter, P. B. (1987). Use of standardized tests with the physically handicapped. In L. King-Thomas & B. J. Hacker, (Eds.), *A therapist's guide to pediatric assessment* (pp. 35–40). Boston: Little, Brown & Co.

Haley, S., Coster, W., Ludlow, L., Haltiwanger, J., & Andrellos, P. (1992). *Pediatric Evaluation of Disability Inventory (PEDI): Development, standardization and administration manual.* Boston: New England Medical Center Hospital.

Hammill, D. D. (1990). On defining learning disabilities: An emerging consensus. *Journal of Learning Disabilities, 23,* 74–84.

Hammill, D. D., Pearson, N.A., & Voress, J. K. (1993). *The Developmental Test of Visual Perception (DTVP-2).* Austin, TX: Pro-ed.

Hammill, D. D., Pearson, N.A., & Voress, J. K. (1996). *The Test of Visual Motor Integration (TVMI).* Austin, TX: Pro-ed.

Harris, S. R. (1988). Early intervention: Does developmental therapy make difference? *Topics in Early Childhood Special Education, 7,* 20–32.

Holloway, E. (1993). Early emotional development and sensory processing. In J. Case-Smith (Ed.), *Pediatric occupational therapy and early intervention.* Boston, MA: Andover Medical Publishers.

Huber, C. J. & King-Thomas, K. (1987). The assessment process. In L. King-Thomas & B. J. Hacker, (Eds.), *A therapist's guide to pediatric assessment* (pp. 3–10). Boston: Little, Brown & Co.

Hypes, B. (1988). A kinesiological analysis of dynamic sitting. In R. Boehme (Ed.), *Improving upper body control* (pp. 189–209). San Antonio, TX: Therapy Skill Builders.

Hypes, B. (1991). *Facilitating development and sensorimotor function: Treatment with the ball.* Hugo, MN: PDP Press.

Jelm, J. M. (1990). *Oral-Motor/Feeding Rating Scale.* San Antonio, TX: Therapy Skill Builders.

Kalscheur, J. A. (1992). Benefits of the Americans with Disabilities Act of 1990 for children and adolescents with disabilities. *American Journal of Occupational Therapy, 46,* 419–426.

Kavanagh, J. F. & Truss, T. J. (Eds.). (1988). *Learning disabilities: Proceedings of the National Conference.* Parkton, MD: York Press.

Kielhofner, G. (1992). *Conceptual foundations of occupational therapy.* Philadelphia: F. A. Davis.

Knobloch, H., Stevens, F., & Malone, A. (1980). *A manual of developmental diagnosis: The administration and interpretation of the revised Gesell and Amatruda Developmental and Neurological Examination.* New York: Harper & Row.

Knickerbocker, B. M. (1980). *A holistic approach to the treatment of learning disorders.* Thorofare, NJ: Charles B. Slack.

Knox, S. A. (1974). A play scale. In M. Reilly (Ed.). *Play as exploratory learning* (pp. 247–266). Beverly Hills: Sage Publications.

Koomar, J. A. & Bundy, A. C. (1991). The art and science of creating direct intervention from theory. In A. G. Fisher, E. A. Murray, & A. C. Bundy (Eds.), *Sensory integration: Theory and practice.* Philadelphia: F. A. Davis.

Latham, P. H. (Fall, 1995). Learning disabilities in the workplace: The legal right to accommodations. *The LD Link, 1,* 8. (Available from Learning Disabilities Research and Training Center, University of Georgia, Athens, Georgia 30602).

Lilly, L. A. & Powell, N. J. (1990). Measuring the effects of neurodevelopmental treatment on the daily living skills of 2 children with cerebral palsy. *American Journal of Occupational Therapy, 44,* 139–136.

Logigian, M. K. & Ward J. D. (1989). *Pediatric rehabilitation: A team approach for therapists.* Boston, MA: Little, Brown & Co.

McEwen, M. (1990). The human–environment interface in occupational therapy: A theoretical and philosophical overview. In S. C. Merrill (Ed.), *Environment: Implications for occupational therapy practice. A sensory integrative perspective* (pp. 3–22). Bethesda, MD: American Occupational Therapy Association.

Magill-Evans, J. E. & Restall, G. (1991). Self-esteem of persons with cerebral palsy: From adolescence to adulthood. *American Journal of Occupational Therapy, 45,* 819–825.

Mason, M. (November 11, 1994). Utilizing metacognitive strategies with learning disabilities. *Occupational Therapy Forum, 4,* 5, 10.

Mathiowetz, V. & Haugen, J. B. (1994). Motor behavior research: Implications for therapeutic approaches to central nervous system dysfunction. *American Journal of Occupational Therapy, 48,* 733–745.

Menken, C., Cermak, S. A., & Fisher, A. (1987). Evaluating the visual–perceptual skills of children with cerebral palsy. *American Journal of Occupational Therapy, 41,* 646–651.

Missiuna, C. & Pollack, N. (1991). Play deprivation in children with physical disabilities: The role of the occupational therapist in preventing secondary disability. *American Journal of Occupational Therapy, 45,* 882–888.

Morris, S. E. (1982). *The normal acquisition of oral feeding skills: Implications for assessment and treatment.* New York: Therapeutic Media.

Morris, S. E. & Klein, M. D. (1987). *Pre-feeding skills: A comprehensive resource for feeding development.* San Antonio, TX: Therapy Skill Builders.

Mulligan-Ault, M., Guess, D., Struth, L., & Thompson, B. (1988). The implementation of health-related procedures in classrooms for students with severe multiple impairments. *Journal of the Association of Persons with Severe Handicaps, 13,* 87–99.

National Advisory Committee on Handicapped Children (1968). *First Annual Report, Special Education for Handicapped Children.* Washington, D.C.: U.S. Department of Health, Education and Welfare.

National Information Center for Children and Youth with Handicaps. (1991). *The educational of children and youth with special needs: What do the laws say?* Washington, DC: National Information Center for Children and Youth with Handicaps.

Neistadt, M. E. (1987). An occupational therapy program for adults with developmental disabilities. *American Journal of Occupational Therapy, 41,* 433–438.

Neville, P., Kielhofner, G., & Royeen, C. B. (1985). Childhood. In G. Kielhofner (Ed.), *A model of human occupation: Theory and application* (pp. 78–98). Baltimore: Williams & Wilkins.

Peacock, W. J. & Stridt, L. A. (1990). Spasticity in cerebral palsy and the selective posterior rhizotomy procedure. *Journal of Child Neurology, 5,* 179–185.

Penso, D. E. (1990). *Keyboard, graphic and handwriting skills: Helping people with motor disabilities.* London: Chapman & Hall.

Penso, D. E. (1993). *Perceptuo-motor difficulties.* London: Chapman & Hall.

Poole, J. L., (1991). Application of motor learning principles in occupational therapy. *American Journal of Occupational Therapy, 45,* 531–537.

Provence, S., Erickson, J. Vater, S., & Palmeri, S. (1995). *The Infant-Toddler Developmental Assessment.* Chicago: Riverside Publishing Company.

Reilly, M. (Ed.). (1974). *Play as exploratory learning.* Beverly Hills: Sage Publications.

Richter, E. & Oetter, P. (1990). Environmental matrices for sensory integrative treatment. In S. C. Merrill (Ed.), *Environment: Implications for occupational therapy practice. A sensory integrative perspective* (pp. 23–44). Bethesda, MD: American Occupational Therapy Association.

Royeen, C. B. & Lane, S. J. (1991). Tactile processing and sensory defensiveness. In A. G. Fisher, E. A. Murray, & A. C. Bundy (Eds.), *Sensory integration: Theory and practice.* Philadelphia: F. A. Davis.

Scherzer, A. L. & Tscharnuter, I. (1990). *Early diagnosis and therapy in cerebral palsy* (2nd ed.). New York: Marcel Dekker.

Schleichkorn, J. (1993). *Coping with cerebral palsy* (2nd ed.). Austin, TX: Pro-ed.

Slavik, B. A. & Chew, T. (1990). The design of a sensory integration treatment facility: The Ayres clinic as a model. In S. C. Merrill (Ed.), *Environment: Implications for occupational therapy practice. A sensory integrative perspective* (pp. 85–101). Bethesda, MD: American Occupational Therapy Association.

Smelt, H. (1989). Effect of an inhibitive weight-bearing mitt on tone reduction and functional performance in a child with cerebral palsy. *Physical and Occupational Therapy in Pediatrics, 9,* 53–80.

Smith, M. A., Connolly, B., McFadden, S., Nicrosi, C. R., Nuckolls, L. J., Russell, F. F., & Wilson, W. M. (1982). *Feeding management of a child with a handicap: A guide for professionals.* Memphis: University of Tennessee.

Stern, F. M. & Gorga, D. (1988). Neurodevelopmental treatment (NDT): Therapeutic intervention and its efficacy. *Infants and Young Children, 1,* 22–32.

Stern, L. (1994). *Pediatric strengthening program.* San Antonio, TX: Therapy Skill Builders.

Stout, J. (1988). Planning playgrounds for children with disabilities. *American Journal of Occupational Therapy, 42,* 653–657.

Taylor, S. & Trefler, E. (1984). Decision making guidelines for seating and positioning children with cerebral palsy. In E. Trefler (Ed.), *Seating for children with cerebral palsy: A resource manual* (pp. 55–76). Memphis: University of Tennessee Center for Health Sciences, Rehabilitation Engineering Program.

Torfs, C. P., Van den Berg, B. J., Oechsli, F. W., Cummins, S. (1990). Prenatal and perinatal factors in the etiology of cerebral palsy. *Journal of Pediatrics, 116,* 615–619.

U. S. Department of Education (1987). *Ninth annual report to Congress of the implementation of the Education of the Handicapped Act.* Washington, DC: U.S. Government Printing Office.

Uzgiris, I. C. & Hunt, J. M. (1975). *Assessment in infancy: Ordinal Scales of Psychological Development.* Urbana: University of Illinois Press.

VanSant, A. (1991). Motor control, motor learning, and motor development. In P. C. Montgomery & B. H. Connolly (Eds.), *Motor control and physical therapy: Theoretical framework and practical applications* (pp. 13–28). Hixson, TX: Chattanooga Group, Inc.

Williams, S. E. & Matesi, D. V. (1988). Therapeutic intervention with an adapted toy. *American Journal of Occupational Therapy, 42,* 673–676.

Williamson, G. G. (1987). *Children with spina bifida.* Baltimore: Paul H. Brookes.

Yasukawa, A. & Hill, J. (1988). Casting to improve upper extremity function. In R. Boehme (Ed.), *Improving upper body control* (pp. 165–188), San Antonio, TX: Therapy Skill Builders.

Yasukawa, A. (1990). Upper extremity casting: Adjunct treatment for a child with cerebral palsy. *American Journal of Occupational Therapy, 44,* 840–847.

Yen, I. H., Khoury, M. J., & Erickson, J. D. (Winter, 1992). The changing epidemiology of neural tube defect: United States 1968–1989. *Matheny Bulletin, 2*(3), 1.

Chapter 30

Orthopedic and Musculoskeletal Problems in Children

Judith Atkins

T he pediatric orthopedic and musculoskeletal conditions discussed in this chapter include congenital
deformities, such as upper extremity amputations, hip dislocation, and arthrogryposis, as well as, conditions that develop or become apparent in infancy and during childhood
such as osteogenesis imperfecta, muscular dystrophy, and juvenile rheumatoid arthritis. Some conditions, such as congenitally dislocated hips, are correctable. Others, such as
arthrogryposis and osteogenesis imperfecta, may improve
with treatment, but will present constant challenges to the
child, parent, and occupational therapy practitioner. Other
disorders are degenerative, most notably Duchenne-type
muscular dystrophy, which ends in death in early adulthood
(Braddom, 1996). Because the causes of these defects are often unknown, parents may feel extremely guilty and grief
stricken. It is very difficult for parents who anticipate a child
who will grow and develop, as do other children, to be faced
with a congenital anomaly or orthopedic diagnosis. Many
times early intervention with a positive approach facilitates
optimum acceptance by the parents and optimal function for
the child. A comprehensive **interdisciplinary** approach can
guarantee a chance for independence and productive living.

This chapter is oriented to interventions provided in
medical model settings, such as hospitals and rehabilitation
centers. The age of the child and severity of the problem influence the evaluation and treatment needed. With each
new developmental change, growth, and maturation, new
problems manifest themselves and require new avenues of
treatment. Despite their degree of severity, all these diag-

noses have significant effects on the lives of all members of
the family and influence the family as a group. Consequently, occupational therapy practitioners must take into
consideration the parents and other family members, their
understanding of the condition and emotional adjustment,
and their ability to cope with the demands placed on them
in caring for their child with orthopedic problems. Children
with orthopedic and musculoskeletal problems may also receive occupational therapy services in public school settings
if their disability interferes with their learning.

Many congenital deformities are recognized at birth and
result in comprehensive evaluation and treatment from the
beginning of the child's life. Other conditions are discovered
when parents seek medical attention because the child is
experiencing **pain**, decreased function, or changes in physical appearance. Pain is a common early complaint, especially
following certain activities. Consequently, a careful history
delineating the onset of pain, its location, character (dull,
sharp), severity, and duration help with diagnosis and treatment. Factors that alleviate and aggravate pain are important
to understand. Decreased ability to use a body part, muscle
weakness, fatigue, instability of a joint, or stiffness of a joint
indicate functional loss. Changes in physical appearance,
such as increase in a curve of a back or a leg length discrepancy, also may be described by parents. Many times musculoskeletal conditions have associated or related problems,
such as heart disease, diabetes, kidney disease, or respiratory
disorders. These may complicate treatment and cause contraindications for certain activities.

▼ EFFECT OF ORTHOPEDIC AND MUSCULOSKELETAL PROBLEMS ON FUNCTION

Orthopedic and musculoskeletal problems result in numerous hospitalizations, surgeries, and therapy sessions. A certain amount of regression and withdrawal occurs with hospitalization and confinement to bed. Parental bonding may be adversely affected because parents may fear handling their children or the casts, splints, and other orthopedic devices make this difficult. Furthermore, developmental delays may occur because the child has diminished opportunity to play. Occupational therapy treatment during hospitalization focuses on developmental assessment and stimulation to mitigate the deprived environment of the hospital.

Hospitalization and treatment has an emotional and financial effect on the family, as well as creating stress for the child. Children are often immobilized for extended periods, negatively affecting development, independence, and play. Loss of days in school may delay their educational progress and inhibit development of peer relationships. Dependency may develop that must later be decreased through occupational therapy treatment and the use of assistive devices and durable medical equipment. Chapter 33 has a section that discusses the influence of chronic illness and disability on psychosocial development.

▼ OCCUPATIONAL THERAPY EVALUATION AND TREATMENT PRINCIPLES FOR ORTHOPEDIC AND MUSCULOSKELETAL CONDITIONS

The occupational therapy practitioner has a great deal to offer the child with orthopedic and musculoskeletal dysfunction. By nature of their disability, these children are at risk for **developmental delay**, **sensory integrative**, fine motor, and behavioral problems. They frequently need help with positioning and development of age appropriate independence in activities of daily living (ADLs). The needs of these children change as they develop; consequently, different evaluations and treatment are indicated during infancy, preschool age, school age, and adolescence.

Evaluation of this type of dysfunction includes active range of motion (ROM), passive ROM, strength, and sensation. Developmental assessment, especially in relation to self-care activities and play and leisure skills, can assist the therapist and family plan treatment that minimize symptoms and maximize function and continued development.

Goals for children with musculoskeletal disorders include such things as gaining, maintaining, and regaining joint motion; increasing muscle strength; and increasing the ability to engage in self-care, play, and school-related tasks and activities. Use of occupational therapy treatment focuses on these goals through activities that promote active, rather than passive, movement. Active movement is safer than passive because pain at the end of the ROM limits movement that might stretch and injure the joint (Salter, 1983). Active exercise, beyond promoting ROM, strengthens muscles and improves coordination. Functional training fosters increased competence, at the same time that musculoskeletal function improves. Splinting, positioning equipment, wheelchairs, and adaptive equipment are used, when needed, to protect joints, maintain posture, and promote mobility and function.

Developmental Evaluation and Treatment

Depending on their problems, children may be evaluated by informal observation and assessment, or by a standardized developmental assessment, such as the Gesell Developmental Test or the Bayley Scales of Infant Development. The findings of this evaluation and normal developmental patterns should be discussed with the family. In collaboration with the family, a home program should be planned to foster development with activities appropriate to the child's needs and the cultural and socioeconomic realities of the child's family. The child should be reevaluated at least every 6 months using the same tool or tools so that a true comparison can be made. Psychometric testing by the school should be recommended at age 5. The tables at the end of this unit list developmental assessment tools used by occupational therapists.

Upper Extremity Evaluation and Treatment

Children with musculoskeletal disorders require a thorough and comprehensive evaluation of their upper extremity strength, coordination, and overall function. Much of the assessment, during infancy and preschool, centers around observation of play and hand function. When the child becomes old enough for more formal assessments, assessments used with any diagnostic group to determine hand function should be considered. Dynamometer and pinch meter readings should be taken regularly to record decreased strength. Goniometry can assess ROM. Hand function and upper extremity use are critical because upper extremity strength and coordination directly affect successful transfer activities, independence in self-care, wheelchair use, and school performance. Functional performance may be assessed using standardized assessment instruments, such as the Functional Independence Measure for Children, the Functional Independence Measure, or the Pediatric Evaluation of Disability Inventory (see Table IX-A at the end of this unit for a complete list of assessment instruments).

TABLE 30-1. Orthopedic and Musculoskeletal Problems in the Newborn

Diagnosis	Clinical Findings Signs and Symptoms	Related Problems
Congenital Amputation of the Upper Extremity (Bayne & Costas, 1990)	Diagnosed immediately at birth. More common in girls. Left below elbow amputation more common than other types.	Usually none. Occasionally associated with a syndrome.
Radial Deformities (Bayne & Costas, 1990)	Unilateral or bilateral. Diagnosed at birth.	Absent thumb or hypoplasia of thumb. Frequently associated with syndromes. Partial or complete absence of radius.
Syndactyly (Bayne & Costas, 1990)	Diagnosed at birth. Webbing of the fingers. May involve skin only or bone.	Often associated with syndromes.
Obstetric Brachial Plexus Injury (Bayne & Costas, 1990)	Nerve injury occurs at birth. Usually due to traction. Isolated to one arm. Pregnancy normal.	Usually none.
Torticollis (Mott, James, & Sperhac, 1990)	Diagnosed at birth.	May be associated with abnormalities of the cervical spine, such as hemivertebrae.
Congenital Hip Dislocation (Herring, 1990; Mott, James, & Sperhac, 1990; Scipien, Chard, Howe, & Barnard, 1990)	Instability in the hip—the femoral head is out of the acetabulum (dislocated) or riding on its edge (subluxed). Difficulty diapering, shortening of one leg, toeing in or toe walking. Early diagnosis reduces risk of hip contractures and poor hip development.	Club feet, arthrogryposis, breech or other traumatic delivery.
Arthrogryposis (Bayne & Costas, 1990)	Apparent at birth. Can be isolated to one joint or many joints. Cause unknown, but may be related to abnormality of hormones, problems with fetal blood supply, in utero infection, neuropathy, and mechanical restrictions.	Usually very bright

ADL = activities of daily living; ROM = range of motion

Functional Implications	Medical/Surgical Treatment	OT Evaluation and Treatment
Loss of function varies. May involve loss of fingers, hand, or all or part of upper extremity.	Fit with a prosthesis early. First prosthesis at 6–9 mo.	Development of trusting relationship with parents is critical to foster child's acceptance of prosthesis. Instruct parents. Developmental assessment. Training with prosthesis.
Hand displaced radially. Stiffness, lack of ROM. Child may use lateral flexion of the hand against the forearm to grasp objects.	Surgery to improve alignment, stability, and function, especially if the child does not use lateral flexion. Index finger may be repositioned to substitute for thumb (pollicization). This enhances prehension.	Evaluate ROM. Stretching exercises. Splinting.
Difficulty with hand function, dependent on loss of ROM.	Surgery to release skin.	Evaluate ROM and development and hand function before and after surgery. Splints may be used after surgery.
Adduction, internal rotation, and contracture of the shoulder. Loss of elbow extension.	Possible surgery. Muscle transfers. 80% recovery without surgery. For children who have residual deformity, surgical correction involving muscle transfers may be used.	Assess ROM and development. Splinting at birth with the arm positioned in external rotation, abduction, humeral flexion, elbow flexion, forearm and wrist neutral and hand in functional position. Passive ROM. As the child improves provide bilateral activities to increase active ROM and use of the extremity. For children who have surgery, it is followed by splinting and muscle reeducation.
Contracture of sternocleidomastoid muscle. Head tilted toward the involved side and chin rotated toward the contralateral shoulder. Limited ROM impairs any activity that requires turning the head.	Referral to occupational therapy. Possible surgery.	Stretching exercises. Splinting with soft or hard collar. Bed positioning. Active ROM. Functional activities to foster movement of the head.
Children with severe dislocation or delayed diagnosis may develop limp or waddling gait. May result in hip problems in later life.	Under 3 mo—abduction harness and splint. 3–18 mo—traction, closed hip reduction, hip spica cast. 18 mo–5 yr—traction closed reduction, surgery.	Development assessment. Age appropriate activities. Adapted equipment to foster independence during period of immobility.
Joint contractures that vary in severity. Poor muscle development and degenerative changes in enervation of these muscles. Limitations in active and passive ROM. Often shoulders adducted and internally rotated. Elbow fixed in extension, the forearm pronated. Hands, wrist flexed and ulnarly deviated. Functional UE activities very difficult for these children (eg, eating, dressing, toileting, and writing).	May benefit from surgery, muscle transfers, contracture releases.	Assessment of ROM, ADL development. Splinting. ROM exercises. Adapted equipment to increase ADL and other functional activities. Power wheelchair for children who cannot walk.

TABLE 30-2. Orthopedic and Musculoskeletal Problems from Infancy through Adolescence

Diagnosis	Clinical Findings Signs and Symptoms	Related Problems
Legg-Calve Perthes disease (Mott, James, & Sperhac, 1990)	Avascular necrosis of head of femur. Occurs between 4 and 10 years of age. Usually boys. Cause unknown. Primary symptoms are limp and pain in knee, thigh, or groin. Children tend to be very active.	None
Osteogenesis imperfecta (Mott, James, & Sperhac, 1990)	Caused by autosomal dominant gene. Blue sclera classic sign of this disorder. Most severe if symptoms occur at birth or during infancy. Fractures at birth, during infancy or later childhood. Bones brittle and osteoporotic. Easily fractures even moving in bed.	Short stature. Scoliosis. Misshapen skull, wide intratemporal measurements, and small triangular face. Teeth also fragile and subject to breaking and cavities. Children may be thought to be battered because of multiple fractures.
Scoliosis, kyphosis, lordosis (Salter, 1983)	Deformities of the spine. May be apparent at birth or may be diagnosed as child grows.	May be associated with other diagnosis such as spina bifida or may be isolated.
Duchenne's muscular dystrophy (Mott, James, & Sperhac, 1990)	Noninflammatory inherited disorder. Most common is Duchenne muscular dystrophy. Transmission by recessive gene. Usually males. Diagnosed between ages 2 and 4 years. Frequent falling; muscle cramps; waddling, lordotic gait, progressive muscle weakness.	Progressive disease. Muscle weakness leads to scoliosis, contractures at the hip and knees, equinovarus deformities in the feet. Heart and respiratory failure eventually lead to death, generally before the age of 20.
Juvenile rheumatoid arthritis (Mosca & Sherry, 1990)	Chronic synovial inflammation of unknown cause. Onset before age 16 yr. Swelling of joints. Exacerbations and remissions. Most children have long remissions, without residual deformity and loss of function.	None

ADL = activities of daily living; ROM = range of motion

Activities of Daily Living Evaluation and Treatment

ADL evaluations, relative to eating, dressing, grooming, and bathing, should be performed at appropriate developmental stages. Oral–motor assessments should be performed when indicated, with treatment dependent on the results of such examinations. Treatment should focus on the acquisition of developmentally appropriate skills. Adaptive equipment may be needed to promote independence because of restricted mobility, decreased muscular strength, pain, fatigue, or combinations thereof. For more detailed information on these assessments refer Chapter 15; for more detailed information about treatment see Chapters 19 and 21.

Adaptive Equipment

Children born with musculoskeletal disorders use many different types of equipment such as braces, wheelchairs, walkers, and crutches. Equipment should be provided to improve function, provide support, help prevent deformity, and ease care for the family.

WHEELCHAIRS

Wheelchairs are necessary to improve the mobility of children who cannot walk. They may also be used by ambulators who are unable to do distance walking. Power wheelchairs may be needed for college or work environment, or when upper extremities are not compatible with manual mobility. High-strength, lightweight wheelchairs are particularly suitable because they are durable and have growth po-

Functional Implications	Medical or Surgical Treatment	OT Evaluation and Treatment
Immobility during treatment. If healing is not symmetrical, degenerative hip disease may develop in adulthood.	Child made nonweight bearing either through traction or casting to enable the acetabulum to heal and maintain the femoral head. Surgery may be used to allow greater mobility during the healing process. Course of the disease lasts 3–4 years.	Developmental assessment. Supportive and developmental activities while in traction. Wheelchair with castboard for independent mobility.
Delayed development secondary to immobility. Refractures secondary to disuse atrophy.	Casting to set fractures	Developmental assessment and intervention. Padded, specially constructed bed to turn prone to supine. Modify car seats wheelchairs for independent mobility. Encourage activity at level that is safe for the child.
Pulmonary restriction, decreasing endurance. May prevent good sitting posture, which impedes upper extremity functional activities.	Exercise, body jacket or positional systems. Surgery may be indicated to fuse spine.	Developmental assessment. Sensory integration testing. Positioning equipment.
Loss of ability to walk. Progressive loss of upper extremity function from proximal to distal, eventually leading to loss of hand function.	Some medications can slow down progression. Treatment of pulmonary problems. Help families and child deal with prognosis.	Stretching to maintain ROM. Muscle strengthening activities contraindicated because they hasten breakdown of muscles. Use of adaptive equipment to maintain independence in ADL and other activities. Power wheelchair for independent mobility. Exercises. As child grows and disease progresses use of lifts to assist with transfers.
Limitation in ROM. Pain and tenderness restricts activities. Fatigue.	Medications	Assess ROM, ADL, and need for adaptive equipment. Intervention involves exercises, splinting, adaptive equipment, joint protection techniques, energy conservation. For children with restricted ambulation, powered tricarts or wheelchairs may be indicated.

tential. Removable armrests and swing-away detachable footrests should always be considered for independent transfers. Elevating leg rests are especially useful for lower extremity fractures. A person prescribing a wheelchair should be knowledgeable about product availability, features, maintenance requirements, and cost. The family and the child should play a key role in the selection process.

ACTIVITIES OF DAILY LIVING EQUIPMENT

Children with orthopedic and musculoskeletal problems benefit from transfer tub seats, handheld shower hoses, and reachers. These needs are identified during the ADL evaluation and in collaboration with the child and the family. Button hooks, built-up handles on eating utensils, adapted writing tools, and such may also be needed for children whose hand function is impaired.

DEVELOPMENTAL AND RECREATIONAL EQUIPMENT

Floor sitters and tables can enhance development of sitting, balance and fine motor skills. Younger children may benefit from a crawler or creeper to enhance prone mobility.

▼ OCCUPATIONAL THERAPY EVALUATION AND TREATMENT FOR SPECIFIC PEDIATRIC ORTHOPEDIC AND MUSCULOSKELETAL CONDITIONS

Occupational therapy evaluation and treatment of specific pediatric orthopedic and musculoskeletal conditions is based primarily on the general principles discussed in the first part of this chapter. However, each diagnosis has unique characteristics that the occupational therapy practitioner must consider. These are outlined in Tables 30–1 and 30–2.

►CONCLUSIONS

Occupational therapy plays a key role in improving function, as well as independence for these children. A comprehensive interdisciplinary approach at the time of birth or onset, can guarantee a more positive outcome, with an increased chance for independence and productive living. It can also further parental understanding, promote parental bonding, and help alleviate many fears. Occupational therapy practitioners, by the nature of their educational background in both physical and psychosocial dysfunction, provide parents with the information and guidance necessary to meet the challenges identified with each developmental age.

▼ REFERENCES

Bayne, L. & Costas, B. (1990). Malformations of the upper limb. In R. T. Morrissy (Ed.), *Lovell and Winter's pediatric orthopaedics* (3rd ed., vol. 2, pp. 563–609). Philadelphia: J. B. Lippincott.

Behrman, R. E. & Vaughen, V. C. (1987). *Nelson textbook of pediatrics* (13th ed., pp. 515–528). Philadelphia: W. B. Saunders.

Braddom, R. L. (Ed.). (1996). *Physical medicine and rehabilitation.* Philadelphia: W. B. Saunders.

Herring, J. A. (1990). Congenital dislocation of the hip. In R. T. Morrissy (Ed.), *Lovell and Winter's pediatric orthopaedics* (3rd ed., vol. 2, pp. 815–850). Philadelphia: J. B. Lippincott.

Mosca, V. S. & Sherry, D. P. (1990). Juvenile rheumatoid arthritis and the seronegative spondyloarthopathies. In R. T. Morrissy (Ed.), *Lovell and Winter's pediatric orthopaedics* (3rd ed., vol 2, pp. 297–324). Philadelphia: J. B. Lippincott.

Mott, S. R., James, S. R., & Sperhac, A. M. (Eds.). (1990). *Nursing care of children and families* (2nd ed.). Redwood City, CA: Addison Wesley Nursing.

Salter, R. B. (1983). *Textbook of disorders and injuries of the musculoskeletal spine* (2nd ed., pp. 77–88, 122–132). Baltimore: Waverly Press.

Scipien, G. M., Chard, M. A., Howe, J., & Barnard, M. U. (Eds.). (1990). *Pediatric nursing care.* St. Louise: C. V. Mosby.

Chapter 31

Cardiopulmonary Dysfunction in Children

Olga Baloueff

Conditions affecting children's cardiac and respiratory systems are either congenital or acquired. They can be a child's primary condition, or they can be associated with other conditions, such as in Down syndrome. Impairments exist in different degrees in children's health and occupational performance according to the severity and chronicity of the condition. This chapter discusses congenital and acquired heart disease and cystic fibrosis, addressing in particular, the role occupational therapy can play in the treatment of children with these conditions.

▼ CONGENITAL HEART DISEASE

All congenital heart defects originate before the end of the first trimester of gestation, as the heart develops early in embryonic life and is completely formed and functioning by 10 weeks (Damjanov, 1996). Congenital heart defects (CHD) involve the heart, or the large arteries and veins, or a combination thereof. The major causes of CHD include maternal infections, drug and alcohol use during pregnancy (eg, rubella; fetal alcohol syndrome), and chromosomal abnormalities (eg, trisomy 21) (Damjanov). The symptoms of CHD become evident at birth or during infancy, or even later in life (Howell, 1994; Moller & Kaplan, 1991). In general, these include cyanosis, heart murmur, heart failure, decreased blood flow to the extremities, failure to thrive, or growth retardation. Diagnoses include septal defects, tetralogy of Fallot, patent ductus aorta, and coarctation of the aorta. Surgical interventions are common for most diagnoses.

▼ ACQUIRED HEART DISEASE

The heart may be vulnerable to a variety of infections (bacterial, fungal, parasitic, and viral), resulting in either, endocarditis, myocarditis, pericarditis, or even in pancarditis (Damjanov, 1996). Rheumatic heart disease (RHD), the most common acquired heart disease, is a sequela of rheumatic fever (RF), a systemic immunological disease, related to streptococcal infections (Damjanov). Rheumatic fever occurs about 2 weeks after an acute streptococcal throat infection (strep throat) which affects children and young adults. It is a multisystemic disease, with the following clinical features: carditis, polyarthritis, chorea, and skin lesions (Damjanov, 1996; Howell, 1994).

Medical treatment consists of bed rest, administration of antibiotics, and anti-inflammatory medications. Complications of RF may involve heart valves becoming calcified and deformed, necessitating surgery at some point, for replacement by artificial valves (Damjanov, 1996; Moller & Kaplan, 1991).

▼ PULMONARY CONDITION: CYSTIC FIBROSIS

Definition of Disease and Disability

Cystic fibrosis (CF) is a biochemical abnormality of the exocrine glands characterized by abnormal cellular chloride transport, resulting in hyperviscous secretions plugging the ducts and tubes of several organs. It affects not only the respiratory system, but also the sweat glands, the gastrointestinal system, and the reproductive organs (Cintas, 1995). It is the most common autosomal recessive disease, affecting 1 in 2500 births in the United States (Damjanov, 1996, p. 119). This lethal genetic disease, which affects chromosome 7, is almost entirely limited to the white population and is extremely rare in other races (Damjanov).

Diagnosis and Medical Management

The clinical manifestations of CF range from mild to severe and from onset at birth to onset years later (Kumar, Cotran, & Robbins, 1992). In about 5% to 10% of cases, CF is diagnosed early in life because the newborn's small intestine becomes blocked by meconium, which leads to a distended stomach and vomiting (Kumar et al, p. 91). If not attended promptly, the child will die of peritonitis.

Food malabsorption is a common sign, reflected in large and foul-smelling stools, abdominal distention, and poor weight gain in infancy (Kumar et al, 1992; Welsh & Smith, 1995). The most important complication of this condition pertains to the hyperviscosity of bronchial mucus, predisposing the child to frequent respiratory infections (Ashwell, Agnew-Coughlin, Boyd, & Brooks, 1994). An analysis of chloride levels in the child's perspiration is used to confirm a CF diagnosis (positive sweat test). Parents will often say their infant tastes salty (Kumar et al). Although CF is still an incurable chronic illness, and most people with it die in young adulthood as a result of pulmonary infections, promising gene therapy research is now being conducted for treating the lung abnormalities (Damjanov, 1996; Welsh & Smith, 1995).

Medical management of CF is largely supportive. It consists of prevention and treatment of upper respiratory infections as well as the administration of nutritional supplements. Antibiotics, vitamins, enzymes, and oral pancreatic supplements are commonly prescribed. Respiratory therapy involving such techniques as postural drainage, percussion and vibration of the chest walls, mist tent, and aerosol therapy are employed for clearing mucus from the airways (Ashwell et al, 1994). Proper intake of fluids and calories are important considerations in the child's daily nutrition (Cintas, 1995).

▼ OCCUPATIONAL PERFORMANCE DEFICITS IN CARDIOPULMONARY DYSFUNCTION

The degree of functional limitations encountered by children with cardiopulmonary conditions and cystic fibrosis (CF) varies greatly from one child to another, ranging from no limitation, to severe limitations with cyanosis at rest (Cintas, 1995). Chronic illnesses have to be considered within a contextual and developmental framework because outcome will emerge as children develop and grow up. In childhood, the most commonly seen deficits are in the performance areas of play and activities of daily living (ADL), particularly feeding and self-care. Performance components most frequently affected are the sensorimotor, especially motor and neuromusculoskeletal.

In adolescence, children with chronic illnesses often experience delayed physiological maturation and are also at greater risk for psychosocial problems, particularly anxiety, depression, poor self-esteem and body-image, and poor social interactions (Patterson, 1985; Rolland, 1994; Sinnema, Bonarius, Van Der Laag, & Stoop, 1988). Adherence to medical treatment, medications, and therapy schedules often becomes an issue for adolescents as the urge for independence, experimentation, and risk-taking behaviors increases (Rolland, 1994; Thompson, Gustafson, Hamlett, & Spock, 1992). Transition to adulthood for children with life-threatening illnesses, such as CF, brings psychosocial issues involving independence from family and choices about education, employment, marriage, and family (Ashwell et al, 1994; Sinnema et al, 1988; Thompson et al, 1992).

▼ FAMILY FUNCTIONING IN CHILDREN WITH CHRONIC ILLNESS

The effect of a child's disability has been discussed earlier in this book (see Chap. 5). However, families of children with chronic illnesses face some specific stresses, such as the financial and physical burdens of care, and frequent hospitalizations. Concerns for their child's mortality and uncertain future (as in CF), as well as their child's and siblings' psychosocial adjustment further contribute to parental stress (Rolland, 1994; Sinnema et al, 1988; Thompson et al, 1992).

Despite these major stressors, many families adjust and contribute to their child's psychosocial adaptation (Patterson, 1991). Optimal function for children with chronic illnesses is rooted in supportive and cohesive families who believe in high but realistic potential for their children and are supportive of their move toward independence (McAnarney, 1985).

▼ EVALUATION OF OCCUPATIONAL PERFORMANCE

Evaluation of health impairments, functional limitations, and strengths in children with cardiopulmonary dysfunction and CF is a family-centered and multidisciplinary approach. Occupational therapy evaluation must take into account the effects of medical and physiological instability, decreased mobility, and contextual situations, such as home environment, hospitalization, and disruptions in typical social, emotional, and physical life experiences (Ashwell et al, 1994; Bozynski, 1989; Kelly, 1994). Ecological assessments are particularly useful with this group of children.

▼ TREATMENT CONSIDERATIONS

The goal of occupational therapy is to facilitate the acquisition of contextual and age-appropriate functional skills. To maximize optimal performance, treatment activities are individualized, family-focused, and graded to the child's level of tolerance. Precautions have to be observed relative to the mode, intensity, and frequency of activities (Howell, 1994). In carrying out treatment, occupational therapy practitioners have to be sensitive to sudden changes in the child, such as pallor or flushing, labored respiration, pulse rate, and decreased stamina. Education and support of the family relative to the child's developmental and special needs are an integral part of the treatment, including environmental adaptations at home and at school to help the child conserve energy.

As children grow older, it becomes important to educate them concerning precautions, energy conservation techniques, responsibilities for following their therapeutic schedule, and to advocate, with confidence, their strengths and limitations.

►CONCLUSION

Cardiopulmonary dysfunction in children has the potential to delay the development of skills related to ADLs and play. School performance may also suffer. Occupational therapy intervention facilitates the development of these functional capacities and supports children and their families as they cope with these potentially life-threatening conditions.

▼ REFERENCES

Ashwell, J. A., Agnew-Coughlin, J. L., Boyd, S., & Brooks, D. (1994). Cystic fibrosis. In S. K. Campbell (Ed.), *Physical therapy for children* (pp. 688–715). Philadelphia: W. B. Saunders.

Bozynski, M. E. A. (1989). Comprehensive management of the infant with bronchopulmonary dysplasia: A growing challenge. *Infants and Young Children, 2,* 14–24.

Cintas, H. L. (1995). Pediatric disorders. In T. M. Long & H. L. Cintas (Eds.), *Handbook of pediatric physical therapy* (pp. 51–99). Baltimore: Williams & Wilkins.

Damjanov, I. (1996). *Pathology for the health-related professions.* Philadelphia: W. B. Saunders.

Howell, B. A. (1994). Thoracic surgery. In S. K. Campbell (Ed.), *Physical therapy for children* (pp. 737–760). Philadelphia: W. B. Saunders.

Kelly, K. M. (1994). Children with ventilator dependence. In S. K. Campbell (Ed.), *Physical therapy for children* (pp. 664–685). Philadelphia: W. B. Saunders.

Kumar, V., Cotran, R. S., & Robbins, S. L. (1992). *Basic pathology.* Philadelphia: W. B. Saunders.

McAnarney, E. R. (1985). Social maturation: A challenge for handicapped and chronically ill adolescents. *Journal of Adolescent Health Care, 6,* 90–101.

Moller, J, H. & Kaplan, E. L. (1991). Forty years of cardiac disease in children. *Minnesota Medicine, 74,* 27–33.

Patterson, J. M. (1985). Critical factors affecting family compliance with home treatment for children with cystic fibrosis. *Family Relations, 34,* 79–89.

Patterson, J. M. (1991). A family system perspective for working with youth with disability. *Pediatrician, 18,* 129–141.

Rolland, J. S. (1994). *Families, illness, and disability.* New York: Basic Books.

Sinnema, G., Bonarius, H., Van Der Laag, H., & Stoop, J. W. (1988). The development of independence in adolescents with cystic fibrosis. *Journal of Adolescent Health Care, 9,* 61–66.

Thompson, R. J., Gustafson, K. E., Hamlett, K. W., & Spock, A. (1992). Stress, coping, and family functioning in the psychological adjustment of mothers of children and adolescents with cystic fibrosis. *Journal of Pediatric Psychology, 17,* 573–585.

Welsh, M. J. & Smith, A. E. (1995). Cystic fibrosis. *Scientific American, 273*(6), 52–59.

Chapter 32

Immune System Dysfunction: Children with HIV or AIDs and Their Families

Jim Hinojosa, Gary Bedell, and Margaret Kaplan

Typical Deficits in Performance Areas and
   Performance Components
Evaluation of Children with HIV or AIDS
Intervention for Children with HIV
   or AIDS
   Psychosocial Skills and Components

Sensorimotor Components
Cognitive Integration and Cognitive
   Components
Performance Areas
Balancing Encouragement and Support
Conclusion

A cquired immune deficiency syndrome (AIDS) was first recognized in children in 1982. Today, most children infected with the human immunodeficiency virus (HIV) acquire it from their mother by vertical transplacental, intrapartum, or postpartum transmission (Mok, 1988). Older children may become infected through unsafe sexual intercourse, intravenous drug use, and sexual abuse (Bartlett, Keller, Eckholdt, & Schleifer, 1995). Frequently, children with HIV infection come from families living in adverse conditions that include poverty and drug use.

The Centers for Disease Control (CDC) classification system for HIV and AIDS in children younger than 13 years of age is based on a continuum of symptomatology, from asymptomatic to symptomatic. The child with HIV or AIDS may have a wide range of clinical manifestations. Neurological deficits include progressive encephalopathy, acquired microcephaly, myelopathy, peripheral neuropathy, pyramidal tract dysfunction, as well as seizure disorders. Opportunistic infections include *Pneumocystis carinii* pneumonia, candidiasis, *Mycobacterium avium intracellulare*, and lymphocytic interstitial pneumonia (Peckham & Gibb, 1995). Thus, the clinical picture includes varying degrees of severity of disabilities, often accompanied by developmental delays (Ultmann et al, 1987). Of particular concern for a practitioner is progressive encephalopathy (ie, impaired brain growth, loss of developmental milestones, and progressive motor dysfunction with pyramidal tract dysfunction). Earlier symptoms may indicate a poor prognosis.

All individuals who live and work with children with HIV infection or AIDS should follow **universal precautions**. These include using gloves, gowns, masks, or goggles during procedures that entail contact or danger of splatter from blood, mucus, and other body fluids (James, 1990). Practitioners may have feelings of fear and anxiety related to exposure to an infectious disease. Universal precautions are effective in preventing transmission of HIV and other infections to others and in protecting children with HIV or AIDS from other people's infections (Centers for Disease Control, 1987; Rango, Burke, & Warren, 1991).

When working with children with HIV or AIDS, practitioners are likely to work with families who have backgrounds quite different from their own. These families may have varying expectations of the practitioner and may react to situations differently than expected. Furthermore, they may have different beliefs about illness and death. A family-centered approach to services as well as an attitude of unconditional positive regard (Rogers, 1961) is essential. Practitioners need to develop strategies to cope with their own grieving and anxiety when working with children with HIV or AIDS and their families. In addition, practitioners need to recognize that they may feel overwhelmed and helpless in the face of the effect of this disease on family function in all areas of life.

▼ TYPICAL DEFICITS IN PERFORMANCE AREAS AND PERFORMANCE COMPONENTS

Children with HIV or AIDS commonly have delays in the development of sensorimotor, cognitive, and language abilities. These delays may be caused by the virus itself, or by the effects of other common risk factors, such as premature birth, multiple drug exposure in utero, and poor prenatal care and nutrition. Neurological symptoms stemming from the virus include muscle tone abnormalities, as well as progressive loss of sensorimotor, cognitive, and language abilities. These losses further complicate the child's development.

Opportunistic infections can also influence the performance of activities. For example, a child with a severe case of candidiasis (thrush) may refuse to eat because of pain and difficulty chewing and swallowing, and may appear lethargic and uncooperative during therapy. A child with chronic lung infection may experience progressive weakness and lethargy caused by decreased oxygen intake and exchange.

A wide range of variation is found for the onset of symptoms and the severity and type of disabilities for children with HIV or AIDS. Abilities can vary on a day-to-day basis owing to effects of opportunistic infections, direct effects of the virus, side effects of medications and medical treatments, and multiple psychosocial issues. Pain can cause further psychosocial issues for the child. Young children have difficulty expressing pain, but may manifest it through an apparent "loss" of abilities, for example, a refusal to walk.

Children with HIV or AIDS often experience extensive loss of primary caregivers, siblings, and other family members. Also, these children may live in multiple foster homes. Repeated hospitalizations and extensive medical procedures contribute to isolation from peers and the community, as well as possible separation from familiar caregivers. Consequently, they may develop separation anxiety, withdrawal, anger, depression, or physical symptoms. These reactions will vary depending on the age, personality, and situation of each child.

Awareness of being different and of society's reaction to HIV and AIDS increases as children grow older. The stigma attached to this infection and related discrimination can foster patterns of secrecy within families. Families may need support in talking to each other, their children, and close friends about their own HIV status and that of their child. Children may need help in coping with the reactions of peers, teachers, and others, especially if they are able to remain in school and participate in community activities.

▼ EVALUATION OF CHILDREN WITH HIV OR AIDS

The evaluation of children with HIV or AIDS is guided by interviews with the caregivers relative to the concerns, priorities, schedules, and other responsibilities of the family as they affect the child. Information from caregivers about the child's developmental history and behavior in different contexts is important as well as determining any difficulties in the performance of self-care, play, and school-related activities. Information about the child's experiences with medical

procedures, hospitalization, and other separations and losses can assist the occupational therapist in gaining a more complete picture of the child.

Observation of the child engaged in play or school activities with peers or family members can contribute information about problems in performance components that may contribute to difficulty in play, self-care, or school. The areas of feeding, mobility, and self-care are often concerns of caregivers, and these can be assessed through observation or with functional assessments such as the Pediatric Evaluation of Disability Index (PEDI) (Haley, Coster, Ludlow, Haltiwanger, & Andrellos, 1992).

Criterion referenced assessments and standardized tests in specific developmental areas can be used in the same manner as they are for other children with developmental delays or disabilities. For the child with HIV or AIDS factors such as fatigue, pain, frustration, irritability, depression, and separation anxiety must be considered during the evaluation process. Also, effects of opportunistic infections such as decreased respiratory capacity, fever, nausea, diarrhea, and dehydration may affect skills and abilities temporarily. Because of the progressive nature of this disease, frequent reevaluations may be needed.

▼ INTERVENTION FOR CHILDREN WITH HIV OR AIDS

Intervention for children with HIV or AIDS is related to the individual child's needs and those of his or her caregivers, and not to the child's diagnosis of this disease. Service delivery that is coordinated, flexible, and interdisciplinary increases the likelihood that the child and caregivers' needs are being met in an efficient manner. For example, if therapy sessions or days of school are missed because of medical appointments or socioeconomic-related issues, then rescheduling appointments and developing alternative service delivery models may be necessary to meet the child's and caregivers' needs.

Psychosocial Skills and Components

Providing a safe and supportive environment is part of every occupational therapy session. This becomes especially important for the child with HIV or AIDS, owing to the unpredictable nature of the syndrome and the child's prior experiences with noxious medical procedures. Often, the child and caregivers are in situations where they have limited control and may feel socially isolated. The child's status may be complicated by pain and just plain not feeling well. Role playing of stressful situations during therapy sessions may allow the child to express feelings and possibly reduce his or her fears, anxieties, and grief. The child can also be provided opportunities to learn new coping strategies to deal with these situations. Some children with HIV or AIDS may have decreased feelings of self-efficacy and have difficulty initiating actions required for need gratification, play, social interaction, activities of daily living (ADL), functional communication, and mobility. This may be due to overprotection or lack of encouragement from caregivers, or to decreased opportunities for the child to influence his or her environment.

Therapeutic relationships with the child and caregivers often need to be reestablished or strengthened because of the increased fear, distrust, and apathy that frequently occurs from prolonged illness, hospitalization, and convalescence at home. Provision of environments where the child and caregivers can express themselves openly, and safely explore and participate in meaningful activities often becomes a primary focus of intervention. Encouraging a child's self-directed actions, choices, and problem solving fosters a heightened sense of control.

Providing occupational therapy in play groups or in the child's classrooms encourages positive social interaction between the child, caregivers, and other children. The natural contexts of home or classroom give the child a real and perceived sense of control, because the child is familiar with the toys, materials, and people within these settings. In natural contexts, the child can learn from modeling other children and by practicing necessary and desired functional skills. Practitioners can demonstrate strategies that can be carried over by the caregivers to reinforce the development of skills.

Sensorimotor Components

Neurodevelopmental treatment is frequently used to address problems related to postural tone, balance, and motor control and coordination. These sensorimotor problems may be related to three conditions: (1) the progressive encephalopathy that occurs when HIV or other HIV infections or cancers enter or develop in the central nervous system (CNS), (2) static encephalopathy that occurs from perinatal factors that are frequently associated with cerebral palsy; or (3) opportunistic infections that do not have a progressive effect on the CNS.

A child may exhibit hyper- or hyporesponsivities to varied sensations in the environment. This can affect how he or she approaches activities or relates to family caregivers and others. Practitioners address these issues by using intervention that uses sensory integration techniques (Kimball, 1993), desensitization procedures, or methods of sensory–affective-regulation (DeGangi, Craft, & Castellan, 1991; Wilbarger & Wilbarger, 1991; Williams & Shellenberger, 1992).

Biomechanical interventions are used to improve the children's strength and endurance, and to provide body and body part positioning (splints, seating, and other adaptive equipment). Energy conservation, work simplification, time management principles, and other adaptive strategies and equipment can be discussed with and used by teachers and primary caregivers to compensate for the children's de-

creased strength, endurance, and mobility. Motor control and learning approaches can also be used for functional skill acquisition (Kaplan, 1994). Many of the aforementioned approaches improve the fine, gross, or perceptual motor abilities needed for ADL, educational activities, play, and leisure.

Cognitive Integration and Cognitive Components

Cognitive–behavioral approaches address deficits in attention, information processing, problem solving, visual perceptual skills, and learning (Todd, 1993). Frequently, a child with HIV or AIDS exhibits forgetfulness or more pronounced memory and orientation problems, disorganization in task performance, and decreased task persistence. These problems may be the result of psychosocial issues, stress, or hectic living situations. They may also indicate CNS damage.

Psychosocial and stress-related cognitive problems can be addressed by using the approaches discussed in the psychosocial section in this chapter and in the text as a whole. Materials, instructions, the physical environment, and the teaching and learning process may need to be modified according to the child's abilities, needs, and learning styles. Smaller groups may be needed for children to attend to important task performance requirements. Classrooms or living spaces may need to be organized in a way that orient and guide the child to specific activity areas and the types of behaviors that are expected and allowed there (eg, academics, free-play, snack time). Providing environmental cues, feedback, reinforcement, and encouraging practice in a variety of contexts may assist the child with learning daily routines and skills needed to function at home, in school, and in the community.

Performance Areas

Intervention to address performance areas, such as bathing and dressing, is similar to that used for other children with disabilities. However, some areas may require special attention. Intervention that addresses oral motor abilities and feeding skills may be complicated by oral thrush, decreased respiratory capacity, sinusitis, malnutrition, and HIV wasting. Food may have to be softer and blander to lesson the discomfort that can occur from oral thrush. More in-depth neurodevelopmental and sensory or physiological state regulation interventions may be required to improve safe and efficient coordination of oral motor abilities with respiration.

Because of frequent absences related to medical illnesses and appointments, the older school-aged child may need assistance with managing daily life routines such as scheduling time needed for taking medications, making medical appointments, studying and doing homework, and pursuing leisure pursuits. Practitioners can also collaborate with the child's teachers and caregivers to develop strategies, environmental modifications, and realistic plans to assist the child with managing an often chaotic daily life.

Because more children with HIV or AIDS are living longer, aspects of adolescent life, such as identity formation, identification with a peer group, grooming and hygiene skills, dating, sexual expression, experimentation with social skills and roles, learning prevocational skills, and exploring vocational or career goals, will become more important. These, as well as other life or death issues, will affect children infected with HIV through unsafe sexual intercourse, intravenous drug use, or sexual abuse. It is important for practitioners to acknowledge these issues when working with children and adolescents with HIV or AIDS and their caregivers.

Balancing Encouragement and Support

One of the most challenging aspects of intervention is knowing how to balance the amount of encouragement and support needed to "push" individuals to "do," and "allow" them to "just be," given their current circumstances. This is especially true when working with a child with HIV or AIDS and his or her caregivers. Because of the chronic and sporadic nature of the disease, it is often difficult or impossible to predict what occupational therapy interventions will be necessary or most effective at any given time.

In general, a child with this disease should be encouraged to be as active as possible. If the child is verbal, practitioners and caregivers should wait and expect the child to ask for what they want or need. Nonverbal communication should be encouraged for the child who does not speak. Practitioners should wait and give the child time to do something themselves before they rush in to help.

If a child is losing abilities owing to illness and not feeling well because of the direct effects of the disease on the neurological system, practitioners may have to assist or do more for the child. It is difficult to know when there is a realistic need for help and when children are using the strategy of getting others to do for them (an often attempted strategy of many children).

►CONCLUSION

Practitioners' judgments and actions taken relative to the issues related to working with children with HIV or AIDS and their caregivers will more likely be effective if they are sensitive to the children's physical conditions, personalities, typical coping styles, and family life circum-

stances. This can also be true if practitioners make a conscious effort to be open and willing to deal with issues by discussing them with the children, family caregivers, other practitioners, and clinical supervisors, and by reflecting on their own practice.

▼ REFERENCES

Bartlett, J. A., Keller, S. E., Eckholdt, H., & Schleifer, S. J. (1995). HIV relevant issues in adolescents. In N. Boyd-Franklin, G. L. Steiner, & M. G. Boland (Eds.), *Children, families, and HIV/AIDS: Psychosocial and therapeutic issues* (pp. 78–89). New York: Guilford.

Centers for Disease Control. (1987). *Recommendations for prevention of HIV transmission in healthcare settings. MMWR 36,* suppl. 25. Atlanta: Author.

DeGangi, G. A., Craft, P., & Castellan, J. (1991). Treatment of sensory, emotional, and attentional problems in regulatory disordered infants: Part 2. *Infants and Young Children, 3,* 9–19.

Haley, S. M., Coster, W. J., Ludlow, L. H., Haltiwanger, J. T., & Andrellos, P. J. (1992). *Pediatric Evaluation of Disability Inventory: Development, standardization and administration manual.* Boston: New England Medical Center Hospitals and PEDI Research Group.

James, S. R. (1990). Principles of nursing care for the hospitalized child. In S. R. Mott, S. R. James, & A. M. Sperhac (Eds.), *Nursing care of children and families* (2nd. ed., pp. 859–904). Redwood City, CA: Addison-Wesley Nursing.

Kaplan, M. (1994). Motor learning: Implications for occupational therapy and neurodevelopmental treatment. *Developmental Disabilities Special Interest Newsletter, 17,* 1–4.

Kimball, J. G. (1993). Sensory integrative frame of reference. In P. Kramer & J. Hinojosa (Eds.), *Frames of reference for pediatric occupational therapy* (pp. 87–175). Baltimore: Williams & Wilkins.

Mok, J. (August, 1988). HIV infection in children [Editorial]. *Journal of the Royal College of General Practitioners,* 342–344.

Peckham, C. & Gibb, D. (1995). Mother-to-child transmission of the human immunodeficiency virus. *The New England Journal of Medicine, 333,* 298–302.

Rango, N., Burke, G., & Warren, B. (1991). Guidelines for the care of children and adolescents with HIV infection. Introduction. *Journal of Pediatrics, 119,* 1–2.

Rogers, C. R. (1961). *On becoming a person.* Boston, MA: Houghton Mifflin.

Todd, V. (1993). Visual perceptual frame of reference: An information processing approach. In P. Kramer & J. Hinojosa (Eds.), *Frames of reference for pediatric occupational therapy* (pp. 177–232). Baltimore: Williams & Wilkins.

Ultmann, M. H., Diamond, G. W., Ruff, H. A., Belman, A. L., Novick, B. E., Rubinstein, A., & Cohen, H. J. (1987). Developmental abnormalities in children with acquired immunodeficiency syndrome (AIDS): A follow-up study. *International Journal Neuroscience, 32,* 661–667.

Wilbarger, P. & Wilbarger, J. L. (1991). *Sensory defensiveness in children aged 2–12.* Santa Barbara, CA: Avant Educational Programs.

Williams, M. S. & Shellenberger, S. (1992). *An introduction to "How does your engine run?" The alert program for self-regulation.* Albuquerque, NM: TherapyWorks.

Chapter 33

Psychosocial Dysfunction in Childhood and Adolescence

Linda Florey

At least 12% of children and adolescents have diagnosable mental disorders, and at least half of them are severely disabled by their disorder (Offord & Fleming, 1996, p. 1167). In addition, many others exhibit broad indicators of dysfunction such as substance abuse, teen pregnancy, and dropping out of school. These are risk factors associated with mental disorders (Zigler & Finn-Stevenson, 1996). Children with chronic medical conditions and brain damage are at increased risk for developing psychiatric disorders (Offord & Fleming). The problem is national in scope and constitutes a major public health concern. The most serious consequences of mental disorders are suicide, serious harm to others, and the need to remove children from their homes (Zigler & Finn-Stevenson).

Children and adolescents with notable psychopathology are identified in the mental health system, and in special education classes in the education system, but they can be found also in the pediatric wards and rehabilitation clinics of the health care system, in foster care and group homes in the child welfare system, and in detention centers in the juvenile justice system (National Mental Health Association Speaks, 1989). This includes children who have suffered bruises, fractures, or head trauma as a result of impulsive or aggressive behavior or as a result of self-inflicted or other abuse. Children with chronic medical conditions may also exhibit behaviors indicative of serious psychopathology.

In the school system, in which nearly 20% of occupational therapy practitioners work (American Occupational Therapy Association [AOTA], 1990, pp. 4–5), there is a large

proportion of children with psychopathology. These youngsters are referred to as seriously emotionally disturbed (SED) and constitute the fourth largest group of children with disabilities served under The Individuals with Disabilities Education Act (IDEA) (US Department of Education, 1995). In addition to the SED population, children with autism and attention deficit disorder are also covered by IDEA, federal legislation that provides for educational services for children with disabilities from 3 to 21 years of age. Yet there may be more children with significant emotional and behavioral problems than are in any of these eligibility categories. There are several reasons for this. There is a lack of systematic identification of this population because of the varied interpretations in definition and eligibility criteria. There is reluctance to label children because of the stigma associated with the label itself. Additionally, school districts may not have the services or may be resistant to paying for services needed for this group of children, owing to funding constraints (Forness, 1988; National Mental Health Association Speaks, 1989). As a result, many children in the school system with significant emotional problems may not be identified at all or may be misidentified as "**learning disabled**."

Occupational therapy practitioners who are working with children and adolescents in various service settings are likely to encounter youngsters with significant emotional problems. The intent of this chapter is to acquaint the reader with typical deficits in performance associated with psychosocial dysfunction, types of assessments and treatment programs that may be used with this population, and features of attention deficit hyperactive disorder (ADHD), conduct disorder, mood disorder, and autistic disorder. Psychosocial implications for children with chronic disabilities will also be discussed.

▼ TYPICAL DEFICITS IN PERFORMANCE AREAS AND PERFORMANCE COMPONENTS FOR CHILDREN AND ADOLESCENTS WITH PSYCHOSOCIAL DYSFUNCTION

Children and adolescents with psychosocial dysfunction may be aggressive, intrusive, disruptive, argumentative, unpredictable, inattentive, bossy, or withdrawn. Some may have difficulty attending to activities and completing tasks, and others may demonstrate a complete lack of interest in or satisfaction with activities. Their deficits pervade all occupational performance areas, although they may do better in some areas than others. Modulating behavior from one context to another or reading cues of expected behavior in a variety of contexts may be difficult for children and adolescents with psychosocial dysfunction. Children with the same diagnostic label may demonstrate their dysfunction differently. Although this is a heterogeneous group, nearly all demonstrate some degree of difficulty in social functioning. Generally, they are not well liked by their peers. The deficits they have in common are "Cub Scout deficits," "not invited to birthday party deficits," "not on the team or liked by the team deficits," "no one to eat lunch, play, or hang out with deficits," or "no best friend deficits."

Occupational Behavior: A Focus for Intervention

The occupational behavior frame of reference targets the broad parameters of play, student role, and socialization as the primary concern of occupational therapy practitioners working with individuals of this age range. A discussion of occupational behavior principles is presented in Chapter 23. The purpose of this section is to present a conceptual map to form the basis for targeting the kinds of deficits identified, the types of assessments to be used, and the formation of treatment principles.

DEVELOPMENTAL PROGRESSION IN OCCUPATIONAL BEHAVIOR

There is a developmental progression in the manner in which work and play are incorporated into an occupational role. An **occupational role** is distinguished from other social roles, such as sexual or familial role, to target the major productive daily activities of individuals. The typical progression is based on those activities that individuals spend most of their time doing. The progression is from player; to

student; to worker, homemaker, or volunteer; to retiree (Moorhead, 1969). The occupational role of preschool children is that of player, as play is the major activity during this period. Work activities emerge through learning the basics of self-care activities and preschool expectations. In middle childhood and adolescence, the major daily activity is attending school, thus the occupational role during this period is student. The dominant theme is work with the emphasis on productive activity in school and on displaying self-reliant behavior and completing chores at home. Paid part-time work may be done during this period. Play activity takes up less time than in early childhood, but is critical for mastering cooperation, teamwork, and competition. During adulthood work predominates, with play serving as a sublatent support, which emerges as leisure pursuits in retirement.

Role behavior involves learning of social expectations and specific ground rules for behavior within different and expanding contexts. For example, children have to recognize and learn the social rules appropriate to the school room, the playground, the soccer team, the sand lot, the church, the camp, and other people's homes. The roles of student and worker emanate largely from the social institutions of school and work, and many expectations are taught through these vehicles. Learning also takes place in families, with peers, and in other groups such as church, clubs, or teams.

DEVELOPMENTAL FOCUS IN PLAY, STUDENT ROLE, AND SOCIALIZATION

A major clinical focus is to determine the extent to which injury or illness has disrupted or impoverished occupational behavior and to identify steps to ameliorate dysfunction and to foster progression. Children and adolescents with psychosocial dysfunction experience difficulty in the social aspects of play and the role of student.

The Occupational Role of Player

The occupational role of player changes throughout development, but it remains as the primary arena in which social relatedness is learned, rehearsed, and mastered. **Play** during infancy and toddler years consists of exploring social influence through playful interactions, intentionally eliciting social responses, and engaging in symbolic social play. Infant games, such as peek-a-boo, are believed to have qualities of social interaction of mutual involvement, alternation of turns, and repetition of sequences (Bergen, 1987). Although toddlers will often approach others and imitate and exchange toys, peers become increasingly more a part of the child's social life during the preschool years. Between the ages of 2 and 5, social interactions are more frequent, more sustained, and more complex (Mussen, Conger, Kagan, & Huston, 1990). In these preschool years, sociodramatic play is prominent, as is constructive play. The use of pretense and pretend play seems to assist children in finding a common ground for interaction among unfamiliar peers (Bergen).

Sociodramatic play permits children to frame play in terms of role expectations, to coordinate these roles, and to communicate within and out of the roles. Simple group and board games allow children to practice rules of reciprocity and taking turns.

The different stages in peer play progression from solitary (no attention to peers), parallel (play next to each other without interacting), associative (play together but uncoordinated), to cooperative (interact in helping one another achieve shared goals) are still mentioned by researchers on play, but there is much more focus on the adaptive elements of different forms of play. Monighan-Nourot, Scales, Van Hoorn, and Almy (1987) caution that solitary and parallel play among preschoolers may represent more maturity than first thought. Solitary play may provide an opportunity for the consolidation and mastery of skills which, in turn, may foster a base for cooperative play and sharing of ideas. Children may use parallel play as a means for entering play or drawing others into play (Figs. 33–1 and 33–2).

Play in middle childhood, ages 6 to 12, is characterized by increasing complexity in peer relationships. During this period, the structure of social groups changes from informal gangs with few formal rules and rapid turnover in membership, to more structured, formal, and cohesive groups, with more elaborate membership requirements. Children form their own clubs, and they are members of many formal organizations, such as Girl and Boy Scouts and various teams. Friendships are prominent, with changes occurring in the basis of friendship formation. Friendship formation moves from friends as those playmates the child sees most frequently, to relationships characterized by cooperation and exchange of deeds and sharing, and lastly to friendship relationships judged in terms of mutual understanding and sharing of thoughts and feelings. Additionally, from the beginning of this developmental period, friendships move from being easily established and terminated to being stable over longer and longer periods (Mussen et al, 1990). Bergen

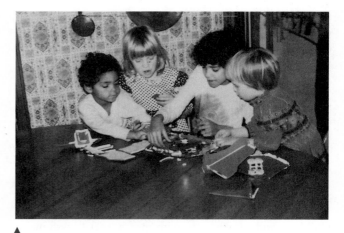

▲
Figure 33-2. Destroying a gingerbread house calls for cooperation.

and Oden (1987) also call attention to activity partnerships that occur during this period. They believe that these partnerships have interactive purposes and characteristics different from friendships. Children converse about activity-related concerns and learn to coordinate their actions toward a common purpose or goal.

This is the age in which the peer culture predominates (Corsaro & Schwarz, 1991; King, 1987). It is estimated that children spend over 40% of their waking time with peers (Cole & Cole, 1993; p. 516). In the peer group, children learn to interact with age mates, deal with dominance and hostility, relate to a leader and be a leader. As more of their allegiance is transferred to the peer group, children derive their sense of self-worth and value from this group. This is the age in which children compare themselves with others and develop images of themselves based on how they "measure up" to others (Mussen et al, 1990). Among themselves, children decide who can play in a game, codes for inclusion and exclusion, how to deal with cheaters, and how to manipulate the situation to one's own and one's friends advantage (Knapp & Knapp, 1976; Slukin, 1981). Mussen and coauthors sum it up this way: "The world of peers is a subculture, influenced in many ways by the larger culture but also having its own history, social organization, and means of transmitting its customs from one generation to the next. Much of the child's understanding of social behavior and how to relate to others is transmitted by peers, not by adults" (pp. 535–536).

Games with rules are dominant. Children go through different stages in their understanding of rules during this period. In the beginning of middle childhood, rules are vague, and children are often unable to put the rules of the game above the need to win. Children think of games such as baseball as action games, with the emphasis on "hitting" the ball and "running" around the bases. Rules such as the numbers of outs in an inning or the numbers of players on a team, are imposed by adults. Toward the end of this period, children become more aware that they can negotiate rules

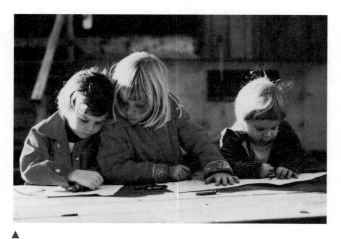

▲
Figure 33-1. Parallel play may facilitate children entering the play of others.

among themselves and determine them by consensus. Games are characterized by competition and often take the form of sports.

Constructive, practice, and symbolic play occur during this period, although the form that is taken is different from that with younger children. Constructive play takes the form of building or creating products, either alone or as part of a group inside or outside of the classroom. This play may include collecting and may form the precursor to hobbies. Practice play is more related to enhancing motor skills needed for competence in games and sports. Children spend a lot of time repeating and varying motor actions such as climbing, shooting baskets, jumping rope, and ball play. Symbolic play often is incorporated into games and the creation of futuristic stories and into language play involving secret codes, jokes, and "just conversation" (Bergen, 1987; Bergen & Oden, 1987).

In adolescence and adulthood, it is believed that the qualities that children exhibit in play are the ones adults continue to seek, although what to call this is up for debate. Whether this is best characterized as **"flow"** as in Csik-szentmahalyi's framework (1990) or how play is manifest may vary. It is believed that the outward manifestations of play continue to change, becoming further miniaturized, socialized, and abstracted as in symbolic board games such as chess (Bergen, 1987). In adolescence, sports and small interest clubs continue to be prominent as does "hanging out." Social relationships continue to be very much in evidence.

Occupational Role of Student

This role is largely defined by the social institutions of the school and the laws regulating schooling. According to Mussen and colleagues (1990), "the school is a small social system in which children learn rules of morality, social conventions, attitudes, and modes of relating to others, as well as academic skills" (p. 519). During middle childhood and continuing through adolescence, individuals spend most of their waking hours in the company of children and adults who are not their family members. In school, children must learn to work with teachers, to whom they must listen, obey, and gain favor with. They are judged against a standard of achievement and measured against their peer group. Grades are the concrete product of that measurement. The fit between the child, the family, and the school is of major importance. This includes the congruence between the expectations of the child and his or her ability, the dominant culture of the family, and the goals for education of the school (Combrinck-Graham, 1996).

In school children must master both academic curriculum and social expectations. The academic curriculum is formally taught: social expectations often are not taught, but must be learned informally. Teachers call social expectations proper classroom behavior. Children learn social behavior outside of the school setting. Families or caregivers refer to these expectations as manners, coaches talk about sportsmanship, Scout leaders refer to citizenship, and camps to

character. Children must be able to recognize and modulate their actions based the particular norms and cues of each environmental context. They must learn "appropriate" actions for different classrooms, the lunchroom, hallway, and playground. This includes how to enter discussions, when to raise hands, how to join a game in progress, how to share the attention of the teacher and classmates, how loud to talk, and when and how silly they can be. They must learn how to read, write, spell, do calculations, and generally master information about the world they live in. They must learn to accommodate to different teachers and different teaching styles.

Typical Performance Deficits in Play, Student Role, and Socialization

Typical performance deficits of children and adolescents with psychosocial dysfunction are in player and student roles because social behavior is embedded within them. The recognition and mastery of social behavior, in addition to the learning, practice, and mastery of sensory, neuromuscular, motor, and cognitive skill components of these roles, are critical. Beyond deficits in social behavior these youths also experience difficulty in their academic performance. Most children designated as severely emotionally disturbed (SED) in the school system fail academically, are socially rejected, have poor self-evaluations and low expectations for their potential contributions to society (Combrinck-Graham, 1996). Data from the National Longitudinal Transition Study of Special Education Students (NLTS) indicate that more than three-fourths of students with SED had failed one or more courses, which was the highest failure rate of any category of students with disabilities. High school students with SED demonstrated a pattern of disconnectedness from school activity. They were the least likely to belong to clubs or social groups at school and had high rates of absenteeism (Wagner, 1995).

▼ EVALUATION OF CHILDREN AND ADOLESCENTS WITH PSYCHOSOCIAL DYSFUNCTION

Occupational therapy evaluation is a comprehensive process of obtaining information that is derived from specific assessment tools and methods. The purpose of evaluation is identification of strengths and weaknesses from which goals and treatment strategies may be drawn. Children and adolescents with psychosocial dysfunction may exhibit a variety of problems stemming from biopsychosocial vulnerabilities. The nature of the disorder implies that problems are focused in the behavioral, affective, or interpersonal areas, and these areas should be evaluated first, relative to individual and interpersonal aspects of play and daily-living routines. Children are screened routinely for visual–motor and motor problems because children with behavior and emotional problems frequently demonstrate deficits in these skill areas. Visual–motor or motor assessments would follow only when the screening indicated that they were necessary.

Typical Evaluation Methods

Four types of evaluation methods are suggested for this population: (1) structured observation, (2) interview, (3) standardized tests, and (4) checklists and inventories. Observation underlies all forms of evaluation. Whether administering a norm or criterion-referenced test or conducting an interview, the occupational therapist is always observing responses to the evaluative situation. It is also a primary way to judge response to treatment.

Structured observations involve either setting up a particular event or activity to be observed or observing in a naturalistic setting and recording, as objectively as possible, the specific behaviors exhibited. An observation guide or checklist is sometimes used to facilitate recording of a specific behavior such as decision making. Play is multidimensional, complex, and inner-directed, and assumes different forms throughout the developmental continuum. Consequently, structured observation is an excellent way to evaluate a child's play, even though it yields at best a snapshot of this area. The therapist can structure the play situations to evoke samples of play that represent a range of the child's performance in this area.

The interview is an important source of information about how children communicate information and how they view their own experiences. How the child chooses to report activities and events should be recorded, even though the accuracy of the report may be questionable. For example, some children report that they have "millions" of friends, but are unable to name any friends or any activities or games they play with these other children. The occupational therapist may wish to verify information by looking through the medical chart or by interviewing the parents or primary caregivers.

Standardized tests provide information on performance with reference to a normal standard. Checklists and inventories are self-administered and provide information relevant to the area being sampled.

EVALUATION OF TODDLERS AND PRESCHOOL CHILDREN

The purpose of evaluation of the toddler and preschool-aged group is to determine the level of function in play and social behaviors, in overall development, and in visual–motor skills.

Play and Social Behavior

With preschool children, two evaluative situations are used: one structured and one unstructured. In structured play, the child is seen alone and is given a sample of a simple project,

such as an animal macaroni collage, and materials to construct one. A choice of animal stencils is provided as well as different kinds of macaroni and beans. Attention span, process–product orientation, attention to detail, and manipulation and construction are assessed here. In unstructured play, the child is provided with a range of toys and materials suitable for sensorimotor, dramatic, and constructive play. The child is seen alone in one session and with a peer in another session. What the child does with materials and how he or she engages with the therapist and a peer are evaluated relative to the Preschool Play Scale developed by Knox (1974) or the developmental play classification developed by Florey (1971).

With children functioning younger than a developmental age of 3, only the unstructured play situation is used because collage construction is too advanced for this age. Interviewing the parents using The Play History (Takata, 1974) is extremely useful in providing a picture of immediate and past play experiences. This yields a perspective on the longitudinal nature of the child's play repertoire and can be helpful in determining the point to start intervention.

Other valuable assessments in this area are The Early Coping Inventory (Zeitlin, Williamson, & Szczepanski, 1988), designed for children ages 4 to 36 months, and The Coping Inventory (Zeitlin, 1985) designed for children ages 3 to 16 years. These are criterion-referenced observational instruments that target the child's coping effectiveness in managing demands and expectations. Children are observed in a variety of naturalistic situations over time to determine the consistency and effectiveness of skills and behaviors the child uses in meeting personal needs and adapting to the demands of the environment.

Developmental Assessments

Developmental assessments provide an indicator of functional level, regardless of chronological age. A number of useful tools are available for this kind of assessment. The Miller Assessment for Preschoolers is a standardized screening tool used to identify children ages 2 years, 9 months to 5 years, 8 months who are at risk for school-related problems. The Gesell Preschool Test yields a developmental level for motor, adaptive, language, and personal–social behavior for children ages 2½ through 6 years (King-Thomas & Hacker, 1987).

Visual–Motor Tests

The Berry-Buktenica Developmental Test of Visual–Motor Integration (VMI) is a developmental test of visual–motor integration that provides age norms and describes the developmental sequence for design copying of geometric forms. It is used with children from 2 through 15 years of age (King-Thomas & Hacker, 1987). If children score below the norm for their chronological age in this area and if they demonstrate motor problems in the developmental testing, the Motor-Free Visual Perception Test (MVPT) is administered if the child is 4 years or older. The MVPT focuses on visual perception not requiring a motor response (King-Thomas & Hacker).

EVALUATION OF SCHOOL-AGE CHILDREN

The purpose of evaluation of school-age children is to determine their level of function in play and social behavior and visual–motor skills. Developmental assessment is done when immaturity in skills is suspected.

Play and Social Behavior

Children are interviewed individually concerning their play interests, play activities, and friends. They are then seen with a peer in game and task or craft activities. Questions target play preferences, interests, friends and playmates, types of activities in which the family may engage, and after-school activities. Children are asked to describe a "typical day" and "typical weekend day" in their living setting. The yield of this information is to gain their perspective of daily living, school, chores, social relationships, and overall time use, in addition to specific play activities. Whenever possible, this information should be validated by the parents or caretaker of the child.

Children are seen alone and are presented with a craft project and evaluated for making decisions, following directions, using tools and materials correctly, and solving problems. They are given a simple two- to three-step project, such as a copper tooling picture with a cardboard frame. Children are then seen with a peer and asked to select and play a board game. They are evaluated for decision making, knowledge of rules and object of the game, and how they accept winning or losing, as well as how they interact socially with the peer. The Coping Inventory (Zeitlin, 1985) described in the previous section is another valuable assessment that yields an adaptive behavior summary and a coping profile.

Visual—Motor and Motor Assessments

The VMI assesses visual–motor integration. If problems are evident in this area, further visual–perceptual assessments are given. The Bruininks-Oseretsky Test of Motor Proficiency (BOTMP) may be administered to assess gross and fine motor skills for children ranging in age from 4½ to 14½ years (King-Thomas & Hacker, 1987).

Developmental Assessment

In working with school-age children and with adolescents, if there is a question of maturity in communication, daily-living skills, socialization, or motor skills, the Vineland Adaptive Behavior Scales (Vineland) should be used. It is not routinely administered owing to time constraints. The Vineland is designed to be used with children from birth to 18 years, 11 months, and employs a semistructured interview administered to the parent or caretaker of the child. This assessment should be administered by therapists with

graduate degrees and experience in assessment and test interpretation (King-Thomas & Hacker, 1987).

EVALUATION OF ADOLESCENTS

The purpose of evaluation with the adolescent age group is to determine level of function in socialization, task performance, daily-living skills, and time management. A cognitive level is also assessed as an adjunct to determining underlying abilities or limitations in task performance and daily-living skills. Visual–motor functioning using the VMI is also routinely assessed. Additional motor and developmental skills are assessed when there is a question of function in these areas. Vocational areas may be evaluated if the adolescent wishes to gain information about him- or herself in this area.

Time Management, Daily-Living Skills, Task Performance, Socialization

Adolescents are interviewed relative to their interests, activity patterns, and friends. This is done using the "typical weekday" and "typical weekend day" semistructured interview format. The interview provides a snapshot of the organization of role behavior relative to daily-living skills, chores and responsibilities, school and after-school activities, and peer and friendship patterns. The adolescents are given a choice of three, two- to three-step craft projects and are asked to complete one project. They are observed for attention span, making decisions, following directions, using tools and materials correctly, and solving problems. Task behavior is also assessed using the Allen Cognitive Level (ACL) Test to provide a quick estimate of the adolescent's current ability to learn. This test, with implications for daily performance activities, has provided valuable information about the kinds of cues the adolescent may need to perform role activities (Allen, Earhart, & Blue, 1992).

The frequency and content of social interactions with peers and adults are assessed by observations made in various settings. They are observed for their ability with respect to initiating and sustaining contact with peers and adults, listening to others, isolating self from others, disrupting or dominating peers.

Vocational Surveys

Adolescents who are interested in learning more about their career interests, skills, and abilities are given career inventories. The COP System Interest Inventory (Edits, 1974) is a self-administered inventory that yields an individual interest profile for 14 career clusters. The Career Ability Placement Survey (Edits, 1976) is a self-administered, timed survey that yields a score in eight primary abilities. These are mechanical reasoning, spatial relations, verbal reasoning, numerical ability, language, word knowledge, perceptual speed and accuracy, and manual speed and dexterity. The scores yield a career profile in which the adolescent's present abilities are compared with those required on jobs in the same 14 career clusters used in the COP System Interest Inventory. The results of these surveys are used to assist the adolescent in identifying and relating current skills and interests to a sample of career clusters.

▼ TREATMENT OF CHILDREN AND ADOLESCENTS WITH PSYCHOSOCIAL DYSFUNCTION

Reilly (1966) developed overall treatment principles to guide the design and provision of services for psychiatric patients. The focal treatment principle is that occupational therapy must build a culture or milieu to examine, evoke, and reconstitute healthy skills and behaviors. This milieu or context must be based on action, rather than discussion. The tasks and behaviors targeted must be tailored to the developmental level, interests, skills, abilities, and occupational roles of the individual. This section focuses on identifying the broad principles of intervention for children and adolescents with psychosocial dysfunction that may be used in a variety of service contexts, such as health care settings and the school system.

An interdisciplinary team approach is typical in psychosocial programs for children and adolescents. The number and composition of the interdisciplinary team varies from setting to setting. Each member of the team contributes a unique focus with the goal of formulating a broad information base and of providing an integrated intervention approach. Members of the team initially meet to develop a treatment plan, or in the school system an individual educational plan (IEP), and meet regularly thereafter to determine progress and the need for revision of the plan. It is important that the occupational therapy practitioner report his or her information in a concise, descriptive manner, free from occupational therapy or psychiatric jargon. When the team is beginning to work with a child, it is much more relevant to know how and under what circumstances a particular behavior is evident than to simply report that the child is angry, depressed, happy, anxious, or out of control.

Another shared focus of the team is the development of some system of managing behavior in group settings. These systems of behavior management range from expectations for behavior within the culture or milieu of the setting, such as school, to formal approaches based on principles of behavior modification, such as a token economy. The occupational therapy practitioner must know the overall system of behavior management and incorporate elements of the system into each person's occupational therapy program.

Characteristics of the Occupational Therapy Treatment Milieu for Children and Adolescents

The treatment milieu for children and adolescents consists of building play and task environments in which there are opportunities for association with peers and adults. Broad features of the play milieu include the provision of toys, craft projects, games, and activities that can be graded in complexity that reflect the events present in typical play. This milieu provides variety and novelty, opportunities for exploration, imitation and repetition, and playful role models. Broad features of the task milieu include the provision of craft projects and activities. This milieu provides systematic instruction that should be within the child or adolescent's cognitive ability, offers a moderate degree of difficulty, and provides knowledge of results or feedback. Models for craftsmanship should be provided (Florey, 1986). Social behavior and learning should be embedded within both the play and task environments. The following are suggestions for constructing a treatment environment for children and adolescents with psychosocial dysfunction.

1. *Play and task environments should be populated with peers.* One-to-one intervention may be desirable and necessary at first, but as soon as feasible, peers should be included. It is within the peer group that the learning and practicing of sharing materials, equipment, space, and the attention of others including the practitioner occurs. It is critical for children with psychosocial dysfunction to be able to function in peer groups. The occupational therapy practitioner grades the learning and practice of social skills within naturalistic play and task domains to facilitate this process.

   One strategy for incorporating peers of different developmental levels within a play or task group is using more mature or older children and adolescents as "helpers" for less mature children. The younger children benefit from learning a task or skill within a "brother or sister" model, and the older children have an opportunity to practice their skills with a less intimidating age group under the supervision of the practitioner.

2. *Social skills learning should be a part of the task and play environments.* Social skills instruction is part of the larger construct of social competence in which social skill is but one component. Social competence refers to mutually reinforcing reciprocal interactions (Cartledge & Milburn, 1995; Cox & Schopler, 1996). There are developmental considerations in selecting social skills to be taught, for certain capacities are believed to change with age. These include the child's ability to take the perspective of another person, the conceptualization of friendship, problem-solving ability, and communication skills. Other areas that should be considered are differences in gender and culture (Cartledge & Milburn).

   Examples of social behavior targeted for preschool and children functioning at lower social levels include proximity to others or being able to work in the same environment, social initiation of reaching out or pointing to objects out of reach, regarding and responding to others, eye contact, simple cause-and-effect sequences, and reciprocal turn taking. Being able to express positive social behaviors such as laughing or smiling and generally giving positive attention, sharing and compromising, and showing affection or acceptance may also be stressed. Targeted areas may include entering ongoing peer activities, sharing, giving affection and praise to others, and laughing with peers (Cox & Schopler, 1996).

Higher-level social behaviors or those for older children involve becoming better able to change behavior in response to the needs of friends and acquaintances. These are subtle and sophisticated skills that include joining groups, being accepted by others, being tactful, giving support, paying attention to others, and helping peers. Good eye contact and the ability to communicate are critical. Targeted areas may include successfully joining a group, sharing and playing cooperatively, and giving compliments (Cox & Schopler, 1996).

A social skills listing offered by Cartledge and Milburn (1995) targets environmental, interpersonal, self-related, and task-related behaviors. Examples of interpersonal behaviors include accepting authority, coping with conflict, gaining attention, greeting and helping others, making conversation, engaging in organized play, playing informally, and demonstrating a positive attitude toward others. Examples of task-related behaviors include asking and answering questions, attending behavior, participating in classroom discussion, completing tasks, following directions, working within group activities, engaging in independent work, engaging in on-task behavior, performing before others, and monitoring quality of work (Cartledge & Milburn).

Social skills training per se is not the complete answer to the performance deficits of children and adolescents with psychosocial dysfunction. Cox and Schopler (1996) caution that there is a big difference between training in controlled settings and the extent to which this can be generalized to the typically spontaneous, fluid and unstructured aspects of the "real world." The important component is that the skill be taught, practiced, and monitored in as naturalistic a manner as possible.

3. *Programs should be conducted within natural childhood activities dominated by toys, crafts, and games.* The overall process of the activity should be emphasized and not the product. The end goal of play with toys or crafts and games focuses on dimensions by which individuals can benefit, such as sharing materials, engaging in social banter, not fighting with others, achieving a sense of pride in task accomplishments, rather than simply making a coin purse or playing a game. Florey and Greene (1997) advocate three major dimensions by which activities should be examined. These are cognitive, motor, and social complexity.

Cognitive complexity refers to the mix of problem-solving processes that involve mastering the steps to complete the activity sequence. Activities should be examined relative to the number of steps required, the sequence and complexity of steps, and the degree of patience and persistence required.

Motor complexity refers to the gamut of fine motor or visual motor skill required for an activity. Children with psychosocial disorders often have learning and other disabilities. These disabilities further compromise their ability to productively engage in typical activities of their age group.

Social complexity refers to the opportunities the situation affords for social exchange, such as sharing and cooperating in the use of space, materials, adult and peer attention and interaction.

Florey and Greene (1997) suggest that activities be analyzed and graded considering these dimensions so that intervention goals can be achieved. Often social goals cannot be realized because the activity itself is too complex or frustrating on other dimensions, and this triggers poor social-coping strategies. The complexity of cognitive and motor components may be simplified initially so that the social features of the situation can be modeled and learned. For example, children often talk with one another and share more frequently when engaged in simple repetitive activities, such as stringing with medium size beads, as they easily master the task requirements.

4. *Intervention should be embedded within natural childhood models for play and school.* In younger childhood, this includes creating a play environment with emphasis on materials for constructive, simple group games and imaginative play. Simple group games lend themselves to taking turns and reciprocity. Imaginative play permits children to engage in a variety of roles and provides a common ground for interaction among unfamiliar peers (Bergen, 1987).

In middle childhood, intervention should emphasize clubs, scouts, or small groups that have a distinctive identity. Children of this age seek to belong and to be part of a larger social environment. Organized groups such as Scouts or informally constructed clubs serve that need. At the UCLA Neuropsychiatric Institute and Hospital (NPI & H), a Cub Scout Den chartered under the Boy Scouts of America has been in operation since 1971. The boys wear scout uniforms to meetings which begin with the scout oath. The scouts engage in earning badges and activities typical of other scout troops. This format models and teaches social skills. A club format may also be used for social and task skill instruction in which children name the club and decide on any special features such as "secret handshakes," code words, or the wearing of special symbols such as a hat or T-shirt. Models for working in the school system may include academic skills, such as a handwriting club, in which part of the agenda can be friendship or activity partnership.

In adolescence, emphasis is on games, sports, and hobbies, as well as activities promoting more independence, such as cooking, vocational exploration, and work skills groups. These groups focus on learning specific skills with more explicit and abstract standards for behavior and outcome. For example, in working on a social goal, treating others "with respect" is emphasized, rather than a concrete behavior such as "waiting one's turn," as might be emphasized with children.

5. *Expectations for behavior should be explicit and known.* These expectations may be part of a larger behavior management system, or they may be specific to the occupational therapy program. Rule behavior is a major focus in childhood, and expectations for behavior can be phrased as specific rules. Rules for safety and the general manner of proceeding should be established by the practitioner, and the consequences of rule following and rule violation should be clearly communicated. Children enjoy constructing rules and can be given an opportunity to contribute to the rules of the group or the use of the play or game space or materials. Adherence to rules may be promoted by verbal praise or concrete symbols for good effort, such as earning stickers or special privileges such as a visit to vending machines. Children and adolescents with behavior or emotional problems often have trouble identifying when they have done something "right," and social feedback or concrete rewards such as a sticker serves this purpose. The children should have a part in identifying their positive behaviors and those they may need to work on so that behavior is a matter under their control.

The intervention principles and characteristics of the milieu establish parameters for the development of programs for children and adolescents. Programs may be individually or group-focused, and if group-focused, individualized goals are implemented within this context. For example, having one child wait his or her turn and follow directions in a game situation and having another child initiate positive social interaction with a peer can both be accomplished within an existing play group. The content of the activities, tasks, and situation in the groups are selected and paced to encourage increasing levels of skill, responsibility, interpersonal responsiveness, and emotional control.

▼ PROMINENT PSYCHIATRIC DISORDERS IN CHILDHOOD AND ADOLESCENCE

Risk factors associated with psychiatric disorders are chronic medical conditions that limit typical childhood activities, brain damage, temperament, poor school performance, and parental psychiatric disorders or deviance (Offord & Fleming, 1996). Social and environmental risk factors, including prolonged separation between parent and child, physical or sexual abuse, poverty, marital discord, and instability in the family environment, also contribute to mental dysfunction (Zigler & Finn-Stevenson, 1996). The causes of disorders are much more difficult to determine. Various theoretical models or perspectives have been advanced to explain causes, and many of these are mutually

exclusive. Etiology is increasing conceptualized from a biopsychosocial perspective, which encompasses both the traditional environmental, interpersonal, and psychological model, and the biological and medical model (Garfinkel et al., 1990). One factor may play a lead role in a specific disorder, but generally, a multiplicity of biopsychosocial vulnerabilities or stressors are implicated. Four disorders will be discussed in this section: attention deficit hyperactivity disorder (ADHD), conduct disorder, mood disorders, and autistic disorder.

Attention Deficit Hyperactivity Disorder

Several overlapping concepts are used to describe key features of this disorder: inattention or attention deficit, overactivity, and impulsiveness. One or more of these features are present in several childhood situations (eg, home and school) and are present to an excessive degree compared with children of the same age (Danckaerts & Taylor, 1995; Taylor, 1994; Weiss, 1996). Inattention or attention deficit refers to orienting briefly to tasks imposed by adults, changing activities rapidly when spontaneous choice is allowed, orienting toward irrelevant aspects of the environment, and difficulty focusing attention generally, although some children may be able to concentrate on activities they find enjoyable. Overactivity refers to an excess of locomotor movements of either the whole body (restlessness) or of purposeless, finer movements irrelevant to the task at hand (fidgeting). Impulsiveness includes behavior that is thoughtless or poorly timed. For example, children with this disorder have difficulty waiting their turn and often interrupt others.

Children with ADHD often have difficulty inhibiting impulses in social behavior and in cognitive tasks. They may be inattentive in games, are often intrusive, and have difficulty getting along with their peers. They are often unpopular with age mates and are underachievers in school (Weiss, 1996). They are at increased risk for behavioral and social difficulties and disabilities. The most prominent features of ADHD vary with age. In preschool children, gross motor overactivity is a common complaint made by parents. In older children, excessive fidgeting, inattentiveness, and restlessness are common. Adolescents with this disorder tend to be more impulsive and display attentional difficulties and motor hyperactivity. They may also display affective lability, hot tempers, impulsivity, disorganization, and intolerance to stress (Greenhill, 1990; Wender, 1990).

ADHD is more prevalent in boys than girls. Prevalence is estimated to be 3% to 5% (APA, 1994, p. 82). The etiology of ADHD is unknown. Children may have a biological vulnerability to this disorder, but psychosocial and environmental factors may also be prominent (Weiss, 1996).

There is a high co-occurrence or comorbidity of ADHD with conduct disorder (Danckaerts & Taylor, 1995; Taylor, 1994; Weiss, 1996). Hyperactivity may be one route into conduct disorder, and it is a risk factor for outcome of aggressive and antisocial behavior and delinquency (Taylor). Many children and adolescents continue to be disabled by the core symptoms of the syndrome and are at risk for developing antisocial personality disorder, criminal behavior, and more psychopathology (Weiss).

Conduct Disorder

The essential feature of conduct disorder is a repetitive and persistent pattern of behavior in which the basic rights of others or societal norms or rules are violated. This pattern of behavior causes clinically significant impairment in social, academic, or occupational functioning (APA, 1994). A pattern of antisocial behavior, usually involving physical aggression, is common, and this behavior is typically considered to be unmanageable by significant others (Earls, 1994). Children with this disorder may display bullying, physical cruelty to people and animals, and may deliberately destroy the property of others. Symptoms vary with age as individuals develop increased physical strength, cognitive abilities, and sexual maturity (APA). There are two subtypes based upon age. Childhood onset occurs before the age of 10 and typically involves physical aggression and disturbed peer relationships. There is an inclination to view oppositional defiant disorder with symptomology of recurrent patterns of negativistic, defiant, disobedient, and hostile behavior as a milder and developmentally related form of this disorder (Earls; APA). Onset in childhood is considered to be the more severe form of the disorder (Kazdin, 1995). Adolescent onset occurs after age 10. These individuals are less likely to display aggressive behaviors and tend to have more normative peer relationships. These youths may engage in illegal and criminal behavior (Kazdin).

Children and adolescents with conduct disorder typically have low self-esteem and, to hide this, may portray themselves as tough and uncaring. Learning disabilities are common with this group of youngsters, and the degree of learning disability often corresponds to their overall degree of maladaptation (Lewis, 1990, 1996). They are likely to show academic deficiencies and diminished social skills in relationship to peers and adults. Different terms may be applied to the same youngster for the same behavior, depending on whether the behavior is defined by the medical or legal system. Lewis (1990) believes that although these children frequently get into trouble with the law, it is important to distinguish conduct disorder, a diagnostic term, from "delinquent," which is a legal term.

Conduct disorder is more common in boys than girls, but the ratio of boys to girls is lower for adolescent than child onset. Overall, for youngsters under 18, the prevalence varies from 6% to 16% for boys and 2% to 9% for girls (APA, 1994, p. 88). There is no single cause of conduct disorder. Children with behavior problems tend to display symptoms that place them on the border of several neuro-logical, psychiatric, and psychoeducational categories (Lewis, 1990, 1996). Prominent risk factors include parental dysfunction and deviance, such as alcoholism and criminal behavior of the father, family characteristics including inconsistent or lax child rearing practices, and contextual conditions associated with a variety of untoward living conditions (Earls, 1994; Kazdin, 1995).

There is a high comorbidity of conduct disorder with ADHD and anxiety disorders. Children with symptoms of ADHD and conduct disorder are at greater risk for poor outcomes than those with either disorder alone. Children with conduct and anxiety symptoms are less likely to have police contacts or be perceived by peers as bullies, for it is believed that the presence of anxiety serves as a "braking system" on the seriousness of antisocial behavior (Earls, 1994; Kazdin, 1995). The course of conduct disorder is variable, but children with early onset are at increased risk for antisocial personality disorders and substance-related disorders (APA, 1994). These youth are at great risk for premature death from violent causes (Earls).

Mood Disorders

Mood disorders in children and adolescents are classified into two major types: unipolar depressive disorders and bipolar disorders. In bipolar disorder, a combination of manic and depressive symptoms are found (Weller, Weller, & Svadjian, 1996). In this section, attention is directed to depression in children, because childhood mania is rare (Harrington, 1994). A brief description of symptoms of manic episodes are given to differentiate them from symptomatology found in children with ADHD.

DEPRESSIVE DISORDER

Until recently, it was believed that depressive disorders could not occur in childhood or could only occur in "masked," form expressed as delinquency or phobias. There is now recognition that disorders, resembling adult depression, can and do occur in childhood and within DSM IV there is one criteria for diagnosis for all ages (Harrington, 1994). Although there are allowances for differences in symptomatology based on age within the DSM IV, there are several developmental studies that substantiate that there are age changes in the frequency and expression of affective phenomena in children. Many clinicians have suggested that these changes might be better addressed by identifying age-appropriate symptoms of depression that account for level of functioning in various cognitive and affective domains (Harrington).

The primary features of a depressive episode are depressed mood for at least a 2-week period and diminished interest or loss of pleasure in most activities. In children and adolescents, mood may be cranky, rather than sad. Somatic complaints, irritability, and social withdrawal are common in children (APA, 1994). Most children describe themselves in negative terms such as "dumb" or "stupid." Adolescents experience hopelessness and feelings that things will never change for the better. The most serious complication is suicidal thoughts, including recurrent thoughts of death or actual attempts at suicide (Weller, Weller, & Svadjian, 1996). The overlap of depression and other psychiatric diagnoses has been one of the most consistent findings of research studies. Depression has been associated with conditions as diverse as conduct disorder, anxiety states, learning problems, drug use, hyperactivity, anorexia nervosa, and school refusal (Harrington, 1994).

The prevalence of depression increases with age. In community studies, the prevalence among preadolescents ranges from 0.5% to 2.5% and from 2% to 8% among adolescents (Harrington, 1994, p. 332). Among depressed children, the sex ratio is nearly equal, but by adolescence, female preponderance is manifest (Harrington). Numerous etiologies may lead to the expression of depressive symptoms. Children with depression usually have multiple problems, such as educational failure and impaired psychosocial functioning. Genetic, biological, psychosocial, and environmental factors have been implicated (Harrington; Weller et al, 1996). Children and adolescents are at high risk for recurrence of the illness. Suicidal behavior remains the most serious aspect of a depressive disorder (Weller & Weller, 1990).

MANIC SYMPTOMS

Symptom patterns of mania vary by age. Young children under 9 years of age present with irritability and emotional lability, whereas older children typically demonstrate euphoria, elation, paranoia, and grandiose delusions. Hyperactivity, pressured speech, and distractibility may be present in both age groups (Weller et al, 1996). Manic children usually display more affect than do children with ADHD and are more euphoric or irritable. They also display a more pronounced shift in mood than do children with ADHD and their activity tends to be more goal-directed (Harrington, 1994).

Autism

Autism is one of the pervasive developmental disorders. It is characterized by a distinctive pattern of deficits in social dysfunction, communicative deviance, and restrictive and repetitive behaviors and interests (APA, 1994; Lord & Rutter, 1994; Volkmar, 1996). Social dysfunction is one of the key features of autism and is manifest primarily in difficulties in reciprocal social interaction and the ability to form relationships. In infancy, there is often lack of eye contact, poor attachments to key individuals, and difficulty with the give and take of social relatedness. In preschool years, children with autism typically demonstrate a lack of interest in other children, and a limited range of facial expression, and unusual eye contact. They may be distressed by separation from their parents, but often do not greet parents in positive ways when rejoined (Lord & Rutter; Volkmar). Communicative deviance is evident in the failure to develop expres-

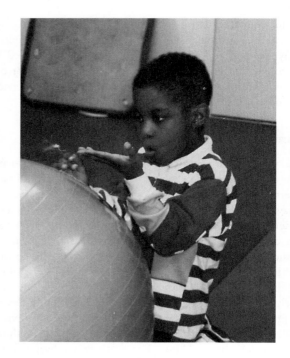

▲
Figure 33-3. Obsessive rituals are common among autistic children; this boy perseverates, to the exclusion of other forms of play, by blowing a piece of string.

sive language. Those individuals who develop speech demonstrate a lack of, or an unusual, social quality. Speech may be characterized by echolalia, pronoun reversal, and failure to use language for social interaction. Restricted and repetitive interests and behaviors (Fig. 33–3) may include preoccupation with a specific part of a toy, such as a spinning wheels on a toy truck, or stereotypical movements such as hand flapping or toe walking. Simple, flexible, imaginative play is rare (Volkmar). Most children with autism show some abnormalities or delays in the foregoing areas before the age of 3.

Autism is more prevalent in boys than girls (Volkmar, 1996). Prevalence rates in general are estimated at 2 to 5 per 10,000 (APA, 1994, p. 69). Autism is believed to have a neurobiological base, although the identification of specific pathology remains elusive (Lord & Rutter, 1994). Autism needs to be differentiated from other psychiatric and developmental conditions that present with abnormalities in language, play, and social development, such as Rett syndrome, disintegrative disorder, and Asperger's disorder. Autism is a lifelong disorder and although many remain severely disabled, about one-third of individuals with autism are able to achieve some level of personal and occupational independence. Volkmar states that important predictors of adult outcome include intellectual level and communicative competence. Lord and Rutter believe that independence often depends on the availability of vocational and residential community resources.

▼ PSYCHOSOCIAL IMPLICATIONS FOR CHILDREN WITH CHRONIC DISABILITIES

Chronic diseases and conditions affect approximately 13% of children in the United States (Wassermann, 1990, p. 487). Psychosocial problems do not automatically occur with a chronic illness, but the presence of chronic illness or disability does increase the risk. The occupational therapy practitioner needs to be aware of illness risk factors, "red flag" periods in development that increase children's vulnerability to negative emotional and social consequences as a result of chronic illness and patterns of poor adjustment, so that he or she can plan effective prevention or remediation along this dimension. Generally, the disability and limitations caused by the illness are two of the greatest factors influencing emotional maladjustment. It is also believed that there is a greater risk of psychological problems if the illness begins at the time of a developmental milestone (Wasserman).

There are illness-related risk factors associated with emotional vulnerability in children. These include the age of the child at the time of illness; parental responsibility related to the illness, such as negligence or genetic or familial influences; the accuracy, certainty, and sensitivity with which the diagnosis is made and transmitted to the child and family; the degree to which the illness interferes with function; the effect on physical appearance; the persistence of symptoms and whether the illness is characterized by periods of remission or increasing discomfort; and the hope for recovery or the degree of uncertainty that may accompany a chronic illness (Mrazek, 1994). Other vulnerabilities of children with chronic illness include the effect of the disability on the total family unit; the side effects of medication that can make the child drowsy, nauseated, depressed, or change their physical appearance; and the need to manage a special diet, as eating is a social activity.

In infancy, there is increased vulnerability if the bonding process between the parents and infant is disrupted. Children may be more irritable, derive no satisfaction from sucking, and may be unresponsive because of a sensory or neurological deficit, thus decreasing parental nurturing and attachment. Parents who feel guilt, anger, and anxiety at first learning the presence of an illness may not be able to invest in the infant. During toddlerhood, adherence to schedules for medication, therapy appointments, and special diets may interfere with the child's normal development of autonomy and control, and toddlers may become apathetic, passive, and clinging. Parents may be reluctant to set limits on the child, which interferes with the development of impulse control. Toddlers tend to see their illness as something that hurts or interferes with their exploration. It is believed that this age child suffers the most from hospitalizations if separated from parents (Wasserman, 1990).

In early childhood, ages 3 to 6 years, children may interpret their pain and other symptoms as punishment. Illness may interfere with the achievements in motor control and social competence. Children may have fewer opportunities for peer interaction and social approval, and school entrance may be delayed, thereby contributing to increased dependency on parents and anger at not being like other children. A chronic illness interferes in several ways with development of school-age children. Children worry about how different they are from their peers and whether they will be accepted. The development of peer relationships is particularly important. School performance may also be limited by stamina, medication side effects, preferential or prejudicial treatment, and excessive time missed from school. Wasserman (1990) believes that when children do poorly in school, they tend to develop emotional problems. During adolescence, particular concerns are with the development of independence and a secure physical and sexual identity. Special diets, medications, therapies, and doctors visits can become a battleground for independence. Whether physical appearance is altered by the pathology of the illness itself or medication is another prominent issue. Adolescents are particularly prone to either overstressing their limitations and succumbing to feelings of futility and despair, or denying their realistic limitations and setting themselves up for unrealistic goals that cannot be achieved.

Children and adolescents with poor adjustment to their chronic disorder tend to exhibit one of three behavior patterns (Wasserman, 1990). The first pattern is characterized by fearfulness, inactivity, lack of outside interests, and a marked dependency on parents. The second pattern is one of overly independent, daring youth, who may engage in prohibited, risk-taking activities. The third pattern seen in older children and adolescents with congenital deformities is a shyness and hostility toward "normal" individuals, whom they see as owing them compensation for their suffering.

►CONCLUSION

Occupational therapy practitioners who work with children and adolescents are likely to come in contact with those who display psychopathology. The occupational behavior frame of reference formed the primary conceptual base for occupational therapy intervention. This frame of reference emphasizes an understanding of normal development and the parameters of play, socialization, and school role in understanding typical performance deficits in working with emotionally disturbed children, in the selection of assessment tools to be used, and in the development of treatment principles for this group of youngsters.

▼ REFERENCES

Allen, C., Earhart, C., & Blue, T. (1992). *Occupational therapy treatment goals for the physically and cognitively disabled.* Rockville, MD: American Occupational Therapy Association.

American Occupational Therapy Association (AOTA). (1990). *Member data survey*. Rockville, MD: Author.

American Psychiatric Association (APA). (1994). *Diagnostic and statistical manual of mental disorders* (4th ed.). Washington, DC: Author.

Bergen, D. & Oden, S. (1987). Designing play environments for elementary-age children. In D. Bergen (Ed.), *Play as a medium for learning and development* (pp. 245–269). Portsmouth, NH: Heinemann.

Bergen, D. (1987). Stages of play development. In D. Bergen (Ed.), *Play as a medium for learning and development* (pp. 49–66). Portsmouth, NH: Heinemann.

Cartledge, G. & Milburn, J. (1995). *Teaching social skills to children and youth* (3rd ed.). Boston: Allyn and Bacon.

Cole, M. & Cole, S. (1993). *The development of children* (2nd ed.). New York: Scientific American Books.

Combrinck-Graham, L. (1996). The development of school-age children. In M. Lewis (Ed.), *Child and adolescent psychiatry, A comprehensive textbook* (2nd ed., pp. 271–278). Baltimore: Williams & Wilkins.

Corsaro, W. & Schwartz, K. (1991). Peer play and socialization in two cultures. In B. Scales, M. Alm, A. Nicolopoulou, and S. Ervin-Tripp (Eds.), *Play and the social context of development in early care and education* (pp. 243–354). New York: Teachers College.

Cox, R. & Schopler, E. (1996). Social skills training for children. In M. Lewis (Ed.), *Child and adolescent psychiatry: A comprehensive textbook* (2nd ed., pp. 902–908). Baltimore: Williams & Wilkins.

Csikszentmihalyi, M. (1990). *Flow: The psychology of optimal experience*. New York: HarperPerennial.

Danckaerts, M. & Taylor, E. (1995). The epidemiology of childhood hyperactivity. In F. Verhulst & H. Koot (Eds.). *The epidemiology of child and adolescent psychopathology* (pp. 179–209). Oxford: Oxford University Press.

Earls, F. (1994). Oppositional-defiant and conduct disorders. In M. Rutter, E. Taylor, & L. Hersov (Eds.), *Child and adolescent psychiatry modern approaches* (3rd ed., pp. 308–329). Oxford: Blackwell Scientific.

Edits (1974). *COP system interest survey*. San Diego, CA.

Edits (1976). *Career Ability Placement Survey*, Dan Diego, CA.

Florey, L. & Greene, S. (1997). Play in middle childhood: A focus on children with behavior and emotional disorders. In L. D. Parham & L. Fazio (Eds.), *Play in occupational therapy for children* (pp. 126–143) St Louis: C.V. Mosby.

Florey, L. (1971). An approach to play and play development. *American Journal of Occupational Therapy, 25*, 275–280.

Florey, L. (1986). Child and adolescent psychiatry. In S. Robertson (Ed.), *Scope: Workbook* (pp. 113–116). Rockville, MD: American Occupational Therapy Association.

Forness, S. (1988). Planning for the needs of children with serious emotional disturbance: The National Special Education and Mental Health Coalition. *Behavior Disorders, 13*, 127–139.

Garfinkel, B., Carlson, G., & Weller, E. (1990). Preface. In B. Garfinkel, G. Carlson, & E. Weller (Eds.), *Psychiatric disorders in children and adolescents* (pp. XV–XVI). Philadelphia: W. B. Saunders.

Greenhill, L. (1990). Attention-deficit hyperactivity disorder in children. In B. Garfinkel, G. Carlson, & E. Weller (Eds.), *Psychiatric disorders in children and adolescents* (pp. 149–182). Philadelphia: W. B. Saunders.

Harrington, R. (1994). Affective disorders. In M. Rutter, E. Taylor, & L. Hersov (Eds.), *Child and adolescent psychiatry modern approaches* (3rd ed., pp. 330–350). Oxford: Blackwell Scientific.

Kazdin, A. (1995). Conduct disorder. In F. Verhulst & H. Koot (Eds.), *The epidemiology of child and adolescent psychopathology*, (pp. 259–290). Oxford: Oxford University Press.

King, N. (1987). Elementary school play: Theory and research. In J. Block & N. King (Eds.), *School play* (pp. 143–165). New York: Garland Publishing.

King-Thomas, L. & Hacker, B. (1987). *A therapist's guide to pediatric assessment*. Boston: Little, Brown & Co.

Knapp, M. & Knapp, H. (1976). *One potato, two potato...the secret education of American children*. New York: W. W. Norton.

Knox, S. (1974). A play scale. In M. Reilly (Ed.), *Play as exploratory learning* (pp. 247–266). Beverly Hills, CA: Sage Publications.

Lewis, D. (1990). Conduct disorders. In B. Garfinkel, G. Carlson, & E. Weller (Eds.), *Psychiatric disorders in children and adolescents* (pp. 193–209). Philadelphia: W. B. Saunders.

Lewis, D. (1996). Conduct disorder. In M. Lewis (Ed.), *Child and adolescent psychiatry: A comprehensive textbook* (2nd. ed., pp. 564–577). Baltimore: Williams & Wilkins.

Lord, C. & Rutter, M. (1994). Autism and pervasive developmental disorders. In M. Rutter, E. Taylor, & L. Hersov (Eds.), *Child and adolescent psychiatry modern approaches* (3rd ed., pp. 569–593). Oxford: Blackwell Scientific.

Monighan-Nourot, P., Scales, B., Van Hoorn, J., & Almy, M. (1987). *Looking at children's play*. New York: Teachers College Press.

Moorhead, L. (1969). The occupational history. *American Journal of Occupational Therapy, 23*, 329–334.

Mrazek, D. (1994). Psychiatric aspects of somatic disease and disorders. In M. Rutter, E. Taylor, & L. Hersov (Eds.), *Child and adolescent psychiatry modern approaches* (3rd ed., pp. 697–710). Oxford: Blackwell Scientific.

Mussen, P., Conger, J. Kagan, J., & Huston, A. (1990). *Child development and personality* (7th ed.). New York: Harper and Row.

National Mental Health Association Speaks. (1989). *Students with serious emotional disturbance underserved in special education*. Alexandria, Va: Author.

Offord, D. & Fleming, J. (1996). Epidemiology. In M. Lewis (Ed.), *Child and adolescent psychiatry: A comprehensive textbook* (2nd. ed., pp. 1166–1178). Baltimore: Williams & Wilkins.

Reilly, M. (1966). A psychiatric occupational therapy program as a teaching model. *American Journal of Occupational Therapy, 20*, 61–67.

Slukin, A. (1981). *Growing up in the playground*. London: Routledge and Kegan Paul.

Takata, N. (1974). Play as a prescription. In M. Reilly (Ed.). *Play as exploratory learning* (pp. 209–246). Beverly Hills, CA: Sage Publications.

Taylor, E. (1994). Syndromes of attention deficit and overactivity. In M. Rutter, E. Taylor, & L. Hersov (Eds.), *Child and adolescent psychiatry modern approaches* (3rd ed., pp. 285–307). Oxford: Blackwell Scientific.

U. S. Department of Education (1995). *Seventeenth annual report to Congress on the implementation of the Individuals with Disabilities Education Act*. Washington, DC: Government Printing Office.

Volkmar, F. (1996). Autism and the pervasive developmental disorders. In M. Lewis (Ed.), *Child and adolescent psychiatry: A comprehensive textbook* (2nd. ed., pp. 489–497). Baltimore: Williams & Wilkins.

Wagner, M. (1995). Outcomes for youths with serious emotional disturbance in secondary school and early adulthood. *The Future of Children, 5*, 90–112.

Wasserman, A. (1990). Principles of psychiatric care of children and adolescents with medical illnesses. In B. Garfinkel, G. Carlson, & E. Weller (Eds.), *Psychiatric disorders in children and adolescents* (pp. 486–502). Philadelphia: W. B. Saunders.

Weiss, G. (1996). Attention deficit hyperactive disorder. In M. Lewis (Ed.), *Child and adolescent psychiatry: A comprehensive textbook* (2nd. ed., pp. 544–563). Baltimore: Williams & Wilkins.

Weller, E. & Weller, R. (1990). Depressive disorders in children and adolescents. In B. Garfinkel, G. Carlson, & E. Weller (Eds.), *Psychiatric disorders in children and adolescents* (pp. 3–20). Philadelphia: W. B. Saunders.

Weller, E. Weller, R., & Svadjian, H. (1996). Mood disorders. In M. Lewis (Ed.), *Child and adolescent psychiatry: A comprehensive textbook* (2nd. ed., pp. 650–665). Baltimore: Williams & Wilkins.

Wender, P. (1990). Attention-deficit hyperactivity disorder in adolescents and adults. In B. Garfinkel, G. Carlson, & E. Weller (Eds.), *Psychiatric disorders in children and adolescents* (pp. 183–192). Philadelphia: W. B. Saunders.

Zeitlin, S. (1991). *Coping inventory.* Bensenville, IL: Scholastic Testing Service.

Zeitlin, S., Williamson, G., & Szczepanski, M. (1988). *Early coping inventory.* Bensenville, IL: Scholastic Testing Service.

Zigler, E. & Finn-Stevenson, M. (1996). National policies for children, adolescents and families. In M. Lewis (Ed.), *Child and adolescent psychiatry: A comprehensive textbook* (2nd. ed., pp. 1186–1195). Baltimore: Williams & Wilkins.

Chapter 34

Child Abuse and Neglect

Debora A. Davidson

Occupational therapy practitioners specialize in helping people of all ages and persuasions to achieve, regain and maintain satisfactory levels of performance in their daily activities (Hopkins, 1993). Practitioners who work in schools, pediatric rehabilitation centers, and early intervention facilities consider helping parents and families a part of their responsibility toward the children who have been referred for service. Families who enact patterns of physical abusiveness toward their children are experiencing dysfunction that results in lasting harm to all members. Consequently, occupational therapy practitioners have a responsibility to be knowledgeable about issues of **child abuse and neglect**, their legal and ethical responsibilities, and their role in providing appropriate therapeutic interventions.

Children whose cognitive, social, or physical development is delayed sufficiently to result in prolonged dependency or in increased demands on adult caretakers are at highest risk for victimization (Frodi, 1981). These characteristics define most of the children who are referred for therapeutic services. Additionally, chronic episodes of abuse place children at increased risk of delayed social, language, and emotional development (Egeland, Sroufe, & Erickson, 1983; Haskett & Kistner, 1991; Hoffman-Plotkin & Twentyman, 1984). Because of these delays, they may be referred to occupational therapy. Consequently, practitioners working with children should be alert to behavior that may indicate child abuse. By developing an awareness of the risk factors for and signs of child abuse, occupational therapy practitioners can use their knowledge base and skills to take an important role in preventing, identifying, and ameliorating this major public health problem.

▼ IDENTIFICATION AND PREVENTION

An understanding of the nature and dynamics of a problem is prerequisite to its prevention. The Child Abuse Prevention and Treatment Act of 1978 (Public Law [PL] 95–266) defines child abuse as "the physical or mental injury, sexual abuse or exploitation, negligent treatment, or maltreatment of a child under the age of eighteen or the Child Protective Law of the State in question, by a person who is responsible for the child's welfare under circumstances which would indicate that the child's health or welfare is harmed or threatened thereby" (U.S. Code Annotated, 1978, p. 228).

The causes of child maltreatment are multiple, and no single feature or condition has been found to be etiological. Research has repeatedly demonstrated that characteristics of the child, the parents, and the social environment affect the level of risk for abuse. Approximately 1.2% of American children have been verified as having been abused, although experts agree that this figure underrepresents actual incidence (Starr, Dubowitz, & Bush, 1990, p. 48). Approximately half of these cases involve primarily neglect of children's basic needs for nutrition, shelter, clothing, medical care, or affection, or some combination thereof, and another 28% involve physical abuse (Starr et al, p. 48).

Children are at greater risk for abuse and neglect if they have increased dependency needs because of medical or developmental problems (Steele, 1987), are the product of an unwanted pregnancy, or are considered by the mother to be of an undesirable gender (Frodi, 1981). Qualities of the parents (particularly the mother, who is usually the primary caretaker) have also been identified as risk factors. These include having histories of being malparented (Main & Goldwyn, 1984; Steele); having a personality disorder that results in behaviors related to immaturity, egocentrism, and impulsivity (Ogata, Silk, Goodrich, Lohr, Westen, & Hill, 1990); and engaging in alcohol or drug abuse (Wolfner & Gelles, 1993).

Another critical set of factors are the larger, community level concerns. Poverty emerges as a predisposing condition for chronic malparenting (Coulton, Korbin, Su, & Chow, 1995). Although poverty is linked to increased levels of child abuse, high levels of social integration and community morale appear to be mediating factors that can reduce levels of child abuse, even in low income neighborhoods (Gabarino & Kostelny, 1992). Social isolation and conflict represent risk factors for abuse and neglect.

Successful intervention and prevention programs will address family and community needs for positive leadership and safe places to gather (Steele, 1987; Vondra, 1990). Occupational therapy practitioners have opportunities to intervene with individuals and families through direct service approaches, and with community agencies and policy making bodies through administration and consultation.

Referral to Protective Agencies

Most states mandate that health care and educational professionals report suspected cases of child abuse and neglect to state protective agencies. Frequently, a decision to refer a family to child protective services is made by a team, and the team's leader actually makes the report. However, in the absence of a team decision, if an individual practitioner has reason to suspect maltreatment, he or she is legally and ethically responsible to make a referral independently. The practitioner's supervisor should be informed of this decision. Referrals involve making a telephone call, followed by a letter that outlines the client's name, age, and address and a summary of the reasons for concern. Reports are categorized according to severity and type, and investigations are scheduled accordingly. Ideally, a referral to child protective services should be made with the parents' knowledge, but this may not be possible if the child's safety or that of others might be jeopardized. Repeated reports should be made if continued observations of the problem behaviors occur; multiple referrals are sometimes needed before a case qualifies for an in depth child protective services evaluation or a legal intervention.

Approximately 25% of reported child abuse and neglect cases reach the courts (Helberg, 1983, p. 239). For documentation to serve as credible evidence in court it must be completed in a reliable and valid manner (Barth, & Sullivan, 1985; Kreitzer, 1981). Reliable evidence is documented close to the event's occurrence and, when possible, by more than one observer. Repeated observations or measures taken over time strengthen the report. Valid evidence is that which employs a variety of direct measures and is based on objective information, rather than the practitioner's interpretation.

Documentation should include a description of the parent's and child's physical appearance, affective behavior, and styles of interacting with one another and the practitioner.

By involving child protective services in a case, the occupational therapy practitioner adds another facet to the treatment team. The role of child protective services in most states is to screen families who have been referred for possible abuse or neglect, to evaluate those whose problems meet intake criteria, and to intervene in identified cases of child abuse. In addition, many child protective services agencies offer an array of services to families who are admitted to the caseload. Services may include: supplemented day care, parent support and education groups, home aides, and transportation to therapy and medical appointments.

Child protective services agencies are frequently recipients of criticism by the media and the community at large. They are traditionally overburdened and underfunded. Child protective services caseworkers typically carry large caseloads that are complex, demanding, and emotionally stressful, and they are usually not child development or mental health professionals by formal education. (Faller, 1985). Occupational therapy practitioners whose clients are involved with child protective services should strive to initiate regular contact with caseworkers to share information that is pertinent to the family's progress, such as indications of the parents' motivation in and use of therapy and updates on the child's developmental progress. Child protective service workers, in turn, can support therapeutic efforts by encouraging parents to attend appointments and to incorporate recommendations into their daily lives, and by assisting with obtaining other needed services.

▼ OCCUPATIONAL THERAPY EVALUATION

The ultimate goals of the evaluation process in cases of known or suspected child abuse and neglect are (1) to help the child and his family by supportively, but objectively, contributing to assessment of the parents' current ability to adequately care for their child; (2) to help determine the child's developmental and functional status and ways to enhance this, and (3) to help the parents identify all available social resources.

The occupational therapy evaluation may identify risk factors related to the parents, child, and environment within the context of a developmental assessment. Qualities of the parent may be ascertained from interviews at intake and while interviewing for developmental history, as well as from observations of the parent–child interaction.

Parenting Evaluation

The development of **rapport** and subsequent progress in treatment requires the therapist to enter the relationship with an attitude of support and a belief that the parents are invested in their children's well-being (Pollack & Steele, 1972). A discussion of the therapist's commitment to confidentiality may help alleviate fears about sharing personal information. Clarification of the child's legal status and subsequent rules of confidentiality should be sought before the session, as needed. If a parent does not have custody, the child protective service caseworker or other legally appointed guardian must grant permission to share information with other individuals or agencies.

An evaluation of parenting skills and practices should include an initial interview and observation of parent–child interactions in structured and unstructured situations. The initial interview is a time to set the tone of the therapeutic relationship, and to observe spontaneous behaviors of the parent and child. Advice or recommendations are generally inappropriate at this stage. Box 34–1 outlines interview questions designed to elicit information on the child, parent, and environment. This interview format may be used as a supplement to gathering traditional developmental data.

Although interviews can quickly provide concentrated information, family relationships are complex and often difficult to characterize adequately in words. A client's ability to report information about family issues may be reduced by limited verbal skills, emotional involvement in the interaction process, the complexity that is present in most family systems, and a desire to limit information to that which will please the therapist. During activities that engage the parents and children, spontaneous and typical interactions can be observed. A parent who gives only socially desirable answers to questions about child management practices may demonstrate during an activities session how difficult it is for her to structure the experience at an appropriate level, how distressed she becomes when the environment becomes messy or unpredictable, or how she tends to compete with her child to get her own needs met.

Evaluation of the Child

Throughout the evaluation process, it is essential to document observations of the child's physical appearance and affective and social behavior. Hygiene, appropriateness of dress, and the presence of bruises or scars should be documented over time through careful written descriptions or photographs, or both. Problematic behaviors that may reflect malparenting include rejection of social contact, clinging, aggression, overactivity, and noncompliance (Hoffman-Plotkin & Twentyman, 1984; Vondra, 1990). Some children from abusive environments develop adult-like skills secondary to assuming caretaking responsibilities in an effort to gain parental approval or to meet family needs (Martin, 1972). Clinical examples of this are a 4-year-old who makes his mother's breakfast before waking her every morning, or a 7-year-old who is primarily responsible for the care of an infant sibling. When evaluating children, a consistent, supportive, and nurturing approach is usually most effective; this is especially true when the child has experienced abuse. Often it helps to observe the child for a series of sessions to establish trust and develop a therapeutic relationship.

A comprehensive developmental assessment provides an excellent opportunity for observing and documenting the problems common to abused and neglected children. Norm-referenced evaluation tools should be employed as much as possible to maximize the credibility of the data if they should ever be used as evidence in court (Helberg, 1983). Developmental assessment of children suspected or identified as being abused can help with securing needed services and designing intervention programs. It may also be of assistance in evaluating the extent to which environmental factors have contributed to delayed development. Standardized developmental assessment before and after therapeutic intervention or foster home placement may indicate rapid developmental spurts that coincide with the intervention. Such findings support a hypothesis for significant environmental contribution to the child's problems (Martin, 1972).

▼ OCCUPATIONAL THERAPY INTERVENTION

Effective intervention of abused children and their families requires an **interdisciplinary team** approach that addresses the needs of the family as a system, as well as the needs of in-

---

▼ BOX 34-1

Developmental Interview Questions for Families at Risk

1. Please tell me about your family. (Listen for adult to child ratio, quantity and quality of social relationships among adults)
   a. Who are the members of your household? What are their ages?
   b. Who does most of the child care in your household?
   c. Do any other family members help? How?
2. How would you describe your child's personality? (Listen for generally positive versus negative outlook, knowledge of the child)
   a. Who is he or she most like?
   b. Who is he or she to live with most of the time?
   c. What are the most effective ways to teach or discipline him or her?
   d. What are your child's most recent accomplishments?
   e. Do you have any concerns or questions about child's development or behavior at this time?
3. Are you experiencing a lot of stress in your life at this time? (Listen for adaptive skills and resources, social support, directly and indirectly communicated concerns.)
   a. Is there someone whom you talk to about problems or concerns?
   b. Are you having any difficulties that I may try to help with?

dividual family members. In most settings that serve children, occupational therapy practitioners function as part of a team that may also include social workers, teachers, psychologists, physicians, nurses, speech therapists, or physical therapists.

Intervention for the Parents

The occupational therapy practitioner can assist parents in two major ways: by facilitating the establishment of a social support system, and by educating them concerning child development and parenting skills. The development of a support system begins with the parent–practitioner relationship, which is facilitated through communication of caring and respect. A milestone in treatment is reached when the parent views the practitioner as someone in whom to trust and confide, and as someone who will try to help. Parent groups may facilitate the formation of helpful social relationships, as participants learn that they are not uniquely troubled, and may discover mutually helpful solutions. More enduring forms of support can be developed by helping parents plan ways to prevent crises by planning ahead and seeking assistance from reliable friends, family, and community resources as needed. Parent education should include nonpunitive behavior management techniques, such as praising approximations of desirable behaviors, sticker charting, and time-out. Information related to normal child development of social, daily living, and safety skills can reduce frustration and danger caused by parents' unrealistic expectations. Role playing and practice of new skills in parent–child activity-based sessions help to consolidate new knowledge and skills. Assertiveness training may help parents develop child management skills, improve general communication abilities, and increase self-esteem.

Carefully timed and tactful referral for further help, such as that afforded by psychotherapists, child care programs, and adult educational or vocational training programs, can also significantly influence family functioning.

Intervention for the Child

Emotional bonding with a caring adult has been postulated to be a prerequisite to healthy personality development (Jernberg, 1979; Martin, 1972.). The practitioner may facilitate relationship building through interactions found in healthy parent–child relationships, including cuddling and holding, feeding, grooming, and teaching developmentally appropriate skills. Reliability, gentleness, and communication of caring are essential features in this kind of therapy. Approaches for addressing the abused child's psychosocial needs may be combined with occupational therapy techniques used in treating other developmental needs, such as motor skills, dressing, and eating. Therapeutic activities based on sensory integration theory, neurodevelopmental treatment, and behavioral approaches are easily performed with attention to the nature and quality of the therapeutic relationship.

Intervention for the Parent–Child Relationship

As the parent and child become better able to receive and respond to nurturance from the practitioner, the likelihood of facilitating their own positive interactions increases. The occupational therapy practitioner can select activities to elicit appropriate caretaking behaviors by grading the amount of interaction and adult-imposed structure required. Activities should be selected for appropriateness in terms of the parent's and the child's developmental levels, and presented in a supportive, nonevaluative mode. The practitioner may need to demonstrate and teach some of the activities initially. In all activities, gentle physical contact, pleasant conversation, and mutual enjoyment are the main goals. The occupational therapy practitioner can also use parent–child sessions to teach concepts of child development. Parent–child sessions can also allow parents to observe and practice behavior management skills, such as praising and correcting behaviors.

▶CONCLUSION

Unlike most of the causes of developmental disabilities, such as prenatal distress and genetic error, child abuse is a common problem that occupational therapy practitioners can help to prevent. Occupational therapy practitioners who work in school- and community-based settings are in a strategic position to routinely screen children for abuse, to provide preventive intervention and referral, and to help ameliorate the consequences of abuse.

The negative effects of physical abuse have been documented as early as infancy and persist through adulthood. Long-term child abuse in families tends to perpetuate an intergenerational cycle of troubled interpersonal relationships, emotional distress, and malparenting (Main & Goldwyn, 1984; Ogata et al, 1990; Prodgers, 1984). Effective intervention with families who engage in violence toward their children is an investment in the occupational performance and well-being of this and future generations.

Acknowledgment

This chapter is based on *Physical Abuse of Preschoolers: Identification and Intervention Through Occupational Therapy*, by Debora Davidson. Copyright 1995. It was revised with permission from The American Occupational Therapy Association.

▼ REFERENCES

Barth, R. & Sullivan, R. (1985, March/April). Collecting competent evidence in behalf of children. *Social Work,* 130–136.

Coulton, C., Korbin, J., Su, M., & Chow, J. (1995). Community level factors and child maltreatment rates. *Child Development, 66,* 1262–1276.

Egeland, B., Sroufe, A., & Erickson, M. (1983). The developmental consequences of different patterns of maltreatment. *Child Abuse and Neglect, 7,* 459–469.

Faller, K.C. (1985). Unanticipated problems in the United States child protection system. *Child Abuse and Neglect, 9,* 63–69.

Frodi, A. (1981). Contribution of child characteristics to child abuse. *American Journal of Mental Deficiency, 85,* 341–345.

Gabarino, J. & Kostelny, K. (1992). Child maltreatment as a community problem. *Child Abuse and Neglect, 16,* 455–464.

Haskett, M. & Kistner, J. (1991). Social interactions and peer perceptions of young physically abused children. *Child Development, 62,* 979–990.

Helberg, J. (1983). Documentation in child abuse. *American Journal of Nursing, 2,* 236–239.

Hoffman-Plotkin, D. & Twentyman, C. (1984). A multimodal assessment of behavioral and cognitive deficits in abused and neglected preschoolers. *Child Development, 55,* 794–802.

Hopkins, H. (1993). An introduction to occupational therapy. In H. Hopkins & H. Smith (Eds.), *Willard & Spackman's occupational therapy* (8th ed., pp. 3–8). Philadelphia: J. B. Lippincott.

Jernberg, A. (1979). *Theraplay.* Washington: Jossey-Bass Publishers.

Kreitzer, M. (1984). Legal aspects of child abuse: Guidelines for the nurse. *Nursing Clinics of North America, 16,* 149–160.

Main, M. & Goldwyn, R. (1984). Predicting rejection of her infant from mother's representation of her own experience: Implications for the abused-abusing intergenerational cycle. *Child Abuse and Neglect, 8,* 203–217.

Martin, H. (1972). The child and his development. In R.E. Helfer &

R.S. Kempe (Eds.), *Helping the battered child and his family* (pp. 93–114). Philadelphia: J. B. Lippincott.

Ogata, S., Silk, K., Goodrich, S., Lohr, N., Westen, D., & Hill, E. (1990). Childhood sexual and physical abuse in adult patients with borderline personality disorder. *American Journal of Psychiatry, 147,* 1008–1013.

Pollack, C. & Steele, B. (1972). A therapeutic approach to parents. In R. Helfer & C. Kempe (Eds.), *Helping the battered child and his family* (pp. 3–21). Philadelphia: J. B. Lippincott.

Prodgers, A. (1984). Psychopathology of the physically abusing parent: A comparison with the borderline syndrome. *Child Abuse and Neglect, 8,* 411–424.

Starr, R. H. Jr., Dubowitz, H., & Bush, B. A. (1990). The epidemiology of child maltreatment. In R.T. Ammerman & M. Hersen (Eds.), *Children at risk: An evaluation of factors contributing to child abuse and neglect* (pp. 23–52). New York: Plenum Press.

Steele, B. (1987). Psychodynamic factors in child abuse. In R.E. Helfer & R.S. Kempe (Eds.), *The battered child* (4th ed., pp. 81–114). Chicago: University of Chicago Press.

United States Code Annotated Title 42: The Public Health and Welfare, Sections 4541 to 6500. (1978). St. Paul, MN: West Publishing Co.

Vondra, J. I. (1990). Sociological and ecological factors. In R.T. Ammerman & M. Hersen (Eds.), *Children at risk: An evaluation of factors contributing to child abuse and neglect* (pp. 149–165). New York: Plenum Press.

Wolfner, G. & Gelles, R. (1993). A profile of violence toward children: A national study. *Child Abuse and Neglect, 17,* 197–212.

UNIT IX
Client Applications

Olga Baloueff

> **Preparing For Patrice's Evaluation: Initial Data Gathering**
> **Theories Guiding the Evaluation Process**
> **Patrice's Occupational Therapy Evaluation**
> **Patrice's Occupational Therapy Intervention**
> **Conclusion**

Patrice is the 9-year-old school boy, introduced in Chapter 27, who told the first part of his story from the perspective of his family background, his performance in school, and his social life in his neighborhood before his traumatic brain injury. Now that you have read the entire unit on pediatrics, you will hear the rest of Patrice's story, and the role occupational therapy and the multidisciplinary team at his school provided in shaping the educational environment to facilitate Patrice's learning.

Preparing For Patrice's Evaluation: Initial Data Gathering

Susan is an experienced occupational therapist with over 10 years of practice in the school system, which

included the Pierce Elementary School (Patrice's school). Over the years, she has built a strong rapport with the school principal, the teachers, and the director of special education. They all value her expertise, and understand the many roles she fills at the school, ranging from consultant to the classroom teacher to providing direct services to the children with special needs. She is assisted by Mary, a certified occupational therapy assistant, with 2 years of experience at the school.

Susan and Mary are well aware that Patrice's return to the classroom setting, in which he is expected to integrate cognitive, social, and neuromotor skills, is not only difficult, but daunting at times. Before formally evaluating Patrice's needs, Susan sets up some time to talk with his classroom teacher and his parents, to understand their perspective on his school reentry. Meanwhile, Mary will observe him in the playground and in the classroom, recording her observations on a checklist she and Susan have developed for all initial data gathering and evaluation at the school.

On the playground Mary sees Patrice playing basketball with his peers. He has trouble making baskets, stumbles, and drops the ball. On several occasions, he lashes out at his friends shouting at them and threatening to hit them. Later in the day, in the classroom during a mathematics lesson, Patrice yawns repeatedly and finally puts his head on the desk. In the reading circle he fidgets more than the other children and needs to be helped to find his place in the book. Mary finds that Patrice is more alert early in the day, but toward the end of the day, he becomes tired and irritable. His behavior is often distracting to the teacher and his classmates.

When talking to his teacher, Susan finds out that on his return to school Patrice has been well received by his classmates. They are generally supportive and helpful, particularly two of the girls who take it upon themselves to redirect him in classroom assignments when he loses his place in the book or in transcribing letters and numbers from the blackboard into his notebook. At times, they also have to show him where his desk is located, because he cannot always remember where it is. The teacher feels that Patrice's attention and his performance are generally better in the early part of the morning, but that he becomes easily distracted, short tempered, and even tired by noon. She knows that he was a good student before his injury, but now, although he seems to understand most of the new materials presented in class, he needs help starting and finishing tasks and he has trouble concentrating and getting organized. She adds that she did not know much about traumatic brain injury (TBI) before Patrice's coming to her class, but that she has begun reading about it and found out that he presents many of the behaviors commonly seen in children with TBI.

She also feels that Patrice at times does not seem to fit in with friends and classmates, particularly at recess, or when the class becomes very animated. She feels sorry for him, and is looking forward to collaborating with the occupational therapy practitioners, the speech therapist, the other team members, and his parents to create strategies and an educational plan suitable to his needs.

When meeting with Mr. and Mrs. Douce, Susan explains to them that her role as an occupational therapist is to help Patrice develop skills and strategies to assist his learning in school. She asks for their input about their goals and what they think are Patrice's present needs. At first, they are surprised by the question and are reluctant to speak up. In trying to put them more at ease, Susan finds out that generally in Haiti professionals are considered to be in charge and tell parents what to do and not the reverse. After awhile, the parents become more comfortable, and they express their joy about their son's recovery, but also bewilderment and sadness about his changed behavior, although the hospital staff had prepared them for that.

When asked about their immediate concerns, they lament that Patrice, who before his injury had been a very good student, is now lazy, stubborn, and unwilling to do his homework. He also frequently interrupts conversations and speaks out of turn. Furthermore, Patrice often fights with his younger brother and appears to act younger than his age. He sleeps a lot, particularly when he comes from school, and he often seems disoriented when he wakes up.

Finally, Susan meets with Patrice. She wants to understand his perspective on the school reentry and on his strengths and needs. By engaging him in a conversation she hopes to open a window on his thinking processes, his feelings, and his speech patterns. She puts the young boy at ease by talking about favorite basketball players and television shows, and about having been herself out of school for a while, owing to an illness, when she was a child.

When asked if he is happy to be back in school, he says, "Oh yes! But it is hard!" When questioned about what is hard, he tells her that he becomes very tired at school, and that he is not able to play basketball with his friends as he used to. "I must also be very dumb now because I forget things, and I often get confused," adds Patrice. Finally, Susan asks him to tell her three things he wants to do better in the future. To that he answers, "Play basketball, not fight with my friends, and make my parents proud of me." Susan tells him that together with him, his teacher, and his parents, they will work at it and find ways for him to become stronger and meet his goals.

Theories Guiding the Evaluation Process

After reflecting on frames of reference to guide Patrice's evaluation, Susan chooses the Model of Human Occupation (MOHO; Kielhofner, 1995), which is holistic and considers the child's total functioning within the environment. To address the movement patterns and sensorimotor characteristics underlining Patrice's production of skilled behavior, she also uses the **neurodevelopmental treatment (NDT)** approach (Dunn & DeGangi, 1993).

Patrice's Occupational Therapy Evaluation

Patrice's occupational therapy evaluation is summarized in Table IX-1. It reflects concepts from the MOHO and NDT frames of reference and the Uniform Terminology for occupational therapy.

TABLE IX-1. Patrice's Occupational Therapy Evaluation

Occupational Performance	Assessment Tools	Principal Findings
Performance Areas Within School Context		
Activities of Daily Living	School Function Assessment (SFA) Coster et al (1995)	Independent in most ADL, but needs a few modifications for full participation in activities such as transitions from one area of school to another; carrying meal tray, books
Educational Activities	School Function Assessment (SFA) Coster et al (1995) and interview or questionnaire of teacher, parents, Patrice	Participates in most activities in regular classroom, with some assistance, such as short breaks, slower pace, redirection, supervision of arithmetic and spelling
Play and Leisure Activities	School Function Assessment (SFA) Coster et al (1995) and interview or questionnaire of teacher, parents, Patrice	Participates in half of the activities he did before; difficulty with running at recess and team sports; tires easily
Performance Components Within School Context		
Perceptual Processing • *Spatial relations* • *Visual discrimination* • *Figure-ground* • *Visual closure* • *Visual memory*	Motor-Free Visual Perception (MVPT-R), Colarusso & Hammill (1995)	Difficulties with visual memory, certain aspects of spatial relations, and visual discrimination; complained of test being hard and of eyes getting fatigued
Motor • *Visual–motor integration*	Developmental Test of Visual Motor Integration (VMI), Beery & Buktenica (1989)	Difficulty with reproduction of diagonals and eye-hand coordination
• *Gross motor* • *Fine motor*	Bruininks-Oseretsky Test of Motor Proficiency (BOTMF) Bruininks (1978)	Poor balance and coordination; difficulty with jumping; slow moving; poor eye-hand and bilateral coordination
Neuromusculoskeletal • *Muscle tone* • *Strength* • *Endurance* • *Postural control* • *Postural alignment* • *Desk and chair support*	Observations from an NDT perspective	Weak postural muscles, leading to increased fatigue; diminished equilibrium reactions in standing; diminished overall strength; slides off his chair easily.
Cognitive Integration • *Attention span* • *Initiation and termination of activity* • *Learning* • *Sequencing* • *Problem solving* • *Generalization*	Teacher's report and School Function Assessment (SFA), Coster et al (1995)	Attention span is poor when tired; easily distracted; needs help in starting and ending activities; irregular performance in class and with homework
Psychosocial Skills • *Self-concept*	Self-Perception Profile for Children (SPPC), Harter (1985)	Feels less worthy than peers in athletic and behavioral conduct
• *Interest* • *Values*	Child's, parents' and teacher's interview	Wants to be a good student, play ball, have friends
• *Social*	Social Skills Rating System (SSRS)—3 versions: child, parents, teacher	Aggressive and acts out when frustrated; impulsive

Assessment tools are listed in Evaluation Tables at the end of this unit.

Patrice's Occupational Therapy Intervention

At the **individualized education program (IEP)** meeting with Mr. and Mrs. Douce, team members present their evaluation results and discuss an education plan for Patrice. The IEP addresses both academic and personal modifications, specific instructional needs, measurements to determine success, and Patrice's present levels of performance. Patrice will receive direct and consultative occupational therapy services twice a week. Mary, the certified occupational therapy assistant, will provide the direct service that will involve working with Patrice during recess, gym, and in his classroom. She will assist the teacher in the classroom in meeting the educational goals for Patrice. She will consult regularly with Susan, the occupational therapist. Susan will also observe in the classroom and consult with the teacher about modifications to the learning environment that will enhance Patrice's learning.

Mr. and Mrs. Douce approve the IEP. To promote communication between the school and home the team and the Douces decide to use a notebook to record observations and strategies relative to Patrice's needs. The Douces agree to contribute to the notebook, so that school personnel can gain an understanding of Patrice's performance at home. This will be sent home daily at the beginning of the school year, changing to weekly when his performance improves and stabilizes. Although Patrice is not at the meeting, Susan gives him feedback on the discussion and reviews the plan designed to help him meet his goals. The team identified the following goals and strategies for Patrice.

1. *Patrice will improve his social skills so that he remains calm in frustrating situations and follows the rules in the classroom, lunch room, and playground.*
   a. To increase Patrice's social skills and promote appropriate behavior, the teacher and the special education team will:
      - Present clear rules of conduct
      - Post classroom rules and review them daily
      - Recognize and reward appropriate behavior immediately
      - Be sensitive to Patrice's cues of confusion and tiredness
      - Prepare Patrice for changes and transitions
      - Model calm, friendly behavior
      - Create opportunities for success each day
2. *Patrice will increase his attention and concentration so that he can remain "on task" for longer periods of time and with fewer modifications in the classroom.*
   a. To increase Patrice's attention and concentration, the teacher will

   - Place Patrice's desk close to her and a well-organized classmate
   - Place Patrice's desk away from the door and other high-activity areas
   - Keep instructions short and concise
   - Keep the environment organized and without excessive distraction
   - Monitor and refocus Patrice as needed
   - Place a symbol or picture card on Patrice's desk, or on the chalkboard, as a reminder and baseline information for task completion (this strategy will be used at home and at school)
   b. The occupational therapist will observe Patrice periodically. Given these observations, the teacher and occupational therapist will develop additional strategies to meet Patrice's needs more effectively.
3. *Patrice will improve his gross motor coordination and endurance so that he can sit comfortably in class and play basketball and other games on the playground*
   a. To enable Patrice to sit comfortably in class, the occupational therapist will
      - Modify Patrice's usual chair in the classroom to include a platform to support his feet, a raised chair back, and arm rests for lateral supports
      - Modify Patrice's desk at school to include raising the desk top and tilting it to 45 degrees to promote upper body stability and wrist extension, and to decrease energy requirements
   b. To develop Patrice's gross motor coordination (postural and trunk control, equilibrium reactions, overall muscle strength) the certified occupational therapy assistant will
      - Provide gross motor activities for Patrice and a small group of children with a large ball, scooter board, and mat equipment
      - Practice basketball-related skills (eg, catching, dribbling, throwing the ball into the basket, and so on)
4. *Patrice will improve his fine motor coordination so that he can engage more successfully in writing and art activities.*
   a. To develop Patrice's fine motor coordination, the certified occupational therapy assistant will work with him on bilateral arm and hand activities during art and writing classes.
   b. The occupational therapist will observe Patrice performing fine motor activities and suggest the above approaches to the certified occupational therapy assistant as Patrice improves.
5. *Patrice will increase his visual-processing skills so that he can read more easily, participate in mathematics activities, and use the computer with less strain.*
   a. To increase Patrice's visual-processing skills, the teacher and the special education team will:
      - Allow extra time for Patrice to examine visual

input, repeat auditory instructions, and when expected to give written and oral responses

- Teach Patrice how to use his finger as a guide to follow information in his book or on the chalkboard
- Teach Patrice to use color cues on the sides of the page for left-to-right cuing
- Use a large-print calculator and large-print books when appropriate
- Teach Patrice strategies for resting his eyes

b. To increase Patrice's visual-processing skills, the certified occupational therapy assistant will
  - Provide activities for Patrice and a small group of classmates to include visual discrimination, spatial relations, and visual figure-ground perception

c. The occupational therapist will observe Patrice and suggest modifications to the above approaches to the certified occupational therapy assistant and teacher as Patrice improves.

During periodic meetings with the Douces the team will address his progress and make suggestions for them to consider implementing at home. These would include reinforcement of the following goals.

1. *To develop Patrice's gross and fine motor coordination*
   - Enroll Patrice in a karate class or other activity that would encourage gross motor development
   - Modify Patrice's usual chair at home to include a platform to support his feet, a raised chair back, and arm rests for lateral supports

2. *To increase Patrice's attention and cooperation*
   - Discuss strategies for keeping Patrice focused on task completion and his ability to comply with directions
   - Help the Douces understand that Patrice's behavior is not always intentional, and that he is not purposely distracting others nor daydreaming

The strategies cited in Patrice's IEP were derived from the following resources: Begali, 1992; Bell, 1994; Dunn & DeGangi, 1992; Savage & Wolcott, 1994; Wolcott, Lash, & Pearson, 1995.

Conclusion

Together with Patrice, Mr. and Mrs. Douce, the classroom teacher, and the rest of the team, Susan and Mary formulated an evaluation process that resulted in an IEP to meet Patrice's educational needs. Because Patrice's needs will change as his brain recovers, the IEP must remain flexible and must be revised regularly. Communication between the family, the classroom teacher, and the team members is very important. Patrice's motivation and involvement are central to the implementation of the plan.

References

Begali, V. (1992). *Head injury in children and adolescents: Resources and review for school and allied health professionals.* Brandon, VT: Clinical Psychology.

Bell, T. A. (1994). Understanding students with traumatic brain injury: A guide for teachers and therapists. *School System, Special Interest Section Newsletter. American Occupational Therapy Association, 1*(2), 1–4.

Dunn, W. & DeGangi, G. (1992). Sensory integration and neurodevelopmental treatment for educational programming. In Royeen, C. B. (Ed.), *AOTA self-study series: Classroom applications for school-based practice.* Bethesda, MD: American Occupational Therapy Association.

Kielhofner, G. (Ed.). (1995). *A model of human occupation: Theory and application* (2nd. ed.). Baltimore, MD: William & Wilkins.

Savage, R. C. & Wolcott, G. F. (Eds.). (1994). *Educational dimensions of acquired brain injury.* Austin, TX: Pro-Ed.

Wolcott, G., Lash, M., & Pearson, S. (1995). *Signs and strategies for educating students with brain injuries: A practical guide for teachers and schools.* Houston, TX: HDI Publishers.

UNIT IX

TABLE IX-A. Selected Pediatric Assessment Tools by Performance Areas

Title, Authors, Publishers	Age Range	ADL	Work or Productive	Play and Leisure
Adolescent Role Assessment. Black, M. (1976). *American Journal of Occupational Therapy, 30,* 73–79.	13–17 y		X	X
Erhardt Developmental Prehension Assessment (EDPA) (prewriting section). Erhardt, R. (1994). San Antonio, TX: Therapy Skill Builders.	1–6 y		X	
Functional Independence Measure (FIM). Hamilton, B. B. & Granger, C. U. (1991). The State University of New York at Buffalo, Buffalo, NY 14214.	8 yr–adult	X		
Functional Independence Measure for Children (Wee-FIM). See above.	6 mo–7 y	X		
Oral–Motor Feeding Rating Scale. Jelm, J. M. (1990). San Antonio, TX: Therapy Skill Builders.	1 y–adult	X		
Pediatric Evaluation of Disability Inventory (PEDI). Haley, S. M., Coster, W. J., Ludlow, L. H., Haltwanger, J. T., & Andrellos, P. J. (1992). San Antonio, TX: Therapy Skill Builders.	6 mo–7.5 y	X		
Play Skills History. Takata, N. (1974). In M. Reilly (Ed.), *Play as exploratory learning* (pp 209–246). Beverly Hills, CA: Sage.	0–16 y			X
Preschool Play Scale. Bledsoe & Shepard (1982); Knox (1974). *American Journal of Occupational Therapy, 36,* 783–788.	0–6 y			X
Self-Help Assessment: Parent Evaluation (SHAPE). Research Edition, Miller, L. J., The KID Foundation, 8101 E. Prentice Avenue, Suite 518, Englewood, CO 80111.	0–6 y	X		
School Function Assessment (SFA). Coster, W. & Haley, S. (1995). Department of Occupational Therapy, Sargent College, Boston University, Boston, MA 02215.	5–11 y (grade K–6)	X	X	X
The Evaluation Tool of Children's Handwriting (ETCH). Admundson, S. J. (1995). Homer, AK: OT KIDS.	6–12 y (grade 1–6)		X	
Transdisciplinary Play-Based Assessment (TPBA). Linder, T. L. (1990). Baltimore, MD: Paul H. Brookes.	6 mo–6 y	X	X	X
Vineland Adaptive Behavior Scales. Sparrow, S., Balla, D., & Cicchetti, D. (1984). Circle Pines, MN: American Guidance Service.	0–18.11 y	X		

TABLE IX-B. Selected Pediatric Assessment Tools by Performance Components

Title, Authors, Publishers	Age Range	Sensorimotor	Cognitive Integration Cognitive	Psychosocial Skills Psychological
Assessment in Infancy: Ordinal Scales of Psychological Development. Uzgiris, I. & Hunt, J. Urbana, IL: University of Illinois Press.	0–18 mo		X	X
Bruininks-Oseretsky Test of Motor Proficiency (BOTMP). Bruininks, R. Circle Pines, MN: American Guidance Service.	4.5–14.5 y	X		
Coping Inventory. Zeitlin, S. Bensenville, IL: Scholastic Testing Service.	5–14 y	X		X
DeGangi-Berk Test of Sensory Integration. Berk, R. & De-Gangi, G. Los Angeles: Western Psychological Services.	3–5 y	X		
Early Coping Inventory. Zeitlin, S., Williamson, G., & Szczepanski, M. Bensenville, IL: Scholastic Testing Service.	4 mo–3 y	X		X
Erhardt Developmental Prehension Assessment (EDPA). Erhardt, R. San Antonio, TX: Therapy Skill Builders.	0–15 mo	X		
Erhardt Developmental Vision Assessment (EDVA). Erhardt, R. San Antonio, TX: Therapy Skill Builders.	0–6 mo	X		
Gesell Preschool Test. Ames, L. B., Gillespie, C., Haines, J., & Ilg, F. L. Rosemont, NJ: Programs for Education Inc.	2.5–6 y	X	X	X
Goodenough-Harris Drawing Test. Goodenough, F. L. & Harris, D. B. San Antonio, TX: Psychological Corporation.	3–15 y		X	
Infant/Toddler Symptom Checklist. DeGangi, G., Poisson, S., Sickel, R., & Wiener, A. San Antonio, TX: Therapy Skill Builders.	7–30 mo	X		
Peabody Developmental Motor Scales (PDMS). Folio, R. & Fewell, R. Riverside Publishing Co.	0–7 y	X		
Piers-Harris Children's Self-Concept Scale. Piers, E. & Harris, D. Western Psychological Services.	8–18 y			X
Quick Neurological Screening Test (QNST). Mutti, M., Sterling, H., & Spaulding, N. Academic Therapy Publications.	5–17 y	X		
Self-Perception Profile for Adolescents (SPPC). Harter, S. University of Colorado.	14–17 y			X
Self-Perception Profile for Children (SPPC). Harter, S. University of Colorado.	8–13 y			X
Sensorimotor Performance Analysis (SPA). Richter, E. & Montgomery, P. PDP Products.	5–21 y	X		
Sensory Integration and Praxis Test (SIPT). Ayres, J. A. Western Psychological Services.	4–8.11 y	X		
Social Skills Rating System (SSRS). Gresham, F. & Elliott, S. American Guidance Service.	5–17 y			X
Tests of Sensory Functions in Infants (TSFI). DeGangi, G. & Greenspan, S. Western Psychological Services.	4–18 mo	X		
Test of Visual–Motor Skills (TVMS). Gardner, M. Psychological and Educational Publications, Inc.	2–13 y	X		
Test of Visual–Perceptual Skills (Non-Motor) (TVPS-R). Gardner, M. Psychological and Educational Publications.	4–12.11 y	X		
The Purdue Perceptual–Motor Survey. Roach, E., Kephart, N., & Charles E. Merrill Publishing Co.	6–10 y	X		
The T.I.M.E. Toddler and Infant Motor Evaluation. Miller, L. & Roid, G. Psychological Corporation.	4 mo–3.5 y	X		

TABLE IX-C. Selected Pediatric Assessment Tools by Performance Contexts: Temporal Aspects

Title, Authors, Publishers	Age Range
Screening	
Bayley Infant Neurodevelopmental Screener (BINS). Aylward, G. San Antonio, TX: Psychological Corporation.	3–24 mo
Denver Developmental Screening Test (DDST-II). Frankenburg, W., Dodds, J., Archer, P., Bresnick, B., Maschka, P., Edelman, N., & Shapiro. University of Colorado, Denver, CO: Denver Developmental Materials, Inc.	0–6 y
FirstSTEP Screening Test for Evaluating Preschoolers. Miller, L. San Antonio, TX: Psychological Corporation.	2.9–6.2 y
Miller Assessment for Preschoolers (MAP). Miller, L. San Antonio, TX: Psychological Corporation.	2.9–5.8 y
Comprehensive	
Battelle Developmental Inventory. Newborg, J., Stock, J., Wnek, L., Guidubaldi, J., & Svinicki, A. Chicago, IL: Riverside Publishing.	1 mo–9 y
Bayley Scales of Infant Development (BSID-II). Bayley, N. San Antonio, TX: Psychological Corporation.	1 mo–42 mo
Developmental Test of Visual–Motor Integration (VMI). Beerry, K. & Buktenica, N.A. Cleveland, OH: Modern Curriculum Press.	2.9–19.8 y
Developmental Test of Visual Perception (DTVP-2). Hammill, D., Pearson, N., & Voress, J. Austin, TX: PRO-ED.	4–10 y
Early Learning Accomplishment Profile (E-LAP). Glover, M., Preminger, J., & Sanford, A. Chapel Hill, NC: Chapel Hill Training-Outreach Project.	0–3 y
Early Intervention Developmental Program (EIDP). Rogers, S., Donavan, C., D'Eugenio, D., Brown, S., Lynch, E., Moersch, M., & Schafer, D. Ann Arbor, MI: University of Michigan Press.	0–3 y
Hawaii Early Learning Profile (HELP). Furuno, S., O'Reilly, K., Hosaka, C., Inatsuka, T., Allman, T., & Zeisloft-Folby, B. Palo Alto, CA: Vort Corporation.	0–3 y
Infant–Toddler Developmental Assessment (IDA). Provence, S., Erickson, J., Vater, S., & Palmeri, S. Chicago, IL: Riverside Publishing.	0–3 y
Neonatal Behavior Assessment Scale (NBAS). Brazelton, B. New York: Cambridge University Press.	0–1 mo
Vineland Adaptive Behavior Scales. Sparrow, S., Balla, D., & Cicchetti, D. Circle Pines, MN: American Guidance Service.	0–18.11 y

TABLE IX-D. Selected Pediatric Assessment Tools by Performance Contexts: Environment

Title, Authors, Publishers	Primary Data Gathering Method
Family Environment Scale. Moos, R. & Moos, B. Palo Alto, CA: Consulting Psychologists Press.	Family self-report
Family Support Scale. Dunst, C., Trivette, C., & Deal, A. Cambridge, MA: Brookline Books.	Family self-report
Home Observation and Measure of the Environment Inventory (HOME). Caldwell, B. & Bradley, R. Center for Child Development and Education, University of Arkansas, Little Rock, AR.	Observation in the home
Nursing Child Assessment Satellite Training: Parent-Infant Interaction (NCAST): Feeding and Teaching. Barnard, K. University of Washington, Seattle, WA: NNCAST Publications.	Observation of parent–child interaction
Parenting Stress Index. Abidin, R. Brandon, VT: Clinical Psychology Publishing Co.	Family self-report
Questionnaire on Resources and Stress for Families with Chronically Ill or Handicapped Members. Holroyd, J. Brandon, VT: Clinical Psychology Publishing Co.	Family self-report
School Function Assessment (SFA). Coster, W., Deeney, T., Haltwanger, J., & Haley, S. Boston University, Occupational Therapy Department, Boston, MA.	Teacher's, school therapist's report

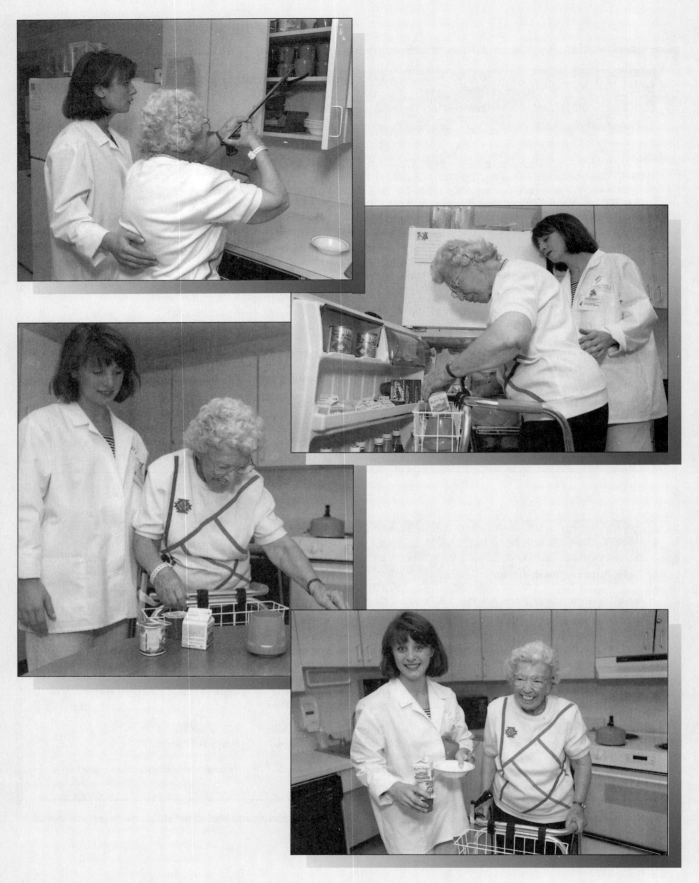

Preparing for discharge after a stroke involves learning new ways to set the table for lunch. (Photos by Gary Samson, Instructional Services, Dimond Library, University of New Hampshire.)

UNIT X

Occupational Therapy: Diagnostic Considerations in Adult and Older Adult Practice

LEARNING OBJECTIVES

After completing this unit, readers will be able to:

▶ Describe the population served by occupational therapy practitioners working with adults and older adults.

▶ Define the diagnoses of adults and older adults receiving occupational therapy and the influence of these diagnoses on occupational performance:

- Neurological dysfunction: cerebral vascular accident, traumatic brain injury, Parkinson's disease, amyotrophic lateral sclerosis, multiple sclerosis, spinal cord injury, Guillain-Barre, and myasthenia gravis
- Orthopedic and musculoskeletal dysfunction: hip fracture, amputations, arthritis, and hand injuries
- Cardiopulmonary dysfunction: myocardial infarction, chronic obstructive pulmonary disease, congestive heart failure, and tuberculosis
- Immune system dysfunction: HIV infection and cancer
- Psychosocial dysfunction: Alzheimer's disease, mood disorders, substance abuse, eating disorders, borderline personality disorder, and schizophrenia
- Skin dysfunction: burns

▶ Define and explain evaluation and intervention strategies for adults and older adults receiving occupational therapy

This unit looks at the ways common medical and psychiatric diagnoses in adults influence occupational therapy evaluation and treatment. Diagnostic conditions are often associated with particular patterns of occupational and component skill dysfunction. For example, a person with a fractured hip could be expected to have difficulty with functional mobility (ie, walking and getting in and out of bed or on and off a toilet). One would not expect this same set of problems for someone with a broken finger. Therapists who are aware of some of the common problems associated with given diagnoses will be able to focus their evaluations quickly. Practitioners aware of common diagnostically related problems will be able to tailor their treatments to those problems.

Moreover, all diagnostic conditions pose certain precautions on occupational therapy intervention. Healing bones, for instance, can be refractured if they are subject to too much pressure, twisting, or compression, early in the healing process before the body has laid down substantial new bone at the fracture site. To keep their clients safe, practitioners need to be aware of precautions associated with (1) given diagnoses, (2) medical equipment related to those diagnoses, and (3) medications frequently prescribed for those diagnoses. Practitioners who are not aware of these precautions can seriously harm clients.

Diagnostic conditions, then, can influence therapists' choice of evaluation methods and practitioners' choice of treatment methods and theories. The occupational therapy intervention is also influenced by treatment settings and professional issues; these topics are covered in the next two units. (*Note*: Words in **bold** type are defined in the Glossary.)

Chapter 35

Introduction to Adult and Older Adult Populations

Betty Risteen Hasselkus

Description of Age Range
    The Concept of Life Span Development
    Occupation and Life Span
      Development
    In Sickness and In Health

Client and Family Narrative
    Disease Progression
    Influence on Life
    Occupational Therapy
    The Turning Point

▼ DESCRIPTION OF AGE RANGE

In recent decades, adulthood and old age have been recognized as complex, dynamic stages of life that offer tremendous challenges and rich contexts of practice for health care professionals in the United States. Approximately half of all occupational therapy services take place with adults and older people. As the demographics of the country shift to a larger and larger proportion of elderly in the population, increasing numbers of occupational therapy practitioners are drawn to geriatrics and its various subspecialties as areas of practice. In a 1995 American Occupational Therapy Association (AOTA) study, 38% of all occupational therapists and 62% of certified occupational therapy assistants reported that they work primarily with older clients (Stancliff, 1996). These numbers represent an increase from 25% of all occupational therapists and 37% of all certified occupational therapy assistants in geriatrics reported in a 1990 survey (Staff, 1990).

In this section of the unit, we will briefly review the many ways that life span developmentalists have characterized adult life and old age. Next, we will examine human occupation during adulthood and aging, focusing on self-care, work, and leisure. Finally, we will discuss adult development and aging within the context of health and illness, focusing on the relationship of adult development to mental retardation, mental illness, and physical disability.

The Concept of Lifespan Development

The term "*human development*" typically refers to a patterned sequence of changes in the human being that occurs over a considerable length of time (Kaluger & Kaluger, 1984; Newman & Newman, 1984). These changes follow system-

atically one after the other, each new change building on the foundation laid by the one that came before it. Developmental changes in the human organism are perhaps most evident in early life, starting with the months immediately after conception, through infancy and childhood, and up until puberty in adolescence. In fact, until the second half of this century, the primary focus of the field of human development was clearly on these early developmental changes (one has only to think of Sigmund Freud's theory of personality development in childhood). In more recent years, however, the emphasis has broadened to a life span view (Erikson, 1959; Reese & Overton, 1970; Vaillant, 1977); adulthood and old age are now firmly ensconced in the concept of human development, extending the study of development throughout maturity to very old age and death.

Human development in adulthood and old age encompasses physiological, psychological, and sociological aspects of change (Dannefer & Perlmutter, 1990). These aspects of development help describe and explain the developmental processes that occur, providing a way to organize the study of life span changes. Attempts to understand the patterns and rhythms of change across the life span have led to the use of several different metaphors to portray development in adulthood and aging. Several of these metaphorical images will be discussed here.

PASSAGES

In 1976, Sheehy introduced the term *passages* to describe critical transitions that define development in adult life. "Life after adolescence is not one long plateau. Changes are not only possible and predictable, but to deny them is to be an accomplice to one's own unnecessary vegetation" (p. 12). Passages are shifts in one's internal self. "Pulling up Roots,"

RESEARCH NOTE

THE FUTURE CHALLENGE FOR OCCUPATIONAL THERAPY RESEARCH IS TO EVALUATE INTERVENTION AT THE LEVEL OF HANDICAP OR SOCIAL WELL-BEING

Kenneth J. Ottenbacher

Traditional medical diagnosis concentrates on the historical clues and physical or psychosocial findings that suggest the correct identification of disease or pathology. Once a medical diagnosis has been established, the occupational therapist must determine the functional consequences of the disease or pathology and establish a treatment plan to reduce or eliminate any functional deficits. The development of an appropriate occupational therapy intervention program requires that the examiner have a clear understanding of the distinctions among disease, impairment, disability, and handicap, as defined by the World Health Organization (WHO, 1980). In the past, intervention and research activities for

adults have focused on impairments and disability; that is, on the physical and organic structures associated with pathology, or on the ability to perform specific activities, such as bathing or dressing. The challenge of occupational therapy research in the 21st century will be to plan, implement, and evaluate intervention at the level of handicap or social well-being. *Handicap* is defined by the WHO as a disadvantage resulting from an impairment or disability that limits or prevents the fulfillment of a role that is normal (depending on age, sex, and social or cultural factors) for that individual. As a profession, occupational therapy is uniquely qualified to address this challenge. ■

WHO. (1980). *International classification of impairments, disabilities, and handicaps: A manual for classification relating to the consequences of disease.* Albany, NY: WHO Publication Center.

for example, is a passage that takes place when young adults gradually shift themselves emotionally and physically away from a self that is centered within the parental home to a new separate self with its own authenticity within its own peer group. The "Urge to Merge" is the passage that leads to coupling and thoughts of marriage. Passages occur across the life span. Sheehy's last life passage, in this 1976 book, is a sort of grand passage titled "Resignation or Renewal" that refers to all development after age 50.

Sheehy wrote another book in 1995 titled *New Passages* in which she discusses the way passages have changed since the decade of the 1970s. For example, Pulling up Roots now occurs several years later than it did 20 years ago. Additionally, Sheehy extends the concept of passages beyond midlife and into older age. In this recent book, having reached the age of 50 herself, she labels this decade of life as the "flaming fifties" (p. 11). She describes it as a time that requires courage and rebelliousness as the person forges ahead into the second half of life. Like the original concept of a passage, the new passage is a conscious shift to another stage of life in which we continue to grow and recreate ourselves.

MARKER EVENTS

Neugarten (1977) discusses the idea of "marker events" across the life span and their relationship to personality development and adaptation. Marker events in life are social occasions such as graduating, marrying, starting a job, or getting a driver's license. Such events trigger periods of change and development in people's lives (Lowenthal, Thurnher, & Chiriboga, 1975). Neugarten (1977) has proposed that the occurrence of a marker event itself does not promote development; rather, it is when such events occur "off-time," rather than "on-time," that major changes occur (p. 639). For example, retirement earlier in life than nor-

mally expected would be off-time and, because of this, the event would generate significant developmental change within the individual; retirement at the usual time in life would not lead to such major adjustment.

Levinson (1978) offers a view of marker events that is similar to Neugarten's idea of on-time and off-time. Levinson agrees with Neugarten that marker events do not, in themselves, cause the stages of adult development. Their significance to development depends largely on *when* they occur in the life cycle. For example, if marriage occurs at ages 18 or 19, its effect as a marker event will be imbedded in the other tasks of that age, such as the process of separation from parents (Sheehy's Pulling up Roots). Alternatively, if marriage occurs in the mid-20s, its effect will be imbedded in the task of launching a career.

SEASONS

In his book on adult development, Levinson (1978) uses yet another image of development, the image of "seasons." Levinson uses the term "life cycle," rather than "life span," intending to convey a sense of a process or journey that has an underlying universal pattern, with a beginning point and an ending. The pattern is made up of periods or stages within the life cycle. These are the seasons of life, metaphorically similar to the seasons of the year with its spring-like beginning and the winter at its end. To Levinson, each season in the cycle of life has its own time and needs to be understood in its own terms. "No season is better or more important than any other" (p. 7). A transition is required for a shift from one season to the next.

LIFE AS A COMPOSITION

Bateson (1989) introduces the themes of composition and improvisation into life span development theory. As adults, we have the capacity to manipulate and recombine familiar and unfamiliar components of our lives, thereby creating new directions for ourselves to take into previously unknown territory. Bateson states that we need to "recognize the value of lifetimes in continual redefinition" (p. 7). Life is like a work in progress; we need to constantly improvise. Life is a composition that we refocus and redefine throughout our lifetimes.

LIFE AS A NARRATIVE

Closely related to the concept of life as a composition is the metaphor of life as a narrative. A narrative is an account of something that contains more than a mere sequence of events; a narrative has a coherence and wholeness (a plot) that binds its components together (Polkinghorne, 1988). According to Bruner (1986), storytelling is one of the ways we create narratives of our lives. We seek to create a wholeness of our lives from beginning to end, to build a coherent narrative across our life spans. Within this metaphor of the life span, adulthood and aging become the middle and ending of the life narrative. Mattingly (1991) introduced the concept of narrative to occupational therapy, suggesting that practitioners use the structure of narrative to make meaning out of our clinical situations. We create *stories* with our clients—stories with specific beginnings, middles, and endings—and we seek to fit these stories into the larger narrative of each client's life, as well as into our own life narratives. Thus, as we work with a person with a disability, our experience together becomes part of both our life stories, contributing to whom we are and what we are still becoming.

These, then, are major images of human development from a life span perspective. Other important frameworks do exist. Continuity, for example, has been posed as an organizer and driving force in development throughout the life span (Atchley, 1989; Kaufman, 1986). Additionally, the examination of gender as it relates to adult development has generated new understandings of developmental processes (Gilligan, 1982; Lerner, 1977; Belenky, Clinchy, Goldberger, & Tarule, 1986), raising our awareness that female and male developmental experiences are both the same and different. Adulthood and aging are, indeed, rich and varied periods of life.

Occupation and Life Span Development

Occupational therapy has been defined as "the use of purposeful activity to achieve a functional outcome" (Punwar, 1994, p. 262). The "outcome" in this definition includes the prevention of disability, the promotion of recovery from disability, and the enhancement of development. Thus, embedded in our professional values and practices are beliefs that occupation—the everyday purposeful activity of human beings—is related to human development. Occupation, then, offers another framework within which to organize and study development in adulthood and aging.

The theories and frames of reference that guide occupational therapy practice have been discussed in Unit VIII of this text. Many of these frames of reference include concepts that link occupation with life span development. Work, play, and self-care are the everyday occupations of life (AOTA, 1995); the activities that make up these occupations and the routines and patterns of these occupations change across the life span. These shifting characteristics and patterns of occupation are linked to human development in two ways: they contribute directly to developmental change and they provide a mirror in which we can see developmental change reflected. For example, a 40-year-old woman who returns to graduate school after years of being at home with two children is experiencing a major shift in the patterns of her daily occupations. The shift in occupations contributes directly to the woman's development; she will be changed during this graduate school experience—intellectually, socially, and psychologically. This shift is also a reflection of much developmental change that has already occurred—the shift from a focus on at-home parenting to a focus on out of the home activities; a newly defined sense of purpose that was not present 5 years before; a heightened level of confidence, and other changes.

The relationship of occupation to life span development has been examined from various perspectives. The traditional concepts of occupation as work, play, and self-care are used here to help us think about occupation within this developmental context.

WORK

Havighurst (1953, 1964) developed a theory of developmental tasks to describe the lifelong process of vocational development. To Havighurst, a developmental task is one "which arises at or about a certain period in the life of the individual, successful achievement of which leads to his [or her] happiness and to success with later tasks, while failure leads to unhappiness in the individual, disapproval by the society, and difficulty with later tasks" (Havighurst, 1953, p. 2). Starting with identification *with* a worker in childhood (mother, father, other significant person), human beings proceed through five other stages of vocational development, ending with the older, retired person who "contemplates a productive and responsible life" (1964, p. 216). Along the way, the individual develops work habits and skills and roles, all of which both contribute to the individual's development and reflect his or her growing mastery and productivity in society.

A different work-related model of development is proposed by Benner (1984) in her study of the acquisition of skills in nursing. Although not life span in scope, Benner's model presents stages of skill acquisition across adulthood, from "novice to expert." On the basis of a model proposed earlier by Dreyfus and Dreyfus (1980), Benner describes the changes in proficiency that occur across time with experience in nursing practice. The novice worker can anticipate gradually shifting to the next developmental stage of advanced beginner; from there, the worker would continue developmentally through three more stages, successively becoming competent, proficient, and finally, expert. The development includes changes within the individual from fragmentary thinking to holistic thinking. The novice nurse relies on the theories and principles learned in the classroom; the expert nurse demonstrates judgment and skill acquired through real-life experience. Presumably, occupational therapy practitioners experience a similar developmental process as they move through their own occupational journeys from student novice to experienced expert.

LEISURE

Leisure, too, may be conceptualized both as an occupation that contributes to development and one that reflects developmental changes throughout adulthood and aging. Kleiber and Kelly (1980) present a persuasive discussion of the strong links between leisure activities and the development of social patterns of behavior across the life span. For example, in young adulthood, shared leisure contributes to the development of intimacy; in middle age, leisure may provide a bridge back to the community for a parent who has been home and family-centered for several years; in old age, leisure may serve increasingly as the vehicle for maintaining social relatedness. Kleiber and Kelly speak strongly about the importance of leisure to socialization across the entire life cycle: "Leisure with its experience of freedom may be the most effective setting for human bonding" (p. 126). From childhood ("Can Molly come out and play?"), to adulthood ("Would you like to go to the concert tonight?"), to old age ("Let's have lunch together.")—leisure serves a purpose for enabling people to get together and to develop patterns of social behavior.

In the past decade, increasing attention has been paid to the gender-specific issues imbedded in the study of leisure (Henderson, Bialeschki, Shaw, & Freysinger, 1989; Henderson, 1990). Before this time, it had been widely assumed that the findings of leisure research involving only male subjects would apply to females. Henderson (1990) argues that the longtime definition of leisure as "nonwork" was derived from the male-oriented model of work as an activity that was separated from the home. Henderson suggests that a redefinition of leisure as a subjective experience is a better fit in the complex world of women today.

In addition to gender, the study of leisure and aging has received increasing attention in recent years (Kelly, 1993). Specific areas of aging concerns include the relationship between leisure and well-being in old age, leisure and friendships among older adults, and leisure opportunities in assisted-living settings. Adding an ethnic research focus, Allen and Chin-Sang (1990) studied the meaning of leisure for aging black women, reporting on the influence of the women's lifetime of work and service on the meanings of leisure in older age. Many of these women said that they had had no leisure in the past. Any "leisure" that they experienced after retirement was imbedded in the work and service context, such as their volunteer activities in the context of their churches or in senior centers. The authors con-

cluded that "the meaning of leisure for these women was revealed by addressing the life course context of work" (p. 739). It can be seen that the leisure of these retired black women reflected their lifelong patterns of behavior while also contributing to their continuing socialization in old age.

SELF-CARE

Activities that individuals engage in on their own behalf to maintain their health and well-being are called activities of self-care (Orem, 1980). Orem states: "Normally, adults voluntarily care for themselves. Infants, children, the aged, the ill, and the disabled require complete care or assistance with self-care activities" (p. 35). Although Orem's statement overgeneralizes people's situations, we know intuitively that self-care capabilities do gradually develop in the child and adolescent, that they continue to shift and change in adulthood (otherwise, why do dental hygienists keep hoping we will start flossing our teeth), and that, for many people, self-care capabilities are diminished in old age. In other words, self-care, too, changes across the life span.

To occupational therapy practitioners, self-care has come to refer collectively to basic personal care tasks, including bowel and bladder management, bathing, dressing, eating, grooming and hygiene, and mobility (Christiansen, 1994). Just as these basic skills develop and change across the life span, so, too, do the more complex instrumental activities of daily living such as meal preparation, medication monitoring, and financial management. The new college student, living away from home for the first time, may dramatically illustrate this development through his or her increasing capabilities and independence in selecting and preparing food, budgeting, and using the laundromat. The new parent calls on existing skills, but also experiences continuing development and change as he or she gradually learns to balance the needs of the newborn infant with the need for continued care of the self.

Much of the emphasis in self-care literature has been on those activities that are related to illness and people's responses to illness. Using a sample of adults from age 20 to 79, Segall (1987) studied the relationship of age to the way people respond to illness symptoms. Segall found age differences in subjects' responses to certain symptoms; for example, for loss of appetite, young adults tended to self-treat and older adults tended to consult a doctor; young and old adults tended to self-treat dizziness and difficulty sleeping, but middle-aged adults tended to seek physician help with these symptoms. People of all ages in the study sought physician help for symptoms such as shortness of breath and frequent headaches.

Self-care may have a very different meaning to elderly people than it does to young adults. Florida Scott-Maxwell (1968), in describing her everyday experiences as a woman in her eighth decade of life, wrote, "I have a duty to all who care for me—not to be a problem, not to be a burden. I must carry my age lightly for all our sakes, and thank God I still can. Oh that I may to the end. Each day then, must be filled with my first duty, I must be 'all right' " (p. 31). The fierce desire "not to be a burden" imbues self-care with a new and different meaning in old age; the focus on the effect of one's self-care capabilities on the lives of others is added to the adult's focus on the effect on self.

We can see that self-care responses to illness include not only the decisions about what actions to take, but also ongoing self-monitoring of health and interpretation of the symptoms (Levin & Idler, 1981). Self-treatment actions require making choices from a wide range of possible home remedies such as self-medication, bed rest, ointments, heating pads, ice packs, and chicken noodle soup. Self-care, defined this way, is a complex activity that both reflects prior life experiences and contributes to new skills and further developmental change.

In summary, the everyday occupations of adults and older people can be used as a framework for understanding the developmental changes of adulthood and old age. Work, play, and self-care are multidimensional categories of activity that reflect aspects of life, including age and developmental stage. The foundations of occupation learned in childhood are expanded and adapted throughout the lifetime, providing support for changes across the life span in human beings. In his delightful short essay on what he learned in kindergarten, Fulghum (1986) summarized his philosophy for daily life as follows: "Learn some and think some and draw and paint and sing and dance and play and work every day some." These are the occupations of life. As occupational therapy practitioners, we use these occupations to guide our therapeutic activities and to enhance life span development in our clients.

In Sickness and in Health

Up to this point, we have primarily addressed everyday occupations and their relationships to life span development within a framework of health and well-being. Now we will examine the meaning of occupation in the development of people with chronic illnesses. Persons who are born with a disability, or who live for years with a long-term illness, experience their everyday occupations in ways that are influenced by the disability. An occupational framework will guide our thinking.

LIFE SPAN DEVELOPMENT AND DEVELOPMENTAL DISABILITIES

Persons with developmental disabilities may have, as part of their life experiences, recurrent hospitalizations, periods of institutionalization, and frequent contacts with health professionals and service agencies in their homes and in the community. Although the goal of all this health care and service is to enhance the person's well-being and ability to have quality of life, paradoxically the disruptions in daily life imposed by this ongoing interaction with special services "can dramatically interfere with the acquisition of adult life

skills" (Neistadt, 1987; p. 433). Disruptions occur in education, social relationships, and family life. Furthermore, living with a chronic disability means living in an environment that is often physically inaccessible and with societal attitudes that are largely patronizing and embedded in negative stereotypes.

Kielhofner (1981), in his research on adults with **mental retardation** (one type of developmental disability), described the altered everyday world of the subjects in his study: "For retarded persons, it is a matter of living in a world that pays a tremendous amount of negative, curious, patronizing, or humorous attention to them and that directs extraordinary social action toward them. . . . In this way, everything about the retarded person's everyday world was altered from that experienced by normal persons" (p. 140).

In this altered world of people who have mental retardation, the typical passages, markers, and seasons of life may not be "typical" at all or may be totally absent. Individuals with mental retardation may never get a driver's license, cast their ballots, "pull up their roots," or establish their own households. Kielhofner's study (1981) focused on the everyday life of residents in a group home. The lack of opportunity for occupation presented by this environment was obvious: "Only a few [of the residents] had any control over their immediate living environment. Almost none of them performed such basic functions as cooking, shopping, traveling, cleaning, laundering, and so forth. . . . Almost all of them had little or nothing to do with their time" (p. 138). In contrast, a study carried out in England (Raynes, Johnson, Sumpton, & Thorp, 1987) compared the daily occupations of two adult men with mental retardation in a large institution with two adults of comparable mental abilities in a group home; the findings revealed significantly more participation in domestic tasks, responsibility for aspects of their own lives, and involvement in community activities for the men in the group home. Thus, being in a group home per se may or may not provide opportunity for occupational role participation; individuals with mental retardation and other developmental disabilities must rely on the people and supports in their environments to facilitate access and provide opportunities for everyday occupational involvement. Without these opportunities, the developmental changes that occupation helps bring about will not occur or will be markedly curtailed.

Another focus of attention related to persons who have mental retardation is on the *aging* sector of this population (Segal, 1990; Seltzer & Krauss, 1987). The number of elderly persons with mental retardation is increasing, and an unfortunate debate exists over whether primary support services and funding for this group of people should come from the associations for people with mental retardation or from associations for the elderly. The provision of residential facilities for older people with mental retardation is a key concern, for many aging adults with mental retardation have lived all their lives with their now aging and dying parents (Seltzer, Begun, Seltzer, & Krauss, 1991; Seltzer & Krauss,

1989; Seltzer, Krauss, & Tsunematsu, 1993). Long-held patterns of dependency and relative isolation may need to be overcome to facilitate new competencies in social skills and activities of daily living (ADLs).

LIFE SPAN DEVELOPMENT AND LONG-TERM ILLNESS

Individuals with long-term illnesses are also vulnerable to being deprived of opportunities for typical occupational daily activities. The deinstitutionalization movement of the 1960s and 1970s led to the discharge of many adults with chronic disabilities and older people from long-term care facilities to community living. Gradually, community-based programs and living facilities began to be developed to support people with chronic illness as they tried to engage in the occupational tasks of independent living.

For persons with chronic mental illness, a new type of supported-living setting emerged called the "halfway house" (Friedlob, Janis, & Deets-Aron, 1986). The mission of a **halfway house** was to provide "a bridge between the hospital and the community via a therapeutic milieu designed to prepare residents for resuming their roles in society. It encourages normal patterns of living, offers support, and supplies opportunities for trying different roles and behaviors in a safe environment" (Freidlob et al, 1986; p. 272). Enabling the residents to learn skills in daily occupations, such as health and hygiene, nutrition, household management, interpersonal relationships, and leisure activities, was a prominent component of the concept as well as vocational training, employment, and eventually moving to more independent settings.

Recognition of the importance of successful engagement in everyday occupations to people with chronic mental illness now permeates mental health practice in most settings. It is probably accurate to state that occupational performance is a highly valued goal of treatment among all disciplines and in all settings—in acute psychiatric care, in home care, in outpatient care, in day care, and in halfway house care. Research in occupational therapy is being carried out on the occupational behavior of clients with depression (Neville-Jan, 1994) and on models of practice used by occupational therapy practitioners as they seek to describe the occupational functioning of their psychiatric clients (Muñoz, Lawlor, & Kielhofner, 1993). The role of work in the lives of people with mental illness has also been the focus of research, as difficulty in maintaining steady employment is viewed as one of the defining features of the illness (Scheid & Anderson, 1995; Sullivan, 1993). Successful vocational activity is most often described as central to community living and as a significant sign of being well.

Chronic physical disability, too, has an impact on a person's occupational life patterns and development. Periods of hospitalization or rehabilitation create interruptions in daily activities and atypical circumstances for occupational and psychosocial development. Neistadt and Marques (1984) described three levels of dysfunction in adults with multiple disabilities: adults with congenital disablement were called "psychosocially deprived"; those with disabilities beginning in adolescence were "psychosocially delayed"; and adults who first experienced their disability after career and family were established were "psychosocially disrupted." These authors described a program aimed at helping adults with disabilities at all three levels overcome deficits in daily-living competencies. The Independent Living Skills Training Program offered training in tasks such as banking, attendant care management, and personal health care for adults with diagnoses such as cerebral palsy, multiple sclerosis, and spina bifida. The persons taking part in the program gained competencies and confidence in their abilities.

As another example of a focus on physical dysfunction and adult development, Quigley (1995) studied the role experience of five women who had sustained traumatic spinal cord injuries in adulthood. Quigley focused on the period after rehabilitation when the women had all returned to community living. Findings revealed that, despite the obvious ramifications of the spinal cord injury, the participants occupied many different roles—both domestic and in the wider society. The women consistently used strategies of adaptation and negotiation to resume their occupations, such as redefining their roles, and adapting their surroundings, daily routines, and relationships. All of the women had developed a new role of self-advocate as they dealt with the barriers imposed by societal attitudes and architectural features. Quigley referred to the adaptation by the women as a process of "recomposing their lives"; the women "accomplished this feat by combining, amending, and contrasting their past lifestyles into their present and anticipatory roles" (p. 784). Quigley concludes that occupational therapy practitioners must assist people with disabilities to reestablish meaningful roles, that is, to reconstruct their lives and facilitate continuing life span development.

In summary, the lack of opportunities for occupational functioning that existed in the prior institutionalized health care system is now recognized as detrimental to an individual's development as a human being within society. Illness and disability are viewed as disruptions in a person's healthful life patterns, disruptions that need to be rectified. In occupational therapy and other health care disciplines, the emphasis has now shifted to teaching life skills and providing a safe environment in which to gradually regain prior occupations and develop new competencies and roles in society.

▼ CLIENT AND FAMILY NARRATIVE

Mr. Henry R. was an older man who had lived his entire life in the midwestern state of Wisconsin. He and his wife lived in a one-bedroom apartment in Madison, having sold their home when Mr. R. was 78 years old. Both a married son and a married daughter also lived in the city.

Mr. R. retired at age 66, after holding a variety of work positions, including those of tavern keeper and telephone lineman. All his life he had enjoyed participating in sports activities such as golfing, fishing, hunting, and bowling; for several years after retirement, his involvement in these activities continued and even increased. He was especially proud of his championship bowling record.

I came to know Mr. R. when I was the occupational therapist with an interdisciplinary geriatric home care program affiliated with the Veterans Administration Hospital in Madison. He was referred to the program when he was 81 years old. The primary medical reason for referral was for management of **rheumatoid arthritis (RA)**, which had been diagnosed when Mr. R. was 77 years old. Mr. R. had experienced persistent inflammation associated with the RA, leading to a daily life of pain, fatigue, and gradually increasing difficulty in carrying out his everyday activities. At the time of referral to home care, he had totally abandoned his previous sports activities, including his much loved bowling. Mr. R. stated that he had not stepped inside a bowling alley for 2 years.

On our early team visits to Mr. R., we learned that he spent his time primarily within the confines of his apartment, taking care of his personal needs, handling the financial aspects of the household, and assisting with some light housekeeping tasks. For leisure, he watched television, did some reading, and worked crossword puzzles. Socialization was limited largely to family visits (which were frequent) and home visits by the home care team. Mr. R. was the driver for himself and his wife for appointments and grocery shopping in the community, thus maintaining a role he had filled throughout their marriage.

Disease Progression

Over the course of the 2 years following referral to home care, Mr. R.'s RA continued to be active. Management efforts included medication trials and adjustments, adapted equipment, splinting, assistive mobility devices, training in joint protection principles, and activity modification. In spite of these carefully planned and monitored health care strategies, Mr. R.'s joint inflammation proliferated, involving his hand joints, wrists, shoulders, cervical vertebrae, knees, ankles, and feet. The persistent swelling from the inflammation began to weaken the periarticular structures of many of his joints. For example, the joint stress from simply using his thumb to push down the heat control lever in his car one winter day ruptured the tendon of his flexor pollicis longus muscle. The metacarpophalangeal joints of his right hand showed increasing ulnar deviation, aggravated by the pressure exerted during use of a cane for walking.

At some point in those 2 years, it became evident that Mr. R. was clinically depressed. His affect became increasingly "flat"; his interest in activities that were still within his capability waned; and he seemed mentally sluggish, giving slow and sometimes confused answers to questions. His wife reported having to prod him repeatedly to get up in the morning. Mr. R., himself, stated that he felt like he was "under a big blanket" for much of the day.

The long-term use of prednisone (a synthetic steroid and anti-inflammatory agent) led to several side effects, including cataracts and general susceptibility to infection. The cataracts affected Mr. R.'s vision to the extent that it was difficult for him to read or do crossword puzzles. The sudden appearance of an infection in his left great toe proved to be a significant turning point for Mr. R.; this situation will be described in some detail later in this narrative.

Influence on Life

The change in Mr. R.'s daily life and activity patterns during these 2 years was marked. His life space became almost totally limited to his apartment except when persuaded and assisted by his wife or children to go on an outing. His daily routine became more and more sedentary, with long periods of time spent just sitting without engagement in any accompanying activity such as watching television or reading. He gave up driving during this period, a decision that seemed necessary, but that obviously contributed to his diminished activity beyond the apartment.

Mrs. R. gradually began to assume responsibility for the financial aspects of their life, feeling defeated in her efforts to persuade "Dad" to continue to take care of these tasks, plus being somewhat concerned about his level of capability, having witnessed the episodes of confusion. His participation in chores around the apartment decreased to the single activity of helping with the dishes. When first referred to the home care team, Mr. R. had been independent in all basic self-care tasks; by the end of 2 years, he needed assistance with tub bathing, dressing, cutting up food, and going up and down stairs. He was still independent in shaving, toileting, transferring onto and off furniture such as the bed and his easy chair, and generally moving about the apartment.

Occupational Therapy

As the occupational therapist on the home care team, I was extensively involved with Mr. R. in his ongoing care. One of my primary responsibilities was to provide support for him as he tried to carry out his usual ADLs. In cooperation with the other members of the interdisciplinary team, I monitored Mr. R.'s functional level, documenting changes in function and planning therapeutic interventions with him and his wife to try to maximize his capabilities in everyday activities. This approach included regular systematic evaluations of his functional performance, combined with planning and carrying out interventions to maintain or increase Mr. R.'s independence.

Over the course of the 2 years, various pieces of adaptive equipment were provided to assist Mr. R. with his daily activities. These included bathing equipment (a bath bench, grab bar, and handheld shower hose), a long-handled shoe-horn and a shoelace adapter, a car door opener and car key holder, a large-handled knife to assist with cutting food, magnifiers for reading, and a medication dispenser to help Mr. R. keep track of his medication schedule. Additionally, Mr. R. was measured for and trained in the use of a cane to assist with walking, and subsequently, the cane handle was padded to reduce the stress to his hand as he used it.

Time was spent helping both Mr. and Mrs. R. gain understanding about the RA disease process and principles of joint protection. This included teaching ways to adapt activity to minimize stress to the joints, such as learning how to get in and out of his easy chair with minimal twisting of the knees. A commercially available resting splint for the right wrist was fitted to Mr. R. to support and reduce stress in those joints during activity. Additionally, a small splint was constructed to support the interphalangeal joint of the right thumb, enabling Mr. R. to continue to use the thumb in activities requiring light opposition in spite of the tendon rupture.

I made an effort to reintroduce some type of leisure sports activity into Mr. R.'s life because it had held such importance to him before the onset of RA arthritis. Initially, I tried to think of different ways that Mr. R. could continue involvement in bowling, such as being a score keeper or even just watching. These ideas were firmly rejected. Ultimately, I talked with him about a swimming program that was available and designed especially for people with arthritis. This idea appealed to him, and I made arrangements for him to attend. Several members of the home care team took turns accompanying him to the swim program once a week for a period of a few months.

Finally, I made a point to encourage Mr. R. to reminisce about his past achievements and experiences in his sporting activities. I had developed a monthly newsletter for the home care program, and each issue featured a story about one of the home care clients. It was easy and delightful to develop a feature story about Mr. R. and his bowling accomplishments. He and his wife searched and found the newspaper clippings, pictures, and trophies that documented Mr. R.'s achievements. They both contributed anecdotes about especially exciting tournaments and scores. I was able to write such details as "High score for a single game was 289 when Henry got nine strikes in a row, then pulled a spare and ended with a strike. He remembers that occasion well as the spectators gathered around in the tenth frame." A sense of accomplishment was strong for Mr. R. during the planning and preparation of the newsletter article; we were all pleased with the end result.

The Turning Point

During the third year of our involvement with Mr. R., a problem arose that seemed initially to be readily manageable, but that, instead, proved to be the trigger for a rapid deterioration in his health status. On one of our home vis-

its, Mr. R. complained of a very sore toe. On examination, the great toe on his left foot was indeed red and swollen around the toenail. After an unsuccessful trial with oral antibiotics, Mr. R. was hospitalized for 6 days for more vigorous treatment of the infection.

During the hospitalization, Mr. R. displayed significant and persistent confusion; I was taken aback one day when I visited him on the ward and found that he did not know who I was. His functional abilities and mobility had declined further so that he needed assistance with all self-care activities and primarily used a wheelchair to get around. After his return home, our efforts to help him regain his pre-hospitalization level of endurance and mobility were not successful, and his cognitive status remained marginal. We introduced a wheeled walker for moving about the apartment and attempted to instruct Mr. R. in its safe use. We arranged for a home health aide to come twice a week to help with bathing. Mr. R.'s days consisted of being helped with his personal care needs, resting, and watching a little television.

Within 3 weeks, it became obvious that the daily care that Mr. R. required was exhausting to both him and his wife. Mrs. R. and the family expressed deep concern about being able to continue to care for "Dad" at home. A meeting was arranged for the family and key members of the home care team to discuss the situation. The family tearfully proposed, and the health team members agreed, that nursing home placement was needed. Mr. R. moved to a nursing home 5 days after the meeting; he died just 2 months later.

From the standpoint of occupation and occupational health, Mr. R. had adapted his lifestyle after his retirement, substituting engagement in outdoor sports and home management activities for previous involvement in work. A few years after retirement, a health problem, in the form of RA, emerged and became a major disrupting factor in his occupational life. During his last few years, Mr. R. experienced a gradual shift from a daily balance of work, leisure, self-care, and rest, to an everyday existence consisting almost entirely of assisted self-care and rest. Through the use of adaptive equipment, modified activity, and new substitute activities, our health care team strove to help Mr. R. maintain a balance of occupation in his life for as long as possible during these years of decline.

▼ REFERENCES

American Occupational Therapy Association (AOTA). (1995). Position paper: Occupation. *American Journal of Occupational Therapy, 49*, 1015–1018.

Allen, K. R. & Chin-Sang, V. (1990). A lifetime of work: The context and meanings of leisure for aging black women. *Gerontologist, 30*, 737–740.

Atchley, R. C. (1989). A continuity theory of normal aging. *The Gerontologist, 29*, 183–190.

Benner, P. (1984). *From novice to expert: Excellence and power in clinical nursing practice.* Menlo Park, CA: Addison-Wesley.

Bateson, M. C. (1989). *Composing a life.* New York: Plume.

Belenky, M. F., Clinchy, B. M., Goldberger, N. R., & Tarule, J. M. (1986). *Women's ways of knowing.* New York: Basic Books.

Bruner, J. (1986). *Actual minds, possible worlds.* Cambridge, MA: Harvard University Press.

Christiansen, C. (1994). A social framework for understanding self-care interventions. In C. Christiansen (Ed.) *Ways of living: Self-care strategies for special needs* (pp. 3–26). Bethesda, MD: AOTA.

Dannefer, D. & Perlmutter, M. (1990). Development as a multidimensional process: Individual and social constituents. *Human Development, 33,* 108–137.

Dreyfus, S. E. & Dreyfus, H. L. (1980). A five-stage model of the mental activities involved in directed skill acquisition. Unpublished report, Air Force Office of Scientific Research, USAF (contract F49620–79–C-0063), University of California at Berkeley.

Erikson, E. H. (1959). Identity and the life cycle. *Psychological Issues, 1,* 1–171.

Friedlob, S. A., Janis, G. A., & Deets-Aron, C. (1986). A hospital-connected halfway house program for individuals with long-term neuropsychiatric disabilities. *American Journal of Occupational Therapy, 40,* 271–277.

Fulghum, R. (1986). *All I really need to know I learned in kindergarten: Uncommon thoughts on common things.* New York: Fawcett Columbine.

Gilligan, C. (1982). *In a different voice.* Boston: Harvard Press.

Havighurst, R. J. (1953). *Human development and education.* New York: D. McKay.

Havighurst, R. J. (1964). Youth in exploration and man emergent. In H. Borow (Ed.). *Man in a world of work.* Boston: Houghton Mifflin.

Henderson, K. A. (1990). The meaning of leisure for women: An integrative review of literature. *Journal of Leisure Research, 22,* 228–243.

Henderson, K. A., Bialeschki, M., Shaw, S., & Freysinger, V. (1989). *A leisure of one's own: A feminist perspective on women's issues.* State College, PA: Venture.

Kaluger, G. & Kaluger, M. F. (1984). *Human development: The span of life.* St. Louis: Times Mirror/Mosby.

Kaufman, S. R. (1986). *The ageless self: Sources of meaning in late life.* Madison, WI: University of Wisconsin Press.

Kelly, J. R. (Ed.). (1993). *Activity and aging.* Newbury Park, CA: Sage.

Kielhofner, G. (1981). An ethnographic study of deinstitutionalized adults: Their community settings and daily life experiences. *Occupational Therapy Journal of Research, 1,* 125–142.

Kleiber, D. A. & Kelly, J. R. (1980). Leisure, socialization, and the life cycle. In J. E. Iso-Ahola (Ed.), *Social psychological perspectives on leisure and recreation.* Springfield, IL: Charles C. Thomas.

Lerner, G. (1977). *The female experience.* New York: Oxford University Press.

Levin, L. S. & Idler, E. L. (1981). *The hidden health care system.* Cambridge: Bollinger.

Levinson, D. J. (1978). *The seasons of a man's life.* New York: Alfred A. Knopf.

Lowenthal, M. F., Thurnher, M., & Chiriboga, D. (1975). *Four stages of life: A psychosocial study of women and men facing transition.* San Francisco: Jossey-Bass.

Mattingly, C. (1991). The narrative nature of clinical reasoning. *American Journal of Occupational Therapy, 45,* 998–1005.

Muñoz, J. P., Lawlor, M., & Kielhofner, G. (1993). Use of the model of human occupation: A survey of therapists in psychiatric practice. *Occupational Therapy Journal of Research, 13,* 117–139.

Neistadt, M. (1987). An occupational therapy program for adults with developmental disabilities. *American Journal of Occupational Therapy, 41,* 433–438.

Neistadt, M. E. & Marques, K. (1984). An independent living skills training program. *American Journal of Occupational Therapy, 38,* 671–676.

Neugarten, B. L. (1977). Personality and aging. In J. E. Birren & K. W. Schaie (Eds.), *Handbook of the psychology of aging* (pp. 626–649). New York: Van Nostrand Reinhold.

Neville-Jan, A. (1994). The relationship of volition to adaptive occupational behavior among individuals with varying degrees of depression. *Occupational Therapy in Mental Health, 12*(4), 1–18.

Newman, B. M. & Newman, P. R. (1984). *Development through life: A psychosocial approach.* Homewood, IL: Dorsey Press.

Orem, D. E. (1980). *Nursing concepts of practice* (2nd ed.). New York: McGraw-Hill.

Polkinghorne, D. E. (1988). *Narrative knowing and the human sciences.* Albany, NY: SUNY Press.

Punwar, A. J. (1994). *Occupational therapy: Principles and practice* (2nd ed.). Baltimore: Williams & Wilkins.

Quigley, M. C. (1995). Impact of spinal cord injury on the life roles of women. *American Journal of Occupational Therapy, 49,* 780–786.

Raynes, N. V., Johnson, M., Sumpton, R. C., & Thorp, D. (1987). Comparison of the daily lives of four young adults who are mentally retarded. *Journal of Mental Deficiency Research, 31,* 303–310.

Reese, H. W. & Overton, W. F. (1970). Models of development and theories of development. In L. R. Goulet & P. B. Baltes (Eds.), *Lifespan developmental psychology: Research and theory* (pp. 115–145). New York: Academic.

Scheid, T. L. & Anderson, C. (1995). Living with chronic mental illness: Understanding the role of work. *Community Mental Health Journal, 31,* 163–176.

Scott-Maxwell, F. (1968). *The measure of my days.* New York: Penguin Books.

Segal, R. (1990). Helping older mentally retarded persons expand their socialization skills through the use of expressive therapies. *Activities, Adaptation, & Aging, 15,* 99–109.

Segall, A. (1987). Age differences in lay conceptions of health and self-care responses to illness. *Canadian Journal on Aging, 6,* 47–65.

Seltzer, G. B., Begun, A., Seltzer, M. M., & Krauss, M. W. (1991). Adults with mental retardation and their aging mothers: Impacts of siblings. *Family Relations, 40,* 310–317.

Seltzer, M. & Krauss, M. W. (1987). *Aging and mental retardation: Extending the continuum.* In M. J. Begab (Series Editor), Monographs of the American Association on Mental Retardation (p. 9). Washington DC: American Association on Mental Retardation.

Seltzer, M. M. & Krauss, M. W. (1989). Aging parents with mentally retarded children: Family risk factors and sources of support. *American Journal on Mental Retardation, 94,* 303–312.

Seltzer, M. M., Krauss, M. W., & Tsunematsu, N. (1993). Adults with Down Syndrome and their aging mothers: Diagnostic group differences. *American Journal on Mental Retardation, 97,* 464–508.

Sheehy, G. (1976). *Passages: Predictable crises of adult life.* New York: E. P. Dutton.

Sheehy, G. (1995). *New passages: Mapping your life across time.* New York: Random House.

Staff (1990). 1990 member data survey: Summary report. American Occupational Therapy Association.

Stancliff, B. (1996, March). OT practitioners work with more elderly patients. *OT Practice,* p. 17.

Sullivan, W. P. (1993). "It helps me to be a whole person": The role of spirituality among the mentally challenged. *Psychosocial Rehabilitation Journal, 16,* 125–134.

Vaillant, G. E. (1977). *Adaptation to life.* Boston: Little, Brown & Co.

Chapter 36

Adult Neurological Dysfunction

Karen Halliday Pulaski

Occupational therapists working with adults with neurological problems must understand clients' neurological dysfunction before beginning evaluation and treatment. The abilities to accurately evaluate clients with neurological deficits, define functional outcomes, and provide efficacious treatment are largely based on a therapist's understanding of how neuroanatomy and neuropathology relate to impairment and disability in functional activity. If a therapist does not understand the functional effect of a neurological deficit, as well as potential secondary problems that might arise, he or she will not be able to either individualize a clients' treatment or help clients set realistic short-term and **long-term goals** achievable within a set time frame.

With the change in the health care reform affecting the total amount of intervention time insurance companies will allow, it is imperative for therapists to be able to effectively and efficiently evaluate clients to help them achieve their highest level of functioning in the least restrictive environment.

A complete review of neuroanatomy and neurophysiology is beyond the scope of this chapter, but a brief review will be provided along with references at the end of the chapter. The main focus of this section is to provide a general overview of neuroanatomy as it relates to function, a description of various adult neurological diagnoses, and a description of "typical" deficits associated with those diagnoses. Prognosis and secondary complications will also be discussed. The occupational therapy interventions within specific settings will be described. Finally, some case examples will be provided to illustrate how specific neurological insults can affect function.

▼ CATEGORIZATION OF ADULT NEUROLOGICAL DYSFUNCTION

There are several ways to categorize or organize specific neurological dysfunction for the adult population: type of onset, upper motor neuron versus lower motor neuron, and hemisphere of lesion are just a few.

Onset

The onset of neurological events can be categorized as sudden and traumatic versus chronic or progressive. Sudden onset or traumatic events are viewed as those insults to the central nervous system (CNS) that occur suddenly or traumatically. Examples of this include **cerebral vascular accident (CVA)**, **traumatic brain injury**, **Guillain-Barré syndrome**, and **spinal cord injury**. Chronic or progressive neurological events are generally viewed as those insults that have a gradual onset during the adult phase (ie, they are not congenital) and may cause a progressive decline in the client's functional ability over time. Examples of this include **Parkinson's disease (PD)**, **amyotrophic lateral sclerosis (ALS)**, and **multiple sclerosis (MS)**. The sudden versus chronic category of neurological diagnosis will affect current and future occupational therapy intervention. For example, short-term treatment for a client with a sudden CVA accident might be focused on muscle reeducation and strengthening during self-care tasks to help the client become more self-sufficient. In contrast, treatment for a client with chronic and advanced MS might be focused on energy conservation and preparing for future wheelchair adaptations to allow the client to remain active in the community as his or her mobility declines.

Upper Versus Lower Motor Neuron

Another way to delineate neurological insults is to categorize them based on the location of the lesion (ie, injured tissue) in terms of upper motor neuron lesions versus lower motor neuron lesions. Upper motor neuron lesions are those lesions that occur within the brain or spinal cord motor tracts. Clients with lesions in upper motor neurons will experience a loss of voluntary muscle control and a loss of inhibition on reflexive movement causing hyperreflexia. This will result in spasticity or excess muscle tone in the affected muscle. Lower motor neuron lesions are those that occur within the cell bodies or axons of the peripheral nerves that innervate or synapse with the muscle fibers. The cell bodies of lower motor neurons are located in nuclei in the brainstem (cranial nerves) or in anterior horn cells of the spinal cord (spinal nerves); the axons are in the peripheral nerves. Clients with lower motor neuron lesions will also experience a loss of voluntary muscle control, but will experience loss of the reflex arc with a consequent decrease in muscle tone. The upper versus lower motor neuron categorization is useful for motor neuron diseases (Kiernan, 1987).

Localization of Lesion

A third way to organize information about neurological dysfunction is to understand how the location of the lesions within the CNS (brain and spinal cord) relates to impairments. It is important to realize first, however, that the function of the brain as a whole is greater than the sum of its parts. In other words, examining various areas of the brain to better understand how the brain functions and affects behavior is valuable, but yields an incomplete picture of how the brain works. Little is known about how the brain functions as a whole. Categorization by lesion site, therefore, is not perfect by any means, but can at least provide some direction to practitioners about the impairments they may be seeing during observations of functional activity. Table 36–1 organizes various diagnoses by site of lesion, type of onset, demographic information, etiology, and functional implications.

Various areas of the brain are involved in controlling different performance components that allow a client to function in different occupational performance areas. When observing a client engaged in a functional activity, such as activities of daily living (ADL), the therapist should be trying to establish hypotheses about why this client is unable to perform independently. Part of formulating these hypotheses is understanding what areas of the brain and what functions have been affected by the neurological event. One way to better understand this is to break the brain down into localized areas and delineate the functions of those areas.

FRONTAL LOBES

The frontal lobes are primarily responsible for executive cognitive functions (ie, ideation and concept formation, judgment, abstract thought, intellectual functions), personality, intention, and execution of voluntary motor function contralaterally (in the area of the precentral gyrus), voluntary eye movements, and programming of the motor component of speech. The frontal lobes are also related to the sequencing, timing, and organization of action and behavior, as well as the initiation and planning of action. These lobes also play a role in emotions.

PARIETAL LOBES

The parietal lobes are primarily involved in reception of somatic sensation (ie, fine touch, pain and temperature, proprioception, kinesthesia) and perception and interpretation

TABLE 36-1. Organization of Diagnoses by Various Factors

Diagnosis	Site of Lesion	Onset	Age Range	Etiologies	Implications
CVA	Brain	Sudden or traumatic	Any age but more common over 60	Embolic, thrombosis, hemorrhage	All performance areas can be affected. All performance components could be affected, dependent on specific location of lesion within the brain.
TBI	Brain	Sudden or traumatic	Any age but most common between 18 and 24 and over 70	Motor vehicle accidents, falls greater than one's own height, sports injuries, work-related injuries, and gunshot wounds.	All performance areas and all performance components could be affected, depending on location and type of injury
Parkinson's disease	Brain	Chronic or progressive	Generally between 50 and 69	Unknown etiology—theories of toxin exposure, sequelae to specific form of encephalitis.	All performance areas and all performance components could potentially be affected.
ALS	Brain and spinal cord	Chronic or progressive	Between 50 and 70	Unknown etiology—theories of toxins, hormonal imbalance, and autoimmune problems.	All performance areas could be affected. Neuromusculoskeletal, motor, temporal, and environmental components could be affected.
MS	Brain and spinal cord	Chronic or progressive	Between 20 and 40	Unknown etiology	All performance areas and all performance components could be affected, depending on site of the lesions.
SCI	Spinal cord	Sudden or traumatic	Any age but most common between 16 and 30	Motor vehicle accidents, falls, acts of violence and sports	All performance areas could be affected. Neuromusculoskeletal, sensory, motor, temporal, and environmental components could be affected.
GB	Peripheral nerves	Sudden or traumatic	Any age	Unknown etiology—theories of exposure to viral infections	All performance areas could be affected. Sensory, neuromusculoskeletal, motor, temporal, and environmental components could be affected.
MG	Myoneural junction	Chronic or progressive	Women generally between 20 and 30, males generally between 60 and 70	Unknown etiology—theories of disturbance in thymus and autoimmune system	All performance areas could be affected. Neuromusculoskeletal, motor, temporal, and environmental components could be affected.

of sensory information. These lobes are also involved in tactile localization and discrimination, as well as stereognosis. The parietal lobes assist with the recognition of tactile, visual, and auditory input. The parietal lobes store motor programs (praxis) as well as an appropriate body scheme and its relationship to the environment. These lobes are also responsible for the comprehension of language and pragmatics (the practical aspects of communication such as turn taking, eye contact, and nonverbal expression).

OCCIPITAL LOBES

The occipital lobes are primarily responsible for visual reception, and integration of visual information. They assist with the perception of visual spatial relationships and the formation of visual memory.

TEMPORAL LOBES

The temporal lobes are primarily involved in auditory reception and comprehension. They assist with the perception of sound and music. The temporal lobes are also responsible for memory, and the learning of visual and auditory patterns. Additionally, these lobes are related to emotions, motivation, and personality.

LIMBIC LOBES

The limbic lobes are intimately involved in emotion and memory through their connections to the medial aspects of the frontal and temporal lobes. The exact function of the limbic lobes is not well understood.

BRAIN STEM

The brain stem (midbrain, pons, and medulla) is responsible for controlling eye movements, facial movements, and spontaneous respiration. The brain stem also has input into the auditory nerve and thus can affect balance and equilibrium.

CEREBELLUM

The cerebellum is the center for controlled coordinated movements. It controls coordination by modulating the synaptic activity that produces movement. The cerebellum makes sure the muscles contract at the right time, with the right amount of force for the activity, to produce the right amount of movement. The cerebellum also is the "storehouse" for remembering motor programs. The cerebellum has direct connections to the vestibular nucleus (through the vestibulocerebellar pathways) and thus also influences balance.

SPINAL CORD

The spinal cord begins at the foramen magnum at the base of the skull and continues to the lower border of the first lumbar vertebrae. Muscle movement (contraction) and sensation are controlled by mixed nerves: efferent fibers control muscle movement and afferent fibers control sensation. These mixed nerves carry the "messages" from the brain to the muscles and also carry sensory information back up to the brain. Efferent myelinated axons synapse with skeletal muscle fibers to produce movement. Axons located medially in the spinal cord control axial muscles, and axons located laterally in the spinal cord control appendicular movement. Afferent sensory axons are both ascending and descending and allow information to flow from the brain to the muscles as well as from the muscles back up to the brain to permit refinement in movement. There are also several spinal reflexes that can be inhibited or facilitated in a mature human to permit purposeful movement. Movement is controlled ipsilaterally in the spinal cord (Arnodottir, 1990; Kiernan, 1987).

Hemisphere of Lesion

Brain functions can also be categorized hemispherically. The left hemisphere of the brain is generally responsible for movement of the right side, processing of sensory information from the right side, perception of the right visual fields, visual and verbal processing, bilateral motor planning or programs (praxis), verbal memory, auditory reception, speech, and processing of verbal auditory information. The right hemisphere is generally responsible for movement of the left side, processing of sensory information from predominantly the left side, left visual fields, visual spatial processing, contralateral motor planning (praxis), nonverbal memory, bilateral auditory reception, processing of pragmatics (nonverbal language), and attention to incoming stimulation and emotion (Adams & Victor, 1989; Arnadottir, 1990; Gilroy, 1990; Kiernan, 1987).

A spinal cord injury is one example of how one might use neuroanatomy functionally to understand the lesions by location. A spinal cord injury will cause sensory or motor impairments, but will not cause cognitive or perceptual impairments. Another example is a left hemisphere CVA. This lesion will cause right, not left hemiplegia. Further use of this classification for improved understanding of impairments will be discussed as it relates to specific neurological diagnoses. I recommend the reader further review a more comprehensive neuroanatomy and neurophysiology review (see references at end of this chapter).

▼ RECOVERY OF FUNCTION

It is possible for many clients with neurological dysfunction to improve their abilities to perform functional activities either through recovery of uninjured neurological tissue or through learning how to compensate for lost neurological function. The amount of recovery will depend on several factors: site of the lesion, size of the lesion, age, and general health of the client.

Relative to the site of the lesion, some recovery of neurological function is possible with brain and peripheral nerve lesions, but not with spinal cord lesions. With brain lesions, recovery of neurological function may be secondary to (1) the brain's ability to use uninjured areas to assume function of injured areas, or (2) the ability of uninjured brain neurons to grow new axonal branches and form new synapses with other intact neurons (Neistadt, 1994). With peripheral nerves injuries, recovery of function is linked to the capacity of peripheral axons to regenerate (Gilroy, 1990).

Relative to size of lesion, larger lesions may cause more damage and will have worse prognoses for recovery than smaller lesions. Older adults or those with poor overall health generally have a poorer prognosis for recovery than younger adults or those in good health (Neistadt, 1994). Occupational therapists need to be aware of the recovery potential of adults with neurological injuries during evaluation and treatment.

▼ OCCUPATIONAL THERAPY EVALUATION AND TREATMENT

Record Review

A complete review of available medical and psychosocial records is a good starting place for an evaluation. One must be very careful not to form a "fixed" picture of the client's functioning based on records, however. Therapists should remain neutral in their clinical impressions of clients until they have the opportunity to complete a thorough evaluation. The medical records can provide therapists with (1) a history of the client's premorbid health problems, (2) a neurological diagnosis, (3) information on the location(s) of the lesion, (4) information on any secondary complications, (5) information on medical precautions and contraindications, (6) a review of the course of the most recent neurological event, (7) a list of medications the client may be taking, (8) psychosocial information and (9) a summary of the client's current life roles and ability to function within those roles. Any information obtained from a client record should always be verified with the client or a significant other if the client can not communicate or has severe cognitive deficits. No information about the client's ability to function should be simply transferred from the medical record onto an evaluation form. A therapist is always responsible for evaluating the client's current level of functioning.

Client Interview and Goal Setting

The next step in evaluation is a client interview. It is essential for therapists to form therapeutic relationships with clients and allow clients to relate, in their own words, what their medical experiences have been like for them. The client interview should focus on the client's understanding of the neurological diagnosis, the client's description of his or her strengths and weaknesses, and the client's goals for rehabilitation. It is important to keep in mind that goal setting may vary depending upon the type of setting in which a client is receiving treatment. A client who is in the acute care or inpatient rehabilitation phase following a CVA may be unable to provide specific goals and may need assistance from the therapist to determine these goals. This same client may be very self-directed by the time he or she reaches outpatient rehabilitation. It is also appropriate and important to involve the client's family or significant other—with the permission of the client if possible—as soon as possible. The family and significant others can be a great resource for further information as well as a resource if the client is unable to provide information for him- or herself.

Therapists must remember that they are not "doing therapy to" a client, but are attempting to form a partnership with the client in order to help the client reach his or her goals. If a client was receiving assistance with dressing before the new neurological event and chooses to continue to receive assistance, then independent dressing goals are not appropriate. It is important that the goals are established with the client, rather than for the client.

Evaluation of Occupational Performance Areas

The evaluation should then proceed to occupational performance areas, ie, ADLs, work and productive activities, and play and leisure (see Chap. 15 for details about evaluations of occupational performance areas). The areas a therapist will evaluate are often determined by the level of recovery a client has reached, as well as by the type of setting in which a therapist practices. An inpatient rehabilitation therapist working with a client who was undergone a new exacerbation of MS may focus on bathing, dressing, transfers, and some light homemaking. A therapist working in an outpatient or home health setting with this same client 4 weeks later may be focusing on work and productive activities (such as full homemaking), advanced ADLs (such as banking and adapted driving), and leisure activities. It is important to keep in mind that many third-party payers will not reimburse for leisure activities because they do not (1) see leisure as a necessity, (2) understand the component skill training that can be accomplished with these activities, or (3) understand the health maintenance benefit of helping people to remain engaged in active lifestyles. Therefore, with leisure activities in particular, occupational therapists need to emphasize the component skill training and time management issues to educate third-party payers about the benefits of these activities.

It is crucial for therapists to have a very clear understanding of their role within a particular setting to maximize a client's benefit from an inpatient rehabilitation stay or a certain number of visits to an outpatient clinic. The overall goal of all therapeutic intervention should be to assist the client to function as independently as possible in the least restrictive environment. An inpatient therapist should be focused on those occupational performance areas, such as mobility and self-care, that affect if and when a client can be discharged from an inpatient setting. An outpatient or group home therapist should be focused on those occupational performance activities, such as homemaking and budgeting, that will enable a client to live as independently as possible in the community. Table 36–2 highlights the focus of treatment based on the setting in which occupational therapy is provided. Failure of therapists to recognize their role within the continuum of care may result in situations where clients must live in more restrictive environments in more dependent lifestyles, such as extended care facilities versus home settings.

Therapists should have a written form for evaluation that reflects the diagnoses as well as the type of setting. For example, an orthopedic evaluation form should be different from a neurological evaluation form, just as a home health form should be different from an acute care one. The occupational therapy evaluations should always focus on occupational performance areas whenever possible, with spaces for evaluation of performance components to reflect a therapist's hypotheses about component deficits. It may be difficult to always start with occupational performance areas (eg, in acute care if a client is medically compromised or if a client with a head injury is in the low-arousal stage of recovery).

TABLE 36-2. Evaluation and Treatment: Focus Throughout the Continuum of Care

Acute Care	Inpatient Rehabilitation	Outpatient/Home Health	Extended Care Centers
Clients are generally not medically stable. Major focus of OT intervention is on evaluation and input for determination of the next most appropriate level of care (ie, inpatient rehabilitation, home with follow-up services, extended care). Those clients who will be going directly home from acute care are priority clients. Treatment for those patients going home often focuses on client and family education, as well as treatment of those activities that client must be able to do (usually with assistance) to go home, such as self-care and basic mobility. Treatment for those patients not going home generally focuses on addressing those performance areas and components that will affect function.	Clients are generally transferred as soon as they are medically stable and can tolerate intensive rehabilitation (usually 3 hrs minimum per day). Focus is to evaluate and assist the client with those performance areas necessary to move on to the next level of care (ie, home) as soon as possible. Good evaluation of the home environment and supports is crucial. Treatment is focused on areas such as bathing, dressing, toileting, eating, functional mobility and light homemaking if necessary. Clients are discharged when they are able to manage safely at home with supports in place. Clients generally require some assistance at home for above activities.	Clients and therapists must work very closely together to establish the specific goals of what activities the client wishes to resume and the purpose of therapy. Treatment may still be focused on ADL performance areas, because many clients are discharged home requiring assistance for these activities. Treatment should also focus on community reintegration, work and productive activities, and play and leisure activities. Home programs should be extremely functionally oriented and the client or family must assume a great deal of responsibility for carrying out the home program and for incorporating what is gained in therapy into everyday life.	Clients are often referred from acute care to an extended care facility if they are not able to tolerate an intensive rehabilitation program, but have the end goal of returning home. Clients may go directly home from this setting or may gain enough strength to be admitted to an inpatient rehabilitation program with eventual discharge home. Focus of treatment is often the same as inpatient rehabilitation, but is provided at a less intensive level. Treatment may also be provided to those long-term residents who have a change in medical status resulting in a decline in ability to function more independently. Treatment would focus on those areas that have been affected by the decline.

Evaluation of Performance Components

During the evaluation of occupational performance areas, the therapist should begin to observe what a client can and cannot complete. The therapist should also begin to observe what performance components may be impaired that prevent a client from completing a performance area. The therapist should then evaluate specific performance components to determine if his or her observations are correct (see Chap. 16 for details about performance component evaluations). The therapist should also use information about the location of the lesion to support his or her observations. It may be difficult to determine exactly why a client is having difficulties completing a task until a therapist can evaluate performance components. By completing an evaluation in this manner, a therapist is also able to observe what strengths and strategies a client may use to compensate for impairments in other performance components.

An example of this evaluation sequence is as follows: A 19-year-old young woman, whose diagnosis is Guillain-Barré syndrome, is seen by an occupational therapist to evaluate homemaking in the client's home. The client has chosen to make a simple meal consisting of baked chicken, a baked potato, and peas. The therapist observes that the client is able to organize the activity and plan the menu. The therapist also notes that the client has difficulty carrying objects within the kitchen, lifting heavy pans, using both upper extremities at the same time (eg, when washing the potato at the sink or opening the package of peas), and maintaining her balance throughout the activity. The therapist may hypothesize that this client has decreased strength in her upper extremities, decreased balance caused by poor trunk control and decreased lower extremity strength, and possible sensory impairments. The therapist would then want to specifically evaluate range of motion (ROM), strength, coordination, and sensation to determine if her hypotheses are correct. The treatment plan would evolve from determining what specific performance components were impaired.

Special Considerations

Many things may impede a therapist's ability to evaluate occupational performance areas or performance components with the neurologically involved client. These may include medical complications, such as uncontrolled blood pressure or seizures; premorbid conditions, such as myocardial infarcts or other disease processes; and current restrictions placed on the client, such as weight-bearing restrictions for a fractured extremity. Clients may also demonstrate behavioral manifestations of the neurological event that interfere with evaluation, such as lethargy, agitation, inattention, or **perseverations**. There may be language deficits, such as an **aphasia**, that make it impossible for clients to provide information or understand the therapist's requests for activities. There may also be perceptual or motor complications, such as a left neglect, a **hemianopsia**, or a premorbid amputation that make evaluation more difficult. Therapists must find a way to modify their evaluations to gain an accurate picture of what the client can and cannot do. A therapist may need to use gestures and the context of a task to accurately evaluate a client with aphasia. The therapist may need to schedule their sessions in the morning, when the client is more alert or less agitated, or to see the client in frequent short treatment sessions, rather than one long treatment session. Any modification made to the "standard" evaluation process should be clearly documented.

Treatment should evolve out of a therapist's evaluation of performance areas and performance components, as well as from the client's input in terms of goals, future performance contexts, and treatment activities. Specific occupational therapy intervention will be discussed within the context of specific diagnoses.

▼ CEREBRAL VASCULAR ACCIDENT (CVA)

Definition, Etiology and Demographics

CVA or cerebral vascular disease (CVD) can be defined as a vascular insult that causes a lesion to the brain resulting in neurological deficits. It is commonly referred to as a stroke or a "shock" because of its sudden onset. A CVA is characterized by an interruption of blood flow to a specific area of the brain, resulting in brain damage due to lack of oxygen. There are many etiologies that cause this interruption but the most common ones are thrombosis, embolism, or hemorrhage.

A thrombosis is a blood clot that forms somewhere in the vascular system and causes a block in the blood supply. In a CVA, the thrombosis occurs somewhere in a cerebral vessel. An embolus is a thrombosis that is formed somewhere else in the vascular system, often the heart, that breaks free and travels to a cerebral vessel, where it becomes lodged and interrupts blood flow. This blockage or interruption causes ischemia or lack of nutrients and oxygen essential to maintaining viable brain tissue. A hemorrhage is a rupturing in the vessel wall causing the vessel to "bleed out" intercerebrally or into the subarachnoid space. This causes pressure on the surrounding tissue and also causes interruption of blood supply to the brain tissue. All three etiologies result in brain damage.

Some clients may experience a transient ischemic attack (or TIA) in which they will experience neurological disturbances similar to a CVA. These disturbances resolve within a short time, usually 24 to 48 hours. A TIA is often a warning or precursor to a CVA.

There are numerous factors that can contribute to CVA. Some of the most common ones include hypertension, obesity, age, diet, sedentary lifestyle, diabetes, and history of vascular disorders and myocardial infarcts. Those clients who have experienced a CVA once are often at higher risk for another one.

In addition to being categorized by etiology, CVA can be categorized by the major cerebral vessel that is occluded. There are six major vessels that may be used as descriptors for diagnosis. They include the internal carotid artery (ICA), the anterior cerebral artery (ACA), the middle cerebral artery (MCA), the posterior cerebral artery (PCA), the basilar artery, and the cerebellar branch. Each of these arteries, along with numerous ancillary arteries, feed various parts of the brain.

The specific effects of brain artery occlusions vary depending on the hemisphere affected. In general, occlusions or hemorrhages of the (1) ICA can result in contralateral hemiplegia, sensory problems, aphasia (usually left hemisphere), and hemianopsia; (2) ACA can result in contralateral hemiplegia, cognitive deficits, sensory deficits, and aphasia (usually left hemisphere); (3) MCA can result in contralateral hemiplegia (primarily the upper extremity), contralateral hemianopsia, sensory deficits, and language deficits; (4) PCA can result in contralateral hemiplegia, ataxia, visual deficits including field cuts, cortical blindness, and normal pursuit eye movements; (5) basilar artery can result in double vision, facial paralysis, visual deficits, and balance or vestibular disturbances; and (6) cerebellar artery can result in vertigo, difficulties in swallowing, ipsilateral ataxia, and changes in sensation (Arnadotiir, 1990; Kiernan, 1987; Wall, 1982).

A CVA is more common in older adults who may have a history of the foregoing risk factors. However, a CVA can strike any age group from newborn up through old age.

Deficits

Lesions from CVA are focal, that is, they are localized in one specific area—the area supplied by the affected blood vessel—and the resulting impairments are directly related to that area of the brain. Common impairments include hemiplegia (on the contralateral side of the lesion), sensory impairment, cognitive disturbances, motor impairments, language impairments, and visual perceptual impairments. Sensory performance component deficits may include impairments of tactile, pain and temperature, proprioception, and kinesthesia. Cognitive component disturbances may include deficits in attention, organization, sequencing, concentration, problem solving, judgment, and safety. Motor component impairments may include changes in tone, disruption of active movement, and apraxia.

Clients may experience language deficits, called aphasias, that may interfere with receptive or expressive language, understanding of pragmatic or nonverbal language, and written expression. Visual component deficits may include visual field cuts, visual field inattention, double vision, problems in scanning or difficulty with depth perception, and figure-ground perception. Clients may also display changes in behavior or personality as well as changes in their affect. These performance component deficits may limit clients' abilities to perform some or all of their ADLs, work and productive, and play and leisure activities (Wall, 1982).

Prognosis

There are many indicators neurologists use to suggest the prognosis for a client with CVA. Indicators include the location of the lesion, the size of the lesion, and the age of the client. The neurologist also takes into account the client's prior health history as well as the course of initial recovery the client exhibits, within the first 72 hours as well as within the first 2 weeks (US Department of Health and Human Services, 1995).

Secondary Complications

The course of recovery varies from client to client depending upon the location of the CVA and the severity. Secondary factors can also affect prognosis. They include edema or swelling within the brain, extensions of the original CVA, or vasospasms that can occur in the vessels surrounding the initial CVA. Clients may also have other medical complications, including pneumonia, uncontrolled diabetes, and cardiac disturbances.

Initial symptoms of oncoming CVA may include incoordination in an extremity, changes in sensation or "tingling" in an extremity or the face, slurred speech, difficulty swallowing, balance disturbances, visual or cognitive disturbances, or severe headache (Fisher, 1995). A CVA may take as long as 48 hours to fully evolve, and clients may eventually become unconscious or unresponsive if the CVA is severe enough.

Stages of Recovery and Occupational Therapy Evaluation and Treatment

Evaluation should begin with performance areas if possible. If a client has suffered a more severe CVA, the acute care therapist may need to begin the evaluation focused on performance components that may eventually affect performance areas. Evaluation at this stage may focus on sensory processing, ROM (both passive and active), tone, and cognitive and perceptual skills. If a client is able to engage in activity, the evaluation should begin with basic performance areas, including self-care activities and basic mobility within functional tasks, such as getting out of bed. Many clients will also experience difficulties with swallowing or dysphagia, and this should be evaluated as soon as possible to pre-

vent possible aspiration. Dysphagia or swallowing evaluations are often performed by both the speech therapist and the occupational therapist.

Clients are generally transferred from acute care to inpatient rehabilitation once they are medically stable and able to participate in intensive rehabilitation. Evaluation at this point should always begin with occupational performance areas that will directly affect the client's ability to return to the community. These areas include (1) self-care activities, such as bathing and dressing, toileting, grooming, and eating; (2) mobility within the context of activity, such as bed, toilet, and tub transfers; and occasionally, (3) homemaking activities, such as meal preparation, laundry, and light housekeeping. The therapist should create hypotheses about why a client is unable to complete a task (ie, hemiplegia, poor trunk control, impaired balance, difficulties with attention, organization and sequencing, or disturbances in visual perception). These hypotheses should then be substantiated by specific evaluation of performance components. The hypotheses should be based on observation and understanding of the neurological basis of impairment. Treatment should focus on improving the areas of impairment to enable a client to perform the various activities he or she must be able to do more independently for a transition into the community.

Once a client is able to make a transition back into the community, the outpatient or home health practitioner will generally focus on ADLs, work and productive activities, and play and leisure activities both within the home and within the community. Attention should be given to the role that the client plays within his or her family context and social network. Evaluation should focus on those activities the client values and is unable to complete, with further evaluation of the impairments that prevent function. Treatment should focus on assisting the client in being able to perform those valued activities within his or her social network, home, and community.

Client and family education is an integral part of the rehabilitation process from the beginning. It is crucial that families and clients understand the changes that have occurred and what the process of rehabilitation can offer. Clients and families may need to receive the same information repeatedly to make sense of all the changes they are experiencing. The earlier families can become involved with the care of a loved one, the easier it is for them to comprehend and become a part of the process. Practitioners can facilitate this by educating families about the causes and sequelae of CVA, as well as about specific interventions families may be able to provide to a loved one, such as ROM, interaction with clients who suffer language deficits, or stimulation for clients with left inattention or neglect. Education should be ongoing in all rehabilitation settings, and families and clients should be made aware of outside opportunities for education and support such as stroke clubs.

CASE STUDY

L J, a 72-year-old retired male, fell one morning getting out of bed. He was brought to the emergency room by his wife. He complained of weakness in his right arm and leg, disturbances in his balance, and problems with his vision. A computed tomography (CT) scan showed a lesion in the left posterior cerebral artery. LJ was admitted to the acute care hospital, but transferred 36 hours later to an inpatient rehabilitation center.

On evaluation in the rehabilitation center, LJ required assistance for all functional tasks, including bathing and dressing, transfers, and simple home-making tasks. The therapist observed that he had difficulty maintaining his balance, using his right upper extremity, and locating objects. The therapist hypothesized that he was experiencing contralateral hemiplegia and ataxia that were affecting his balance and ability to use his right upper extremity; and a right hemianopsia that was affecting his visual abilities in locating items during functional activity. She tested this hypothesis by further evaluating the client's active ROM, muscle strength, coordination, and visual fields.

Treatment focused on improving strength and ROM, improving coordination, and teaching the client compensatory strategies for the hemianopsia. Treatment was provided through functional activities, including bathing and dressing, grooming, homemaking, and leisure activities.

▼ TRAUMATIC BRAIN INJURY

Definition, Etiology, and Demographics

Traumatic brain injury can be defined as any injury resulting from a traumatic event that causes direct or indirect damage to the brain. The most common causes of traumatic brain injury are high-speed motor vehicle accidents (often involving alcohol, drugs, or both) and falls from heights greater than that of the person. Other common causes include sports injuries, injuries resulting from violence, gunshot wounds, and work-related injuries.

Traumatic brain injuries are generally categorized into two different types, based primarily on their etiology. A focal contusion is a bruising of the brain as a result of a direct blow to the head. This can occur, for example, from a fight or sports injury. Diffuse axonal damage is damage resulting from twisting, tearing, or stretching of the axons of the nerve fibers throughout the brain. This primarily occurs because of velocity when the brain and body are moving forward at a certain speed and are suddenly stopped short. This causes the brain to bounce back and forth within the skull, leading to diffuse damage. These may also be called shearing injuries. This type of injury can occur in a motor vehicle accident or a fall from greater than one's own height. Some clients may suffer both focal contusions as well as diffuse axonal damage, as in a motor vehicle accident when a client may hit his head on the windshield (focal), but also suffer damage from the impact of velocity (diffuse). Focal contusions are visible on specialized-imaging studies called magnetic resonance imaging (MRI) and on CT scans, once the bruising or lesion has formed. Diffuse axonal damage is not visible on imaging studies and is generally diagnosed through medical history and evaluation of the client's behavior. Factors that suggest diffuse axonal damage include causes of injury that involve velocity, loss of consciousness, and cortical posturing (specific body tonal postures that occur as a direct result of severe injury).

The most "common" profile of a person with a head injury is generally young (ages 15 to 24) and male, with a history of high-risk behaviors (Winkler, 1995). The second most common profile is an elderly person (over 70) with either balance or cognitive difficulties, whose injury results from a fall within the home. Obviously these are merely profiles and there are many survivors of traumatic brain injury who do not fit either profile.

Deficits

Traumatic brain injury affects all performance areas including ADLs, work and productive activities, and play and leisure activities. Clients can experience impairments in every performance component because of the nature of traumatic brain injury. Clients often have motor disturbances with abnormal tone resulting in hemiplegia, paraplegia, triplegia, or quadriplegia. They may have restricted ROM, poor postural control, and poor motor control. Often, clients experience sensory disturbances. They may also suffer from cognitive impairments in level of arousal, orientation, attention, memory, sequencing, and organizing. They may be unable to problem solve effectively or to learn new information. Clients often display visual perceptual deficits and may have problems with spatial relations, position in space, figure-ground, and depth perception. Many clients have language deficits that interfere with their abilities for self-expression and socialization. Oftentimes, clients have a great deal of difficulty controlling their emotions and can easily become overwhelmed (Winkler, 1995).

Specific impairments in performance components are directly related to the location of the lesion(s). If a client suffers unilateral or bilateral frontal contusions, he or she may not experience any motor or sensory deficits at all, but may have significant problems in cognitive, psychological, and social performance components. If the client suffers significant diffuse axonal damage he or she may have deficits in performance areas because of impairments in all of the performance components. It is the therapist's job to determine what performance areas are affected, develop hypotheses based on the neurological diagnosis as well as observation about what performance components are affected, and then substantiate these hypotheses with thorough evaluation. Treatment should consist of using functional activity to address both performance areas and performance components that may be affected by the traumatic brain injury.

Prognosis

Prognosis for individuals who suffer traumatic brain injury is dependent on several things. Neurologists usually evaluate the client's age, the size and location of the injury, the type of injury, the level of consciousness at the time of injury, and the length of coma if loss of consciousness occurs. The Glascow Coma Scale is a scale generally used at the scene of the accident and frequently thereafter to monitor a client's level of consciousness. Prognostic indicators that support a favorable outcome include a young age, a small lesion in a noncritical part of the brain, focal rather than diffuse injury, and a short episode of loss of consciousness (ie, less than 1 day) (Katz, 1992).

Secondary Complications

Secondary complications that can arise will also affect prognosis. These include edema or swelling of the brain (which can increase the pressure on the brain and, therefore, cause more damage), hygromas (collections of cerebral spinal fluid that pool due to a tearing of the membranes that surround the brain), hematomas (a collection or pooling of blood that can increase intercranial pressure), or infections of the brain or of the membranes that surround the brain. Intercranial pressure caused by any of these can often be monitored and controlled by medications as well as by pumping mechanisms or surgery to remove the fluid and reduce the pressure. Another secondary complication that can occur is anoxia or loss of oxygen to the brain. This may be caused from bleeding, a severe drop in blood pressure, or respiratory failure. All of these secondary complications can cause fur-

ther damage to the brain; therefore, they have a direct influence on prognosis.

Stages of Recovery and Occupational Therapy Evaluation and Treatment

There are many different descriptions about the stages of recovery through which clients with traumatic head injury may pass. Most descriptions center around the client's cognitive status as an indicator for recovery. It is important to remember that not all clients will experience all stages and that clients can become "fixed" in any stage along the road of recovery. It is also important to remember the stages are merely descriptions and that some clients at various points in their recovery will exhibit characteristics of more than one stage.

In general, clients will initially suffer a loss of consciousness, during which they may not respond to any stimulus at all. Often clients at this stage require a **tracheostomy** as well as a ventilator to assist them in respiration. Clients at this stage of recovery receive their nutrition through a feeding tube (either a nasal gastric or gastric tube) and are obviously dependent for all care. They may experience changes in their muscle tone (either hypotonic or hypertonic), which may limit their ROM. An occupational therapist who works with clients at this stage of recovery (acute care) will not be able to begin his or her evaluations focusing on occupational performance areas, but will need to evaluate performance components such as neuromusculoskeletal that may affect future performance areas. Therapists will also want to provide controlled stimulation and an opportunity for purposeful response to stimuli such as deep touch, pain, light touch, gustatory, olfactory, visual, and kinesthetic stimulation. The purpose of sensory stimulation is not to "speed up" a client's recovery, but rather, to determine when a client makes a transition from coma level to a low-arousal level. Treatment at this stage often focuses on preserving ROM, tone management, providing opportunities for purposeful response, positioning for skin and respiratory preservation, and family education.

The next, low-arousal level is generally characterized by spontaneous eye movement, visual tracking of objects or people in the room for very brief periods (2 to 3 seconds), and some type of purposeful response to stimulation, such as eye opening to auditory stimulation or withdrawal from painful stimulation. Therapists who provide evaluation and treatment at this stage of recovery (acute or inpatient rehabilitation) will continue to monitor musculoskeletal, cognitive, and sensory performance components, but will also begin to try to elicit even more purposeful response, especially in terms of following one-step commands or spontaneously attempting basic performance areas; for example, washing one's face or combing one's hair, within a structured context. Practitioners should provide treatment in a quiet environment and keep verbalizations to a minimum. Tasks can be introduced through objects, such as handing the client the wash cloth or comb and pairing it with a simple one-step command. Evaluation and treatment can be graded up depending on the client's ability to arouse, attend, and participate. The client who begins to follow one-step commands with any consistency is usually transitioning to a **posttraumatic amnesia** state.

Clients in the posttraumatic amnesia (PTA) stage usually experience a state of confusion or disorientation, with no awareness of time or place. Clients at this stage have extremely impaired attentional skills and an inability to form memories secondary to severe inattention. Clients may be agitated and restless, or lethargic. They may exhibit uninhibited behaviors, such as using inappropriate language. Therapists working with clients in this stage (usually inpatient rehabilitation) will want to begin to evaluate what performance areas clients can accomplish, how much assistance they need, and why they require assistance. The performance area evaluated may be determined by how confused the client is, and the tasks may need to be broken down into smaller tasks, such as combing one's hair, instead of full bathing and dressing. Although clients in this stage cannot form memories as we know them, they are often able to relearn commonly performed tasks such as bathing and dressing, through a process known as procedural learning or procedural memory (Giles & Shore, 1989; Miller,

1980). Therapy focuses on basic performance areas, including mobility, as well as basic play and leisure skills. Treatment also focuses on evaluating and improving those performance components, such as ROM, that may prevent a client from being able to complete these tasks. The length of this stage is often directly related to the length of the client's coma stage; that is, the longer the coma, the longer the period of posttraumatic amnesia. As clients become less confused, they move into a postconfusional state.

Clients in a postconfusional state may demonstrate impairments in higher-level attention and concentration, as well as impairments in memory. Clients at this stage may still be agitated or disinhibited, with an inability to control frustration or anger. They may also have the opposite problem, displaying difficulty initiating activity or interaction, and showing little or no affect. Most higher-level cognitive skills, such as reasoning, concentration, problem solving, safety, and judgment, are also usually impaired. Practitioners who provide intervention at this stage of recovery (inpatient rehabilitation or outpatient or home health) will focus on more advanced ADLs, both in the home and in the community, work and productive activities, and play and leisure. Clients will make the transition to outpatient or home health therapies when they can safely return to community living with existing supports: family, sitters, or group homes.

CASE STUDY

TR, a 17-year-old senior in high school, was involved in a high-speed motor vehicle accident. He was the driver and collided head-on with another vehicle. The passenger in his car was killed instantly. At the scene, TR was unconscious and unresponsive, even to painful stimulation. His respiration was labored, and his blood pressure was dropping. He was intubated at the scene and rushed to the hospital emergency room. A CT scan showed multiple contusions in both frontal lobes, as well as in the right fronto parietal-temporal region. He was later placed on a ventilator to assist his breathing.

During his intensive care stay, TR suffered from intracranial pressure, secondary to edema and multiple infections. He first showed signs of arousal—spontaneous eye opening and tracking people in his room—27 days after the accident, and followed his first command 35 days after injury.

He was transferred to inpatient rehabilitation, where he presented with poor attention, agitated behavior, and left hemiplegia. He required assistance with self-care activities, mobility, and play and

leisure activities. His ability gradually improved during his inpatient stay, so that he could complete basic self-care and was able to participate in work and productive, as well as play and leisure activities.

When he made the transition to outpatient therapies, he was independent in basic selfcare, and able to initiate and participate in other activities with minimal assistance. He continued to experience difficulties with higher-level cognitive functions, such as concentration, judgment, and problem solving, and had diminished use of his left upper extremity.

Currently TR is in outpatient therapies. He becomes easily frustrated and states he feels as if "life has gone on without him." Many of his friends have gone to college or are working. The outpatient therapist is helping TR to set realistic goals in terms of education and vocation, as well as advanced ADLs home and within the community, such as cooking, shopping, and banking. She is also working with TR to improve the functional use of his left upper extremity. TR is involved in many groups at outpatient therapy to help him reestablish leisure interests and a social network.

Many clients experience depression and isolation because of the change in their abilities to independently manage occupational performance areas and function in previous life roles as family members, workers, and friends. Traumatic brain injury severely interrupts clients' place in their life phases, whether that be a senior in high school preparing for college, or a wife who has two children at home and an active career.

▼ PARKINSON'S DISEASE (PD)

Definition, Etiology, and Demographics

PD is a progressive degenerative disease, characterized by the degeneration of dopaminergic neurons in the substantia nigra, deep in the brain (Gersten, 1990). Dopamine is an inhibitory neurotransmitter that greatly affects motor control. Clients with PD experience a reduction of available dopamine within their CNS. This causes an imbalance between the inhibitory and the excitatory effects of the neurotransmitters used for motor control. The exact etiology of PD is usually unknown, although it can be caused in a few by toxic poisons, or as sequelae to a specific form of encephalitis.

Deficits

Performance areas that can be affected by PD include ADLs, work and productive areas, and play and leisure activities. Performance components that may be impaired include (1) sensory, including vestibular and perceptual processing; (2) neuromusculoskeletal, such as ROM, reflexes, muscle tone, strength, endurance, postural control and alignment, and soft-tissue integrity; (3) motor, such as gross and fine coordination, motor control, oral–motor control; and (4) eventually, cognitive performance components, including short-term memory. It is unclear exactly how PD affects a client's cognitive skills, but these changes are thought to be related to the connections of the substantia nigra to other areas of the cortex (Gersten, 1990).

Prognosis

PD is progressive, and there is no cure for it. Numerous medications can be used to slow the progression of the disease. These medications are generally dopamine agonists used to increase the amount of available dopamine within the CNS. Surgery may also be used to reduce some of the motor manifestations, including tremor and rigidity; however, PD is eventually fatal.

Clients with a diagnosis of PD will initially often experience a tremor of the hand or foot that may be present only with intentional movement. As the disease progresses, this tremor may spread to include all extremities, as well as the trunk and head, and be present at all times, or absent only during sleep. Clients experience increases in muscle tone, rigidity that may lead to "cogwheeling" (intermittent resistance to passive movement), decreased ability to initiate movement, disturbances in postural control and alignment, alterations in gait, fatigue, and decreased control of motor output. The onset of PD is usually gradual and generally occurs between the ages of 50 and 69 (Gersten, 1990).

Secondary Complications

Secondary complications arising from PD may include changes in soft-tissue integrity, reduced passive and active ROM leading to contractures, reduced muscle strength, skin and respiratory problems, infections, dysphagia, and disruptions in speech production. Clients may also experience "masking," or an inability to produce facial expression, secondary to the weakness of facial muscles. Eventually in the late stages of PD, clients may experience changes in cognition and perceptual skills. Also, depression is often part of the clinical presentation, although it is difficult to know if this is a clinical manifestation of the disease itself, or is simply an understandable psychological reaction to issues of loss and change.

Occupational Therapy Evaluation and Treatment

Clients with PD may be provided with occupational therapy on either an inpatient rehabilitation or outpatient basis, depending on the progression of the disease. Therapists who provide evaluation and treatment for clients with PD must keep in mind that this disease is progressive and that extreme fatigue can exacerbate the symptoms. Evaluation should be focused on specific activities that have become difficult for the client to accomplish. Treatment should include both remediation of sensory, neuromusculoskeletal, and motor components, as well as assisting the client with adapting his or her current lifestyle. A practitioner must be sure to focus on remediation only of those performance components that can be changed. Use of adaptive equipment may enable a client to remain more independent for a longer time. Environmental adaptations and recommendations may also permit a client to function within the home over a longer time frame. Energy conservation is another avenue of education the practitioner should provide for the client.

A further focus of treatment should be on education for the client and his or her family to facilitate understanding and acceptance of the disease process. As the disease progresses and the client loses his or her ability to communicate or facially express emotions, the ability to connect with loved ones may be greatly strained. By assisting the client in remaining in his or her own environment for as long as possible and as independently as possible, a practitioner can have a great influence the client's quality of life as well as that of the family.

▼ AMYOTROPHIC LATERAL SCLEROSIS (ALS)

Definition, Etiology, and Demographics

ALS, or "motor neuron disease," more commonly known as "Lou Gehrig's disease," is a degenerative process that destroys motor neurons in the cortex, brain stem, and spinal cord. It affects both upper and lower motor neurons. This disease causes massive loss of anterior horn cells in the spinal cord as well as in the lower brain stem, leading to weakness and muscle atrophy (ie, amyotrophic) (Hallum,1995). It also causes demyelinization of corticospinal and corticobulbar tracts, secondary to the degeneration of the motor cortex, resulting in upper motor neuron lesions (ie, lateral sclerosis) (Hallum, 1995). The etiology of this disease is unknown, although research has investigated various possible causal factors, including exposure to toxins, exposure to viruses, hormonal imbalances, and autoimmunity problems (Hallum, 1995).

Most clients who have a diagnosis of ALS are between 50 and 70 years of age and more men are affected than women (Hallum, 1995). There is no specific medical test for ALS; a diagnosis is based on clinical manifestations. Onset is gradual, and often the client has adapted to the slow loss of muscle strength long before noticing significant changes and seeking medical assistance.

Deficits

Initial symptoms often include complaints of an inability to perform functional tasks, such as buttoning buttons or climbing stairs. Another symptom may be cramping or muscle twitching in the muscle groups that are weakened. These are often described as "fasiculations." Upper motor neuron problems may include hyperreflexia and spasticity. Weakness can occur anywhere in the body, but first, is slightly more common in the lower extremities, rather than the upper extremities, and is more distal, rather than proximal. Onset of weakness is also usually asymmetrical. Clients may experience involvement of the cranial nerves, resulting in poor oral motor and facial control, with eventual dysphagia and speech disturbances (Hallum, 1995).

Prognosis

ALS is fatal, and death is usually the result of respiratory failure, secondary to weak musculature and eventual paralysis. The average life span following diagnosis is approximately 4 years. There is no medical treatment for ALS itself, but many interventions may allow the client to remain as active as possible and, eventually, as comfortable as possible. These include therapy, pain medications, alternative nutritional sources (including diet alteration and feeding tubes if the client wishes), and use of mechanical ventilation (again, if the client so wishes).

Secondary Complications

Secondary complications can include infections, changes in soft-tissue integrity, skin breakdown, and respiratory complications, such as dyspnea. Clients may also understandably experience depression and fear. Depression and fear may lead to a less active lifestyle that can result in further muscle atrophy (Hallum, 1995).

Occupational Therapy Evaluation and Treatment

Clients with ALS may be seen by occupational therapy practitioners in an inpatient rehabilitation setting, but more likely will be seen in an outpatient or home health setting. It is crucial for the therapist to have a clear understanding of the etiology of the disease and the prognosis assist the client in setting realistic goals and to develop an appropriate treatment plan. Practitioners must be careful not to cause a client to overexert, and thereby, cause an overuse syndrome. Should clients engage in activities that cause an overuse syndrome, they may actually lose muscle strength.

Evaluation should begin with a thorough look at what the client is able to do in terms of functional activities within the context of the client's home and work environment. Thorough evaluation of ADLs, work and productive activities, and play and leisure activities is necessary for the therapist to gain a clear understanding of what difficulties the client may be experiencing. The therapist will have a generalized idea of what impairment is contributing to any disability, such as decreased muscle strength, but will want to further evaluate specific impairments in neuromusculoskeletal and motor components. This will include a thorough evaluation of ROM, muscle tone, strength, endurance, and soft-tissue integrity. The therapist will also want to evaluate gross and fine motor coordination, motor control, and oral–motor control, especially as it relates to eating and basic communication.

Treatment should be focused on improving impairments in performance components through use of functional activities, such as increasing upper extremity strength through self-care activities. As the disease progresses, the client may benefit from adaptive equipment to maintain independence for as long as possible. This may include equipment for bathing and dressing, eating, and mobility. It may also include adaptation of the home and work environment, as well as adaptations to leisure activities.

Client and family education are essential, from the time of diagnosis, to assist the client and family in making decisions, especially about quality of life issues, such as tube feedings and use of mechanical ventilation. As the client becomes more dependent in ADLs, education should focus on teaching the family to assist the client, as well helping the client learn to direct his or her caregivers. Teaching caregivers how to perform ROM and how to position the client may also help with pain management and skin issues in the later stages of ALS.

As with any progressive degenerative disease that is eventually fatal, clients may experience depression and feelings of loss of control over their lives. Many clients also experience anger, denial, and apathy. It is important for the practitioner to recognize that many of these emotions are an anticipated part of adjusting to living with ALS. Support groups and one-on-one counseling may be helpful, as well as informal networking with other clients and families dealing with ALS. Educating the client and family and allowing the client to remain as independent as possible, for as long as possible, will help to reduce the feelings of loss of control. It is also essential to allow clients to make their own end of life decisions with dignity.

▼ MULTIPLE SCLEROSIS (MS)

Definition, Etiology, and Demographics

MS is a progressive disease with gradual onset that is characterized by a demyelinization or destruction of the myelin sheath that covers the nerve fibers within the CNS. The myelin sheath allows nerve impulses to be carried from the brain to various parts of the body. As the myelin sheath is destroyed, so is the body's ability to send messages via the nervous system. The destroyed myelin sheath is eventually replaced by "plaques" or sclerotic (hard) patches within the white matter of both the brain and the spinal cord; hence, the name multiple sclerosis.

The etiology of MS is unknown. This disease is characterized by a series of exacerbations and remissions, with each exacerbation potentially resulting in some residual loss of function. Many factors are thought to contribute to an exacerbation, including fatigue, increased physical demand, stress, poor nutrition, and cold weather. The average age for diagnosis of this disease is usually between the ages of 20 and 40 (Spencer, 1988).

Deficits

Clients with MS may experience difficulty in all of the performance areas of their lives. Consequently, clients often experience changes in their ability to complete self-care activities, work and productive activities, and play and leisure activities. Clients' abilities to actively engage in these tasks often fluctuate, depending on whether or not they are in acute exacerbation. Ongoing evaluation of the client's ability to perform various activities is required as the client passes through an acute exacerbation into remission. The therapist must be able to evaluate and help the client understand any residual disability that may exist following an exacerbation. Impairments in performance components are directly related to where in the CNS the disease strikes.

Clients may experience impairments in sensory processing (any sensation or vestibular changes), neuromusculoskeletal (ROM, muscle tone, strength, endurance, postural control, postural alignment, and soft-tissue integrity), motor (gross and fine coordination, motor control, praxis, and oral–motor control), cognition (memory, organization, sequencing, problem solving, insight, judgment, and new learning), and psychosocial skills (potential psychotic episodes, mood swings, and depression). Multiple sclerosis has the potential to affect every performance component because it can attack any part of the CNS. Initially, clients may experience only incoordination of a limb, parasthesias of the limbs, trunk or face, and fatigue. Exacerbations may resolve in as little as 1 to 2 weeks. Exacerbations generally leave behind some residual impairment. Over time, with multiple exacerbations, the client is less and less able to recover from each exacerbation and return to his or her baseline functioning abilities (Spencer, 1988).

As with any progressive disease, clients often experience feelings of hopelessness, anger, denial, and depression. Many clients describe feelings of losing control over their lives as well.

Prognosis

Eventually, MS is fatal. The life span for someone diagnosed with MS varies tremendously, depending on how frequent and severe the exacerbations are. Life spans can be as long as 40 years after the initial diagnosis (Spencer, 1988).

Secondary Complications

Secondary complications can be extremely varied, often depending on what part of the CNS is affected. They may include contractures, compromised respiratory system, infections, and skin breakdown.

Occupational Therapy Evaluation and Treatment

A large part of treatment must focus on providing the client with education about the disease process and assisting the client in adjusting to the ongoing, degenerative nature of the disease. Treatment must include a way for a client to learn to grade activities, based on their current level of functioning. Treatment should also focus on teaching energy conservation, work simplification, and safety awareness. Clients must learn to identify for themselves when they are becoming too fatigued, for the fatigue itself can trigger an exacerbation. By working with the client to provide avenues to adjust activities, the practitioner also helps the client to retain control over his or her daily life. As the disease progresses, the practitioner may need to introduce adaptive equipment and environmental adaptation to allow the client to continue to function as independently as possible.

Clients with a diagnosis of MS may be seen in any type of setting, depending on how significant their exacerbations are. Some clients may be able to remain at home, and even continue to work a modified schedule, if their exacerbations are not severe. Other clients may experience exacerbations so severe or so debilitating that they require inpatient rehabilitation attention. Practitioners who provide treatment in the acute or inpatient rehabilitation phase should be focused on evaluating what functional activities a client is able or unable to perform that will influence discharge to the home environment. Practitioners must be very careful not to cause overexertion or undue fatigue for the client during evaluation and treatment.

Treatment in an inpatient rehabilitation phase may include focusing on ADLs, such as bathing, dressing, grooming, and eating. Functional mobility will also be a focus, including toilet transfers, bed transfers, and tub transfers. If the exacerbation is severe enough, an alternative method of mobility, such as a wheelchair, may need to be introduced. Special attention should be given when ordering a wheelchair for a client with MS, for the wheelchair should be one that can be easily adapted and modified in anticipation of further decline (ie, manual to power chair, additions of head support, lateral supports and tilt in space mechanisms, or other). Further adaptation of the home environment may be needed for such things as transfers, safety, and mobility.

Once the client can be safely managed at home, he or she will transfer to outpatient or home health therapies. The practitioner in these settings should focus on the client's ability to manage functional activities within the home and the community. This may include home management, child care, banking, and adaptation of the work place.

Because the average age of diagnosis is between 20 and 40 years of age, many clients are in a highly productive phase of their lives. They may be engaged in various roles in life, including spouse, worker, and parent. The therapist must work to help the client remain active in these important life roles in whatever capacity possible. Evaluation of functional activity should be completed as it relates to the individual client's life roles, and treatment should focus on the same activities.

Ongoing client and family education is absolutely necessary to assist the client and the family in understanding the disease process and in helping the client and the family adapt as the disease progresses. A good understanding of the possible consequences of the disease process will permit the client and the family to plan in advance for those future activities that the client may no longer be able to do because of physical or mental decline. This planning can significantly affect the quality of life for both the client and the family as the disease progresses. Referral to support groups, such as those sponsored by the Multiple Sclerosis Society may also be of great benefit.

▼ SPINAL CORD INJURY

Definition, Etiology, and Demographics

Spinal cord injury can be defined as any traumatic event that causes damage to the spinal cord. Spinal cord injury can be caused by laceration, puncture, or compression of the cord. This injury is often caused by a fracture in the vertebral column. Common causes of spinal cord injury include motor vehicle accidents, falls, acts of violence, and sports injuries such as diving accidents. The most "common" profile of a person with spinal cord injury is a single male between the ages of 16 and 30 who is either a student or employed (Trieschmann, 1988; Zejdlik, 1992).

Spinal cord injuries may result in damage that is permanent or temporary. Damage may further be defined as complete, incomplete, or transient. A complete lesion is characterized by complete loss of function below the level of the lesion. Incomplete lesions are those that result in partial loss of function below the level of the lesion. Transient injuries are usually due to compression from a fracture or edema; as the pressure is removed, function eventually returns. Transection or partial transection of the spinal cord causes spinal shock, loss of motor control and sensation, and alterations in muscle tone (initially flaccid and then spastic).

Deficits

Deficits resulting from spinal cord injury are directly related to the site of the lesion. Function is impaired below the level of the lesion. Clients can experience impairments in sensation, motor, and neuromusculoskeletal performance components. They usually experience impairments in psychological, social, and self-management areas as well. It is important for the clinician to understand what function to expect based on the level of the lesion. This is more difficult if a lesion is incomplete. Clients with lesions below C8 or T1 will have full use of their upper extremities and will be considered to have paraplegia. Clients with lesions above this level will have impairment in the function of their upper extremities and will be considered to have quadriplegia. Table 36–3 shows what movements can be expected at various levels, how that can affect function, and what the goals might be given the level of innervation.

Practitioners who provide treatment for clients with spinal cord injury must also be fully aware of the psychological, social, and self-management disabilities a client may experience. Common stages of adjustment may include denial, anger, bargaining, depression, and acceptance. Clients may also experience feelings of isolation, despair, frustration, and hopelessness. It is often extremely beneficial for clients to receive therapy in a rehabilitation center that offers a dedicated spinal cord injury program so that the client is able to interact and gain psychological and social support from other people with similar experiences. Other clients

TABLE 36-3. Implications of Innervated Spinal Cord Levels

Last Innervated Level	Active Movement	Affected Performance Areas	Possible Treatment
C1–C3 Key muscles: Sternocleidomastoid Possibly partial trapezius Possibly partial diaphragm	Can assist with respiration Neck movement Partial scapular elevation	Dependent in self-care activities. Functional and community mobility needs may be met through use of power wheelchair. Communication and leisure activities may be met through adapted equipment. Work and productive activities may be met through some adaptive equipment. Dependent in home management tasks. Able to engage in educational and vocational tasks within limits.	Use of power wheelchair controlled by head or chin control units. Client to use portable respirator. Mouthstick for use of computers, tape recorders, and for educational, leisure and vocational activities. Use of environmental control units (ECUs) for controlling things in the environment as well as for leisure activities. Able to direct direct caregiver.
C4 Key muscles added: Full innervation of diaphragm Trapezius	Full respiration Neck movements Scapula movement Scapula retraction	Dependent in self-care. Client may be able to use adaptive equipment for drinking. Functional and community mobility needs met through use of power wheelchair. Communication and leisure activities may be met through use of adapted equipment as well as work and productive activities. Dependent in home management tasks. Able to engage in educational and vocational tasks within limits.	Use of power wheelchair controlled by head, chin, or sip and puff control units. Client no longer reliant on portable respirator. Long straw for drinking. May use externally powered arm supports for UE use in activities. Continued use of adapted equipment as stated for C1–C3. Client generally with better endurance and more options for educational, leisure, and vocation.
C5 Key muscles added: Partial deltoid Partial biceps Rhomboids Partial rotator cuff	Shoulder flexion and abduction to 90 degrees Partial elbow flexion Supination	Can participate in ADL activities, such as bathing, dressing, grooming, and eating with adapted equipment. Functional and community mobility still most practical with power wheelchair. May assist with transfers. Continued participation in education, vocational, and play and leisure activities with adapted equipment. Client may now be able to engage in wider range of activities.	Use of secure shower seat, washcloth mitt, and adapted shower head for ADL. Dynamic tenodesis splint and long opponens splint with mobile arm support for eating, typing. More options for wheelchair and ECU controls. More options for educational, vocational, and leisure activities as well as more options in how to engage.
C6 Key muscles added: Partial serratus anterior Partial pectoralis Partial latissimus dorsi Deltoid Biceps Carpi radialis	Scapula adduction Shoulder flexion and extension Weak trunk control Elbow flexion Wrist extension (tenodesis for grasp)	Able to complete self-care activities independently with adapted equipment, including bathing, dressing, grooming, eating. Able to use communication devices without adaptation. Can engage in light homemaking tasks. Increased variety for educational, vocational, and leisure activities. Can use manual chair with adaptations for mobility. Can drive with adaptations. Can assist in sliding board transfers.	Tenodesis splints for activities requiring hand grasp. Adaptive ADL equipment, including razor holders, eating utensils, dressing loops, and friction pads, adapted long-handled sponge and washmitt, adapted leg bag for continence. Knobs on wheelchair rims and on steering wheel with hand controls. Return to work environment that is wheelchair accessible.
C7 Key muscles added: Triceps Extrinsic finger flexors and extensors Partial wrist flexors	Moderate trunk control Elbow extension Functional grasp and release	ADL-independent in all areas of self-care. Client requires less use of adapted equipment. Can use manual wheelchair and transfer independently to most surfaces. Light home management tasks in wheelchair accessible home. Return to many educational, leisure, and work, and productive activities without requiring as much adapted equipment. Environment must be wheelchair-accessible.	Equipment may still be needed, such as buttonhook or pant loops, but less adaptation or effort required. May still require bathing equipment. Less adaptation for eating required. May still require adaptive equipment for toileting. No longer require splinting for UE use.
C8–T1 Key muscles added: Intrinsics of the hand Including thumb	Full use of upper extremities	Independent in all ADL activities. Can participate in numerous educational, leisure, and work activities in wheelchair-accessible environment.	Use of manual wheelchair that should be adapted to client's lifestyle. May still use some adapted equipment for self-care, such as long-handled sponge, suction for soap. Client often can engage in numerous activities without further adaptation.

(Physical Therapy Section, University Hospital, 1988; Spencer, 1988).

may be able to offer encouragement and motivation in a way that a health care professional cannot. The ability for clients who are in the early phases of rehabilitation to interact with a client who is more independent often can have a major influence on the total rehabilitation process. Individual and group counseling may also be beneficial.

Prognosis

Fifty years ago, most people with spinal cord injuries died, either immediately or within a year of injury. Owing to the tremendous advances in the medical management for persons with spinal cord injury, people now experience a full life expectancy following injury. There are still numerous secondary complications that can cause disruption in a client's life, and a great deal of responsibility lies with the client to safeguard against these complications (Zejdlik, 1992).

Secondary Complications

Because of the way in which spinal cord injuries occur, co-existing problems may include head injury and fractures. Further damage may be caused at the scene of the injury by failure to stabilize the vertebral column while moving the injured person. Secondary complications may also include respiratory distress or arrest, problems with skin maintenance, urinary tract infections, and problems with blood pressure (ie, autonomic dysreflexia) (Zejdlik,1992).

CASE STUDY

MJ is a 32-year-old man who was involved in a motor vehicle accident that resulted in spinal cord injury at the C-6 level. X-ray films showed that the spinal cord injury was a complete transection and was caused by severe displaced fractures of the vertebral column. Initially, MJ experienced a great deal of swelling in the spinal cord due to the traumatic nature of the injury.

When the acute-stage therapist initially evaluated MJ, he demonstrated an ability to breathe on his own (C1-C3), and some ability to demonstrate shoulder flexion, abduction, and elbow flexion; however, he had no sensation below the level of the lesion. The acute-stage therapist focused on ROM, increasing MJ's ability to be more upright both in bed and eventually in a wheelchair; bed and wheelchair positioning to preserve respiratory status and to prevent decubitus; and introducing adaptive equipment for eating and leisure activities.

When MJ was medically stable and able to tolerate a more intensive rehabilitation setting, he was transferred to an inpatient rehabilitation center with a dedicated spinal cord injury program. The inpatient therapist again evaluated MJ's active and passive ROM and found that he could now also demonstrate shoulder extension, forward reach, internal rotation, adduction, and wrist extension. This active movement was now consistent with the initial diagnosis of complete transection at the C-6 level and indicated that MJ's initial edema had resolved. The inpatient therapist focused on upper extremity strengthening, endurance (especially respiratory), and on assisting the client in becoming more independent in mobility (bed mobility, transfers, wheelchair mobility), self-care activities (eating, bathing, dressing, and grooming), and leisure and work activities. MJ had been employed as a computer analyst before the accident and enjoyed using computers for leisure as well.

The therapist determined that MJ could use **tenodesis** for functional activities and so provided him with a universal cuff for eating, writing, bathing, and grooming. The therapist also worked with him on (1) learning to use a sliding board for transfers, (2) using compensatory techniques and adapted equipment for dressing and bathing, and (3) resuming use of his computer. The therapist provided education and referral to a specialist when MJ and his wife began to seek information about sexuality. The therapist also provided a home evaluation before discharge to assist MJ, his wife, and their 2-year-old child in adapting the house for a wheelchair.

When MJ reached a level at which he and his wife could manage safely at home, he was discharged from the inpatient setting and began therapies at a local outpatient center. The outpatient therapist focused on assisting MJ in reintegrating into the community and back into the life roles that he had previously enjoyed, including computer analyst, husband, and father. The therapist assisted him in community mobility, community accessibility, adapting his work environment to permit use of his wheelchair, and adapted driving. She also focused on adaptations to allow him to participate in child care. She referred MJ for participation in several groups with other clients to assist him in his adjustment. MJ and his wife also received one-on-one counseling.

Stages of Recovery and Occupational Therapy Evaluation and Treatment

Evaluation will need to start with an understanding of what functional movement and sensation a client has. This can be achieved through consideration of diagnosis as well as specific manual muscle testing and sensory testing. This testing may need to be done in an ongoing fashion for incomplete or transient lesions because as the swelling and edema subside, more function returns.

The role of the acute and inpatient practitioner is to maintain passive and active ROM, strengthen the remaining motor function, provide appropriate wheelchair and bed positioning to preserve respiratory and skin functions, and evaluate the need for adaptive equipment and methods to allow a client to function as independently as possible. Splinting and fabrication of adaptive equipment may be used to meet these goals. Some examples of equipment may include the use of universal cuffs, self-care adaptive equipment, and long opponens splints that allow the client to independently perform bathing, dressing, eating, and work activities.

The outpatient practitioner or home health practitioner should assist the client in focusing on activities occurring within the home and community. Every practitioner who interacts with the client needs to have a clear understanding of what the client's goals are, as well as the life roles the client was engaged in before injury and what life roles the client wishes to engage in after injury. Environmental adaptations in the home and workplace may allow a client to function independently in both of these arenas.

Again, client and family education are essential throughout the entire rehabilitation process. A major focus of education includes teaching the client how to direct a caregiver in assisting him or her in daily activities if the client requires this help. Family involvement at an early stage helps both the client and the family to cope with the numerous changes that are occurring as a result of the spinal cord injury.

▼ GUILLAIN-BARRÉ SYNDROME

Definition, Etiology, and Demographics

Guillain-Barré syndrome is generally characterized by an acute inflammation of multiple peripheral nerves, leading to rapid progressive muscular weakness, potential paralysis, and sensory disturbances or loss. In some cases, the onset of inflammation may be more gradual, although this is rare. The exact etiology of the Guillain-Barré syndrome is unknown, although it often occurs after recovery from or exposure to an infectious viral disease, such as chickenpox. Diagnosis is made based on the client's clinical presentation of the foregoing characteristics as well as an elevated protein level in the cerebrospinal fluid, determined by spinal tap. Guillain-Barré may result in death from respiratory failure caused by paralysis or secondary complications from paralysis, but is usually a transient motor unit disease that generally results in full recovery. Some clients may experience residual weakness, which may be a result of prolonged hypoxia in the acute phase. This syndrome may occur in a mild form, causing some paresis in only the lower extremities, or in a severe form causing quadriplegia and respiratory failure. The extent of the disease is directly dependent on which nerves are involved, as well as how many nerves are involved. It can attack all people at all stages of life (Spencer, 1988).

Deficits

Clients may experience impairments in sensory processing, neuromusculoskeletal, and motor components. Clients may have no sensation or may be hypersensitive. They may experience parasthesias that can be particularly painful. Clients may have disturbances in ROM, muscle tone, strength, endurance, postural control and alignment, or soft-tissue integrity. They often present with poor coordination and motor control from both proximal and distal motor weakness as well as sensory changes. They may also have impairments in their oral motor control, resulting in swallowing deficits and placing them at risk for aspiration. These impairments will have a tremendous influence on the client's ability to participate in ADLs, work and productive activities, and play and leisure activities (Spencer, 1988).

Prognosis

Clients are often treated with steroids to reduce the inflammation. As the inflammation recedes, muscle activity and sensation gradually returns. Complete recovery may take as little as 2 months or as long as 2 years. More acute onset generally results in a more rapid recovery, whereas a slower onset may take longer to recover or may leave the client with permanent residual weakness. Aggressive exercise programs or interventions that place a great physical demand on the client are contraindicated, for this may cause an increase in muscle weakness or even a relapse (Spencer, 1988).

Secondary Complications

Secondary complications may include respiratory failure, unstable blood pressure, skin breakdown, urinary tract infections, muscle atrophy, soft tissue shortening, and extremely poor endurance. Clients may also be depressed, angry, apathetic, or frustrated. Clients often also experience a great deal of pain caused by the inflammation of the sensory axons in the nerves. This pain can be medically controlled to a certain point and also improves over time (Spencer, 1988).

Stages of Recovery and Occupational Therapy Evaluation and Treatment

The role of the acute-stage therapist is to determine at what level the client is able to participate. Often, these therapists may intervene while clients are still being maintained on a ventilator, which limits their ability to participate. Evaluation would then focus on passive and active ROM, strength, bed positioning for skin and respiratory maintenance, soft-tissue integrity, muscle tone, coordination, and sensation. Therapists may need to provide splinting and specialized positioning to prevent loss of ROM and changes in soft-tissue integrity as well as to help decrease the amount of pain a client is experiencing. If a client is no longer ventilator-dependent, it may be feasible to complete a bedside evaluation for swallowing and oral motor impairments that would affect a client's ability to eat. If a client is able to tolerate a diet by mouth, the practitioner can also begin to assist the client to self-feed. Acute-stage practitioners may need to provide adaptive equipment for this. A client may be transferred to an inpatient setting before being able to tolerate a diet by mouth, and self-feeding would then become a focus for the inpatient practitioner.

A client will be transferred to an inpatient rehabilitation setting once he or she is medically stable and can tolerate more intensive rehabilitation. The inpatient rehabilitation therapist will focus evaluation on (1) self-care activities, such as bathing, dressing, grooming, eating, and toileting; (2) functional mobility, including bed mobility, transfers, wheelchair mobility, and functional ambulation; (3) productive activities, such as meal preparation, laundry, and house cleaning; and (4) leisure activities. Further evaluation will be based on developing hypotheses about what performance component deficits are causing a client's difficulty with these tasks. Possible deficits include sensory, neuromusculoskeletal, and motor impairments. Practitioners may need to provide specialized splinting or adaptive equipment for this client to allow him or her to be as independent as possible during this transitional stage. It is important to remember, however, that most clients with Guillain-Barré syndrome make a complete recovery. This will affect what equipment a therapist recommends for this client. A therapist would not, for example, want to recommend a power chair for a client in the earlier stages of the disease, even if that client is presenting with quadriplegia. Therapists should consider the cost of equipment and how long a client may use that equipment before recommending that the client purchase that equipment. A therapist may be able to loan a piece of adaptive equipment to a client or to fabricate an inexpensive piece of equipment if the client will not be using it over an extended time period. Once a client has reached a level at which he or she can be safely managed at home, the client would then make a transition to outpatient or home health services.

Practitioners working with clients at the outpatient or home health stage of recovery would focus evaluation and treatment on community reintegration, work and productive activities, including educational activities and vocational activities, and resumption of leisure tasks. Again, hypotheses should be developed to determine why the client needs assistance, and then treatment should be focused on remediating or providing compensatory strategies for performance component deficits so a client can become fully functional again.

Throughout the rehabilitation process, practitioners who provide treatment for clients recovering from Guillain-Barré syndrome will need to have an excellent ability to grade activities, as well as teach the clients to grade their own activities to prevent too great a demand on the client. Overexertion can cause further muscle weakness or a relapse. Client and family education should be ongoing throughout the rehabilitation process.

▼ MYASTHENIA GRAVIS (MG)

Definition, Etiology, and Demographics

MG is a progressive, degenerative muscle disease that occurs at the site of the myoneural junction. Specifically, there is a degeneration of the terminal nerve and a reduction of the postsynaptic region, resulting in a decrease of the numbers of receptors for neurotransmitters (acetylcholine) necessary for muscle contraction (Adams & Victor, 1989). The etiology of this is unclear, although most research suggests it is a result of disturbances in the thymus and the body's immune system (Adams & Victor, 1989). It is important to understand that there is no actual lesion within the brain or the spinal cord. Muscle weakness occurs because of changes occurring at the myoneural junction.

MG can attack anyone at any age, but usual onset for women is between the ages of 20 and 30 years; onset for men is generally between 60 and 70 (Adams & Victor, 1989). A diagnosis of MG is more likely to be made in women.

Deficits

There is no common course of MG. Each client may experience different symptoms, different rates of progression, and different outcomes. Initial symptoms may include fluctuating weakness of the eyes, face, jaws, and throat. This may result in drooping eyelids, decreased oculomotor control of the eyes, decreased ability to chew and swallow, changes in the ability to speak or in voice quality, and difficulty holding up one's head. This disease also affects those facial muscles responsible for facial expression, such as smiling. As the disease progresses, it may include weakness of the shoulder girdle muscles, hip musculature, and trunk muscles responsible for flexion and extension. In the latter stages of the disease, muscles responsible for respiration, such as diaphragm and intercostal muscles, are affected.

A major characteristic of MG is the fluctuating nature of the weakness. As a muscle group is used repetitively, as in chewing, it fatigues. With rest, strength returns, at least in part. There is little actual atrophy of the muscle and rarely any pain. There has been little documented in terms of sensory loss, but some clients have complained of parasthesias (Adams & Victor, 1989).

Clients suffering from MG may experience problems in ADLs, work and productive activities, and play and leisure activities. Initially, a client may need assistance with eating and swallowing. A client may be experiencing diplopia (double vision), and this could affect any number of functional activities. If the disease has affected shoulder or trunk musculature, clients may need assistance in bathing, dressing, grooming, and functional mobility. They may also lose their independence in homemaking tasks, such as meal preparation, shopping, and laundry. If balance and functional mobility are significantly impaired, clients may not be able to participate in community activities or continue with work or leisure activities. Severe fatigue can greatly affect a client's functional abilities.

Prognosis

Myasthenia gravis is also characterized by remissions and progressions. Remissions generally last only a few months to a year, but the disease itself can remain stable for years before beginning to progress (Adams & Victor). Full progression of the MG results in severe permanent paralysis. Death from MG generally results from respiratory complications, such as aspiration pneumonia or other infections (Adams & Victor, 1989).

Secondary Complications

Secondary or coexisting complications may include thymic tumors, rheumatoid arthritis, lupus, and aplastic anemia (Adams & Victor, 1989). Clients are also at risk in the later stages for aspiration, skin breakdown, changes in soft-tissue integrity, infections, and depression.

Occupational Therapy Evaluation and Treatment

Clients with MG will usually receive services on an outpatient or home health basis. The therapist should begin evaluation based on the client's lifestyle and life roles, such as worker, husband, wife, father, and such. Evaluation should be focused on what activities the client is able to complete and for which activities he or she requires assistance. Further evaluation and development of hypotheses about performance component deficits by the therapist should incorporate understanding of the neurological changes the client is experiencing. The therapist should be careful not to fatigue the client in either evaluation or treatment because this can cause further decline of the client's functional capacities. Specific component evaluation should focus on strength, ROM, endurance, postural control, and soft-tissue integrity. It should also include evaluation of coordination and oral motor control, especially as it relates to eating, swallowing, and communication.

Treatment should be focused on using those activities the client wishes to perform to strengthen muscles as much as possible. Treatment should also include a strong educational component, centered on energy conservation and work simplification techniques. Education should also focus on helping the client and the family understand the course of the disease and teaching the client to grade activities to avoid overuse or fatigue. As the disease progresses, the practitioner may want to introduce adaptive equipment to assist the client in maintaining independence for as long as possible. This equipment may include bathing and grooming equipment, eating equipment, a wheelchair with adaptable features for further decline, and equipment for leisure activities. Specialized splinting may also assist a client in functional activity. Adaptation of the home and work environment may also assist the client in independence. As severe permanent paralysis sets in, practitioners may want to educate the client and the family on environmental control units (ECUs) to permit the client's continued independence in some activities, such as turning on lights, switches to turn on radios and televisions, and communication devices.

The practitioner should ultimately focus on quality of life for the MG client. This disease can be a slowly progressing or a rapidly progressing disease. The practitioner can assist the client and the family in adjusting to this progression by providing activity-directed treatment to maintain current strength and adaptation to the progression of the disease to maintain independence.

►Conclusion

Occupational therapy practitioners who provide rehabilitation services to adult clients with neurological impairment in the current health care environment are faced with a great challenge. It is crucial for practitioners to have a working knowledge of neuroanatomy and neurophysiology as it relates to neurological insult if clients are to receive the maximum benefit from therapeutic intervention. Therapists must be able to observe clients performing valued functional activities, quickly develop hypotheses about why clients may have difficulty performing these tasks, and develop a treatment plan using functional activity to address performance component deficits that affect independence in occupational performance areas.

Practitioners must be extremely focused in their treatment and make sure they have a specific goal for every interaction that occurs with clients. Practitioners must also be constantly re-evaluating the treatment they are providing to make sure they are truly assisting clients in reaching their goals in the most efficacious way. Practitioners must always remember that the focus must be on goals that clients value, which may not always be the same goals that practitioners value.

▼ REFERENCES

Adams, R. & Victor, M. (1989). *Principles of neurology*. New York: Mc-Graw-Hill.

Arnadottir, G. (1990). *The brain and behavior*. St. Louis: C.V. Mosby.

Fisher, M. (1995). *Stroke Therapy*. Boston: Butterworth & Heinemann.

Gersten, J. (1990). Rehabilitation for degenerative diseases of the central nervous system. In F. Kottke, G. Stillwell, & J. Lehman (Eds.). *Krusen's handbook of physical medicine and rehabilitation* (pp. 778–791). Philadelphia: W. B. Saunders.

Giles, G. & Shore, M. (1989). A rapid method for teaching severe brain injured adults how to wash and dress. *Archives of Physical Medicine and Rehabilitation, 70*, 156–158.

Gilroy, J. (1990). *Basic neurology* (2nd ed.). New York: McGraw-Hill.

Hallum, A. (1995). Neuromuscular diseases. In D. A. Umphred (Ed.), *Neurological rehabilitation* (pp. 375–393). St. Louis: Mosby-Year Book.

Katz, D.J. (1992). Neuropathology and neurobehavioral recovery from closed head injury. *Journal of Head Trauma Rehabilitation, 7*, 1–15.

Kiernan, J. (1987). *Introduction to human neuroscience*. Philadelphia: J. B. Lippincott.

Miller, E. (1980). The training characteristics of severely head injured patients: A preliminary study. *Journal of Neurology, Neurosurgery and Psychiatry, 43*, 525–528.

Neistadt, M. E. (1994). The neurobiology of learning: Implications for treatment of adults with brain injury. *American Journal of Occupational Therapy, 48*, 421–430.

Physical Therapy Section, University Hospital (1988). *Functional significance of spinal cord levels*. Unpublished.

Spencer, E. (1988). Functional restoration: Neurological, orthopedic, and arthritic conditions. In H. Hopkins & H. Smith (Eds.), *Willard and Spackman's occupational therapy* (pp. 483–502). Philadelphia: J. B. Lippincott.

Treischmann, R. B. (1988). *Spinal cord injuries: Psychological, social, and vocational rehabilitation* (2nd ed.). New York: Demos Publications.

US Department of Health and Human Services. (1995). *Clinical practice guideline: Post stroke rehabilitation*. Rockville, MD: AHCPR.

Wall, N. (1982). Stroke rehabilitation. In M. Logigan (Ed.), *Adult rehabilitation: A team approach for therapists* (pp. 225–275). Boston: Little, Brown & Co.

Winkler, P. (1995). Head injury. In D. A. Umphred (Ed.), *Neurological rehabilitation* (pp. 421–453). St. Louis: Mosby-Year Book.

Zejdlik, C. P. (1992). *Management of spinal cord injuries* (2nd ed.). Boston: Jones and Barlett Publishers.

Chapter 37

Orthopedic and Musculoskeletal Dysfunction in Adults

Section 1: Adult Orthopedic Dysfunction

Section 2: Musculoskeletal Dysfunction in Adults

Section 1

Adult Orthopedic Dysfunction

Elizabeth Newman

Typical Deficits
Occupational Therapy Evaluation and Treatment
Hip Fracture

Orthopedic conditions encompass dysfunctions of bones, joints, and their related structures: muscles, tendons, ligaments, and nerves. These conditions can be due to injuries, developmental deformities, or a disease process. An **orthopedic** condition can be caused by a sudden traumatic event, such as motor vehicle, sports, or work-related accident. Conditions may be cumulative, such as carpal tunnel syndrome, or they may result from congenital anomalies, such as a limb length discrepancy or scoliosis.

▼ TYPICAL DEFICITS

There are typical deficits in performance areas and performance components for those with orthopedic dysfunction (Goldstein, 1995). Typical deficits are functional impairments in mobility, self-care and community living skills due to limitations caused by (1) pain, (2) immobilization, or (3) decreases in range of motion (ROM), sensation, strength, or some combination thereof (Goldstein, 1995). Limitations may also occur as a result of precautionary movement restrictions or limited weight bearing for extended periods. Deficits in functional performance may be temporary, long-

term, or become progressively more severe. Although the performance deficits may be typical, the causes may vary greatly. Evaluation and intervention may differ according to the medical history, onset of limitations, and prognosis.

Developmental orthopedic dysfunction may be a result of an abnormality in bone or muscle growth and development. These conditions often require intervention to increase mobility, increase function, correct deformity, or decrease pain.

Trauma to bones, joints, and related structures may also result in orthopedic dysfunction. Fractures are classified by the extent of bone damage, type of bone tissue damaged, angle of the fracture, and amount of soft tissue damage around the fracture site (Apley & Solomon, 1988). For example, a partial, closed fracture, refers to a fracture that looks like a crack in the bone, with minimal soft tissue damage, no break in the skin, with a low chance of infection. In contrast, in a complete, open fracture, the bone shaft is completely broken, with substantial soft tissue damage, and the bone is exposed through the skin, increasing the risk of infection. The type of fracture and method of reduction are predictors for rehabilitation potential, recovery time, and risk of infection.

The method of fracture reduction is dependent on the type, severity of bone fracture, and the extent of soft tissue damage (Heppenstall, 1980). With open reduction internal fixation (ORIF), the fracture is stabilized surgically with a bone plate or screws. A severe open fracture may require an external fixator, which is a device composed of a series of bars and clamps attached to threaded percutaneous pins inserted into the bone. This device is used to stabilized the fracture. It allows excellent access for wound care and observation, as well as client mobility. Occupational therapy evaluation for clients with fractures must be a continuous process that is carefully coordinated with the stage of bone healing, the chosen method of reduction and stabilization, and the surgeon's protocol for immobilization or movement parameters during healing (Heppenstall, 1980).

Precautions and protocols from the physician may include: (1) restrictions in active range of motion (AROM) or weight bearing, (2) immobilization, or (3) a structured increase in range of motion (ROM). Occupational therapy practitioners need to watch for signs and symptoms of complications such as (1) deep vein thrombosis, (2) pulmonary emboli, (3) infection, (4) decreased circulation, or (5) decreased sensation. Severe pain should also be monitored. The practitioner should notify the physician immediately about severe pain or other signs and symptoms suggesting complications.

Orthopedic dysfunction can also be the result of disease processes that damage bones, joints, and related structures. With these diseases, a gradual decline in ROM and strength and an increase in pain can result in significant deficits in functional mobility, activities of daily living (ADL), and work and productive activities. A disease that causes orthopedic dysfunction presents with a decrease in function over time (Felsenthal, Garrison, & Steinberg, 1994). For example, an person with osteoarthritis, develops increasing pain in both knees over many years as a result of degenerative deterioration of the knee joints. The person presents with decreased functional mobility, and decreased ability to complete day-to-day activities. A joint replacement or **arthroplasty** followed by rehabilitation is recommended. Joint arthroplasty replaces the damaged joint, or portion of the joint, with a prosthetic joint. Immediately following surgery, the same deficits are seen in performance areas, with more severity owing to post-surgical edema and pain. The rehabilitation goal would be to increase mobility, and performance of ADL, work and productive activities. Treatment protocols are specific to the type and method of arthroplasty (Felsenthal et al, 1994).

▼ OCCUPATIONAL THERAPY EVALUATION AND TREATMENT

Occupational therapy evaluation and treatment of orthopedic dysfunction will vary depending on the medical intervention and the individual's precautions and limitations. For those with orthopedic dysfunction from developmental or disease processes that does not require surgical intervention, evaluation and treatment may emphasize adapting the environment to maximize function and education for problem solving and prevention of further deformity. For those with orthopedic dysfunction from trauma or following a surgical intervention, protocols and precautions are followed to progress the client through the recovery process. The goal is to progress the client toward maximal function of the affected extremity in the context of functional activities.

Occupational therapy evaluation for clients with orthopedic dysfunction includes AROM, sensation, strength, skin, circulation, pain, functional mobility, self-care, home management, positioning, home accessibility, community reentry, and driving, if appropriate, along with a cognitive assessment to determine the individual's ability to follow precautions

(see Unit VI for details about evaluation procedures). Precautions may require modification of evaluation procedures.

Treatment is usually to get the client up and moving as soon as there are doctor's orders to do so. This prevents complications from immobilization and improves healing (Goldstein, 1995). Treatment protocols may include, immobilization, early mobilization, exercise program, positioning, edema control, weight bearing, scar management, modalities, adaptation of the environment, and ongoing education (see Unit VII for details about treatment procedures). Complications can and do occur relatively quickly, requiring an immediate review and possible alteration of treatment plans.

▼ HIP FRACTURE

The method of reduction and stabilization of a hip fracture is dependent on several factors: (1) the age of the client, (2) severity of pain, (3) presence of disease process, and (4) premorbid activity level. For a younger, more active client with an otherwise healthy joint, the surgical intervention will be ORIF. This will require few precautions, most commonly weight-bearing limitations. With these clients, therapists will evaluate ADL, home management, safety, and the need for assistive and adaptive equipment.

For an 85-year-old client with osteoarthritis who presents with a hip fracture, the surgical intervention most likely will be a cemented total hip arthroplasty (THA). Weight-bearing status following a THA depends on the procedure. If the arthroplasty is cemented, weight bearing is usually permitted as tolerated; a THA using a noncemented technique requires non–weight-bearing for a designated amount of time (Wixson, Stulberg, & Mehlhoff, 1991). The noncemented technique requires the bone to knit to the prosthetic device and will be stronger than a cemented THA.

There are precautions about how to move the operated on leg to decrease the chance of dislocation for 6 weeks or longer. Hip precautions consist of (1) no hip flexion beyond 90 degrees, (2) no hip rotation, (3) no crossing legs, (4) no adduction, and (5) no bending or bringing foot close to hands. Occupational therapy evaluation consists of ADL, home management, functional mobility, safety, and a cognitive assessment to determine the client's ability to adhere to the precautions and learn adaptive techniques. Treatment includes teaching clients to (1) incorporate hip precautions into ADLs and home management, (2) use adaptive equipment, and (3) adhere to precautions. Common recommendations are a pillow between the knees in the sitting and supine positions to maintain the proper position of the femur. Adaptive equipment recommendations often include (1) a long-handled sponge, (2) dressing stick, (3) reacher, (4) long-handled shoehorn, (5) nonskid bath mat, (6) grab bars, (7) bath bench, and (8) raised toilet seat. Practitioners might also suggest elevating seat surfaces in the home (Seeger & Fisher, 1982). Treatment is performed one-on-one or in group settings (Cedar, Thorngren, & Wallden, 1980).

Section 2

Musculoskeletal Dysfunction In Adults

Elinor Anne Spencer

This section presents a brief introduction to musculoskeletal injuries of the upper extremities (UEs) as related to occupational therapy intervention. The specific conditions of amputation, arthritis, and hand injuries are discussed.

▼ TYPICAL DEFICITS IN UPPER EXTREMITY INJURIES

Trauma and disease of the musculoskeletal system result in direct or indirect physical and mental disability. Onset may be sudden or gradual; the course may be nonprogressive or progressive; disability manifestations may be temporary or permanent. Secondary effects such as muscle contractures or atrophy, limitations in joint mobility, deformity in alignment, weakness, sensory dysfunction, and chronic pain can occur.

Performance Areas

UE dysfunction can result in limitation or loss of independence in activities of daily living (ADL). This loss affects self-esteem and motivation and may impose changes in family roles. An adult may need to adjust to accepting assistance with personal tasks from a child, family member, or stranger. Dependence on others may extend to household tasks, driving, shopping, caretaking, and other significant duties.

UE dysfunction can also lead to disruption of work and productive activity. This disruption can tax the psychological-coping skills of the injured worker and others around him or her. The family may or may not be capable of adjusting to the daily effects of disability on the client. Loss of work time and the possible need for vocational redirection also has economic implications.

UE dysfunction can limit play or leisure activities, resulting in loss of previously enjoyed activities. Time away from work may not transfer to enjoyment in forced or extended leisure time. Choices of activity become dependent on disability and adaptation. The work and play and leisure activity balance is affected. Changes in the daily pattern become necessary. Exploration of methods to provide motivation and satisfying activity for recuperation becomes important (Trombly, 1995).

Performance Components

Performance components affected by UE injury or illness include sensory, neuromuscular, motor, or psychological. In addition, developmental and cultural aspects of activity can be affected. Laceration, penetration, or compression of tissue can cause discontinuity of nerve pathways, resulting in temporary or permanent change in *sensory awareness* and *sensory functions*. Loss of pain and touch sensations is a safety hazard; without this sensory feedback clients may burn or scrape themselves without knowing it. Persistent pain contributes to fear and reluctance to move the extremity or part, hindering return of mobilization and function. There may be specific deficits in tactile discrimination, localization, and stereognosis. These deficits affect the motor functions of grasp, release, coordination, and reach.

Disruption of nerve pathways interferes with the nervous system's control of movement. Limitation or loss of ROM, strength, and endurance results from a disruption of this essential neuromuscular integration. This loss of neuromuscular integration also hinders postural control, body alignment, and motor control of isolated muscles and joint movements. The injured extremity may lack motor power for gross and fine coordination tasks requiring strength against gravity or other forms of resistance. Limitations may affect bilateral capabilities by necessitating compensatory strength and coordination from the unaffected extremity (Praemer, 1992; Trombly, 1995).

The *psychological* effect of disease or injury on the client will vary. In some situations, long-term functional potentials may not initially be recognized or accepted by the client and family because of feelings of confusion, fear, insecurity, anger, inadequacy, and disequilibrium. These clients and families see the injury suddenly replacing previous levels of life adjustment and activity with unfamiliar, unknown, and unacceptable conditions or situations. Other clients and families will be able to recognize potential functional gain and work toward recuperation and positive outcomes.

Injury and disease interfere with the *developmental* process. Age, gender, education, work experience, lifestyle, and family involvements affect the client's attitude toward dysfunction. The adolescent or adult who has experienced life as an able-bodied person, with few or no physical limitations, may meet sudden debilitating trauma with shock, disbelief, anger, and denial.

Perceptions of illness and disability vary within *cultures* and socioeconomic groups. The functional restoration program provided to the client must be geared toward the context of the individual to be acceptable and appropriate to his or her particular motivations, interest, abilities, and goals.

▼ EVALUATION FOR UPPER EXTREMITY INJURIES

Evaluation procedures must be understood and tolerated by the client to ensure participation in the occupational therapy program. The more the client understands and becomes involved in the procedures, the better the rapport between therapist and client, and the more complete the progress. Evaluation methods include observation, interview, standardized and nonstandardized testing, and performance tasks. The evaluation provides objective feedback to the client on his or her present functional levels, and encourages discussion of treatment priorities and potentials. Please refer to Unit VI for information on specific evaluation methods.

Performance Areas

Evaluation of performance of ADLs identifies self-care potentials, need and potential for use of adaptive methods and assistive devices, level of dependence in self-care and daily activity responsibilities, and the pretrauma daily activity pattern. Methods of evaluation may include check-lists for self-evaluation, interviews with the client concerning the home environment, therapist observation of ADL functions, and discussion of feasible alternatives to present task approaches.

Evaluation of work and productive activities includes discussion of (1) the daily work context and schedule, (2) work demands and pretrauma performance capabilities, (3) imposed changes in daily routine relative to family relationships and responsibilities, (4) options for temporary adjustment in work patterns, and (5) alternatives for vocational training. Interviews with the client concerning general occupational history, the effect of the injury or condition on daily work activity, financial effect, and goals indicate the client's expectations, needs, and priorities. Performance tests indicate work readiness, endurance, and functional capacity related to job requirements. Evaluation of safety and the client's awareness of precautions and limitations are important aspects of assessing the clients' abilities to perform home tasks, child care, general daily activities, and job-related work.

Identification of play or leisure activities in which the client habitually engages for individual enjoyment or social pleasure and interaction is essential in the initial contact with the occupational therapist. Check-lists or the development of an activity schedule of the daily or weekly pattern can be helpful in planning home programs to gain functional ability through these types of activities during recuperation and time off from work.

Performance Components

Evaluation of performance components begins with assessment of the client's *sensation*, including (1) sensory awareness of the extremity, (2) positioning of the extremity at rest and with movement, (3) functional ability, and (4) subjective feelings regarding the injured extremity. Visual attention to and verbal discussion of the extremity may be diminished owing to limitations in sensation or hypersensitivity to the injury or disability. Specific levels of sensory disturbances in tactile localization, static and moving stimulus perception, one- and two-point discrimination, sensory discrimination, and stereognosis are determined. The cause, location, and extent of pain are also evaluated to learn precautions and limitations.

Evaluations of *neuromuscular* performance include tests of (1) ROM of both upper extremities, (2) strength of both upper extremities, (3) endurance in general movement and activity, (4) pain, (5) postural control and alignment, and (6) the effect of the injury on the soft tissue. During evaluations the extremity should be positioned in optimum alignment in pain-free positions as much as possible.

Evaluations of *motor* control include standardized tests for gross and fine motor movements, and observation of these movements in ADL, work, or leisure activities. The injured extremity is evaluated, using the noninjured extremity as a guide for normal function of the individual. Bilateral limitations are also evaluated, with particular attention to the hand dominance of the client.

Evaluation of *psychological* aspects begins with developing rapport with the client and identifying the client's behavior and feelings about the injury. Feelings might include anxiety, impatience, anger, fatigue, distractibility, or sadness. Personal concepts of functional and cosmetic damage can positively or negatively affect the client's motivation for recuperation.

Developmental aspects of the client's life experience also influence attitudes toward injury and illness and the ability to cope with adverse conditions. It is essential that the adult be recognized as having a developmental history. Disability brings dependence, which is often a difficult reminder of the dependency of childhood. The dependent adult must be treated as an adult in all aspects of therapeutic intervention. Collaborating in setting treatment objectives based on evaluation results enables the adult client to take an adult role.

During the evaluation process, the occupational therapist and the occupational therapy assistant maintain an attitude of flexibility and openness in meeting the variety of *cultural* variables that are found in individual clients and families. Changes from premorbid pattern of behavior are noted as early as possible.

▼ TREATMENT FOR UPPER EXTREMITY INJURIES

Functional restoration is the primary objective of rehabilitation. Assisting a person to build or restore his or her life to its fullest use and satisfaction is a philosophical mandate of occupational therapy (Spencer, 1993c). Therapeutic intervention can reverse disability, improve ability, and prevent further disability.

Performance Areas

The client learns to minimize the disruption of established routines of self-sufficiency by setting priorities for ADL functions and problem solving. The client learns to (1) apply and remove splints and prostheses, (2) perform tasks with adaptive devices, (3) develop adaptive techniques for temporary use, and (4) work toward maximal functional independence. The client also learns precautions relevant to deficits and practices techniques at home while receiving treatment on an outpatient basis following acute care.

Treatment programs related to work and productive activities include training in (1) adaptive techniques for homemaking and other daily activities, (2) energy conservation and work simplification procedures, (3) use of adaptive equipment to improve skill levels, (4) work capacity, and (5) use of long-term splints and prostheses. Additionally, occupational therapy practitioners provide assistance in redirecting vocational interests and skills as necessary.

Play or leisure activities are used to foster positive involvement, enjoyment, family, and community participation. The client may discover new economic benefits from avocational interests.

Performance Components

Treatment of *sensory* deficits includes (1) reduction of and adaptation to pain, (2) training in sensory awareness and discrimination, (3) desensitization, (4) sensory stimulation, (5) facilitation of body image adjustment and acceptance, and (6) facilitation of positive social interaction. It is particularly important to teach the client the safety hazards of decreased sensation.

Treatment of *neuromuscular* deficits includes (1) passive and active ROM, (2) movement and function in activities to encourage extremity control and trunk alignment, (3) activities to improve general endurance, (4) methods to adjust to pain and limitations, (5) strengthening of affected areas and extremities, and (6) involvement in overall body movement.

Performance component treatment also includes *motor* exercises and activities, bilateral functions of extremities, and involvement in task performance to develop gross and fine motor coordination and dexterity. The occupational therapist must make every effort to involve the client in planning and executing appropriate progressive exercises and activities both in the clinic and at home.

The *psychological* aspect of the treatment program involves patient education about (1) potentials of function and the value of adaptations, and (2) current limitations and treatment objectives. Practitioners also address psychological issues by collaborating with clients to determine treatment priorities, focusing treatment on clients' goals.

Successful treatment helps clients develop or regain pretrauma skills and accept functional limitations for a temporary or permanent period. Changes in activity competency or method require adjustment and adaptation. Participation in a functional activity program individually and with others contributes to this adjustment and aids the individual to view himself or herself as a valuable functioning member of adult society.

Before the injury, the person may have been a high-functioning member of a family and neighborhood, known to have certain interests, skills, and roles, within a unique *culture*. Following injury, disability, and recuperation, the person must be equipped to reenter that familiar community and lifestyle, perhaps with a brace, a splint, a prosthesis, assistive device, or a significant scar. The client will be the one to educate the community about his or her personal challenges, limitations, and potentials.

▼ UPPER EXTREMITY AMPUTATION

To have an amputation is to be without a limb or part because of congenital anomaly, injury, or disease. Common causes of amputation in the UE are external trauma, prolonged infection, severe neuromuscular impairment, and tumors. Typical signs and symptoms include loss or impairment of bone, neurovascular tissue, muscle tissue, functions of the extremity, distal sensations, and cosmesis. The higher the level of the amputation, the greater these losses will be (Fig. 37–1).

Early fitting of a prosthesis (1) hastens psychological adjustment, (2) reduces pain and edema, (3) facilitates healing, (4) limits phantom sensations by early prosthetic contact and function, and (5) introduces prosthetic adaptation to the amputee and his or her family. The prosthesis is prescribed by the medical team and fabricated by a certified prosthetist. The occupational therapist performs a check-out of fit and function and educates the client in the wear, operation, precautions, and functions of the prosthesis in daily activity.

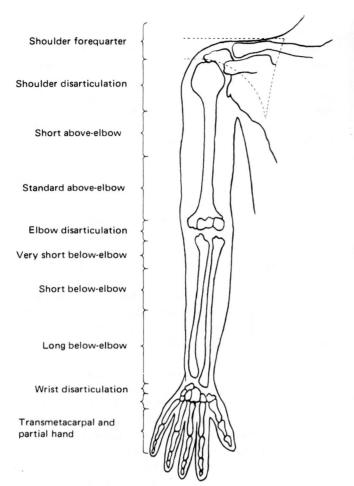

Shoulder forequarter

Shoulder disarticulation

Short above-elbow

Standard above-elbow

Elbow disarticulation
Very short below-elbow

Short below-elbow

Long below-elbow

Wrist disarticulation

Transmetacarpal and
partial hand

▲
Figure 37-1. Amputation levels of the upper extremity.

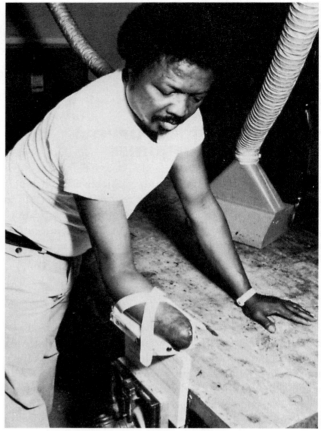

▲
Figure 37-2. Below-elbow amputee benefits by early active use of the amputated extremity in sanding with an adapted sanding block. The patient gains early awareness of the use of his arm, and pressure on the sanding block helps desensitize the stump.

Deficits in Performance Areas

Independent functions in ADL are affected by partial or complete lack of hand and perhaps arm function; loss of bilateral functions; and effects of the amputation on body image, cosmesis, personal care, and functional lifestyle. The client must adjust to the care of the stump and the prosthesis, as well as to the appearance and use of the prosthesis in the environment. Assistive devices enhance early preprosthetic use of the stump in bathing and hygiene as well as other self-care tasks. Use of the extremity enhances integration of the stump and the prosthesis into the body image for independent daily activity (Figs. 37–2 and 37–3).

Functions in work and productive activities are affected by (1) loss or change in UE unilateral and bilateral functions, (2) change in postural control, (3) loss in work time, (4) change in job capability, and (5) change in daily activity routine and future planning. The amputee learns preprosthetic and prosthetic use of the affected area in coordination and grasping activities (Figs 37–4 and Fig. 37–5). A prevocational assessment assists the clients in recognizing capabili-

ties related to feasibility of either a safe return to the former occupation, or to vocational redirection. Specific tasks such as safe and efficient tool, equipment, and material handling are used in prevocational evaluation (see Figure 37–4). Assessment of attitudes, aptitudes, work habits, work tolerance, and skills using standardized tests and work-simulated tasks are included, as well as observation of household tasks, driving, and child care.

Participation in previously enjoyed individual and social play and leisure activities may require adapted equipment or techniques. Resumption of these activities during treatment assists in general body conditioning, integration of the prosthesis into the person's lifestyle, and the development of a positive image. Avocational and sports activities provide motivation, social interaction, daily coordination, and strength development.

Deficits in Performance Components

Amputation results in pathological changes in body image and awareness. Sudden trauma results in localized pain from

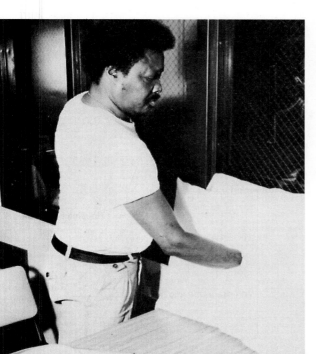

▲

Figure 37-3. To desensitize and improve pressure tolerance of the distal stump in preparation for socket contact, the amputee punches a soft pillow with increasing arm force.

the injury or surgery. Because *sensory* representation of the limb remains in the brain after the limb has been removed, sensation of the missing part (phantom sensation) can be triggered or reinforced by sensory input from elsewhere in the body (Cummings, Alexander, & Gans, 1984). Painful phantom sensations (phantom pain) may be experienced by the amputee as tingling, gripping, clenching, burning, or cramping. Pain can also result from edema, infection, or neuroma in or around the amputation. Postsurgical scar tissue, fragile skin areas, and bony prominences can hinder sensory tolerance of socket contact and the prosthetic control system. The client is educated to monitor the skin on the stump to prevent secondary sensory deficits, caused by pressure from ill-fitting prostheses.

Loss of *neuromuscular* tissue results in limitations in (1) passive and active ROM relative to the site and type of amputation, (2) strength of the extremity, (3) general functional endurance, and (4) postural alignment. After the amputation, changes in weight, sensation, and use of the missing part cause a shift in the amputee's center of gravity. Atrophy of the musculature on the side of the amputation, scoliosis, and compensatory curves may occur without appropriate overall body exercise in both isolated and integrated movement patterns.

With loss of body tissue, there is loss of sensory, *motor*, and coordination functions in both the directly affected and surrounding tissue of the limb. The higher the amputation, the more the amputee must depend on the prosthesis for replacement of bodily function. The shorter the stump the greater the coverage of the stump socket which adds weight, limits proximal joint functions, and limits sensory

▶

Figure 37-4. The below-elbow amputee is able to position the carpenter's hook to hold a nail for hammering.

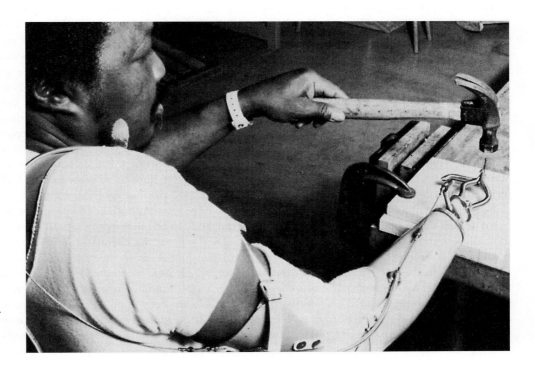

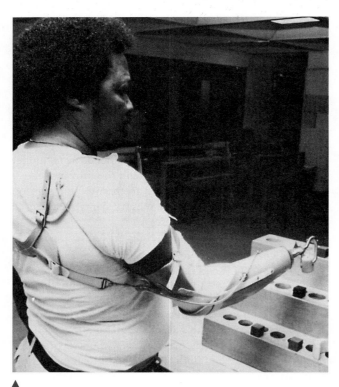

▲
Figure 37-5. Amputee practices control of book opening and closing in grasp, release, and placement of blocks of various shapes.

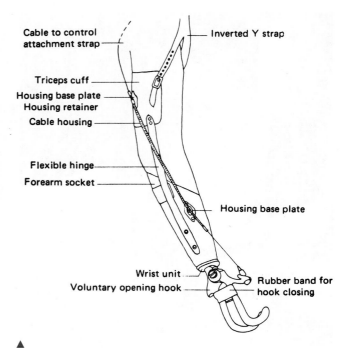

▲
Figure 37-6. Conventional right, below-elbow prosthesis.

contact of the extremity. Before the client receives the prosthesis he or she must develop strength and tolerance in the stump for prosthetic operations (see Figures 37–2 and 37–3). Preventing faulty body mechanics, developing sufficient ROM and strength for prosthetic operation, and maintaining optimum body alignment are goals for training. Motor control of the prosthesis involves learning the control motions for the hook or the hand (terminal device) for grasp and release combined with reach (see Figures 37–4 and 37–5; Fig. 37–6).

The *cognitive* challenge of accepting and functioning with a changed physical body requires productive sensory and motor activity with and without the prosthesis (see Figures 37–2 and 37–4). To be functionally useful, the prosthesis must be integrated into the functional body schema and become a viable part of the person's functional perspective. With trauma resulting from electrical accidents or crush injuries, the client may show signs of cognitive dysfunction caused by the trauma. The occupational therapist assists the client in understanding and accepting the functions and limitations of the prosthesis.

Becoming familiar with the prime psychological concerns of the client is an essential part of the initial contact. Guilt, shame, depression, anger, or impatience about the amputation may be expressed. The person may have lost a dominant hand. It is essential to provide opportunities to work through emotional and physical adjustment through activity, individually and in groups. Involvement of family members in the training program can be beneficial. Participation of the client in the choice of the prosthesis is also important; views of the importance of functional (hook, gripper) and cosmetic (prosthetic hand) prostheses vary among persons with amputations (Spencer, 1993a).

Adjustment to potential changes in ability and performance are affected by premorbid *developmental* factors. A child born with a congenital anomaly generally develops body functions and a body image incorporating that anomaly during the growth process. The older child, adolescent, or adult, having passed this developmental period in physical performance, suffers the traumatic amputation as a loss that disrupts both the body image and the integration of previously developed and habituated functions and skills. The prosthesis is an addition to the natural developmental process and must be incorporated into a meaningful relationship with the body to become an acceptable functional part of it. People with either traumatic or congenital amputations must adapt to the mechanical or electronic replacement of natural functions.

Adjustment to prosthetic wear and use can be enhanced or hindered by *cultural* views and expectations. Preparation of the client for prosthetic wear begins with orienting the client to the functional and cosmetic options of prostheses relative to the client's needs and expectations. The need for and potential value of the prosthetic replacement will partly depend on the client's limitations as a result of the amputation, avocational and vocational needs and interests, and personal attitude toward prosthetic potential. The latter begins with the person's attitude toward the loss of the limb, meaning of the loss, and the perspectives and influence of family and friends. The priorities of the client's personal habits, homelife, work, hobbies, social life, and aspirations will affect the choice of prosthetic components and success of prosthetic wear and operation .

▼ ARTHRITIS

Arthritis is a common chronic condition of the joints that results in pain, loss of motion, deformity, and associated functional deficits. Arthritis is caused by joint disease or direct trauma to bone and soft tissue. Rheumatoid arthritis (RA) is a progressive systemic disease characterized by remissions and exacerbations of destructive inflammation of connective tissue, particularly synovial membranes in synovial joints; RA results in limitations in ROM and deformity. Connective tissue changes may cause sensory impairments in the hands and feet. The disease can occur at any age and is manifested by swollen, reddened, and painful joints during and after excessive use. Rheumatoid arthritis affects the client's functional ability, physical appearance, and mental and physical tolerance (Kelley, 1993; Springhouse Corporation, 1995).

Osteoarthritis (OA) or degenerative joint disease (DJD) is a slowly progressive joint disease that commonly affects the joints of the fingers, elbows, hips, knees, and ankles. Osteoarthritis is characterized by degeneration of the articular cartilage and swelling in the joints. It generally accompanies the aging process, affecting the weight-bearing joints. It is also experienced by people who have been active in sports or by those whose jobs have caused strain in their fingers and legs. Traumatic injury to bone or joints may result in chronic intermittent joint pain exacerbated by heavy use of the extremity or changes in temperature or humidity (Maher, 1993; Springhouse Corporation, 1995).

Deficits in Performance Areas

The person with arthritis pain and deformity develops difficulties in ADL owing to changes in sensation, ROM, and strength in the upper and lower extremities and trunk. Decreased comfort, speed of movement, and endurance in daily task completion result in physical dependence and loss of self-esteem. Adaptations are available to simplify physical challenges, decrease pain in grip, and extend grip and reach. For example, an adolescent with arthritis can continue to write in school by using custom-made hand, wrist, or finger splints and large rough or rubber-textured pencils and pens for easy traction grip, even with hand deformities and pain. Patient education and practice in activity analysis, work simplification, and energy conservation aid the client in daily pacing of tasks to prolong activity.

The problems of arthritis affect the work and productive activity of the person by limiting the timely independent accomplishment of specific job tasks and responsibilities, often requiring job sharing, if available, in the home or in the workplace. Certain tasks may exacerbate the painful condition by requiring repetitive motions or prolonged resistive force of movement without rest. With decreases in sensitivity, grip strength, and ROM, tolerance for the physical forces in tool and material handling is lowered, rendering the person vulnerable to further joint damage and inability to meet work demands. Change in work capability may lead to wage loss.

A change in play or leisure activities may result from decreased facility in activities requiring strength and coordination, along with the social loss from decreased participation in activities with family and friends. This can affect self-esteem, relaxation, and general enjoyment. Change of position or methods of performing activities of interest can facilitate continued participation. The balance of work, play, rest, and leisure is vitally important within the daily activity pattern, particularly when disability interferes with past or future independent activity.

Deficits in Performance Components

A prime *sensory* deficit for individuals with arthritis is intermittent or chronic pain; this pain can temporarily or permanently affect physical functions needed for task accomplishment. Perception and tolerance of pain vary with individuals. When joint inflammation is active, the client may complain of severe pain, and there may be visible inflammation of the joints. During this time joint protection is essential. Restricting mobility during inflammation promotes function following this period. Improper use of joints and lack of attention to therapeutic positioning of the body can cause or increase pain. Denial, frustration, or tension may result in improper use of joints, which puts undue stress on them. When there is a reduction of swelling and inflammation, rehabilitation procedures can begin. A second sensory deficit is decreased sensory perception in the hands and feet, particularly with RA. Numbness, tingling, or decreased coordination in object handling may indicate the possibility of sensory deficits.

Neuromuscular deficits in arthritis include limitations or loss in ROM, strength, and endurance, leading to abnormal postural alignment and joint deformities. Malalignment or deformities in positions of hyperflexion, hyperextension, abduction, adduction, and ulnar deviation may be present. Improper fit of wheelchairs and crutches, walkers, splints, and other tools and utensils exacerbates misalignment of joints and overuse of muscles in resistive activity. Deformities may prevent functional use of muscles. Functional hand splints can assist in alignment of muscles, tendons, and bones. Activities requiring strength are used carefully in the therapeutic program; too much resistance can cause joint pain and fatigue. In the presence of subluxation or dislocation, it is important to avoid overactivity of the affected joints and excessive resistive exercise and activity of the muscles controlling these joints. Muscle atrophy is prevented by passive and active joint ROM (Sobel & Klein, 1993).

Deficits in the *motor* components of function include limitations in gross and fine motor coordination, awkward dexterity, decreased movements in hands and arms, decreased speed of movement, and limitations in task completion and endurance. Functional problems may be caused by internal joint damage, fear of pain, actual pain, decreased strength and sensation, and deformity. When presenting functional challenges, the practitioner must remain alert for signs of mental, psychological, and physical fatigue, as well as the client's subjective responses to the treatment process. The most effective way to prevent deformity is to incorporate therapeutic positioning and movement into daily-living activities. Clients need education in (1) joint protection, (2) use of adaptive equipment, (3) conservation of energy, (4) therapeutic use of joints through balance of activity and rest, and (5) pacing of daily activities and exercises. Assistive devices should be used only to increase function or to protect impaired joints. They should be lightweight, comfortable, and simple to use. If the client cannot use or accept the device easily he or she will soon discard it. Splinting may be used with arthritis to (1) provide support to diseased joints, (2) alleviate pain, (3) prevent deformity, (4) maintain and promote function, and (5) establish functional alignment of bones.

Psychological adjustment to progressive disability and augmentation of natural ability with splints and assistive devices challenges both the individual and his or her family. Because the disease is progressive, the client experiences a gradual decrease in functional ease and capacity owing to decreasing strength, mobility, coordination, and pain-free movement. Because of pain and instability, some clients with arthritis fear further damage to the joints; therefore, they avoid using them. On the other hand, a client may deny the disability and avoid preventive precautions, caus-

ing joint destruction and deformity. Treatment must be geared toward assisting the client to combat the debilitating effects of the disease and to maintain maximal independent functions. The occupational therapist and occupational therapy assistant aid the client in developing a self-directed program of joint protection and function to continue at home (Spencer, 1993b).

Developmentally progressive limitations in independent functions in self-care, work, and play activities hinder the self-esteem of young and older adults. Arthritis may cause lifestyle changes.

Alternating the degree of physical and mental stress in a daily plan of scheduled activities enables the client to engage in both work and rest activities, both gross and fine motor functions, in both sitting and standing positions. Daily plans similar to this help adults maintain activity tolerance, and realistic productivity according to their needs, desires, and abilities (Fries, 1995).

The *cultural* aspects of the client's home environment and general routine influence his or her willingness to adapt to change. For example, concern about appearance may keep people from accepting home adaptations such as entrance ramps. Perceptions of illness and disability may vary between the client and family; each may have different ideas about how much assistance is needed. The family may err in giving too much assistance to the client, building dependence, and depriving the client of the needed exercise of independent daily choices of functions through exercise and activities.

▼ HAND INJURIES

The degree of dysfunction related to hand injuries depends on the type of trauma, location of trauma, and the extent of the injury. Direct trauma may result in sprains, strains, frac-

---

HISTORICAL NOTE
DUNTON'S REFLECTIONS ABOUT ADULTS: COLLABORATIVE CARE

Suzanne M. Peloquin

William Rush Dunton, Jr. described an early encounter with adult clients when he was an assistant physician at Sheppard and Enoch Pratt Hospital in Towson, Maryland. At the time, Dunton (1943) organized dramatic plays for the clients. He remembered:

We had a scene painter as a patient and I was able by much bossing to make him paint some attractive sets. Each morning, he would say: "Won't you let me off today?" And I would harden my heart and refuse.. . . It is probable that in later years I would not have been so brutal in my treatment of my scene-painter patient and I

would have drawn him back to his vocation by easy stages, but experientia docet and I wanted new scenery. (p 245)

Dunton's reflection that experience teaches (experientia docet) reminds us that we can welcome the opportunities for learning—about occupation, about illness, and about people—that present themselves in practice. Dunton's story also seems a plea that we treat adults as such, engaging with them in the collaborations and personal reflections that turn mistakes into the wisdom of maturity. ■

Dunton, W. R. (1943). How I got that way. *Occupational Therapy and Rehabilitation, 22,* 244–6.

tures, and dislocations of bone. Repeated trauma may result in inflammation of muscles, tendons, or nerves. Severe lacerations and bone injuries may result in structural and functional damage to skin, nerves, muscles, tendons, and other soft tissue. The course of the injury may be limited to the immediate and residual effects of direct trauma, or it may result in progressive symptoms of dysfunction from **cumulative trauma** related to occupational illness or injury (Pascarelli, 1995).

A common environment for hand injuries is in the workplace where injuries occur from overexertion of the body, blows from an object, or a fall. Hand injuries also may be caused by tools, machinery, or tasks in the home.

Typical signs and symptoms of hand injury include (1) disruption of skin integrity, (2) localized pain, (3) decreased ROM, (4) possible sensory loss, (5) decreased functional use, (6) a period of immobilization or limited use of the extremity, and (7) fear and denial of the functional prognosis.

Deficits in Performance Areas

Injury to the hand affects independence in ADL because of temporary or permanent disruption of hand dominance, dependence in bimanual hand use, and decreased comfort, function, and endurance in task performance. The daily and economically significant functions of work and productive activities may be affected by loss or limitation in hand use, temporary or permanent disruption of hand dominance, loss or limitation in bimanual functions, and use of splints or assistive devices to augment or substitute for functions. Workers may be excused from work with compensatory financial assistance, but if disability from the injury is permanent, the worker may be unable to return to the former job. The financial loss for both the client and the family can be significant.

Loss of ability to participate in play and leisure activities occurs with forced change in physical functions. Clients may experience imposed leisure time without the ability to perform activities habitually enjoyed. If participation in effective individual and social leisure activity is not available, clients' psychological health may suffer.

Deficits in Performance Components

Deficits in *sensory* functions of the hand include changes in overall sensory awareness of the hand or extremity, changes in sensation, and increases in pain levels. Changes in sensory functions can significantly affect the neuromuscular functions of movement and coordination (Cailliet, 1994).

Because pain is a subjective response, the therapist evaluates the presence of pain through the client's ability to tolerate palpation, movement, force, and object manipulation. Edema and swelling affect the sensory response of the client because the edema chemically irritates and compresses nerve endings. A volumeter is commonly used in hand clinics to measure changes in hand mass caused by edema in comparison with the uninjured hand. Circumference measurements are also obtained by using a tape measure or calipers. Following identification of sensory deficits, the occupational therapist works out a functional program to limit pain, increase the client's pain tolerance and increase sensory awareness (see Chap. 20; Sec. 1).

Impairments in *neuromuscular* functions include effects of sensory and motor disturbances on postural alignment and control, limitation or loss in ROM, limitation in extremity strength and endurance, and development of positive or negative compensatory positions. Neuromuscular functions are generally limited by restrictions of surgery, pain, and the client's fear of moving the hand or arm.

Static splints are used to position the hand or arm in optimum alignment for tissue healing preparatory to passive and active programs. Ideally these should be put on and removed by the client, according to therapist instructions. They may be prescribed by the physician for therapeutic exercise following casting and healing periods. Dynamic or functional splinting allows and encourages joint movement against progressive resistance and may be used in light and graded activities. A splint can help or hinder motion or function. It must be augmented by exercise and activity, as medically and functionally appropriate (Boscheinen-Morrin, Davey, & Conolly, 1995).

Limitations in *motor* components include limitations in gross motor and fine motor coordination, limitations in dexterity, decreased functional ability in the extremity, limitation in endurance and strength, and dependence on adaptive functioning and assists.

Psychological issues in hand injury include (1) the emotional response to trauma, (2) the ability to adapt to restrictions in function, (3) adjustment to the disability and prognosis, (4) the effect on family roles, and (5) the effect on vocational expectations and potentials. Attention to the priorities of the client is crucial in developing the treatment program and assisting the client to accept long-term limitations of cosmesis and function if this is necessary. Assistance in vocational redirection, referral to interdisciplinary personnel, and therapeutic involvement in work-simulated tasks, as appropriate, assists the client in progressing positively, even with the adjustment to splints or assistive devices to substitute for lost functions.

In the *developmental* continuum, the hand injury often occurs to the working age male or female, due to direct or cumulative trauma. The effect of a hand injury on the daily lifestyle and future planning of the client varies with the seriousness of the injury. The working adult who has lost economic security at the beginning or prime of occupational accomplishment and advancement may or may not have the tolerance, interest, or ingenuity to redirect avocational and vocational efforts purposefully.

Cultural and personal perceptions of illness and disability affect individual motivations toward benefiting from therapeutic intervention. The family's attitudes and behaviors also influence the client's progress positively or negatively. It is important to consider the treatment program of the client within the context of his or her lifestyle to ensure maximum participation.

►CONCLUSION

Orthopedic conditions, amputation, arthritis, and hand injury have been presented here to introduce some of the variations of treatment relative to each condition. All of these conditions are common in adults and the student's preparation for clinical entry will require further reading of technical material. Each client is unique, presenting a personal situational context. Although prognoses may be generally assessed, success in recuperation depends on the attitude and effort of the client. Occupational therapists and assistants provide an essential service by progressively involving the client in ADLs, work and productive activities, and play and leisure activities.

Acknowledgments for Section 2

With heartfelt thanks I acknowledge the encouraging contributions of Florene Black, Jane Horton, Mary Katsiaficas-Libby, Kathy A. Long, Gigi Leonard, Peg MacDonald, Barbara Ramsey, Lois Rosage, Blue Hill Memorial Hospital, and the spirit of ewsPatricia Curran to these pages.

▼ REFERENCES

Apley, A. G. & Solomon L. (1988). *Concise system of orthopaedics and fractures*. Cambridge, UK: Butterworth.

Boscheinen-Morrin, J., Davey, V., & Conolly, W. B. (1995). *The hand: Fundamentals of therapy* (2nd ed.). Boston: Butterworth-Heinemann.

Cailliet, R. (1994). *Hand pain and impairment* (4th ed.). Philadelphia: F. A. Davis.

Cedar, L., Thorngren, K. G., & Wallden, B. (1980). Prognostic indica-

tors and early home rehabilitation in elderly patients with hip fractures. *Clinical Orthopedics and Related Research, 152,* 173–184.

Cummings, V., Alexander J., & Gans, S. O. (1984). Management of the amputee. In A. P. Ruskin (Ed.), *Current therapy in psychiatry* (pp. 212, 213, 219). Philadelphia: W. B. Saunders.

Felsenthal, G., Garrison, S. J., & Steinberg, F. U. (1994). *Rehabilitation of the aging and elderly patient*. Baltimore: Williams & Wilkins.

Fries, J. F. (1995). *Arthritis: A take care of yourself health guide for understanding your arthritis*. Reading, MA: Addison-Wesley.

Goldstein, T. S., (1995). *Functional rehabilitation in orthopaedics*. Gaithersburg, MD: Aspen Publishers.

Heppenstall, R. B. (Ed.). (1980). *Fracture treatment and healing*. Philadelphia: W. B. Saunders.

Kelley, W. N. (1993). *Textbook of rheumatology*. Philadelphia: W. B. Saunders.

Maher, A. B. (1994) *Orthopedic nursing*. Philadelphia: W. B. Saunders.

Pascarelli, E. F. (1994). *Repetitive strain injury: A computer user's guide*.

Praemer, A. (1992). *Musculoskeletal conditions in the U. S.* Park Ridge, IL: American Academy of Orthopaedic Surgeons.

Seeger, M. S. & Fisher, L. A. (1982). Adaptive equipment used in the rehabilitation of hip arthroplasty patients. *American Journal of Occupational Therapy, 36,* 503–508.

Sobel, D. & Klein, A. C. (1993). *Arthritis: What exercises work*. New York: St. Martins Press.

Spencer, E. A. (1993a). Functional restoration: Amputation and prosthetic replacement. In H. L. Hopkins & H. D. Smith (Eds.), *Willard and Spackman's occupational therapy* (8th ed.; pp. 656–674). Philadelphia: J. B. Lippincott.

Spencer, E. A. (1993b). Functional restoration: Neurologic, arthritic, orthopedic, cardiac, and pulmonary conditions. In H. L. Hopkins & H. D. Smith (Eds.), *Willard and Spackman's occupational therapy* (8th ed.; pp. 621–656). Philadelphia: J. B. Lippincott.

Spencer, E. A. (1993c). Functional restoration: Preliminary concepts and planning. In H. L. Hopkins & H. D. Smith (Eds.), *Willard and Spackman's occupational therapy* (8th ed.; pp. 605–621). Philadelphia: J. B. Lippincott.

Springhouse Corporation. (1995). *Professional guide to diseases* (5th ed.). Springhouse, PA: author.

Trombly, C. A. (Ed.). (1995). *Occupational therapy for physical dysfunction* (4th ed.). Baltimore: Williams & Wilkins.

Wixson, R. L., Stulberg, D., & Mehlhoff, M. (1991). Total hip replacement with cemented, uncemented and hybrid prostheses. *Journal of Bone and Joint Surgery, 73 A,* 257–269.

Chapter 38

Cardiopulmonary Dysfunction in Adults

Regina Ferraro

The purpose of this chapter is to help occupational therapy practitioners understand basic cardiopulmonary diagnoses and their implications for occupational therapy treatment. This information is important even for those practitioners who do not specialize in cardiopulmonary rehabilitation. Many clients have cardiopulmonary disease either in their past medical history, or secondary to multiple trauma, multisystem failure, or neurological injury. Consequently, all occupational therapy practitioners working in physical dysfunction settings should be knowledgeable about the medical and surgical interventions used in the care of clients with cardiopulmonary dysfunction.

▼ PERFORMANCE AREA AND COMPONENT DEFICITS

There are many functional limitations experienced by clients with cardiopulmonary dysfunction. These clients are typically (1) impaired by disease for prolonged periods, as in the client with chronic obstructive pulmonary disease (COPD); or (2) impaired by sudden onset, as in the client with acute myocardial infarction (MI). In both of these scenarios, the client with cardiopulmonary dysfunction is expected to undergo lifestyle and role changes that, in turn, affect occupational performance.

Activities of daily living (ADLs), work, and play or leisure activities are the occupational therapy performance areas that are affected by cardiopulmonary dysfunction. The performance components that contribute to these performance area deficits are found in sensory motor, psychosocial and psychological, and at times, cognitive integration categories. Within those categories, the components of endurance, activity tolerance, gross motor coordination, roles, values, and coping skills are particularly affected.

Cardiopulmonary disease is a somewhat unique disorder in that it imposes multiple lifestyle changes on clients and their families. Noncompliance with cardiopulmonary activity limitations, medications, and diet can lead to worsening of disease processes, severe medical complications, and sometimes death. Occupational therapy practitioners, because of their training in the psychosocial as well as the physical frames of reference, play a key role in the treatment of this client population. Our foundation in activity analysis and activity adaptation, allows occupational therapy practitioners to be vital and integral members of the cardiopulmonary rehabilitation team.

▼ EVALUATION

Evaluation of clients with cardiopulmonary dysfunction can be broken down into four essential components: medical chart review and history taking, client interview, functional evaluation, and physiological evaluation.

History Taking

It is critical to do a detailed medical chart review before beginning an interview or evaluation with a client. The occupational therapy practitioner should look for the following information during this chart review: (1) the client's presenting primary diagnosis, (2) the secondary diagnosis, (3) past medical history, (4) surgical procedures, (5) medications, and (6) results of laboratory or other diagnostic tests. In addition, information about the client's work history and social support system should be noted. Physician recommendations relative to activity levels are also important. The occupational therapy practitioner is responsible for understanding the medical information in the chart. Any terminology that is unfamiliar should be looked up in a medical dictionary, or discussed with the client's medical team before evaluation.

The primary precaution for clients with cardiopulmonary disease is the risk of fatal cardiac or respiratory arrest. Activity levels that overtax clients' diseased cardiac or pulmonary systems can trigger those arrests. The chart review should give the occupational therapy practitioner an idea of what activity levels are safe for particular clients.

Client Interview

The initial interview for clients with cardiopulmonary disease can begin with a discussion about their functional performance levels. The occupational therapist also needs to ask clients about their preadmission roles and coping skills. Because stair climbing requires a lot of cardiopulmonary work, it is also important to ask clients about the number of stairs in their work and home environments. During the interview, the occupational therapist should observe the client's breathing patterns, level of comfort or discomfort, posture, and information-processing skills. Chapter 13 contains more detail about interviewing techniques.

Functional Evaluation

An initial occupational therapy evaluation for this population includes evaluation of the client's current level of functioning in ADLs, with particular attention to the client's physiological response to functional activity. These physiological responses are an indication of the client's activity tolerance or endurance. Psychological coping skills also need to be assessed. Chapters 15 and 16 contain more information about ADL and psychosocial assessments, respectively.

Clients with cardiopulmonary dysfunction may also be screened for upper extremity range of motion (ROM), strength, gross and fine motor coordination, and sensation. Chapter 16 offers details about these evaluation techniques.

Therapists need to check with medical staff about any special precautions before performing these evaluations.

Physiological Evaluation

VITAL SIGNS MONITORING

Clinicians working with clients with cardiopulmonary disease need to be competent in monitoring vital signs, because these are indicators of a client's physiological status. Vital signs require monitoring during evaluation and treatment, both at rest and in response to therapeutic activity. Clinicians need to keep a watchful eye on the clients and monitor how they are physiologically responding to given activities. Clinicians also need to identify cardiopulmonary distress quickly. Cardiopulmonary distress is defined by Krider (1995) as labored, rapid, irregular, or shallow breathing that may be accompanied by coughing, choking, wheezing, dyspnea, anxiety, chest pain, or cyanosis of the oral mucosa, lips, and fingers.

Vital signs are often the first and most important indicator that a client's condition is changing (Krider, 1995). The **vital signs** most commonly monitored in the cardiopulmonary population are **pulse** (heart rate; HR), **respiratory rate (RR)**, and **blood pressure (BP)**.

Pulse

Pulse is the rhythmical dilation of arteries, produced by the blood being pumped into the arteries by the contractions of the heart. Therefore, pulse is an indication of heart rate—the number of times the heart contracts or beats per minute. The normal pulse, or HR for adults ranges from 60 to 100 beats per minute (bpm), with an average of 72 to 78 bpm. A pulse rate higher them 100 bpm is termed **tachycardia** (abnormally fast HR). A pulse rate less than 60 bpm is termed **bradycardia** (abnormally slow HR). Pulse is evaluated for rate, rhythm, and strength. The most common location to palpate the pulse is at the site of the radial artery in the wrist. Once palpated, the number of beats per minute is counted and recorded. If a client is suffering from a low BP, pulse is more easily palpated from a carotid artery in the neck, because these arteries are closer to the heart than the radial arteries.

Respiratory Rate

Respiratory rate (RR) is counted by watching the abdomen or chest wall move in and out with breathing, a motion caused by the expansion and deflation of the lungs. Each full cycle of chest or abdominal movement (in and out) counts as 1 breath. The normal range for the adult RR is 12 to 22 breaths per minute. Tachypnea refers to a RR above normal. This rate can be the result of exercise, fever, pain, or anxiety. **Bradypnea** refers to a slow RR rate. This rate is the less common of the two, yet may occur as a side effect of medication or in a client with central nervous system damage. It is important for the practitioner to count the RR without letting the client know this is being done. If the client is aware that he or she is being monitored, he or she can alter the rate. Movement of the supraclavicular fossae, at the union of the neck and the shoulders, may be used in those cardiopulmonary clients whose chest or abdominal movements are difficult to see.

Blood Pressure

Blood pressure (BP) is the force exerted against the walls of the arteries as the blood moves through the arterial vessels. BP is measured with a sphygmomanometer, and is recorded in millimeters of mercury (mm Hg). The BP cuff of the sphygmomanometer is wrapped around the client's brachial artery and inflated to a pressure 30 mm higher than the client's average, which results in temporary obliteration of the pulse. This obliteration creates turbulence in the brachial artery. The turbulence creates sounds (Korotkoff sounds) that can be heard with a stethoscope held over the brachial artery as the cuff is deflated. Systolic blood pressure (SBP) is the peak force that occurs when blood is circulated through the systemic and pulmonary systems during contraction of the heart. It corresponds to the first sound heard in the brachial artery as the BP cuff deflates. The normal adult range for SBP is 90 to 150 mm Hg, with the average being 120 mm Hg. Diastolic blood pressure (DBP) is the force that occurs in the blood vessels when the heart is relaxing. It is during this period that the heart is filling with blood. The normal adult range for DBP is 60 to 90 mm Hg, with the average being 80 mm Hg. This corresponds to the last sound heard in the brachial artery as the BP cuff deflates. BP consistently greater than 140/90 is referred to as hypertension (high BP). BP consistently lower than 90/60 is referred to as hypotension (low BP).

OTHER ASSESSMENTS

Additional diagnostic tests are used to assess physiological and cardiopulmonary function. One of the most commonly used laboratory tests to assess respiratory function is arterial blood gases (ABGs). The ABGs are measured from the arterial blood supply, which contains oxygen and carbon dioxide levels indicative of lung function. Measurements of ABGs provide us with information on the oxygenation status of the blood and the acid–base balance in the blood (Wilkins, 1995). Three relevant measurements of oxygenation provided by ABGs are PaO_2, SaO_2, and CaO_2. PaO_2 is the partial pressure of oxygen in plasma and reflects the ability of the lungs to transfer oxygen from the environment into the circulating blood. The normal adult range for PaO_2 is 75 to 95 mm Hg on room air. A PaO_2 less than the predicted range is an indication of hypoxemia (abnormally low O_2 levels in the blood). PaO_2 has clinical significance because clients who sustain a low PaO_2 are at risk for cognitive compromise because the brain is not receiving adequate oxygen. These clients are generally in need of oxygen therapy, which is discussed later in this chapter.

SaO_2 is the amount of oxygen bound to hemoglobin. The normal value of SaO_2 is greater than 95%. CaO_2 is the total content of oxygen in arterial blood and is one of the most important blood gas determinations because it influences tissue oxygenation. The normal range for CaO_2 is 16 to 20 mL/dL blood. CaO_2 levels need to be stable prior to treatment so that exercise does not further compromise tissue oxygenation.

EQUIPMENT

There are many different types of medical equipment used to monitor a client's physiological status in cardiopulmonary dysfunction settings. Equipment used with this population extends from the inpatient setting to the outpatient arena and is vast and ever developing. Practitioners who wish to specialize in this treatment area should be thoroughly oriented in the purpose, operation, and precautions for the equipment housed on their particular unit. Some frequently used equipment is described here.

Arterial Pressure Line

An **arterial pressure line** (A-line or art-line) is a catheter that is inserted into an artery, most commonly the radial artery in adults, to monitor BP and provide blood gas measurements. Usually the reading is projected onto a monitor at or above the clients bedside. Clinicians should use caution not to confuse an A-line with an intravenous line, because the two entail different precautions for movement and activity.

Oximeter

An **oximeter** is a noninvasive instrument that measures the percentage of hemoglobin saturated with oxygen. The normal adult value for O_2 saturation is greater than 95%. Oximetry is often used during occupational therapy treatment sessions to monitor a client's physiological response to activity (Fig. 38–1). When clients are unable to maintain adequate oxygenation with activity, they are said to be in desaturation.

Electrocardiogram

An electrocardiograph (ECG or EKG) is a machine that graphically records the heart's electrical activity through electrodes, or leads, placed over the chest. ECG monitoring can be performed on a continuous basis in the intensive care unit (ICU), or by a portable 12-lead ECG. The purpose of performing a 12-lead ECG is to obtain 12 different views of the electrical activity in the heart. These electrical currents are then recorded, or traced, by the ECG on specialized graph paper. The ECG tracings are clinically evaluated for abnormalities in several different variables. Abnormalities in ECG tracings are termed dysrhythmias. Dysrhythmias, or **arrhythmias**, are any abnormality in the rate, regularity, or sequence of cardiac electrical activity. Occupational therapists working with those clients with cardiopulmonary dis-

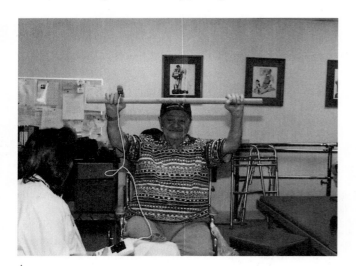

▲
Figure 38-1. This client performs upper extremity (UE) active range of motion (AROM) activities while being monitored via oximetry.

ease who require 12-lead ECG monitoring with activity, should pursue continuing education in this area.

Holter Monitor

A **Holter monitor** is a small recording unit that stores a client's ECG tracings from surface electrodes for a preprogrammed time period. It is, in essence, a portable ECG unit. Clients wear the unit and electrodes while keeping a diary of activities. Later a cardiologist can interpret the tracings to see if (1) arrhythmias occur over time, and (2) particular activities cause abnormalities in the electrical activity of the heart. The ability to link specific activities to heart function helps determine safe activity levels for clients with cardiopulmonary dysfunction. Holter monitors are also sometimes used with clients who do not have a primary diagnosis of cardiac dysfunction. For example, many clients who are admitted to acute-care hospitals for cerebral vascular accidents are placed on Holter monitors. The monitors identify the presence of an arrhythmia, which assists in the confirmation of an embolism as a stroke's cause. In total, cardioembolic phenomena cause about 15% to 20% of all strokes (Roth, 1993).

Other Monitors

Many medical devices that can monitor HR, oxygen saturation, BP, and ECG concurrently are commercially available. Use of this type of equipment is helpful during the early phases of activity progression. It is critical that in the initial evaluation of the client with cardiopulmonary dysfunction, close attention is paid to the physician-directed activity level and vital signs limitations. Contrary to previous beliefs, there is no longer a role for rest therapy, or prolonged bed rest, in the management of the client with cardiovascular disease (Kottke, Haney, & Doucette, 1990). Early mobilization is pro-

moted in acute hospitalization and has been deemed beneficial to the client's recovery process (Wegner et al., 1984).

▼ TREATMENT

The ultimate goal of occupational therapy treatment for adults with cardiopulmonary disease is to help them resume their valued life activities and reduce their disease-related risk factors, such as cigarette smoking. To accomplish these goals, occupational therapy practitioners use activity grading and monitoring, energy conservation and work simplification, relaxation and stress management, and prevention and home programs.

Activity Grading and Monitoring

ACTIVITY GRADING

Treatment of clients with cardiopulmonary disease begins in the acute care setting and extends to rehabilitation hospitals, skilled nursing facilities, outpatient clinics, and the home. Once a client's functional and physiological status is evaluated and documented, treatment begins. Clients with cardiopulmonary dysfunction require regulated activity during the rehabilitative process. The main reason for regulating activity is to reduce or control the stress or workload placed on the heart. The greater the cardiac workload, the greater the oxygen demand of the myocardium.

Because of the need for regulated activity, an essential component of treatment for the client with cardiopulmonary disease is the use of graded activity. Clients who have experienced prolonged hospitalizations because of cardiopulmonary instability are, for the most part, largely deconditioned and significantly impaired in ADL performance. For these clients a simple bathing activity, such as face washing, may cause desaturation. It is essential that activity implementation with this population be modified and graded according to client progress. Progression through graded activities enables the client with cardiopulmonary disease to regain or enhance activity tolerance.

ACTIVITY MONITORING

As an upper extremity exercise program or an ADL activity is graded, the clients physiological tolerance of these activities must be monitored and documented (Fig. 38–2). At the beginning of each treatment the occupational therapy practitioner should take the clients' vital signs at rest. Pulse or HR, BP, RR, and oxygen saturation should be measured and recorded. If the client's resting vital signs are not within the ranges considered medically safe for him or her, the treatment session should be discontinued. If the client's resting vital signs are within a medically safe range, then treatment can continue. Vital signs should be measured again 5 to 10 minutes into the treatment session. The meaning of changes in vital signs is different for each client: for some, a

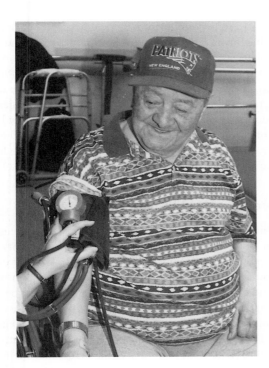

Figure 38-2. This client has his blood pressure monitored after activity.

small change indicates physiological instability; for others, this is not true. Therefore, physician-guided vital sign limitations are helpful.

In general, oxygen saturation should be maintained at 90% or greater during functional activity, and HR should be limited to an increase no more than 20 to 30 bpm above the resting rate. A HR of less than 50 bpm is considered an inappropriate response, and the activity being performed should be terminated. Afterward the client should be monitored, and the physician notified (Shanfield & Hammond, 1984). BP responses can be variable even in healthy individuals, so medical guidance relative to safe parameters for individual clients is advisable. As a general rule, BP should be limited to an increase or decrease of no more than 15 to 20 mm Hg (Kottke et al., 1990; Krider, 1995; Ogden, 1979; Shanfield & Hammond, 1984).

If the cardiovascular response to activity is deemed appropriate by the monitoring clinician, the activity is continued, and the vital signs are recorded again 5 minutes after completion of activity. The occupational therapist should record the client's vital signs in graph form on initial evaluation and treatment notes. Doing so will assist the client and the therapist in recognizing progress. Initial cardiopulmonary response to activity may be demonstrated by elevated HR and BPs, because of the increased work required by the heart. As the conditioning effect occurs, the resting and working HR and BP should decrease to more appropriate levels.

Clients with cardiopulmonary dysfunction require education about the symptoms of increased cardiac work before activity progression. This teaching is needed in advance so that feedback may be adequately provided to the practitioner by the client in the event of a nonadaptive physiological response. Physiological signs and symptoms of cardiopulmonary distress include dizziness, fatigue, chest pain, palpitations, headache, nausea, shortness of breath, diaphoresis (profuse sweating), and anxiety. Clinicians should also be alert to the nonverbal signs of client discomfort. The principles of activity gradation and monitoring are clearly illustrated in cardiac rehabilitation programs.

CARDIAC REHABILITATION

There are four phases of cardiac rehabilitation. Phase I is the acute hospitalization period. Activity during this stage is limited to bed to chair transfers, basic ADLs, and slow walking. Orthostatic intolerance and sinus tachycardia are often present during activity progression in phase I. Phase II begins at the time of discharge and extends 12 weeks after the cardiac event. Phase II focuses on regaining endurance and improving activity tolerance. Reconditioning and risk modification programs are implemented. No isometric exercise is permitted at this time. Mild endurance exercise training is begun to increase aerobic capacity. In phase III, rigorous risk factor modification is begun, strength training is performed to induce physiological adaptations to exercise, and the client is prepared for return to work. Exercise training is aimed at lowering BP and HR to decrease myocardial workload. Phase IV is considered the maintenance phase. During this phase exercise habits are established, and risk factor modification is ongoing.

As clients proceed through the phases of cardiac rehabilitation, activity levels are increased, based on the client's physiological responses to activities. All purposeful tasks place an energy demand on the cardiopulmonary system. The metabolic equivalent (MET) is considered the unit of choice to measure energy expenditure in the cardiopulmonary population (Ogden, 1979). The MET is the energy expended in a resting state: 1 MET is equal to 3.5 mL oxygen per kilogram of body weight per minute. The energy cost of activities is then rated based on the resting MET. For example, if an activity is rated as 5 METs, that means that it requires five times the oxygen expended at rest.

Minimal or very light cardiac activity is considered to require 1 to 2 METs; light cardiac activity requires 2 to 3 METs; moderate cardiac activity requires 3 to 4 METs; and heavy cardiac activity requires 4 to 5 METs. Table 16–22 (p. 255) provides examples of appropriate functional activities for distinct levels of cardiac activity. The MET levels appropriate for a given client in a given phase of cardiac rehabilitation should be determined in conjunction with the client's physician.

Energy Conservation and Work Simplification

The principles of work simplification for energy conservation are fundamental to the treatment of clients with cardiopulmonary dysfunction. Work simplification is the performance of a task in an organized, planned, and orderly way, such that body motions, work load, and fatigue are reduced to a minimum. Energy conservation is essential for clients with cardiopulmonary dysfunction because it enables them to save their energy for fundamental tasks or for times during the day when more energy is needed. The following work simplification and energy conservation techniques are recommended:

- Balance work and rest. For example, if a client has a social function to attend in the evening, recommend resting in the afternoon. Clients are advised to take frequent rest breaks to prevent fatigue and by all means avoid rushing.
- Maintain good posture. Be especially cautious of prolonged stooped posture. Avoid reaching and bending by prearranging work at comfortable levels.
- Whenever possible perform a task in a sitting, instead of a standing, position.
- Avoid lifting and holding. Use a rolling cart, or slide items when possible.
- Rest for at least 60 minutes after meals so that the blood needed for digestion will not be interrupted by exercise.
- Work in a properly lit and well-ventilated environment.
- Prioritize tasks, practice delegation, and eliminate steps that are unnecessary to task completion.

Clients with cardiopulmonary disease may need assistance in deciding how to conserve energy. They should be guided in their decision-making process about how they wish to use their energy. An interest checklist may be helpful for these clients. For example, a client with limited activity tolerance may choose to employ a homemaker for housecleaning tasks to save energy to perform an alternative task. A different client may take great pride in his or her role as a homemaker and, hence, employ work simplification techniques for the successful performance of this task. Adaptive equipment plays a role for clients with cardiopulmonary dysfunction, especially in the home environment. Long-handled sponges and tub seats increase bathing independence in the client with limited activity tolerance.

Relaxation and Stress Management

Principles of stress management and relaxation are appropriate for integration into occupational therapy treatment protocols for clients with cardiopulmonary dysfunction. Clients with cardiopulmonary dysfunction have, at times, been mandated by physicians to make what they would consider to be drastic lifestyle changes. They require education in the physiological effect that stress has on their body, the warning signs of stress, and methods to reduce stress. The stress induced flight-or-fight response stimulates the release of a variety of hormones, including epinephrine and norepinephrine. These hormones can increase BP and cholesterol levels. Epinephrine may cause constriction of the coronary arteries, reducing blood flow to the heart (Stuart, Deckro, DeSilva, & Benson, 1993). Instruction in the relaxation response and cognitive behavioral stress management techniques (see Chap. 20, Sec. 9) serve to significantly lower rates of coronary disease and increase coping skills. The carryover of these techniques is essential to lifestyle modification in the client with cardiopulmonary dysfunction.

Prevention and Home Programs

Prevention education and home program implementation for the promotion of healthy lifestyle changes in clients with cardiopulmonary dysfunction is essential. Risk factor modification needs to begin in the rehabilitative program structure and be carried out into the home. Clients must be educated in the coronary and pulmonary risk factors that they can control. Coronary disease factors that clients can control are smoking, high BP, sedentary lifestyle, overweight, high cholesterol, and stress. Pulmonary risk factors that clients can control are smoking and environmental conditions. Clients may be at a point at which role performance is rapidly altered by physical limitations or physiological impairments. Because of this, a key to the success of disease management is for the client to gain a sense of control.

During acute hospitalization, clients retain little information concerning their conditions. Education must include written handout materials, and demonstrative learning when possible. Education of cardiac clients cannot be considered complete without the inclusion of their partners and family members, owing to the high anxiety they experience and the important role they play in caring for the cardiac client (Tooth & McKenna, 1995). Clients with **chronic obstructive pulmonary disease (COPD)**, who suffer from anxiety coupled with dyspnea (shortness of breath), also benefit from having procedures written down. Education should bridge the gap between hospital and home.

Pederson states that "a successful home care plan depends on careful assessment and planning before discharge" (Pederson, 1993; p. 24). Compliance with home programs should be fostered by the client keeping a journal and by partner and family encouragement. The positive effects of exercise and diet change, such as feeling better and having more energy, should be emphasized to the client during this difficult lifestyle change. The following sections deal with specific cardiopulmonary diagnoses.

▼ MYOCARDIAL INFARCTION

Demographics

All occupational therapy practitioners who work with adults will encounter clients at one time or another who suffer from coronary artery disease (CAD). One of the most frequently seen clinical manifestations of CAD is myocardial infarction (MI). Nearly 1.5 million Americans sustain an MI, or heart attack, each year. Of these 500,000 episodes are fatal (Wegner et al., 1995). MI is not an affliction of the elderly population alone; 45% of MIs occur in persons younger than 65 years of age. MI occurs more frequently in men than in women.

Definition

The heart is a muscle that receives its vascular blood supply from the coronary arteries and their respective branches. Inadequate blood supply, or sudden interruption of blood flow to the myocardium leads to ischemia (tissue damage). If the blood supply does not resume, then infarction (tissue death) develops. The most common cause of inadequate blood flow is narrowing of the coronary arteries by atherosclerotic disease, or by thrombotic or embolic occlusion. Acute ischemic syndromes include acute MI, angina, and sudden ischemic death.

Signs and Symptoms

The primary presenting symptom for the diagnosis of MI is usually a pressure like chest pain that is unrelenting and severe. The pain is located substernally, and can radiate to the arms, back, or upper jaws. Secondary symptoms are dyspnea (shortness of breath), nausea and vomiting, and confusion, particularly in the elderly. Some people present with only these secondary symptoms.

MIs are classified according to which coronary artery is occluded and which ventricle is involved. Most frequently, they affect the left ventricle. The different types of left ventricular MIs are classified according to which wall of the left ventricle has been affected—the anterior, inferior, septal, posterior, or anterolateral (Miracle, 1988). There are differences in the medical management of the different types of MI, which are beyond the scope of this chapter. In general, after a left ventricular MI, a client is more likely to develop dysrhythmias; whereas, after a right ventricular MI, a client is more likely to develop decreased cardiac output.

Angina is sometimes associated with MI. Angina is a transitory syndrome characterized by episodic pain when the oxygen supply to the heart is insufficient to meet the heart's needs. It can occur as a result of an increased oxygen need in high-cardiac–output conditions (Klein, 1988).

Medical Interventions

MEDICATIONS

During the acute hospitalization period, pharmacological treatment of acute MI is used to relieve pain and anxiety, limit the extent of heart muscle necrosis, and prevent complications. The following lists some of the common medications used for the acute MI population:

- Nitrates—used to improve myocardial oxygen supply by dilating the coronary arteries and collateral vessels (eg, nitroglycerine).
- β-Adrenergic blockers—used to decrease HR, BP, and the force of contraction, thereby decreasing the myocardial oxygen demand and preventing ischemia (eg, metoprolol [Lopressor]).
- Calcium channel blockers—a group of organic compounds that inhibit calcium entry into smooth muscle and myocardial cells. They decrease the BP by peripheral vasodilation and relieve coronary vasospasm by dilating the coronary arteries (eg, verapamil and nifedipine).
- Inotrophic agents—used to increase cardiac output and increase blood flow (eg, dopamine).

SURGERY

There are different types of surgical procedures used in people after an MI to restore myocardial profusion. Thrombolytic therapy is an early treatment used to improve the survival rate of MI clients. It is started, within the critical time frame of 0 to 6 hours after symptomatic onset, by direct infusion of a thrombolytic agent into an occluded or infarct-related artery. Examples of thrombolytic agents are tissue plasminogen activator (tPA), urokinase, and streptokinase. This procedure can dissolve some or all of the blockage in the infarct-related artery, which limits the infarct size and improves outcome. The smaller the area of myocardial damage, the better the heart's overall functioning will be.

Percutaneous Transluminal Coronary Angioplasty (PTCA)

This procedure involves dilation of the affected, or acutely occluded, coronary artery by balloon angioplasty to open the vessel for myocardial profusion. The PTCA has the advantage of not requiring clients to undergo open-heart surgery. It is most indicated for those with proximal, single-vessel coronary artery disease (Halperin & Levine, 1985; Tommaso, Lesch, & Sonnenblick, 1984).

Intraaortic Balloon Pump (IABP)

The IABP is a mechanical support device used for acute myocardial reperfusion. The balloon device is inserted into the femoral artery and passed to the ascending aorta. While using ECG or hemodynamic monitoring, the balloon is inflated with helium during diastole and deflated during systole. This serves to increase cardiac output and decrease myocardial oxygen consumption (Gersh & Rahimtolla, 1991).

Coronary Artery Bypass Graft (CABG)

The CABG is a surgical procedure that was devised for the treatment of coronary artery disease in the late 1960s. It is currently one of the most commonly performed major surgical operations, and holds only a 1% to 2% risk of mortality (Tommaso et al., 1984). During this procedure a vein from another part of the body, usually the saphenous vein in the lower extremity, is grafted onto the heart surface, to bypass, or detour the atherosclerotic narrowing of a coronary artery. This creates a patent (open) artery and, thereby, permits improved blood flow to the myocardium.

Occupational Therapy Treatment

The principles of cardiac rehabilitation are used in the occupational therapy treatment of clients following an acute MI or after cardiac reperfusion surgery. The client is gradually progressed through the appropriate activity level, as described earlier in this chapter. These clients are seen in a variety of treatment settings, ranging from acute-care hospitals to outpatient clinics. The role of the occupational therapy practitioner in the treatment of the client with cardiac dysfunction is to maximize independence, increase activity tolerance and psychosocial skill performance, while promoting reintegration into work, productive, and leisure activities within established activity limitations.

▼ CONGESTIVE HEART FAILURE

Demographics and Definition

The National Heart, Lung, and Blood Institute estimates that over 2 million Americans have heart failure and that about 400,000 new cases are diagnosed each year (Konstam et al., 1994). Congestive heart failure (CHF) is a clinical syndrome in which the heart fails to maintain an adequate output, resulting in decreased blood flow to the tissues and congestion in the pulmonary or the systemic circulation, or both. A client who is experiencing heart failure has a weak heart, with reduced pumping power.

Signs and Symptoms

For most clients, heart failure is a chronic condition, which means that it can be treated and managed, but not cured. The most common causes of heart failure are CAD (usually with previous MI), cardiomyopathy, hypertension, and heart valve disease. The signs and symptoms of CHF are difficulty breathing, especially on exertion or when lying flat in bed (nocturnal dyspnea); waking up breathless at night; frequent dry, hacking cough, especially when lying down; fatigue, weakness; dizziness or fainting; edematous (swollen) feet, ankles, and legs; and nausea with abdominal swelling, pain, or tenderness. These signs and symptoms occur because the heart is pumping with less power and force than normal.

Medical Treatment

MEDICATIONS

Initial medical management of congestive heart failure includes rest to decrease cardiac work, and initiation of pharmacological agents. The following lists some of the common medications used with the congestive heart failure population:

- Diuretics are started immediately when the client presents with symptoms of volume overload. Diuretics are often referred to as "water pills" because they help remove excess fluid and salt from the body. An example of a commonly used diuretic is furosemide (Lasix).
- Angiotensin-converting enzyme (ACE) inhibitors relax the blood vessels, making it easier for the heart to pump. An example of a commonly used ACE inhibitor is captopril.
- Digitalis increases the force of ventricular contraction; because it strengthens each heart beat, more blood can be pumped. Digitalis is commonly prescribed as digoxin.

SURGERY

Some clients with CHF benefit from surgical revascularization. Clients with CHF are generally candidates for revascularization if they have viable myocardium fed by stenotic arteries (Konstam et al., 1994). Two types of surgical revascularization procedures considered for clients with CHF are CABG and balloon angioplasty. Use of CABG prolongs life in clients with worsening heart failure. Valve replacement or valve repair is undertaken if the cause of CHF is valvular dysfunction.

Heart transplantation is also considered for those clients who continue to have repeated hospitalizations despite aggressive medical therapy. Cardiac transplantation recipients must meet specific selection criteria. Clients with end-stage coronary disease or idiopathic cardiomyopathy, a condition that affects the muscular function of one or both ventricles, and who have a potential of survival of less than 12 months, are appropriate candidates for transplantation (Myerowitz, 1987) .

Practitioners working with the heart transplant population must be aware of precautions for clients with compromised immune systems. To prevent a transplant recipient from rejecting the tissue transplant or graft, the client is treated with immunosuppressive therapy. This therapy includes antirejection drugs, such as azathioprine and cyclosporine. These drugs inhibit the immune response and serve to prevent tissue rejection, but also increase the client's risk of contracting infection. A simple cold can not be fought off by the immunocompromised client. Practitioners working with this population are required to follow institution-guided precautions, including treatment in isolation rooms during early stages, gowning, gloving, and masking. Clients who have undergone cardiac transplantation are appropriate for cardiac rehabilitation with slight modifications. Clinicians must remember that clients undergoing cardiac transplantation have been debilitated for prolonged periods. They may have presurgical functional and MET capacity limitations influencing the initial phases of cardiac rehabilitation.

CLIENT EDUCATION

Heart failure is one of the most common causes for hospital readmission. Proper discharge planning and client education is essential to prevent unnecessary readmissions. Education of this client population should include general counseling about the disease process, symptoms of worsening heart failure, risk factor modification, prognosis, activity recommendations, dietary restrictions, and medication management. Clients with CHF are advised to keep a diary of their daily weights and to inform their physician if a weight gain of 3 to 5 lb or more occurs within a week. This weight gain means that the client is retaining fluids and medication regimens may need to be altered.

Occupational Therapy Treatment

Occupational therapy treatment of the client with CHF uses principles of cardiac rehabilitation, with a focus on ADL training and maximizing activity tolerance. Energy conservation and work simplification techniques need to be integrated into clients' daily living skills and work and productive activity performance to facilitate psychosocial adaptation in the face of physiological limitations and altered role performance.

▼ CHRONIC OBSTRUCTIVE PULMONARY DISORDER

Demographics and Definition

Chronic obstructive pulmonary disorder (COPD) affects 9 million Americans. It is the fifth leading cause of death in the United States and is 1.8 times more prevalent in men than in women (Fishman, 1988; Johannesen, 1994). COPD is the term used to describe a variety of pulmonary disorders, including **chronic bronchitis**, asthma, **emphysema**, and **bronchiectasis**. It is, however, generally restricted to chronic bronchitis and emphysema, because unlike asthma, COPD implies irreversible airway damage (Fishman, 1988). COPD is characterized by progressive limitation in the flow of air into and out of the lungs.

Emphysema is the destruction of the walls of the bronchioles and alveoli, resulting in abnormally enlarged air spaces. The most common cause of emphysema is the inhalation of tobacco smoke, which induces an imbalance between protease and antiprotease activity in the lung, resulting in a destruction of the elastic fibers in the alveolar walls.

Chronic bronchitis is characterized by excessive mucous secretion in the bronchial tree, which leads to obstruction of airflow and mucous plugging. It is manifested by persistent productive cough. Chronic bronchitis is diagnosed when cough and symptoms are present on most days for a minimum of 3 months, for at least 2 successive years or 6 months during 1 year.

In COPD, the walls of the small airways and alveoli lose their elasticity. The alveolar walls become thickened and the air passageway becomes plugged with mucus. Air enters the alveoli during inhalation, but may not be able to escape during exhalation because the air passages collapse, trapping stale air. This leads to decreased gas exchange, tiring of respiratory muscles, increased CO_2 accumulation, and hypoventilation.

As COPD progresses, the disease process places a large burden on the heart. The right side of the heart needs to produce high pressures to force blood through the narrow blood vessels to the lungs. This causes the right chambers of the heart to enlarge and thicken. Cor pulmonale is a condition in which the right ventricle of the heart is hypertrophied secondary to lung disease.

Signs and Symptoms

The client with COPD usually presents with the following symptoms: dyspnea (difficulty breathing), morning cough, expiratory wheeze, and in the later stages of the disease, breathlessness that prevents them from lying down. Dyspnea is the hallmark of COPD and is often viewed as the single greatest contributor to functional difficulties (Leidy, 1995).

Medical Treatment

There is presently no cure for COPD; however, positive lifestyle changes can result in a longer, more comfortable life (Johannsen, 1994). In many instances, some irreversible damage has already occurred by the time COPD is diagnosed. Management of COPD is through health care education, smoking cessation, pharmacological therapy, supplemental oxygen, infection protection, nutritional therapy, and pulmonary rehabilitation.

HEALTH EDUCATION

General health education is needed in the COPD population to promote healthy lifestyles. In addition to general health practices, this population is advised to avoid exposure to dust and fumes, curtail physical activities during air pollution alerts, and to avoid extremes in temperature and humidity, because these conditions trigger hyperreactivity in their irritated airways (Johannsen, 1994). Smoking cessation is essential in preventing the progression of COPD. Cigarette smoking results in destruction of lung tissue. Clients should be referred to smoking cessation programs for assistance with this lifestyle change.

MEDICATIONS

Pharmacological therapy for the client with COPD includes the use of bronchodilators, steriods, antibiotics, diuretics, and mucolytics. Bronchodilators, such as ipratropium bromide, act as anticholinergic agents. Once inhaled, they block the muscarinic cholinergic receptors, decrease vagal tone, increase smooth muscle contraction, and decrease mucous secretion. Corticosteroids are used in the treatment of COPD to decrease airway inflammation.

An example of a corticosteriod is prednisone. Antibiotics are used in clients with COPD, usually during acute exacerbation to decrease the duration of the episode and improve expiratory flow rates. Antibiotic prophylaxis (given in anticipation of infection) is also used with this population. Examples of antibiotics include tetracyline and amoxicillin. Diuretics, such as furosemide (Lasix), are used with the COPD population to prevent water retention. Mucolytics, such as guaifenesin, are used in clients with COPD to decrease the viscosity of the mucus to facilitate mucociliary clearance. Clients with COPD are also encouraged to keep airways clean by mobilizing secretions with aerosol treatments, chest percussion, and postural bronchial drainage.

SURGERY

There is an new surgical technique being used for the client with chronic emphysema This technique is lung volume reduction surgery (LVRS), during which part of the diseased lung tissue is removed. LVRS allows the chest wall and diaphragm to resume a more normal position to improve the mechanics of breathing, and allow the client to take a deep breath. Clients who have had this surgery show a marked decrease in dyspnea, an increased activity tolerance, and report a better quality of life (Lavell & Richardson Higgins, 1995). Research into LVRS is ongoing because the effect the surgery has on the ultimate progression of emphysema is unknown. However, many end-stage emphysema clients wish to pursue the surgery, and it compares favorably with lung transplantation—another surgical treatment.

OTHER MEDICAL TREATMENTS

Oxygen

Supplemental oxygen reduces mortality in clients with COPD. Continuous oxygen therapy generally is reimbursed for clients with a sustained PaO_2 of less than 55 mm Hg, or an oxygen saturation of less than 88% and evidence of cor pulmonale. Intermittent oxygen therapy is reimbursed for clients with a PaO_2 of less than 55 mm Hg or oxygen saturation of less than 88% during exercise or sleep.

Infection Protections

The excess thickened mucus in the lungs of clients with COPD is an excellent growth medium for bacteria. Infection protection in the COPD population includes prophylactic vaccination against influenza and pneumococcal pneumonia, avoidance of exposure to persons (especially children) with respiratory infection, and maintaining adequate hydration to thin mucous secretions.

Nutritional Therapy

Nutritional therapy in the COPD population is essential because weight loss and nutritional deficiencies decrease respiratory muscle strength. A high fat, reduced carbohydrate diet is recommended.

Occupational Therapy Treatment

EDUCATION

Clients with COPD require considerable education in proper breathing techniques to facilitate improved oxygenation, increase ventilatory muscle endurance, and promote relaxation. Clients with COPD are educated in the use of the pursed-lip breathing technique. In this technique the client breathes in slowly through the nose, purses lips as if to whistle or kiss, and breathes out very slowly through the pursed lips. The pursed lips serve to control the flow of air with exhalation. Rehearsal of this technique can lead to better-breathing patterns in clients with cardiopulmonary dysfunction.

PULMONARY REHABILITATION

Pulmonary rehabilitation is implemented for clients with stable COPD. Its goal is to return the client to the highest level of functional capacity through education, exercise training, and psychosocial support. The demonstrated benefits of pulmonary rehabilitation are reduction of respiratory symptoms, reversal of anxiety and depression, improved self-esteem, enhanced ability to carry out ADLs, increased exercise tolerance, and improved quality of life (Johannsen, 1994; Shanfield & Hammond, 1984).

Occupational therapy treatment in pulmonary rehabilitation programs should include the use of (1) graded activities; (2) ADL training; (3) **instrumental activities of daily living (IADL)** training; (4) exercise training programs to increase activity tolerance; (5) education in principles of energy conservation, work simplification, stress management and relaxation techniques, and pursed-lip breathing; (6) family education; and (7) establishment of home programs. During the rehabilitation process, clients with COPD need to learn problem-solving skills that they can use in the home environment.

▼ TUBERCULOSIS

Demographics and Definition

Tuberculosis (TB) is a major world health problem. It is estimated that there are 1 billion persons infected with TB worldwide, making it one of the most prevalent infections in the world (Fishman, 1988). TB is more prevalent in urban areas. It is also more common among Hispanics, African-Americans, Asians, Native Americans, drug-dependent individuals, the homeless, persons in residential care facilities and other closed institutions, alcoholics, prison inmates, and individuals with **human immunodeficiency virus (HIV)** (Rieder, Kelly, Bloch, Cauthen, & Snider, 1991). Tuberculosis is an infectious disease that is caused by *Mycobacterium tuberculosis*, or rarely in the United States, *M. bovis*. This infectious bacterium is airborne, acid-fast, and slow-growing.

The TB infection is transmitted primarily by inhalation of contaminated droplets of respiratory secretions dispersed through the air by coughing, sneezing, or talking. There are three types of TB: primary TB, reactivation or postprimary TB, and extrapulmonary TB. In adults, reactivation TB is the most common form of clinical disease. Extrapulmonary TB is the infection's involvement in any organ outside the lung. Extrapulmonary TB involvement occurs in two-thirds of clients infected with HIV. Low CD4 cell counts are associated with greater probability of extrapulmonary TB in clients with HIV (Friedman, 1994).

Signs and Symptoms

The classic symptoms of TB are cough, hemoptysis (spitting up blood), fever, night sweats, and weight loss.

Medical Treatment

HOSPITALIZATION

Medical management of TB is centered on eradicating the infecting organism and preventing the emergence of drug-resistant strains. Clients with active TB are hospitalized and kept in respiratory isolation during the initial phase of therapy. Two weeks of therapy greatly decreases the infectiousness of clients with pulmonary TB. However, occupational therapy practitioners working with this population should adhere to respiratory precautions, as dictated by the institution in which they practice. Generally, these clients are bedded in private, reverse air pressure rooms with antichambers. Clinicians involved in direct contact with these clients are required to wear specialized masks to comply with Occupational Safety and Health Administration (OSHA) requirements for prevention of disease transmission.

MEDICATIONS

The pharmacological management of TB involves the administration of multiple medications. The current acceptable minimal duration of therapy is 6 months; this is greatly shortened from the 1970s when 18 months was the norm. HIV-infected clients with TB should be treated for a minimum of 9 months. A typical medication regimen for the treatment of TB would include medication with isoniazid, rifampin, and pyrazinamide. There has been an increase in the number of persons with multidrug-resistant TB (MDR-TB). MDR-TB is caused by strains resistant to two or more drugs. These clients require the use of second-line TB drugs, and drug therapy for 13 months to 2 years may be necessary. Lung resection surgery may also be used in the advanced treatment of drug-resistant TB.

Occupational Therapy Treatment

Occupational therapy has historically maintained a place in the treatment of clients with TB. Occupational therapy was one of the first programs instituted in TB sanitariums, where reading, entertainment, and the development of craft activities were therapeutically used to make the prolonged hospital stay of the client more tolerable (Northrop, 1978). The concept of graded activity may have originated in German tuberculosis sanatoria in the late 1300s (Creighton, 1993). At present the effectiveness of medications has made it possible for shortened lengths of stay in the hospital and earlier return to work for the client with tuberculosis. However, occupational therapy treatment continues to be an essential service to clients who experience functional limitations secondary to infection with *M. tuberculosis*. The elderly and immunocompromised with TB are appropriate for occupational therapy intervention focused on education concerning energy conservation, work simplification, and graded activity to maximize endurance.

▶CONCLUSION

Occupational therapy practitioners play a vital role in the rehabilitation of the client with cardiopulmonary dysfunction. This is a growing client population, and occupational therapy practitioners are involved with these clients in a variety of settings. Occupational therapy practitioners need to have a comprehensive understanding of the cardiopulmonary disease process and its wide-reaching implications. The use of activity gradation and adaptation, which remains unique to the occupational therapy profession, significantly enhances the quality of life in persons afflicted with these illnesses. Occupational therapy practitioners bring together function and physiology to compliment the cardiopulmonary rehabilitation team.

▼ REFERENCES

Creighton, C. (1993). Graded activity: Legacy of the sanatorium. *American Journal of Occupational Therapy, 47,* 745–748.

Fishman, A. P. (Ed.). (1988). *Pulmonary diseases and disorders* (2nd ed.). New York: McGraw-Hill.

Friedman, L. N. (Ed.). (1994). *Tuberculosis current concepts and treatment.* Ann Arbor, MI: CRC Press.

Gersh, B. J. & Rahimtolla, S. H. (Eds.). (1991). *Acute myocardial infarction.* New York: Elsevier Science Publishing.

Halperin, J. L. & Levine, R. (1985). *Bypass.* New York: Times Books.

Johannsen, J. M. (1994). Chronic obstructive pulmonary disease: Current comprehensive care for emphysema and bronchitis. *Nurse Practitioner, 19*(1), 59–67.

Klein, D. (1988). Angina. *Nursing, 18*(7), 44–46.

Konstam, M. Dracup, K., Baker D., Brooks, N., Dacey, R., Dunbar, S., Jackson, A., Jessup, M., Johnson, J., Jones, R., Luchi, R., Massie, B., Pitt, B., Rose, E., Rubin, L., & Wright, R. (1994). Heart failure: Management of clients with left ventricular systolic dysfunction. *Quick reference guide for clinicians No. 11.* Rockville, MD: U.S. Department of Health and Human Services, Public Health Service, Agency for Health Care Policy and Research and National Heart, Lung and Blood Institute (AHCPR Publication No. 94 0613).

Kottke, T. E., Haney, T. H., & Doucette, M. M. (1990). Rehabilitation of the patient with heart disease. In F. J. Kotte and J. F. Lehmann (Eds.), *Krusen's handbook of physical medicine and rehabilitation* (4th ed.; pp. 874–903). Philadelphia: W. B. Saunders.

Krider, S. J. (1995). Vital signs. In R. L. Wilkins, S. J. Krider, and R. L. Sheldon (Eds.), *Clinical assessment in respiratory care* (3rd ed.; pp. 35–46). Boston: C.V. Mosby.

Lavell, D. R. & Richardson Higgins, V. (1995, July). Lung surgery, when less is more. *RN*, pp. 43–45.

Leidy, N. K. (1995). Functional performance in people with chronic obstructive pulmonary disease. *IMAGE: Journal of Nursing Scholarship, 27,* 23–34.

Miracle, V. (1988). Understanding the different types of MI. *Nursing, 18* (1), 53–56.

Myerowitz, P. D. (1987). Selection and management of the heart transplant recipient. In P. D. Myerowitz (Ed.), *Heart transplantation* (pp. 73–88). Mount Kisco, NY: Futura Publishing.

Northrop, C. (1978). Pulmonary disease: a. Tuberculosis. In R. Goldenson (Ed.), *Disability and rehabilitation handbook* (pp. 525–540). New York: McGraw-Hill.

Ogden, L. D. (1979). Activity guidelines for early subacute and high risk cardiac patients. *American Journal of Occupational Therapy, 33,* 291–298.

Pederson, B. (1993). Home care management of the chronic obstructive pulmonary disease patient increases patient control and prevents rehospitalization. *Home Healthcare Nurse, 10,* 24–30.

Rieder, H. L., Kelly, G. D., Bloch, A. B., Cauthen, G. M., & Snider, D. E. (1991). Tuberculosis diagnosed at death in United States. *Chest, 100,* 678–681.

Roth, E. (1993). Heart disease in patients with stroke: Incidence, impact, and implications for rehabilitation part I: classification and prevalence. *Archives of Physical Medicine and Rehabilitation, 74,* 752–757.

Shanfield, K. & Hammond, M. A. (1984). Activities of daily living. In E. Hodgkin, J. E. Zorn, & G. Long Connors (Eds.), *Pulmonary rehabilitation: Guidelines to success* (pp. 171–193). Philadelphia: J. B. Lippincott.

Stuart, E. M., Deckro, J. P., DeSilva, R. A., & Benson, H. (1993). Cardiovascular disease: The heart of the matter. In H. Benson, & E. M. Stuart (Eds.), *The wellness book* (pp. 363–398). New York: Simon & Schuster

Tommaso, C. L., Lesch, M., & Sonnenblick, E. H. (1984). Alterations in cardiac function in coronary artery disease, myocardial infarction, and coronary bypass surgery. In N. K. Wenger & H. K. Hellerstein (Eds.), *Rehabilitation of the coronary patient,* (2nd ed.) (pp. 41–65). New York: John Wiley & Sons.

Tooth, L. & McKenna, K. (1995). Cardiac patient teaching: Application to patients undergoing coronary angioplasty and their partners. *Patient Education and Counseling, 25,* 1–8.

Wegner N. K., Froelicher, E. S., Smith, L., Ades, P., Berra, K., Blumenthal, J., Certo, C., Dattilo, A., Davis, D., DeBusk, R., Drozda, J., Fletcher, B., Franklin, B., Gaston, H., Greenland, P., McBride, P., McGregor, C., Oldridge, N., Piscatella, J., & Rogers, F. (1995). Cardiac rehabilitation as secondary prevention. *Clinical practice guideline, No. 17.* Rockville, MD: U.S. Department of Health and Human Services, Public Health Service, Agency for Health Care Policy and Research and National Heart, Lung and Blood Institute (AHCPR Pub. No. 96–0673).

Wegner, N. K. (1984). Early ambulation after myocardial infarction: Rationale, program components, and results. In N. K. Wenger & H. K. Hellerstein (Eds.), *Rehabilitation of the coronary patient* (2nd ed.; pp. 97–110). New York: John Wiley & Sons.

Wilkins, R. L. (1995). Interpretation of blood gases. In R. L. Wilkins, S. J. Krider, & R. L. Sheldon (Eds.), *Clinical assessment in respiratory care* (3rd ed.; pp. 103–124). Boston, MA: C.V. Mosby.

Chapter 39

Occupational Therapy for Adults with Immunological Diseases

Michael Pizzi and Ann Burkhardt

The immune system defends the body against microorganisms, such as bacteria and viruses, and destroys abnormal cells produced by dysfunctions in cellular DNA. When the immune system is impaired, the body is especially susceptible to (1) infection from microorganisms and (2) the unchecked proliferation of abnormal cells. Two common adult immunological diseases are (1) human immunodeficiency virus (HIV) infection, which leads to **acquired immunodeficiency syndrome (AIDS)**; and (2) cancer. In HIV infection, a virus directly attacks the immune system, rendering it ineffective in fighting off infections from microorganisms. In cancer, the immune system is ineffective in controlling the growth of abnormal cells. This chapter will describe occupational therapy evaluations and treatments specific to adults with these two diseases.

▼ HIV INFECTION AND AIDS

Etiology and Demographics

HIV infection is caused by a retrovirus known as human immunodeficiency virus (HIV). Retroviruses contain RNA, but not DNA; they use their RNA to produce DNA once they have gained entry to a host cell—a reversal of the usual sequence during which DNA directs the production of RNA. HIV specifically targets cells in the body that have CD4 receptors on their surface membranes: the T4 helper lymphocytes (also known as $CD4^+$ cells) and some cells in the central nervous system (CNS), gastrointestinal tract

(GI), and uterine cervix. HIV ultimately destroys its target cells causing immune, CNS, GI, and uterine dysfunctions. The damage to the immune system makes people vulnerable to a wide range of **opportunistic infections** (microorganisms that take advantage of the opportunity afforded by a compromised immune system). Death from HIV infection is usually due to these opportunistic infections (Kassler, 1995; Springhouse Corp., 1995).

HIV is transmitted by exposure to blood or body secretions of persons who are infected with the virus. This can occur through sexual transmission, blood transfusion, sharing of needles, and gestation (mother to child). AIDS was first described in the homosexual populations in New York and California in 1981. Soon thereafter, it was found among intravenous drug users, hemophiliacs and other individuals who had received blood transfusions, and children. The disease is now becoming especially prevalent in heterosexual women and young adults with no known risk factors other than their sexual behavior(s) (Kassler, 1993; Springhouse Corp., 1995).

Stages of HIV Infection: Signs and Symptoms

There are four stages of HIV infection: (1) acute infection—the body's initial short-lived flulike response to the virus; (2) asymptomatic disease—HIV continues to replicate in the body and affect the immune system, but not enough to cause signs and symptoms; (3) symptomatic—HIV has done enough damage to the immune system to cause signs and symptoms; and (4) advanced disease or AIDS—the immune system is severely compromised. Beginning in the asymptomatic stage the CD4+ cell count begins to drop from normal levels of more than 1000/mm³ of blood; in AIDS, CD4+ counts are fewer than 200/mm³. Diagnosis of any stage depends on both laboratory and clinical findings (Kassler, 1993; Springhouse Corp., 1995).

There are a variety of sequelae associated with the symptomatic and advanced stages of HIV infection. One common sign is generalized lymphadenopathy, or enlargement of the lymph nodes. People with lymphadenopathy often complain of fatigue and weight loss. They may find it difficult to participate in all the activities they normally would have in the course of a day and or evening. They may also complain of general malaise. The weight loss may be associated with malabsorption of nutrients or with a loss of nutrient to the metabolism of the virus itself.

Other signs include fever and diarrhea. These problems can also deplete one's energy and tolerance for activity. Neurological disorders often accompany advanced stage disease-AIDS. Cognitive impairment, affective, and sensory changes owing to dementia, myelopathy (pathology of the spinal cord), and peripheral neuropathies can occur as a direct result of the disease itself or as side effects of pharmaceutical treatments. Cognitive impairment that leads to poor safety may limit the choices for home care. Affective changes interfere with communication and expression. Personality is often altered. Interpersonal relationships are often changed. Sensory changes can interfere with the simplest of basic activities of daily living (ADLs), especially if an individual cannot hold onto tools and implements we all use daily: feeding utensils, combs, tissues, money, and the telephone. If hyperesthesia (unusual sensibility to stimuli) is part of the sensory change, touch can be painful and aversive. Visual changes can occur because of some opportunistic infections. For example, cytomegalovirus infection can cause retinopathy and result in low vision or blindness. When both vision and somatic sensation are impaired, engaging in and successfully completing simple daily tasks becomes problematic. Life roles are adversely changed.

Occupational Considerations for People with HIV Infection and AIDS

PHYSICAL CONSIDERATIONS

Fatigue, shortness of breath, visual impairments, peripheral and central neuropathies, various forms of cancer, opportunistic infections, cardiac problems, and the wasting syndrome, all may develop over the course of infection with HIV. Physical pain may occur from a variety of causes including peripheral nervous system (PNS) damage. Postural changes, with or without a formal underlying neurological diagnosis, may occur in association with extreme weight loss. These postural changes can also result in pain (Galan-

tino, Mukand, & Freed, 1991). The CNS damage results in dementia, spinal cord dysfunction, and stroke. Both PNS and CNS dysfunctions may be accompanied by gait disturbances, balance impairment, and restricted mobility, as well as changes in muscle tone. Range of motion (ROM), strength, coordination, and sensation can be affected, resulting in mild to severe changes in function. Physical problems must be fully assessed for their effect on occupational roles (Galantino & Pizzi, 1991).

PSYCHOSOCIAL CONSIDERATIONS

The disease caused by HIV is often viewed only in terms of its progressive course. The psychosocial effect of hearing the diagnosis may result in depression, anxiety, and guilt. People infected with the disease may become preoccupied with death and the process of dying. Anger accompanies the adjustment process—anger at the disease, the prospect of a lonely and painful death, the lack of available medical treatment, the medical staff, and oneself.

Anxiety, manifested as tension, stress, tachycardia, agitation, insomnia, anorexia, and panic attacks, serves to perpetuate an already maladaptive cycle of behavior. Neuropsychiatric symptoms, such as forgetfulness, lack of concentration, apathy, withdrawal, and decreased alertness, can occur. In the later stages of disease, confusion and disorientation may become evident.

Physical disfigurement caused by AIDS often leads to problems with self-image. This coupled with neuropsychiatric dysfunction may result in limited social and occupational activity. Feelings of lost control over one's life and loss of mastery of the self may lead persons with AIDS to state that the disease seems to be controlling their life. This idea usually contributes to the development of feelings of helplessness and hopelessness; thus, to clinical depression. The meaning of activity is often critically overanalyzed; occupational therapy practitioners need to help clients rediscover meaning in the presence of such life-altering change (Pizzi, 1991). Adaptation of life roles is needed. Grief and bereavement issues related to the loss of prior life roles should be considered by the occupational therapy practitioner in conjunction with other team members.

ENVIRONMENTAL CONSIDERATIONS

The inability of family members and significant others to cope with revelations concerning disease-related risk behaviors of a loved one can lead to alienation of the individual with HIV infection. Partners may leave the relationship because of fear, guilt, illness, or perceived inability to care for a person with a chronic illness. Occupational therapy practitioners must be aware of how these possibilities can affect the occupational therapy process and the client's functioning.

The physical environment may become too challenging for people who have fatigue, shortness of breath, visual or somatic sensory losses. Their restricted mobility at home, work, or in the community may make it difficult for them to balance the activity demands of self-care, work, and leisure. Visual and somatic sensory problems may also make it difficult to negotiate physical environments.

Physical and social environments may be affected by a change in job status and income. Individuals who do not have adequate disability coverage can lose their homes, families, and friends. The threat of homelessness may be very real. Once pleasurable avocational activities, such as going to the movies or out to dinner, may be beyond their current economic resources. The occupational therapist must consider the economic situation of clients before making treatment recommendations, particularly if clients must purchase equipment and materials to maintain productivity (Pizzi, 1991a).

Occupational Therapy Assessment

Clients with HIV will need to prioritize their goals. Longer-term goals may become shorter-term ones, necessitating shifts in habits, time management, and engagement in productive pursuits. Personal values become more meaningful, and they often shift from concrete materialism to more spiritual values. Symbolism, control, temporal rhythms, occupation, and occupational role and environment are themes that guide occupational therapy practice for persons with HIV and AIDS (Clark & Jackson, 1990).

Before an assessment, therapists must determine the need to observe any special infection precautions. If a therapist has a cold or the flu, he or she should wear a mask to avoid infecting the person with HIV. Therapists should follow infection control precautions (**Universal Precautions**) with all persons, regardless of their HIV status. In addition, special infection control precautions should be followed when these are posted outside a client's room.

Relative to universal infection precautions, all practitioners should be familiar with the infection control procedures at the facilities and agencies in which they work. Generally, occupational therapy practitioners need to wash their hands before and after seeing each client. Gloves are worn when assisting with ADL, if it is likely that the occupational therapy practitioner is coming into contact with body fluids or blood. Gowns, masks, and goggles are worn if there is risk of body fluid splashes (eg, a client who is spitting up sputum or experiencing diarrhea).

Because people with HIV infection have specialized problems and needs, it is advisable to use specific assessment batteries created for this population. One such assessment is the Pizzi Assessment of Productive Living for Adults with HIV Infection and AIDS (PAPL: Box 39–1; see Pizzi, 1993, for more detail). This assessment was developed to holistically assess all domains of function and occupational behaviors in a short time (Pizzi, 1993). The time variable is important, for many people with HIV and or AIDS have limited endurance. In addition, because managed care will limit our ability to provide more that a prefixed amount of care, time management is essential.

For ADL, work, and leisure, therapists must weigh the importance of activity participation for the person involved. If basic ADLs are overly time and energy consuming, the therapist may recommend that the person allow a caregiver to do one activity, so the person has the energy and time to participate in an activity of greater meaning. It is also important to assess if there are particular times in a day when a person feels more energetic, so activities can be planned to make use of the enhanced tolerance at those times. Consideration of stress triggers are also important for evaluation, case management, and treatment planning, because stress contributes to immunosuppression.

Occupational Therapy Treatment

The purpose of occupational therapy treatment with adults with HIV infection is to enhance competent performance of self-chosen occupations that contribute to valued roles. Data from assessments, such as the PAPL, outline problem areas to be addressed in treatment.

There are several special considerations for therapists when developing treatment plans and goals for the person with HIV infection:

1. Some of the medical conditions that accompany HIV infection are infectious processes and require special isolation procedures. In a hospital setting, the isolation procedure is often posted at the door of the room, or available in the nursing station. If there are no special precautions, the practitioner should use universal precautions with all clients, regardless of their HIV status.
2. Subtle cognitive and physical changes can occur rapidly, so frequent informal re-evaluation of these areas is important.
3. Discrimination against and negative social judgments of people with HIV infection are inappropriate. All clients are entitled to nonjudgmental care and acceptance as persons.
4. Many persons with this disease have dealt with a number of personal losses during their illness. Mourning is a natural reaction to loss.
5. The lack of a cure for HIV infection, at the time of this writing, affects the hope and the reality that will be faced in the future.
6. Alternatives and modifications to allow one to continue working are valuable.
7. Fatigue and weakness will limit activity tolerance and ability to participate. Energy conservation, work simplification, and occupational adaptations can enhance productivity.
8. Although adaptive equipment and positioning may enhance activity participation and preserve skill, a person who is in denial may not be able to accept these alternatives psychologically at the point they are needed. This denial must be respected until the person can deal with the underlying issue.

(text continues on page 710)

BOX 39-1

Pizzi Assessment of Productive Living for Adults with HIV Infection and AIDS (PAPL)

Demographics

Name _____ Age _____ Sex _____

Lives with (relationship) _____

Identified caregiver _____

Race _____ Culture _____ Religion _____ Practicing? _____

Primary occupational roles _____

Primary diagnosis _____

Secondary diagnosis _____

Stage of HIV _____

Past medical history _____

Medications _____

Activities of Daily Living (use ADL performance assessment)

Are you doing these now? _____

Do you perform homemaking tasks? _____

(For areas of difficulty) Would you like to be able to do these again like you did before? Which ones? _____

Work

Job _____ When last worked _____

Describe type of activity _____

Work environment _____

If not working, would you like to be able to? _____

Do you miss being productive? _____

Play/Leisure

Types of activity engaged in _____

_____

Are you doing these now? _____

If not, would you like to? _____ Which ones? _____

Would you like to try other things as well? _____

Is it important to be independent in daily living activities? _____

Physical Function

Active and Passive range of motion:

Strength:

Sensation:

Coordination (gross and fine motor or dexterity):

Visual–perceptual:

Hearing:

Balance (sit and stand):

Ambulation, Transfers, and Mobility:

Activity tolerance/endurance:

Physical pain:

Location: _____

(continued)

▼ **BOX 39-1** (Continued)

Does it interfere with doing important activities? _____

Sexual function:

Cognition
(Attention span, problem solving, memory, orientation, judgment, reasoning, decision making, safety awareness)

Time organization
Former daily routine (prior to diagnosis) _____

Has this changed since diagnosis? _____ If so, how? _____

Are there certain times of day that are better for you to carry out daily tasks? _____

Do you consider yourself regimented in organizing time and activity or pretty flexible? _____

What would you change, if anything, in how your day is set up? _____

Body image and self-image
In the last 6 months, has there been a recent change in your physical body and how it looks?

How do you feel about this?

_____

Social Environment (Describe support available and utilized by patient)

Physical Environment (Describe environments where patient performs daily tasks and level of support or impediment for function)

Stressors
What are some things, people, or situations that are/were stressful? _____

What are some current ways you manage stress? _____

Situational Coping
How do you feel you are dealing with:

a) your diagnosis _____

b) changes in the ability to do things important to you _____

c) other psychosocial observations _____

Occupational Questions
What do you feel to be important to you right now? _____

Do you feel you can do things important to you now? In the future? _____

Do you deal well with change? _____

What are your hopes, dreams, aspirations? What are some of your goals? _____

Have these changed since you were diagnosed? How? _____

Do you feel in control of your life at this time? _____

What do you wish to accomplish with the rest of your life? _____

Plan:

STG:

LTG:

Frequency:

Duration:

Therapist:

copyright 1991 Michael Pizzi, MS, OTR/L, CHES; reprinted with permission
Note. STG, short-term goals; LTG, Long-term goals

9. Self-esteem can be enhanced when clients are given some control over their schedule and routine. As skill competence is challenged with disease progression, control through choices facilitates positive feelings of self-worth and empowerment.

10. Complementary and alternative medical techniques may enhance the quality of life and decrease pain and dependency on drugs. Some of the techniques used include progressive relaxation, biofeedback, prayer, therapeutic touch, Chinese traditional medicine, energy work, myofascial release, craniosacral therapy, imagery, and visualization.

11. Wellness is inextricably connected with nutrition. Occupational therapy practitioners can collaborate with a nutritionist to develop strategies clients can use to follow a sound nutritional program. Sometimes assessing the safety of oral feeding and recommending alternative nutritional methods is best. For example, feeding tubes can assist the individual to achieve caloric requirements and feel stronger, if eating by mouth becomes too energy consuming or painful. Oral candidiasis (yeast infection) can cause dysphagia. Neurological manifestations of AIDS can also contribute to dysphagia. Sometimes a feeding tube gives someone a "new lease on life." If the person regains the ability to swallow, oral feeding can be resumed. For people with loss of appetite, the tube can be used to supplement caloric intake. If they recover from the dysphagia or loss of appetite, the tube can be pulled.

The treatment focus will change and require modification throughout the course of HIV infection. For persons who are symptomatic, the treatment will be tailored to the sequelae exhibited. Persons with neurological sequelae may benefit from compensatory training, caregiver education, and adaptive equipment. In general, energy conservation, health promotion, and wellness strategies can enhance immunocompetence and physical and psychosocial well-being. As the disease progresses, adaptive strategies, environmental modification, and modification of ADL techniques can be added to preserve a sense of mastery and self-control (Denton, 1987; Gutterman, 1990; Pizzi, 1988, 1989, 1990, 1991; Weinstein, 1990). Pain management also becomes increasingly important over time. Myofascial release, craniosacral therapy, acupressure, biofeedback, imagery, and visualization may be useful (Galantino, et al., 1991)). As the disease progresses, the strategies used should be adapted to the level of participation and understanding of the recipient.

In the later stages of the disease process, adjustment to dying, grief, loss, and bereavement become central issues during daily life. The theme of therapy may shift to focus on projects with inherent symbolism for the client. Often projects such as a memory book or a time capsule to leave behind for friends and loved ones are valuable. Spiritual needs are expressed. A sense of accomplishment with ones life is key to issues of self-esteem and feelings of self-worth. Assis-tance with the achievement of comfort during all occupations, including sleep, supports the quality of life.

At this time, therapeutic use of self will be individualized and dependent on the level of comfort of the practitioner given the situation. Some practitioners will want to support the family through the death experience. For others, this is too intense or draining. Those who are less comfortable with spirituality and the concept of death may withdraw or take a respite from the case at this time. Teaching and training caregivers may be the most effective use of treatment time as the disease progresses (see Pizzi, 1990; pp. 260–263, for a detailed case study).

▼ CANCER

Etiology

Cancer is a malignant **neoplasm**. Neoplasms are proliferations of abnormal cells in the body. These abnormal cells usually form a solid mass or tumor, as in breast cancer. Sometimes neoplasms do not form solid tumors, as in leukemia in which the abnormal cells are lymphocytes. Neoplasms are characterized as malignant when they invade surrounding cells, disrupting the function of those cells. Malignant tumors can also metastasize or send abnormal cells to other parts of the body through the blood or lymph systems. The branch of medicine that deals with cancer is called oncology.

Cancers may be low grade or high grade. Low-grade tumors tend to be slower growing, and their cell structures are more uniform and consistent. They often respond well to surgery, chemotherapy, hormone treatment, or radiation. One example of a low-grade tumor is prostate cancer. Adenocarcinoma (malignancy of epithelial tissue of a gland) of the prostate is very slow growing and not highly metastatic. In contrast, high-grade tumors are rapidly growing and tend to metastasize to other organs. They tend to be more resistive to conventional oncological treatment. One example of a high-grade tumor is inflammatory breast cancer. It is aggressive, resistive to chemotherapy and radiation treatment, and metastasizes readily to other areas of the body, such as the lung, brain, liver, or bone.

Cancers are staged from the time of the diagnosis through progression of the disease. There are many staging systems in use. Perhaps the easiest to understand is the tumor, metastasis, node system (TMN). The presence of tumor(s) and number of primary tumors is representative of the "T." The number of metastases is represented by the "M," and the number of positive lymph nodes is represented by the "N." For example, a person who presents with T1, M0, and N0 has a detectable tumor that has not spread. The general prognosis will still be dependent on the virulence of the tumor type itself, but the staging tells us the cancer has been detected before any perceivable spread of the disease. In contrast, someone with T1, M2, and N12 has more advanced disease (Burkhardt & Joachim, 1996).

Demographics and Sequelae

People of all ages, from infancy through old age, can develop cancers. When people develop cancer, they often lose a significant amount of body weight, even though they are not dieting. This is because tumors have a higher metabolic rate than normal tissues. Many cancers grow extensive circulatory networks around themselves and withdraw nutrients from the bloodstream, which leads to weight loss. This increased metabolism of tumors allows them to grow and replace themselves more rapidly than normal tissue.

Other sequelae experienced by clients with a diagnosis of cancer are caused by (1) the effect of the primary cancer itself on normal tissues, (2) the extent and location of the surgery performed to resect or bypass the tumor, (3) the side effects of the chemotherapy, (4) the side effects of hormonal therapy, and (5) the side effects of radiation therapy.

CANCER

Primary tumors can develop in virtually any organ of the human body. The sequelae from a primary tumor may be related to the function of the primary organ. For example, in liver cancer the liver enzymes may become elevated and the person may become jaundiced. The increase in liver enzymes makes the person fatigue easily, complain of arthralgias or "joint pains," and have a low tolerance for activity.

SURGERY

Many tumors can be completely resected from the body. That is, the tumor is removed en bloc, in a whole piece. With limb tumors, if the tumor has not entangled itself with the nerves or blood vessels (the neurovascular bundle), removal of the the limb by amputation can often be spared. These surgeries are referred to as "limb sparing." If the tumor involves the neurovascular bundle, an amputation may be the only recourse. If internal organs, such as the pancreas or the liver, are involved, it may be necessary to remove part or all of the organ. If tumor resection is not possible, sometimes bypass surgery is done to bypass a tumor-related obstruction and allow the affected organ to continue functioning as the disease advances.

CHEMOTHERAPY

The high metabolism of tumors is helpful in controlling them with chemotherapy, because tumors absorb the chemotoxins before normal tissues. Consequently, the concentration of chemotoxins in the blood used by tumors is higher than the concentration in freely circulating blood. The sequelae associated with chemotherapy is dependent on the type of chemotherapy used and its effect on normal tissues of the body. Some chemotherapy drugs are mild, with side effects often imperceptible or identifiable only by minor changes in constitutional symptoms, such as changes in bowel activity. Other chemotherapy agents cause highly perceptible changes, such as hair loss, paresthesias (sensory changes characterized by tingling and numbness of the dis-

tal extremities), muscle weakness, or vascular changes in the limbs, resulting in increased incidence of orthostatic hypotension or permanent nerve damage.

HORMONES

Use of hormones in treatment can produce premature menopause or accentuation of secondary sexual characteristics. For example, diethylstilbestrol (DES), a synthetic estrogen used in the treatment of prostate cancer, can cause enlargement of the breasts in men being treated with the hormone. Some hormones used to treat prostate cancer produce a chemical orchiectomy: render the testes inactive. In women, a hormone used to block bonding of estrogen to estrogen-dependent breast tumors causes premature menopause and weight gain and can lead to the development of primary cancer of the ovaries or uterus.

RADIATION

Radiation kills tumor cells by raising their temperature above the tumor tolerance level. Radiation, however, also affects normal tissues. Near the end of several weeks of radiation treatment, soft tissues become erythematous (red); the skin may be painful, often sustaining the equivalent of a superficial second-degree burn; and local edema is present. While the person is actively undergoing radiation treatment, the use of lotions and topical ointments may be restricted, because lotions and creams change the surface tension of the skin and, in doing so, can enhance the action of the radiation, rather than soothing the sequelae.

Once the radiation treatment is completed and the skin heals, the soft tissues in the path of the radiation will continue to change. This process, known as radiation fibrosis, lasts for several years. During this time, the person will report feeling tightness of soft tissues with movement. This sensation is associated with a loss of elasticity and resultant tightening in the soft tissues. People with this problem are at risk for losing movement, particularly when the radiation was given over or adjacent to a joint. For instance, clients with head and neck cancer or breast cancer may have radiation involving their glenohumeral joint. Their shoulder may progressively stiffen, and they can develop adhesive capsulitis as part of the fibrosis. Range of motion (ROM) and soft tissues mobilization techniques, such as myofascial release, may preserve or restore normal movement. These techniques may be needed for the 3-year window of time in which the fibrosis is active. Once the fibrosis settles down, clients can generally keep the motion they have without further exercise. Therefore, ROM and mobilization techniques are strategic during and following radiation therapy treatment while radiation fibrosis is occurring. Scar management, especially using silicone gel pads, can assist by softening the irradiated tissues and preserving the elasticity of the soft tissues during the postradiation phase of recovery (Burkhardt & Weitz, 1990).

Another unfortunate side effect of radiation treatment is the loss of myelin from nerves, resulting in decreased sensory and motor nerve function of the demyelinated nerves. One common example is brachial plexopathy (demyelinization of the nerves branching off from the brachial plexus). Clients who receive radiation for breast or lung cancer may develop brachial plexopathy.

Radiation-induced plexopathy is a permanent loss of nerve function. It is often progressive and results in significant functional loss for the affected upper extremity. The associated sensory changes may or not result in pain. If the person experiences burning hyperesthesias that interfere with sleep and significantly impair quality of life, the affected nerve may be blocked to remove the sensation of pain (eg, phenol block or electrical stimulation blocks), or the client may be placed on specific drugs to diminish the neuropathic pain. Transcutaneous electrical nerve stimulation (TENS) may be used near the origin of the point of pain to block pain messages. TENS should never be used on a limb in which lymph nodes have been removed or irradiated. Sometimes use of superficial vibration can positively influence the hyperesthesia. When sensation is impaired, safety is an issue that will need to be addressed in therapy. Functional changes will be managed with positioning and use of adapted ADL devices or treatment techniques to compensate for lost function (Cook & Burkhardt, 1994).

Occupational Therapy Evaluation of the Person with Cancer

Evaluations should encompass physical, psychological, and social aspects of living, because all of these areas affect our occupations in life. Evaluations should be done for (1) mobility, including all of the usual subsets of movement (ROM, muscle strength, dexterity, coordination, speed of movement, and purpose of movement); (2) sensation (protective and discriminative); (3) cognition; (4) vision (acuity and visual perception); (5) ADLs; (6) work (including homemaking); and (7) leisure activities.

Occupational Therapy Treatment

The type of occupational therapy intervention will depend on the course of the disease and treatment and the person's medical status at the time of referral. In a hospital setting, immediately after surgery, or during chemotherapy or radiation treatment, the purpose of an occupational therapy referral may be to improve general mobility and basic self-care ability. Swallowing may also be an issue if the person develops dysphagia from neurological damage, surgical resection involving the oral or oral pharyngeal cavity, or fungal infections of the oral pharyngeal cavity. (Fungal infections commonly occur in all immunosuppressed people.)

Following initial staging and treatment of the disease, referrals are often for (1) limitations in joint mobility (eg, early onset of adhesive capsulitis); (2) lymphedema (edema caused by obstruction of the lymphatics); (3) difficulty eating or swallowing; (4) instability involving the trunk or a limb(s); (5) loss or impairment of hand or upper extremity function; (6) scar management, splinting, and positioning; (7) fabrication of cosmetic devices (in the event of soft tissue compromise); (8) alterations in body image; (9) depression; (10) an adjustment disorder; or (11) somatosensory pain syndromes.

With progression of the disease, or in the event of progressive conditions associated with treatment, such as radiation-induced brachial plexopathy, the emphasis of treatment shifts to supportive care: positioning to optimize functioning or to reduce pain, or rehabilitative approaches to substitute for lost function (Dietz, 1974). Counseling concerning changes in life roles is important at this point. Some practitioners fail to recognize the value of counseling at this juncture. Developing support for self-esteem and engendering hope can make the difference between a feeling of well-being or an assumption of the sick role. Also, other health professionals may not be aware that these issues are addressed by occupational therapy practitioners.

With advancing disease, palliative or comfort care becomes the focus of intervention (Dietz, 1974). The occupational therapy practitioner's role in palliative care is to help the client (1) maintain some degree of mastery over the environment, and (2) meet emotional needs. Sometimes clients only need low-technology equipment, such as a long-handled reacher, to control their environments. When the cancer has caused severe disability, technologically advanced equipment, such as computerized communication and environmental control systems may be needed. For emotional needs, occupational therapy practitioners can empower individuals by helping them successfully complete activities of importance to them. Practitioners can also interact in ways that tell clients they are valued. For instance, accepting compliments from clients with advancing disease allows them to realize that their opinion still matters. Sharing something they love, such as a piece of literature, a poem, or music, communicates respect and appreciation. Allowing reminiscence and formulating tapes or writings of things remembered can also be helpful. The use of techniques such as a massage or the use of guided imagery may promote a sense of well-being or pleasure.

Preventative care is also an important aspect of any rehabilitation program (Dietz, 1974). In reference to cancer, providing wellness strategies while intervening with a population at risk for cancer is important. For instance, smoking tobacco leads to lung cancer, breast cancer, head and neck cancer, and cardiovascular disease. Working on smoking cessation, in all occupational therapy settings, is a viable form of preventative care (Williams, Burkhardt, & Royce, 1995). Another example of prevention is teaching stress reduction techniques with all populations of clients, because stress can lead to other risk behaviors that can contribute to cancer, such as poor diet and abuse of drugs or alcohol.

Factors Influencing Treatment

There are several precautions that are important to consider when treating clients with cancer. When someone has had surgery, initial precautions will include protection of the incision or resection site and mobility limitations. With skin incisions, practitioners need to be careful not to pull the incision open during procedures such as ROM. Once the incision is healed, full movement should resume, unless there was reconstruction to the site. Reconstructive procedures will have highly specific mobility allowances that should be obtained directly from the surgeon(s). For example, if a tendon transfer or a flap has been done, the surgeon may wish to ensure the reconstruction is stable before movement training is begun. Although similar to reconstructive procedures done with hand injuries, the orders for these cases may need to be individualized, because there is greater tissue compromise associated with the tumor resection. Radiation may have further influence on the site, as well.

Chemotherapy can cause several conditions that warrant treatment precautions. The first and foremost of these is thrombocytopenia, a diminished platelet level. Platelets assist the blood to clot and are important in terms of recovery from trauma. When the universal platelet level dips to low levels, such as below 45,000 to 50,000 units, resistive activity should be avoided (Burkhardt & Joachim, 1996). Care should be taken to avoid cuts and bruises when platelets are low, because bleeding can readily result and may require extensive time to be controlled.

Myelosupression is also a concern with clients receiving chemotherapy or undergoing bone marrow transplantation. Myelosupression predisposes individuals to infections. Sometimes common infections can be fatal for a person with myelosupression because the immune response is severely suppressed. Anemia, another side effect of chemotherapy, lowers tolerance for activity, because often, even basic ADL may result in shortness of breath and ease of fatigue. Pacing and conservation of energy are important with all of the aforementioned complications. Arrhythmias may also occur in response to chemotherapy; in these clients occupational therapy treatment should be avoided until the arrythmia is stabilized with medication.

Orthopedic precautions are a concern if the individual is at risk for a pathological fracture owing to bony metastases or if there has been bony resection of a limb. Often, clients are encouraged to use their limbs for light ADL activities, despite the risk of a pathological fracture, because disuse leads to significant decreases in limb function. The presence of metastases to bone may limit tolerance for activities with inherent torsion and torque, for these activities may result in a fracture. When a client has had resection of a bony lesion, the precautions will depend on the presence of a joint replacement, bone graft, or fusion. Limb-sparing procedures may have a different outcome than noncancer arthroplasty surgeries, for resection of soft tissue may be necessary, depending on the infiltration of the tumor. Specific postoperative protocols should be obtained from or developed in collaboration with the surgical team.

Swelling of a limb(s), may occur due to (1) compression of the lymphatics, (2) lymphatic invasion by tumor, (3) decreased functioning of the lymphatics associated with lymph node resection or irradiation, or (4) cellulitis (inflammation of the involved limb) (Burkhardt & Joachim, 1992). With lymphedema the person may have pain and decreased use of the arm or leg. Energy conservation and work simplification may be important aspects to consider in developing a treatment plan.

Issues of Death and Dying

People's concepts of death and their spiritual beliefs will influence their abilities to cope with the diagnosis of cancer, especially if the disease is likely to be progressive. Adults may find spirituality for the first time when they are dealing with a diagnosis of cancer. Some people tell of renewed faith and strong beliefs in the power of prayer. Guilt may be expressed concerning the suspected influence past behaviors may have contributed to the development of a diagnosis of cancer (such as smoking for a person with lung cancer).

Many people do not reach a level of acceptance concerning death. The greatest challenge is for the individual to remain hopeful, despite the progressive nature of the disease. Other clients, who actually have a good prognosis, need education and reassurance to accept the reality that many people today have such a diagnosis, are treated, and continue to survive some cancers, without any shortening of their lifespans.

Consistently doing what you promise to do, making repeat visits, listening, and generally demonstrating a caring attitude engender trust and a sense of well-being between practitioner and cancer survivor. Accountability is the underlying issue supporting the development of trust (Burkhardt & Joachim, 1996). Some practitioners will wax and wane in their ability to work with people facing life decisions. In your own practice as an occupational therapy practitioner, it may be something about which you are introspective and acutely aware. On the other hand, attempting to treat someone may unexpectedly awaken your own fears and pain of past or recent loss. Using supervision to manage a case, and your own issues, is important under these circumstances. Each client we interact with throughout our careers adds new dimensions to our observations and understanding. As we grow and experience life, our coping abilities change, as well. Sharing in a person's fears can be threatening to the unprepared or spiritually challenged practitioner. The strength of practitioners to confront their own issues head on is crucial and the core of therapeutic use of self.

CASE STUDY

Evaluation

Valerie, a 42-year-old woman with a diagnosis of breast cancer, was referred to occupational therapy for management of her left arm lymphedema. She had recently had a recurrence of her breast cancer. The initial diagnosis of breast cancer was made 3 years earlier. At the time of diagnosis, Valerie had a modified radical mastectomy. Five months before the recurrence, she underwent reconstructive surgery: a transrectus abdominis mammoplasty (TRAM). She was last seen by the plastic surgeon 2 weeks before referral for an episode of cellulitis in the involved arm. At that time she was treated with a broad-spectrum antibiotic and was started on a diuretic regimen. She continued to have swelling and also complained of reflex muscle spasm in her shoulder and upper back.

On evaluation, it was noted that Valerie had erythema of her breast and chest wall. Her sensory evaluation was significant for intermittent tingling, in a glovelike distribution, of her left arm. Her shoulder ROM was severely limited in a capsular pattern of mobility. Her strength was diminished in a pattern consistent with upper brachial plexopathy involvement. On palpation, an enlarged, hardened cervical lymph node was felt. The client stated she refused chemotherapy with this exacerbation, because she had doubts that the chemotherapy had helped the first time. She had been seeing a homeopathic physician and practiced chelation therapy.

Valerie was fitted with a tubular support bandage and a wrist support. She was provided with several items of adapted equipment, including Dycem, a bath sponge, a buttonhook, and a dressing stick. She was given resources and recommendations for additional items she might find useful. A referral was made back to her primary oncologist for further workup relative to the erythema and the neurological findings.

Valerie's primary oncologist diagnosed metastases to the skin and brachial plexopathy and referred her for emergent radiation therapy. She complained of discomfort positioning her arm. The paresthesias worsened and were disrupting her sleep, as well. The doctor placed the client on a regimen of amitriptyline (Elavil) to decrease the neuropathic pain, decrease the edema, and enhance relaxation for sleep (the medication is taken at night).

Treatment

Valerie purchased a reclining lounge chair, to sleep in at night. She continued to complain of pain in her arm. A program of TENS was begun to control the discomfort. Also, Valerie was fitted with a swathe and sling of foam construction, to support the arm during ambulation. She was advised to stop taking the diuretic, because her lymphedema had hardened with its dehydration effect. Valerie was instructed in the positioning of her arm during ADL, for maximum comfort and function. She was advised not to massage her arm until her medical treatment was completed (because of the degree of lymphadenopathy). Valerie reported her sleep pattern improved.

Valerie was also a mother of three children. She verbalized her concerns over the progression of the cancer and the effect it would have on her boys and her husband. She was concerned how her husband would manage when she was gone. Valerie verbalized that she was desirous of continuing her sexual relationship and sought advice on positions that would allow maximum comfort and pain relief during the activity. She was grateful for the recommendations made and reported they helped her to continue her relationship with her husband, which she continued to value.

She was encouraged to begin memory books for her family and to write a series of letters to her family and friends, to gain some control and closure over her fear of leaving everyone behind. She did not want her children to think she had not fought her disease hard enough. The oldest was 14 years old and the youngest was 3. Her husband and parents were supportive of her throughout the advancement of the disease. She wanted so much to be able to give back something to each of them.

Spirituality was extremely important to her. She joked, "my sister-in-law took me off the prayer list because I was doing so well. I called and asked her to put me back on and never to take me off of it again." Valerie stated that prayers others said for her were very important to her. She said it made her feel less alone, facing metastatic cancer. It was important to her to have her caregivers understand these feelings and values. She asked everyone she met to keep her in their prayers. It gave her hope. That hope spurred her on to do her best to live as normal a life as her progressing disease allowed.

Valerie was admitted to the hospital one more time, 4 months before her death. She was able to manage her edema and position her arm for maximal comfort. She continued to be able to participate in her ADLs and homemaking with one person's assistance. She was able to have **hospice** care

(Continued)

home, so she could be with her family throughout the remainder of her life. Occasionally, she would call her occupational therapist for advice concerning positioning, her lymphedema, or with questions that arose concerning daily activities. When she had a doctors appointment at the medical center, she would schedule a therapy appointment to upgrade her home program, as well. The family, in particular her father and husband, always accompanied her and listened to or were trained to assist with the advice and home program prescribed or upgraded. Valerie freely expressed her concerns over the effect her death would have on her family. Despite her concerns, she almost systematically continued to develop reminiscence strategies to communicate her feelings to her family and to put them at ease about her

death. She had a calm perspective concerning her own short yet meaningful life. Valerie was grateful for her family and she was able to use each moment to the fullest, to show her appreciation to them.

Although the practice of the occupational therapist was hospital-based, the approach to case management (balancing visits in person with phone communication) was more of a community-based model. The occupational therapist served as a consultant on lifestyle adjustment and modifications in activities defining Valerie's roles as homemaker, wife, mother, and independent person, always in charge of her own personal care. The choices she made were somewhat unorthodox, from an allopathic medical perspective, but they were her choices—for better or worse.

▼ REFERENCES

Burkhardt, A. & Joachim, L. (1996). *A therapist's guide to oncology: Medical issues affecting management.* San Antonio: Therapy Skill Builders, Psychological Corporation, Harcourt-Brace.

Burkhardt, A. & Joachim, L. (1992). Occupational therapy techniques used in the treatment of the edemas. *Occupational Therapy Practice, 4*(1), 8–21.

Burkhardt, A. & Weitz, J. (1990). Oncological applications for silicone gel sheets in soft-tissue contractures. *American Journal of Occupational Therapy, 45,* 460–462.

Clark, F. & Jackson, J. (1990). The application of the occupational science negative heuristic in the treatment of persons with the human immunodeficiency infection. *Occupational Therapy in Health Care, 6*(4), 69–91.

Cook, A. & Burkhardt, A. (1994). The effect of cancer diagnosis and treatment on hand function. *American Journal of Occupational Therapy, 48,* 836–839.

Denton, R. (1987). AIDS: Guidelines for occupational therapy intervention. *American Journal of Occupational Therapy, 41,* 427–432.

Dietz, J. H., Jr. (1974). Rehabilitation of the cancer patient: Its role in the scheme of comprehensive care. *Clinical Bulletin, 4,* 104–107.

Galantino, M. L., Mukand, J., & Freed, M. M. (1991). Physical therapy management of patients with HIV infection. In J. Mukand (Ed.), *Rehabilitation for patients with HIV Disease* (pp. 257–282). New York: McGraw-Hill.

Galantino, M. L. & Pizzi, M. (1991). Occupational and physical therapy

for persons with HIV disease and their caregivers. *Journal of Home Health Care Practice, 3*(3), 46–57.

Gutterman, L. (1990). A day treatment program for persons with AIDS. *American Journal of Occupational Therapy, 44,* 234–237.

Kassler, W. (1993). *An introduction to HIV.* Redwood City, CA: Benjamin Cummings Publishing.

Pizzi, M. (1988, Aug. 18). Challenge of treating AIDS patients includes helping them lead functional lives. *OT Week, 31,* 6–7.

Pizzi, M. (1989). Occupational therapy: Creating possibilities for adults with HIV infection, ARC and AIDS. *AIDS Patient Care, 3,* 18–23.

Pizzi, M. (1990) The model of human occupation and adults with HIV infection and AIDS. *American Journal of Occupational Therapy, 44,* 257–264.

Pizzi, M. (1991). HIV infection and occupational therapy. In J. Mukand (Ed.), *Rehabilitation for patients with HIV disease* (pp. 283–326). New York: McGraw-Hill.

Pizzi, M. (1993). HIV infection and AIDS. In H. L. Hopkins & H. D. Smith (Eds.), *Willard and Spackman's Occupational Therapy* (8th ed.; pp. 716–729). Philadelphia: J. B. Lippincott.

Springhouse Corp. (1995). *Professional guide to diseases.* Springhouse, PA: Author.

Weinstein, B. (1990). Assessing the impact of HIV disease. *American Journal of Occupational Therapy, 44,* 220–226.

Williams, V., Burkhardt, A., & Royce, J. (1995) Helping you call it quits: O.T. practitioners are in a unique position to help clients quit smoking successfully. *OT Week, 9*(9), 18–20.

Chapter 40

Psychosocial Dysfunction in Adults

Judith D. Ward

T he following psychiatric diagnoses were selected for discussion because occupational therapy practitioners encounter them in their work in mental health settings and in physical rehabilitation and long-term care. Although many diagnoses were left out, the ones that are included exemplify cognitive, behavioral, and psychosocial problems associated with most psychosocial and many physical disorders seen by occupational therapy practitioners. Depression is everywhere. Substance abuse is the cause of problems occupational therapy practitioners see in nursing homes, trauma centers, and in physical and cognitive rehabilitation settings. The people occupational therapy practitioners treat in these settings may also suffer the effects of dementia. And, finally, people with severe and persistent mental illness share many of the problems discussed in the sections on borderline personality disorder and schizophrenia

Although these psychosocial problems are seen in a variety of settings, they will be discussed here, primarily, from the perspective of psychosocial practice in mental health setting; each disorder will be examined in terms of the American Psychiatric Association (APA) diagnostic criteria. However, it is hoped that enough information is given to show the implications for occupational therapy in a variety of practice situations.

▼ THE *DIAGNOSTIC AND STATISTICAL MANUAL OF MENTAL DISORDERS*

The **Diagnostic and Statistical Manual of Mental Disorders,** 4th edition (DSM-IV) is the American Psychiatric Association's guide to the diagnosis of mental disorders. It provides the criteria for diagnosis, description of symptoms, information on familial patterns, and the prevalence and course of the disorders.

The manual provides International Classification of Diseases (ICD) codes for most diagnoses (American Psychiatric Association [APA], 1994). DSM-IV is descriptive and does not discuss theories about causation unless specific biological factors are known. "The purpose of DSM-IV is to provide clear descriptions of diagnostic categories in order to enable clinicians and investigators to diagnose, communicate about, study, and treat people with various mental disorders" (APA, 1994, p. xxvii). Because the manual is used to provide a means of communication among a diverse population of mental health and legal professionals, work on the latest revision included liaison with organizations interested in its construction. Among them was the American Occupational Therapy Association (APA, 1994).

The Diagnostic and Statistical Manual of Mental Disorders: A Multiaxial System for Assessment

The DSM-IV provides a multiaxial system for assessment. Each axis provides domains of information that guide the gathering of data on a client so that a comprehensive picture can be obtained. The five axes are:

Axis I   Clinical disorders
Other conditions that may be a focus of clinical attention
These include all mental disorders except personality disorders and mental retardation.

Axis II   Personality disorders
Mental retardation

Axis III   General medical conditions
These include any medical conditions, such as diabetes or heart disease, that may be relevant in managing the client's mental disorder.

Axis IV Psychosocial and environmental problems
Any life events, familial circumstances, economic, environmental circumstances that are relevant to the client's mental illness or recovery are noted on this axis.

Axis V   Global assessment of functioning
A Global Assessment of Functioning (GAF) Scale is provided that rates the individuals current functioning in social, occupational, and psychological functioning.

(American Psychiatric Association, 1994)

▼ THE MENTAL STATUS EXAMINATION

The mental status examination is a formal procedure used to examine and diagnose the mental functioning of a person. It serves the same function in psychiatry as the physical examination does in medicine. A psychiatrist or psychologist conducts the mental status examination and occupational therapy practitioners may contribute information about their observations of the client to enable a diagnosis to be made.

The mental status examination is conducted through an interview in which the examiner considers the clients verbal responses and observes related psychomotor behaviors and appearance to evaluate and diagnose the individual. A *general description* of the client is recorded. This includes appearance, motor behavior, speech, and attitude. The *emotional expression* is noted, and equally important is the observation of the context in which the emotions are expressed. For example, if the client laughed while describing the death of a close family member, the examiner would attempt to determine the significance of this inappropriate response. *Perceptual disturbances, such as* **hallucinations**, illusions,

and depersonalization, are identified, and the *thought processes* and *thought content* are explored. During the interview, the examiner assesses the client's *intelligence* by noting vocabulary and level of *education*. If problems are suspected, the client will be given a standardized intelligence test. *Orientation* to person, place, and time indicates our ability to know who we are, where we are, and the date and time. Remote, recent past, and short-term *memory* are also assessed (Scheiber, 1988).

A knowledge of the client's social history, as well as information from the mental status interview, help the examiner assess the *impulse control* and *judgment* of the client. And finally, the individual's *insight,* his or her understanding of the extent and origination of the problem, is explored (Scheiber, 1988). Many of the functions noted in the mental status examination are interrelated. For example, perceptual disturbances can interfere with thought process and content. Memory loss results in disorientation.

▼ ALZHEIMER'S DISEASE AND OTHER DEMENTIAS

Alzheimer's disease is classified by the APA as a dementia. The DSM-IV uses to term **dementia** to designate cognitive disorders that are caused by a general medical condition or the persistent effects of a substance (APA, 1994).

The Dementias
- Dementia of the Alzheimer's type
- Vascular dementia
- Substance-induced persisting dementia
- Dementia of multiple etiologies
- Dementia caused by
  HIV disease
  Head trauma
  Pick's disease
  Parkinson's disease
  Huntington's disease
  Creutzfeldt-Jakob disease (APA, 1994)

Regardless of cause, the dementias present common symptoms. These always include impairment of memory and may include the inability to think abstractly or plan and carry out complex actions. **Apraxia, aphasia**, or **agnosia** may also be present. These symptoms are severe enough to impair social or occupational functioning in a individual who, earlier in life, was unimpaired (APA, 1994).

Alzheimer's Disease

Alzheimer's disease is the most prevalent dementia. Its onset is insidious and occurs mainly in the aged, but can have an early onset. The initial signs of Alzheimer's are memory impairments, social withdrawal, apathy, and sleep disturbance.

The individual may be unable to concentrate and may have hypochondriacal complaints. Early signs of dementia can be difficult to distinguish from depression. In dementia and depression, thinking is slowed and recall is difficult. To complicate matters, people with dementia may also be depressed about their condition (Update on Alzheimer's Disease—Part II, 1995).

Symptoms of Dementia

- Memory impairment—affects the ability to learn new information (registration) and remote memory, remembering old information (retention and recall).
- Confabulation—reciting imaginary events to fill in for gaps in memory
- Aphasia—impairment of language
  Receptive aphasia—the inability to understand spoken or written language
  Expressive aphasia—impairment in the use of verbal and written language
- Apraxia—inability to perform motor activities, although sensory motor function is intact and the individual understands the requirements of the task.
- Agnosia—inability to recognize familiar objects in spite of intact sensory capacities (APA, 1994)

Short-term memory is the first cognitive function to be lost in Alzheimer's. This loss may not be noticeable if individuals live in familiar surroundings and do the same jobs or activities they have done for years. Sometimes the first symptoms noticed by the family are emotional. People with dementia may be frustrated and depressed about their failing abilities and become irritable and withdrawn. One man who was upset about his trouble with work, was testy at home. When his wife engaged him in marital counseling, things got worse because the Alzheimer's was not identified. He said: "I knew something was wrong. I could feel myself getting uptight over little things. People thought I knew things about the plant that I . . . I couldn't remember. The counselor said it was stress. I though it was something else, something terrible. I was scared" (Mace & Rabins, 1991, p. 9). The emotional reactivity may not be only in response to the condition. It may be a function of the brain changes that occur with Alzheimer's. In these cases the behavior cannot be controlled.

Initially, people with Alzheimer's can accommodate to their memory impairment by creating systems for remembering but, as deterioration progresses, the adaptations no longer work. Even in the early stages, symptoms become more pronounced if there is extreme stress or change in the usual environment. For example, a woman who functions well in her own home may become disoriented during a weekend stay with relatives. When the familiar landmarks and routines are absent, the dementia is revealed. She is unable to become accustomed to (learn) the new environment, and her ingrained habits do not serve her well in new routines.

In more advanced stages, the person with Alzheimer's is unable to hold a job that demands organization of thought and recent memory. The inability to remember recent events can cause disorientation and paranoia. For example, the man who forgets that he just paid for groceries may accuse a family member of stealing the money from his wallet. Memory loss can be dangerous if the person forgets she has lit a burner on the stove, or if she takes a walk and gets lost. Memory impairment also sabotages one's sense of time:

The other day I walked out of the room and returned in less than a minute. She looked at me accusingly and said, 'Where have you been? I've been waiting hours for you to come back.'. . . I don't argue because her sense of time is gone. For her to understand how much time has passed means she must also remember what she did in the immediate past. She can't do that because she can't recall the immediate past and has no concept of time (Murphey, 1988, p. 39).

It can be frustrating and exhausting to live with a person who has Alzheimer's. As memory deteriorates, long-term memory is affected and the individual may not recognize family members. Alan Bennett (1995) noted the magnitude of memory loss in his mother, when he visited her in a nursing home:

Mam's memory has almost gone, leaving her suffused with a general benevolence. . . It is a beautiful day and we walk on the sands. 'Has Gordon been to see you?' I ask. 'Oh yes,' she says, happily. 'Though I'm saying he has, I don't know who he is.' 'Do you know who I am?' She peers at me. 'Oh yes, you're. . . you're my son, aren't you?' 'And what's my name?' 'Ah, now then.' And she laughs, as if this is not information any reasonable person could expect her to have (Bennett, 1995, pp. 76–77).

Bennett's mother is cheerful and easygoing. Not everyone is. Alzheimer's affects the individual's personality, as well. People who were kind and gentle souls all their lives may turn surly and aggressive. A person who had been fastidious may become sloppy and disheveled. The person who was always self-reliant and independent may now follow the caretaker around like a shadow. Confusion can result in socially inappropriate behavior: "One teenage boy came home to find his father sitting on the back porch reading the newspaper. He was naked except for his hat" (Mace & Rabins, p. 130). This man stripped because he was hot, unaware of his public display.

Psychotic symptoms can also accompany Alzheimer's. The delusional thinking can be a function of memory impairment, or it can arise unrelated to forgetfulness. The behaviors stimulated by the **delusions** can be difficult to manage, as Bennett described in his diary:

This evening Mam is convinced that there are people outside the house and that they are waiting to take me away. I get her off to bed but she keeps coming down, anxious to be taken away in my place. At one point she gets outside in the bitter cold, and eventually I go to bed in order to stop her coming downstairs. I drift off to sleep three or four times, but each time she wakes me, wanting to know if I am all right (Bennett, 1995, p. 70).

Some individuals become worse in the evening, or they may awaken in the night and become disoriented. This is called **sundowning.** It is not known what causes this phenomenon. Some have attributed the confusion to waking in the dark and being unable to get one's bearings. A nightlight sometimes helps these people. For others, sundowning may be a sign of fatigue and lowered stress tolerance at the end of the day (Mace & Rabins, 1991). Alzheimer's clients may become agitated and anxious for no apparent reason, and they will sometimes overreact to seemingly inconsequential things. This is known as catastrophic reaction, and occasionally, the individual will strike out at others. Sometimes one can identify a reason for the reaction:

Mother hit me. She isn't strong enough to hurt me physically. But, along with the verbal tirade, I reacted badly. I yelled back and she got worse. . . . Mother wasn't angry at me even though she shouted when she struck me. She gets that way when the TV gets loud, a lot of action takes place, or when several people come into the room. Even if she used to know them, they are strangers now and their presence confuses her (Murphey, 1988, p. 128).

Family members need to understand the limits Alzheimer's disease places on the client. And health care professionals need to understand the stress families endure as they live with someone whose brain is slowly dying.

Communication becomes more and more difficult with time. Problems with verbal expression can start with getting words mixed up. For example one woman said "You know I don't like to eat carburetors," when discussing cauliflower with her daughter (Murphey, 1988). It is often the names of things that go first. Bennett's mother stood before the mantelpiece staring at the clock, trying to name it: "It's one of those things," she said, "with things that go round, and then when they get there they've had it for a bit" (p. 75). Some people ramble on, talk and talk without making sense, others revert to silence.

Motor abilities are affected as the disease progresses. Sometimes motor planning is impaired so the person might lie the wrong way, across the bed or try to sleep standing up. One woman said of her husband: "He's had trouble opening his eyes lately. He will complain, 'Fern, I can't see,' but when I explain to him that he has his eyes closed, he counters with, 'I can't open my eyes.'. . . And later, he opens his eyes without effort" (Konek, 1991, p. 88). The simple task of dressing may be impossible. This is not because people lose the ability to move their arms or fingers, but because they do not know how to accomplish these tasks (apraxia).

Alzheimer's ultimately ends in death, but the client could live as long as 20 years with the disease (Update on Alzheimer's Disease—Part I, 1995). Some people die of other diseases of aging. Those who do not, may progress to a vegetative state and require constant care until they die.

TREATMENT AND IMPLICATIONS FOR OCCUPATIONAL THERAPY

Dead brain cells cannot be revived, and there is no cure for Alzheimer's disease. It is important, however, to differentiate Alzheimer's from dementias that have a treatable cause. For example, if the dementia is caused by cerebrovascular disease, it is possible to intervene in the progress of dementia by treating the vascular disease. Occupational therapy practitioners should, nonetheless, consider the implications of dementia when treating clients who have had strokes.

GENERAL GOALS IN THE MANAGEMENT OF ALZHEIMER'S

The goals in treatment of Alzheimer's disease include medical treatment of physical problems, provision of nutrition, and maintenance of health. The symptoms of dementia are managed by providing an environment that supports function and facilitates social interaction. Psychotic symptoms, agitation, and depression can be treated by medication. However, care must be taken because older people are more susceptible to the side effects of these drugs (Levy, 1987a).

Occupational Therapy for Dementia

Occupational therapy practitioners, in most areas of practice, will be faced with working with the symptoms of dementia. **Cerebral vascular accidents (CVA), Parkinson's disease, meningitis, human immunodeficiency virus (HIV)** infection, all can result in temporary or permanent dementia. The therapist must evaluate the cognitive abilities of clients for whom dementia may be a complication of their condition. Instruction in treatment activities must be geared to cognitive abilities with consideration of deficits. If the problem is irreversible and progressive, this must be taken into account.

Structure and predictability are important aspects of the living situation for people with dementias. The performance skills of the person with dementia depend not only on cognitive abilities, but also on the individual's motivation and the nature of the environment. People with Alzheimer's may be unable to learn new skills, but old skills and habits remain deeply ingrained, and these can be used, long into the disease (Borell, Sandman, & Kielhofner, 1991).

People with Alzheimer's are likely to live with their families during some of their illness. Education and support of the family is critical. Families need to understand the disease and learn what they can expect in terms of confusion and apparent inconsistencies of behavior. There are a several excellent books about living with and caring for Alzheimer's clients that give examples of the variety of problems that can be encountered and how to manage them (Mace & Rabins, 1991; Murphey, 1988). Families can be helped to identify resources such as support groups for caregivers and respite care services.

Occupational therapy practitioners can help families identify those environmental factors that will facilitate maximum function and support peace of mind. The individual's capacities, including communication skills, are assessed to determine current strengths and limitations. Whether individuals are living with families or in institutions, they require appropriate sensory and social stimulation in an environment that supports function and minimizes disabilities. Because sensory abilities become impaired, environmental stimulation needs to be intensified (Levy, 1987a). Care must be taken, however, because overstimulation can cause agitation, confusion, and catastrophic reaction.

Daily routines that are predictable and reflect the rhythm of the larger society, with the opportunity for activity and a chance to rest, help keep the person in touch. Familiar objects and lifestyle also help keep one grounded in reality. A sense of autonomy can be maintained if people are given the freedom to choose their activities with a variety of options (Levy, 1987a).

Levy (1987b) recommends Allen's Cognitive Disability approach to the management of Alzheimer's. This approach, described elsewhere in this text, measures the cognitive level of the individual and identifies the sensory cues to which the individual, at a particular level, is able to attend. Once the family and practitioner understand the cognitive level of the client, they are able to understand how to provide the correct stimulation to engage the client in activity. They will also understand the cognitive limitations of the client and provide stimulation for only those responses that are possible. One can fashion the environment to the person's abilities, interest, and comfort level, and help maintain his or her dignity (Levy, 1987b). Because in Alzheimer's and other degenerative dementias, cognitive abilities decrease over time, the environment must be adapted accordingly. Even when abilities are very simple, it is possible to provide occupation:

Grandpa's fascination with paper helped him to pass the time. We now put colorful advertising supplements from the newspaper, old catalogs, and junk mail on the table in the family room for him. These were his playthings for hours because he could no longer do more complex things (Honel, 1988, p. 187).

▼ MOOD DISORDERS

The **mood disorders** are classified in two major categories: **depressive disorders** and **bipolar disorders**. Depressive disorders are those in which there is a prolonged emotional state of sadness. Bipolar disorders have periods of mania and periods of depression, the two poles. All the mood disorders have the following:

1. Disturbance of mood
2. Psychomotor symptoms which affect:
   Thought processes
   Attention
   Activity level
3. Disturbance of sleep and appetite

Depressive Disorders

Depression is pervasive in our society—17 % of Americans will suffer severe depression in their lifetime (Update on

---

American Psychiatric Association Classification of Mood Disorders
Depressive disorders
Major depressive disorder
Dysthymic disorder
Depressive disorder NOS
Bipolar disorders
Bipolar I disorder
Bipolar II disorder
Cyclothymic disorder
Bipolar disorder NOS
(American Psychiatric Assoc., 1994)

Mood Disorders—Part I, 1994). All the depressive disorders share similar symptoms, but the degree of severity varies. A depressed mood has many faces. The person may feel tired, sick, heavy, hopeless, or sad. But depression can also manifest itself as irritability and anger. Depression depresses function as well as mood. To the depressed person everything seems harder to do. People with depression may feel life is not worth the effort. In her autobiographical novel, *The Bell Jar*, Sylvia Plath describes the depression of her main character, Esther, who has not slept for a week. She had not washed her hair and has worn the same clothes, without washing them, for 3 weeks "because it seemed so silly":

I saw the days of the year stretching ahead like a series of bright white boxes, and separating one box from another was sleep. . . . It seemed silly to wash one day when I would only have to wash again the next. It made me tired just to think of it (Plath, 1971, pp. 104–105).

Esther, similar to many depressed people, cannot find meaning in life, and this attitudes colors her perceptions. Why should she care for her grooming when life is an "infinitely desolate avenue"? She is not even able to escape this desolation through sleep, a common problem in depression. Depression kills the ability to experience pleasure (anhedonia) and even those things that were enjoyed in the past no longer hold meaning.

The APA describes two types of depressive disorders: **major depressive disorder** and **dysthymia**. These disorders have many of the same symptoms, but the onset, duration, and severity of the depression differs (APA, 1994).

MAJOR DEPRESSIVE DISORDER

Major depressive disorder is severe depression that is present almost all of every day for at least 2 weeks. There is a noticeable change in the person's usual mood which is evident through sadness, and a loss of pleasure in almost everything. People with major depression lose their appetite and often cannot get a full night's sleep. Some people suffer from hypersomnia. There is frequently an overwhelming fatigue that immobilizes the person. This inertia is so paralyzing that it is impossible to pull oneself together to do the simplest activities. Percy Knauth (1975) describes this phenomenon as he hears his visiting son's footsteps:

It was my son returning unannounced from Vietnam. . . . If ever there was a situation in which a man would do everything possible to pull himself together, this was it. But although I felt this overwhelmingly, there was absolutely nothing I could do. I sat rooted in my chair and waited, trembling like a man condemned. I heard the footsteps stop outside the door; I saw the handle turn. I shrieked inwardly at myself: 'Get up! *Get up* !' Then he was there. . . .

To me he looked seven feet tall. The brass on his uniform glittered, the ribbons were flashes of color on his chest, his boots shone like twin mirrors. He was everything I was not—strong, healthy, alive. . . . I don't believe I will forget that moment, or my own dreadful sense of helplessness, until the day I die (Knauth, 1975, p. 93).

Knauth was not physically paralyzed, but he was unable to respond. This inertia is called psychomotor retardation. Everything slows. It is hard to concentrate, thoughts and actions are sluggish. Making decisions becomes an impossible hurdle, and self-esteem plunges. Irrational thoughts of worthlessness and guilt may become obsessive. Knauth explains:

In my own eyes I became worthless. . . . I reviewed my life and saw everything that I had done wrong. Not even the most trivial detail escaped this deadly scrutiny. . . . I realized what a poor excuse for a father I had been. I recalled the details of my divorce, and I understood precisely why my first wife had left me for another man. Viewed in the merciless gloom of this early-morning self-analysis, even my work appeared to me to have been a fraud. At last I was being showed up for the hapless faker that I was and this was my punishment (Knauth, 1975, pp. 35–36).

In some people the feelings of guilt and worthlessness may take on the severity of psychotic delusions or other psychotic features. A major depressive episode can develop in a day or over weeks. It may last for months. If untreated, it can last longer than 6 months. In most cases, with remission, the individual returns to premorbid functioning (APA, 1994).

Depression is Ubiquitous

In addition to depression classified under mood disorders, depression can be associated with:

Adjustment disorder with depressed mood
Alzheimer's and other dementias
Depression associated with a medical condition
General anxiety disorder may co-occur with major depressive disorder
Posttraumatic stress disorder has increased risk of major depressive disorder
Schizoaffective disorder—depressive type
Substance-induced depression

(American Psychiatric Assoc., 1994)

DYSTHYMIA

Dysthymia has a slower onset than major depression and it lasts longer. Its symptoms are not as pronounced as those in major depressive illness, and the individual is usually able to work and does not need to be hospitalized. It is a serious disease, however, and most people with dysthymia go on to develop major depression (Dysthymia and Other Mood Disorders, 1991). To make the diagnosis, the individual must be depressed "for most of the day, for more days than not" (APA, 1994, p. 349) for at least 2 years. This depression takes the form of fatigue, listlessness, and blunted pleasure. The individual may carry out essential activities, but with great effort and without enjoyment. Self-esteem is low, and function may be impaired by poor concentration or the inability to make decisions. Appetite and sleep are affected. People with dysthymia may be so accustomed to being depressed that they take it for granted (APA, 1994). It took Pat Love, a psychologist, years to recognize her own depression. She says: "The way it affects me is that I have a gloomy outlook on life. . . Life doesn't excite me. It puts a negative slant on life for me....It's difficult to think positively. This is like having a really bad hangover. It feels almost like a physical residue of a drug in my tissues. . . It's in your cells. . . My body feels gloomy. But when you feel that way, the inclination is to start thinking that way" (Love, in Cronkite, 1994, p. 49).

Bipolar Disorder

Bipolar disorder is sometimes called manic–depression because people with the disorder go through cycles of both moods. The depression associated with bipolar disorders is similar to the depression described in the depressive disorders. Mania is the polar opposite of depression. Mania is characterized by excessive energy with flight of ideas associated with an elevated, expansive, or irritable mood. This mood must persist for at least a week or be severe enough to require hospitalization for the diagnosis to be applied (APA, 1994).

Additional symptoms of mania include sleeplessness, and grandiose thinking, with inflated self-esteem. The person may dress flamboyantly, behave in a dramatic manner, may spend money lavishly, running up huge credit card or phone bills. Speech is often pressured, loud, and nonstop. Individuals with mania seem to talk to hear themselves talk, punning and singing without listening to others. Their judgment is impaired, and they may be sexually overactive and promiscuous (APA, 1994). During manic episodes clients may have, as APA puts it: "excessive involvement in pleasurable activities that have a high potential for painful consequences" (APA, 1994, p. 335). These behaviors are calamitous to families and are the cause of humiliation and regret when the individual is in **remission**.

There are degrees of mania. Fieve describes the extreme delirious mania of one of his clients:

On the psychiatric ward she developed a great excitement and overactivity. She said she had so much to do that she no longer had time to eat. After five days of starvation she required tube feeding.... She entered a phase of great physical activity. She paced the floor, and went into patients' rooms, causing considerable disturbance. She was distractible, mis-identified people, and was disoriented in time and place. Her condition seemed to approach a state of ecstasy when she sang religious hymns and unabashedly stripped in front of everyone. Once she became violent and struck another patient. On another occasion she broke the window in her room (Fieve, 1975, p. 23).

This is an extreme case of mania. Others are milder and less destructive, but would be considered mania if they are intense enough to impair social or occupational functioning (APA, 1994).

MIXED EPISODES

Associated with bipolar I disorder are mixed episodes that present concurrent symptoms of mania and depression. The individual may have flight of ideas and grandiose thinking while breaking into sobs or feeling "despairing anxiety," all at the same time (Duke & Hochman, 1992). These mixed episodes are severe enough to interfere with social and occupational functioning or to require hospitalization.

BIPOLAR I AND BIPOLAR II DISORDERS

The DSM-IV distinguishes two bipolar disorders. The difference between them is that, although both have episodes of major depression, bipolar I disorder has occurrences of full-blown mania or mixed symptoms. Bipolar II disorder has recurrent depressive episodes with *hypomania*. Hypomania is a persistent state of inflated or irritable mood that is distinctly different from the individual's usual nondepressed behavior. During the hypomanic episode the individual may have any of the symptoms described for mania, but these symptoms are milder and do not impair social and occupational functioning and do not require hospitalization (APA, 1994).

CYCLOTHYMIC DISORDER

Cyclothymia is a chronic mood disturbance in which there are periods of hypomania and periods of depressive symptoms. The symptoms are less severe than, or do not meet all the criteria for manic episode or major depressive episode, but last for, at least, a 2-year period. Cyclothymia has a slow, gradual onset in adolescence or early adulthood, and it appears to predispose the individual to other mood disorders (APA, 1994).

Mood Disorder Specifiers

A. The specifiers for the severity of the current episode **are:**

Mild	**Severe with psychotic features**
Moderate	**Partial remission**
Severe without psychotic features	**Full remission**

B. Specifiers to describe the nature **of the** current or most recent episode.

Chronic: This specifier is applied to the Depressive Episodes of Major Depression and the Bipolar Disorders. All the criteria for a Major Depressive Episode must be present for 2 years, at least.

Catatonic features: Refers to psychomotor disturbance in which the individual motorically immobile or excessively overactive for no apparent purpose.

Melancholic features: Applied to the most recent *Major Depressive Episodes* of the Mood Disorders. Loss of pleasure or lack of reaction to pleasurable stimuli. Frequently depression is worse in the morning and sleep disturbance is characterized by early morning awakening. Excessive or inappropriate guilt, loss of appetite, and psychomotor retardation or agitation may be present.

Atypical features: The *Depressed* individual's mood lightens in response to pleasurable stimuli (mood reactivity). May also include increase of appetite, excessive sleeping, and a feeling of heaviness in arms or legs. Some have social sensitivity, which impairs social or occupational functioning.

C. Specifiers to describe the course **of** recurrent episodes **are:**

With or without full interepisode recovery: This describes the *most recent* period between episodes of Recurrent Major Depression, Bipolar I or Bipolar II Disorders. Sometimes there are prominent symptoms present between episodes of the disorder; if this is the case it is noted as Without Interepisode Recovery. Other cases show full remission between episodes and this is noted.

Seasonal pattern: In some individuals the Major Depressive Episodes of the Mood Disorders have a seasonal pattern, the most common is that which begins in fall or winter and ceases in the spring. This is sometimes known as Seasonal Affective Disorder, SAD.

Rapid cycling: When an individual with Bipolar Disorder has at least four episodes of Major Depression, Mania, Mixed or Hypomanic Moods in the last year the specifier rapid cycling can be applied.

(American Psychiatric Association, 1994)

Causal Factors and the Course of Mood Disorders

External stress, such as job loss, death of a loved one, or illness, can lead to depression. However, it appears that these stressors are more important in the first episode of depression than in subsequent ones. This has led to the theory that the original stressors produce changes in brain cells, thereby creating long-term susceptibility to depression (Update on Mood Disorders—Part II, 1995). If one is female and has a family history of depression, there is a two to three times greater risk for depression than the general population (Hirchfeld & Goodwin, 1988). Sixty to sixty-five percent of people with bipolar disorder have family members with a history of major depression (Hirchfeld & Goodwin, 1988).

A National Institute of Mental Health (NIMH) study found that 89% of people with bipolar disorder had further manic or depressive episodes after their first hospitalization (Bipolar Disorder: Outcome, 1994). Mood disorders may become chronic and worsen over time. More than half of the people who suffer from one major depressive episode will have another. And those who have two episodes have an 80% chance of a third. On average, an episode of major depression will last 4 months (Update on Mood Disorders—Part I, 1994).

Treatment of Mood Disorders

Treatment for depression depends on the severity, persistence, and cause. If the depression is associated with a medical disorder or is substance-induced, these factors must be addressed. Psychotherapy is effective for some people, but there needs to be more research to identify the more effective methods. A study conducted by the NIMH, found that interpersonal therapy that examines the social context of the depression was slightly more effective than **cognitive behavioral therapy** for clients with major depression. However, cognitive therapy is very effective for people with depression who are not excessively guilty or pessimistic (Update on Mood Disorders—Part II, 1995). If mood changes are seasonal, the systematic, controlled use of bright light is effective (Seasonal Affective Disorder, 1993). The NIMH study found that medication worked better and faster than other treatments. Psychotherapy and medication are frequently used together, with the medication lightening the mood and the therapy used for support and stress management.

Electroconvulsive therapy (ECT) is helpful for at least half of depressed clients who do not respond to medication. It is most valuable for cutting short a depressive episode (Update on Mood Disorders—Part II, 1995).

Medication is an important treatment for mood disorders. Antidepressant medications, which affect the biochemistry of the brain, fall into three major categories of drugs: (1) the tricyclic antidepressants (TCAs), which block norepinephrine reuptake; (2) selective serotonin reuptake inhibitors (SSRIs); and (3) monoamine oxidase inhibitors (MAOIs), which prevent norepinephrine and dopamine from being broken down. All three types of drugs are effective treatments for depression. The SSRIs have the fewest side effects and fluoxetine (Prozac), one of the them, is the most widely prescribed psychoactive drug in the United States (Update on Mood Disorders—Part II, 1995).

The antimanic medications include lithium carbonate, antipsychotic medications, and anticonvulsants (Hirchfeld & Goodwin, 1988). Lithium carbonate is a major treatment for bipolar disorder. It is successful in shortening and lessening mood swings and decreases the number of depressive and manic episodes in 70% of cases. Twenty percent of clients become completely symptom-free when taking lithium (Treatment of Mood Disorders: Part III, 1988). Lithium can curtail a manic episode and, when used regularly, can prevent future manic and depressive episodes. It is not always effective in curtailing a developed severe depressive episode and may be used in conjunction with an antidepressant in that event (Hirchfeld & Goodwin, 1988). Antipsychotic medications are used for psychotic symptoms of depression and mania, sometimes in combination with other medications.

Implications for Occupational Therapy

DEPRESSION AND DEPRESSIVE EPISODES OF BIPOLAR DISORDERS

Depending on the degree of severity, depression affects all areas of performance. The individual with dysthymia can often carry on necessary activities, but without enjoyment. The severely depressed person may actually be in a state of catatonia (APA, 1994) in which they do nothing for themselves, or they are occupied with purposeless excessive motor activity.

When working with the depressed individual it is important to consider the psychomotor retardation that slows motor and cognitive functioning. One may need to give directions in simple, one-step fashion, and give the person plenty of time to respond. During conversation the practitioner must be able to tolerate the time required for the clients' cognitive integration of information received and their verbal response. The psychomotor retardation alters social functioning. Depressed people become isolated and may even be unable to ask for help or convey the magnitude of their depression.

There is always a risk of suicide with depression. Ironically, it is more likely to occur after a deep depression has somewhat lifted, and the individual gains the energy to carry out the act.

One walks a fine line when working with depressed people. Care must be taken not to insult their intellects while grading activity for psychomotor retardation. The practitioner may feel the need to provide the energy for the interaction, but that also may engender what Styron described as "humiliated rage" when his art therapist conducted sessions that he called "organized infantilism." He says:

Our class was run by a delirious young woman with a fixed, indefatigable smile, who was plainly trained at a school offering courses in Teaching Art to the Mentally Ill; not even a teacher of very young retarded children could have been compelled to bestow, without deliberate instruction, such orchestrated chuckles and coos (Styron, 1990, p. 74).

On the other hand, it is also important to help depressed people mobilize themselves. When Knauth (1975) reflected on his depressive illness, he realized that the most elementary actions helped him survive. Each morning he forced himself to get out of bed, make coffee, and make his bed.

If this sounds too trivial to mention, it is not. It proved to me, day after day, that I was still able to accomplish something, even though my mind was telling me I was a total loss. By the act of getting out of bed I proved that I could still command my body and had at least a semblance of free will. By the act of making coffee I proved that I could still do something to preserve myself and thus deny my growing wish for death. By the act of making my bed I proved that I had not fallen completely into the state of sloth and disarray that my disorganized mind constantly told me I was in: I still cared (Knauth, 1975, pp. 87–88).

Because stress can precipitate depression, it is valuable to address its management. There is a link between stress, depression, and physical illness, and between mood disorders and alcohol and substance abuse. If the occupational therapy practitioner is aware of the client's medical and social history these factors can be addressed.

MANIA

Hypomanic and manic individuals may be exceptionally productive or creative (Richards, 1992). This does not mean that all people with mania are creative. Nor does it mean that it is easy to work with the manic or hypomanic client. The description of Dr. Frieve's deliriously manic client illustrates how these individuals can lose control and present danger to others. It may be impossible for them to engage in purposeful activity.

During a manic episode people are likely to be disruptive of groups because of their verbal or motor overactivity. They can take over a group, intimidating other clients and subverting the practitioner. Manic clients can be dangerous to themselves, careless with tools, without regard for self-injury. It is unwise to foster excessive activity in people who are manic because they may be unable to recognize their own physical exhaustion.

When the manic symptoms fade, the occupational therapy practitioner and client can address the daily living patterns to mutually assess routines and habits for stressors that might precipitate future relapses. People who have had chronic mood disorder for most of their adult lives may not have developed mature occupational skills and may need help learning time management, parenting skills, and other adult roles. This instruction is more effective when the disease has responded to medication and the manic symptoms are modified enough for the individual to attend and be able to concentrate.

When a person is suffering from a mood disorder, judgment is impaired. The depressed person has an exaggerated gloomy outlook, and the person with mania may not feel that anything is wrong. Thus, it is helpful to assist the client and family members to recognize precursors of the manic or depressive episodes so that prompt intervention can be arranged. Even if clients respond well to medication, it is important for them to know how to maintain balanced lives to prevent relapse. The actress Patty Duke, who has learned to live with her bipolar illness, which is well controlled by lithium, says:

You still have to deal with reality. And reality is hard. . . . It takes practice to do it differently than you used to, and to recognize your norm for tolerance of aggravation, or of stress, or of sleep deprivation, or hunger (p. 248). I'd be less than honest if I said that manic depression is not part of my life today. . . . I am who I am, with behavior patterns that have been going on for years. Just taking a pill doesn't mean I'm going to become a different person. The whole world doesn't immediately turn rosy. So I keep working really hard to break behaviors I don't like in myself. I practice. . . It is a question of relearning—or maybe learning for the first time—how to behave the way you want to behave (Duke & Hochman, 1992, pp. 239–240).

▼ SUBSTANCE ABUSE

When people use drugs in a compulsive or self-destructive way they are said to abuse substances. In this discussion of substance abuse, the terms drug and substance will be used interchangeably to refer to any psychoactive chemical, including alcohol, inhalants, or illicit or prescribed drugs and medication.

Substance Dependence and Abuse

When describing the effects of the misuse of psychoactive drugs the DSM-IV (APA, 1994) distinguishes between **substance dependence** and **substance abuse**. Substance *dependence*, often called drug addiction, refers to repeated self-administration of drugs that leads to significant cognitive, behavioral, and physiological problems. Included among the problems of dependence may be the development of drug tolerance and unpleasant withdrawal symptoms. Those who are addicted to substances spend a great deal of time obtaining the drugs or recovering from the effects. Thus, social and occupational function is impaired. Often, addicted individuals want to control their use of drugs, but they are unable to regulate the amount used or they use the substance over a longer period than intended. People who are substance dependent will continue maladaptive patterns of use, even when they know that they have physical or psychological problems associated with abuse (APA, 1994).

In substance *abuse* individuals do not develop tolerance or withdrawal symptoms, but experience social consequences of drug use, which lead to failures in fulfillment of role responsibilities and poor school or work performance. Abusers will use a drug, in spite of engaging in activities, such as driving, that are hazardous when impaired by such substances. When abuse results in legal problems, the individual may continue the abuse, in spite of the problems (APA, 1994). The distinction between substance abuse and dependence "is neither precise nor fixed for any given person" (Treatment of Drug Abuse and Addiction—Part I, 1995, p. 1).

Drug abuse and dependence are not simple problems. In the American population, 39% of alcohol abusers and 50% of persons who have other drug problems have a second psychiatric disorder. Antisocial personality disorder, borderline personality, anxiety, and mood disorders are the most common problems in these people with a dual diagnosis. Although it is unclear which problem came first, the consensus among experts is that the drug abuse must be treated before other psychiatric problems can be addressed (Treatment of Drug Abuse and Addiction—Part II, 1995).

Additional complications in the treatment of drug addiction are that many users are involved with more than one drug and there is a high incidence of acquired immunodeficiency symdrome (AIDS) among intravenous drug users. Approximately 30% of new cases of HIV infection in the United States are, directly or indirectly, due to intravenous drug use (Treatment of Drug Abuse and Addiction—Part II, 1995).

Drug Tolerance and Withdrawal

Tolerance occurs when individuals require increasingly more of the drug to obtain the desired effect; or, when continuing to use the same amount of the substance, experience a diminishment of effect.

Withdrawal symptoms are behavioral, cognitive, and physiological changes that occur in an individual who has used a substance regularly, over a prolonged period, and then ceases to use the drug. These symptoms will abate when drug intake is resumed. The degree of tolerance and the severity of withdrawal symptoms vary with the substance (APA, 1994).

Causes of Drug and Alcohol Abuse and Dependence

There is no single cause that can be attributed to all substance abuse. Even when considering a single substance one cannot isolate a single cause.

BIOLOGICAL FACTORS

There is some evidence of a genetic predisposition to alcoholism. Studies have reported that a third of alcoholics have an alcoholic parent. And over 40% of males who have two alcoholic parents develop alcoholism. However, these studies did not rule out the environmental factors, such as mod-

eling, that could take place in alcoholic families (Carson & Butcher, 1992). Other substances, too, are thought to have biological or genetic factors in their use. However, Goldstein (1994) cautions against misunderstanding the genetic vulnerability to drug addiction. He says, "Drug addiction differs from clearcut genetic diseases, which do not depend on external factors. The position may be closer to that of diseases with strong hereditary influences, like the common kinds of heart disease or like colon and rectal cancers, in which environmental factors play a major role" (Goldstein, 1994, p. 87).

PSYCHOSOCIAL FACTORS

The three most commonly cited reasons for using heroin are pleasure, curiosity, and peer pressure (Carson & Butcher, 1992). This seems to fly in the face of theories that drug abusers are responding to environmental stress and unhappy childhoods. Studies of alcoholics have found that as children and adolescents they were more active, self-confident, rebellious, and aggressive than average. (Alcoholism—Part II, 1986). And, there is little evidence to suggest that alcoholism is caused by being raised in unhappy families or that alcoholics have a particular alcoholic personality (Alcoholism—Part II, 1986).

ENVIRONMENT

Environment does influence drug abuse. There can be a vicious cycle in substance abuse during which people who enter the drug culture become so immersed in it that they are isolated from the larger world. This often happens at a young age; hence, the individual develops a sense of inadequacy at dealing with the adult world. This can be a self-perpetuating dilemma in which the addict then uses drugs and alcohol to escape personal anxieties (Carson & Butcher, 1992). Some people become hooked on drugs when they are prescribed for pain during illness or after surgery. This is more common in middle-aged and older people who use alcohol and pills for sleeping as well as pain.

Treatment of Drug Abuse and Dependence

Whatever the cause of substance abuse, it is agreed that the first step in treatment is to stop using the substances. This begins with the acknowledgment that there is a problem. There is much denial associated with substance abuse. Betty Ford, in her book, *A Glad Awakening* describes her denial:

My makeup wasn't smeared, I wasn't disheveled, I behaved politely, and I never finished off a bottle, so how could I be alcoholic? And I wasn't on heroin or cocaine, the medicines I took—the sleeping pills, the pain pills, the relaxer pills, the pills to counteract the side effects of other pills—had been prescribed by doctors, so how could I be a drug addict? (Ford, 1987, p. 7).

Sometimes problems with the law, such as drunk driving charges, will awaken the individual to the seriousness of their use. In Betty Ford's case the family held an "intervention," during which they carefully confronted her with the effect her abuse had on them. This was done in the company of professionals and the opportunity for help (Ford, 1987).

DETOXIFICATION AND THE USE OF DRUGS FOR TREATMENT

Addiction to opiates, alcohol, and other sedatives may require supervised withdrawal from the drug. In the case of severe withdrawal symptoms—delirium and seizures—hospitalization may be required. Detoxification is the beginning, not the end, of treatment. Ironically, drugs with effects similar to the abused drug are sometimes used to ease the detoxification process. In opiate addiction the drug methadone, a synthetic opioid, is prescribed for long-term use. This replaces addiction to an illegal, self-administered drug with a supervised, orally administered addictive drug. Methadone maintenance programs are controversial and regulated by law and health agencies. But for people who were living in crime and completely involved in obtaining drugs for the next fix, methadone provides stability and enables the addicted individual to maintain a job (Treatment of Drug Abuse and Addiction—Part I, 1995).

The drug disulfiram (Antabuse), is prescribed for regular use by some alcoholics. If alcohol is ingested after taking disulfiram the individual becomes nauseous (Treatment of Drug Abuse and Addiction—Part I, 1995). This negative reinforcement of drinking is only as successful as the individual's resolve to stay with the Antabuse program.

GROUP TREATMENT OF SUBSTANCE ABUSE

Individual therapy is part of many treatment programs, but is seldom used alone. Most drug treatment programs employ various forms of group treatment. Substance abusers tend to isolate themselves and feel they are alone with their problem; groups help them find those who have been through the same experiences.

RESIDENTIAL THERAPEUTIC COMMUNITY

These residential programs, which are staffed by former drug addicts, are for individuals whose lives have been consumed by their addiction. The life of the community is highly structured and all members engage in household and other responsibilities required to maintain the environment. The community is monitored closely and residents have little contact with outsiders. Standards of behavior are clearly defined and regimented. Through regular individual and group therapy sessions residents continuously confront their drug use and the concomitant problems. An important element in such a program is the learning gained from formerly addicted staff members. The philosophy behind the therapeutic community (TC) is: "Drug abuse is regarded as a disease of the emotions that requires a transformation in thinking, feeling, and behavior leading to the development of self-reliance, a sense of responsibility, and a work ethic" (Treatment of Drug Abuse and Addiction—Part I, 1995, p. 3).

CHEMICAL DEPENDENCY PROGRAMS

These programs usually take place in a special unit of psychiatric or general hospitals and are run by professionals with some inclusion of ex-addicts (Treatment of Drug Abuse and Addiction—Part I, 1995). The length of stay can vary from a matter of days to a month, and treatment is usually reimbursed by private insurers. Various aftercare follow-up programs are included, and clients are encouraged to join a 12-step program, such as Alcoholics or Narcotics Anonymous.

TWELVE-STEP PROGRAMS

These are self-help programs fashioned after Alcoholics Anonymous (AA) in which abstinence is the goal. In all these programs members acknowledge their inability to control their addiction and refer to themselves as "recovering," rather than recovered. AA and Narcotics Anonymous emphasize seeking help from a higher power. Newer 12-step groups have a more secular approach while acknowledging the need for help from others.

Occupational Therapy for Substance Abuse

Occupational therapy practitioners who treat substance abuse work in psychiatric and specialized drug treatment centers. However, in other settings, practitioners work with problems that are the result of substance abuse. Dementia and amnestic disorder are psychiatric disorders caused by prolonged use of substances, and 68% of disabilities caused by trauma are a result of risk-taking behavior while under the influence of drugs or alcohol (Heinemann, 1993).

Occupational therapy practitioners who work in substance abuse programs do so as part of a team that may consist of psychiatric social workers, nurses, physicians, drug counselors who may be recovering addicts, and recreation therapists. The problems occupational therapy addresses are those having to do with life management (Raymond, 1990). Skills in daily living are likely impaired in anyone who abuses substances. The following description of the effect of abstinence on the recovering alcoholic aptly describes the difficulties encountered by any substance abuser.

Alcoholics in the first few years of abstinence have been compared with returning prisoners of war. Their world is unfamiliar, because they have been living in an environment created by alcohol. Feelings that have been blunted or suppressed come back to trouble them. They have lost a great deal of time and must start where they left off. Being sober, like being free after imprisonment, entails new responsibilities. Thus alcoholics in the early stages of abstinence often suffer from anxiety and depression and may find it difficult to hold a job or preserve a marriage. The resolution of these problems comes when they establish new personal relationships, rebuild old ones, and begin to develop confidence in their power to control their lives (Treatment of Alcoholism—Part II, 1987, p. 2).

Perhaps the greatest contribution occupational therapy can make to the lives of recovering substance abusers is the refinement or acquisition of practical skills of life management that will meet their immediate and long-term needs and develop a sense of control over their lives (Raymond, 1990). In doing so the following problems are addressed:

SOCIAL ISOLATION

Substance abusers often feel alienated from the outer world. Their lives are lonely and consumed by otaining drugs and getting high (Robak, 1991). Callahan (1989) describes this situation:

All that winter and into the spring I lost ground to booze. I was now drinking a maintenance fifth, usually of tequila, plus 'social' drinks amounting to another fifth. Gradually I stopped going out and just drank my two fifths at home. I avoided situations where being drunk would seem inappropriate and I avoided people who weren't also drunks—99 percent of the real world. . . (p. 106).

Group activities help recovering abusers cut through their loneliness and, in drug treatment units, occupational therapy programs usually consist of groups in which recovering addicts help each other. These groups promote drug-free socialization and create a climate of mutual understanding that may ease the transition to self-help programs in the larger community.

Some addicts benefit from groups that are directly related to the development of social competence. Many people lack the very foundation of social competence, that of trusting others.

I feel I need to mention the importance of relationships—friendships as well as intimate relationships. As I began my recovery, for a long time I couldn't allow someone to love me. If somebody wanted to do something for me. I would instantly ask myself, 'What do they want?' It felt like a set-up. You see, the street is a place where everybody takes advantage of everybody else. If I help you on the street and you accept that help, you instantly owe me. And every time we look at each other we both know it. I had to come to terms with the fact that everyone needs help. . . (Gorman, 1993, p. 16).

Social skill development includes assertiveness training, development of communication skills, and interpersonal and social responsiveness training. All of these are done in a reflective manner in which the addict learns to think before acting. Psychoeducation techniques are often used in these groups in which life skills are learned through information sharing, practicing skills, role playing, and homework assignments (Raymond, 1990).

BASIC LIFE SKILLS

Raymond (1990) found that money management was the topic most requested for occupational therapy groups when she surveyed clients in an inpatient drug and alcohol abuse unit. Users are often surprised to discover how much money they spent on their drugs, or they never learned to manage money because it was consumed by their drug use. One cannot assume that clients possess the most ordinary habits of daily living. The administration of an activities configuration to identify use of time may reveal other basic skills that have fallen into disuse, or were never acquired.

TIME, LEISURE, AND STRESS MANAGEMENT

Substance abuse leads to a narrowing of life and time. With abstinence, time takes on new dimensions. The individual needs to find satisfying ways to fill leisure time that, in the past was spent using a substance. A new, clean, and sober, social network is needed. And recovering addicts need to identify times they are likely to use, and develop ways of coping with stress and boredom, without resorting to psychoactive substances. Occupational therapy groups that can address these needs include those in stress management, relaxation training, social recreation, and leisure planning.

WORK

Vocational planning and the assessment of work skills is not an area that can be addressed in a short-term, inpatient treatment environment. But employment issues cannot be ignored, and may be addressed briefly in basic life skills groups.

PROBLEM SOLVING AND GOAL SETTING

These are skills needed to address the larger issues that come with recovery. The recovering abuser needs to learn to approach problems in a thoughtful, structured way. Often individuals who abuse have very low self-confidence and do not believe they will be successful. They avoid problems for fear of failing to overcome them (Robak, 1991). By learning to formulate attainable goals and to approach problems proactively, people gain psychological strength while learning practical approaches. Problem solving and goal setting can be offered as separate groups dealing with these concepts, or they can be structured into all functional groups as part of the goals of the group (Raymond, 1990).

DUAL DIAGNOSIS

Special consideration may need to be given to clients who have a dual diagnosis of substance abuse and another psychiatric disorder or mental retardation. Raymond (1990) reported that in her work with inpatient clients with psychiatric disorders and substance abuse she preferred to colead her occupational therapy groups with another staff member who was familiar with the clients' psychiatric symptoms. She also found that these clients needed more specific skill training and practice than her clients whose sole problem was substance abuse. The psychiatric clients had a more difficult time conceptualizing their life outside the hospital and would want to focus on current problems and events on the inpatient unit.

Substance Abuse and Physical Disability

In the psychiatric literature, it is difficult to find a discussion of the problems of people with physical disabilities and drug addictions. This is a significant omission because drug use is a likely cause of traumatic brain and spinal injuries, but the treatment of drug abuse is usually neglected in physical rehabilitation centers. Also, drug treatment programs often do not consider the physical accessibility to their activities (Gorman, 1993). Professionals in physical rehabilitation medicine often avoid confronting the substance abuse of their clients, yet it is likely that those who abused substances before their injuries will abuse them after rehabilitation (Heinemann, 1993). Gorman, a paraplegic who was injured when driving under the influence says:

The loss of both my legs was not even enough to make me give up my drugs and alcohol. My friends smuggled booze to me in the intensive care unit at the hospital. I watched the clock waiting for my morphine shot every three hours. I didn't have much pain, but I liked the morphine high. Pain was an excuse to get high and I used it. A doctor at the rehabilitation hospital asked if I liked beer. I told him, 'No, but I like hard liquor every once in a while.' So he wrote in my chart that I could drink while in rehabilitation. (I remember how he wrote it. . . 'Let Ken have his spirits.') (Gorman, 1993, pp. 12–13).

▼ EATING DISORDERS

Anorexia nervosa and **bulimia nervosa** are eating disorders found primarily in women of modern industrialized societies (Luder & Schebendach, 1993). The onset for both disorders is in adolescence and early adulthood (APA, 1994)

Anorexia Nervosa

Anorexia nervosa is self-induced starvation, often a chronic condition with medical and psychological components. It affects 1% of women between the ages of 12 and 40.

American Psychiatric Association Diagnostic Criteria for Anorexia Nervosa

1. Because of purposeful restriction of food intake the person weighs less than 85% of what is considered normal for height and age.
2. Obsessive concern with weight and fear of becoming fat. Self-esteem is tied to thinness, and weight loss is considered an achievement.
3. Distortion of body image and denial that there is a problem.
4. Amenorrhea for at least three menstrual cycles in postmenarcheal women. (APA, 1994)

Although anorexics may hide their shape under baggy clothes, they are severely emaciated. They often have yellowish dry skin and fine downy hair (lanugo) over their bodies (Luder & Schebendach, 1993). Bruch describes her 20-year-old client, Alma:

When she came for consultation she looked like a walking skeleton, scantily dressed in shorts and a halter, with her legs sticking out like broomsticks, every rib showing, and her shoulder blades standing up like little wings. . . Alma's arms and legs were covered with soft hair, her complexion had a yellowish tint, and her dry hair hung down in strings. Most striking was the face—hollow like that of a shriveled-up old woman with a wasting disease, sunken eyes, a sharply pointed nose on which the juncture between bone and cartilage was visible. When she spoke or smiled—and she was quite cheerful—one could see every movement of the muscles around her mouth and eyes, like an animated anatomical representation of the skull. Alma insisted that she looked fine and that there was nothing wrong with her being so skinny. 'I enjoy having this disease and I want it. I cannot convince myself that I am sick and that there is anything from which I have to recover' (Bruch, 1979, pp. 2–3).

Anorexia nervosa is a paradox. People with this disease starve themselves, even though they are skeletal. They become obsessed with their weight and claim not to be hungry, although those who recover say that they thought about food all the time while anorexic. In their effort to control food intake, people with eating disorders develop rituals around eating, cutting food into tiny pieces or eating very slowly (Luder and Schebendach, 1993).

There are two types of anorexics, those who achieve their excessive thinness through severe restriction of eating and excessive exercise. And those who binge and purge or starve and purge to achieve weight loss. About 50% of anorexics induce vomiting and use laxatives (Brotman, 1994).

People with anorexia often resist treatment and deny that they have a problem even as they suffer medical consequences. Menstruation ceases, and in 25% of cases does not resume when normal eating is reinstituted. This results in sterility and osteoporosis. People with anorexia may develop cardiac arrhythmias, and the death rate is as high as 20% (Brotman, 1994).

Along with the physical problems of anorexia nervosa are the cognitive and emotional problems associated with starvation. Thinking becomes distorted and may exacerbate the anorexic's irrational fears of getting fat. Luder and Schebendach (1993) describe this distorted thinking: "Personal encounters with patients who would not converse over the phone, fearing caloric transmission if the other party was eating while conversing; would not watch television commercials, fearing transmission of calories through the television screen; and would not eat off of glass dinnerware, convinced that it retained calories from previously eaten foods, all illustrate just how bizarre these fears can be" (p. 55).

After recovery, one woman noted: "Instead of feeding my brain, I was starving it. This is where the distorted thinking took over. When I saw I was twenty pounds underweight, I was so frightened, I became thirty pounds underweight. The thought of gaining twenty pounds was overwhelming. I felt locked in with no options, and unable to change" (Meyers, 1989, p. 36).

One woman described her state of mind: "I had begun to feel that there was some sort of glass partition between me and the rest of the world" (MacLeod, 1981, p. 106). In fact people with both anorexia and bulimia become isolated from the rest of the world (APA, 1993). Their eating disorders can take over their lives leaving little time for fun and social activities.

Bulimia Nervosa

Bulimia nervosa consists of binge eating followed by self-induced vomiting—or use of laxatives, excessive exercising, or fasting to compensate for the binge. Unlike those with anorexia nervosa, those with bulimia have normal weight and regular menstruation.

American Psychiatric Association Diagnostic Criteria for Bulimia Nervosa

1. Binging is characterized by a lack of control over eating that lasts for a discrete time period. During that period bulemics eat more than most people would eat, and they can neither stop eating nor control what they eat.
2. To compensate for overeating, bulemics engage in excessive exercise, vomiting, and overuse of laxatives, enemas, or diuretics to prevent weight gain.
3. This binge and purge behavior occurs at least twice a week for 3 months.
4. The person with bulimia nervosa's self-esteem is unreasonably tied up in weight and body shape.
   (APA, 1994)

The prevalence of bulimia among females is 1% to 3% (APA, 1994). One cannot identify bulimia by appearance, for weight is usually normal. But as with anorexia, people with bulimia are preoccupied with their weight and exercise excessively. They can become socially isolated because they are secretive in their episodes of overeating and vomiting. Medical complications of bulimia are a result of the vomiting and laxative abuse. These include fluid and electrolyte imbalance, sore throat, abdominal pain, and esophageal or gastric rupture caused by frequent vomiting. People who engage in vomiting also have dental enamel erosion and may exhibit "Russell's sign," skin changes on the dorsum of the hand from rubbing against the teeth when inducing vomiting. Laxative abuse causes dehydration and electrolyte depletion; and there may be irregular menstruation (Luder & Schebendach, 1993).

Forty percent of people with severe bulimia have a history of anorexia (Eating Disorders—Part I, 1992). Bruch describes Celia who, when hospitalized for anorexia began to binge and purge. Celia said that the hospitalization took away her anorexic behavior, which was her only source of feeling strong and independent.

She began to have eating binges, eating out of a sense of panic, or out of emptiness; she denied that they ever occurred out of feelings of hunger, 'I don't eat when I feel an inner strength derived from being independent, but when this independence is destroyed, my defenses against eating also are.' Sometimes she would throw up after such eating binges, usually she refused meals for several days.

Though she never had been heavy, she was preoccupied with the fear of getting fat and fear of being rejected. Paradoxically, she also felt that food gave her a sense of security. 'I feel always more secure when I have eaten a lot, when I have a full stomach. It is just as I would be gratified from getting attention, socializing successfully. Quantity is an important element; the more I can get into my stomach the safer I feel.'. . .

But when she ate she felt exceedingly guilty, full of self-contempt and disrespect for herself which contributed to her sense of worthlessness, 'because food has become my only source of satisfaction; because I can't control my eating or my feelings...' When she could control her eating and would lose weight, she felt strong and cheerful. When she gave in to the urge for food she became depressed and suicidal (Bruch, 1973, pp. 268–269).

Causal Factors, Onset, and Course

People with eating disorders can sometimes pinpoint the event that triggered their problem. For some, it may have been incidental weight loss that elicited praise and compliments. Some feel pressure from those around them to lose weight. They may have been brought up in families who are excessively weight conscious and gradually develop an eating disorder. Celia, like most people who develop anorexia nervosa, was not obese before beginning to diet. But, when her 130-lb boyfriend remarked that she weighed almost as much as he did, she started to diet (Bruch, 1973). What starts as "normal" dieting becomes an obsession in people with eating disorders.

BIOLOGICAL FACTORS

Eating disorders run in families, and there is some suggestion, from twin studies that heredity is partly implicated. There are abnormalities in hormone and neurotransmitter regulation in people with eating disorders, and they also have trouble interpreting internal sensations of hunger and fullness (APA, 1993). However, when examining biological factors, cause and effect are hard to determine. (Eating Disorders—Part I, 1992).

PSYCHOLOGICAL FACTORS

Psychological theories about causation include the idea that people with eating disorders use dieting and weight control measures to compensate for feelings of personal ineffectiveness and low self-esteem (APA, 1993). The personalities of anorexic females are depicted as "shy, serious, neat, quiet, conscientious, perfectionistic, hypersensitive to rejection, and inclined to irrational guilt and obsessive worrying" (Eating Disorders—Part I, 1992; p. 3). They have a desire for control and a need to feel special. The eating disorder is viewed as a means of gaining control when the individual feels that she lacks autonomy.

Some feel that anorexia is the response of young women to the pressures of sexuality and adult independence (Eating Disorders—Part I, 1992). Women with anorexia feel that they do not know their own desires and live to please others.

The obsessive control of eating is an area in which they express their independence (Eating Disorders—Part I, 1992).

People with bulimia are more outgoing than anorexics. They are also more emotional and impulsive. Some theorize that, as children, bulemics were fed to soothe them or to put them to sleep and were encouraged to eat when they were not hungry. Others propose that food takes the place of love (Eating Disorders—Part I, 1992).

FAMILY FACTORS

Some suggest that families of people with eating disorders are pathological (APA, 1993). The family member with the eating disorder is viewed as exhibiting a pathology that is really family dysfunction. However, it may be the stress of having a child with an eating disorder that creates family problems (Eating Disorders—Part I, 1992).

SOCIOCULTURAL FACTORS

The foods eaten, patterns of food consumption, and body image are influenced by culture. Ninety percent of anorexics are women (Brotman, 1994), and there is a great deal of social pressure on women to be slender.

The more intense the social pressure for slimness, the more likely it is that a troubled girl or young woman will develop an eating disorder rather than some other psychiatric symptom—especially if she also regards self-control in eating as a sign of the discipline needed for high achievement and social success. In our society richer and better-educated women tend to be thinner than average, and they may also be at higher risk for eating disorders. Anorexia and bulimia are especially common among women athletes and ballet dancers. One survey found that 15% of female medical students have had an eating disorder at some time; another study found bulimia to be five times more common in college women than in working women of the same age (Eating Disorders—Part II, 1993, p. 1).

OTHER FACTORS

Depression is associated with eating disorders and some conceive of eating disorders as a variant of depression. Serious depression is found in 40% to 80% of anorexic clients. And women who suffer from severe depression have double the rate of bulimia and eight times the rate of anorexia than the general population. It is not clear if depression is the effect of dieting, or if depressed people develop eating disorders (Eating Disorders—Part I, 1992).

Treatment

TREATMENT GOALS

For Anorexia

1. Restore weight to within 10% to 15% of ideal (Brotman, 1994).
2. Restore menstruation.

For Anorexia and Bulimia

1. Address physiological factors associated with eating disor-

der effects of starvation—emotional and cognitive—personality changes.
2. Restore normal eating patterns.
3. Address the psychological, social, and behavioral factors which may underlie the problem.
4. Treat associated mood disorders.
5. Challenge distorted cultural values. (APA, 1993; Brotman, 1994)

TREATMENT OF MALNUTRITION AND OTHER BIOLOGICAL PROBLEMS

Hospitalization is not required for uncomplicated bulimia (APA, 1993). However, hospitalization is required for anorexics if weight is less than 30% of minimal healthy weight or if medical complications, such as slow pulse, low blood pressure causing dizziness, loss of potassium, or cardiac arrhythmias, are present (Brotman, 1994). Although longer stays are more beneficial, insurance will currently not pay for more than a few days (Brotman, 1994). Because starvation brings about distorted thinking, it is difficult to address the psychological factors when the individual is not thinking well. The goal of hospitalization is weight gain and medical stabilization. Weight gain is not the cure, but it is necessary to clarify thinking, which is distorted by starvation, so that underlying factors can then be addressed.

MEDICATION

Medication is used if there are accompanying problems: antidepressants for depression or obsessive—-compulsion, and antianxiety medication for anxiety. Medication will help the anorexic with depression and anxiety, but does not address the eating disorder (Brotman, 1994). In bulimia, even when depressive symptoms are not evident, antidepressant medication may reduce binge eating and purging (APA, 1993).

TREATMENT OF PSYCHOLOGICAL, BEHAVIORAL, AND SOCIAL PROBLEMS

Anorexia is a complex, life-threatening illness and requires ongoing attention. Currently, the best, immediate results come from a combination of weight restoration, followed by individual and family psychotherapy (APA, 1993). The goal of psychotherapy is to address the psychological issues that are at the foundation of the eating disorder. Psychodynamic therapies are helpful in facilitating insight, and sometimes the subject of food and weight is avoided (Comparing Treatments for Bulimia, 1994). In this noncoercive approach, clients with anorexia do not feel that their need for control is being threatened (APA, 1993). Bulimia, also, "can be treated without direct attention to eating habits and weight, simply by relieving depression and improving the patient's social life" (Comparing Treatments for Bulimia, 1994).

Often, the onset of anorexia occurs in girls young enough to be living with their family of origin, and family therapy is included in the treatment regimen. Whether families have a major role in the cause of the eating disorder, or are suffering the effects, the family is involved. Family therapists view the family as a system in which the roles, rituals, and rules are addressed (Eating Disorders—Part I, 1992).

Cognitive behavioral treatment is effective for both anorexia and bulimia (Brotman, 1994; Comparing Treatments for Bulimia, 1994). This treatment addresses the client's attitudes and is especially effective in bulimia to change eating habits and body image, reduce perfectionism, and enhance self-esteem. In one study cognitive therapy was most effective at changing attitudes of bulemics toward food and weight and 36% effective in addressing binging and purging (Comparing Treatments for Bulimia, 1994). Other facets of treatment may include nutritional counseling (Brotman, 1994) and expressive therapies for people who have trouble with verbal communication (APA, 1993). Group interpersonal therapy has been found to be 44% effective for binging and purging symptoms of bulimia (Comparing Treatments for Bulimia, 1994).

OUTCOME

Most people with bulimia respond to individual and group therapy (Eating Disorders—Part II, 1993). Anorexia tends to be a chronic problem, requiring years of treatment. "The anxiety and frustration of caregivers and family members is extraordinary. It is painful to watch helplessly as a young woman starves herself to death" (Brotman, 1994, p. 8).

Occupational Therapy Treatment Considerations: Anorexia and Bulimia

People with eating disorders are usually able to function in work or school (Shimp, 1989) unless they are suffering from starvation effects. At first glance these women appear to be very competent and functional because they are often perfectionistic, high achievers. However, there are psychosocial areas that can be addressed by occupational therapy practitioners.

Occupational Therapy Assessments for People With Eating Disorders

Occupational history
Activity configuration
Self-image
    Self-portrait
    String test, estimation of body size
Interest inventory
Locus of control
Physical assessment
    Muscle strength
    Balance
    Endurance

(Bridgett, 1993)

One of the first goals of treatment articulated by Bridgett (1993) is to gain physical, cognitive, and social awareness. A step toward identifying internal cues of hunger and satiation and gaining a more realistic body image can include activities that involve multisensory stimulation of visual, tactile, and proprioceptive receptors. This may include the appropriate use of exercise (Bridgett, 1993).

People with eating disorders are not only out-of-touch with their bodies, they are also out-of-touch with their own psychological and social needs and desires. Particularly those with anorexia, may not be in touch with what they want for themselves because they are so eager to please others. Bruch (1979) tells the story of a girl who was always trying to second-guess what her parents wanted of her, so she could satisfy them. This included trying to find out what they had gotten her for Christmas, so she could express an interest in it. Assertiveness training may be a good addition to the treatment regimen for these women and girls to help them identify their own needs and ways to fulfill them.

Because many anorexic clients have trouble talking about their problems (APA, 1993) expressive activities, such as art, dance, expressive crafts, and music, may help with self-expression. The occupational therapy practitioner must recognize the multiple benefits of expressive activities. They provide multisensory input and can address self-assertion. They promote self-awareness through emotional expression and sensory stimulation (Bailey, 1986). The practitioner can implement expressive activities in ways that address all of these elements.

Time management, to include leisure activities and social contact in life routines, is another occupational therapy goal (Bridgett, 1993). People with eating disorders often become so preoccupied by exercise, food rituals, and work or school performance that they do not include leisure in their lives. If they do engage in recreation it takes on a pressured feeling from which they derive little enjoyment. Bridgett (1993) described the activity configuration of one of her clients with anorexia. This 17-year-old woman's typical day consisted of 8 hours of school or school work, 6 hours on the job, 6 hours of sleep, and 2 hours of exercise. She neglected meals, spent little time with her family, and increasingly avoided involvement with peers.

Psychoeducational groups to develop stress management skills are helpful. The goals of such groups are to seek ways to broaden leisure and social activities by examining current activities and interests, exploring community resources, and developing a plan of action to broaden and balance life activities (Bridgett, 1993).

There remains the question of food, nutrition, cooking, and eating. Should this be an occupational therapy activity? Shimp (1989) reports on an occupational therapy program in a short-term treatment program for eating disorders which consisted of a "family-style meal group." In these groups clients planned, shopped for, prepared, and ate a meal. The purpose of these groups was to channel the need for control of eating into healthy functional control, rather than the unhealthy behaviors associated with eating disorders. Each individual formulated personal goals for the meal: "'To eat without panicking,' 'not to worry about amounts so much,' 'to eat without anger,' and 'to be cooperative in preparing the meal instead of just doing things my own way'"(Shimp, 1989, p. 2).

Shimp reports "Eating the meal is hard, but the patients learn to take their own adequate portions and complete their meals in 30 min. without negative statements (although initially seldom without tears). In this high-stress area, the patients also find it difficult to get the 'right' amount of food without measuring portions, to eat with others (especially for those who are new to the unit), and to deal with the temptation to binge with the extra food on the table while they are waiting for the others to finish. Some patients even have trouble sitting down with others and then not getting up to clean the kitchen without eating as they have done in the past (especially those with families)" (Shimp, 1989, pp. 2–3).

Occupational therapy practitioners who engage in cooking and nutrition groups should heed the following caution from a nutritionist and her colleague who work with eating disorders: "Nutrition plays an important role in eating disorders, for it is as much a part of the symptom as the cure. The patient's obsession about nutrition issues often makes the nutritionist a popular member of the treatment team. However, care must be taken to avoid a proselytizing attitude about 'good' versus 'bad' nutrition. Indeed, the concept of nutrition as a process that transcends a specific food, food group, or daily intake must be clearly conveyed and continually reinforced" (Luder & Schebendach, 1993, p. 61). It is also important to remember that studies have found that people with eating disorders can be treated without direct attention to eating habits (Comparing Treatments for Bulimia, 1994; APA, 1993).

▼ BORDERLINE PERSONALITY DISORDER

Borderline personality disorder is classified on Axis II of DSM-IV. It is one of many personality disorders; these disorders are among the most ambiguous in the spectrum of mental illness. Personality traits are the characteristic way in which people think, feel, and act. They are enduring qualities that persist over time and people who have personality disorders suffer from long-standing, maladaptive personality traits. Borderline personality was not classified by the APA until 1980 and is not considered a highly reliable diagnosis. The term borderline refers to the characteristics that border on psychosis and neurosis. Sometimes it is difficult to distinguish personality disorders from depression, anxiety disorders, schizophrenia, or adjustment disorders (Borderline Personality—Part I, 1994).

Characteristics of Borderline Personality

People with borderline personality disorders share one or more of the following characteristics:

1. Instability of thought, mood, and behavior
2. Unstable interpersonal relationships
3. Problems with self-image
   (APA, 1994)

INSTABILITY OF THOUGHT, MOOD, AND BEHAVIOR

People diagnosed with borderline personality tend to be impulsive. They are quick to anger and likely to abuse drugs and alcohol. There is a 60% rate of major depression in people with borderline personality. Their depression is qualitatively different from others who suffer from chronic depression. In borderline personality disorder there is less guilt, lethargy, and appetite loss than in mood disorders. Instead, people with borderline personality disorder complain of loneliness, boredom, and a feeling of emptiness (Borderline Personality—Part I, 1994). Self-mutilation and suicide attempts are serious problems in people with borderline personality. Some people engage in cutting themselves claiming that it "makes me feel real." Others have chronic suicidal tendencies that are sometimes viewed, by their therapists, as bids for attention. However, suicidal gestures cannot be dismissed because people with borderline personality are impulsive and have the same rate of suicide as people with schizophrenia and bipolar disorder (Borderline Personality —Part III, 1994).

UNSTABLE INTERPERSONAL RELATIONSHIPS

People with borderline personality disorder can be a challenge for those who work and live with them. Their instability of thought and mood causes them to be unpredictable in their behavior. They appear to overreact to events that others find unremarkable. They invest a great deal of importance and intensity in relationships, but inexplicably reject the individual they once idolized. It is thought that this occurs because the people with borderline personality have such an intense need for others that it is impossible for others to live up to their expectations. This causes the person with borderline personality to feel betrayed and angry when their unreasonable demands of others are not met. For example, Mary, a 30-year-old woman with borderline personality disorder felt rejected and angry when her friend canceled a lunch date because of a death in the family. A psychotherapist reported that in therapy with his client, "Miss N," she "let me know that she wanted me to say only perfect and precise things that would immediately and clearly reflect how she was feeling and would reassure her that I was really with her. Otherwise I should say nothing but listen patiently to her attacks on me" (Kernberg, 1984, p. 129).

Another factor in the relationships of people with borderline personality is their use of splitting. Splitting is a primitive defense mechanism in which individuals view themselves and others as all good or all bad (Carson & Butcher, 1992). Cognitive therapists call splitting dichotomous thinking which is thinking that places everything in discrete categories, black or white, rather than on a continuum of reality (Beck & Freeman, 1990). This kind of all-or-nothing thinking may explain why the person with borderline personality seems to quite suddenly turn against a friend or a therapist. It may be that their perfect image of the friend was marred, in some way, and instead of being able to acknowledge that no one is perfect, the friend is now conceptualized as completely bad.

In therapeutic situations the consequences of dichotomous thinking are that the client might classify staff as either good or bad and, if care is not taken, staff and other clients may be drawn into this splitting. This produces division among staff and among staff and clients and damages the therapeutic environment. It is important to recognize this phenomenon and maintain good communication.

PROBLEMS WITH SELF-IMAGE

People with borderline personality disorder have not achieved an integrated sense of self, or they have a sense of "impaired self" (Miller, 1994). They may express their feelings of inadequacy:

It has always been there, for as long as I can remember, even back in school, even in middle school. . . it is like a rating scale. . . I don't give people numbers. I just rate them against me and I never met anyone that I was equal to or better than, no matter what. . . Even if it is a bum on the street, there is something that makes him better than me (Miller, 1994, p. 1217).

Feeling inadequate leads to estrangement and despair. One person with borderline personality disorder said she feels ". . . separated in a way, not quite in there with the rest." "I think it is because I already feel I'm different, so I feel I should separate myself from everyone else in some way" (Miller, 1994, p. 1217). A study in which people with borderline personality disorder were interviewed found that "Each person revealed an ever-present wish not to be alive" (Miller, 1994, p. 1217).

People with borderline personality disorder are not always in turmoil (Beck & Freeman, 1990). They go through periods of holding jobs and maintaining relationships. In social situations they do best in settings, such as work, where the structure permits them to maintain control. Mental health workers see borderline clients when they are feeling out of control and decompensated, but for some, there are periods of high functioning.

Cause

The cause is unknown, but many people with borderline personality disorder have a history of persistent abuse in childhood. Other theories about cause include a biological deficit in the regulation of affect or mood, and inconsistent parenting. It is primarily a diagnosis of women, who make up 70% to 77% of all those diagnosed (Linehan, Tutek, Heard, & Armstrong, 1994), and is found in 2% of the general population (APA, 1994).

BIOLOGICAL THEORIES

There is a hereditary component to personality, and some have proposed that borderline personality disorder may be caused by an inherited brain malfunction, for there is a higher rate of borderline personality in certain families. Limited research has found brain damage or injury to the limbic system or frontal lobes in some clients with borderline disorders. These areas of the brain modulate impulses and emotions (Borderline Personality—Part I, 1994).

PSYCHODYNAMIC THEORIES

The psychoanalyst Otto Kernberg attributes borderline personality disorder to the use of immature defense mechanisms: "splitting, poor reality testing, a weak ego, and inadequate integration of identity—inability to make sense of the contradictory aspects of oneself and others" (Borderline Personality—Part I, 1994, p. 3). These attributes are caused by the unstable early childhood interactions with the caretaker, which have been characterized as unpredictable, alternately smothering and rejecting. Psychodynamic theories consider the first 2 years of life significant in the development of borderline. It is thought that during these years those parenting practices that foster aggression and frustration interfere with the child's development of a stable ego identity. Later in life, the person with borderline personality disorder may reenact this childhood relationship, resulting in reinforcement of maladaptive interactions (Borderline Personality—Part II, 1994).

ASSOCIATED FACTORS

There is a high rate of substance abuse among those diagnosed as having borderline personality disorder, and other forms of self-destructive behaviors are common. About 25% of people with borderline personality disorder also have a diagnosis of posttraumatic stress disorder that is the result of persistent abuse as a child (Herman, 1992).

Post-traumatic stress disorder is a condition of anxiety, flashbacks, and problems with interpersonal relationships resulting from a highly traumatic experience in which one's life or well-being has been threatened. It can also occur in an individual who witnessed the traumatic experiences of another. The symptoms usually have their onset after the trauma and can cause severe debilitation of social and occupational function (APA, 1994).

Treatment of Borderline Personality

Treatment of borderline personality disorder follows the frame of reference of the practitioner and the setting. Sometimes people with borderline personality require hospitalization when there is danger of suicide or severe regression. It is advised that hospitalization be kept brief and that the individual understand that the purpose of the protective environment is not to foster the sick role, but to help the person regain control of his or her life.

PSYCHOTHERAPY

A variety of psychotherapies, from psychoanalytic to supportive psychotherapy, have been used for borderline personality disorder. Evaluations of treatment approaches are inconclusive because there has been little systematic research done. It is thought that it is difficult to change personality which is, by definition, ingrained, enduring patterns of thought and behavior (Borderline Personality—Part II, 1994).

DIALECTICAL BEHAVIOR THERAPY

Dialectical behavior therapy is a cognitive behavioral technique that has been helpful in treating important symptoms of borderline personality disorder. It combines individual and group therapy using methods to help the borderline client control impulses and soothe herself or himself. The theory behind this treatment is that people with borderline personality disorder have problems with regulation of impulses and emotions. They lack skills in stress tolerance and self-regulation, which interfere with interpersonal relationships. It is believed that this maladaptive behavior is caused by a combination of personal factors and an environment that fosters and reinforces these characteristics (Linehan et al, 1994).

Dialectical behavior therapy methods include "psychoeducation, problem solving, social skills training, modeling, homework assignments and behavioral rehearsal" (Borderline Personality—Part III, 1994, p. 1). These methods address problems with impulsive responding and the inability to modulate feelings, anger, and self-destructive behavior.

The goals of dialectical behavior therapy are to

1. Reduce suicidal and other life-threatening or self-mutilative behavior
2. Lessen noncompliant behaviors that interfere with treatment
3. Change behavior patterns that lead to inpatient psychiatric care and interfere with quality of life
4. Enhance coping skills (Linehan et al, 1994)

MEDICATION

In the past, drug therapy was avoided, but now medication is used for the symptoms the individual exhibits. Thus medication can include that for anxiety, depression, mania, and psychotic symptoms. Antipsychotic medication appears to be effective for many of these symptoms when found in borderline personality disorder (Borderline Personality—Part III, 1994).

Implications for Occupational Therapy

Because people with borderline personality disorder may be depressed and suicidal and they may also abuse substances, occupational therapy practitioners should consider the implications of those problems when working with these people.

It is important for all who work with people with borderline personality disorder to be consistent and trustworthy. This can be a challenge because the person with borderline personality has such difficulty trusting others and seems to sabotage relationships (Beck & Freeman, 1990). On one hand, people with this disorder have great dependency needs. They feel empty and inadequate and wish that others could help them. On the other hand, they are terrified of intimacy for fear of rejection and abandonment.

Kernberg, a psychoanalytically oriented psychiatrist, suggests that the treatment setting provide a homelike environment in which work and leisure routines can be maintained. Task groups are important as a means to gain leadership and collaborative skills and to test ego function; they are not a time to explore feelings and intrapsychic conflict (Kernberg, 1984). In inpatient settings or day treatment "bridges between hospital life and the external social environment" (Kernberg, 1984; p. 344) are created while individual and group therapy is carried out. Kernberg stresses the importance of the personal, as well as professional attributes of staff, because staff use their interpersonal interactions with the clients to work through borderline issues. It is important that the analysis of client–staff interaction stick to here-and-now events. Staff are cautioned to "consistently preserve socially appropriate behavior toward clients and clearly delimit their personal boundaries from their professional functions. To be spontaneous and open in their interactions with clients does not mean that members of staff should talk about their personal lives"(Kernberg, 1984, p. 345). Communication among staff is critical to support the therapeutic community and to prevent splitting (Kernberg, 1984).

Because people with borderline personality disorder who are in crisis are so difficult, there is the danger that staff will despair of satisfactory recovery. One woman with the disorder articulated the effect this had on her:

I know that things are getting better about borderlines and stuff. Having that diagnosis resulted in my getting treated exactly the way I was treated at home. The minute I got that diagnosis people stopped treating me as though what I was doing had a reason. All that psychiatric treatment was just as destructive as what happened before . . . Denying the reality of my experience—that was the most harmful. Not being able to trust anyone was the most serious effect . . . I know I acted in ways that were despicable. But I wasn't crazy. Some people go around acting like that because they feel hopeless. Finally I found a few people along the way who have been able to feel OK about me even though I had severe problems. Good therapists were those who really validated my experience (Herman, 1992, p. 56).

Outcome

Borderline personality disorder appears to be a chronic problem that may require long-term, intermittent therapy during periods of crisis. Therapy is supportive to help the individual regain some equilibrium and to intervene in self-destructive behavior. The Harvard Mental Health Letter (Borderline Personality—Part III, 1994) sums up the outcome of the disorder:

If they live through their 20's without disaster, persons diagnosed as borderline often reach a kind of equilibrium. Their extremes of mood and impulsive behavior are moderated and suicide attempts almost cease. Several studies of long-term outcome in formerly hospitalized borderline clients have come to the same conclusion: Little change over a 5-year period, but much improvement after 15 years and more . . . Most had freed themselves of their worst addictions, married, become parents, and kept jobs. They were doing about as well as patients committed to the same hospital at the same time for depression. . . . In middle age most patients in the outcome studies no longer qualify for a diagnosis of borderline personality (p. 3).

In the outcome studies, those people who fared best were those who were more intelligent, who found satisfaction in work, and who had special talents (Borderline Personality—Part III, 1994).

▼ SCHIZOPHRENIA

Schizophrenia is probably a group of related psychotic disorders, rather than a single entity. The disturbed thought processes and psychotic symptoms associated with schizophrenia lead to difficulties with communication, interpersonal relationships, and reality testing.

Schizophrenia is found in 1% of the population and is equally common in males and females. The age of onset is typically early adulthood, but schizophrenia may appear in adolescence. For the diagnosis to be made, the symptoms must be severe enough to impair social or occupational function and must be present for at least 6 months (APA, 1994).

Characteristic Symptoms

Characteristic symptoms of schizophrenia include disturbances of (1) thought content, (2) process (form) of thought, (3) perception, (4) affect, (5) volition, and (6) sense of self. There may also be social withdrawal and disturbed psychomotor behavior. No single feature is always present, but there are likely to be delusions, hallucinations, and disorganized speech and behavior (APA, 1994).

POSITIVE AND NEGATIVE SYMPTOMS OF SCHIZOPHRENIA

Positive symptoms are those that are conspicuously disturbing to others. Symptoms are active, florid, characterized by excessive or peculiar activity. The individual experiences bizarre delusions and insulting or commanding auditory hallucinations. They may go into sudden, unexplained rages, and their speech and thinking are incoherent.

Negative symptoms are less conspicuous than positive symptoms. The individual is passive, speaks with a toneless voice, and exhibits little facial expression (flat affect). They avoid eye contact and rarely smile or return greetings. They do not initiate activity and make few spontaneous movements. Speech is empty and thoughts obscure. They have trouble concentrating and seem to take little pleasure in anything. Negative symptoms can be confused with depression and look like the side effects of antipsychotic medication.

Often, negative symptoms are the prevailing condition, with positive symptoms periodically emerging. People with positive symptoms are more likely to be hospitalized (APA, 1994)

DISTURBANCE OF CONTENT OF THOUGHT

Delusions are false ideas that may be fragmented and bizarre, or organized and systematic. Common schizophrenic delusions are *thought broadcasting* during which individuals believe that they are able to send out their thoughts to others. Sometimes they believe someone is putting thoughts into their heads; this *thought insertion* can consist of very unpleasant and disturbing delusions. *Thought withdrawal* is when it seems that thoughts have been removed. This may be an expression of the impoverished thought associated with schizophrenia. Sometimes there are delusions of being controlled, during which persons are being given instructions that they feel impelled to follow.

DISTURBANCE IN FORM OF THOUGHT

Schizophrenia has been referred to as a formal thought disorder. This refers to the impairment of thinking in which the individual does not exhibit an organized, coherent pattern of thought. This is known as loose associations and is observed through the person's speech patterns or writing. People with schizophrenia may have vague, overly abstract, or overly concrete speech. Some speak in repetitive stereotyped phrases.

North describes her thought processes during a psychotic episode. We can see how her incoherent associations are related to her delusional thinking, when she describes the result of her attempt to keep her thoughts from being broadcast to others.

Most of all, I wanted to keep my mother from hearing my thoughts. Whenever it seemed she was tuning in on my thought waves, I purposely substituted nonsense words for my true thoughts, or intentionally scrambled the words as they came to me. But in the process, my thoughts sometimes got so hopelessly jumbled that I needed to write them down to straighten them out for my own comprehension. To keep anyone from being able to read the thoughts I was writing, I invented a private code of original characters symbolizing letters, words, phrases, and tenses all mixed up in such a way that no one could possibly read it. On paper it looked like endless columns of nonsensical symbols (North, 1989, p. 37).

PERCEPTUAL DISTURBANCES

People with schizophrenia experience all kinds of hallucinations, but the most common type are auditory, in the form of voices or sounds. Tactile hallucinations can take the form of burning, tingling, "electrical" sensations. Some feel their body mysteriously change and may actually envision the changes. Others may have exceptional sensitivity to sound, sight, or smell.

North describes her visual hallucinations:

My thoughts weren't the only thing giving me trouble. My perceptions had changed. I had become vaguely aware of colored patterns decorating the air. When I first noticed them, I realized I had actually been seeing them for a long time, yet never paid attention to them before. I thought that everyone saw them, that they were a visual equivalent of background noise, like a fan's hum that goes unnoticed. These patterns, composed of tiny spicules and multicolored squiggly lines, wiggled and wormed their way around and through each other like people milling in a crowd. The patterns looked like what I imagined the visual equivalent of radio static to be, so I called them Interference Patterns (North, 1989, p. 37).

North's term "Interference Pattern" is wonderfully descriptive and apt. Hallucinations, of every kind, interfere with schizophrenic clients' perceptions of the world. Whether they hear voices, or see, or feel these sensory misperceptions they are distracted and impaired by these phenomena. It is difficult to think straight, to organize and carry-out purposeful action, and to relate to people in the face of these distractions.

DISTURBANCES OF AFFECT

Affect refers to the emotional tone of individuals demonstrated by their facial expressions and voice inflections. When the affect lacks intensity, it is called blunt. If there is no emotional expression, the person is said to have a flat affect. Sometimes people with schizophrenia have an inappropriate affect during which they, for example, laugh or smile when talking about sad events; or they look terrified when there is nothing obviously frightening.

All of the symptoms of schizophrenia are interrelated. Hallucinations pull people with schizophrenia away from reality, and their affect reflects their perceptions, rather than those of the observer. When clients are preoccupied with their inner reality, their cognitive and motor responses to the external environment slow or are bizarrely irrelevant. To the observer, the clients' thought processes, their affect, and behavior seem inappropriate. North describes:

Dr. Hemingway had no idea of the high activity level of the voices as we talked, and he didn't know that the voices were heavily influencing me. To him I looked flat, vacant, catatonic. I moved slowly, and left giant gaps between my words. I talked very little as far as he could tell, but *I* felt I was talking a lot. After all, I was carrying

on simultaneous conversations with him and the voices (North, 1989, p. 187).

DISTURBED SENSE OF SELF

It seems reasonable that if one is hallucinating and delusional one might be perplexed about one's identity. One woman said that her schizophrenic son kept asking her if he was Jesus. He'd say: "I'm not Jesus. I'm not Jesus, am I Mom?" The person might know that the delusion does not make sense, but cannot get rid of it. Some have no doubts about their delusional thinking and hallucinations.

A disturbed sense of self can also become evident when the individual becomes obsessed by the meaning of life or feels controlled by outsiders. There may be a loss of ego boundaries where the client does not have a sense of self. Mark Vonnegut describes how his delusional thinking led him to question how he could negotiate his way with his new view of the world:

When I looked at someone they were everything. They were beautiful, breathtakingly so. They were all things to me. The waitress was Eve, Helen of Troy, all women of all times, the eternal female principle, heroic, beautiful, my mother, my sisters, every woman I had ever loved. Everything good I had ever loved. Simon was Adam, Jesus, Bob Dylan, my father, every man I had ever loved . . . They were whatever I needed and more. I loved them utterly. . . .

I worried about how complicated this could make my life. Maybe it was enlightenment but it brought up not inconsequential problems of engineering. Who sleeps with whom was one, but there were lots of others. Like what if two people I loved wanted me to do different things? Who would I spend time with, who would I talk with, who would I dedicate my life to? If I loved everyone there was no way to focus any more, no reason to spend time with anyone in particular (Vonnegut, 1975, p. 117).

DECREASED VOLITION

People with schizophrenia have trouble initiating action and engaging in goal-directed activity. Their interest in the world is muted, and they often lack the drive to follow up a course of action to its conclusion. This makes it difficult to live independently, because they have trouble with the most mundane tasks. To the outsider this appears as "laziness," but as Vonnegut said he sometimes "had trouble walking and remembering to breathe" (Vonnegut, 1975, p. 112). Here is how Maxine, a woman who suffered from schizophrenia all her adult life is described:

Maxine had never been able to survive on her own, even in a room at the Y. She was careless and lazy. The neighbors came over one day after Maxine had put all the dirty dishes in the kitchen sink and turned the water on—'so the dishes would wash themselves'—and found water all over the floor (Sheehan, 1995, p. 205).

Maxine was not a stupid woman but her schizophrenia impaired her judgment. Vonnegut describes some of the psychotic perceptions and thoughts that interfere with completing a task.

Small tasks became incredibly intricate and complex. It started with pruning the fruit trees. One saw cut would take forever. I was completely absorbed in the sawdust floating gently to the ground, the feel of the saw in my hand, the incredible patterns in the bark, the muscles in my arm pulling back and then pushing forward. Everything stretched infinitely in all directions. Suddenly it seemed as if everything was slowing down and I would never finish sawing the limb. Then by some miracle that branch would be done and I'd have to rest, completely blown out ... Then I found myself being unable to stick with any one tree ... I began to wonder if I was hurting the trees and found myself apologizing. Each tree began to take on a personality. I began to wonder if any of them liked me. I became completely absorbed in looking at each tree ... (Vonnegut, 1975, p. 99).

WITHDRAWAL

Because people with schizophrenia are preoccupied with delusions and hallucinations they seem to have withdrawn from the world. If their delusions are paranoid, they do not trust others and avoid the dangers interaction would foster. For some the withdrawal seems emotional, they appear detached and unconcerned.

DISTURBANCE IN PSYCHOMOTOR BEHAVIOR

Disturbance in psychomotor behavior can take many forms. When Vonnegut describes pruning the trees, he probably appeared as slow moving and preoccupied as he felt. He worked slowly, resting between the cutting of each branch as he closely examined each tree. Some people with schizophrenia engage in bizarre posturing or excessive motor activity, pacing, rocking, and other excited actions that seem unrelated to environmental stimuli.

OTHER FEATURES

People with schizophrenia may be disheveled or eccentrically groomed. They are not socially adept, but rather, withdrawn and isolated; some are obnoxious. Depression, anxiety, and anger sometimes accompany the disorder.

Sylvia Frumpkin (Sheehan, 1983) was angry a lot of the time and people found her aggressive and difficult. Her attire was interesting:

Miss Frumpkin seemed unaware of the [hot and humid] weather that morning, she was wearing a blouse, a vest, a pair of blue jeans, and a quilted jacket. She had tied another pair of bluejeans around her neck. She also wore around her neck a chain with a pop top from a soda can on it. On her feet were a pair of socks and the high heeled gold sandals. On her head was a bandanna. Knotted into the bandanna was a spoon (Sheehan, 1983, p. 104).

Causal Factors Associated with Schizophrenia

What causes schizophrenia is unknown. There is a familial predisposition to schizophrenia, and adoption studies suggest a biological, rather than environmental connection in these cases. A disproportionate number of people with schizophrenia are born in the late winter or early spring, which fosters the theory that infectious diseases may have a prenatal effect (Schizophrenia: The Present State of Understanding—Part I & Part II, 1992).

Brain-imaging technology, which enables researchers to view the structure and activity of the living brain, has revealed that people with schizophrenia show pathology in a number of brain functions. However, there is no single pathology common to all. Some have enlarged ventricles. Some have an increased number or increased sensitivity of dopamine receptors (Schizophrenia: The Present State of Understanding—Part I & Part II, 1992). The latter theory is based on the fact that antipsychotic medications, used to treat the symptoms of schizophrenia, successfully reduce hallucinations and delusions, in a variety of diagnoses. These drugs alter the activity of dopamine, a neurotransmitter.

Outcome of Schizophrenia

30% Recover—remain symptom-free for 5 years
60% Respond to medication and other treatments and live in the community with outpatient treatment. They have varying degrees of social and occupational impairment and personality impoverishment. They may need brief hospitalization for psychotic behavior, often due to failure to comply with medication regimen.
10% Remain profoundly disabled

(Carson & Butcher, 1992)

Treatment and Implications for Occupational Therapy

The first-line treatment of schizophrenia is medication. The examples given here to illustrate the symptoms of schizophrenia are of people who were not being treated by medication, at the time. Antipsychotic medication intervenes in most of the psychotic symptoms, for many people. However medication, alone, is not enough to ensure a good quality of life for most individuals. Psychosocial management is equally important. The management and rehabilitation goals are:

1. Prevent relapse.
2. Reduce the symptoms such as thought disorder, delusions and hallucinations.
3. Remedy social and vocational disabilities.
4. Remove or compensate for environmental impediments to functioning. (Liberman, 1988)

Even with successful response to medication, the individual with schizophrenia is still left with little experience dealing with the world. The disease strikes so early in adulthood that the client may not have ever experienced normal adult life. An important role of occupational therapy is to assess the client in terms of adult, occupational roles. Instruction in everyday activity may be required to help clients organize their lives and alleviate stress. Relapse can be caused by stress, and the person with schizophrenia is less resilient than others.

STRESS MANAGEMENT

When thinking about schizophrenia and stress it helps to keep in mind Vonnegut's claim that he had trouble walking and remembering to breathe. The claims of everyday life are magnified by the impairments of schizophrenia. For the person with schizophrenia, stress may be having to smile at the customer while handing him his change at Burger King, or sorting laundry and remembering to put the soap in the washing machine.

The intelligence and verbal skills of some people with schizophrenia may mislead one to believe they can hold jobs and maintain multiple life roles. This is not true, for all. They may need to work in an environment that is quiet and not socially demanding. Occupational therapy practitioners work with the 60% of those who have only partial recovery and live marginal lives.

Stress management includes staying healthy, clean, and sober. Street drugs and alcohol can bring relapse. In Vonnegut's case, drugs triggered his psychosis. Occupational therapy practitioners teach people with schizophrenia to recognize early symptoms of relapse, how to respond, and how to get help.

Often the occupational therapy practitioner, more than any other mental health professional, is aware of the discrepancy between verbal proficiency and functional performance skills of people with mental illness. Even those people with schizophrenia who have good verbal skills cannot be assumed to be capable of organizing thought and action. Studies have shown that people with schizophrenia have trouble with tasks that require problem solving and novel thinking (Schizophrenia: The Present State of Understanding—Part I, 1992). The implications for occupational therapy are that people with schizophrenia must be carefully taught strategies for solving everyday "problems." They need to learn to anticipate predictable difficulties so that they will be prepared, for example, to phone the doctor, or arrange for transportation. Practice of skills and rehearsal of social behaviors are critical for learning. Liberman (1988) recommends periodic "booster sessions" of instruction to successfully maintain skills.

Studies have also shown that people with schizophrenia have trouble with the coordination and integration of multisensory information and have difficulty grouping objects and ideas by form and meaning or emotional relevance (Schizophrenia: The Present State of Understanding—Part I, 1992). Thus, when introducing new learning, occupational therapy practitioners must break down activities to manageable components and give concrete instruction. Even social skills need to be specifically taught and re-

hearsed. Some need explicit instruction on affiliative skills, holding a conversation, being a friend, or dating. Behavioral approaches to learning are effective with the practitioner acting as teacher, prompter, coach, and reinforcer (Liberman, 1988).

SENSORY INTEGRATION AND ACTIVITY

There are mixed reports about the effectiveness of sensory integration treatment for adults with schizophrenia. There appears to be a temporary effect on motivation and affect, but no permanent restoration of function (Hayes, 1989). Structured group activity programs, in any treatment setting, improve bizarre behaviors and obsessive ruminations (Hayes, 1989). In spite of the difficulty people with schizophrenia have with multisensory integration, one study of activity and verbal groups found more verbal interaction among people with schizophrenia engaged in a group construction task than in a verbal group (Odhner, in Hayes, 1989). In some activity groups the occupational therapist acts as a facilitator of social interaction and problem solving while the clients work cooperatively or in parallel (Hayes, 1989). Other groups are geared to learning specific skills, and in those groups the practitioner acts as teacher and coach.

FAMILY EDUCATION AND SUPPORT

People with chronic schizophrenia need supportive living environments and may live with their families. Family members benefit from learning management skills that help reduce the stress of living with a person with schizophrenia. They need education about the disease and its management; how to communicate, verbally and nonverbally with the client, and how to deal with problems (Liberman, 1988).

CREATING A FUNCTIONAL SENSE OF SELF

The psychiatrist, Larry Davidson, engaged in phenomenological research that examined interviews of 74 people with schizophrenia who had been hospitalized for severe psychotic symptoms. Davidson says: "We have come to understand that reconstructing a functional sense of self in the midst of persisting psychotic symptoms and dysfunction is an important aspect of the improvement process in schizophrenia" (Davidson, 1994, p. 113). Here is how one of the client's in his study talked about her improvement:

It is being active, and I take pride and I'm independent to a certain extent . . . like in my jazz music, like I'll turn on my jazz radio, and I'll love it . . . it's *my* interest. I turn the radio on myself, no one had it going to nourish *them*selves, to entertain *them*selves, like parents would at a house. *I* turn it on, *I'm* responsible, I enjoy the music, I make notes and draw while I'm hearing it . . . then I turn it off, then I have some evidence, I've got something done, I've been productive, I have the drawings to look at. Maybe they're damn fine drawings . . . It was for me and by me. My own nurturing. So I'm proud of this effort, but I do need that active state of mind to be steady, to be constant. (Davidson, 1994, p. 109).

Schizophrenia and Other Psychotic Disorders

Schizophrenia Subtypes

Paranoid type:
  Persecutory or grandiose delusions or hallucinations
  Speech and behavior is more organized than other types
  Affect and cognition relatively well preserved
Disorganized type:
  Flat or inappropriate (silly) affect: Marked disorganization of speech and behavior
Catatonic type:
  Disturbed psychomotor behavior either excessive activity or immobility
Undifferentiated type:
  Symptoms meet the general criteria described in the text
Residual type:
  No current hallucinations or delusions, but a history of at least one episode of schizophrenia and continuing evidence of negative symptoms

Other Psychotic Disorders

The following disorders share most of the characteristics of schizophrenia with differences in duration, cause, or concurrent symptoms. The treatment and management of the psychotic symptoms are similar, and occupational therapy considerations are often the same if functional impairment accompanies the disorder.

Schizophreniform disorder
Schizoaffective disorder
Delusional disorder
Psychotic disorder due to general medical condition

Brief psychotic disorder
Substance-induced psychotic disorder
Shared psychotic disorder (folie à deux)

(American Psychiatric Association, 1994)

►CONCLUSION: DOES DIAGNOSIS MATTER?

In this chapter, mental illness has been discussed according to diagnosis. The diagnosis helps us communicate by naming the condition. Diagnostic categories give us consistent terminology and criteria with which to discuss particular disorders and lend baseline information for research. The beginning of the **clinical reasoning** process may start with the diagnosis because it places the problem in a particular domain of practice. When practitioners know their clients' diagnoses they bring particular expectations about symptoms and prognosis to the treatment arena. One can expect to use specific assessments and precautions, based on diagnosis. Even when practitioners do not know the diagnosis, they make assumptions as they interact with each client and get clues that might point to a diagnosis.

The use of diagnosis can enhance communication and facilitate the treatment process, but it can also stereotype people. The assumptions we make about a diagnosis may not hold true for a particular individual. And, although we cannot work without the shared language that a diagnosis provides, it is ultimately the individual who is our concern. The individual transcends the diagnosis.

▼ REFERENCES

Alcoholism—Part II. (1986, May). *The Harvard Medical School Mental Health Letter, 5*, 1–4.

American Psychiatric Association (APA) (1993). Practice guidelines for eating disorders. *American Journal of Psychiatry, 150*(2), 212–223.

American Psychiatric Association (1994). *Diagnostic and statistical manual of mental disorders* (4th ed.). Washington, DC: Author.

Bailey, M. K. (1986). Occupational therapy for patients with eating disorders. *Occupational Therapy in Mental Health, 6*(1), 89–116.

Beck, A. T. & Freeman, A. (1990). *Cognitive therapy of personality disorders.* New York: Guilford Press.

Bennett, A. (1995, May, 22). Notes from offstage. *The New Yorker*, pp. 68–78.

Bipolar disorder: Outcome and treatment effects. (1994, Oct.). *The Harvard Mental Health Letter, 11*, p. 7.

Borderline personality disorder—Part I. (1994, May). *The Harvard Mental Health Letter, 10*, pp. 1–3.

Borderline personality disorder—Part II. (1994, June). *The Harvard Mental Health Letter, 10* pp. 1–4.

Borderline personality disorder—Part III. (1994, July). *The Harvard Mental Health Letter, 11* pp. 1–3.

Borell, L., Sandman, P. O., & Kielhofner, G. (1991). Clinical decision making in Alzheimer's disease. *Occupational Therapy in Mental Health, 11*(4), 111–124.

Bridgett, B. (1993). Occupational therapy evaluation for clients with eating disorders. *Occupational Therapy in Mental Health, 12*, 79–89.

Brotman, A. W. (1994, Jan.). What works in the treatment of anorexia nervosa. *Harvard Mental Health Letter, 10*, p. 8.

Bruch, H. (1973). *Eating disorders: Obesity, anorexia nervosa, and the person within.* New York: Basic Books.

Bruch, H. (1979). *The golden cage: The enigma of anorexia nervosa.* New York: Vintage Books.

Callahan, J. (1990). *Don't worry, he won't get far on foot.* New York: Vintage Books.

Carson, R. C. & Butcher, J. N. (1992). *Abnormal psychology and modern life* (9th ed.). New York: HarperCollins.

Comparing treatments for bulimia. (1994, May). *Harvard Mental Health Letter, 10,* p. 8.

Cronkite, K. (1994). *On the edge of darkness: Conversations about conquering depression.* New York: Doubleday.

Davidson, L. (1994). Phenomenological research in schizophrenia: From philosophical anthropology to empirical science. *Journal of Phenomenological Psychology, 25*(1), 104–130.

Duke, P. & Hochman, G. (1992). *A brilliant madness: Living with manic–depressive illness.* New York: Bantam Books.

Dysthymia and other mood disorders. (1991, May). *The Harvard Mental Health Letter, 7,* pp. 1–3.

Eating disorders—Part I. (1992, Dec.). *Harvard Mental Health Letter, 8,* pp. 1–4.

Eating disorders—Part II. (1993, Jan.). *Harvard Mental Health Letter, 9,* p. 1–4.

Fieve, R. R. (1975). *Moodswing.* New York: Bantam Books.

Ford, B. & Chase, C. (1987). *Betty: A glad awakening.* New York: Doubleday.

Goldstein, A. (1994). *Addiction: From biology to drug policy.* New York: W. H. Freeman & Co.

Gorman, K. K. (1993). Addicted and disabled: One man's journey from helplessness to hope. In A. W. Heinemann (Ed.), *Substance abuse and physical disability* (pp. 11–20). New York: Haworth Press.

Hayes, R. (1989). Occupational therapy in the treatment of schizophrenia. *Occupational Therapy in Mental Health, 9*(3), 51–68.

Heinemann, A. W. (1993). An introduction to substance abuse and physical disability. In A. W. Heinemann (Ed.), *Substance abuse and physical disability* (pp. 3–9). New York: Haworth Press.

Herman, J. L. (1992). *Trauma and recovery.* New York: Basic Books.

Hirchfeld, R. M. A. & Goodwin, F. K. (1988). Mood disorders. In J. A. Talbott, R. E. Hales, & S. C. Yudofsky (Eds.), *Textbook of psychiatry.* Washington, DC: American Psychiatric Press.

Honel, R. W. (1988). *Journey with Grandpa.* Baltimore: Johns Hopkins University Press.

Kernberg, O. (1984). *Severe personality disorders: Psychotherapeutic strategies.* New Haven: Yale University Press.

Knauth, P. (1975). *A season in hell.* New York: Harper & Row.

Konek, C. W. (1991). *Daddyboy: A memoir.* St. Paul, MN: Graywolf Press.

Levy, L. L. (1987a). Psychosocial intervention and dementia, part I: State of the art, future directions. *Occupational Therapy in Mental Health, 7*(1), 69–107.

Levy, L. L. (1987b). Psychosocial intervention and dementia, part II: The cognitive disability perspective. *Occupational Therapy in Mental Health, 7*(4), 13–36.

Liberman, R. P. (1988). Psychosocial management of schizophrenia: Overcoming disability and handicap. *The Harvard Medical School Mental Health Letter, 5*(5), 4–6.

Linehan, M. M., Tutek, D. A., Heard, H. L., & Armstrong, H. E. (1994). Interpersonal outcome of cognitive behavioral treatment for chronically suicidal borderline patients. *American Journal of Psychiatry, 151,* 1771–1775.

Luder, E. & Schebendach, J. (1993). Nutrition management of eating disorders. *Topics in Clinical Nutrition, 8,* 48–63.

Mace, N. L. & Rabins, P. V. (1991). *The 36-hour day* (revised ed.). Baltimore: Johns Hopkins.

MacLeod, S. (1981). *The art of starvation.* London: Virago.

Meyers, S. K. (1989). Occupational therapy treatment of an adult with an eating disorder: One woman's experience. *Occupational Therapy in Mental Health, 9*(1), 33–47.

Miller, S. G. (1994). Borderline personality disorder from the patient's perspective. *Hospital and Community Psychiatry, 45,* 1215–1219.

Murphey, C. (1988). *Day to day: Spiritual help when someone you love has Alzheimer's.* Philadelphia: Westminster Press.

North, C. S. (1989). *Welcome silence: My triumph over schizophrenia.* New York: Avon.

Plath, S. (1971). *The bell jar.* New York: Harper & Row.

Raymond, M. (1990, Sept.). Life skills and substance abuse. *American Occupational Therapy Association: Mental Health Special Interest Section Newsletter,* pp. 1–2.

Richards, R. (1992, April). Mood swings and everyday creativity. *The Harvard Mental Health Letter, 8,* pp. 4–6.

Robak, R. (1991). *A primer for today's substance abuse counselor.* New York: Lexington Books.

Scheiber, S. C. (1988). Psychiatric interview, psychiatric history, and mental status examination. In R. E. H. J. A. Talbott & S. C. Yudofsky (Eds.), *Textbook of psychiatry* (pp. 163–194). Washington, DC: American Psychiatric Press.

Schizophrenia: The present state of understanding, Part I. (1992, May). *The Harvard Mental Health Letter, 8,* pp. 1–4.

Schizophrenia: The present state of understanding, Part II. (1992, June). *The Harvard Mental Health Letter, 8,* pp. 1–5.

Seasonal affective disorder. (1993, Feb.). *Harvard Mental Health Letter, 9,* pp. 1–4.

Sheehan, S. (1983). *Is there no place on earth for me?* New York: Vintage.

Sheehan, S. (1995, Feb. 20 & 27). The last days of Sylvia Frumkin. *The New Yorker,* pp. 200–211.

Shimp, S. L. (1989). A family-style meal group: Short-term treatment for eating disorder patients with a high level of functioning. *Mental Health Special Interest Section Newsletter, 12,* pp. 1–3.

Styron, W. (1990). *Darkness visible: A memoir of madness.* New York: Random House.

Treatment of alcoholism—Part II. (1987). *The Harvard Medical School Mental Health Letter, 4,* pp. 1–3.

Treatment of drug abuse and addiction—Part I. (1995, Aug.). *The Harvard Mental Health Letter, 11,* pp. 1–4.

Treatment of drug abuse and addiction—Part II. (1995, Sept.). *The Harvard Mental Health Letter, 11,* pp. 1–3.

Treatment of mood disorders—Part III. (1988, Nov.). *The Harvard Medical School Mental Health Letter, 5,* pp. 1–4.

Update on Alzheimer's disease—Part I. (1995, Feb.). *The Harvard Mental Health Letter, 11,* pp. 1–5.

Update on Alzheimer's disease—Part II. (1995, Feb.). *The Harvard Mental Health Letter, 11,* pp. 1–5.

Update on mood disorders—Part I. (1994, Dec.). *The Harvard Mental Health Letter, 10,* pp. 1–4.

Update on mood disorders—Part II. (1995, Jan.). *The Harvard Mental Health Letter, 11,* pp. 1–4.

Vonnegut, M. (1975). *The Eden express.* New York: Bantam Books.

Chapter 41

Skin System Dysfunction: Burns

Elizabeth A. Rivers and Cheryl Leman Jordan

The skin injuries most frequently seen by occupational therapists are burns. Burns affect people of all ages. The annual incidence of burn-related injuries in the United States is estimated at 1.25 million, of which over 51,000 require hospitalization and 5,500 die (Brigham & McLoughlin, 1996). The results of a 1988 survey of burn facilities in the United States indicated that about 55% of all burns treated were the result of flame or flash exposure. Hot liquids and immersion scalds accounted for 35% of the injuries. Electrical contact and chemical burns were each about 5% of all admissions (M. Lewis and M. Jordan, personal communication, August 1991).

▼ REVIEW OF SKIN ANATOMY AND FUNCTIONS

The skin is the largest organ in the body. Its structure and appendages provide an extensive, complex, flexible, physical barrier for protection from environmental stresses. Skin functions include (1) thermoregulation; (2) sensation; (3) prevention of water loss; (4) protection from chemical, bacterial, and other foreign body invasion, ultraviolet (UV) rays, and mechanical trauma; and (5) provision of form, shape, and color to body areas. Skin damage results in a complex myriad of systemic, physiological, and functional problems (Falkel, 1994). The complex and life-threatening systemic effects of burn trauma in the cardiovascular, respiratory, endocrine, central nervous, gastrointestinal, genitourinary, and metabolic systems are beyond the scope of

this chapter. Readers should consult burn or wound texts for further details because assessment and treatments are based on an in-depth understanding of the total extent of anticipated burn responses.

Skin has two distinct layers: the epidermis and dermis. The epidermal cells originate in the basal layer and undergo a process of keratinization as they migrate to the surface to form a protective barrier of keratin. Melanocytes, found at the dermoepidermal junction, produce melanin to provide protection from the UV rays of the sun (Falkel, 1994). Epidermal cells lining the hair follicles and sweat glands (epidermal appendages embedded in the dermis) serve as a source of epithelium for healing wounds. Sebaceous glands, other epidermal appendages embedded in the dermis, are found in most areas, except where there is no hair. The secretion from sebaceous glands, sebum, moves toward the surface and probably enhances barrier properties by moisturizing the skin (Johnson, 1994).

The dermis is made up of vascular connective tissue. Interlacing collagen fibers interspersed with elastic fibers in this layer give the skin strength and elasticity. Dermis does not regenerate. It heals by scar formation.

▼ BURN CLASSIFICATION

The signs and symptoms of burns relate to the classification of the burn. Burn centers classify the seriousness of injury by the cause of injury, depth of injury, the percentage of total body surface area (TBSA) involved, location of the burn on the client, and age of the client.

Depth

The depth is estimated from clinical observation of the appearance, sensitivity, and pliability of the wound (Wachtel, 1985). Superficial—historically called first-degree—burns involve only the outer layers of the epidermis. The skin is red, but never blisters. These burns are painful briefly but heal uneventfully in 4 to 8 days. A sunburn is a good example of a superficial burn.

Partial-thickness (historically called second-degree) burns can be superficial or deep. Superficial partial-thickness wounds involve only the epidermis and generally blister. When a blister is removed, the wound is erythematous (red), weeping, and very painful. Superficial partial-thickness wounds generally heal in 10 days to 2 weeks with minimal permanent changes. Deep partial-thickness burns involve the epidermis and varying depths of the dermis. Hair follicles, sweat glands, and sebaceous glands are spared to some extent. These wounds are either hemorrhagic or waxy white in appearance. They are generally soft, dry, edematous, and occasionally insensate, with pain increasing as wound healing occurs. A deep partial-thickness wound can convert to full thickness by bacterial proliferation and infection. Deep partial-thickness wounds require more than 3 weeks to heal and nearly always result in some amount of scar as well as poor skin quality. The surgeon generally applies skin grafts early in areas that affect function.

Full thickness (historically called third-degree) burns involve the epidermis, dermis, and the epidermal appendages. Full-thickness burns are dry, tan, or deep red, with thrombosed vessels visible. The skin is cold, hard, and insensate. Edema is present owing to capillary damage causing fluid shifts from the intravascular to extravascular space. Edema, eschar (burned tissue) tightness, and wound inelasticity restrict movement and circulation. The surgeon may cut through the eschar (escharotomy) to improve circulation. Surgical treatment with skin grafts speeds wound closure. Scarring and disfigurement are frequently the outcome (Johnson, 1994).

Body Surface Area Involved

The extent of the burn is classified as a percentage of the TBSA. Two methods for estimating burn size are the rule of nines and the Lund and Browder chart. The rule of nines is simple and quick, but relatively inaccurate. It divides body surface into areas comprising 9%, or multiples of 9%, with the perineum making up the final 1%. The head and neck are 9%, each upper extremity (UE) is 9%, each leg is 18%, and the front and back of the trunk are each 18%. This method is modified for children up to 1 year of age, with the head and neck being 18% and each lower extremity (LE) 14%. The percentages for the head and neck and lower extremities are gradually modified from ages 1 to 10 years. The Lund and Browder chart provides a more accurate estimation of the TBSA (Lund & Browder, 1944). This chart as-signs a percentage of surface area for more specific body segments by equating proportions of each segment to the TBSA. An example of body segments is the division of the arm into the upper arm, forearm, and hand. (Because of the chart's detail, the reader is referred to the original reference to gain an understanding of it: Lund & Browder, 1944.) A client's palm print, excluding the fingers, is about 0.5% of the TBSA, and may be used as a quick estimate of burn surface area involvement (Sheridan et al., 1995).

Severity of the Burn and Location of Burn on Client

In 1995 the American Burn Association (ABA) listed 139 burn centers in the United States, about 10 of which have successfully completed verification by the ABA. Clients with the following burns should be treated in a specialized burn facility after initial evaluation and treatment at an emergency department: (1) partial- and full-thickness burns greater than 10% of TBSA in clients younger than 10 or older than 50 years old; (2) partial- and full-thickness burns greater than 20% TBSA in other age groups; (3) partial- and full-thickness burns with serious threat of functional or cosmetic impairment that involve face, hands, feet, genitalia, perineum, and major joints; (4) full-thickness burns greater than 5% TBSA in any age group; (5) electrical burns or chemical burns with serious threat of functional or cosmetic impairment; (6) inhalation injury with burn injury; or (7) circumferential burns of the extremity and chest. All of the foregoing are considered major or severe.

In addition to the area exposed, the severity of a burn injury depends on the duration and intensity of thermal exposure. Therefore, ambulance emergency medical technologists or hospital staff immediately identify the mechanism of the burn injury. Superficial partial-thickness burns typically occur after a brief contact with hot liquids or flames. Deep partial-thickness burns are caused by longer exposure to intense heat, such as with hot water immersion scalds or contact of flaming materials with the skin. Full-thickness burns result from longer exposure to flames, prolonged immersion scalds, contact with hot oil, tar, or chemical agents, and electrical contact.

Age of the Client

Age is an important variable in hospital course and prognosis after a burn. Babies and older adults generally are more fragile physiologically. Thin skin and slow circulation allow them to absorb more heat than they can dissipate. Complications associated with the burn (eg, massive fluid shifts and infections) and surgical procedures are poorly tolerated. Donor areas heal poorly. Acceptable pain management is difficult for these frail individuals, their families, and the burn care staff (Rivers & Fisher, 1997). Age, burn size, severity of injury, and severity of associated problems, such as an inhalation injury and head injury, are all considered in predicting prognosis.

▼ FLUID RESUSCITATION

A burn injury causes translocation of body fluids. With large burn injuries, burn shock can occur because of extensive intravascular fluid loss that causes decreased plasma volume, blood volume, and cardiac output. If fluid resuscitation is inadequate or the client does not respond to the resuscitative efforts, acute renal failure and death ensue (Wachtel, 1985). Several formulas are available for calculating fluid requirements for burn clients; however, the specifics for the type of fluid, hourly rate, and amount used are determined by the individual physician's philosophy.

▼ WOUND CARE

Various topical agents are available to treat burn injuries. Their purpose is to delay colonization and reduce bacterial counts on or in the wounds. Silver sulfadiazine, silver nitrate soaks, and mafenide (Sulfamylon) are just a few examples (Richard & Staley, 1994; Weber & Thompkins, 1993). Although all burn wounds are generally treated with some type of topical antibacterial agent, these agents do not substitute for surgical treatment if the need is indicated. When the depth and extent of the wound are known to require 3 or more weeks for healing, surgery is generally needed to decrease burn morbidity and mortality (Heimbach & Engrav, 1984).

Surgical treatment for burn wounds consists of excision (removal) of the burned tissue (eschar) and placement of skin grafts. Transplantation of the person's own skin from one site to another is referred to as an autograft. Split-thickness skin grafts (STSG) are either meshed to expand the coverage and assist drainage and wound adherence, or applied in sheets. Meshed grafts leave a permanent mesh pattern on the mature wound. Microvascular skin flaps (full-thickness skin graft) are used when the wound is limited in size, but the defect is so deep that tendon survival or graft adherence is doubtful. When an adequate autograft is unavailable because of the extent of body surface area involvement, or when wound depth is such that graft take is questionable, a temporary biological dressing is frequently used.

Biological dressings, either viable or nonviable, can be used as a temporary wound covering (Heimbach & Engrav, 1984). The proposed benefits of biological dressings are that they reduce fluid loss, decrease pain, inhibit bacterial growth, and protect the wound until autografting is possible. Examples of these dressings are (1) homografts, which are made from processed cadaver skin, (2) xenografts, which are made from processed pig skin, (3) synthetic products such as Biobrane, a nylon–silicone mesh coated with colla-

gen, or (4) artificial skin substitutes (Saffle & Schnebly, 1994).

▼ HYPERTROPHIC SCARS

Burn scar and contracture are common sequelae after a deep burn injury, with collagen being the primary structural component. The quality of burn wound maturation is affected by numerous factors, some of which occur during the early phases of burn care. A significant determinant in potential for scar development is the number of days required to achieve wound closure. Bacterial infection in a burn wound can increase the inflammatory response and delay healing. Spontaneous healing of full-thickness burns is a prolonged process that contributes to collagen overgrowth. Strict adherence to infection control procedures, the use of topical antibiotics, scrupulous cleansing of the burn wound, and early surgical burn wound repair minimizes the potential for burn scar contracture (Johnson, 1994). Despite these procedures and surgical interventions, scarring continues to be a major deterrent in recovering full function after a major burn injury.

Race, age, anatomical location, and depth of the burn wound can influence scar formation. **Hypertrophic scars** rise above the skin surface anytime from 4 to 12 weeks after wound closure. Initially the hypertrophic areas appear thick, rigid, and hyperemic (congested with blood). Their functional or cosmetic significance varies with the anatomical location of the wound. Hypertrophic scars that cross joints can limit range of motion (ROM) and function. Collagen contraction or skin shortening over the joint also limits ROM. If contractures are left untreated, shortening of the muscle and fibrous contraction of the joint capsule eventually occur. Scars on the face distort facial features and also limit jaw, lip, and eyelid function.

Numerous anecdotal reports of successful scar treatments are available, but few randomized, prospective, controlled studies have been published. With maturation, the hypertrophic scar softens, thins, and flattens, with collagen synthesis and degradation becoming balanced. Surgeons generally agree that hypertrophic scars will not develop in wounds that epithelialize and are becoming lighter in color 2 to 3 weeks after the injury. The process of collagen degradation in hypertrophic scar is still not fully understood (Chang et al., 1996; Fisher, Patterson, & Peltier, 1996; Laubenthal et al., 1996)

▼ EVALUATION

Burn occupational therapists evaluate, treat, and reevaluate clients of all ages, as ordered by the physiatrist or surgeon, from the time of the burn injury until all wounds are mature and the client has returned to preburn family, home, work, school, and community life. Wounds are mature when they are durable, soft, mobile, of proper color, and as flexible as possible. All phases of burn healing overlap because an injury is rarely of a single depth and varying parts of the body heal at different speeds (Rivers & Fisher, 1991).

A client with a severe burn injury, admitted to the hospital, experiences a multitude of emergency procedures by many personnel. Doctors place endotracheal airways and intravenous fluid lines, do escharotomies, estimate burn size, and order medications, activity, diet, x-rays, and analgesics. Nurses cleanse the wounds and apply a topical antimicrobial agent and dressings, place tubes to decompress the stomach and bladder, and weigh the client. When possible, the occupational therapist views the client's wounds during these initial procedures and determines areas of involvement that may require positioning or splints or both. Therapists do this initial therapy evaluation in hydrotherapy if possible. If the client is alert and willing, evaluate functional motions. Although it is easier for some clients to move without their dressings, with adequate analgesia, it is possible to evaluate active ROM when dressings are in place (Helm & Fisher, 1993). Goniometer measurements over dressings are possible by making allowances for the bandage thickness. Document active ROM of uninvolved areas also. Although it is difficult to objectively evaluate strength at this time because of edema and pain, note whether the client can move each joint through a full ROM against gravity. Obtain hand dynamometer and pinch gauge measurements if the hand is not involved, or if the burn is only a superficial partial-thickness burn with minimal surface area involvement, and no edema is present.

Obtain the client's preinjury level of function through interview with the client. When this is not possible, or when the client is intubated (using an oral or nasal airway for breathing), a close family member may be able to provide this information. Determine previous musculoskeletal injuries, sensory deficits, hand dominance, self-care function, job title, and a basic description of work skills, educational level achieved, personality traits, cultural requisites, and recreational activities. Maximizing client choice and control in the care plan increases client motivation (Law, Baptiste, & Mills, 1995). However Caplan (1988) noted that the capacity for voluntary autonomy must be re-created in clients who experience sudden, severe, and incurable impairments. Spiritual components (Egan & DeLaat, 1992) and cultural influences (Leslie, Blakeney, Moore, Desai, & Herndon, 1996) also sway client participation. For example, some people from Southeast Asia may refuse operations, based on the belief the spirit escapes from the client during surgery. During the interview, the occupational therapist indicates respect for all unique characteristics of the client. All of this information becomes the basis for an individualized treatment plan.

When interviewing or working with the client, all staff observe universal infection control precautions, according to the hospital's procedures. The following are included in most universal precaution protocols. Wash hands before and after each client contact; don protective garb, aprons, caps, or gloves before client contact and discard immediately after leaving the bedside or room; change gloves whenever contaminated with secretions or excretions from one site before contact with another site; and decontaminate all equipment, materials, and surfaces between client contacts (Weber & Thompkins, 1993).

Burn occupational therapists evaluate wound condition, scar density, ROM, strength, endurance, and function at frequent intervals during hospitalization and after hospital discharge to identify specific problem areas and decreases in function that commonly occur. Although changes in function are generally attributed to the scarring associated with burn wound healing, hospitalization and the metabolic effects of a burn injury also contribute to decreases in strength, endurance, and functional activity performance. In addition to the physical components of function, monitor skin and scar status, sensation, emotional responses, and coping skills (Leman & Ricks, 1994). The client's collaboration, understanding of recovery needs, and ability to assume responsibility for long-term care are important considerations. Although basic splint designs, specific resting positions for burned body areas, and exercise techniques frequently are taught as the standard for burn rehabilitation, every treatment plan should be developed by determining the specific needs of each particular client.

▼ PHASES OF RECOVERY

Burn care techniques and the focus of the burn team change with the phase of recovery. There are essentially three phases of burn recovery: (1) the burn shock (acute care) phase, (2) the wound surgery (and postoperative) phase, and (3) the rehabilitation (wound maturation) phase. Whether the client goes through all three phases depends on the depth and extent of the burn injury. Because of the mixed nature of the burn injury, these stages usually overlap.

The burn shock or acute care phase consists of fluid resuscitation, client stabilization, and initial wound care procedures. With superficial or partial-thickness wounds that heal without surgery, the acute care phase is also considered the period from the date of injury until epithelial healing. When the wounds are superficial, this is the only phase the client experiences. When the wounds are partial thickness in depth, do not require surgery, but take more than 2 to 3 weeks to heal, the client may also require treatment that is associated with the rehabilitation phase.

After acute resuscitation and stabilization of major burn injuries, the second phase is the wound surgery and postoperative phase. During this phase, the client undergoes multiple surgical procedures and immobilization periods. This is also the period when infections and other medical complications can occur.

The third phase is the rehabilitation phase. This phase begins with wound closure and continues through wound maturation. After severe burn injuries, therapy assumes the primary role during the rehabilitation phase.

▼ TREATMENT GOALS RELATED TO PHASES OF RECOVERY

The burn occupational therapist must constantly integrate and use physical, environmental, and psychosocial treatment skills. The physical and cosmetic disabilities that are often the sequela of a burn injury, challenge the family, client, and therapist. Although specific rehabilitation goals may be the primary responsibility of certain burn team members, depending on individual burn center policies, everyone focuses on restoring or maximizing the client's functional capacity. Therefore, the burn rehabilitation goals that follow are also goals of the occupational therapist. In the following sections, there may be overlap of other disciplines with occupational therapy, and the goals will be referred to as rehabilitation goals (Richard & Staley, 1994).

Burn Shock or Acute Care Phase

During the acute care phase, resuscitation and wound care are the foci of the burn team. When the wounds are superficial, the goal of rehabilitation therapy is to prevent loss of strength and endurance by promoting normal function. Limb elevation decreases the risk of edema and alleviates pain. Skin care education includes moisturizing to combat the itching and dryness frequently experienced with epithelial healing.

When burn wounds are partial thickness or full thickness, the acute care rehabilitation goals are to (1) control edema; (2) prevent loss of joint mobility, functional strength, and endurance; (3) promote self-care skills; (4) provide orientation activities and stimulation; and (5) begin client and family education about rehabilitation.

Wound Surgery (and Postoperative) Phase

During the surgical phase of care, immobilizing the grafted area in prescribed positions for prescribed amounts of time enhances graft adherence. Immobilization is necessary to prevent displacement of skin grafts during their vascularization. The position and length of immobilization time vary with the body area treated, the depth of the excision, the type of surgical procedure performed, and the physician's preference. The range of time for postoperative immobilization is generally 3 to 7 days. Joints are generally immobilized one joint proximal and one joint distal to the grafted joint.

During this phase, occupational therapy goals are to (1) design splints and implement positioning techniques for immobilization in consultation with the surgeon; (2) teach the family to provide appropriate sensory stimulation to prevent client disorientation; and (3) provide adaptive devices to increase self-care skills when appropriate. Other rehabilitation goals at this time are to (1) continue client and family education, and (2) prevent thrombophlebitis, skin tightness, and disuse atrophy of areas not immobilized, by implementing a controlled exercise plan for areas proximal and distal to the grafted site.

Rehabilitation Phase

The rehabilitation phase starts during wound closure. A client with a severe burn can enter this phase before all wounds are healed. Many times, on entering the rehabilitation phase, a client with a severe burn injury needs one or two more surgical procedures or has certain small areas still requiring topical antibiotics.

The rehabilitation phase is the most challenging of all for burn clients and their families. It is the period when burn scar and contracture can be recognized, and the client must assume responsibility for self-care. The need for care does not end with hospital discharge when wounds are often still flat and mobile; it continues until wound maturation is complete. This is difficult for some clients because they usually view hospital discharge as the end of the discomfort, pain, and burn care.

Although burn wound maturation may take several years after injury, every client is unique. The time needed for wound maturation varies from 9 months in a light-pigmented adult up to 5 years in a growing or darkly pigmented child. Client perseverance, patience, and a sense of humor can defuse anger during this rigorous, prolonged phase.

▼ TREATMENT

Client and Family Education

Education about burn care is a crucial basis to help the client, family, and community contacts cope with the multiple facets of burn care. Education starts at the beginning of the recovery process to ensure the client and family's understanding of the long-term needs associated with burn recovery. Pain, immobilization, and lengthy hospitalization often alter the thought processes of a burn client. The appearance of his or her wounds at varying stages of recovery is disconcerting. A burn team member saying that the wound looks good is depressing if the client does not understand that this is only one phase in the healing process. Experience shows that clients can cope more easily with the constant changes when they learn what to expect.

Family education and understanding occur at a slower pace than that of the clients (Jordan, Allely, & Gallagher, 1994.) The client speaks to the burn team constantly, whereas the family may see a burn team member for a few minutes during visiting hours. Convening family groups to discuss nutrition, exercise, pain, wound changes, and other common topics augments learning and maximizes staff time. Talking about the frustration of watching a family member struggle to function independently may comfort relatives. The recovery process is shorter when staff, clients, and family share outcome goals and clearly record progress. Discharge should never be a surprise.

Functional recovery after a burn injury is a dynamic process, considering the scarring and deconditioning that occur during hospitalization and bed rest. Because burn recovery is a painful process, it is important that clients become actively involved with their rehabilitation program at the beginning. A client who learns and uses pain and stress management techniques early often carries out a successful outcome. Advances in client-centered pain management continue with improved understanding of drugs and physiology (Pain management of the burn client, 1995). Successful clients allow the accident to become a part of their unchangeable past and assume responsibility for their long-term recovery. They understand the purpose of specific treatments, potential outcomes if they avoid or discontinue treatment, the prolonged burn recovery time, pain management techniques, and methods for independently assessing scar maturation.

Exercise

The goal of exercise is to improve physical function through increased muscle strength, endurance, flexibility, and power. A thorough history helps determine the type of range of motion that will safely meet the mutual goals of the client, physician, and therapist. Although clients tend to avoid movement in general, when they do move, it is painful, slow, and labored. As the burn wound closes, scar tightness, hypersensitivity, pain and discomfort experienced when stretching scars, the client's emotional adjustment, and a generalized feeling of fatigue often limit a burn client's willingness or ability to exercise. During this period, motions often appear robotlike, with fluidity of movement absent; spontaneity is absent, normal motions and joint ROM are limited. If these movements are allowed to persist, functional limitations develop.

Clients will develop painful joints if they do not regain full active ROM quickly after the burn. Pain can be the result of tight contractures of soft tissue, tendons, ligaments, blood vessels, and nerves surrounding the involved joint. It can be from skin contractures or hypertrophic scar bands. Pain also develops from cartilage deterioration owing to poor joint nutrition caused by lack of complete joint gliding. If joints remain stiff, clients may have difficulty with self-care activities or returning to work. Clients may also experience postural strain from substitution patterns when they are not able to move their extremity in a full arc of motion. Although activity and active exercise are needed for muscle strength and endurance, continuous passive motion

(CPM) devices can be used as an adjunct to the exercise regimen (Covey, Dutcher, Marvin, & Heimbach, 1988). Covey and associates (1988) demonstrated increased recovery and no tissue damage with CPM machines. CPM devices are beneficial when the client's active motion is limited secondary to pain, edema, or anxiety. Although the therapist must monitor the client's response when initially using the device, a CPM device is an extension of treatment when the therapist is not available. It is especially appropriate for use when the client is resting or sleeping.

Free weights using the Delorem method (see Chap. 20, Sec. 3) or electronically controlled dynamometers are examples of strengthening techniques. Use of a bicycle ergometer for endurance is also appropriate in burn rehabilitation. Although exercise tolerance in the hypermetabolic client is a concern, there are methods for assessing exercise response. Monitoring pulse rate, blood pressure, and respiration are just a few of the techniques that assist in safely grading exercises.

Stretching exercises are important before exercising during burn recovery, to prevent injury. Before stretching, massage a lubricating cream into the maturing tissues. This prevents skin rupture from dryness and scar rigidity. Add complex motions and resistive exercises during the rehabilitation phase of recovery. Flexibility exercises, or combined joint movements, are complex motions. Although a burn scar can limit motion of the joint it crosses, it can also affect those proximal and distal to it. Therefore, it is important to provide exercises that require concurrent joint motions. For example, an exercise program for an UE burn may emphasize elbow function, but should also incorporate coordinated movements of the shoulder, elbow, and hand. In designing an individualized exercise plan, it is important to analyze the total effect of the scar, while also considering the functional and vocational needs of the client. Burn occupational therapists use functional, vocational, and leisure activities to stretch contractures. Because burn contractures are dynamic, fluidity of full motion is more pivotal to recovery than regaining early function with adapted equipment or substitution of motions.

Positioning

Positioning techniques were first developed for the acute phase of burn care. In response to fear of pain, the burn client frequently assumes a protective childlike posture of adduction and flexion of the upper extremities, flexion of the hips and knees, and planar flexion of the ankles. Hand burn pain causes clients to hold their hands in a dysfunctional thumb adducted, wrist flexed position. Using a pillow when there are neck burns and resting with the head of the bed in an upright position when there are trunk burns contribute to inappropriate posturing. If the burn client remains in a flexed, fetal, withdrawal position as wound healing progresses, contractures develop and limit function. In general, therapeutic burn positioning entails encouraging some degree of extension of all involved areas when resting. Therapeutic positioning of a cooperative burn client aids in edema control and reduction, maintains normal muscle length when resting, ensures wound coverage immediately after placement of skin grafts, limits the degree of scar contracture, and teaches the client methods for combating the skin tightness that affects function.

During the acute phase of care, the main purpose for positioning is to limit edema formation (Helm & Fisher, 1983). Although there is an initial diffuse capillary leak with a severe burn, the severity or consequences of distal extremity edema formation can be limited with elevation of the limb at or slightly above heart level. For hand and arm burns use foam wedges or pillows. In these cases, extension of the elbows is important to prevent restriction of venous return. Raise the foot of the bed to reduce foot or leg edema. Do not flex the hips more than 30 degrees when the legs and hips are burned and keep the knees extended. With face and neck burns, raise the head of the bed at least 30 degrees or use a foam elevation wedge for edema management.

As wound closure begins and progresses, address more proximal positioning concerns. When the axillae and anterior trunk are involved, abduct the arms to 90 degrees using armboards attached to the side of the bed or overhead suspension. Blanket rolls placed along the upper trunk also promote shoulder abduction. If any portion of the neck is involved, the client should not use a pillow for head support. Use a small towel roll behind the neck instead.

Postoperative immobilization positions may entail many of the techniques already described, but may also be specific for the type of procedure used or area treated. When a skin graft is used for wound coverage, the body area or joint treated is usually held in some degree of extension or abduction. When a skin flap is performed, positioning specifics change to prevent stress on the suture lines. Knowledge of the surgical procedure performed and determination of potential postoperative complications, such as suture-line stresses or graft shifting, enable the therapist to institute effective, safe positioning techniques. If functionally limiting contractures develop from poor positioning at home, use splints for positioning.

Activities of Daily Living (ADL)

When medically stable, the client begins independent eating, although dressings and edema may alter performance. Adapted utensils to improve grasp may be needed temporarily. Avoid extending utensils and straws because using the elbow at the habit level promotes more normal ROM. Remember that ADL independence is one of the least painful methods to achieve full active ROM. Therefore, remove adaptive devices as soon as possible to avoid dependence on them.

Clients usually receive hydrotherapy on a daily basis as part of wound care. Nurses cleanse the wounds, but client participation in bathing and grooming should be encour-

aged. Although it is difficult for clients to reach all body areas, becoming involved in bathing is a beginning point for wound healing education while fostering independence in self-care. Overall, ADL practice during this early phase of care focuses the client toward recovery, emphasizes abilities, and provides a means for discharge education.

As wound closure is achieved and the client nears discharge from the hospital, normal independent self-care proceeds. Independence in bathing, grooming, eating, toileting, and dressing skills should be evaluated. Perform bathing and grooming in a bathroom with appliances similar to those used at home. Practice dressing skills with clothes from home so the client and family realize that adapted clothing is rarely necessary. With major burn injuries, adaptations may be needed to encourage self-care independence. Use a mirror to assess self-care skills. The client observes scar stretching and understands the benefit of improved function.

Experience has shown that many clients fear hot water, especially if they were injured in the shower or bath tub. These clients are eager to learn how to safely test water temperatures and to set the thermostat of their hot water heater below 120°F. Cooking is another activity that many clients avoid at home because they fear heat or were injured while cooking. Cooking activities in the clinic decrease fears and teach safe cooking procedures to be used at home.

Educate the client in skin and scar care, including home wound care, skin moisturizing and lubrication, and independent donning of vascular support or compression garments. Performance with a therapist brings an awareness and understanding of the time and benefits of ADL activities, developing patience, and planning time to perform tasks independently.

Unprotected sun exposure to a healed wound results in blotchy, unpredictable tanning. If pigment is absent in the healed wound, severe tissue damage can result from sun exposure. Teach the client to avoid sun exposure injuries. Wearing a wide-brimmed hat is recommended for any one with maturing face and neck burns. Clients exposed to sun and heat learn to work in shaded areas; wear light-colored, lightweight, nonrestrictive clothing and a cool flap hat or wide-brimmed hat; use a battery fan; spray bottle; sunglasses; drink more fluids; and avoid vasoconstricting drugs such as cigarettes (Rivers & Fisher, 1997). Skin protection using a sunscreen with a 30-rated sun protection factor (SPF) should be recommended. Sunscreens should be applied anytime a client is in the sun, even if simply riding in a car.

Because circulation is permanently changed in scarred areas, and sweat glands may be absent, heat exposure is a problem. Injured skin is very sensitive to temperature extremes. Severely injured clients may need to remain in air-conditioned areas if the temperature is above 70°F. Often a fan and spray bottle of water will be adequate coolant. The clients also learn to prevent frostbite and cold injuries in the outdoor environment. Teach them to keep their vehicles well maintained, use a cell phone, stay with vehicle during breakdowns, and keep blankets, extra mittens, warm clothing, boots, flash lights, and snacks inside. At work, clients should use (1) insulated, waterproof boots; (2) safety shoes with fiberglass toe and shank if approved by employer; (3) flap hats or insulated hood; (4) multiple layer, nonrestrictive clothing of wind-resistant fabric; and (5) avoid vasodilating drugs such as alcohol, and vasoconstricting drugs such as cigarettes (Rivers & Fisher, 1997).

Splints

The use of splints in burn care varies with the phase of wound healing, but more importantly, with the philosophy of the burn center. Traditionally, in acute care, splints were taken off only for meals, dressing changes, and exercise. Today, splints are used less often during acute care. Acute care splints are generally static in design and used at night or for short periods, with activity and exercise emphasized during the day.

The primary splint still used in acute burn care is the burn hand splint. The time of application differs. Some therapists begin the splints only when ROM becomes limited. Others wait 48 to 72 hours after injury to apply the hand splint (Miles & Grigsby, 1990). This is because the extreme fluid shifts that occur during acute resuscitation can greatly affect splint fit. The purposes of the burn hand splint are to prevent ligamentous stress at the interphalangeal joints, to assist in edema reduction, and to allow flow to the intrinsic muscles of the hands by emphasizing the distal transverse arch of the hand. This splint prevents the burn claw deformity, which is flexion of the wrist, hyperextension of the metacarpophalangeal joints, and flexion of the interphalangeal joints.

The burn hand splint differs from other hand splints by the position of its components. Usually made out of a low-temperature thermoplastic material, the splint positions the wrist in about 30 to 35 degrees of extension, the metacar-

pophalangeal joints are flexed 50 to 70 degrees, the interphalangeal joints are held in extension, and the thumb is abducted (Fig. 41–1). These positions vary with the surface area burned, with the preceding design being used for dorsal hand burns. When there are circumferential hand burns, the positions can be modified. Usually secure the acute hand splints with gauze or disposable elastic wraps. Do not use straps because of infection control concerns and the possibility of distal edema. When an acute splint is used, it is usually a conformer splint that has total contact with the surface area being treated and generally places the body area in an extended position (Helm et al., 1983). Frequent evaluation of fit and readjustments are needed with these types of splints to accommodate fluid volume changes in the extremity and variations in dressing bulk.

A conforming positioning splint may be needed after skin grafts are applied. Because of the bulk of the postoperative dressing, plaster strips are frequently used for splinting during operations. Most postoperative splints hold the joint or limb in extension, with the exception of a foot splint, which positions the ankle in dorsiflexion, and the airplane splint, which positions the shoulder in about 90 degrees of abduction (Fig. 41–2).

Although static splints may be needed during burn wound maturation, do not restrict activity if possible. Low-temperature thermoplastic dynamic splints may be appropriate when scar contracture is present. The purpose of a dynamic splint is to assist or regain function or to provide slow dynamic stretch to contracting tissues. When fabricating and fitting a dynamic splint, use caution to prevent the splint components from exerting ligamentous stress, friction, or joint compressive forces. There are a few commercially available dynamic splints for elbows, knees, and ankles, but these should be used with caution. Whenever a commercial splint is used, frequent evaluation of fit is necessary to prevent edema, to accommodate volume changes in the extremity, and to avoid joint compressive forces.

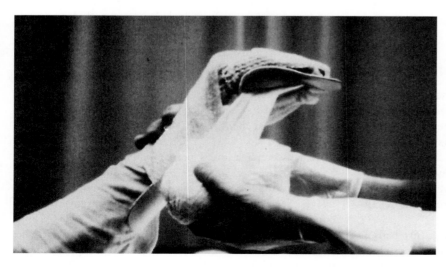

◄

Figure 41-1. Gauze and elastic wraps are used to maintain hand position on a burn hand splint.

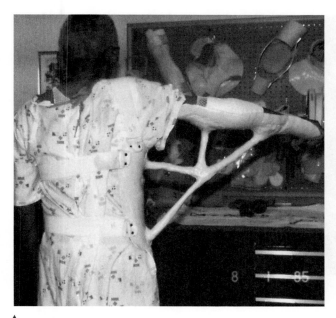

▲
Figure 41-2. An airplane splint allows mobility while maintaining the shoulder in 90 degrees of abduction.

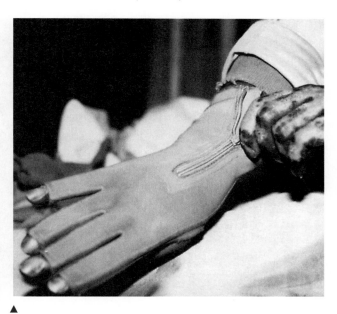

▲
Figure 41-3. A custom-fitted external compression and vascular support glove is worn 23 hours a day to minimize scarring, edema, and vascular pooling. Open fingertips in gloves can improve fingertip prehension and sensation.

Plaster casts maintain correct positions or stretch and soften contractures. Advantages of plaster casting are the low cost of materials and the characteristics of accurately conforming, nonremovable circumferential contact. Plaster, as with all circumferential wrappings, should be applied distal to proximal on the limb to assist venous return. Serial casting and a dynamic plaster casting technique have both been described for treatment of scar contractures of the hand, wrist, elbow, knee, and ankle (Ridgeway, Daugherty, & Warden, 1991).

In many instances, it is difficult to discuss burn splinting as separate from scar management (Daugherty & Carr-Collins, 1994; Leman, 1992). Splints such as the total contact transparent face mask and neck splints are more appropriately presented as methods of scar management, with positioning techniques used during the acute phase. Splint design should be specific for the particular wound healing problem. (See Chap. 20, Sec. 4 for more details on splinting.)

Scar Management

Mechanical pressure has long been advocated as a way to influence scarring and has been used as treatment for or prevention of hypertrophic scars (Carr-Collins, 1992). As a scar develops, it becomes hyperemic (red), raised and rigid (Johnson, 1994). Long-term scar care includes the use of splints and compression or external vascular support garments (Fig. 41–3).

The purpose of using elastic compression garments and splints on maturing burn wounds is to apply perpendicular pressure that approximates capillary pressure because it has been postulated that wounds mature more rapidly with fewer scars when deprived of circulation and oxygen. Elastic wrap supports prevent dependent edema under grafts on dependent extremities. When the healed wound tolerates the shear of donning a sleeve, the wraps can be replaced with cotton and rubber tubes or custom measured garments. Providing for normal motions while maintaining adequate scar control and coverage is difficult. Creativity, skill, perseverance, and always questioning what else can be done are needed qualities for the occupational therapist. No pressure appliance or garment is perfect, and frequent reevaluation is needed to ensure appropriate pressure and fit.

Numerous pressure dressings and techniques are available for use early during wound healing (Ward, 1991, 1993). Although scar hypertrophy and collagen contraction generally are not noted until after wound closure, some vascular support and compression techniques are applied early. Vascular supports control edema, minimize vascular and lymphatic pooling in the extremities, and condition the new skin for the shear force demands of commercial garments. Interim pressure garments begin skin desensitization and sensory reeducation, teach independent dressing or garment-donning skills, and provide timely compression therapy education.

Elastic wraps applied over gauze dressings in a figure-eight, gradient fashion are the initial treatment choice in most burn centers. They are also considered the first stage of graded pressure therapy. As the wounds heal and dressing needs diminish, compression therapy can be progressed to using tubular elastic dressings that are pulled on. Elastinet and Tubigrip, available in rolls of various circumferences, are frequently

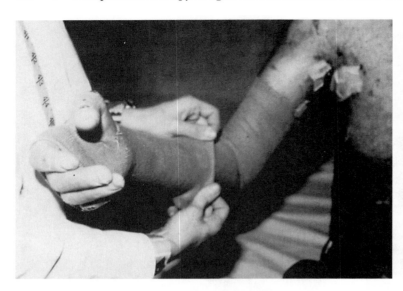

◄ *Figure 41-4.* Tubular elastic dressings are used for skin conditioning on the extremities. The hand or foot must be included in the dressing to prevent distal swelling.

used for intermediate compression therapy on the extremities (Fig. 41–4). Interim pressure on the hand can be accomplished by progressing to an intermediate Spandex glove that is made by the therapist, by using manufactured presized gloves such as Isotoner or Hatch, or by applying a total–contact Coban wrap (Fig. 41–5). Consider the cost and purposes for using interim pressure when choosing a method. Skin condition, the need to decrease edema, and the client's functional abilities and understanding are a few of the important points. The overall goal is to prepare the client, both physically and psychologically, for custom–fitted garments.

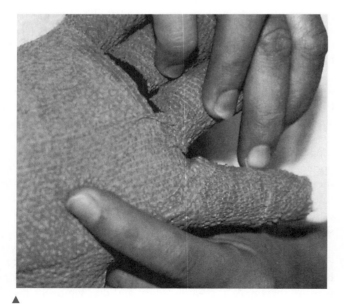

▲ *Figure 41-5.* Coban wraps are used to minimize edema and to prepare the hand for a custom-fitted glove. A strip placed dorsal to volar provides web-space control. –

Although custom garments are made from sequential measurements of the client, actual garment fit is not perfect. To be effective, the elastic garment must exert equal pressure over the entire area. This is not always possible because of body contours, bony prominences, and postural adjustments by the client. When the garment does not fit consistently, a therapist adds inserts or overlays to distribute pressure uniformly. Areas frequently needing inserts are the superior anterior chest, breast areas on women, web spaces on the hand, anterior surface of the toes, the upper and lower lip areas, and nasolabial folds on the face. Inserts are also needed to prevent garment overlap and folding in the antecubital areas of the elbows, posterior aspect of the knees, axillary folds, and anterior aspect of the ankle.

Pressure inserts were originally made from thermoplastics, but problems of skin maceration under the inserts were common. Today, thermoplastics are used only for fairly large surface areas for which positioning is also needed, such as the anterior chest, or areas in which there is minimal motion, such as between the breasts. Most inserts are now made from more flexible materials, such as orthopedic felt, Plastazote, silicone gel, Aliplast, silicone elastomer, or a closed cell foam (Miles & Grisby, 1990; Van den Kerckhove, Boeckx, & Kochuyt, 1991). Friction or skin maceration are not common with these materials because they are flexible. The material chosen depends on the function of the area being treated. If the insert is needed to provide gentle positioning at rest, along with being flexible to allow some motion, Aliplast, or silicone elastomer can be used (Van den Kerckhove et al., 1991). When flexibility and pressure distribution in smaller areas are the primary needs, Plastazote, silicone gel, or a closed cell foam is used. Many of the materials for pressure inserts are subject to tearing and eventual compression; therefore, frequent evaluation and replacement are necessary. The client's ability to keep the insert in the correct position under the garment, skin reaction, cost, safety, and wound changes influence insert use.

Despite advances in scar control using garments and inserts, splints may still be needed for certain body areas. There are also areas where effective pressure distribution is not possible with elastic garments. The neck, face, and mouth are good examples of areas for which an alternative method for pressure therapy is needed. Preventing scar contracture of the neck is difficult, owing to neck mobility, ineffectiveness of elastic garments, and dysfunctional postural adjustments that the client may make in response to scar tightness and discomfort. Scar involvement of the neck region can extend from the face to the superior aspect of the chest, causing distortion of the lower face and lip commissures, eversion of the lower lip, limited neck rotation and extension, and shoulder protraction (Fig. 41–6).

Early splint designs for neck contracture prevention consisted of a total-contact neck conformer made from a thermoplastic material (Willis, 1970). Problems encountered with this neck conformer are mandibular retraction, minimal to no neck rotation allowed, and decreased surface contact with neck motion. An advancement of this splint design is a rigid, total-contact, transparent chin and neck orthosis (Rivers & Fisher, 1991) (Fig. 41–7). Fabricating a transpar-

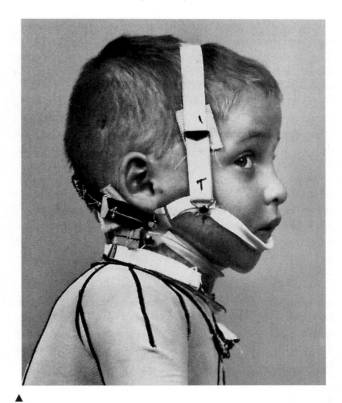

▲
Figure 41-7. A profile of a transparent chin and neck orthosis worn with a presized external vascular support garment.

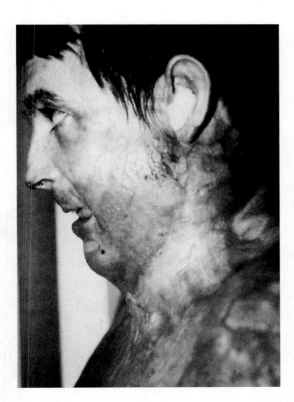

▲
Figure 41-6. Scar contracture of the neck. When the scar shortens by contraction, the chin shelf and cervicomental angle are lost, and range of motion is restricted.

ent plastic splint is an involved process, but allows more precise alterations and evaluation of fit compared with opaque thermoplastic materials. An alternative splint design is the triple-component neck splint, which consists of a chin cup, chin strap, and modified neck conformer (Leman & Lowery, 1986). It is basically a two-piece neck conformer with an elastic chin strap. Its design allows neck rotation and some extension and flexion, preserves the cervicomental angle of the chin, and provides compression to supraclavicular scar.

Burn scar contracture of the perioral facial region may lead to cosmetic and functional impairment. Microstomia, or contracture of the oral commissures, affects intubation for surgery, eating skills, oral hygiene, dental care, facial expression, and sometimes speech. Because of the structure of the perioral region and the need for stretching pressure when scar is developing, an elastic hood without an insert increases circumoral contractures. A microstomia-prevention appliance is commercially available for preventing or decreasing microstomia during wound healing (Carlow, Conine, & Stevenson-Moore, 1987). The commercial microstomia-prevention appliance is effective in preserving the horizontal width and can be adapted to increase vertical stretching by molding a piece of thermoplastic to its acrylic sections. Problems with this approach are distortion of the tissues surrounding the oral commissures and potential pressure sores of the oral mucosa. A modified microstomia-prevention splint is constructed by the therapist (Fig. 41–8). The advantage of this design is its flexibility in allowing modification of the splint's commissures, without adding additional material.

In the face, it is difficult to exert adequate pressure to all involved areas using elastic garments. This is due to its multiple contour changes and soft tissue planes. Facial pressure devices include elastomer inserts under elastic garments, low-temperature thermoplastic masks, and total-contact, transparent face orthoses (Figs. 41–9 and 41–10). The advantages of a transparent mask are that more precise alterations are possible, the amount of scar contact can be easily evaluated, and facial contours can be emphasized. Many clients prefer the transparent mask because it is simple to don and doff, is less obtrusive, and the hair is uncovered, allowing some identity.

Scar management is a long-term process requiring frequent assessment and adjustment of garment and splint fit. Increasing the person's ability to don and doff garments and splints is an important objective in design selection (Fig. 41–11). In most cases, success is dependent on the person's creativity and ability to assume responsibility for self-care.

Skin Care

Whether or not scar contracture develops during burn wound maturation, the new skin (epithelium) will never look or react to exposure or contact the same as it did be-

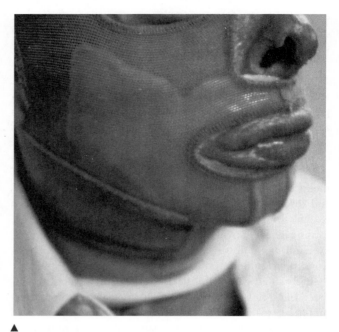

▲
Figure 41-9. Elastomer insert worn under an external compression and vascular support face mask distributes pressure more uniformly.

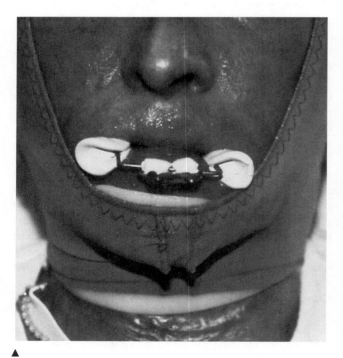

▲
Figure 41-8. A therapist-made microstomia-prevention splint. A thermoplastic chin cup, worn under the elastic chin strap, is molded to the patient to preserve the cervicomental angle and chin shelf.

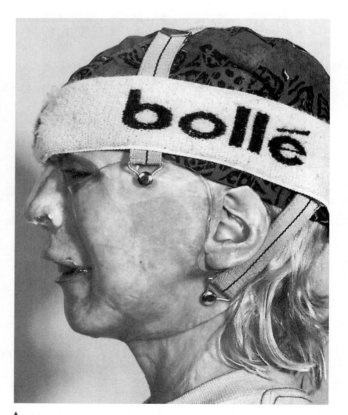

▲
Figure 41-10. Side view of a transparent facial orthosis. Headbands are frequently used for forehead scar control.

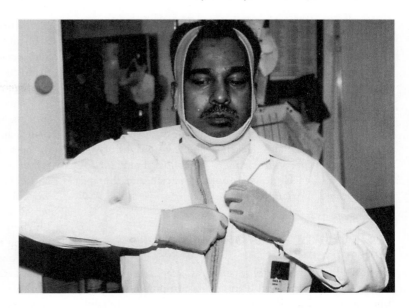

▶ *Figure 41-11.* A patient independently donning a triple-component neck splint and external compression and vascular support garment.

fore injury. Common problems include edematous, insensate or hypersensitive, dry, and unusually fragile skin (Fig. 41–12). Newly healed skin is also vulnerable to exposure to UV light, extremes of temperature, and chemical irritation (Rivers & Fisher, 1997). Because of changes in elasticity, shear tolerance, sensation, and pigmentation, skin care and conditioning should be part of self-care education in every burn treatment plan.

Before discharge from the hospital, the client should learn how and when to lubricate the skin. This is necessary because most deep partial-thickness and full-thickness burns frequently damage epidermal appendages that contribute to the skin's moisture balance. Lubrication should be performed every day after bathing and at intervals during the day when the skin feels exceptionally dry, tight, or itchy. Massage, using a non–water-based cream, should always precede stretching exercises to prevent the dry skin from rupturing (Jordan, Allely, & Gallagher, 1994; Miles & Grisby, 1990).

Improving skin tolerance and sensitivity to friction or trauma is also part of skin care. Scratching, rubbing, bumping into something, and the shearing forces of custom-made, external vascular support garments can cause blisters. Clients should be taught not to be alarmed when blisters occur and to leave small blisters intact. If the blister is large, it should be drained, and mercurochrome and dry gauze should be applied. Spenco dermal pads, other gel pads, or extra linings in garments over areas prone to trauma, such as the knees, can be used for its prevention. A disposable contact layer of gauze, cloth, Webril (if no open areas are present), or paper towel under the pad decreases perspiration and contact dermatitis. Interim pressure dressings and pre-sized garments, massage, exercise, and activity while wearing interim garments, and desensitization activities are also effective in increasing skin tolerance and decreasing sensitivity. Vibration or tapping with a cool pack decreases itching.

It is important for the therapist to be aware of possible complications of contractures and scar control devices. De-

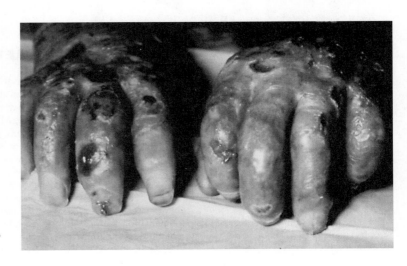

▶ *Figure 41-12.* Burn wounds that heal without surgery are frequently edematous, fragile, and prone to blistering. Skin conditioning and intermediate garments are used to prevent this type of problem.

formities such as delayed skeletal growth from the scar management devices have been reported (Leung, Cheng, Ma, Clark, & Leung, 1983). In 1985 Robertson, Zuker, Dabrowski, and Levinson reported sleep apnea as a complication of burns to the head and neck of children, especially children who wore chin straps at night. In 1995 Nahieli, Kelly, Baruchin, Ben-Meir, and Shapira, reported oromaxillofacial skeletal deformities resulting from burn scar contractures of the face and neck in a client who did not wear support or compression garments or splints. Frequent follow-up in a burn clinic with both physician and therapist evaluation is important for safety.

▼ RETURN TO WORK

Physical demands of jobs, such as reaching, stooping, pulling, lifting, and manipulating, are components of many functional activities. Because the emphasis of burn rehabilitation is on functional recovery, a resourceful occupational therapist uses activities and exercises for dual purposes—both functional and work-related (Fig. 41–13).

Identifying and integrating job skills in the acute care treatment plan decreases the potential for loss of skills and fosters the client's realization that he or she is going to be okay. Returning to work before final scar maturation pre-

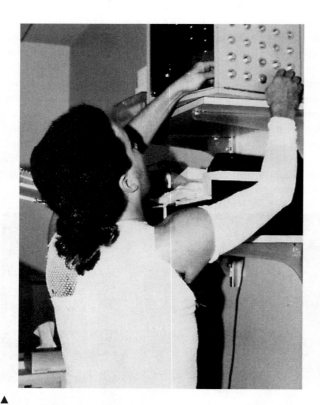

▲
Figure 41-13. Work samples, such as the Valpar Small Tools Work Sample, can be used to simulate both functional motions and work skills during acute care.

serves function and improves the client's self-concept. This is possible, however, only after reintegration into the family and socialization concerns are resolved. Mutual expectations from the surgeons, nurses, social workers, and therapists encourage early return to work.

Preparing a burn client for return to work is a shorter process when treatment plans incorporate both job demands and basic functional needs. Include a job description in the activity needs analysis. If the client was injured on the job or is lacking confidence in his or her abilities, many psychosocial issues may emerge when discussing return to work. Fear, anger, and pain need to be addressed early and, when needed, with a psychologist (Watkins, Cook, May, & Ehleben, 1988). The person may not feel capable of performing the job again, may be anxious about being injured again, or may be self-conscious about appearance. Job desensitization can take place when the client goes to the workplace, observes the job and discusses concerns with coworkers and a supervisor, and later with the therapist. Group sessions that include both inpatients and outpatients have also had positive results in resolving return to work issues (Leman, 1987). Work provides distraction, control, and independence desired by a burned client.

►CONCLUSION

Advances in burn care have improved burn injury outcomes. Today, most clients recovering from a burn injury can expect to return to a near-normal life, including return to school or work early during the recovery process. To achieve this goal, a team approach to client-centered care is necessary.

Therapists refer clients to numerous burn-related programs. School reentry programs (Blakeney et al, 1995; Doctor, 1995), burn camps (Rosenstein, 1986), and recovered burn groups are just a few of those programs for recovering burn clients. For health care professionals, the American Burn Association, a national organization, is dedicated to burn rehabilitation, education, research, and burn prevention.

▼ REFERENCES

American Burn Association. (1995). *Burn care services in North America.* (Available from the American Burn Association. 800–548–2876).

Blakeney, P., Moore, M. A., Meyer, W. III, Bishop, B., Murphy, L., Robson, M., & Herndon, D. (1995). Efficacy of school reentry programs. *Journal of Burn Care and Rehabilitation, 16,* 469–472.

Brigham, P. A. & McLoughlin, E. (1996). Burn incidence and medical care use in the United States: Estimates, trends, and data sources. *Journal of Burn Care and Rehabilitation, 17,* 95–107.

Caplan, A. L. (1988). Informed consent and provider–patient relationships in rehabilitation medicine. *Archives of Physical Medicine & Rehabilitation, 69,* 312–317.

Carlow, D. L., Conine, T. A., & Stevenson-Moore, P. (1987). Static orthoses for the management of microstomia. *Journal of Rehabilitation Research and Development, 24*(3), 35–42.

Carr-Collins, J. A. (1992) Pressure techniques for the prevention of hypertrophic scar. In R. E. Salisbury (Ed.), *Clinics in Plastic Surgery, 19*, 733–743.

Chang, P., Laubenthal, K. N., Lewis, R. W. II, Rosenquist, D., Lindley-Smith, P., & Kealey, G. P. (1996, March). Prospective randomized study of the effect of pressure garment therapy on the rate of wound maturation in burn patients [Abstract]. *Proceedings of the American Burn Association Annual Meeting, 28*, 83.

Covey, M., Dutcher, K., Marvin, J., & Heimbach, D. (1988). Efficacy of continuous passive motion (CPM) devices with hand burns. *Journal of Burn Care and Rehabilitation, 9*, 397–400.

Daugherty, M. B. & Carr-Collins, J. A. (1994). Splinting techniques for the burn patient. In R. L. Richard & M. J. Staley (Eds.), *Burn care and rehabilitation: Principles and practice* (pp. 242–323). Philadelphia: F. A. Davis.

Doctor, M. E. (1995). Commentary. *Journal of Burn Care and Rehabilitation, 16*, 466–468.

Egan, M. & DeLaat, M. D. (1992). Considering spirituality in occupational therapy practice. *Canadian Journal of Occupational Therapy, 61*, 95–101.

Falkel, J. E. (1994). Anatomy and physiology of the skin. In R. L. Richard & M. J. Staley (Eds.), *Burn care and rehabilitation: Principles and practice* (pp. 10–28). Philadelphia: F.A. Davis.

Fisher, S.V., Patterson, R. P., & Peltier, G. (1996, March). Effect of pressure on hypertrophic scars secondary to burns [Abstract]. *Proceedings of the American Burn Association Annual Meeting, 28*, 85.

Heimbach, D. M. & Engrav, L. H. (1984). *Surgical management of the burn wound.* New York: Raven Press.

Helm, P. A. & Fisher, S.V. (1993). Rehabilitation of the patient with burns. In J. A. Delisa (Editor in Chief), *Rehabilitation medicine principles and practice* (2nd ed.). Philadelphia: J. B. Lippincott.

Helm, P., Kevorkian, G., Lushbaugh, M., Pullium, G., Head, M., & Cromes, F. (1983). Burn injury: Rehabilitation management in 1982. *Journal of Burn Care and Rehabilitation, 4*, 411–422.

Johnson, C. (1994). Pathologic manifestations of burn injury. In R. L. Richard & M. J. Staley (Eds.), *Burn care and rehabilitation: Principles and practice* (pp. 29–48). Philadelphia: F.A. Davis.

Jordan, C. L., Allely, R., & Gallagher J. (1994). Self-care strategies following severe burns. In C. Christiansen (Ed.), *Ways of living* (pp. 305–332). Bethesda, MD: American Journal of Occupational Therapy.

Laubenthal, K. N., Lewis R. W. II, Rosenquist, D., Lindley-Smith, P., Chang, P., & Kealey, G. P. (1996, March). Prospective randomized study of the effect of pressure garment therapy on pain and pruritus in the maturing burn wound [Abstract]. *Proceedings of the American Burn Association Annual Meeting, 28*, 161.

Law, M., Baptiste, S., & Mills, J. (1995). Client-centered practice: What does it mean and does it make a difference? *Canadian Journal of Occupational Therapy, 62*, 250–257.

Leman, C. (1987). An approach to work hardening in burn rehabilitation. *Topics in Acute Care and Trauma Rehabilitation, 1*(4), 62–73.

Leman, C. J. (1992). Splints and accessories following burn reconstruction. In R. E. Salisbury (Ed.), *Clinics in Plastic Surgery, 19*(3), 733–743).

Leman, C. & Lowery, C. (1986). The triple-component neck splint. *Journal of Burn Care and Rehabilitation, 7*, 357–361.

Leman, C. J. & Ricks, N. (1994). Discharge planning and follow-up burn care. In R. L. Richard & M. J. Staley (Eds.), *Burn care and rehabilitation: Principles and practice* (pp. 447–472). Philadelphia: F. A. Davis.

Leslie, G., Blakeney, P., Moore, P., Desai, M. H., & Herndon, D. N. (1996, March). Native Americans: A challenge for the pediatric burn team [Poster]. *Proceedings of the American Burn Association Annual Meeting, 28*, 147.

Leung, K. S., Cheng, J. C. Y., Ma, G. F. Y., Clark, J. A., & Leung, P. C.

(1983). Complications of pressure therapy for post-burn hypertrophic scars: Biochemical analysis based on 5 patients. *Burns, Including Thermal Injury, 10*, 434–438.

Lund, C. & Browder, N. (1944). The estimation of area of burns. *Surgical Gynecology and Obstetrics, 79*, 352–355.

Miles, W. & Grigsby, L. (1990). Remodeling of scar tissue in the burned hand. In J. Hunter, L. Schneider, E. Mackin, A. Callahan (Eds.), *Rehabilitation of the hand: Surgery and therapy* (3rd ed.; pp. 841–857). St. Louis: C.V. Mosby.

Nahieli, O., Kelly, J. P., Baruchin, A. M., Ben-Meir, P., & Shapira, Y. (1995). Oro-maxillofacial skeletal deformities resulting from burn scar contractures of the face and neck. *Burns, Including Thermal Injury, 21*, 65–69.

Pain management of the burn patient. (1995). *Journal of Burn Care and Rehabilitation, 16*, (3, Pt. 2), 343–376.

Richard, R. L. & Staley, M. J. (1994). *Burn care and rehabilitation: Principles and practice.* Philadelphia: F.A. Davis.

Ridgeway, C. L., Daugherty, M. B., & Warden, G. D. (1991). Serial casting as a technique to correct burn scar contractures. *Journal of Burn Care and Rehabilitation, 12*, 67–72.

Rivers, E. & Fisher, S. (1997). Burn Rehabilitation. In B. O'Young & M. A. Young (Eds.), *Physical medicine and rehabilitation secrets* (pp. 418–428). Philadelphia: Hanley & Belfus.

Rivers, E. A. & Fisher, S.V. (1991). Advances in burn rehabilitation. In F. J. Kottke & E. A. Amate (Eds.), *Clinical advances in physical medicine and rehabilitation* (pp. 334–357), Washington, DC: Pan American Health Organization, Pan American Sanitary Bureau, Regional Office of the World Health Organization. (also available in Spanish as *Adelantos clinicos en medicina fisica y rehabilitacion.* 1994.).

Robertson, C. F., Zuker, R., Dabrowski, B., & Levinson, H. (1985). Obstructive sleep apnea: A complication of burns to the head and neck in children. *Journal of Burn Care and Rehabilitation, 6*, 353–357.

Rosenstein, D. (1986). Camp celebrate: A therapeutic weekend camping program for pediatric burn patients. *Journal of Burn Care and Rehabilitation, 7*, 434–436.

Saffle, K. R. & Schnebly, W. A. (1994) Burn wound care. In R. L. Richard & M. J. Staley (Eds.), *Burn care and rehabilitation: Principles and practice* (pp. 119–176). Philadelphia: F.A. Davis.

Sheridan, R., Petras, L., Basha, G., Salvo, P., Cifrino, C., Hinson, M., McCabe, M., Fallon, J., & Thompkins, R. G. (1995) Should irregular burns be sized with the hand or the palm: A planimetry study [Abstract]. *Proceedings of the American Burn Association Annual Meeting, 27*, 262.

Van den Kerckhove, E., Boeckx, W., & Kochuyt, A. (1991). Silicone patches as a supplement for pressure therapy to control hypertrophic scarring. *Journal of Burn Care and Rehabilitation, 12*, 361–369.

Wachtel, T. (1985). Epidemiology, classification, initial care, and administrative considerations for critically burned patients. In T. Wachtel (Ed.), *Critical care clinics* (pp. 3–26). Philadelphia: W. B. Saunders.

Ward, R. S. (1991) Pressure therapy for the control of hypertrophic scar formation after burn injury: A history and review. *Journal of Burn Care and Rehabilitation, 12*, 257–262.

Ward, R. S. (1993). Reasons for the selection of burn-scar-support suppliers by burn centers in the United States: A survey. *Journal of Burn Care and Rehabilitation, 14*, 360–367.

Watkins, P. N., Cook, E., May S. R., & Ehleben, C. M. (1988). Psychological stages in adaptation following burn injury: A method for facilitating psychological recovery of burn victims. *Journal of Burn Care and Rehabilitation, 9*, 376.

Weber, J. M. & Thompkins, D. M. (1993). Improving survival: Infection control and burns. *American Association Critical Nursing, 4*, 414–423.

Willis, B. (1970). The use of orthoplast isoprene splints in the treatment of the acutely burned child. *American Journal of Occupational Therapy, 24*, 187–191.

UNIT X
CLIENT APPLICATIONS

Betty Risteen Hasselkus

Evaluation and Treatment of Mr. R Using Two Theoretical Perspectives

Mr. R, the man with rheumatoid arthritis who was described in the narrative on pages 656–658, was referred to the home care team when he was 81 years old. In the Model of Human Occupation, it is a general therapeutic principle that therapy is an event that comes into a life that has both a history and a future that extend beyond the therapeutic experience. In Mr. R's situation, we, as team members, would be described as coming "into a life in progress" (Kielhofner, 1995, p. 253). In this model, appreciation of the life that has been lived before and that will be lived in the future should always be a part of the therapeutic process. This principle is imbedded in the concept of life as a narrative or story.

In the Model of Human Occupation, disease or injury are viewed as disruptions in a person's life story; when such disruptions occur, it is necessary to reorganize one's life into a new or modified story. The reorganization represents the healing process that is needed after illness or injury, enabling the individual to re-create meaningful new directions for the life that lies ahead. Therapy represents a process that facilitates the reorganization of the life story into a new plot (Kielhofner, 1995).

In the narrative in Chapter 35 at the beginning of this unit, I tried to enter Mr. R's life with an appreciation for his history and for the life that lay ahead of him. To enter a life that is in old age is very different from entering at other life stages. Mr R's history was long and rich with many life roles, experiences, and personal accomplishments. At 81 years old, Mr. R's future was likely to be short by comparison. With that in mind, the challenge for me, when working with this older person, was to fit occupational therapy into that long and rich life in a way that would facilitate a reorganization and meaningful continuation of his life narrative, for as long as that narrative lasted.

Perhaps the therapeutic activity that fit most powerfully with Mr. R's personal narrative was the development of the feature story for the monthly home care newsletter. In creating the story, Mr. R reconnected with his past and brought selected experiences from that past story into the present; in the process, he also connected with many other people through the sharing of that part of his history. Ideally, then, engagement in the newsletter story served to help restore a sense of wholeness to Mr. R's life narrative, a wholeness that had been disrupted by the rheumatoid arthritis. The newsletter activity provided a way to link the present with the past, and vice versa. The rheumatoid arthritis, in fact, served as a vehicle that brought Mr. R access to the newsletter because of his need for home health care. Up until that point in time, the disease had been linked only to giving up important parts of his life—the hunting, fishing, and bowling. Alternatively, in the development of the newsletter article, the disease provided the entreé to an occupation that helped reorganize his life in such a way that the past was not discarded; rather, it continued to offer meaning to the present.

Another principle of the Model of Human Occupation is the following: "The only tool which therapists have at their disposal is to change the relevant environment to support or precipitate a change in the human system" (Kielhofner, 1995, p. 261). Much of the occupational therapy focus with Mr. R was on modifying his environment. Examples are the assistive devices that became a part of his life space, such as the bathing equipment, magnifiers, medication dispenser, car door opener, and cane. In tandem with these environmental changes, the emphasis in therapy was on Mr. R's skills and functional performance, that is, his ability to get in and out of the bathtub, to take his medication independently, to continue to drive, to be able to do crossword puzzles and read. This is in contrast with other theoretical frameworks that focus on bringing about change in the underlying neurophysiological capacities of the mind–brain–body performance subsystem.

"The loss of roles and habits requires swift replacement" (Kielhofner, 1995, p. 264). This is a third principle in the Model of Human Occupation. Kielhofner likens a person's loss of roles and habits to the collapse of the scaffolding that holds up much of everyday life. Such losses can lead to strong emotional reactions and disorganization of a person's way of life. Mr. R's role losses were numerous, including the roles of hunter, fisherman, champion bowler, driver, and keeper of the financial records, to name only a few. He also experienced losses in his daily routines and habits as the arthritis gradually necessitated modifications and changes in the way he carried out his self-care and household activities. It is probable that Mr. R's depression was a reaction to these losses of roles and habits.

The assistive devices described in Chapter 35 served to help support Mr. R's continuation of familiar daily activities and routines. Participation in the arthritis swim program provided Mr. R with a new role and new routines as partial replacement for the losses. As the occupational therapist, I negotiated with Mr. R to help bring about this opportunity for a new social role. In this process of negotiation, I respected Mr. R's choice not to take part in former activities such as bowling, even in a modified way; he was clearly telling me that this previous highly valued activity was no longer desirable under the new conditions of his life. It was my challenge to provide the opportunity for replacements, ones that fit into the narrative of Mr. R's life—past, present, and future.

The occupational therapy engaged in with Mr. R might also be described within the Rehabilitation Frame of Reference. The strong emphasis in therapy with Mr. R on the maintenance of independent function in daily activities and the use of compensatory techniques and equipment to facilitate function are part of the philosophy and goals of rehabilitation. Within this framework, the changes in functional performance secondary to the rheumatoid arthritis are viewed as occupational dysfunction, for which compensatory methods are needed.

In my occupational therapy evaluation of Mr. R, I focused on monitoring his function in work, self-care, and leisure over time. I administered the Barthel Index at 6-month intervals to monitor Mr. R's functional performance in daily self-care activities (Hasselkus, 1982; Mahoney & Barthel, 1965). The Barthel Index is an evaluation of basic self-care and includes the following ten items: eating, transferring, toileting, ambulation, personal hygiene, bathing, dressing, going up and down stairs, and continence of bowel and bladder. Mr. R's score on referral to the home care team was 90, meaning he was independent in all self-care items except eating and bathing, for which he needed minimum assistance. At the time he was discharged from home care to nursing home care, his score had dropped to 45; Mr. R was wholly or partially dependent in all but toileting and bowel and bladder continence. The Barthel Index provided a systematic method of monitoring for changes in function; when changes were detected, compensatory techniques and equipment were introduced in an effort to restore previous levels of competence and independence or increase safety during the activity.

The Rehabilitation Frame of Reference is strongly associated with the biomedical view of health and illness. In the biomedical view, the human being is viewed as an organism made up of organ subsystems and physiological processes. One understands illness by understanding the pathologies represented in these subsystems and processes. Rheumatoid arthritis represents pathology in the musculoskeletal subsystem. As the occupational therapist, in addition to monitoring function as described earlier, I watched carefully for signs of periarticular changes in Mr. R's involved joints. I was especially attentive to his hands and wrists, examining him regularly for signs of active inflammation such as swelling, redness, fever, tendon or ligament damage, early deformities. I questioned him about the duration of his morning stiffness and about his level of pain. I taught him joint protection techniques to "protect" his joints from undue stress that might exacerbate the disease activity and put his joints in further jeopardy. I constructed a small splint to support the damaged IP joint of his thumb; I fitted Mr. R with a commercially available splint to put his right wrist at rest, thus helping to control the inflammation in the carpal joints.

All of this therapy was carried out within the context of medical management of the rheumatoid arthritis. I was part of Mr. R's medical management, along with the physician and pharmacist who also monitored the disease activity and regulated his medications, the nurse who monitored his general health, the physical therapist who evaluated and treated his gait and mobility problems, and the social worker who attended closely to the family needs. Although this was a very interdisciplinary team, and we all tried to be holistic in our approach to the home care clients, nevertheless, much of our activity was governed by the rehabilitation model, emphasizing the body systems and their pathologies. With Mr. R, the team focused strongly on the pathology of rheumatoid arthritis and the need for compensation in his daily life.

Occupational therapy with Mr. R, thus, represented more than one theoretical frame of reference. The Model of Human Occupation and the Rehabilitation Frame of Reference are both represented in the occupational therapy process that evolved with this older person. The two frameworks overlap and complement each other in several ways. Both emphasize function in activities of daily living. The Rehabilitation Framework also emphasizes the capacities that underly that function, those that are more at the level of the body organ subsystems and physiological processes. Both emphasize the importance of the environment as a modality that can be modified to enhance function; the Rehabilitation Framework refers to the environment as a source of compensation and the Model of Human Occupation refers to it more as a resource to support the reorganization of the person's narrative of life. Different forms of clinical reasoning seem to be emphasized in each framework. Procedural reasoning is evident in the rehabilitation framework, especially in the therapy that focused on the pathology of rheumatoid arthritis and in the therapeutic skills such as splint-making and teaching joint protection. Narrative reasoning fits well with the therapy that was guided by the principles of the Model of Human Occupation; conceptualizing Mr. R's life as a narrative and searching for ways to fit into that narrative and help with its reorganization led to the idea for the feature story in the newsletter. The swim program was the result of more narrative reasoning, but also conditional reasoning and interactive reasoning: as the therapist, I was able to imagine Mr. R in the new role of a swimmer and I reasoned together with him to create a shared view of him in that role.

Near the end of the story of Mr. R, conditional and interactive reasoning were strongly emphasized as the team worked together—with other community health workers, with Mrs. R, and with the rest of the family—to imagine what his future would be and then to agree on the appropriate plans to bring that future about. The move to a nursing home was another major disruption in Mr. R's life narrative. Perhaps his death two months later is testimony to the magnitude of the shattering effects of the move. For a person's life story must somehow maintain a wholeness and integrity to the end. Occupational therapy practitioners must continue to seek ways to make that possible.

References

Hasselkus, B. R. (1982). Barthel self-care index and geriatric home care patients. *Physical and Occupational Therapy in Geriatrics, 1*(4), 11–22.

Kielhofner, G. (1995). Change making: Principles of therapeutic intervention. In G. Kielhofner (Ed.), *A model of human occupation: Theory and application* (2nd ed.; pp. 251–270). Philadelphia: Williams & Wilkins.

Mahoney, F. & Barthel, D. (1965). Functional evaluations: The Barthel index. *Maryland State Medical Journal, 14*, 61–65.

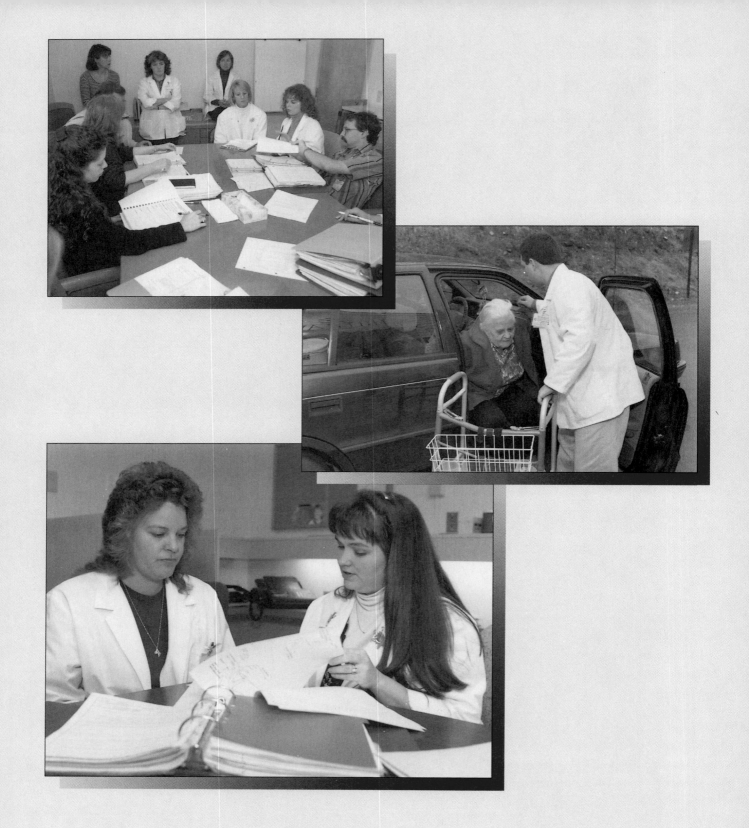

(top) Team meetings foster interdisciplinary collaboration; (middle) The ability to safely transfer in and out of a car is an essential aspect of community reentry; (bottom) Supervision and collaboration are important aspects of the role of occupational therapy practitioners (Photographs by Gary Samson, Instructional Services, Dimond Library, University of New Hampshire).

Unit XI

Environments for Practice

LEARNING OBJECTIVES

After completing this unit, readers will be able to:

▶ Explain how legislation and reimbursement mechanisms influence occupational therapy practice.

▶ Describe the differences between acute care, rehabilitation, and chronic or subacute care settings relative to goals, staff, documentation, reimbursement issues, and occupational therapy roles.

▶ Describe the differences between community-based settings in relation to goals, staff, clients, and occupational therapy roles.

▶ Discuss occupational therapy management issues relative to planning, budgeting, marketing, policies and procedures, productivity, clinical documentation, and quality assurance.

▶ Define and discuss communication relative to interdisciplinary teams, supervision of occupational therapy personnel, and fieldwork supervision.

The day-to-day practice of occupational therapy is influenced by administrative, reimbursement, and legislative issues. Federal legislation may constrain or expand practice opportunities. Third-party payers and their requirements control the availability of reimbursement of our services and shape our documentation. Occupational therapy department managers must be proactive in a rapidly changing health care environment that seems to be changing every day. The planning and supervisory functions of department managers enable occupational therapy practitioners to work effectively, despite the uncertainty that surrounds them. This unit reviews these issues and closes with two chapters that describe current occupational therapy practice settings. (*Note*: Words in **bold** type are defined in the Glossary.)

Chapter 42

Legislative and Reimbursement Influences on Occupational Therapy: Changing Opportunities

Diana M. Bailey

The principle that competition within a free market will lead to the most efficient provision and distribution of health care services guides the delivery of health care in the United States. The forces of supply and demand do not always allocate resources according to social need. This has led to government intervention in the form of market controls, reimbursement by **Medicare** and **Medicaid**, and direct provision of health care by federal programs, such as the Veterans Administration, and state-supported services, such as psychiatric hospitals and community mental health programs. This chapter will delineate the legislative and reimbursement changes in health care and the influence of these changes on the delivery of occupational therapy services.

▼ EVENTS SHAPING HEALTH CARE

Rapid improvement in medical care, rising costs leading to cost-containment measures, and the aging of the population have influenced health care and occupational therapy prac-

tice. The development of **neonatal intensive care units** has enabled premature babies to live, and many Americans survive serious accidents because of improved emergency care. Expansion of rehabilitation programs are a direct outcome of these medical advances.

Following the initial implementation of Medicare and Medicaid, pressure for more entitlements led to a dramatic rise in health care costs. This has led to increasingly frequent and urgent attempts at cost containment by federal legislators. For example, the Tax Equity and Fiscal Responsibility Act (TEFRA) of 1982 introduced cost caps and the 1983 Prospective Payment System dictated that only a preapproved dollar amount would be paid for each condition. Stringent cost containment has resulted in shorter hospital stays and a reduction in services provided in the hospital. Although **managed care** has recently been embraced as a cost-saving mechanism, Congress and President Clinton have tried to further tighten federal health care spending and to ensure that federal dollars are spent more effectively. Attempts continue as this book goes to print.

In 1970, 9.8% of the population was 65 years or older; by 1994 this percentage had increased to 12.8% (US Bureau of the Census, 1995, p. 15). The number of people aged 85 years and over is expected to increase by 40% this decade, and those 65 to 85 years will be the fastest-growing segment of the population for years to come (Health Care Financing Administration, 1994, p. 14). People over the age of 65 years have various chronic conditions and require more health care. Occupational therapy practitioners are particularly well prepared to work with this population because they can assist elders in maintaining their independence, despite chronic illness and age-related changes.

▼ LEGISLATION THAT HAS AFFECTED HEALTH CARE SERVICES

From the passage of the workers' compensation legislation in 1910 to Medicare and Medicaid, US legislative acts have changed the face of health care and have directly influenced the delivery of occupational therapy services.

Workers' Compensation Plans

Signed into law in 1910, the Workers' Compensation Plan was designed to cut down on court trial costs resulting from employee injuries at work. Today it also provides temporary income while the employee is out of work and encourages employers to take some responsibility for the safety of their employees. Plans are administered by the states. They pay for medical costs related to the injury, vocational rehabilitation, and weekly compensation. Occupational therapists are qualified care providers under most state workers' compensation laws. Many of these laws have utilization guidelines for each diagnosis to which care providers must adhere.

Medicare

As passed in 1965, Medicare provides health care coverage for persons 65 years and older, people on kidney dialysis, and people receiving social security because of disabilities (SSDI). At that time, Medicare paid for inpatient care at reasonable cost. It was based on a retrospective payment system, meaning that any service deemed necessary was provided, then billed and reimbursed. Costs soon escalated because no controls on the type and quantity of services provided to individuals existed. Medicare is now the largest single health care expense in the United States, and Medicare recipients make up the largest group of clients seen by occupational therapy practitioners.

Medicare has two parts: Part A covers inpatient care in hospitals and skilled nursing facilities, home health, and hospice care; Part B covers outpatient services, long-term care in skilled nursing facilities, and assistive devices. In 1987,

legislative changes made in Part B allow occupational, physical, and speech therapists to join physicians as the only providers able to bill Medicare as independent providers.

Medicaid

Medicaid began in 1967 as a stepchild to Medicare, to provide health care for women and children receiving Aid to Families with Dependent Children (AFDC). It is a matched program—every 200,000 dollars a state spends is matched with 100,000 dollars of federal money. States administer the program. Some are more generous in their Medicaid programs than others. Coverage for occupational therapy varies from state to state. In some states, occupational therapists can obtain a provider number and independently bill Medicaid for services.

Other recipients were soon added to the Medicaid program: the disabled, the blind, and the poor elderly. Although originally few, these groups have increased so that as of 1994, 75% of Medicaid was spent providing for their health care needs (US Bureau of the Census, 1995, p. 116). Nursing home care for the poor elderly accounts for 47% of Medicaid expenditures (Dorgan, 1995, p. 170). Medicaid is now the second largest health care expense in the United States.

Section 223, Medicare Amendments, 1972

In 1972, in response to rapidly rising costs, Congress made major revisions in Medicare (Somers & Somers, 1972). These revisions included limits on charges for certain inpatient services, most notably nursing services. Commonly called the Section 223 limits, these changes were contained in Section 223 of Public Law 92–603, the Medicare Amendments of 1972. They set the stage for subsequent cost caps on most patient care provided in hospitals, including occupational therapy.

Tax Equity and Fiscal Responsibility Act

Despite the Section 223 limits, between 1971 and 1982 health care costs rose approximately 390%, far more than the general inflation rate of approximately 240% (Dorgan, 1995, pp. 402–403). A succession of regulatory policies was introduced in an attempt to contain costs. The Tax Equity and Fiscal Responsibility (TEFRA) Act of 1982 (Public Law 97–248) introduced new limits on payment for hospital costs, by establishing limits on a per case, rather than on a per diem basis. Occupational therapy services were often included in the per case rate. TEFRA adjusted each hospital's reimbursement limit to reflect its mix of cases and clinical problems and provided hospitals with financial incentives when they spent less than their limit. Hospitals eliminated services perceived to be less essential as a way to limit their costs. Occupational therapy was sometimes seen as a nonessential service. Most significantly, TEFRA mandated the development of a legislative proposal for a prospective payment system for Medicare.

Prospective Payment System

When Medicare was introduced in 1965, health costs amounted to 6% of the Gross National Product; in 1982 that percentage was 10.4% (Dorgan, 1995, p. 327). At that rate, the Medicare Trust Fund would have been insolvent by 1990 (Primus, 1982). Clearly, something had to be done. Thus, in 1983, the Prospective Payment System (PPS) was introduced (under the Medicare Prospective Payment Law, Public Law 98–21). Touted as the ultimate method for cost containment, PPS completely overhauled Medicare. Services previously reimbursed by a retrospective method (in which services were provided first and billed later) were now reimbursed prospectively by preestablished rates. That is, hospitals are paid per admission according to the rates for each of 471 diagnosis-related groups (DRGs). These rates are based on type and amount of treatment needed for each diagnosis. They also consider regional variability in cost and include an allowance for teaching hospitals. The hospital is reimbursed this fee regardless of the actual costs incurred in treating a particular individual. Consequently, it is in the hospital's financial interest to keep the costs incurred within the established rate. Certain facilities, such as psychiatric hospitals, children's hospitals, and freestanding rehabilitation hospitals, are currently exempt from the Medicare prospective payment system. However, they are similarly affected, because most other third-party payers demand data that show the cost effectiveness of treatment and many have adopted payment rates similar to the DRGs. Because most occupational therapy practitioners work in exempt facilities, it has taken longer for them to feel the consequences of the PPS. More recently, occupational therapy practice has changed as cost-containment measures spread from PPS to other forms of health care coverage.

The PPS has been directly responsible for shortened hospitalizations. In 1984, the first full year of the PPS, the length of stay for Medicare patients dropped 9%, the single largest drop in its 20-year history (Dorgan, 1995, p. 437). Length of stay has been shortening ever since. This means that patients are often not ready to receive occupational therapy before they are discharged, making it a service more appropriately provided at home or in community-based facilities. The result has been an exodus of practitioners from acute inpatient settings into home health care and facilities such as rehabilitation hospitals, subacute units, and transitional care units.

Surprisingly, fewer people have been admitted to hospitals because of the PPS. In 1984, Medicare admissions dropped 3.5%, marking the first admissions decline in Medicare's history (Dorgan, 1995, p. 437). Hospital occupancy fell from 72.6% in 1983 (the year the PPS was introduced) to 67.1% in 1984 and to 63.6% in 1985 (Pew Health Professions Commission, 1993, p. 83). The Health Care Financing Administration, the agency responsible for administering the PPS, expects that the PPS will eventually close one of every six US hospital beds. The closing and downsizing of hospitals have contributed to the move of rehabilitation professionals to community health care facilities.

Health Maintenance Organization Act and Managed Care

Although managed care plans were in place during the 1940s, expansion of this type of health program was slow until the passage of the **Health Maintenance Organization (HMO)** Act of 1973. This act provided financial incentives for the development of the HMO type of managed care plan. Soon after, a variety of new ways to deliver health care services were developed using the concepts of managed care. Today, an estimated 75 million Americans are in some type of managed care plan, up from 15 million in 1984 (Dorgan, 1995, p. 514). The Pew Health Professions Commission estimates that up to 90% of Americans will receive health care through some form of managed care by 2005 (1993, p. 71). This rapid rise is due to more people enrolling in HMOs and **Preferred Provider Organizations (PPOs)**, and to a move by government insurers toward managed care systems. For example, some states now take a managed care approach to administer their Medicaid programs. Today, consumers must choose among complex managed care plans and consider such things as coverage, cost, ability to select providers, and access to providers.

Managed care is the term used for programs that seek to control the patients' use of physicians and other health care providers and services. Managed care systems integrate the financing and delivery of health care services. All such programs have the common goal of reducing health care expenditures while maintaining the quality of care. Participants prepay for their care with an organization such as an HMO or a PPO, and the payment covers all the services they receive with few deductibles and no hidden costs. Each member has a primary care physician who coordinates all of the member's care and refers him or her to specialists within the network of providers in the organization. Typically, a utilization reviewer must approve care by specialists and nonemergency hospital admissions.

Occupational therapy practitioners have been slow to join managed care networks, yet it is crucial that they do so because of the many people who receive their health care from these programs. The challenges to practitioners include the following: (1) consistently achieving expected functional outcomes at or before the patient's maximum length of stay; (2) ensuring that the functional outcome is durable over time and does not require additional intervention; (3) defining critical pathways (typical expected course of treatment leading to a specific outcome for a particular diagnosis); and (4) identifying difficult or exceptional cases early (Foto, 1995). Because of these managed care requirements, outcomes research is essential for the profession (Ellenberg, 1996; Rogers & Salta, 1994).

Omnibus Budget Reconciliation Acts of 1987 and 1990

The Omnibus Budget Reconciliation Acts (OBRA) of 1987 and 1990 have had the largest influence on the long-term care industry since the inception of Medicare. These new requirements have turned long-term care into one of the most highly regulated industries in the United States and have forced the industry to reevaluate its environmental conditions and caregiving practices. OBRA emphasizes the individual rights, autonomy, and quality of life of nursing home residents. Its goals include more and better qualified staff, humanistic and individualized care, and elimination of physical and chemical restraints. Recognition of residents' rights, including free choice, privacy, confidentiality, visitation, work, self-administration of drugs, and the rights of married couples are important aspects of OBRA (Goldman, 1995). OBRA mandates formal occupational therapy screenings for all residents annually and informal screenings once per quarter. Requirements for occupational therapists entail consultation with staff on issues such as positioning, eating, and freedom from restraint, and consultation with activities directors relative to the activities program in the facility.

The Americans With Disabilities Act (ADA)

Although the aim of the **ADA** of 1990 was not cost control, no list of laws having an effect on occupational therapy would be complete without it. The ADA is a civil rights law intended to bring men, women, and children with disabilities into the mainstream of American life. It was enacted because of pressure from people with disabilities and their advocates. Its main thrust is to alter society's attitudes toward people with disabilities. Title I of the act addresses employment discrimination and reasonable accommodations within the work setting. Title II addresses access to public services (including transportation), programs, and facilities under the administration of state and local governments. Title III requires all public accommodations and services operated by private entities to be accessible to persons with disabilities. Title IV addresses telecommunications and devices for persons with speech or hearing impairments. The law has provided many consultative opportunities for occupational therapists to help local public authorities and private business owners accommodate persons with disabilities.

Recent Health Care Reform Proposals

The health care industry is reshaping itself in the face of managed care, massive cost-cutting, privatization of services,

and hospital mergers and closings. In 1993 and 1994, President Clinton and various members of Congress made a series of legislative proposals to address major issues in the health care system. Unfortunately, most of these proposals were not passed into law and the issues remain largely unresolved. These include access to care, universal coverage, comprehensive benefits, prevention, and financing.

ACCESSIBILITY

In 1994, over 37 million Americans were uninsured and, therefore, had no access to covered health care (Pew Health Professions Commission, 1995, p. 5). About 50 million people are underinsured (Richmond & Fein, 1995, p. 69); consequently, their health care needs are only partially covered (Harrington, Cassel, Estes, Woolhandler, & Himmelstein, 1991; Saltman, 1992; Schramm, 1991). The Clinton health care plan proposed that all Americans should have free access to health care services.

UNIVERSAL COVERAGE

The current system is multitiered, resulting in different degrees and types of care for different people. Over the past 5 years, approximately 63 million people have lost their health insurance when they changed jobs (Richmond & Fein, 1995, p. 69). In August 1996 President Clinton signed the Kassenbaum–Kennedy bill that created portable health insurance for workers who change jobs and imposed limits on denial for preexisting conditions. Despite this legislation, President Clinton's goal of universal coverage for all Americans still has not been achieved.

COMPREHENSIVE BENEFITS

Many insurance programs do not cover all needed services, such as mental health, long-term care, home care, hospice, vision, dental, medications, and assistive devices. A comprehensive minimum benefits package for all has been recommended.

PREVENTION

Some health care plans, notably HMOs, are better at providing coverage for prevention than others. All health care providers must be concerned with prevention as well as intervention, and reimbursement mechanisms for preventive care should be included in all insurance programs.

FINANCING

A hodgepodge of private and public agencies funded by a mix of taxes, individual out-of-pocket payments, and employee or employer payments finance health care. Recent bills have proposed a single-payor system in which consumers would be taxed and a central agency would administer the entire health care program. Despite protracted debate, Congress did not enact a comprehensive reform bill for health care financing.

▼ ORIENTATION TO HEALTH CARE REIMBURSEMENT STRUCTURE

The reimbursement structure is changing as fast as changes in the provision of health care services. Reimbursement mechanisms for occupational therapy are no exception. Studying current reimbursement methods can lead to a general understanding of policy that will form a foundation for understanding the changes that will continue to evolve. Reimbursement mechanisms beyond the publicly funded Medicare and Medicaid include (1) traditional indemnity insurance, (2) health maintenance organizations, and (3) preferred provider organizations.

Indemnity Insurance Plans

These are the health insurance plans offered by freestanding insurance companies that have operated under the "old" rules of retrospective reimbursement. Consumers, either as individuals or as part of a group through their employer, pay a premium to the insurance company for a specified set of benefits. Consumers may visit any providers they wish. These providers bill the insurance company after services have been rendered. In the past, there were few, if any, checks on whether the services were necessary or of acceptable quality.

This system of unchecked retrospective reimbursement led in large part to enormous cost increases for health care. Now, many indemnity plans include some managed care elements, such as requiring a utilization reviewer to verify that hospitalization and certain procedures are necessary.

Health Maintenance Organizations

The nation's 550 HMOs are both insurers and providers of care. Consumers pay a flat fee to the HMO to cover all services and then must receive those services from providers at that HMO. HMOs provide each consumer with a primary care physician who manages the consumer's care within the HMO. Built-in aspects of HMO services include quality control and utilization review.

There are two main structural models for HMOs: the staff model and the individual practice association (IPA). In the staff model, the HMO is freestanding and owns its own hospital, pharmacy, and other service organizations. The HMO hires all personnel, including physicians, as staff members. In contrast, HMOs using the individual practice association model, create a network of services including contracted hospital beds, existing group practices, and individual providers. Occupational therapists are gradually being hired by staff model HMOs, while therapists in private practice are contracting with IPAs to provide occupational therapy services (VanDeusen, 1995).

Employers and employees join HMOs to cut their own costs. In 1992, employers paid 23.2% less per employee for HMO coverage than for traditional indemnity plans (Dorgan, 1995, p. 260). Individuals typically pay lower monthly fees and little or nothing when they visit providers for services.

Preferred Provider Organizations

A form of managed care, a PPO is a network of providers who compete to provide services to members of an existing group (such as an employed group receiving care from an HMO) for a fixed monthly amount. They give a discount to the group (usually through the employer) to encourage them to buy health services from the PPO. PPOs operate on a capitation system, under which members pay a fixed monthly amount, determined by the number of members in the group and the services they are estimated to need. The network negotiates a contract with employers to provide a given package of services to a guaranteed number of employees. Consumers can go to other providers, but must pay an additional fee to do so, the provider within the PPO network is the "preferred provider." Quality assurance and utilization review mechanisms are built into the network.

▼ COMPARISON WITH HEALTH CARE IN OTHER COUNTRIES

Passage of the Medicare and Medicaid Acts is considered by some as the most significant contribution to health care policy in the United States. They were landmarks in paying for basic health care for Americans over 65 and the medically indigent. This legislation, in combination with existing private health insurance plans that evolved during the Great Depression and World War II, has resulted in a health care system dominated by third-party reimbursement, both public and private. In contrast, the governments of other countries organize health care delivery and finance it through taxation.

For instance, the British National Health Service (NHS), the world's first comprehensive government health care system, provides most health services free of charge to all British subjects and legal residents. Services not provided free, such as medication and dentistry, are provided for a fee that is lower than actual cost. The recipient's ability to pay does not restrict access to services. Despite universal coverage, only 6% of Britain's Gross Domestic Product is spent on health care, compared with an estimated 14% in the United States (Dorgan, 1995, p. 923), whereas mortality and morbidity levels are the same or better (Dorgan, 1995, pp. 936–937). Much of this difference is accounted for by lower administrative and legal costs.

Canada provides another distinct contrast to the United States in national health policy (Redelmeier & Fuchs, 1993). For almost half a century, Canada has enjoyed a publicly funded health system funded primarily through taxation. Canada's constitution gives its ten provinces and two territories jurisdiction over health and social services. The constitution gives the federal government the power to influence health priorities by placing conditions on cost-sharing agreements and through its authority to collect taxes (Quinn, 1993). The Canadian health care system may be characterized as comprehensive, universal, accessible, portable, and publicly administered. Yet, unlike the British system, Canada does not have socialized medicine: 95% of physicians are self-employed, and 90% of hospitals are private, nonprofit organizations (Dorgan, 1995, p. 947).

Field's (1989) typology of health care systems describes the health care system of the United States as pluralistic. The term system is misleading, however, because diversity in funding and service provision has resulted in what may be better described as a conglomerate of health care subsystems—or as a nonsystem. Opponents of US health care delivery criticize it as chaotic, uncoordinated, and overlapping, and point to inequities in access for consumers and treatment standards (Fackelman, 1986; Richmond & Fein, 1995). The complexity of the system has also produced high administrative costs.

▼ DELIVERY OF OCCUPATIONAL THERAPY SERVICES

The traditional role of occupational therapy practitioners, that of evaluation and treatment, continues in rehabilitation hospitals, schools, skilled nursing facilities, adult day care, partial hospitalization, clients' homes, outpatient facilities and, to a lesser extent, in acute care hospitals. Occupational therapy practitioners work increasingly in subacute and transitional care units, new types of facilities that provide rehabilitations services at a lower cost than acute care or rehabilitation hospitals. Although most practitioners still provide direct treatment, new roles are available because of changes in legislation and reimbursement mechanisms. Some of these include consultation, private practice, quality assurance, and case coordination.

Movement to Subacute and Transitional Care Units

Insurers now favor subacute care and transitional care, less medically intensive and, therefore, less costly alternatives to acute hospital care. For example, during 1995 in Massachusetts 27 such units opened and 40 more are being planned (Somers, Pontzer, & Metzler, 1996, p. 141). Transitional care units are usually found in converted units of local acute care hospitals, whereas subacute units are more often found in skilled nursing facilities or sometimes in rehabilitation hospitals.

Transitional care units and subacute units both provide less intensive therapy than that provided in rehabilitation hospitals

because their patients are more acutely ill. Units often specialize in a specific disability, such as hip replacement, and provide a place following acute hospitalization where patients can recover from surgery and prepare to go home. Because insurers consider rehabilitation services essential for discharge, these as well as other necessary care, are reimbursed.

The Consultative Role

Opportunities for occupational therapy practitioners to consult to schools, businesses, public agencies, and nursing homes continue to expand. Although **PL 94–142** mandated that all children, including those with disabilities, were entitled to a public education, **IDEA (PL 101–476)** has led to a new understanding of the concept of "inclusion." This has prompted many occupational therapy practitioners to take a consulting role in public schools to ensure that children with disabilities are fully included in the life of the school (See Chap. 27 in this volume for a discussion of IDEA and PL 94–142). Because of ADA, practitioners also have new opportunities to consult with local authorities on such issues as transportation, recreation, and adult education. They also can help towns, other government agencies, and businesses to provide accessibility for people with disabilities.

In long-term care, the OBRA requires occupational therapy consultation in skilled nursing facilities. Additionally, occupational therapy practitioners have found opportunities to consult to psychiatric hospitals, nursing homes, and home care companies, among others. Because of rapidly changing methods for delivering health care services, these facilities are seeking help in deciding where and how to fit occupational therapy into their spectrum of services.

Private Practice

With legislation enabling occupational therapists to bill third-party payers, particularly Medicare and Medicaid, the number of therapists opening their own private practices burgeoned in the late 1980s and early 1990s. These practices are typically freestanding corporations in which therapists obtain provider numbers and bill Medicare and Medicaid directly for their services. Numbers of private practices peaked around 1994 and have begun to decline because of the move to managed care and the different strategies needed for doing business with HMOs and PPOs (Landry & Knox, 1996). However, some entrepreneurial occupational therapists are now developing contracts with managed care companies. It is possible that private practices may flourish again (Foto, 1995).

To gain contracts with HMOs and PPOs, occupational therapists must be an integral part of a chain of services, because the managed care company needs to buy a spectrum of services for them to be cost effective. Consequently, many occupational therapy private practitioners aim to write affiliation agreements with other care providers to become part of a service network large enough to provide services for a managed care company.

Over the past five to ten years while freestanding private practices were developing, many other occupational therapists became independent contractors. These therapists contract individually or as groups to provide occupational therapy services on a per diem basis in agencies such as schools, nursing homes, skilled nursing facilities, and community or neighborhood facilities for elders or people with disabilities. Therapists find this work appealing because of the variety of the clients on their caseload and the flexibility of work hours.

Changes in Psychiatric Care

Changes in insurance coverage have also resulted in shortened stay—or no inpatient treatment at all—for people with mental illness. Services, instead, concentrate on very short-term hospitalization and follow-up care in the community. Occupational therapy practitioners have been slow to move into community mental health settings, yet will need to do so if they are to remain viable members of rehabilitation teams in psychiatry (Van Leit, 1996). Because administrators of **community mental health programs** are still unfamiliar with the services occupational therapy practitioners offer, they have not created occupational therapy positions in these programs. Some practitioners have created jobs for themselves by educating employers in partial hospitalization programs, mobile treatment teams, day treatment centers, homeless shelters, clubhouse model programs, community residences, and sheltered workshops. It is generally not cost-effective to hire occupational therapy practitioners solely for direct treatment in these settings because neither the clients nor the facilities where they receive services tend to be eligible for insurance coverage. The community-based practitioner's primary role is consultative, providing needs assessment and program development.

Quality Assurance and Case Coordination

Because of requirements from the Joint Commission on the Accreditation of Health Organizations, the Commission on the Accreditation of Rehabilitation Facilities and managed care companies, quality assurance and coordination of client care are playing a more important part in service delivery. Occupational therapists are well qualified to take these positions and are doing so in increasing numbers.

▼ CHALLENGES TO OCCUPATIONAL THERAPY PRACTITIONERS IN AN EVER-CHANGING HEALTH CARE ENVIRONMENT

Health care legislation, the multitiered health care system, and the changing demographics of the US population have influenced the practice of occupational therapy in several ways.

Some challenges to practitioners include working with clients who are older, adapting to new service delivery locations, increased intensity of rehabilitation, and threats to practitioners' professional autonomy and traditional belief system.

Aging Population

The American population is growing older, which means that many of our clients are older adults. Because Medicare or Medicaid pays for most older people's health care, practitioners need to have a clear understanding of how these methods of insurance work and how to obtain the best possible care for the client. The adoption of the PPS by Medicare has led to shortened hospital stays. Consequently, hospital-based occupational therapy services are now delivered to only acutely ill patients. Occupational therapy continues in rehabilitative, subacute, outpatient or in-home settings. Care in these settings is covered by Medicare for clients who meet certain criteria. Occupational therapy practitioners must know the requirements for coverage at each level of care so that appropriate and reimbursable services are provided to meet clients' needs (Howard, 1991).

A top priority for the health care team is feeling confident that the older client will be safe after returning home. Because occupational therapy practitioners are knowledgeable about function and safety issues, their expertise is especially important in discharge planning. Treatment in inpatient settings focuses on assuring that safety needs are adequately met before discharge. In contrast, outpatient and home-based services focus on aspects of therapy such as cooking, shopping, and self-care skills. These were formerly addressed in the hospital.

Changes in Location of Occupational Therapy Services

Medicare's PPS and DRG mandates have led to greatly reduced lengths of stay in acute care hospitals. Consequently, inpatients often do not have time to reach the point in their recovery at which they can benefit from occupational therapy. This has resulted in a dramatic exodus of practitioners from acute care hospitals into rehabilitation hospitals, subacute facilities, transitional care units, and home health care agencies. Many feel that this change has been auspicious because our major treatment role is rehabilitative, and we can perform this role for our clients best in rehabilitation settings and even more beneficially in the clients' own homes.

How an insurance policy is written can also influence where clients receive their care. Because of reimbursement criteria day surgery is now common for many operations. Psychiatric clients receive treatment in community settings, such as day treatment programs, rather than as inpatients. Clients, who have been treated by occupational therapy practitioners in a particular setting in the past, may no longer be reimbursed for care in that setting.

Increased Intensity of Rehabilitation

With the introduction of DRGs and critical pathways, reimbursement is now based on an established number of inpatient days per diagnosis. This reimbursement rate assumes the provision of certain treatments and services. For hospitals to meet the goals of critical pathways, some provide rehabilitation services 7 days a week. This means that rehabilitation can begin when the client is admitted and that weekends are now used for treatment.

Intensity of treatment may also be affected when private practitioners contract with HMOs or PPOs. Managed care plans usually cover only short-term rehabilitation, typically 2 months with 30 to 36 visits, so occupational therapy must be offered frequently throughout a short time span. If a longer period of treatment is needed, it must be justified during a case review.

Threats to Professional Autonomy

Occupational therapy practitioners have fought and continue to strive for autonomy within the health care system. An ongoing challenge to this autonomy is our dependency on physicians for client referrals. This is especially true in medical model settings. However, the spread of HMOs threatens the professional autonomy of all health care providers from physicians who previously enjoyed almost complete autonomy to rehabilitation personnel. This threat is posed by a transfer of clinical decision-making power from health care service providers to case managers in insurance companies. Case managers are the gatekeepers to further services and require prior approval for many procedures and interventions.

Although the extent to which managed care will affect occupational therapy practitioners' independence is not yet clear, there are indications that the repercussions will be profound. Productivity quotas, reduced choices for reimbursable treatment methods, and standardized documentation, all reduce the self-determination of practice, as well as placing enormous personal pressure on practitioners. To some practitioners, the need to generate an expected number of treatment units per day to keep their employers financially solvent seems to supersede clients' needs (Burke & Cassidy, 1991; Howard, 1991).

Conflicts with Occupational Therapy Practitioners' Expectations for Care

There has been considerable fallout from cost-containment measures on the manner in which occupational therapy is practiced. Practitioners have had to rethink previously stated principles about their services—where services are offered, under what conditions the services are provided, who delivers the services, and who receives them (Brayman, 1996). The recent drive for cross-training and for multiskilled providers (Foto, 1996) are two examples of the push for cost-effective therapy. Typically, the conflicts resulting from differences between practitioners' notions of what makes good treatment and expectations from cost-containment efforts raise not only pragmatic questions, but ethical ones. Practitioners feel that their traditional **fiduciary** relation with the client has been compromised by their recently added role of "gatekeeper" to services. They have also expressed concern that administrators increasingly influence clinical decisions based on financial and reimbursement considerations—decisions that used to be made by clinicians (Burke & Cassidy, 1991).

The market-driven health care system in the United States has always required practitioners to adapt their services to survive and to meet the changing demands of the marketplace. Recently, pressure from insurers to treat clients and predict outcomes according to protocols and diagnoses has resulted in extreme conflict for occupational therapy practitioners whose approach is humanistic and individualized (Abreu, 1996; Peloquin, 1993). A similar conflict has arisen because of incentives within the market to specialize in treating one part of a disability and to abandon the professions' holistic approach to client treatment (Burke & Cassidy, 1991). These two pressures have resulted in whole areas of unmet client needs, a situation most practitioners find distressing.

▶CONCLUSION: NEW OPPORTUNITIES FOR OCCUPATIONAL THERAPY PRACTITIONERS

In reaction to conflicts with the basic belief system of occupational therapy practitioners, some have suggested that practitioners cease compromising the tenets of their profession and look for practice settings outside the insurance-driven health care system (Kornblau, 1995; Scott, 1995). Others view these developments as opportunities for growth, encouraging practitioners to be creative and proactive in marketing their skills, so that they become important service providers within the evolving system (Christiansen, 1996; Foto, 1995; Rosenfeld, 1990).

Whichever path individuals choose, many challenging new opportunities exist. Occupational therapists can become medical case managers or serve as expert witnesses in ADA, Social Security, disability, personal injury, or medical record review cases. They can explore self-employment options, such as home assessments paid for privately by the families of elders or persons with disabilities. They can develop consumer-financed wellness and prevention classes, or programs such as stress management, relaxation, time management, or smoking cessation (Sorensen, 1996). Occupational therapy practitioners may operate children's activities centers or they may develop partnerships in the work place as "productivity enhancers," facilitating an employee's return to or reassignment at work (Kornblau, 1995; Scott, 1995). Today's fast-paced and rapidly changing health market is a challenge. Occupational therapy practitioners will need to continually reassess and adapt to remain vital health care providers.

▼ REFERENCES

Abreu, B. C. (1996). Occupational therapy in a managed care environment. *American Journal of Occupational Therapy, 50*, 407–408.

Brayman, S. J. (1996). Managing the occupational environment of managed care. *American Journal of Occupational Therapy, 50*, 442–446.

Burke, J. P. & Cassidy, J. C. (1991). Disparity between reimbursement-driven practice and humanistic values of occupational therapy. *American Journal of Occupational Therapy, 45*, 173–176.

Christiansen, C. (1996). Managed care: Opportunities and challenges for occupational therapy in the emerging systems of the 21st century. *American Journal of Occupational Therapy, 50*, 409–412.

Dorgan, C. A. (1995). *Statistical record of health and medicine.* Detroit, MI: Gale Research.

Ellenberg, D. B. (1996). Outcomes research: The history, debate, and implications for the field of occupational therapy. *American Journal of Occupational Therapy, 50*, 435–441.

Fackelman, K. A. (1986, Oct. 20). A fragmented mental health system. *Medicine and Health* (Suppl. *Medicine and Health Perspectives*), pp. 1–4.

Field, M. G. (Ed.). (1989). *Success and crisis in national health systems: A comparative approach.* New York: Routledge.

Foto, M. (1995). [Nationally speaking] New president's address: The future—challenges, choices, and changes. *American Journal of Occupational Therapy, 49*, 955–959.

Foto, M. (1996). [Nationally speaking] Multiskilling: Who, how, when, and why? *American Journal of Occupational Therapy, 50*, 7–9.

Goldman, B. (1995). Omnibus Budget Reconciliation Act. In D. Bailey & S. Schwartzberg (Eds.), *Ethical and legal dilemmas in occupational therapy* (pp. 113–130). Philadelphia: F. A. Davis.

Harrington, C., Cassel, C., Estes, C., Woolhandler, S., & Himmelstein, D. U. (1991). Caring for the uninsured and underinsured: A national long-term care program for the United States. *Journal of the American Medical Association, 266*, 3023–3028.

Health Care Financing Administration. (1994). *The acute-care hospital industry: Recommendations for 1995 and beyond.* Author.

Howard, B. S. (1991). How high do we jump? The effect of reimbursement on occupational therapy. *American Journal of Occupational Therapy, 45*, 875–880.

Kornblau, B. (1995). *Creating new practice areas in an age of health care reform.* 13th Annual Great Southern Occupational Therapy Conference, Little Rock, AR. November 2–4.

Landry, C. & Knox, J. (1996). Managed care fundamentals: Implications for health care organizations and health care professionals. *American Journal of Occupational Therapy, 50*, 413–416.

Peloquin, S. M. (1993). The patient–therapist relationship: Beliefs that shape care. *American Journal of Occupational Therapy, 47*, 935–942.

Pew Health Professions Commission. (1993). *Health professions education for the future: Schools in service to the nation.* San Francisco: Author.

Pew Health Professions Commission. (1995). *The future of allied health: Perspectives from the field.* San Francisco: Author.

Primus, W. E. (1982). Financing Medicare through 1995. *National Journal, 14*, 789–793.

Quinn, B. (1993). Community occupational therapy in Canada. *AOTA Mental Health Special Interest Section Newsletter, 16*(2), 1–4.

Redelmeier, D. A. & Fuchs, V. R. (1993). Hospital expenditures in the United States and Canada. *New England Journal of Medicine, 328*, 772–778.

Richmond, J. B. & Fein, R. (1995). The health care mess: A bit of history. *Journal of the American Medical Association, 273*, 69–71.

Rogers, J. C. & Salta, J. E. (1994). [Case report]. Documenting functional outcomes. *American Journal of Occupational Therapy, 48*, 939–945.

Rosenfeld, M. S. (1990). A mid-career perspective of mental health practice. *Occupational Therapy in Mental Health, 10*, 47–61.

Saltman, R. B. (1992). Caring for the uninsured and the under-insured. Single source financing systems: A solution for the United States? *Journal of the American Medical Association, 268*, 774–779.

Schramm, C. (1991). Caring for the uninsured and the under-insured. Health care financing for all Americans. *Journal of the American Medical Association, 265*, 3296–3299.

Scott, P. (1995). *Creating new practice areas in an age of health care reform.* 13th Annual Great Southern Occupational Therapy Conference, Little Rock, AR. November 2–4.

Somers, F., Pontzer, K., & Metzler, C. (1996). *National policy forum.* AOTA's Annual Conference and Exposition, Chicago, IL. April 19–23.

Somers, H. R. & Somers, A. R. (1972). Major issues in national health insurance. *Millbank Memorial Fund Quarterly, 1*, 177–210.

Sorensen, J. (1996). These ladies turn trial into triumph. *Advance for Occupational Therapists, 12*, 4.

U.S. Bureau of the Census. (1995). *Statistical abstract of the U.S.: 1995* (115th ed.). Washington DC: Author.

VanDeusen, J. (1995). What is the role of occupational therapy in managed care? *American Journal of Occupational Therapy, 49*, 833–834.

Van Leit, B. (1996). Managed mental health care: Reflections in a time of turmoil. *American Journal of Occupational Therapy, 50*, 428–434.

Chapter 43

Management of Occupational Therapy Services

Judith M. Perinchief

M anagement in health care, from the organizational level to the department level, is increasingly important because of recent trends in cost containment, quality assurance, and competition. Administration is defined as the management of institutional affairs. Organization is defined as a body of people organized for the attainment of a specific goal. In this context, the organizational environment must be conducive to assisting people reach and maintain their maximum potential. The director of an occupational therapy department engages in management of the resources of the department, these include the staff that work in the department, supervision of their work, as well as overseeing the planning, documentation, and fiscal functions of the department.

▼ MANAGERIAL FUNCTIONS

The key to effective management is understanding what organizational behavior is all about, understanding styles and philosophies of management, and selecting those with whom one feels most comfortable. Historically managers have had designated functions, primarily planning, organizing, directing, controlling, and evaluating. All administrative aspects of the managers job fall into one of these categories.

Organizing

The managers role as an organizer encompasses activities aimed at creating and maintaining a formal structure for accomplishing tasks within a system. Professional management developed early in the 1900s. Between 1935 and 1955 the

"science" of management began to develop. In health care, integrated hospital care grew, and practitioners focused their activity on the hospital setting. Things began to be measured and counted. During this period the pressure of World War II was very influential on medical organization and the delivery of care. The systems movement of the period from 1955 to 1970 created the expectation that the health care system would deliver limitless quality care. Organizational structures stressed accountability, and planning processes became formalized during this period. In the 1970s networking took on greater importance, as regulation took a firmer hold on the health care industry. It was during this period that for-profit health care systems began to develop. During the 1980s high technology, costs, and expectations drove change in the health care industry. Managers began to downsize operations and build management teams to contend with the demand for more rapid decision making. Internal conflict within organizations increased in an attempt to determine managerial direction, to increase bureaucratic control, or to open the decision-making process to more people. This caused stress on the managers and tested the organizational ability to implement change. In the 1990s economic competition has continued to affect managerial practices. Focused management teams have replaced more traditional management structures. Managers today must be willing to take risks and must have a vision for the future, for it is through their leadership that the organization will founder or flourish.

MANAGEMENT PRINCIPLES

Over the years, a variety of principles and styles of management have evolved. Studies of organizations and managers have identified that no one style or theory is the definitive or correct way to manage an organization. A manager will work with the style that is most comfortable and protective for that manager in the given environment. Different environments and situations call for different approaches on the part of a manager. Therefore, it is important for managers to recognize their capabilities as they consider their management style.

The factors that affect a management style include the environment in which the individual manages, the beliefs and value system of the manager, the personality characteristics of the individual manager, and an element of chance. Management styles are not fixed. They are subject to modification through formal education or self-training and in response to environmental change.

Managerial Grid

The Managerial Grid (Blake & Mouton, 1964) is a theory of managerial behavior based on degrees of concern for people and concern for production. Attitudes that demonstrate concern for people include the amount of attention ascribed to accountability, self-esteem, the degree of personal commitment to completing a job, the establishment and maintenance of working conditions, the importance of equitable salary structure and benefits, and social relations with associates. Those attitudes that demonstrate concern for production include attention to the quality of policy decisions, procedures, or processes; the number of creative ideas an individual may have; the quality of services staff provide; and the workload and efficiency of individual workers. The relative value a manager places on concern for people and concern for product will influence the management style he or she uses. These styles change in popularity over time, but most can be seen to one degree or another in managers today.

The Country Club Style. A country club manager acts on the assumption that production requirements are contrary to people's needs. A manager that uses this style feels that the attitudes and feelings of people are important and supersede the production goals of the organization. The manager plans, directs, and controls activities of subordinates, but does not push them to accomplish organizational goals. This type of manager will demonstrate and support staff and may, under certain circumstances, pitch in to assist them. Because country club managers value the attitudes and feelings of their staff, they are likely to expect devoted loyalty in return.

The Laissez-Faire Style. A laissez-faire manager acts on the assumption that there is a basic incompatibility between the production requirements of the organization and the needs of personnel. This type of manager has low involvement with personnel and contributes minimally toward organizational purpose. This style may result in lack of accomplishment of organizational goals because little leadership is exerted to facilitate and support the staff in achieving these goals. This style is most common in bureaucratic, noncompetitive organizations with routine operations and repetitive actions.

The Authoritarian Style. Authoritarian managers act on the assumption that organizational goals are quotas for the personnel to meet. Human relationships have low priority in this style of management, whereas productivity has high priority. Work conditions emphasize efficiency and minimize the interference of human elements in the work environment.

The Participative Style. A participative manager acts on the assumption that people want to work and assume responsibility for achievement of the goals of the organization. Managers believe that if people are treated properly, they can be trusted and will put forth their best effort. Participative managers motivate by use of factors intrinsic to the worker, such as satisfaction with assigned tasks, self-esteem, and recognition for a job well done. Delegation is an important factor in this managerial style.

The Rules-Oriented Style. A rules-oriented manager acts on the assumption that people require reinforcement from the manager to function. This type of manager believes that things must be done by the book. Consequently, enforcement of policies, rules, and procedures is thought to facilitate motivation and achievement. These managers tend to be highly bureaucratic; that is, they focus much of their efforts on the hierarchical structure of the organization and its rules and regulations.

None of these styles is inherently better than another. In certain situations, a participative style is most appropriate because it fosters involvement of all personnel and provides for greater control of the work environment by those responsible for the work itself. However, a new manager may decide to follow a country club style if personnel do not feel valued. This approach is useful to develop a sense of support and trust so that a participative style can be used at a later date. If the group were so demoralized, beginning with a participative approach might not work because inadequate trust had not been established. Clearly, in some situations, especially when efficiency is essential for the continuing survival of the organization, an authoritarian style may be the best approach.

Planning

Planning is the process of making decisions in the present to bring about an outcome in the future. Planning is inherently systematic and is characterized by a cyclical process in which goals and specific objectives are periodically reviewed, evaluated, and modified to meet the evolving needs of the organization. It is the most fundamental management action and precedes all other management functions. Planning is also one of the more complex and frustrating aspects of managing in the health care industry because the health care system is, by nature, nonsystematic. Health care managers employ planning processes in an attempt to promote order in what is frequently viewed as a disorganized system.

Any planning undertaken by an organization should directly relate to its mission. In establishing this link at the outset of organizational planning, diversions and extraneous elements can be avoided. The goals of an organization originate in the mission statement that defines the purpose or philosophy of the organization. Goals are the ends toward which activity is directed. In a sense a goal is never completely achieved, but rather, it is in a continuing ideal state, to be attained. Organizational goals may be found in the charter, articles of incorporation, the mission statement, or official bylaws of the organization.

ORGANIZATIONAL PLANNING

Planning takes many forms within an organization. Planning may be formulated around a program, such as in a new service or an extension of an existing service, or in the physical arrangement of either new or renovated space. In any event, planning is based on the philosophy, goals, and objectives of the organization, and these must be reviewed in the initial considerations of the planning process. Regardless of the program to be developed and the setting, certain principles are involved in devising the plan of action.

In approaching organizational planning there are three major elements that must be considered: (1) surveys, (2) interviews, and (3) evaluations. A survey is used to identify the need for the program. The population to be served, the source of referrals, the needs of the staff, the treatment methods and the anticipated caseload all must be identified through this survey. Interviews with top-level administrators should be conducted to determine their perception of the nature and extent of the program being planned. Fiscal considerations and administrative restrictions must be accommodated. Interviews should be conducted with potential consumers to determine the appropriateness of the program and with community leaders in which the program is to be located. The evaluative phase of planning is the translation of all of the information gathered into a workable plan. At this stage, personnel and facilities are matched with the needs of the organization and the program.

PARTICIPANTS IN PLANNING

Top-level managers set the basic tone for planning. They determine the overall goals for the organization and give direction on content of policies and planning documents. The board of trustees, managers, chief executive officers (CEOs), or presidents are considered top-level managers within the overall organization. At a departmental or program unit level, directors or chiefs of service are considered the top level of management. These individuals are responsible for the planning process in their areas. They identify goals and set policies for their individual departments or services. As a result of federal legislation, specifically the Rehabilitation Act of 1973 and subsequent legislation in 1974, consumers

also participate in planning, particularly in federally funded programs. Within an individual institution, department, or program, others may participate in planning as delegated by top-level management. The use of staff planners or planning consultants to initiate planning within a health care service has become more or less obsolete. These individuals are now more effectively used as facilitators of a planning process that seeks to establish organizational direction.

PLANNING FOR GROWTH

As health care organizations intensify their competitive strategies and move into new markets, planning for organizational growth becomes more important. Understanding the strengths and weaknesses of the organization is a necessary first step in planning for growth. Despite the competition and cost constraint pressures, the expansion of health care systems is projected into the 21st century. The demand for medical care programs will continue, with emphasis on community-based programs in the areas of outpatient services and new technology sectors. The retrofitting of inpatient facilities that began in the 1990s will continue, as evidenced in the development of freestanding alternative health care centers. Generally speaking, these delivery centers have been and will continue to be designed for ambulatory, non–life-threatening conditions that need not be treated in a hospital. Careful, cost-effective planning is essential to meet the projected needs of the health care consumer. All members of the health care profession will need to be prepared to participate in meeting these planning demands.

PLANNING IN AN OCCUPATIONAL THERAPY DEPARTMENT

Occupational therapy managers are involved continuously in planning both within the department and across program lines. At this level, managers need to be intimately aware of the resources necessary for various programs and the financial implications of providing these resources. The department manager must analyze the costs and benefits of programs, including comparing expenses with projected revenues. The manager must also identify the probability of securing the staff necessary for expanding or new programs. An analysis of space and equipment needs must also be conducted by the manager to identify provision of resources in a cost-effective manner. The occupational therapy manager should be well versed in the various provisions for reimbursement of occupational therapy services. Because coverage varies dramatically, depending on the services rendered, this information is paramount in planning. The occupational therapy manager should be involved in initial planning meetings and should submit a report to top-level management based on data, revenue, and expense projections for resources that are necessary for expanding or new occupational therapy programs.

Planning takes many forms within an occupational therapy department (eg, planning for program, planning for physical arrangement of space and equipment, or for development of service within an existing agency). Regardless of the purpose of planning there are factors that must be considered. These include (1) the type of institution, agency, or service needed; (2) the principal diagnoses to be treated; (3) the bed capacity devoted to the service; (4) the projected average monthly census and rate of turnover; and (5) the eligibility of patients by payer mix. In addition, personnel requirements must be determined; namely, the number of registered occupational therapists, certified occupational therapy assistants, and support staff that will be needed, and the ratio of clients per practitioner. The number of professional and support staff needed to adequately staff a department is difficult to ascertain. Many variables must be considered (eg, diagnoses, complexity of problems, size of institution or service, referral rates, and average length of stay). Very little reliable data is available to assist a manager in planning for staffing. A general guideline for a client/staff ratio is 10:1 for individual treatment caseload and 15:1 for group treatment. In addition, a manager should consider current staff patterns and use of space in making future projections.

In determining space allocation, the basic areas to be considered are: (1) the primary treatment areas for assessment, work stations and specialized treatment rooms; (2) support areas for reception and waiting, storerooms, dressing rooms; and (3) administrative areas for management and staff offices, clerical staff, conference and classrooms. Factors that influence space requirements include: (1) the client load at any one time, (2) the number of personnel using the area at one time, (3) the work flow, and equipment and storage needs. Safety features should also be considered in planning space, including provision of panic bars on doors, sprinkler systems, fire extinguishers, emergency alarm systems in secluded treatment areas, storage for flammable materials, and proper receptacles for disposal of materials. Accessibility of communication systems, whether they be telephones, intercoms, or paging systems, should also be included in space planning.

STRATEGIC PLANNING

Regardless of the purpose of planning, a systematic approach is strongly recommended. Strategic planning relates to goals that are essential, basic, or critical to the continuation of an institution or organization and involves the allocation of resources to achieve an organization's long-range goals. Strategic planning deals with three basic questions: (1) Where are we? (2) Where do we want to be? (3) How do we get there? These questions are asked throughout the planning process.

Planning tests managers. All planning, regardless of the system used, involves the expenditure of effort to collect data to identify trends, and then, project this into the future. Countless meetings among those involved in the planning process are required. Good planning mandates close interrelations between the planners and executives, but also requires participation from all levels in the organization. A participatory management style that values the input of all personnel facilitates commitment to the planning process.

Strategic planning entails five steps: (1) assessment, (2) analysis, (3) decision making, (4) implementation, and (5) evaluation.

Assessment

Assessment involves the construction of a thorough assessment of the current and future state of the organization. At this stage there is the opportunity to involve many managers and employees with special expertise. By involving groups of employees in the development of assessments, these groups will feel a sense of ownership of the strategic plan. Through the assessment phase, issues will be identified and can then be ranked in order of priority.

Analysis

To develop focus, issues are selected from the assessment that could influence the organization's response. A literature review is essential at this point in the process. Trends should be analyzed, and brainstorming of implications for the future should take place.

Decision Making

During this phase, advantages and disadvantages are discussed concerning each of the issues that were analyzed. At this stage, preferred options are determined and ranked; these become the actual objectives of the strategic plan.

Implementation

Methods to implement the plan must be developed. Because this is the stage at which failure commonly occurs, it is advantageous to determine action steps, set timetables, and allocate resources for each step.

Evaluation

At this step, the outcome of the planning process is evaluated. The usual way is to measure the actual outcome against a standard. Questions should be asked to determine when an issue is resolved and how this can be measured. If the plan is not working within a particular parameter, then the individuals involved in planning should return to the decision-making phase to consider ways of improving or eliminating the action plans, or to develop new ones.

Successful strategic planning results in values and themes that guide and strengthen an organization's ability to succeed in changing environments. There are, however, potential pitfalls of the process. The process has been criticized in the past for requiring too much time and losing the original focus of the strategic-planning process (Hayes, 1985). Research has shown that problems develop in strategic planning if inadequate time is allocated to the process, if planners are hired, which minimizes staff involvement and commitment, or if goals are not tested adequately to be sure that they are appropriate ones to pursue. Furthermore, because planning is a creative process, finding the right balance for the process is essential. Too much structure stifles creativity, whereas too little leads to lack of focus, which impedes task completion (Steiner, 1979).

MARKETING

A discussion of planning would be incomplete without inclusion of an overview of marketing issues and strategies. Strategic planning asks what are the organization's mission and goals and considers economic alternatives in planning services. In contrast, marketing asks what are the needs and desires of the consumer and is concerned with public relations and sale methods. Marketing is not just advertising a product; it is identifying and serving the evolving needs of the consumers and the public. Both marketing and strategic planning are inextricably linked, because there must be a match between the goals and mission of the institution and the needs of the consumer in the development of any new service.

Marketing experts suggest that the health care professions have neglected market research, and have overlooked the development of market strategies, in their pursuit of methods to produce quick results. Marketing in health care is a growing discipline that combines a knowledge of health care, its environment, and analytic design, with a study of their interactions. Analysis of consumer behavior, attitudes, knowledge, and beliefs are changing the way some health care systems are planning for new services. The number of new programs being offered that emphasize lifestyle change, disease prevention, and alternatives to hospital care reflects this consumer orientation.

Occupational therapy service managers can successfully incorporate marketing into their administrative practices by combining proved marketing strategies with traditional practice methods. Such a combination maintains professionalism, delivers high-quality care, and satisfies the needs of potential clients, at the same time ensuring the viability of the program. Marketing concepts can be used effectively to demonstrate occupational therapy services to others within the organization. Methods of internal marketing strategies might include a departmental open house, inservices for nursing or social service personnel, or feature articles in employee newsletters. Progress notes and service reports, as well as participation in case conferences, are other methods that demonstrate the benefits of occupational therapy and, therefore, can be construed as marketing tools. Marketing can also be used externally to educate consumers to the need and availability of occupational therapy services, such as community newsletters, workshops for special disability groups, and participation in health fairs within the community.

The occupational therapy manager must educate staff about the merits of marketing to the well-being of the organization. Many staff members do not perceive themselves as having a role in marketing occupational therapy. Staff can be reminded that the impression they create with clients or visitors in a clinical setting is, in fact, a marketing measure. Staff can also be reminded that marketing is necessary to create public awareness of occupational therapy and to differentiate occupational therapy practitioners from competing health care providers.

Directing

LEADERSHIP AS A MANAGEMENT FUNCTION

A basic responsibility of a manager is to shape and modify employee behavior through directing, so that an employee can acquire the necessary knowledge and skill to perform assignments in compliance with policies and procedures of the institution. An individual in a management position must blend and adapt leadership styles and strategies to the organizational environment. Leadership is a process of influence between one who leads and those who follow. Leadership may be formal or informal; that is, influence by legitimate authority or the strength of personality.

Managers exert their power through the use of influence and formal authority. Formal authority is power that is legitimized through an individual's organizational role. Influence differs from formal authority in the manner in which compliance is evoked. Through the use of influence a leader may elicit compliance without relying on formal action, rules, or force. Formal authority carries with it the power to mandate action, and it is reinforced by organizational charts, job descriptions, procedure manuals, and work rules. Formal authority differs from influence in that it is clearly vested within the organizational structure. Effective managers use both forms of power to achieve organizational goals. Too great a reliance on formal authority, without the use of influence, may leave personnel feeling that they are working in a coercive, bureaucratic environment that is more concerned with rules than relationships. A manager who relies predominantly on an authoritarian or rules-oriented style may evoke this feeling.

Giving orders is a major function of a manager's daily role. It is often taken for granted that every manager knows how to give orders. Issuing effective orders requires attention to timing and language. Leaders must prepare employees in many ways so that when orders are actually given, they are both acceptable and effective in terms of essential communication. Leaders must also be prepared to discipline. Disciplining is more likely to address behavior than to address work results. Discipline may, however, have a connotation of punishment; discipline should be used by a leader to improve employee behavior. A manager can discipline by calling attention to correct behavior in an effective manner; by calling attention to responsibilities and by making suggestions. An employee should be treated as a person with a problem, not a problem employee. Leaders are dealing with people and, in this capacity, must develop skills in negotiating to assist people in dealing with their differences. The objectives of good leaders include raising the level of member motivation, improving quality of all decisions, developing teamwork and morale, furthering individual development of members, and increasing readiness to accept change. This requires a balance in the use of formal authority and influence.

DECISION MAKING

Regardless of the management position (ie, department chief or staff supervisor), the process of making decisions is a key component of the position. There are two elements to decision making; the quality of the decision and the acceptance of the decision by those it affects. Many daily decisions that managers face must be made on the spot. Most decisions are based on intuition as well as logic and experience. When time permits, a manager may involve subordinates in the decision-making process and may involve others through group consensus. This is a common practice in decentralized decision making, when the process is moved from the top level of management to incorporate involvement by those on lower levels of the hierarchy. This process is more likely to be comfortable for participative managers. The brainstorming technique used in the team approach to problem solving is often a helpful technique. Regardless of the style of decision making, the traditional approach to problem solving is an effective tool for use in this process.

SUPERVISION

A supervisor is any individual having authority in the interests of the employer to hire, transfer, lay off, recall, promote, assign, reward, or discipline other employees. The primary duties of a supervisor consist of the management of a unit and the direction of two or more employees to promote the growth of the supervisee. Contact between a supervisor and supervisee may vary from close daily interaction to only monthly contact. A line-staff member in an occupational therapy department may have daily contact with a supervisor; on the other hand the unit supervisor in the occupational therapy department may have only weekly or biweekly contact with the next level of management. Supervisors are middle managers, those who represent the administration to employees and employees to the administration. Almost every technique of supervision can be learned, and the basic principles can be transferred from one work place to another. (See Chap. 44 for more information about this topic.)

Controlling

ORGANIZATIONAL HIERARCHIES AND PATTERNS

Management takes place within an organization. Several universal characteristics are present, to some degree, in all organizations, regardless of their product or setting. The three universals are purpose, people, and hierarchy. By effectively managing the universals, efficient production results, and the organization remains sound. The purpose of a health care organization is to supply quality health care at a cost-effective level. Purpose cannot be achieved without people. The process of achieving purpose through the efforts of several people results in some people attaining authority to supervise, plan, control, and direct others through a hierarchy.

Relationships in formal organizations are highly structured in terms of authority and responsibility. The flow of authority and responsibility that can be observed in a hierarchy constitutes a chain of command. Chain of command is defined as an organizational pattern that links the highest manager in the hierarchy to the lowest in an unbroken chain of authority, responsibility, and accountability. A clear chain of command shows who reports to whom, who is responsible for the actions of an individual, and who has authority over the worker. According to classic organization principles, an individual supervisor can direct only a limited number of subordinates, this is referred to as span of control. Generally, organizational theories hold that the more efficient organizations have a smaller span of control. To further understand these concepts a discussion of organizational patterns is helpful.

Organizational patterns are schematic renderings that arrange positions in the organization in a hierarchical pattern. These patterns illustrate the chain of command within the organization or department. They are schemes of planned interaction and indicate responsibilities of individuals working within a structure. The patterns may be vertical, horizontal, pyramidal, or matrical. In a vertical pattern, the chain of command proceeds from top to bottom in a straight chain. The horizontal pattern proceeds from left to right. The pyramid pattern proceeds from top to bottom, becoming more diversified as it proceeds down the chain. The matrix pattern is a combination of the vertical and horizontal patterns. The matrix pattern allows for the simultaneous existence of both the hierarchical (vertical) association through departmental organization and lateral (horizontal) association across departments. The horizontal associations are typically called programs and are illustrated in patient care teams. Within this pattern, the program manager is responsible for overall management of the program group and, therefore, is responsible for results. The department manager retains responsibility for the functional department and, therefore, is responsible for providing resources to attain results.

TABLES OF ORGANIZATION

From the schematics just described, an organization or manager develops a table of organization or organizational chart. The structure of any organization is a device that has been designed to assist management in achieving various objectives. A table of organization or organizational chart depicts major functions, specific relations, lines of communication and formal authority, and positions by title. No table of organization or organizational chart is static; it changes as the organization grows and changes. Usually, only major functions are shown, except at a departmental

Small Occupational Therapy Department

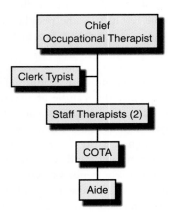

▲
Figure 43-1. Table of organization of a small occupational therapy department.

level, for which greater detail of individual relationships may be illustrated. Only formal lines of authority and communication are shown. Tables of organization or organizational charts cannot be properly interpreted without reference to policy manuals or job descriptions. Figure 43–1 depicts a small occupational therapy department, displayed in a vertical chain. Figure 43–2 shows a table of organization of a large occupational therapy department, with multiple programs in which the unit supervisor reports to a program manager as well as the director of occupational therapy.

CONTROLLING FUNCTIONS

Job Descriptions

A job description is a written statement of a single position. The purpose of a job description is to identify, define, and describe the position. A job description is a tool for controlling by clarifying the role of the position within the organization. A job description should cover every aspect of the job. It should be reviewed with prospective candidates for a position and reviewed annually with personnel holding the position. Because a job description enumerates all aspects of a job, the employee is assured that significant elements of the job are known to all parties and that the job is correctly described. As a result of the Americans with Disabilities Act (ADA) of 1990, job descriptions must be specific in the physical and mental requirements of a job (ADA, 1991).

A job description assures employees that the jobs of greater difficulty and value receive greater remuneration or pay. It also provides a means of performance appraisal as an on-going part of self- and supervisory evaluation. Each individual organization or institution has its own method of writing job descriptions. A job description typically contains the following elements: (1) job title, (2) department, service or work area, or unit, (3) qualifications, (4) basic functions and duties, and (5) specific duties. Figure 43–3 il-

lustrates a typical job description for an entry-level position for an occupational therapist in a rehabilitation hospital.

Policies and Procedures

Policies and procedures are necessary to effectively control administrative management of a service, department, or organization. The extent of the policies or procedures is dictated by the size and complexity of the organization, and they exist to greater or lesser degrees, depending on the level of bureaucracy within the organization. Typically policies and procedures are not transferable from one organization to another.

Policies. Policies are a set of criteria of what is to be done and what activities will be carried out within the organization, department, service, or program. Policies are controlling, in that they set forth regulations. They are never established on a verbal basis and should be written and approved at top administrative levels. Policies should be reviewed regularly, updated, or revised according to changing conditions or new regulations. There is no universal guide that applies to the development of policies. In writing specific policies at a departmental level, the first consideration should be the way in which the departmental policy will blend or relate to those of the organization. The second consideration should be to reflect the philosophy of the department.

Policies should provide the user with information about action to be taken, action to be avoided, and when and how to respond. Once policies are written and reviewed by top management, they should be permanently filed in a policy manual. New policies should be distributed to all staff levels to which they apply. Review of new policies with personnel assures that all staff members understand them and, thus, improves compliance.

The following is representative of the types of policies that would be found in most institutions today:

- Personnel: Salary administration, work schedules, vacation allowances, sick leave, personal time off, probationary periods, employee separation, benefits, transfer, and promotions.
- Institutional: Interview of applicants, preemployment and annual physical examinations, performance appraisal, fire and safety, medical records, quality assurance.
- Departmental: Treatment, referral, equipment maintenance, fees and charges, documentation, safety, dress code.

Procedures. Procedures are set criteria of how things are to be done, a course of action or way of doing something. Procedures are more detailed than policies; they should state precisely how and in what specific order an activity is to be carried out. Generally, a procedure is developed for each regulating policy if the policy requires certain activities to be fulfilled. Once procedures have been written, authorized, and implemented, they are assembled in manageable form,

Large Occupational Therapy Department

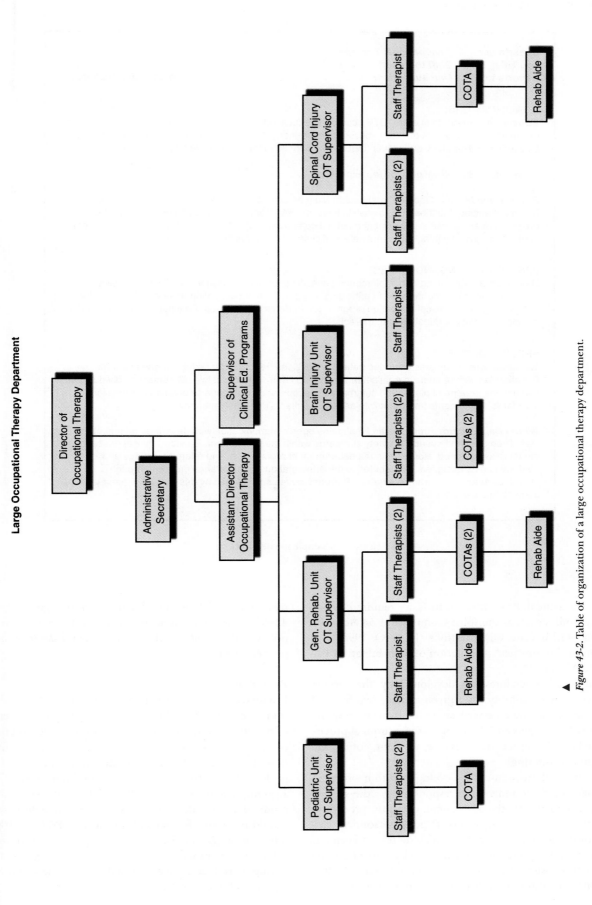

Figure 43-2. Table of organization of a large occupational therapy department.

Department:	*Occupational Therapy*		
Job Title:	*Staff therapist*		
Reports to:	*Unit supervisor*	Supervises:	*Unit technician*

QUALIFICATIONS:
Education: Graduate of an ACOTE accredited educational program in occupational therapy with a minimum of a bachelor's degree in occupational therapy. Certification by the National Board of Occupational Therapy Certification (NBCOT). Licensed in the State of New York.

Experience: Entry-level position, no experience.

Physical and Mental: Good general health. Must be able to access a variety of heights within the treatment setting. Must be able to assist clients in ambulation, transfers, and positioning. The presence of any physical impairment must not compromise client care and safety. Must be mentally alert and cognitively intact to assure safety of clients and others in the treatment setting.

BASIC FUNCTIONS AND DUTIES:
Responsible for planning and implementing specific treatment programs for both individual and groups of patients according to the principles and practices of occupational therapy. Responsible for contributing to the clinical education program for students as assigned. Functions in a collaborative manner with the coordinating staff therapists.

SPECIFIC DUTIES:
With Patients: Evaluates assigned patients. Develops treatment plans for assigned patients. Collaborates with patients in goal setting, including family when possible. Documents individualized evaluations, treatment plans, and summaries in accordance with departmental and professional standards. Implements treatment with assigned patients in a timely manner.

Within Department: Promotes and maintains open communication with departmental and other staff. Promotes and maintains safety standards within the department. Provides clinical education to students as assigned. Represents the department at professional and related meetings and conferences as assigned. Contributes to departmental quality assurance program through outcomes studies, program evaluation. Performs duties as assigned by department director or immediate supervisor.

▲

Figure 43-3. Sample job description.

usually in a manual. Procedure manuals are required by accrediting bodies such as the Joint Commission on Accreditation of Health Care Organizations (JCAHO, 1995) and the Commission on the Accreditation of Rehabilitation Facilities (CARF, 1994).

Institutional procedures are developed by the service with specific responsibility for a given activity (eg, fire and safety procedures would be written by the manager responsible for risk management). Examples of institutional procedures include fire, evacuation, disaster, accident, communication, and accounting.

Departmental procedures are developed within a specific department by those individuals responsible for the service (eg, an occupational therapy documentation procedure would be written by occupational therapy personnel). Examples of departmental procedures include record keeping, equipment and supplies, maintenance and repair of equipment, quality assurance, staff orientation, referral, scheduling, client evaluation or assessment, tests and measurements, treatment modalities, and documentation. Figures 43–4 and 43–5 are examples of an occupational therapy department policy and procedure related to fire and disaster training of new employees.

Productivity

Productivity is the ratio between the output and the resources expended to obtain the desired output. A given level of quality is always implied for any output. The importance of obtaining productivity data relates to the cost effectiveness of a program. It is not unusual for administrators to set goals for productivity and strive for a minimal goal of 5% to 15% improvement annually. It is highly unlikely that 100% productivity would ever be achieved, and administrators should not strive for percentages beyond 80% to 90%. The information gathered in productivity studies can assist in planning new programs, making personnel projections, balancing work loads, improving staff effectiveness, and reducing or containing costs.

Newway Health Care Institution Administrative Policy

All new employees will receive training in and demonstrate back proper procedures to be followed in the event of fire or disaster within the institution. Training will be scheduled by immediate supervisor at the time of initial orientation and will be completed within 3 weeks of employment.

Effective: 10/1/94
Reviewed: 6/95; 9/96

▲
Figure 43-4. Sample policy.

If an occupational therapy program is not cost-effective, the service will not be competitive in the health care industry of the future. By evaluating productivity data, a manager can evaluate how much time is spent in direct and indirect service. The data may be reported by individual practitioner (registered occupational therapist or certified occupational therapy assistant), by diagnosis, by modality, or by treatment outcomes. Productivity data can assist the occupational therapy manager to improve efficiency by integrating planning information to ensure fiscally viable products and services, without sacrificing the quality of care. It is important that an occupational therapy manager inform the staff about the purposes of productivity studies. This is a very sensitive topic, and staff tend to react negatively to this type of study if they are not informed of its purpose. The involvement of staff in data collection and analysis can help alleviate fears of loss of position or major changes occurring within the department. If handled well by the manager, productivity studies can be extremely beneficial to the department and may even result in increased staff, space, support personnel, or financial resources.

Evaluating

For the manager, evaluation may assume many names, but essentially it is the managerial function that assures quality of service. Quality assurance lies at the heart of the basic purpose of health care. Beyond our ethical responsibility to provide optimal care, consumers demand that excellent health care is excellent. From the perspective of a manager, quality assurance is a method for assessing program delivery and outcomes, personnel performance, and staff productivity. As such, managers place emphasis on achieving the highest possible quality of care and quality of service. In assessing health care outcomes, quality assurance deals with aggregates, not individual clients. Quality assurance is not voluntary, it is mandated by federal legislation and accreditation standards. The JCAHO (1988) includes quality assurance, utilization review, and program evaluation within its criteria for accreditation.

Quality assurance begins with inquiry into three elements of quality of care: (1) structure, (2) process, and (3) outcome (Donabedian, 1982).

Newway Health Care Institution Procedure for Fire and Disaster Training for New Employees

1. Immediate supervisor will provide new employee with written procedures for fire and disaster as part of the initial employee orientation.
2. Supervisor will schedule training session with Plant and Risk Management Supervisor.
3. Immediate supervisor will note date and time of training in writing and provide the employee with a written schedule. Schedule for training will be noted in employee's departmental record.
4. Upon successful completion of training, the Plant and Risk Management Supervisor will notify the employee's supervisor in writing that training has been completed. The employee will be given a certificate indicating satisfactory completion of training.
5. A copy of the certificate will be forwarded to the Human Resources Department to be placed in the employee's permanent record.

Effective: 10/15/94
Reviewed: 6/95; 8/96

▲
Figure 43-5. Sample procedure.

1. *Structure.* Structure refers to the institution and the way in which it is organized and the resources used to provide care. Questions about structure would deal with issues such as the organization of the occupational therapy department, how personnel are scheduled, and whether the department has sufficient supplies, equipment, and space to meet the needs of its clients.
2. *Process.* Process refers to the totality of interaction between the consumer and the provider of care, including what is and what is not done. In other words, process is concerned with the interactions between occupational therapy practitioners, clients, and in many instances, the clients' family.
3. *Outcome.* Outcome refers to the results of intervention and interaction with the system. In this case, outcome studies are concerned with such issues as the functional status of clients after discharge and the clients' satisfaction with their care.

QUALITY ASSURANCE PROGRAMS

Quality assurance involves defining quality by continuously measuring outcomes against standards and then taking corrective action when problems are identified. This may be measured concurrently when the care is being delivered and retrospectively after discharge. A quality assurance program includes the following components: (1) quality assurance, (2) utilization review, and (3) program evaluation.

Quality Assurance

Quality assurance identifies problems in health care service delivery and corrective actions to be taken. Criteria that are considered achievable that have not been achieved are the focus of quality assurance. These problems could be in the areas identified by Donabedian (1982): structure, process, or outcome. The quality assurance process starts by asking and answering questions. These questions address structure, process, and outcome and might include any or all of the following:

- What would I see if my department were providing quality care?
- Do all the clients return home?
- Do clients participate in setting their own goals for treatment?
- Are clients able to participate and perform certain tasks? How many?
- How many hours a day do practitioners provide client care?
- What are the costs of this care?

These questions can be answered through quality assurance monitoring by continuously measuring outcomes against standards that have been set within the department, the institution, or the profession. When a problem is identified, corrective action is taken. For instance, the problem may be cause by structural difficulties, such as inadequate equipment, or by procedures that do not meet client needs.

New equipment purchases can be justified because a problem has been identified related to the quality of service. Likewise, identification of procedural problems directs occupational therapy personnel to examine the procedure and revise it to alleviate the problem. The problem may be related to the competence of occupational therapy practitioners. This process issue can be addressed by training programs for these individuals. New programs may also evolve from the process.

There are five stages in quality assurance monitoring.

Stage 1. In stage 1, the indicators of quality care are identified. The indicators should be those aspects of care that have high priority, high risk, high volume, and are perceived as solvable should a problem occur.
Stage 2. In stage 2, data is collected that is measurable (ie, standardized performance measures that will reflect the indicators).
Stage 3. In stage 3, cause is determined, and if a problem is found, remedial action is indicated.
Stage 4. In stage 4, the remedy is implemented. This is a very important step, and it is sometimes overlooked. The remedy should be short and simple and should not be too costly to implement.
Stage 5. In stage 5, the measurement process is performed again to determine if the problem has been solved. If the problem has not been solved, the process reverts to stage 3, and the cause is reinvestigated. If the problem is solved, it should be monitored periodically with lengthened measurement intervals to determine that no further complications have occurred.

Depending on the size of the occupational therapy department, quality assurance monitoring may be carried out by an individual or a committee. Regardless of how the monitoring is managed, the study must be documented and reported to top-level management and, ultimately, to the governing body of the organization.

A discussion of quality assurance monitoring would not be complete without discussion of other important elements of the process. The JCAHO requires that studies be documented and reported through the chain of command to the board of trustees. Because the ultimate responsibility for quality assurance rests with the board of trustees, all services should be involved in monitoring studies, even contract services such as joint ventures for the supply of equipment to clients. Written documentation of monitoring studies should be forwarded through the department head to the Quality Assurance Committee or similar committee or department with review authority, to the chief executive officer (CEO), and finally, to the board of trustees in a report format usually drafted by the CEO.

The American Occupational Therapy Association (AOTA) has produced several excellent resources on quality assurance (AOTA, 1990; Forer, 1996; Ostrow, Williamson, & Joe, 1983). These are updated regularly to reflect the requirements of accrediting bodies.

Utilization Review

Utilization review is a hospital- or facility-wide function. It is a program that monitors the use of facilities and services. Utilization review assures that the client receives only those services that are medically necessary and no more. In addition, utilization review assures the payer that the care is delivered economically and conforms to criteria determined by peers within the facility.

Utilization review programs are coordinated by an individual who has extensive knowledge of all aspects of patient care. These coordinators are often nurses or health information managers. Utilization review coordinators are responsible for certifying admission, reviewing for length of stay, and notifying the attending physician of any problem that occurs or issues that might warrant the discharge of a client. The implications for occupational therapy practitioners are that documentation must be accurate, timely, and understandable in terms of goals and progress, because it is the record that is reviewed for utilization of facilities and services. It is important for occupational therapy practitioners to be aware of admission certification dates and approved lengths of stay, for these may have an influence on projected treatment program and goals.

Program Evaluation

Program evaluation defines and reviews the results achieved following the provision of care; it is an outcome-monitoring system that reflects the results of services on consumers. Continuous quality improvement (CQI) is an example of the system frequently used by teams in a rehabilitation setting (Slater, Evans, & Small, 1993). The actual method of evaluation varies from one program to another and from one department to another. Accrediting agencies such as JCAHO and CARF require that each institution has a system for evaluating its program of care.

The methods for program evaluation are generally guided by diagnosis or service rendered (eg, individuals with myocardial infarction or neurosurgical intervention in individuals with parietal lobe trauma). As in other quality assurance programs, program evaluation studies involve the identification of goals, purpose, indication for treatment, recommended services, the clients status at discharge, and the need for follow-up or community level services. Data on outcomes are related to those consumers who achieved the goals or have demonstrated change as a result of receipt of service. A committee reviews data collected retrospectively and determines the strengths, weaknesses, and shortcomings of the program being evaluated. The results of the study are shared with those involved with the program, and plans are made for implementing any changes to improve the program or service. Another method for evaluating a program is to conduct a client satisfaction survey. This is a common practice in evaluating specially funded programs, such as those financed by a grant.

Either of the preceding methods may be used to evaluate an occupational therapy program. The studies would be conducted within the department by management-level staff or their designees. An occupational therapy department might evaluate the following: (1) achievement of functional goals for head trauma clients, (2) evaluation of levels of self-care skills, as measured by the Barthel Index, of clients with left hemiplegia, (3) examination of parallel group participation in individuals performing on an Allen Cognitive level 4, or (4) client and family satisfaction with training programs in occupational therapy. Program evaluation in an occupational therapy department may be used to communicate to third-party payers, meet accreditation standards, assist in marketing, plan new programs, and improve benefits to consumers.

PERFORMANCE APPRAISAL AND CREDENTIALING

A discussion of the evaluating function of a manager would be incomplete without including issues of performance evaluation. In contrast with the preceding components of quality assurance, the evaluation of job performance relates specifically to an individual and the assurance that the individual is qualified and performing his or her duties at a determined level of quality. Performance appraisals are formal mechanisms used by managers to provide positive and constructive feedback to a supervisee on performance, in comparison with prescribed expectations. The criteria for evaluations are described in job descriptions and in department and institutional policies and procedures. It is generally assumed that in using these measures, a level of objectivity can be assured in the process. As a result of performance appraisals, training needs can be identified, areas of noncompliance can be remediated, and staff development can be determined. In addition, areas of strength can be identified so that these can be used more effectively to build on the practitioners areas of competence and to meet the needs of the program. The issues identified through this portion of the evaluation will become criteria for future evaluations. (See Chap. 44 for more information on supervision.)

Credentialing through certification and licensure assures the public that the personnel who provide care are qualified to do so. It is the responsibility of a manager to verify credentials on employment and to assure that employees maintain appropriate credentials on an ongoing basis.

▼ DOCUMENTATION

Documentation is one of the most important functions performed by occupational therapy practitioners that supports intervention with clients. In other words, next to treatment, documentation accounts for a major portion of time in the daily schedule of practitioners. Documentation is the key to communicating occupational therapy services to others on the professional team and to the reimbursement agency. The relation of documentation in professional practice to reimbursement issues cannot be stressed enough. In addition, documentation is the basis for measuring quality assurance throughout the organization or system. Records and reports generated at various levels in a department or institution reflect the quality of activity taking place.

Because documentation is a form of communication, issues of language and the correct use of terminology are paramount. Complicating this issue is that standards and expectations for language are constantly changing. In documentation it is crucial to use the terminology appropriate to the setting (ie, medical terminology in a medical setting and educational terminology in a public school). Jargon should be avoided, most especially when documenting for audiences that are unfamiliar with this more specialized vocabulary. Although jargon should be avoided, efforts to standardize terminology have increased. Two systems that practitioners should be familiar with are the AOTA Uniform Terminology and the ICIDH Codes.

Uniform Terminology

In 1977 the Secretary of Health and Human Services was required by legislation (PL 95–142) to establish regulations for uniform reporting systems in hospitals. The AOTA developed a uniform reporting system in 1979 for use throughout the profession. Despite the fact that the Department of Health and Human Services never adopted the system, due to concerns about price fixing and antitrust issues, the *AOTA Uniform Terminology for Occupational Therapy Services*, third edition (1994), is widely used by occupational therapy practitioners (see Appendix F for the Uniform Terminology and Chap. 12 for expanded explanations of the terms).

Because all occupational therapy services collect data on attendance, intervention, and treatment results, it is beneficial for information collected to be compared and contrasted from one setting to another. The use of an agreed on standard terminology can assist in avoiding disparity in the types of coverage from one region to another. The use of the Uniform Terminology in reporting service will facilitate review for reimbursement, in that the reviewers will be accustomed to the terminology from one setting to another. The use of uniform terminology can have a positive influence on standards, reimbursement, management, and research.

International Classification of Impairments, Disabilities, and Handicaps (ICIDH) Codes

Within the last few years, reimbursers have shifted from approving therapy claims based on impairments to those based on functional limitations. This change has implications for occupational therapy documentation. The AOTA is currently recommending that the World Health Organization's (WHO) ICIDH be used in documentation of occupational

therapy outcomes (WHO, 1980). The classification system provides a uniform language for documentation of services and assists in tracking outcomes. Similar to the Uniform Terminology, use of ICIDH codes creates a common language for all practitioners to use, improving and clarifying communication.

Purposes of Documentation

The documentation of the evaluation and treatment data is the only evidence of professional decision making. It is the only method that assures that something has taken place in the eyes of reimbursement agencies and accrediting bodies. Occupational therapy practitioners have been known to say, "if it is not documented, it did not happen." Not surprisingly, this statement is used as a guideline for documentation considerations.

Documentation has four major purposes: (1) it facilitates effective treatment, (2) it justifies reimbursement, (3) it stands as a legal document, and (4) it provides communication among the client, the treatment team, and the family (AOTA, 1986; Tiffany, 1983). Therefore, documentation has legal, ethical, and financial ramifications.

Documentation is not a simple skill that can be acquired in one setting and transferred to another. Although skill in documentation may be acquired in terms of use of terminology, legibility, structure, and phraseology, additional knowledge must be constantly updated in terms of standards set forth by reimbursement agencies, regulators, and accreditors. The AOTA has published numerous documents as reference material for the documentation process. These include *Practice Guidelines* (AOTA, 1996), *Managed Care: An Occupational Therapy Sourcebook* (AOTA Managed Care Project Team, 1996), and *Guidelines for Documentation* (AOTA, 1986).

Guidelines for Documentation

The guidelines for documentation vary in accordance with state and federal laws and regulations, accreditation standards, and institutional requirements. In considering the diversity of documentation requirements mandated by the variety of populations treated by occupational therapy practitioners it is small wonder that many consider it a chore or overwhelming task. The following suggestions may assist in organizing the thought process in approaching documentation and in reducing the negative connotations associated with it.

WHO IS THE AUDIENCE?

First, the practitioner should consider the audience for whom the documentation is intended. It is important to know who will read this documentation and who will benefit from it. Answers to this question will depend on the setting, the consumer, the payer, and the providers. That is to say, the rules for documentation in any work setting must be built on an understanding of (1) the needs of the consumer (the client, the family, or significant others), (2) the other team members (nurses, physical therapists, physicians, social workers, teachers) who will be reading the documentation, (3) the requirements of reimbursers (Blue Cross/Blue Shield, Medicare, Medicaid, HMOs, or commercial insurance companies) who will be making decision about reimbursement and continued care, and (4) the accreditation and governmental regulations (JCAHO, CARF, federal, state, and local government agencies) which will provide the standards for continuing accreditation of the institution. For example, JCAHO prescribes the information that the client treatment record must contain. Their inpatient requirements are extremely detailed and can be found in a current copy of the Accreditation Manual for Hospitals.

HOW CAN DOCUMENTATION BE EVALUATED?

Beyond the evaluation standards of the institution, third-party payers, and accrediting agencies, occupational therapy practitioners can use the RUMBA test. This was originated by AOTA in the 1970s for quality assurance. The use of RUMBA has been developed further as a method of self-assessment in documentation, intervention, and research. The RUMBA test can be applied to documentation by asking the following questions:

Is It RELEVANT?

Reports should reflect functional goals and achievement, for this is the true relevance of whether intervention is meaningful. The sheer reporting of measurements taken on a weekly basis does not reflect meaningfully to members of the audience who will read the report. An increase in grip strength of 5 lb, or an increase of 15 degrees of ROM in the elbow with a muscle grade of 3 (good) in the triceps, is meaningless other than to demonstrate that the client has greater strength or ROM than last week. These facts, standing alone, are not relevant to function. When accompanied by statements that reflect that the client is able to feed himself or herself a full meal independently as a result of improved grip strength, or a client is able to transfer safely using a transfer board as a result of improved strength and increased ROM in the elbows, the reader has a more complete understanding of the relevance of the documentation.

Is It UNDERSTANDABLE?

First, documentation must be readable; therefore, the writing must be legible. Jargon should be avoided. Other professionals, clients, and families do not understand the jargon of occupational therapy and thus would not understand what it is the occupational therapy practitioner is discussing. Sentences should be concise, succinct, and constructed using proper grammar and spelling. Contrary to early professional standards in documentation, it is now becoming more acceptable to use the first person in sentence structure; that is,

"this therapist applied" or "I have determined." It is no longer acceptable to use noncommittal language; that is, "it seems or appears." A client does not appear depressed, he or she either is or is not, as evidenced by his or her behavior and the observations and judgments of the practitioner. A client does not seem to be independent in donning a shirt: the client either does or does not require assistance.

Is It MEASURABLE?

Goals and statements should be written in measurable terms. Once these have been documented in such a way, other professionals will be able to understand the measures that are being used. Measurements should be reported in terms of frequency and duration; that is, how long something occurred, or how many times something was done. For example, "Millie is able to legibly write her first name, five times on wide-lined paper and then, because of fatigue, must refrain from any fine motor activity for 3 to 5 minutes" or "John is able to feed himself breakfast, lunch, and dinner independently after his place is set." Readers have a common understanding of how long it takes to write the word "Millie" or to eat a meal, which John is able to do three times a day. If time was a relevant issue, that is, if Millie or John took longer than would be expected to meet their goals, then this should be noted as well.

Is It BEHAVIORAL?

Occupational therapy practitioners are trained to be fine observers of behavior. Behaviors are those occurrences that are seen and can be measured as well. We can count how many times a child loses his or her balance to the right, or how many times a client loses control during a group activity, whether someone cries, or whether a client reaches for an object. Friendly, depressed, appropriate, and unmotivated are descriptors of attitudes not behaviors. They cannot they be measured. Therefore, references to these labels should be avoided, and descriptions of behaviors that indicate these attitudes are essential. For example, depressed clients are likely to complain of sadness and lack of hope about the future. They may refuse to participate in activities, explaining that it is takes too much effort to get involved. It is these behaviors that should be documented.

Is It ACHIEVABLE?

Third-party payers and accreditors are concerned with the achievement of goals. Consequently, one aspect of the evaluation of documentation is to determine if these agencies will consider the plan or goal to be achievable given the time constraints imposed by reimbursement or regulatory standards. If the answer is no, then the goal is not a realistic one, given the treatment setting and constraints, and the goal and plan should be revised so that it is achievable. The resulting documentation should reflect this change. Figure 43–6 shows a SOAP note that is a good example of documentation that passes the RUMBA test.

Patient Name: James Jones

Date: 6/19/96   **Time:** 1:45 PM

Problem #3 Lower Extemity Dressing

S: "Ever since my surgery to replace this left hip, I need help putting on my pants and shoes. They won't let me bend to reach my feet 'cause it will damage the hip."

O: Mr. Jones is 48 hours postsurgery for left total hip replacement. He is limited in active and passive left hip flexion to 90 degrees and left hip abduction at neutral by postsurgical precautions. Right hip ROM is WNL. He has normal upper extremity strength and ROM bilaterally. Sitting balance and posture in wheelchair are good. He is able to sit at the side of the bed unsupported, with good balance. Patient can transfer from wheelchair to bed independently, non–weight-bearing on left LE.

Mr. Jones can dress his upper extremities independently. He requires assistance to place underwear and trousers over his feet, but can pull the clothing up from his knees. He is unable to put on shoes and socks.

A: Mr. Jones will be independent in all lower extremity dressing, observing postoperative hip precautions, within 2 days.

P: Secure long-handled dressing stick, sock donner, long shoehorn, and stretch shoe laces for Mr. Jones. Train Mr. Jones with adapted equipment during two treatment sessions. Educate Mrs. Jones in the use of equipment so that she may support her husband's level of independence.

▲

Figure 43-6. Sample SOAP note.

Documentation Systems

PROBLEM-ORIENTED MEDICAL RECORD

The problem-oriented medical record (POMR) was developed by Lawrence Weed (1971) as a means of providing structure for progress note writing. The problem oriented model has become the standard method of client care documentation used in many health care settings today. The system is based on a list of problems that is generated by assessing the client's abilities and limitations. This is a master list developed by the treatment team collectively. These problems are numbered and each subsequent progress note, called SOAP notes, is written with reference to the problem list. The structure of a SOAP note is as follows:

S = Subjective. This is the section of the note where the practitioner records information as reported by the client, the family, or significant other. This information might include what a client says that cannot be measured.

O = Objective. In this section of the note, the practitioner records measurable, observable data, usually obtained through formal evaluation or assessment tools. Specific medical information and history would also be included here.

A = Assessment. This is the section of the note in which the practitioner records his or her professional judgment or opinion on functional expectations or limitations, given the objective data noted in the previous section.

P = Plan. In the last section of the note, the practitioner records a specific plan of action to be followed to resolve problems. This section may include short-term or long-term goals, how long treatment should be provided, and how often the client should receive treatment.

In some settings, outcome criteria or goals of treatment are added to the SOAP format. The use of G = Goals is becoming a common practice. This section would reflect the long-term and short-term goals of the particular health care practitioner writing the note.

The SOAP format may be used for initial notes, interim or progress notes, and discharge notes. The determination to use the POMR is generally an institutional one. Each SOAP note written in the client care record must refer to a problem that is on the list, thus any reader tracking a particular problem can readily see progress from all treatment areas surrounding that problem. These notes are written in an integrated section of the chart to which all disciplines contribute, rather than in discipline-specific sections. The provider writes SOAP notes to those problems that are appropriate to their intervention.

SEQUENTIAL CLIENT CARE RECORDING SYSTEM

Llorens and Shuster (1977) developed this system in response to the needs of researchers as well as clinicians. This system combined developmental theoretical components, evaluation and intervention strategies, and the POMR. They found that the sequential client care recording system was more efficient than other more traditional documentation methods. This system has been adapted and used in clinical settings with individuals with developmental disabilities.

COMPUTERIZED DOCUMENTATION

Computerized medical records are now a reality in many health service organizations. The POMR lends itself very well to computerization because it is a standardized system. Similar to the Uniform Terminology and ICIDH Code, computerization facilitates standardization, which has the potential to improve consistency in documentation. Computerized systems for the reporting of statistical data have been a part of the health care industry since the mid-1970s.

Computerization has evolved to include standardized assessment tools. For example, the Occupational Therapy Functional Assessment Compilation Tool (OT FACT) is a computerized method for documentation that generates a profile of an individual's abilities and limitations using the Uniform Terminology (AOTA, 1990). This software was developed by AOTA in 1990 and is becoming more widely used in practice today. The Medical University of South Carolina has developed a computerized system that uses small bar code scanners that have limited word-processing capabilities. Practitioners record all aspects of evaluation using the scanner and then download the information to the main computer to generate reports. Greenleaf Medical Systems (in California) has developed EVAL, which is a computerized evaluation system for the spine and extremities. Currently in development, in collaboration with the American Society of Hand Therapists (ASHT), is a system for evaluation and ongoing documentation using a handheld processor that is subsequently downloaded to produce progress reports.

These systems are constantly being updated to meet the demands of administrators, payers, and governing bodies. In consideration of documentation requirements and the professional time spent to meet these requirements, computerization has the potential to become a cost benefit measure within the health care organization.

Documentation Practices

Documentation requirements vary substantially from one setting to another. These variations stem from the differences in the mission of the organization, the needs of its consumers, as well as reimbursement and regulatory requirements. These issues are addressed in this section as well as in Chapters 45 and 46.

HOSPITALS

Within a hospital organization, the occupational therapy practitioner is guided in documentation by departmental policies and procedures and by requirements of accrediting bodies, such as the JCAHO, and the CARF. Within acute care settings, the SOAP note system is commonly used. In a psychiatric unit, the individual treatment plan (ITPs) is the most frequent form of documentation. In longer-term care institutions, the documentation system may change in accordance with the requirements of individual reimbursers. The requirements of reimbursers must always be taken into considera-

tion, regardless of the setting. Institutions generally tailor their documentation techniques to comply with JCAHO-monitoring standards. Despite this fact, there continues to be a question of accountability for determining quality of medical care and good documentation. Because JCAHO defines occupational therapy services, the provision of services should be retained within the scope of practice delineated by this organization. If services are provided outside the scope of practice or documentation is incomplete, accreditation can be jeopardized. Likewise, noncompliance can jeopardize reimbursement. For those institutions or units that are accredited by CARF or any other accrediting body, their documentation standards should also be reviewed and adhered to, so that one can avoid loss of accreditation or reimbursement.

COMMUNITY AGENCIES

Within community agencies, documentation is governed by policies and procedures within the agency and by various regulators of the agency at a local, state, or federal level. The types of practice that would be considered here include home health agencies, public health agencies, outpatient clinics, and private practice. Reimbursement for services rendered in these agencies might include commercial insurance providers, Medicaid, HMOs, Easter Seals, public schools, or the Division of Services for Crippled Children (DSCC). With such diversity in reimbursement organizations, it is not surprising that documentation standards vary considerably. The occupational therapy practitioner in these settings must review the guidelines for each reimburser so that the documentation meets reimbursement requirements. For example: Medicaid guidelines are state-specific within the federal guidelines, but cannot be generalized from one state to another. In some states occupational therapy services are not even funded by Medicaid.

RESIDENTIAL AGENCIES

Within residential agencies, documentation is regulated by federal and state laws. Medicaid guidelines have the greatest influence on documentation in residential settings as a result of the Department of Health and Human Services Health Care Financing Administration Rulings (Conditions of Participation, 1988). Those occupational therapy practitioners in mental health facilities should be informed about current local and state regulations, but should keep in mind that these facilities may be accredited by JCAHO. In this instance, the practitioner must meet those documentation standards as well.

SCHOOLS

Within school systems, documentation is guided by local educational agencies that must meet state and federal regulations. Public Law (PL) 94–142, the Education for All Handicapped Children Act and Amendments (1977, 1989) continues to be the guide for documentation procedures in the schools. In addition, the U.S. Department of Education regulations for implementation are a valuable resource relative to the influence of legislation on documentation. The AOTA incorporated the federal guidelines in the Guidelines for Occupational Therapy Services in School Systems (1989). Individual education programs (IEPs) (U.S. Department of Education, 1981) must be completed for any child to receive special services within the school setting. The IEP is a collaborative plan put in writing as a commitment of resources and services, and it serves as the evaluation device for use in determining a child's progress toward meeting proposed outcomes. Current performance levels, annual goals and short-term objectives, the involvement of special education and related services, the amount of regular class placement, projected dates for initiation and anticipated duration of services, and evaluation criteria and schedules for measurement on an annual basis, all must be included in each IEP (Montgomery County Association for Retarded Citizens, 1978).

▼ FISCAL MANAGEMENT

Fiscal management is an activity concerned with discovering, developing, defining, and evaluating the financial goals of the organization, department, or program. It is linked with all aspects of the manager's role because the financial well-being of the occupational therapy department is essential for its long-term survival. This activity is usually the responsibility of administrators or managers; however, the success of fiscal management is often dependent on combined efforts at all levels of staff. If sound financial management is in its proper perspective, it can do much to augment the quality, quantity, and effectiveness of health care by providing a system that makes service available and accessible at a reasonable cost. Table 43–1 provides a list of key terms and definitions for fiscal issues.

Table 43-1. Financial Management Terminology

Term	Definition
Balance sheet	Portrays the assets, liabilities and fund balances at a particular time within the fiscal year.
Budget period	A time frame for budgeting purposes. The time frame may be 12 mo, as in a calendar or fiscal year, or 3, 5, or 10 yr depending on the purpose of the budgeting function. Longer time frames are frequently used for depreciation or capital equipment budgets.
Capital budget	The capital budget is used to reflect anticipated expenses to be incurred for the purchase of major equipment or improvements to the facilities. A capital budget often covers more than the fiscal year; usually a budget period of 2–5 yr. Items included in a capital budget are generally those items that have at least a 5 yr life expectancy and cost more than $300.
Chart of accounts	This is a basic accounting method for organizing data in reference to costs. Most charts of accounts are number-coded for ease of identification and organization. These charts should allow for expansion and contraction to accommodate changes in goals, but should maintain basic uniformity for recording and reporting information.
Cost accounting	The theories, methods, and procedures for identifying, measuring, and reporting the cost of obtaining or providing services. The principle objective of cost accounting is to measure the resources used to produce a service.
Cost centers	The segments of activity for which costs are collected. The cost centers in each service are numbered for accounting purposes.
Departmental budgets	These budgets are working, detailed budgets for each unit and are usually developed by the unit manager in collaboration with individuals from the fiscal or financial department. Departmental budgets tend to be highly specific and permit identification of line items as well as close coordination and monitoring of revenues and expenses.
Direct costs	Costs that can be traced to a specific unit or activity. Direct costs are reimbursable.
Fiscal year	The usual accounting period for an annual or operating budget.
Indirect costs	Costs that cannot be specifically traced to a particular service. Indirect costs are more difficult to justify for reimbursement purposes.
Master budget	The central, composite budget for the entire organization. This budget is usually provided to top-level management and the board of trustees. The revenues and expenses of individual units are reflected in the master budget.
Operating budget	The operating or department budget reflects anticipated revenues and expenses for a given fiscal year. It delineates revenues expected from payment of services rendered, endowments, special funds, grants, and other special sources. Anticipated expenses are enumerated in terms of personnel, equipment, supplies, and benefits.
Tax-exempt status	The tax status of an organization is determined by the ownership and control classification of the organization. Health care organizations are classified as nonprofit, for-profit, or government controlled. Nonprofit organizations are usually determined to be tax exempt by government standards. For-profit organizations are owned by a group or individual for the care of their own consumers. These include investor-owned facilities that provide services with the anticipation that a profit will be made and distributed to investors.

Budgeting

Budgets ensure that program objectives are formulated with financial realities in mind. Budgeting is a planning and controlling tool. As a plan, a budget is a specific statement of anticipated results, expressed in numerical terms, covering a specific time period. It is the basis of continuing and future financial planning. When administered properly, a budget controls. The organizational structure based on department goals and functions is reflected in a budget. A budget is an educated estimate of future needs and is based on past records, personal experience, knowledge, and projected planning. Budgets are generally fixed, but should have some flexibility to respond to unforeseen demands on the organization or individual departments.

BUDGETING PROCESS AND METHODS

To establish a budget, specific information about direct and indirect costs must be gathered. There are various formulas used for determining revenue and expenses. Any manager would check with fiscal advisers within the organization to determine the formulas to be used for budgeting purposes.

The first step in the budget process is to identify the direct costs. Direct costs include salaries, payroll taxes, overtime, vacation relief, supplies, student programs, educational expenses, inservice, and reimbursable equipment. The expenses in each category are listed separately and then totaled. The next step in the process is to determine the indirect costs. Indirect costs include administrative support for personnel, accounting, purchasing; cleaning and maintenance of department, laundry, and plant operations, including utilities. The determination of indirect costs is based on the percentage of usage or percentage of space allotment. A formula to determine indirect costs would be as follows:

$$\frac{\text{Departmental square footage}}{\text{Total facility square footage}} = \frac{\text{\% square footage allotted}}{\text{to department}}$$

When applied to an occupational therapy department that is 54×40 ft, the following would result:

$$\frac{2,100 \text{ ft}^2}{120,000 \text{ ft}^2} = 0.0175$$

Therefore, if the cost to the facility for utilities is 8000 dollars, the portion allocated to the occupational therapy department would be 8000 dollars $\times$ 0 .0175 or 140 dollars. The direct and indirect costs are then totaled for the total budget figure. If the organization includes a bad debt allowance in the operating budget, this figure would be added to the total.

The next step in the process is the determination of the treatment costs once the total budget has been ascertained. The formula for this process is to divide the total budget by the number of projected treatment procedures for the budget period. For example:

$$\frac{\text{Total budget} = \$378,234}{\text{Tx. procedures} = 24,750} = 15.282 \text{ cost per procedure}$$

Thus, the cost for each treatment procedure is 15 dollars. Because fee for service is becoming obsolete in health care reimbursement, this figure is used by financial administrators to justify allocation of income.

In final form, the budget includes all of the data gathered through methods outlined in the foregoing. Once the budget has been struck, it is approved through administrative channels and becomes part of the Master Budget. Through review of the Monthly Cost Center Report, a report generated by the financial department, ongoing monitoring of revenues and expenses is possible.

Reimbursement

Any discussion of fiscal management must include issues surrounding coverage for services. It is vital that an occupational therapy manager be knowledgeable about reimbursement issues in relation to the programs that are being administered. This knowledge base should include existing coverage for occupational therapy services, the terminology used by third-party payers, current federal legislation concerning services and reimbursement for given populations, denials for reimbursement within the institution or organization in which occupational therapy services are provided, reasons for rejections of reimbursement, and appeal mechanisms. An overview of reimbursement legislation and its influence on delivery of services is included in Chapter 42.

▶ CONCLUSION: IMPLICATIONS FOR MANAGEMENT IN THE PRACTICE ENVIRONMENT

This chapter has described the issues of managing an occupational therapy department. These include the roles of organizing, planning, directing, controlling, and evaluating in departmental administration. Issues related to documentation and fiscal planning were also discussed. Today, entry-level practitioners must have an awareness of administrative and management functions and their effect on the organization and management on the settings in which they are employed. The occupational therapy manager provides an image of the profession among peers in the health care delivery system and thus must be highly qualified as an administrator. The need for qualified, effective occupational therapy managers is essential for the future growth of the profession. In a time when occupational therapy is considered an expanding field, the profession, through education and professional standards, must be prepared to meet the need.

▼ REFERENCES

American Occupational Therapy Association (AOTA). (1986). Guidelines for occupational therapy documentation. *American Journal of Occupational Therapy, 40*, 830–832.

American Occupational Therapy Association. (1989). *Guidelines for occupational therapy services in school systems* (2nd ed.). Rockville, MD: Author.

American Occupational Therapy Association. (1990). *OT FACT.* Rockville, MD: Author.

American Occupational Therapy Association. (1994). Uniform terminology for occupational therapy—third edition. *American Journal of Occupational Therapy, 48*, 1047–1054.

American Occupational Therapy Association. (1996). *Practice guidelines.* Bethesda, MD: Author.

Americans with Disability Act of 1990 (ADA), Public Law 101–336, 104 Stat. 327–378. (1991).

AOTA Managed Care Project Team (1996). *Managed care: An occupational therapy sourcebook.* Bethesda, MD: American Occupational Therapy Association.

Blake, R. R., & Mouton, J. S. (1964). *The managerial grid.* Houston, TX: Gulf Publishing.

Commission on Accreditation of Rehabilitation Facilities (CARF). (1994). *Standards manual for organizations serving people with disabilities.* Tucson, AZ: Author.

Conditions of Participation for Intermediate Term Care Facilities, 42 C.F.R. Ch. IV, Part 483 Subpart I (1988).

Donabedian, A. (1982). *Exploration of quality assessment and monitoring: Vol. 2: The criteria and standards of quality.* Ann Arbor, MI: Health Administration Press.

Education for All Handicapped Children Act of 1975, Public Law 94–142 89, Stat. 773–796 (1977).

Education for All Handicapped Children Act Amendments of 1986, Public Law 99–457, 100 Stat. 1145–1177 (1989).

Forer, S. (1996). *Outcome management and program evaluation made easy: A toolkit for occupational therapy practitioners.* Bethesda, MD: American Occupational Therapy Association.

Hayes, R. (1989). Strategic planning—forward in reverse? *Harvard Business Review,* Nov/Dec.

Joint Commission of Accreditation of Healthcare Organizations (JCAHO). (1988). *The quality assurance guide.* Chicago: Author.

Llorens, L. A., & Shuster, J. J. (1977). Occupational therapy sequential client care recording system: A comparative study. *The American Journal of Occupational Therapy, 31*, 367–371.

Montgomery County Association for Retarded Citizens (1978). *IEP: Individualized educational program. What is it/how does it work?* Silver Spring, MD: Author.

Ostrow, P.C., Williamson, J.W., & Joe, B.E. (1983). *Quality assurance primer.* Rockville, MD: American Occupational Therapy Association.

Slater, C. A., Evans, R. W., & Small, L. (1992). Clinical program evaluation: An example of continuous quality. Presented at the American Speech and Hearing Association Annual Symposium. Anaheim, CA.

Steiner, G. A. (1979) *Strategic planning: What every manager must know.* New York: Free Press.

Tiffany, E. G. (1983). Psychiatry and mental health. In H. L. Hopkins & H. S. Smith (Eds.), *Willard and Spackman's occupational therapy* (6th ed., pp. 267–334). Philadelphia: J. B. Lippincott.

U.S. Department of Education (1981). Assistance to states for education of handicapped children. *Federal Register, 46*(12), 5460–5473.

Weed, L. L. (1971). *Medical records, medical evaluation and patient care.* Chicago: Yearbook Medical Publishers.

World Health Organization (WHO) (1980). *International classification of impairments, diseases and handicaps: A manual of classification relating to consequences of disease.* Geneva, Switzerland.

Chapter 44

Interdisciplinary Communication and Supervision of Personnel

Ellen S. Cohn

▼ TEAMS AND TEAMWORK

In the often cited poem about Hinduism, *The Blind Men and the Elephant*, John Godfrey Saxe described the plight of six men, all blind, who happened on an elephant. The first man, feeling the elephant's side, reported it was like a wall. The second, feeling the tusk, interpreted the creature to be like a spear. The third, finding its trunk, declared it to be like a snake, and so on. Thus, when each observer stated his opinion of the elephant, "each was partly in the right, and all were in the wrong!" (Saxe, 1871, p. 260). Herein lies the concept underlying the use of the interdisciplinary team communication. Although each member, representing a different perspective, is hardly blind, a single way of observing limits the ability to comprehend the whole. It is the combined vision, evaluation, and coordinated plan that provides a complete picture of the "whole" person receiving occupational therapy intervention.

For most areas of practice, interdisciplinary team interactions are the norm. Successful intervention involves a collaborative and mutual process during which practitioners and clients develop the care plan together (Case-Smith & Wavrek, 1993; Golin & Duncanis, 1981; Humphry, Gonzalez, & Taylor, 1993; Leff & Walizer, 1992). According to Parham (1987), occupational therapists are "concerned with understanding the occupations of human beings, the ways in which people organize the activities that fill their lives

and give their lives meaning" (p. 555). To understand how a particular client experiences illness or disability within the context of his or her occupations and daily life, the occupational therapy practitioner will need to collaborate with other members of the team involved in providing care for that client. The team comprises a variety of different specialists who have different backgrounds, training, values, world views, and sometimes different goals. These specialists work together in different configurations, depending on the needs of the client. Each team member addresses the client's concerns from a unique perspective, and these perspectives are then coordinated to structure the client care plan. It is assumed that this coordinated perspective will make a difference in the ultimate outcome for the recipient of the care plan (Crepeau, 1994a, 1994b; Unsworth, Thomas, & Greenwood, 1995).

Ideally, interdisciplinary team members (1) share a common concept of the client's concerns and a common philosophy of care management; (2) synthesize the diverse information gathered from their own evaluations and those of outside consultants; and (3) work together to formulate and implement a comprehensive care plan based on the available data. Most importantly, the team should act as a functional unit whose members are willing to learn from each other and modify, when appropriate, their own opinions, based on the combined observations and expertise of the entire group (Turk & Stieg, 1987). The advantages of a team approach are (1) a more holistic approach to client care, (2) integrated interventions, (3) the reduction or elimination of duplicated services and fragmentation or gaps in care, and (4) quicker and more informed decisions for client plans (Stancliff, 1995).

Historically, health care teams have generated a client's care plan behind closed doors, without the client's input and then shared their plans with the client. In current practice, however, additional voices are influencing the team process. Incorporation of the client as a member of the team is now espoused by health professionals and is viewed as crucial to the eventual success of the care plan (Case-Smith & Wavrek, 1993; Crepeau, 1994a, 1994b; Intagliata, 1993; Turk & Stieg, 1987). In the managed care environment, which focuses on both cost containment and quality of care, the third-party payer's perspective is increasingly considered another crucial factor in the team's decision-making process.

An understanding of the potential contributions of the various people and professionals involved in the client's life will enable the occupational therapist to develop a more meaningful plan for each client. The members of the team have interrelated functions. Depending on the practice environment, the occupational therapy practitioner's interactions with other professionals and with the important people in the client's life will vary. In a medical setting, such as an acute care hospital or a rehabilitation unit, the team members may operate under a physician's order, and practitioners might interact with team members numerous times a day. Alternatively, a practitioner in private practice or employed by a home care agency might not have frequent contact with other specialists, but may have more frequent contact with family members or other significant people in the client's life.

Regardless of the environment, occupational therapy practitioners need to be aware of the roles of the other members of the team, so practitioners may be clear about the contributions occupational therapy can make and how everyone can work together for the client's benefit. Therefore, occupational therapy practitioners will need to interpret their role and contribution to the treatment team, for it is never safe to assume that other members of any particular treatment team will have a full understanding of the potential contributions of occupational therapy. Consider, for example, Rose's story.

Rose is a 72-year-old woman who recently received a total hip replacement and is now receiving occupational therapy services in her home. Although her husband is devoted to her, he is unable to help her maintain the home. A social worker is available to consult with the intervention team. Together, the occupational therapist, the client, her husband, and the social worker determined that seeking the services of a meals-on-wheels program would alleviate the pressure of preparing meals. This team decision-making process helped the occupational therapist determine the focus of occupational therapy intervention. With Rose's homemaking duties alleviated, the occupational therapist

was able to focus on helping Rose regain and monitor her strength and endurance so that she had the resources to again join her husband at their weekly singing group. With the assistance of the intervention team, occupational therapy was focused on a meaningful activity for Rose and her husband.

Although practically every medical and allied health professional may be called on to provide services to address the range of client conditions seen by occupational therapy practitioners, the professionals listed in Box 44–1 may be especially relevant (Allen, 1996; Goldenson, 1978).

Team Interaction Models

Each client usually has an identified case manager or team leader. The case manager is the designated person on whom clients and their family can consistently rely to explain, clarify, or acquire necessary information. This case manager may also serve the role of the client ombudsman. The leadership of the team or the case management may change over time, according to the identified concerns of a particular client, the members of a team, the nature of the task, and the structure of the organization. In a traditional medical model, the physician is often the leader of the team. Today, especially in community-based settings, a therapist, special service coordinator, or teacher may lead or coordinate the team and simultaneously serve as the case manager.

Teams may be organized into multidisciplinary, interdisciplinary, or transdisciplinary models. Often, however, a team moves from one model to another and functions in its own unique variation of the classic models. In the multidisciplinary approach, team members work side by side, and each member has a clearly defined role with specific areas of responsibility. Evaluation, planning, and therapy take place independently. Generally, families and clients meet with the team members of each discipline separately. In an interdisciplinary approach, team members share responsibility for providing services, often sharing roles. Team members conduct separate evaluations, but share the results to develop an integrated and coordinated care plan. Clients and families or other significant people in clients' lives meet with the team or a representative of the team, such as the team leader or case manager. In a transdisciplinary team, members commit to teaching, learning, and working across disciplinary boundaries to plan and provide integrated services. The team assimilates the perspectives of the various team members to make joint decisions, traditional role boundaries are crossed, and the skills of other disciplines are integrated into a total care plan.

Creating Shared Meaning and a Common Language

Professionals and clients may have different viewpoints or priorities for the care plan; or they may have the same

▼ **BOX 44-1**

Medical, Rehabilitation, and Educational Professionals

Adapted physical educator: adapts sporting equipment and games for individuals with special needs.

Administrator: applies and enforces federal, state, and local laws that regulate finances, standards, and environments for most health and educational programs; has valuable expertise in management of personnel, space, and finances.

Audiologist: specializes in diagnosis and treatment of hearing impairments; administers a variety of tests to determine hearing level and site of damage to the auditory system; recommends hearing aid and other assistive devices to enhance residual hearing loss or the need for special training.

Biomedical engineer: specializes in the application of scientific theory and technology to the development of devices and techniques for medical treatment, rehabilitation, and research; provides technical expertise in recommendation of commercial products and the modifications of existing devices or the design and fabrication of custom equipment or adjusted environments.

Chaplain: focuses on religious and spiritual needs of clients, provides nondenominational individual and family counseling, as well as special services.

Orthotist and prosthetist: the prosthetist designs and fabricates artificial limbs, with special attention to enhancing fit, function, and appearance, while the orthotist makes and fits braces to (1) support or correct body parts weakened by disease, injury, or congenital deformity, or (2) to help prevent deformities.

Physical therapist: evaluates physical capacities and limitations, and administers treatment designed to alleviate pain, correct or minimize deformity, increase strength and mobility, and improve general health.

Physicians: Consulting physicians are usually specialists to whom a client has been referred by the primary care physician. They may include orthopedists, ophthalmologists, neurologists, cardiologists, physiatrists, or psychiatrists.

Psychologist: provides psychological, projective, and behavioral assessments; provides individual, couple, family, and group psychotherapy related to behavioral or adjustment issues.

Therapeutic recreation specialist (recreation therapist): facilitates the enjoyable use of leisure time to promote mental and physical well-being; uses social and recreational activities to aid in adjustment to disability and participation in community activities.

Rehabilitation nurse: provides goal-directed, personalized care that encompasses preventive, maintenance, and restorative aspects of nursing; administers medication and instructs client and significant others in care management and health maintenance programs.

Respiratory therapist: (also known as inhalation therapy), administers oxygen and mists for medical purposes, provides oxygen assessment programs and client education.

Social workers: assists client, family, or other important people in the client's life to achieve a maximal level of social and emotional functioning; provides client and family counseling, discharge planning, and education on entitlements and other available resources; assists in identifying transportation and attendant care resources.

Special educator: serves as a teacher of children with either unusually high intellectual potential or children who are handicapped by mental illness, learning disabilities, or developmental deviations. May have advanced skills in teaching children who are blind, deaf, emotionally disturbed, mentally retarded, or physically handicapped.

Speech and language pathologist: specializes in speech disorders, the development of language and speech production, the physiology of speech, theories and measurement of hearing and phonetics.

Teacher: certified to provide education at the early childhood, kindergarten, elementary, secondary, or high school level.

Vocational counselor: provides diagnostic evaluation of transferable skills, achievement levels, aptitudes, and interests to determine employability and job placement potential; works with employers to facilitate successful work placements.

---

goals, yet differ in the meaning of the goals or the approach for reaching goals. Therefore, it is essential for the team members to develop shared meaning about the client's entire condition. For the intervention to be effective, the treatment team must understand clients' (1) beliefs, (2) attitudes, (3) ways of making meaning of their life-world, (4) knowledge of their condition, (5) expectancies for the future, and (6) expectancies about treatment (Crepeau, 1994a; Salisbury, 1992; Turk & Stieg, 1987). The constructionist process, as described by Buckholdt and Gubrium (1979) and Crepeau (1994a, 1994b), involves the individual clinical reasoning of the team members and the collective reasoning of the group. Formal lines of communication and methods for sharing these interpretations often develop through team meetings, collaborative intervention sessions, written evaluations, or progress notes. Each team member makes his or her own interpretation of the client's lived experience and then articulates this interpretation to the other team members. The team collectively reconstructs the interpretation to create a unified image from the diversity of their individual perspectives. Through this constructionist process team members discover, interpret, and negotiate their understanding of the client by "sorting out conflicting data to arrive at a common definition of the problems faced by the patient" (Crepeau, 1994b, p. 161).

To develop a cohesive treatment team that uses a constructionist process, the team must focus their energy and creativity to establish a shared mission (Dudgeon, 1996). Only in a climate of mutual trust and respect can a group of people with diverse perspectives develop into a cohesive team (Zenger, Musselwhite, Hurson, & Perrin, 1994). Thus, it is important to acknowledge that team building is a developmental process; it takes time and energy to learn about each member's values, goals, and communication style (Blechert, Christiansen, & Kari, 1987). Although teams may have different needs at different times, Blechert and her colleagues have found that team development can be described in terms of life stages. In the first stage, team members explore and define their roles within the context of the team and work setting. Each team member identifies his or her area of expertise and interest, thereby defining the unique contribution of each team member. Once the team has worked together, adjustment and rearrangement of roles may be necessary to progress to the next stage. Finally, as team members redefine their roles and learn to value each other, they begin to think about issues from multiple points of view. When functioning well, the team members are able to see the issues as a "whole." Similar to the blind men with the elephant, the image developed by the team is broader and richer when multiple perspectives are shared to construct a unified image.

▼ SUPERVISION

Supervision Story

Barbara, an occupational therapist with 3 years of experience, has just started working in a day school program for children with developmental disabilities. Within 4 weeks of her involvement in the program, Barbara is required to complete annual evaluations for five children. Barbara is unfamiliar with the assessment tools used by the occupational therapy department in the day school program, yet believes she should know how to administer them. Initially, Barbara is reluctant to reveal to her supervisor that she is unfamiliar with the assessments, because she perceives the lack of this knowledge as incompetence and fears her supervisor's disapproval. Nonetheless, she understands the purpose of supervision, and challenges herself to seek the guidance she needs. Barbara's supervisor is pleased that Barbara was able to identify her learning needs, and together they develop a learning plan for Barbara. This situation highlights the complexity of the supervisory process. Tasks include ensuring quality while teaching and developing skills, all within the context of an interpersonal relationship. This occurs among all levels of occupational therapy personnel, from aides, students, staff therapists, to all occupational therapy practitioners. The following section addresses definitions, the supervisory relationship, functions, goals and components of the supervisory process, and staff development.

Definition of Supervision

Supervision is a dynamic, interactive process in which the supervisor has been assigned or designated to assist in and direct the work and growth of the supervisees. The word supervisor is derived from the Latin word *super*, "over," and *videre*, "to watch, to see" (Harel, 1994). Therefore, the supervisor is assigned or designated by the organization administration to oversee or watch over the work of another, and the supervisee is expected to be accountable to the supervisor. The supervisory process, as defined by the American Occupational Therapy Association (AOTA), is "a process in which two or more people participate in a joint effort to promote, establish, maintain, and/or elevate a level of performance and service" (1994a, p. 1045). Supervision is viewed as a mutual process that "fosters growth and development; assures appropriate utilization of training and potential; encourages creativity and innovation; and provides guidance, support, encouragement, and respect while working toward a goal" (AOTA, 1994a, p. 1045). These definitions of supervision all identify the supervisor as a person who has some official responsibility to direct, guide, and monitor the supervisee's practice. These authority, evaluation, and accountability functions distinguish supervision from consultation or mentorship. In the mentorship or consultative role, the more experienced practitioner guides or coaches the apprentice, without the authority function of evaluating performance and maintaining the standards and viability of the organization.

Supervisory Relationship

The importance of the relationship between supervisors and supervisees is inherent within the supervisory context. Christie and coworkers (1985), in their study of 65 fieldwork centers, confirmed the longstanding belief that the relationship between students and fieldwork educators is the most significant aspect of the fieldwork experience. In the study, both students and educators perceived the supervisory process as the most critical element in distinguishing good from poor fieldwork experiences. Furthermore, communication and interpersonal skills were identified as distinguishing characteristics of an effective supervisor. These characteristics are essential to any supervisory relationship.

Each member in the supervisory relationship enters with his or her own assumptions and expectations. These expectations are based on the supervisee's past experiences with other supervisors, parents, and other authority figures. These experiences, together with supervisee's emerging images of occupational therapy and professional goals, provide the foundation for the supervisory relationship. Supervisors, in turn, have a notion of the behaviors, skills, and attitudes necessary for effective practice in their settings. Initially, the delineation of expectations of both supervisors and supervisees is a primary focus of supervision. Later, the focus shifts to providing feedback related to the stated expectations.

The feedback provided by supervisors is critical to supervisees' development. Feedback is defined as sharing knowledge of the results of an individual's performance with the intent of changing that individual's behavior in a desirable direction. It refers to a particular aspect of behavior, to a total behavioral sequence or performance, or to the nature of the message itself. For example, the message may convey information about supervisees' attitudes toward clients. This definition connotes an expectation that "some change will occur in the supervisee's understanding, attitude, or behavior in response to feedback" (Freeman, 1985, p. 5). Feedback can help (1) identify the next step in the change process, (2) clarify steps that have taken place, (3) evaluate whether a particular step meets performance criteria for a specific task and whether it relates to or achieves the overall goals, and (4) clarify or modify those goals or expectations as needed. One of the key sources for feedback is the supervisor. It is important for supervisees to recognize that supervisors are not judging the supervisee's worth or goodness, but assessing how well the supervisee is performing. Crist (1986) suggests that supervisees be willing to try new suggestions, while evaluating their own biases and preferences. "Feedback, given honestly and sincerely is often the most valuable change agent" (Freeman, 1985, p. 109).

Functions of Supervision

Supervisors assume multiple roles as they promote the growth of their supervisees. These roles have been described by Harel (1994) as being distinct, yet overlapping, functions. The educational role focuses on learning and performing. In this role, the supervisor acknowledges that the supervisee is an adult learner and assumes the supervisee will take an active role in the supervisory process. Drawing on the principle of adult learning that learners should be empowered to share responsibility for planning and evaluating their learning experiences, the supervisor works with the supervisee to plan and achieve acceptable goals (Knowles, 1980). The learning may begin with the direct transmission of information essential to perform one's job responsibilities, such as orientation to the organization of the facility and department, including structure, function, policies, and procedures. The supervisor then teaches or coaches the supervisee to explore the range of possibilities to promote quality delivery of services. As in Barbara's situation, the supervisor may negotiate a learning contract that outlines specific skill and theories to be mastered and delineates a plan to meet specific objectives.

In the administrative function, the performance of the supervisee is observed to ensure the maintenance of job requirements and professional standards. The supervisor evaluates and documents the supervisee's ability to meet these requirements and standards. If the job requirements and standards that are consistent with professional, state, and department guidelines have not been achieved, the supervisor will assume the teaching role to promote successful performance.

Both the administrative and educational roles require the supervisor to be a supportive role model. The role model is widely recognized as central to assisting others in the traditions and standards of practice (Rogers, 1982). Many clinical situations provoke reflection on complex, intense issues of life and death, personal loss, disease, or disability. Given the potential for personal responses to the complex issues practitioners encounter, the supervisor must attend to the supervisee's responses to these issues, and to his or her ability to cope with the situations present. The supervisor can help the supervisee identify behavior and feelings that may affect his or her interactions with clients or his or her ability to provide quality care. However, it is beyond the role of the supervisor to provide psychotherapy to a supervisee. When psychotherapy is indicated, supervisors should make the necessary recommendation.

Components of the Supervisory Process

Anderson's (1988) analysis of the supervisory process identified the following components:

UNDERSTANDING THE SUPERVISORY PROCESS

For the supervisory process to be effective, both the supervisor and supervisee need to be prepared for their roles. Thus, the supervisory process should include ongoing discussions relative to expectations, concerns, needs, learning styles, and perceptions of the supervisory experience. Through these ongoing discussions, expectations, goals, and approaches may be modified in response to the evolving process.

PLANNING

Planning begins as soon as the supervisory process begins. It is a joint process in which the supervisor and supervisee identify (1) the supervisee's ability to problem solve, (2) the degree of involvement each participant desires, (3) the ability of the supervisee to observe and analyze his or her behavior, and (4) the supervisor's flexibility in adapting his or her style to the supervisee's needs. Together, the supervisor and supervisee determine the objectives and methods for accomplishing the given objectives.

OBSERVING

The observational component of the supervisory process involves data collection and recording by both supervisor and supervisee for further analysis and interpretation, which can then lead to performance evaluation. The most traditional form of observation is for the supervisor to watch the supervisee perform a given task and simply to write evaluative statements reflecting his or her perceptions of the appropriateness of the supervisee's performance. Other forms of observation include tallies of specific behaviors, use of specific rating scales, verbatim recording, selective recordings, observing nonverbal behavior, and audiotaping or videotaping the therapy sessions.

Goals of Supervision

The goal of supervision "is the professional growth and development of the supervisee and the supervisor, which it is assumed will result ultimately in optimal service to clients" (Anderson, 1988, p. 12). Subsumed in this broad goal emphasizing learning and service are the following subgoals:

- To develop a sense of professional identity
- To increase theoretical knowledge and apply this knowledge to the complexities inherent in practice
- To develop reflection on practice
- To name, frame, and solve problems in an organized, thorough, and analytical fashion
- To make thoughtful decisions in a reasonable time period
- To be objective, flexible, and independent in thought and action
- To develop self-awareness and make changes in behavior on the basis of such awareness
- To cultivate individual abilities

To achieve these goals, the supervisor will need to establish a safe and trusting relationship with his or her supervisee. This type of relationship will foster a mutual sharing of questions, concerns, observations, speculations, and identification of alternative or multiple approaches to solving the complexities of practice. Some of the goals of supervision are similar to those we might think of as the role of staff development. Indeed, as we will see in the following section, supervision is an essential component in any comprehensive staff development program.

Staff Development

Staff development is critical to achieving and maintaining quality delivery of services in any organization. Although the components of a staff development program are highly dependent on the nature and resources of that particular facility, most organizations take a performance-oriented approach. When viewed from this perspective, the purpose of staff development is to facilitate the growth of employees such that they can achieve the highest performance possible. An effective staff development program should focus on the integration of the organization's and the employee's goals (Lieberman & Miller, 1979). However, the increasingly complex climate of managed health care, which emphasizes productivity and meaningful outcomes, may leave managers with less time to establish clinical competence in their employees. The health care environment of today demands that practitioners be competent and ready to provide quality services as soon as possible.

Traditional staff development programs generally consist of formal courses, workshops, conferences, or a series of in-service training units that teach specific skills and procedures. Orientation programs to introduce new staff members to its policies, procedures, evaluation tools, and documentation requirements are common in many settings. A more highly developed program for new staff members may include lectures on topics specific to the clinical population receiving services. These programs focus on immediate skill development and establish facility standards.

To address employee personal and professional goals from a developmental perspective, Smith and Elbert (1986) recommend using a self-appraisal approach. That is, employees complete an assessment of their competence and then write objectives for future learning. Self-appraisals include content relative to clinical knowledge and skills as well as professional development content, such as time and stress management, communication skills, interdisciplinary communication, and professional standards and ethics. Once employees identify their goals, they can develop an individualized development program by drawing on the resources of the facility, their supervisors, and the educational opportunities in their community and the broader professional communities.

Lieberman and Miller (1979) recommend using the work itself to stimulate and reinforce professional growth and development. Drawing on Schon's (1983) notion of reflection-in-action, in which practitioners critically examine or reflect on the reasoning processes used in everyday practice, Slater and Cohn (1991) advocate videotaping and analyzing therapy sessions in either peer-learning or small-group situations. While examining the videotapes, learners

ETHICS NOTE

WHO SHOULD BE RESPONSIBLE FOR ASSURING COMPETENCE?

Penny Kyler and Ruth A. Hansen

Tom, who is a registered occupational therapist, has worked in acute physical rehabilitation for the last 12 years. During the recent reorganization of the hospital many staffing changes have occurred. Tom now is working half-time in adolescent psychiatry. He has no previous experience working with adolescents with a primary psychiatric diagnosis. He will be working alone on the unit.

1. Does Tom have the credentials and the competence to provide services in adolescent psychiatry?
2. Does Tom have the right to refuse to work in adolescent psychiatry?
3. Does the employer have the right to expect that Tom can provide occupational therapy services on this unit?
4. What actions should the employer and Tom take to assure that he can deliver competent services for the patient? ■

and supervisors can stop the action and discuss the various approaches used and explore new interpretations to address therapy from a broader perspective.

▼ SUPERVISION OF OCCUPATIONAL THERAPY PERSONNEL

Supervision Guidelines and Standards for Occupational Therapy Practitioners

The amount and nature of supervision in a particular setting are closely determined by the structure of the setting, the role functions of the practitioner, and the practitioner's expertise in his or her various roles. AOTA (1993) provides guidelines for supervision that indicate patterns and types of supervision. The guidelines describe supervision along a continuum that includes close, routine, general, and minimal levels of supervision. Close supervision requires daily, direct contact at the site of work. Routine supervision requires direct contact at least every 2 weeks at the site of work. Interim supervision occurs through indirect methods, such as telephone or written communication. General supervision requires at least monthly direct contact, with supervision available as needed by other methods. Minimal supervision is provided only as needed, and may be less than monthly (AOTA, 1993).

The AOTA document entitled *Occupational Therapy Roles* (1993; see Appendix C) makes a distinction between formal supervision, which includes the oversight or accountability responsibility; and functional supervision, which implies that supervisors have specialized knowledge as a result of their experience and expertise. Barbara, cited in the earlier example, requires functional supervision to assist her in learning needed skills. A functional supervisor provides information and feedback relative to a particular function, such as implementing a particular intervention technique or learning a particular assessment.

The AOTA (1994a) maintains the principle that occupational therapy practice should be supervised by trained and qualified occupational therapy practitioners. Administrative supervision can be provided by others, such as special education directors, principals, facility administrators, or other health care providers (AOTA, 1994a). (See Appendix D for the AOTA *Guide for Supervision of Occupational Therapy Personnel*.) Entry-level practitioners require close supervision of their occupational therapy practice by intermediate-level practitioners for service delivery aspects, and routine supervision for administrative aspects of their work. Intermediate-level practitioners who have mastery of basic role functions require routine to general supervision from advanced practitioners, and advanced practitioners require minimal supervision within their area of expertise and general supervision for the administrative aspects of their work (AOTA, 1993).

Although professional guidelines recommend minimal levels of supervision, the consumers of occupational therapy

and occupational therapy practitioners have a certain amount of faith in the occupational therapy process, without much empirical evidence to document the efficacy of a given intervention. As a profession, we are just beginning to measure therapy outcomes. In this context, supervision becomes a critical mechanism to encourage occupational therapy practitioners to examine the underlying assumptions and postulates for changes that guide our therapy process. Supervision then becomes a vehicle to examine the reasoning behind the daily actions of practice. Thus, supervision is a valuable and often overlooked process for even the most experienced practitioner.

Supervision of Occupational Therapy Students

The consensus within the occupational therapy profession is that the fieldwork experience plays an integral role in professional development. In 1923, the first standards requiring fieldwork experiences were approved by AOTA (Pressler, 1983). Fieldwork continues to function as the critical link between the academic world of theory and the clinical world of practice (Cohn & Crist, 1995). This component of education functions as the gateway into our profession, because all students must complete fieldwork requirements to become eligible to take the certification examinations for occupational therapists and occupational therapy assistants.

The process and content of fieldwork experiences have been debated over the years. Yet the value of having an opportunity to integrate academic knowledge with application skills at progressively higher levels of performance and responsibility has always been acknowledged as important (Pressler, 1983). Christie, Joyce, and Moeller (1985) highlight that value by documenting the fieldwork experience as having the greatest influence on the development of a therapist's preference for a specific area of clinical practice. Of the 131 therapists surveyed, 55% indicated that clinical practice preferences were either formed or changed during the fieldwork experience, and another 24% noted that fieldwork experience expanded their interests to other areas of practice (Christie, Joyce, & Moeller, 1985, p. 673). Thus, the fieldwork experience can be rich and rewarding, and as such, it is likely to have a tremendous bearing on a student's career choices.

PURPOSE AND LEVELS OF FIELDWORK

The *AOTA Essentials and Guidelines of an Accredited Educational Program for Occupational Therapist and Occupational Therapy Assistants* (AOTA Essentials) (AOTA, 1991a, 1991b) outline the general fieldwork requirements for all students. The requirements are divided into two classifications, Level I and Level II fieldwork. Level I fieldwork offers students practical experiences that are integrated throughout the academic program. The AOTA Essentials describe Level I fieldwork as "experiences designed to enrich didactic course work through directed observation and participation in selected aspects of the occupational therapy process" (1991a, p. 1082; 1991b, p. 1090). The ultimate goal of Level I fieldwork is "to enhance an understanding of the developmental stages, tasks, and roles of individuals throughout the life span" (COE, 1992, p. 1). Through Level I fieldwork experiences, students are exposed to the values and traditions of occupational therapy practice and have the opportunity to examine their reactions to clients, systems of service delivery, related personnel, and potential role(s) within the profession. Because the academic level performance expectations and specific purposes of the Level I fieldwork experience vary in each occupational therapy curriculum, the timing, length, requirements, and specific focus of the experience are negotiated with each academic program on an individual basis (COE, 1988).

The purpose of Level II fieldwork for the occupational therapy student is to "promote clinical reasoning and reflective practice; to transmit the values, beliefs, and ethical commitments of the field of occupational therapy; to communicate and model professional behaviors attending to the developmental nature of career growth and responsibility; and to develop and expand a repertoire of occupational therapy, assessments and treatment interventions related to human performance" (AOTA, 1991a). For occupational therapy assistant students the purpose of Level II fieldwork is "to provide in-depth experiences in providing occupational therapy services and to develop and expand a repertoire of occupational therapy practice" (AOTA, 1991b, p. 1090). Under close supervision students test firsthand the theories and facts learned in academic study, and refine skills through interaction with clients.

The requirements established by AOTA include a minimum of the equivalent of 6 months, or 960 total hours, of Level II fieldwork for occupational therapy students (AOTA, 1991a) and a minimum of 12 weeks, or 440 hours, for occupational therapy assistant students (AOTA, 1991b). To offer occupational therapy students experience with a wide range of client ages and a variety of physical and mental health conditions, the 6 months are usually divided into two 3-month experiences in different clinical facilities. Alternatives to full-time fieldwork, such as part-time models or 12-month experiences, are becoming more common (Adelstein, Cohn, Baker, & Barnes, 1990; Phillips & Legaspi, 1995). Successful completion of Level II fieldwork is a requirement for **certification** as a registered occupational therapist (OTR) or certified occupational therapy assistant (COTA). Fieldwork provides students with situations in which to (1) practice interpersonal skills with clients and staff and, (2) develop characteristics essential to productive working relationships (AOTA, 1988).

For students, the overall purpose of the fieldwork experience is to gain mastery of occupational therapy clinical reasoning and techniques to develop entry-level competence. Effective oral and written communication of ideas and objectives relevant to the roles and duties of an occupational

therapist or occupational therapy assistant, including professional interaction with clients and staff, is expected of all students. Students are responsible for (1) demonstrating a sensitivity to and respect for client confidentiality, (2) establishing and sustaining therapeutic relationships, and (3) working collaboratively with others. Another expectation—more internal to the students' development of positive professional self-images—includes taking responsibility for maintaining, assessing, and improving self-competence. Students are responsible for articulating their understanding of theoretical information and identifying their abilities to implement assessments or treatment techniques. Moreover, the ability to benefit from supervision as a resource for self-directed learning is critical to professional development. Thus, understanding and articulating one's individual learning style becomes essential to the supervisory process (Schwartz, 1980).

TRANSITION FROM STUDENT TO PROFESSIONAL

The shift from the academic setting to the fieldwork setting is an obvious, yet often underestimated, life change. Occupational therapy students are making the environmental transition from the classroom to the fieldwork setting while simultaneously emerging from the role of student to the role of occupational therapy practitioner. As with any transition, occupational therapy students leaving academia face a process of change from one structure, role, or sense of self to another. The struggle to assimilate into a new environment and to develop a new role may jolt students into disequilibrium, and some may have trouble adjusting to the new role. As is true of all life changes, this disequilibrium can be an opportunity for growth, especially in the context of a supportive supervisory relationship.

This time of transition for students results in changes in assumptions about themselves and the world and requires a corresponding change in behaviors, relationships, learning styles, and self-perceptions. As they move into fieldwork settings, students may begin to reassess their suppositions about occupational therapy, the theories they learned in school, and their views of themselves as practitioners, learners, and individuals. Because individuals differ in their ability to adapt to change and because each student will be placed in a different fieldwork setting, the transition will have a different effect on each student.

The nature of the fieldwork environment is fundamentally different from that of the academic environment. Knowing and acknowledging some of the distinctions between the two settings may ease the transition and provide students with support to accept the challenges of fieldwork experiences (Table 44–1).

Within the fieldwork environment, the learning focus shifts to the application or implementation of therapy techniques in an applied interpersonal context. Techniques that were introduced in a simulated context now must be mastered and applied with attention to the client's emotional

Table 44-1. Distinctions Between Academic and Fieldwork Settings

Characteristic	Academic Setting	Fieldwork Setting
Purpose	Dissemination of knowledge, development of creative thought and student growth, award degrees	Provide high quality client care
Faculty/supervisor accountability	1. To student 2. To university/college	1. To client and significant others 2. To fieldwork center 3. To student
Student accountability	To self	To clients and significant others, supervisor, and fieldwork center
Pace	Dependent on curriculum; adaptable to student and faculty needs	Dependent on clients' needs; less adaptable
Student/educator ratio	Many students to one faculty member	One student to one supervisor; small group of students to one supervisor; one student to two supervisors
Source of feedback	Summative at midterm or end of term; provided by faculty	Provided by clients and significant others, supervisor, and other staff; formative
Degree of faculty/supervisor control of educational experience	Able to plan; controlled	Limited control; various diagnoses and length of client stay
Primary learning tools	Books, lectures, audiovisual aids, case studies, simulations	Situation of practice; clients, families, significant others, and staff
Conceptual learning	Abstract, theoretical	Pragmatic, applied in interpersonal context
Learning process	Teacher directed	Client, self, peer. Or supervisor directed
Tolerance for ambiguity	High	Low
Lifestyle	Flexible; able to plan time around class schedule	Structured; flexible time limited to evenings and weekends

needs. Abstract questions appropriate in the academic environment shift to pragmatic questions to reduce the possibility of error in one's thinking. For example, rather than thinking about a client's function in the kitchen from an abstract perspective, the student has to think about the client's function in the context of a specific kitchen in a certain small apartment and to attend to the client's concerns about his or her family. Because the student recognizes that his or her actions will have an influence on the client's life, tolerance for ambiguity or uncertainty declines during fieldwork.

In the academic setting, students are accountable to themselves, and performance is evaluated on a summative basis through tests, assignments, and grades. Students choose whether to disclose their grades to family or peers, and their performance does not affect others. In the fieldwork center, a student's performance is evaluated on a formative basis and may be observed by the entire health care team, especially at team meetings. Performance is no longer the private matter it was at school, but is publicly observed, because it has direct and critical consequences for clients. Colleagues, clients, and their families then may offer meaningful feedback. Although all these opportunities may create disequilibrium or tension, they likewise constitute new ways in which students learn about themselves and their profession. The broad and diverse experience within the fieldwork setting challenges students to redefine their sense of self.

Fieldwork takes place in a situation over which fieldwork educators have little control. The organizational factors of the health care setting, combined with client care factors,

such as the nature and complexity of the client's problem, the length of stay, and fluctuation in client load, make planning difficult, especially in acute care settings. In settings that provide extended care for clients, however, the fieldwork educators are able to plan ahead because the client population is more constant, and the fieldwork educator knows which clients will be available during student placements.

The fieldwork educators' primary responsibility is client care; they have an ethical imperative to ensure the welfare of clients. This appropriate professional ethic may constrain activities that may be desirable from the standpoint of education. However, the supervisory relationship allows fieldwork educators to adapt to the constraints of the setting. This unique relationship is a positive aspect of the fieldwork environment, because fieldwork educators can adapt the fieldwork experiences to meet the needs of the learner.

ROLES AND RESPONSIBILITIES

After completion of the prerequisite academic course work, occupational therapy and occupational therapy assistant students are eligible to begin their fieldwork experiences. Clearly defined objectives and guidelines help students organize their efforts toward achieving clinical competence. Working toward mastery of the entry-level skills required for high-quality client care is a mutual undertaking between the fieldwork educators and students. Both are responsible for the process of evaluating student progress and modifying the learning experience within the environment.

Students are responsible for fulfilling all duties identified by the fieldwork educators and academic fieldwork coordinators within the designated times and complying with the professional standards identified by the fieldwork facility, the education program, and the *Occupational Therapy Code of Ethics* (AOTA, 1994b; see Appendix B). The people responsible for the fieldwork education program and direct supervision of occupational therapy students must be registered occupational therapists, with a minimum of 1 year of experience in direct client service. For occupational therapy assistant students, direct supervision can be provided by a registered occupational therapist or certified occupational therapy assistant, also with a minimum of 1 year of experience. Although the minimum requirement is 1 year of experience, fieldwork educators should be competent clinicians who can serve as good role models or mentors for future practitioners. As stated in the Essentials (AOTA, 1991a, 1991b) these people are formally titled "fieldwork educators," although "clinical educators," "fieldwork supervisors," and "student supervisors" are interchangeable titles (COE, 1988). Two areas of responsibility of fieldwork educators are administrative functions and direct day-to-day supervision. The administrative responsibilities of the fieldwork educator include, but are not limited to, collaborating with the academic fieldwork coordinator to develop a program that provides the best opportunity for the implementation of theoretical concepts offered as part of the academic educational program, and creating an environment that facilitates learning, clinical inquiry, and reflection on one's practice.

Each education program has an academic fieldwork coordinator who functions as a liaison between the academic setting, the fieldwork educators, and the students. The academic fieldwork coordinators assign eligible students to fieldwork experience and is available for consultation with both students and fieldwork educators.

FIELDWORK EVALUATION

Frequently, students receive informal feedback during supervision meetings; however, formal mechanisms for providing feedback and evaluation of a student's performance, judgments, and attitudes are built into the fieldwork experience. There are two distinct purposes in fieldwork evaluation. One is the formative, ongoing process of directing student learning throughout the fieldwork experience; the other is summative, documenting the level of skills attained at the completion of the fieldwork experience. Although these two processes are different, they are not mutually exclusive. The formative process occurs throughout the fieldwork experience so that students and fieldwork educators can compare perceptions, assess which student activities are important and which are less so, review objectives, plan new learning opportunities, and make necessary modifications in behaviors. The second process, which is cumulative, requires documentation of a student's performance after completion of the fieldwork experience.

The Fieldwork Evaluation (FWE) is the instrument adopted by the AOTA for evaluating performance of professional-level occupational therapy students in all fieldwork education centers (COE, 1986). The FWE consists of two sections. The first section has 51 behavioral statements depicting competent performance in five areas: evaluation, planning, treatment, problem solving, and administrative or professionalism. The student is evaluated in each area on the basis of performance, judgment, and attitude on a rating scale, ranging from excellent to poor. The second section is a written summary of performance, indicating particular strengths and weaknesses and any other information useful in documenting professional growth and learning. This form should serve as a summary of what students already know of their performance. Completion, administration, and subsequent use of the FWE should be conducted with consideration of all legal and ethical implications for each student assessed. Such consideration includes the right to nonprejudicial evaluation, the right to privacy of information, and the right for students to appeal (COE, 1986).

The Fieldwork Evaluation Form for the Occupational Therapy Assistant Student (FWE/OTA) is the instrument adopted by AOTA for evaluating performance of occupational therapy assistant students in all fieldwork centers. Developed in 1983, this instrument contains 24 competency items, divided into four sections: evaluation, treatment, communication, and professional behavior. Each of the 24 items on the FWE/OTA is rated on a scale of 1 to 5, with criteria stated for each level. The FWE/OTA is used in a formative manner at midterm to provide students with feedback and to develop strategies for improving performance. It is used in a summative manner after completion of the fieldwork experience, because the AOTA states that the FWE/OTA final scores be based on the last 2 weeks of the fieldwork experience (COE, 1983).

Finally, the intent of the fieldwork evaluation is not to differentiate between students, but to measure their achievement of specific competencies. Future employers will want assurance that students satisfy the entry-level requirements. The FWE data may be synthesized to provide the foundation for employment references.

Students also have the opportunity to provide the fieldwork educators and fieldwork facility with feedback. The Student Evaluation of Fieldwork Experiences form (SE-FWE) is recommended for use by the Commission on Education (COE, 1995). This form allows students to provide feedback about the orientation process, supervisor interaction, and the entire learning experience. The fieldwork sites will use this information to improve fieldwork programs, and the academic programs share the information with future students who are interested in training at these sites.

A profession usually defines its boundaries by setting up criteria for entry. In occupational therapy, the fieldwork experience is an essential component of the entry criteria. Fieldwork is the beginning of a lifelong process of connecting theory with practice. The depth of the experience is highly dependent on the degree to which students and fieldwork educators share the responsibility for teaching and learning.

Supervision of Occupational Therapy Aides

To provide efficient and cost-effective occupational therapy services, many occupational therapy departments are employing occupational therapy aides. An occupational therapy aide is an individual assigned by an occupational therapist to perform delegated, selected, skilled tasks in specific situations under intense close supervision of occupational therapy practitioners. Ultimately, the occupational therapist or assistant is responsible and accountable for the overall use of aides in implementing services. The use of occupational therapy aides must be conducted in accordance with state laws and regulations, and practitioners must use professional judgment to determine which tasks to delegate to an occupational therapy aide in each particular situation. Finally, site-specific training must be provided along with appropriate supervisory mechanisms to continuously monitor competency (AOTA, 1995).

Supervision of Certified Occupational Therapy Assistants

The *AOTA Guide for Supervision of Occupational Therapy Personnel* (1994a) states that a certified occupational therapy assistant must receive supervision from a registered occupational therapist and that all occupational therapy practitioners shall practice and manage occupational therapy programs in accordance with applicable federal and state laws and regulations. These regulatory mandates often identity specific standards for supervision. Most of the state regulatory boards include provisions for the regulation of occupational therapy assistants. Therefore, the registered occupational therapist has a legal and ethical responsibility to provide supervision of the certified occupational therapy assistant. Supervision must be an interactive process to establish service competence. That is, whenever an occupational therapist delegates a task to an occupational therapy assistant, he or she must ensure that the assistant can perform the same or equivalent procedures with the same results. The supervisor will need to consider the setting and the client population. For example, the certified occupational therapy assistant who is working with a person whose condition is rapidly changing will require more supervision because of the need for frequent evaluation, reevaluation, potential therapy modifications, and the amount of potential risk involved. Regardless of the setting and formal qualifications, the supervisor and supervisee have mutual responsibility to understand each other's educational backgrounds, role competencies, and responsibilities to work as a team (Fenton & Alicandro, 1995). For more information about the roles of certified occupational therapy assistants see Chapter 8 in this volume.

Supervision of Entry-Level Registered Occupational Therapists

The *Guide for Supervision of Occupational Therapy Personnel* (1994a) recommends that entry-level therapists receive close supervision by an intermediate-level or advanced-level registered occupational therapist. It is essential for individuals with limited clinical experience to obtain appropriate supervision and to negotiate for this level of supervision during the initial job interview. Valuing and directly requesting appropriate levels of supervision will help ensure quality care.

►CONCLUSION

Today's health care environments are becoming more and more complex. To be successful in these complex situations, practitioners must be able to make judgments based on thoughtful inquiry, analysis, and reflection on practice. All occupational therapy practitioners, regardless of their job title or years of experience, deserve and can benefit from the opportunity to reflect on and analyze their practice. It is through the telling of their experience to others that practitioners can become aware of their unshared biases and presuppositions that affect every interaction with clients. Indeed, clinical supervision is a precious gift that we must give to ourselves and each other.

▼ REFERENCES

Adelstein, L. A., Cohn, E. S., Baker, R. C., & Barnes, M. A. (1990). A part-time level II fieldwork program. *American Journal of Occupational Therapy, 44,* 60–65.

Allen, A. S. (1996). Relationships with other service providers. In J. Case-Smith, A. Allen, & P. N. Pratt (Eds.), *Occupational therapy for children* (pp. 18–24). St. Louis, MO: C.V. Mosby.

American Occupational Therapy Association. (1991a). Essentials and guidelines of an accredited educational program for the occupational therapist. *American Journal of Occupational Therapy, 45,* 1077–1084.

American Occupational Therapy Association. (1991b). Essentials and guidelines of an accredited educational program for the occupational therapy assistant. *American Journal of Occupational Therapy, 45,* 1085–1092.

American Occupational Therapy Association. (1993). Occupational therapy roles. *American Journal of Occupational Therapy, 47,* 1087–1099.

American Occupational Therapy Association. (1994a). Guide for the supervision of occupational therapy personnel. *American Journal of Occupational Therapy, 48,* 1045–1046.

American Occupational Therapy Association. (1994b). Occupational therapy code of ethics. *American Journal of Occupational Therapy, 48,* 1037–1038.

American Occupational Therapy Association. (1995). Position paper: Use of occupational therapy aides in occupational therapy practice. *American Journal of Occupational Therapy, 49,* 1023–1025.

Anderson, J. L. (1988). *The supervisory process in speech-language pathology and audiology.* Boston, MA: Little, Brown & Co.

Blechert, T. F., Christiansen, M. F., & Kari, N. (1987). Intraprofessional team building. *The American Journal of Occupational Therapy, 41,* 576–582.

Buckholdt, D. R. & Gubrium, J. F. (1979). Doing staffing. *Human Organization, 38,* 255–264.

Case-Smith, J. & Wavrek, B. (1993). Models of service delivery and team interaction. In J. Case-Smith (Ed.), *Pediatric occupational therapy and early intervention* (pp. 127–159). St. Louis, MO: C.V. Mosby

Christie, B. A., Joyce, P. C., & Moeller, P. L. (1985). Fieldwork experience 1: Impact on practice preference. *American Journal of Occupational Therapy, 39,* 671–674.

Cohn, E. S. & Crist, P. (1995). Back to the future: New approaches to fieldwork education. *American Journal of Occupational Therapy, 49,* 103–106.

Commission on Education (COE). (1983). *Fieldwork evaluation for the occupational therapy assistant.* Rockville, MD: American Occupational Therapy Association.

Commission on Education. (1986). *Fieldwork evaluation for the occupational therapists.* Rockville, MD: American Occupational Therapy Association.

Commission on Education. (1988). *Guide to fieldwork education.* Rockville, MD: American Occupational Therapy Association.

Commission on Education. (1992). *Guidelines for occupational therapy fieldwork—level I.* Rockville, MD: American Occupational Therapy Association.

Commission on Education. (1995). *Student evaluation of fieldwork experience.* Bethesda, MD: American Occupational Therapy Association.

Crepeau, E. B. (1994a). Three images of interdisciplinary team meetings. *The American Journal of Occupational Therapy, 48,* 717–722.

Crepeau, E. B. (1994b). Uneasy alliances: Belief and action on a geropsychiatric team. (Doctoral dissertation, University of New Hampshire, 1994). *Dissertation Abstracts International, 9506410.*

Crist, P. (1986). *Contemporary issues in clinical education.* Thorofare, NJ: Slack.

Dudgeon, B. (1996). Pediatric rehabilitation. In J. Case-Smith, A. Allen, & P. N. Pratt (Eds.), *Occupational therapy for children* (pp. 777–795). St. Louis, MO: C.V. Mosby.

Fenton, E. C. & Alicandro, S. (1995, April). *COTA supervision.* Paper presented at Administration and Management class at Tufts University–Boston School of Occupational Therapy, Medford, MA.

Freeman, E. (1985). The importance of feedback in clinical supervision: Implications for direct practice. *Clinical Supervisor, 3,* 5–26.

Goldenson, R. M. (1978). Rehabilitation professions. In R. M. Goldenson, J. R. Dunham, & C. S. Dunham (Eds.), *Disability and rehabilitation handbook* (pp. 716–761). New York: McGraw-Hill Book Co.

Golin, A. K. & Duncanis, A. J. (1981). *The interdisciplinary team.* Bethesda, MD: Aspen.

Harel, B. H. (1994). Supervision. In K. Jacobs & M. K. Logigian (Eds.), *Functions of a manager in occupational therapy* (pp. 67–97). Thorofare, NJ: Slack.

Humphry, R., Gonzalez, S., & Taylor, E. (1993). Family involvement in practice: Issues and attitudes. *The American Journal of Occupational Therapy, 47,* 587–593.

Intagliata, S. (1993). Rehabilitation centers. In H. L. Hopkins & H. D. Smith. (Eds.), *Willard and Spackman's occupational therapy* (8th ed., pp. 784–789). Philadelphia: J. B. Lippincott.

Knowles, M. (1980). *The modern practice of adult education.* New York: Association Press.

Leff, P. T. & Walizer, E. H. (1992). *Building the healing partnership: Parents, professionals, and children with chronic illnesses and disabilities.* Cambridge, MA.: Brookline Books.

Lieberman, A. & Miller, L. (1979). *Staff development: New demands, new realities, new perspectives.* New York: Columbia University Press.

Parham, D. (1987). Toward professionalism: The reflective therapist. *American Journal of Occupational Therapy, 41,* 555–561.

Phillips, E. C. & Legaspi, W. S. (1995). Brief or new—a 12 month internship model of level II fieldwork. *American Journal of Occupational Therapy, 49,* 146–149.

Pressler, S. (1983). Fieldwork education: The proving ground of the profession. *American Journal of Occupational Therapy, 3,* 163–165.

Rogers, J. C. (1982). Sponsorship: Developing leaders for occupational therapy. *American Journal of Occupational Therapy, 36,* 309–313.

Salisbury, C. (1992). Parents as team members—inclusive teams, collaborative outcomes. In B. Rainforth, J. York, & C. Mac-donald (Eds.), *Collaborative teams for students with severe disabilities* (pp. 43–68). Baltimore: Brookes.

Saxe, J. G. (1871). *The poems of John Godfrey Saxe.* Boston: Fields, Osgood, & Co.

Schon, D. (1983). *The reflective practitioner: How professionals think in action.* New York: Basic Books.

Schwartz, K. B. (1980). *Fieldwork policies and procedures.* Medford, MA: Tufts University–Boston School of Occupational Therapy.

Slater, D.Y. & Cohn, E. S. (1991). Staff development through analysis of practice. *American Journal of Occupational Therapy, 45,* 1038–1044.

Smith, H. L. & Elbert, N. F. (1986). *The health care supervisor's guide to staff development.* Rockville, MD: Aspen Systems.

Stancliff, B. L. (1995, Nov.). Rehabilitation teams versus individual departments. *OT Practice,* p. 21.

Turk, D. C. & Stieg, R. L. (1987). Chronic pain: The necessity of interdisciplinary communication. *The Clinical Journal of Pain, 3,* 163–167.

Unsworth, C. A., Thomas, S. A., & Greenwood, K. M. (1995). Rehabilitation team decisions on discharge housing for stroke patients. *Archives of Physical Medicine and Rehabilitation, 76,* 331–340.

Zenger, J. H., Musselwhite, E., Hurson, K., & Perrin, C. (1994). *Leading teams: Mastering the new role.* Homewood, IL: Business One Irwin.

Chapter 45

Facility-Based Practice Settings

Maureen Freda

This chapter addresses facility-based occupational therapy practice settings and the differences between them. Physical medicine rehabilitation facilities include community or teaching hospitals, rehabilitation hospitals, and subacute facilities. Mental health settings include psychiatric units in community or teaching hospitals, free-standing psychiatric hospitals, and state-supported psychiatric hospitals. All may provide inpatient and outpatient services. Each setting varies in requirements relative to length of stay. More acute settings, such as community and teaching hospitals, have very short lengths of stay, whereas subacute facilities provide care over a longer time span. Each has a unique culture and treatment environment. Additionally, each setting has very specific requirements for documentation, reimbursement, service delivery, and practice parameters. Because the cost of care is so critical in today's health care environment, case managers are expecting services in lower-cost settings. This means that third-party payers exert pressure to transfer clients as soon as possible to less acute inpatient settings or to outpatient or community-based programs.

▼ COST CONTAINMENT AND CHANGES IN THE DELIVERY OF SERVICE

The delivery of occupational therapy services has responded to these cost-containment pressures by (1) increasing the use of certified occupational therapy assistants and **occupational therapy aides**,(2) maximizing use of professional personnel, and (3) using group treatment.

Increasing Use of Certified Occupational Therapy Assistants and Occupational Therapy Aides

Because of cost-containment efforts, there is mounting pressure to use certified occupational therapy assistants and occupational therapy aides in most settings in which occupational therapy is practiced. Certified occupational therapy assistants have completed an accredited educational program, typically in a junior or technical college. These programs include approximately 2 years of academic work and fieldwork experiences. Certified occupational therapy assistants must pass a national certification examination administered by the National Board of Certification for Occupational Therapy. Occupational therapy aides, in contrast, generally receive specific job training in their work settings. Certified occupational therapy assistants serve as collaborators in the occupational therapy treatment process and can assist in carrying out specific occupational therapy interventions based on **service competencies** established in their work sites. In many instances they assume primary treatment responsibility for client care. The type of work and level of supervision depends on the complexity of clients' problems and the level of competence of the certified occupational therapy assistant (AOTA, 1994). Occupational therapy aides, in contrast, must work with much closer guidance and supervision.

Therapists supervising these certified occupational therapy assistants and occupational therapy aides must be knowledgeable about supervision policies and procedures in their facilities as well as the licensure laws within their states. In addition, they need to develop skills in evaluation and training so that they can adequately supervise and manage others providing care to clients (The evolution of rehab, 1996). Establishing collaborative relationships between and among all occupational therapy personnel enhances the provision of services to clients. Chapter 8 discusses the interdependence between occupational therapy practitioners.

Maximizing the Use of Professional Personnel

One way to reduce costs is to create efficiencies in the treatment process. "Doubling" or "tripling" is one way of doing this. In doubling or tripling, occupational therapists are expected to treat more than one client simultaneously to maximize the number of interventions per hour. In this model a therapist may see two or three clients during the same treatment hour. The multiple clients may be seen simultaneously or may be staggered so that treatment overlaps during part of the hour. Treating two clients during the same hour may be accomplished by a single therapist; however, to do so, the hour must be organized so that the needs of both clients can be met. This can be done by having two clients of similar diagnoses and comparable levels share the same treatment hour using a common activity or intervention. Two clients with dissimilar diagnoses could be treated at the same time by alternating direct treatment with one and supervised practice with the other.

Certified occupational therapy assistants can be very helpful in situations that call for doubling or tripling. This "teaming up" becomes essential for treating three clients during the same period, if each client is to receive adequate attention and supervision. Occupational therapy aides may also be used for assistance, provided they have been adequately trained for the tasks they are asked to assume and are closely supervised. Sound clinical reasoning and the skills of an experienced therapist are needed for this model to work. Good communication with the certified occupational therapy assistant or occupational therapy aide is essential.

Because this model is a departure from the one-to-one model practiced in the past, many therapists may feel that they are not giving enough individual attention to their clients. Therapists must prioritize the needs of each client and design the treatment plan to meet those needs. Individual treatment can be interspersed as deemed clinically necessary. In addition, clients can receive individual attention during morning activities of daily living (ADL) training sessions. Quality is not analogous with individual treatment. Chapter 8 delineates how occupational therapist and certified occupational therapy assistant teams can provide excellent care while maximizing the use of personnel and controlling costs.

Use of Group Treatment

Group treatment, long the standard in mental health settings, is being used increasingly in physical rehabilitation.

Traditionally, group treatments have been used as an adjunct to other more intense interventions. Groups may focus on exercise, cooking, or other life skills, preparation for return to work, or the development of new leisure options. Certified occupational therapy assistants are often employed for the group treatments and may be paired with a registered occupational therapist for groups that are large or require a lot of individual attention (Freda & Rao, 1995).

▼ TYPES OF FACILITIES

Physical Medicine Settings

ACUTE CARE MEDICAL FACILITY

Community and teaching hospitals are typical acute care medical facilities. People usually enter these hospitals for conditions that require the highly skilled care of doctors, nurses, and allied health professionals. Laboratory, x-ray, and other diagnostic and treatment services are an inherent part of the hospital setting. People are discharged to their homes or to other less acute settings as quickly as possible. For example, the length of stay for someone who has had a stroke is about 7 days. Because length of stay is so brief, occupational therapists spend much of their day evaluating clients and preparing them for discharge. This may involve education of clients and their families if they are expected to go home directly from the hospital. This may frustrate some practitioners because they rarely see the long-term results of their therapeutic interventions. In the past the first session was reserved for comprehensive evaluation. Managers now expect therapists to combine initial treatment with the first session. As a result, the evaluation process has been streamlined, and occupational therapists have learned to quickly prioritize treatment and articulate discharge-planning goals.

Because of the higher level of skill required to evaluate acute clients in such a short time, occupational therapy managers are reluctant to use less-skilled personnel, despite cost-containment pressures (Is there an OT role, 1996). Certified occupational therapy assistants working in acute care settings can play a valuable role by working in partnership with a registered occupational therapist. For example, the occupational assistant can provide valuable assistance in client education, ADL training, as well as some of the routine care provided to people in the intensive care unit, such as carrying out sensory stimulation and passive range of motion (ROM) programs. In some settings the certified assistants may participate in parts of the evaluation process.

PHYSICAL DYSFUNCTION REHABILITATION

Rehabilitation occurs in freestanding rehabilitation hospitals or in rehabilitation units in community or teaching hospitals. Because the goal in these settings is rehabilitative, people must be medically stable and able to tolerate a total of 3 hours of therapy a day. Additionally, to obtain Medicare reimbursement, a client must have measurable goals and must be making measurable progress for the duration of the admission. Excellent documentation is essential, because if the requirements are not clearly documented, reimbursement may be denied for part or all of the stay.

Evaluations should be short, objective, concise, and very clearly state the goals to be attained in treatment. Many rehabilitation facilities use an integrated evaluation for all services to avoid duplication and decrease time spent evaluating the client. The ongoing record of progress must relate explicitly to the stated treatment goals. Weekly progress notes are typical in inpatient settings. A daily log supplements these notes and records daily attendance, interventions, and client response. In outpatient settings, documentation standards vary from daily to weekly notes. Discharge summaries should describe the status of all goals set at admission and reasons for any differences between the goals set and those attained.

SUBACUTE MEDICAL OR REHABILITATION FACILITY

The number of subacute facilities is expanding rapidly in response to the goal of managed care companies for a lower-cost alternative to rehabilitation settings. Because many subacute facilities are located in long-term care settings and offer less intense rehabilitation programs, they are able to charge a much lower daily rate than an acute rehabilitation setting. Subacute units must meet very specific standards for both Joint Commission of Accreditation of Healthcare Organizations (JCAHO) or Commission on Accreditation of Rehabilitation Facilities (CARF) accreditation in addition to meeting the stringent Medicare guidelines for long-term care.

Two major sources of reimbursement for subacute care are Medicare and managed care. Per diem rates are negotiated with managed care companies. Their goal is to keep the volume high, that is keep the beds filled so that they can maximize the use of personnel and keep their daily rates as low as possible.

Occupational therapy documentation follows a pattern similar to documentation in acute rehabilitation. Evaluations, initially and at discharge, are performed for all clients. Progress notes are usually written on a weekly basis, with a daily log kept of attendance and specific treatment modalities. Medicare guidelines do require that progress be evident in these weekly notes. Reimbursement may be denied if documentation standards are not met. Table 45–1 summarizes information about each setting.

Mental Health Settings

ACUTE PSYCHIATRIC FACILITY

Similar to all other aspects of health care, psychiatry has also been affected by managed care. The acuity level of clients is often high and the approved length of stay shorter and shorter. The typical length of stay is now only 7 to 15 days. Crisis stabilization is the most frequent goal for inpatient settings. Treatment focuses on the crisis that precipitated this admission. Both group and individual treatments help the client develop strategies to prevent future crises. These may include education about the role of medication in their care, stress management, use of community supports, and life skills training. Occupational therapy is part of the multidisciplinary team. Groups are a frequent mode of treatment, supplemented by individual sessions for people who cannot tolerate a group environment or who need more individualized intervention. Examples of groups led by occupational therapy practitioners include community reintegration, assertiveness training, anger management, self-esteem, task-oriented groups, and stress management. Discharge planning begins immediately, with an emphasis on use of outpatient or community-based services to prevent future admissions. Daily notes are common following an initial assessment and treatment plan.

LONG-TERM PSYCHIATRIC FACILITY

As in other settings, the decreased length of stay in long-term psychiatric facilities has increased the emphasis on evaluation and referrals to the community settings. In this instance, it is imperative to have accurate assessment data to make the most appropriate community referral (ie, community-based group homes, day treatment, or other). This shift to community-based treatment has come about in two segments. First, the deinstitutionalization movement of the 1970s and 1980s resulted in massive discharges from state psychiatric hospitals. Second, managed care has dramatically shortened the length of stay as a way to reduce costs.

People who are so incapacitated that they cannot live in the community, even in a supported-living arrangement, remain in long-term care psychiatric settings. Many state hospitals have nursing home units to care for people with chronic mental illness who also have other medical conditions. These individuals often cannot be cared for in other nursing home settings.

Occupational therapy is frequently delivered in groups that may be led or coled by occupational therapists, certified occupational therapy assistants, or other members of the team. Occupational therapists frequently are case managers within the team. In this role they ensure that the appropriate treatment is rendered and that all necessary paperwork is completed to provide for continued treatment for the client. Weekly progress notes, with daily attendance logs, are customary in long-term care facilities. Documentation is extremely crucial to the continued payment for services in mental health. The necessity for ongoing treatment must be well defined within the documentation of all team members. Table 45–2 provides additional information about mental health facilities.

Table 45-1. Physical Medicine Facilities

	Acute Medical	Physical Dysfunction Rehabilitation	Subacute Medical/Rehabilitation
Client Population			
Age	All ages	Pediatric: 0–21 yr; adult: 14 yr–geriatric	Adult to geriatric
Diagnoses	Orthopedic surgery, neurosurgery, pulmonary, cardiac oncology, burns trauma, ob/gyn, neurology medical/surgical, organ transplants, AIDS	CVA (complex), TBI, MS, SCI (high lesions), amputations (with co-morbidities), joint replacements (complex), multiple trauma, severe arthritis, other neurological conditions, and ventilator-dependent clients	CVA (simple, joint replacements, MS, amputations, general musculoskeletal disorders, AIDS, medical diagnoses
Typical Length of Stay	Depends on DRG (eg, CVA = 7 days)	2–6 wk (eg, CVA = 18 days)	1–3 wk (eg, CVA = 15 days)
Delivery of Services			
Types of Services	Evaluation, client education, discharge planning, skill training, adaptive equipment	Evaluation; training in ADL, functional skills, community reintegration, compensation techniques, and use of adaptive equipment; cognitive retraining	Evaluation; training in ADL, functional skills, adaptive equipment, motor development, compensation techniques and use of adaptive equipment; splinting
Number of hours of occupational therapy per day	1/2–1 hr	1–2 hr: part individual and part group	1–1 1/2 hr: groups interspersed as appropriate
Goals	Client will understand postoperative precautions and limitations. Prepare client to attain short-term goals at rehabilitation or subacute setting.	Client will increase independence in ADL (eg, move from moderate to minimal assistance). Prepare client to attain long-term goals in outpatient setting or home.	Client will increase independence in ADL (eg, move from moderate to minimal assistance). Prepare client to attain long-term goals in outpatient setting or home.
Documentation	Brief evaluation, daily notes, discharge summary	Inpatient: evaluation, weekly notes, daily graphics, discharge summary. Outpatient: evaluation, daily notes, weekly summary, monthly summary, recertifications, discharge summary.	Evaluation, weekly notes, daily graphics, discharge summary.
Typical Day for Occupational Therapy Personnel	Check the previous day's admissions, pick up referrals from the various units, schedule new clients, run a patient education group for preop clients, evaluate new clients, perform morning ADL activities, treat clients at the bedside or in the clinic, participate in rounds on the units, cotreat a client with another team member, take part in supervision meetings, take part in a family meeting regarding a discharge issue, schedule new referrals that came in late in the day	Meet to discuss coverage for unplanned absences of occupational therapy personnel, ADL training on the unit, treatment of caseload in the main clinic area, attendance at a team or family conference, meet with aide to discuss treatment plan of a specific client, document evaluation of a new client, lead a group treatment with the assistance of an occupational therapy aide, review paperwork of a new client assigned by supervisor, design schedule for new client in cooperation with other team members, take part in supervision meeting, fill out charge tickets for all clients treated that day, make phone calls to families or vendors regarding specific issues for individual clients.	Check for admissions, ADL training on the units, group treatment (some coled with physical therapist), doubled sessions with clients (2 per occupation therapist per hour), evaluate clients, reschedule to evaluate newest admissions, write notes, meet with occupational therapy aide, meet with case manager about hours of therapy approved, meet with certified occupational therapy assistant.

CVA = cerebrovascular accident; AIDS = acquired immune deficiency syndrome; DRG = diagnosis-related group; MS = multiple sclerosis; TBI = traumatic brain injury; SCI = spinal cord injury, ADL = activities of daily living

Table 45-2. Mental Health Settings

	Acute Psychiatric	Long-term Psychiatric
Client Population:		
Age	Pediatric to geriatric	Adolescence to geriatric
Diagnoses	Depression and other affective disorders, borderline disorders, attention deficit disorder, schizophrenia, addictions/detoxification, polysubstance abuse, acute psychotic episode	Chronic schizophrenia, bipolar disorders, brain disorders, such as Alzheimer's disease
Typical Length of Stay	7–15 days	Generally longer than 15 days, dependent on reimbursement and mental status
Delivery of Services		
Types of Services	Assessment, prevention strategies, community reeducation, stress management, discharge planning	Assessment, occupational therapy case management, community reentry planning
Methods	Individual and group	Predominantly group
Typical Goals	Crisis stabilization strategies to prevent reoccurrence or readmission, understand the role of medication, accessing community resources	Appropriate community referrals
Documentation	Initial assessment, treatment plan, daily notes, discharge plan	Initial assessment, daily activity log, weekly notes, discharge plan
Typical Day	Attend report regarding the previous night's activities, review daily list of new admissions, get notes and charge tickets ready for the day, attend team meeting (often with clients), process the team meeting, note writing, write up assessments, lead a group treatment, do an individual treatment session, check midday admissions, in the afternoon repeat the morning activities	Staff meeting, preparation time for the day's activities, lead morning group treatment sessions, team meeting, phone conversation regarding a community referral, discharge planning meeting, lead afternoon group treatment sessions, in-service training or supervision meeting, documentation time, charges and other miscellaneous paperwork

CASE STUDY

PHYSICAL REHABILITATION

This example illustrates how a person moves from acute care through long-term care. Pay special attention to how many times Mr. Thompson has to change primary therapists and environments and how quickly a primary therapist must discharge him to another setting.

Five months ago, Mr. Thompson suffered a right **cerebrovascular accident (CVA)**, resulting in a dense left sided hemiplegia. At the time he was 70 years old and lived with his 72-year-old wife in a ground floor condominium. Before his stroke, Mr. and Mrs. Thompson led an active life. They walked their dog several times a day, had a small garden around their deck that was the showplace for the condominium, volunteered in the literacy program at the library, and visited often with family and friends. Initially, Mr. Thompson was admitted to the local community hospital, an acute care facility. The occupational therapist evaluated him on his fourth day in the hospital. She was unable to conduct the evaluation sooner because he was not medically stable. Her

evaluation revealed that Mr. Thompson had a flaccid left upper extremity, with moderate shoulder **subluxation** and a moderate facial droop. She found that he had decreased sensation, particularly proprioception. He also appeared to have a moderate left-sided neglect and some spatial orientation problems. He required maximum assistance in bed mobility and for bed to wheelchair transfers. During the evaluation Mr. Thompson said that he wanted to return home and was very concerned that he would not be able to walk his dog or take care of the garden. The occupational therapist decided that day's priority was to make certain he was positioned properly in his bed and in his wheelchair. The next day the occupational therapist began to see Mr. Thompson at his bedside for passive ROM, training in how to range himself, and initial ADL training focusing on grooming. Because the occupational therapist knew that she would have only a few days with Mr. Thompson before he would be transferred to the rehabilitation

(continued)

(Continued)

hospital, she focused on preparing him for the rehabilitation program there. Consequently, she focused on maintaining his ROM, developing his bed mobility, and beginning ADL training with simple grooming. The acute care occupational therapist knew that she would not be the one to see Mr. Thompson meet any of his long-term goals. On the eighth day, Mr. Thompson was transferred to a rehabilitation hospital. The occupational therapist summarized her evaluation and Mr. Thompson's progress on the discharge summary.

With the information from the hospital discharge summary as the baseline for her evaluation, the registered occupational therapist evaluated Mr. Thompson within 24 hours of his admission. From this evaluation she formulated short-term and long-term goals. Short-term goals included (1) increased independence in grooming, hygiene, dressing, bed mobility, and transfers; (2) control of edema in the affected extremity and self-awareness for proper positioning; and (3) increased attention to the left side of the environment and an understanding of how the spatial relations deficits affect daily life activities. Her initial treatment included ADL sessions with Mr. Thompson each morning. Once Mr. Thompson understood the techniques, the registered occupational therapist delegated this aspect of his care to an occupational therapy aide for several days of the week. Mr. Thompson received 30 to 60 minutes occupational therapy treatment every day. Part of the time his registered occupational therapist doubled his treatment with another person. In doubling, an occupational therapy aide may be the extra pair of hands enabling the occupational therapist to treat two people in the same time span. This aspect of his rehabilitation focused on edema control, positioning, perception, and spatial relations. The occupational therapist guided some of the conversation to gardening so that they could explore ways for him to continue with this activity when he returned home. The occupational therapist showed him the raised beds outside the dining room as an example for him to consider. Mr. Thompson also spent 2 to 4 hours each week in groups. These groups were led or coled by an occupational therapist and a certified occupational therapy assistant. They included ROM, mobility, and leisure skill development.

Mrs. Thompson was included in these interventions. She observed and assisted with the ADL and transfer training so that she and Mr. Thompson felt secure about him returning home. This also provided the staff with the opportunity to evaluate the level and type of home health care that Mr. Thompson

might need. Mr. and Mrs. Thompson attended a discharge-planning group coled by an occupational therapist and social worker. This group addressed issues related to assuring safety, articulating needs, directing care, and resuming roles within the family. Mr. Thompson was discharged from the inpatient rehabilitation hospital on the 18th day following admission. He was scheduled for his first outpatient appointment 5 days after his discharge from the hospital. The inpatient therapist communicated his current status and long-term goals to the outpatient therapist to ensure continuity of care. Additionally, the inpatient therapist prepared Mr. Thompson for the outpatient experience by showing him the outpatient area, introducing some of the staff, and explaining the therapy he would be receiving over next 6 weeks.

Mr. Thompson achieved his long-term goals during the outpatient component of his care. He learned to walk with the four-prong cane and became independent in bathing, dressing, using the toilet, and grooming. Although full function did not return to his right arm, he developed sufficient control to use it to assist with some activities. A driving evaluation determined that Mr. Thompson had not recovered sufficiently to drive safely. Because Mrs. Thompson does not drive, occupational therapy intervention involved learning how to use public transportation, focusing especially on Mr. Thompson's ability and comfort getting on and off the bus. Mr. Thompson did not recover his balance sufficiently to walk his dog, but he and his wife began to take short walks with the dog as part of Mr. Thompson's physical therapy. They are exploring having raised beds built for the deck so that he can continue gardening in the spring. The condominium manager has approved these plans. The Thompson's sons have promised to make them by the time the danger of frost has passed.

During Mr. Thompson's rehabilitation, he received occupational therapy from three registered occupational therapists, two certified occupational therapy assistants, and two occupational therapy aides. His care was facilitated by the awareness of all practitioners of the need to focus on short-term goals that would prepare him for discharge to the next level of care. Their ability to delegate aspects of his care to the certified occupational therapy assistants and occupational therapy aides substantially reduced the cost of his care without jeopardizing its quality. Their ability to communicate important information about Mr. Thompson, his functional status, and his goals facilitated excellent continuity of care between settings.

HISTORICAL NOTE
THE STORY OF JOHNNIE ON THE S.P.O.T: THE PROFESSION'S VIEW OF ENVIRONMENTS

Suzanne M. Peloquin

Although the founders of the Society for the Promotion of Occupational Therapy (SPOT) held singular views, they shared the common perspective that occupation could help individuals in a variety of circumstances. The letters that abbreviated the Society's name pleased George Edward Barton:

I am strongly in favor of the National Society for the Promotion of Occupational Therapy as a title. I know that it is long but it does tell the story and the S.P.O.T. suggests the ever alert "Johnnie." (as cited by Licht, 1967; p. 272)

Some among us may not recall that the early-century phrase "Johnnie-on-the-spot" designated a person in the right place with the just-right timing and ever-handy tool. Many late-century therapists enjoy a similar reputation. Barton's reference to the "spot" in question reveals the long-standing interest that occupational therapists have had in the environments, or spots, within which individuals find and occupy themselves. The continuity of the profession, embedded within the larger issue of its relevance, hinges on the degree to which therapists stay alert to the environments within which they practice. ■

Licht, S. (1967). The founding and founders of the American Occupational Therapy Association. *American Journal of Occupational Therapy, 21,* 269–277.

▶CONCLUSION

Facility-based occupational therapy practitioners face many challenges. They must balance professional and ethical practice issues with cost containment, efficiency, productivity, and stringent oversight by managed care providers. The practice environment is fast paced, demanding, and ever changing. Practitioners working in inpatient facilities also have many wonderful opportunities for learning from others, working side by side with master clinicians, and being on the cutting edge of designing service delivery models that work from both a client care and business perspective.

Acknowledgments

The author gratefully acknowledges the following individuals for sharing their expertise as this chapter was being written: Jinny Racine, Senior Therapist at Montgomery General Hospital, Olney, MD; Ronnie Schein, Outpatient Clinical Supervisor, and Jill Schie, Acute Care Program Manager, National Rehabilitation Hospital, Washington, DC; and Mary Taugher, Director Rehabilitative Services/ Program Administrator of Medical Day Treatment, Milwaukee County Mental Health Division, Wauwatosa, WI.

▼ REFERENCES

American Occupational Therapy Association. (1994). Guide for supervision of occupational therapy personnel. *American Journal of Occupational Therapy, 48,* 1045–1046.

Is there an OT role in acute care. (1996, Feb. 8). *OT Week,* pp. 12–13.

The evolution of rehab. (1996, March 7). *OT Week,* pp. 20–21.

Freda, M., & Rao, P. (1995, Oct.-Nov.). Rehab's sea change. *Rehab Management,* pp. 62–67.

Chapter 46

Community-Based Practice Arenas

Lou Ann Sooy Griswold

The community provides a context for learning, playing, working, and experiencing life (Grady, 1995). Each community setting in which occupational therapy practitioners work has a unique mission that fosters the ability of clients to live optimally. Often, community settings are based on models other than a medical model. For example, public schools are organized within an educational model, whereas early intervention and hospice care use a family-centered model. Community-based practitioners must use a variety of intervention approaches: establishing or restoring skills, altering or finding a different setting so that there is a better match between skills and expectations, adapting the task demands or context, preventing additional problems, and creating circumstances that enhance task performance (Dunn, Brown, & McGuigan, 1994).

This chapter describes occupational therapy practice in the following community-based areas: early intervention, schools, work hardening, home health care, community mental health, adult day care, and hospice. Each section describes the setting, its goals, staff, and clients, and ends with a description of a typical "day in the life" of a practitioner working in the setting.

▼ EARLY INTERVENTION

Early-intervention programs address the developmental, educational, and social needs of children, up to the age of 3, who have a disability or developmental delay (Case-Smith

& Wavrek, 1993; Hanft, 1988). Services are family-centered, focusing on the needs of the family unit, not just the child's (Leviton, Mueller, & Kauffman, 1992). An early-intervention team typically includes an early childhood educator, speech and language pathologist, physical therapist, occupational therapy practitioner, social worker, and family members. In a family-centered model, family members are considered to be equal members of the team and participate in all aspects of planning the child's care (Leviton, Mueller, & Kaufman).

Occupational therapy includes promoting development and function for typical play and self-care skills (Case-Smith, 1993). Goals may include gaining motor skills; adapting to and responding to environmental stimuli, such as noises, touch, and movement; developing appropriate feeding skills; and acquiring adaptive skills such as recognizing cause and effect.

Day in the Life of an Occupational Therapy Practitioner Working in Early Intervention

Joan has a car full of toys as she travels from house to house to provide services to children and their families. Joan usually visits six to eight children in a day. Her first stop is Sam's house, where she helps Sam's mother give him a bath. Joan makes suggestions to decrease the stiffness in his body for easier bathing and dressing. Joan then spends 20 minutes talking with Sam's mother about how the family is adjusting to Sam's diagnosis of cerebral palsy. Other children Joan sees include a 15-month-old toddler who is blind, two children with Down syndrome, a girl who had neurological damage after falling into a lake, and two more children with cerebral palsy. Joan provides play activities that focus on developing each child's movement patterns and cognitive skills. She includes older brothers and sisters in these activities and even a family dog who retrieves a ball kicked by a 2-year-old as Joan facilitates balance reactions. She also talks with the parents to be sure that the interventions fit with the feelings, needs, and goals of the family.

▼ SCHOOL SYSTEMS

Schools teach children how to read, write, and understand and use mathematical concepts. They also socialize students to function with others and to become aware of the world around them to prepare the children for their future roles as community members.

Children who have disabilities that prevent or inhibit them from learning may receive special services. These students may have difficulty moving within their environment, using their hands to write, or taking in, processing, and using information. Teachers (classroom, physical education, and special education), the student's parents, speech and language pathologist, occupational therapy practitioner, psychologist, and guidance counselor form the school placement team. The team determines if the student has a disability that interferes with learning. If so, the team members develop an **individual education plan (IEP)** to meet the student's educational needs and goals. This plan addresses the child's learning needs in an environment most typical for all students at that age (Giangreco, 1995).

Occupational therapy enhances skills that provide a foundation for learning, such as developing trunk stability to sit in a chair, or developing fine motor skills to write with a pencil. The practitioner may also suggest a particular classroom and teaching style that would enable the student perform optimally (Dunn, 1990; Dunn, Brown, & McGuigan, 1994).

Day in the Life of an Occupational Therapy Practitioner Working in a School Setting

Mike begins his work day at 7:45 AM with a team meeting to discuss Rachel, a 10-year-old with learning disabilities. Together, the team of eight members discuss modification of classroom activities that will enhance Rachel's learning, but are similar to those of her classmates. Mike then provides four children with 20 minutes of sensorimotor activities to improve their attention abilities in the classroom. Mike observes a student's performance in class and during recess. He also leads class activities to promote gross motor

or fine motor development and attends two gym classes, adapting the activities for children with disabilities. During lunch, Mike meets with a teacher about the child he had observed, to develop strategies to help the student stay on task. He spends an hour after lunch evaluating a student's motor abilities and the next half an hour working on the report, which he will finish at home that evening. He ends his day in an after-school meeting with a group of first grade teachers to discuss prerequisite skills for handwriting and introduces them to activities that enhance fine motor development.

▼ WORK-ORIENTED REHABILITATION PROGRAMS

Work-oriented rehabilitation programs enable people who have been injured return to the work force, often to the job held before the injury or diagnosis. Clients may have a wide range of disabilities, the most common being lumbar spine injuries, carpal tunnel syndrome, cervical spine injuries, shoulder injuries, and tendinitis (King, 1993). The majority of clients are men between 26 and 46 years of age (King, pp. 597–599). The team in work programs generally consists of a physician, physical therapist, and occupational therapy practitioner. Employment supervisors work with the team to coordinate the rehabilitation goals and program with the client.

Occupational therapy goals relate specifically to each person's job and injury or diagnosis. Typical goals are reconditioning, controlling symptoms, stress management, and education for injury prevention (King, 1993). Occupational therapy services include evaluation of physical capacity and functional limitations, graded work simulation, and work adaptations or assistive devices to enable the client to return to work. Occupational therapy also addresses the psychosocial issues related to the disability (Biernacki, 1993).

Day in the Life of an Occupational Therapy Practitioner in a Work-Oriented Program

Catherine begins her day by registering clients as they report to the simulated work program. Many clients are paid by their employers if they verify their participation through this registration process. She leads a group of clients in flexibility and warm-up exercises. After the exercise group she sets up a "work-circuit system" that includes a series of work-related tasks to address individual client's goals (Niemeyer, 1989). With colleagues she monitors clients' progress. Catherine then assesses a new client for his strength and work capacity using job-related functions. She continues her day working with clients using aerobic training equipment and work simulators to duplicate the physical demands of their jobs (Wyrick, Niemeyer, Ellexson, Jacobs, & Taylor, 1991). Later,

Catherine meets with a young man to discuss how he can use leisure activities to reduce the stress, anxiety, and depression he is experiencing because of his disability. Catherine ends her day with a job-site analysis for a client who had been injured on the job. She assesses the work environment, physical demands of the tasks, machines, tools and equipment used, and worker traits required for the job (McCormack, 1990; Niemeyer, 1989). Catherine's job analysis has a dual purpose: (1) adapting the job tasks for the client referred for therapy and (2) preventing future injuries for him as well as his colleagues. She will report her recommendations to the factory supervisor next week.

▼ HOME HEALTH CARE

Home health care promotes independent functioning to enable people to live at home. It blends the medical and family-centered models, as services are medically determined, yet provided with sensitivity to the physical and emotional needs of clients and their families. It serves those who need support or assistance in performing self-care, home-making, or leisure tasks independently and safely. Although any age group can receive home health care, most clients are elderly. Some clients have rehabilitation goals, whereas others need modification of daily tasks to foster greater independence (Brittingham & Dempster, 1990; Clark, Corcoran, & Gitlin, 1995). Team members include nursing personnel, physician, physical therapist, speech and language pathologist, occupational therapy practitioner, social worker, and home health aide.

Occupational therapy services are designed to promote the person's occupational roles at home by facilitating self-care and household tasks and leisure activities (Brittingham & Dempster, 1990). Practitioners may work on specific skills, such as motor coordination, strength, or sensation, through the use of meaningful activities, or may suggest equipment to adapt the task to the person's ability.

Day in the Life of an Occupational Therapy Practitioner in a Home Health Program

Renee has learned to be very flexible in her role as a home health occupational therapy practitioner. As she travels around the city to clients' homes, she never knows what issues might arise, and which professional and personal skills she will need to use. Her days begin at various times, depending on the clients she visits each day. Today, Renee begins her day at 9:00 A.M. to assist Mr. T in daily living skills. Mr. T has **Parkinson's disease** and is experiencing rigid movements and decreased mobility. Renee observes Mr. T as he showers and dresses himself. She recommends modifications to the bathroom and shows Mr. and Mrs. T some safety hazards they need to consider relative to Mr. T's shuffling gait. They discuss these hazards and potential solutions. Mr.

and Mrs. T. decide to remove the scatter rugs in the hallway. Something they all agreed was the greatest hazard. Next, Renee assesses Mrs. G, who has just been discharged from the hospital, after having hip surgery. Renee considers Mrs. G's leisure interests and suggests activities with some adaptations that would maintain Mrs. G's involvement with her friends. On her third visit for the day, Renee works with Mr. and Mrs. W. Mr. W is recovering from a stroke that has left him with severe right-sided hemiplegia and little speech. Consequently, he is dependent on his wife for his care. Renee helps Mrs. W devise a new routine so that she can tend to her husband's needs and yet have a more balanced life herself. They discuss the possibility of a home health aide to reduce some his Mrs. W's responsibilities. Renee calls the nursing supervisor to request these services before she leaves. Renee dictates notes in her car about each of the therapy sessions, which a secretary will transcribe for her. Her day ends with another home evaluation and an hour in the office to order equipment and call clients whom she will see tomorrow.

▼ COMMUNITY MENTAL HEALTH

Community mental health programs support people in the community with chronic psychiatric illnesses, such as **schizophrenia**, and with major affective disorders, such as **bipolar disorder** (Richert & Merryman, 1987; Wilberding, 1991). Because most people with chronic psychiatric illness have difficulty living independently in the community, these programs are designed to prevent decompensation and subsequent inpatient hospitalization (Richert & Merryman). Some community mental health settings include room and board for clients, others provide day services for clients who live nearby.

Community mental health teams include psychiatrists, psychiatric nurses, rehabilitation workers, social workers, occupational therapy practitioners, and other therapists providing art, music, or movement therapy. Frequently, paraprofessionals or personnel without specific mental health education provide the daily care and structure for clients, particularly in programs offering board and care.

Occupational therapy services focus on teaching and promoting basic-living skills for work, self-care, and leisure (Wilberding, 1991). Personal hygiene, housework, interpersonal skills, coping strategies, job readiness, money management, using public transportation, and participation in leisure are some of the skills practitioners address (Azok & Tomlinson, 1994; Earle-Grimes, 1994; Richert & Merryman, 1987; Wilberding).

Day in the Life of an Occupational Therapy Practitioner Working in Community Mental Health

Karen works in a **half-way house** in which 15 clients live and approximately 20 other clients come for the day program. Karen typically works from 8 A.M. to 5 P.M. However, one day a week, she works from 12 P.M. to 8 P.M. to provide therapeutic activities in the evening. When she comes in at noon, Karen reviews the report prepared by the night counselor and talks with another staff member about the morning events to learn about the residents' current function. At 1 P.M. Karen coleads a self-awareness group using art as the therapeutic media. At 2 P.M. she leads the weekly meal-planning group. Residents each select a lunch and dinner to prepare with a partner. Karen incorporates nutrition, budgeting, and time management as ideas for meals are discussed and a grocery list developed by the group. Tomorrow she will take the group to the grocery store to purchase the food. At 4 P.M., Karen works with two residents as they make dinner, assisting only when necessary. Karen joins the group for dinner, modeling social interactions and communication skills. After the dishes are done, Karen leads an evening relaxation group using guided imagery. She checks on hygiene needs before residents retire to the television room and documents her therapy sessions in the house journal and residents' charts before leaving for home.

▼ ADULT DAY CARE

Adult day care provides meaningful, structured activities, assisting people with physical or cognitive disabilities to remain living at home. Clients have a range of diagnoses including cerebrovascular accident (CVA), rheumatoid arthritis, Parkinson's, multiple sclerosis, or senile dementia of the Alzheimer type. Beyond its goal to improve and maintain functional abilities and prevent additional losses, adult day care provides respite for primary care givers (Hasselkus, 1992). Team members include nurses, nurses aides, social workers, and physical and occupational therapy practitioners, therapeutic recreation specialists, and paraprofessionals and aides.

Occupational therapy focuses on a person's ability to engage in self-care and leisure activities while maintaining or enhancing perceptual, motor, cognitive, and psychological skills (AOTA, 1986a).

Day in the Life of an Occupational Therapy Practitioner Working in Adult Day Care

Susan greets participants and their caregivers as they arrive at the center. Many move slowly as they enter on foot or by wheelchair. She begins with a morning meeting, in which she orients participants to the day, date, current events, and activities for the day. She then coleads an exercise group to improve range of motion (ROM), motor planning, coordination, and endurance. Later Susan helps interested participants do a simple craft activity to promote cognitive, perceptual, and social skills. After the crafts group, she consults

with an aide who is helping a group of participants fold and staple the monthly newsletter for the center. Susan continues to consult with others in the kitchen, where a group of people are preparing a midmorning snack for everyone. She suggests some adaptive equipment to enable one woman to participate more fully. In the afternoon, Susan leads a group discussion on strategies for greater independence in self-care. She ends her day with a team meeting to review participants' progress and activity levels. Before leaving, she makes some calls to locate information on bathroom adaptations needed by a caregiver (AOTA, 1986b; Hasselkus, 1992).

▼ HOSPICE CARE

Hospice programs provide care to enhance the quality of life for people who are dying and for their families. Goals include controlling pain, providing health care services, and helping clients to control their lives as much as possible until their death (Pizzi, 1992). Hospice personnel also work closely with caregivers, helping them with the practical aspects of providing care to a terminally ill person, and with the emotional stress the illness and his or her death entails. People with any terminal illness who have 6 months or less to live can receive hospice care. Cancer is the most frequent diagnosis. However, people who are dying from diseases such as kidney failure, **emphysema**, and **acquired immunodeficiency syndrome (AIDS)** may also receive hospice care (Pizzi). The hospice team consists of a physician, nurse, and social worker, in addition to other necessary rehabilitation professionals, such as physical, occupational, or respiratory therapists.

Beyond services designed to sustain as much independence as possible, occupational therapy intervention assists a person who is dying realize the meaning his or her life has had and to feel good about that life. Occupational therapy facilitates continued participation in activities that enhance quality of life through grading and adapting valued activities to the person's current functional level. Additionally, occupational therapy practitioners work closely with family members by providing information and helping them with the inevitable role transitions terminal illness brings to the family unit (Pizzi, 1992).

Day in the Life of an Occupational Therapy Practitioner Working in Hospice Care

Unlike many occupational therapy practitioners who work in 15-minute to half-hour units, Ken schedules his time in several-hour blocks and sometimes whole days. This enables him to attend to the multiple needs of clients at a pace they can tolerate. Ken begins his day by helping Mr. Q perform his morning care tasks. He spends the morning with Mr. Q in his raised-bed garden, which Ken helped design so that

RESEARCH NOTE
RESEARCH SHOULD ESTABLISH THE COMMUNITY-BASED EFFECTIVENESS OF OCCUPATIONAL THERAPY

Kenneth J. Ottenbacher

Dramatic changes are occurring in the American health care system. These changes have a direct influence on *who provides* health care services, *what* services are provided, *who pays* for them, and *where* the services are provided. All these changes will influence the way occupational therapy is delivered in the next decade and also determine how students are educated. In a Health Policy Report published in the *New England Journal of Medicine,* Iglehart (1995) speculated that, by the year 2005, the majority of all health care services in this country will be provided outside traditional hospital and rehabilitation facilities. This migration to home and community-based service delivery represents an unprecedented research opportunity for occupational therapists. Occupational therapy interventions, when properly planned, implemented, and evaluated, should have their greatest effect in the clients natural (home or community) environment. The next decade will present clinicians and researchers with a unique opportunity to establish the community-based effectiveness of occupational therapy. ■

Iglehart, J. K. (1995). Health policy report: Rapid changes for academic health centers. *New England Journal of Medicine, 332,* 407–411.

Mr. Q could garden in his wheelchair. During the gardening, Mr. Q reminisces about raising nearly all of the fruits and vegetables for the family when his children were growing up. Ken recognizes the value of the discussion as well as the continued involvement in gardening activities for Mr. Q. He spends a few minutes talking with Mrs. Q to make sure that she is coping well with her husband's increasing dependence. Ken then attends a team meeting to discuss a new client and to plan for a vigil for Mrs. J, who is very near death. Ken's last 2 hours of the day are spent interviewing Mrs. M, a new client, in her home about her social history, work and leisure interests, and goals and desires during her last few months of life.

►CONCLUSION

Work in community settings is extremely rewarding, for it enables occupational therapy practitioners to help clients continue to live in their homes surrounded by their family, friends, pets, gardens, and mementos. Practitioners working in community settings must have a strong sense of what they have to offer, because they usually work without contact with other occupational therapy personnel. Working in these settings requires practitioners to collaborate with other team members and know when and how to seek support and supervision from others.

▼ REFERENCES

American Occupational Therapy Association (AOTA). (1986a). Occupational therapy in adult day-care [Position paper]. *American Journal of Occupational Therapy, 40,* 814–816.

American Occupational Therapy Association. (1986b). Roles and functions of occupational therapy in adult day-care. *American Journal of Occupational Therapy, 40,* 817–821.

Azok, S. D. & Tomlinson, J. (1994). Occupational therapy in a multidisciplinary psychiatric home health care service. *Mental Health Special Interest Section Newsletter, 17*(2), 1–3.

Biernacki, S. D. (1993). Reliability of the worker role interview. *American Journal of Occupational Therapy, 47,* 979–803.

Brittingham, K. M & Dempster, M. (1990). Occupational therapists in home health care: Ensuring positive outcomes through collaboration. *Occupational Therapy Practice, 2*(1), 32–44.

Case-Smith, J. (1993). Defining the early intervention process. In J. Case-Smith (Ed.), *Pediatric occupational therapy and early intervention* (pp. 31–61). Boston: Andover Medical Publishers.

Case-Smith, J. & Wavrek, B. B. (1993). Models of service delivery and team interaction. In J. Case-Smith (Ed.), *Pediatric occupational therapy and early intervention* (pp. 127–160). Boston: Andover Medical Publishers.

Clark, C. A., Corcoran, M., & Gitlin, L. A. (1995). An exploratory study of how occupational therapists develop therapeutic relationships with family caregivers. *American Journal of Occupational Therapy, 49,* 587–594.

Dunn, W. (1990). A comparison of service provision models in school-based occupational therapy services: A pilot study. *The Occupational Therapy Journal of Research, 10,* 300–320.

Dunn, W., Brown, C., & McGuigan, A, (1994). The ecology of human performance: A framework for considering the effect of context. *American Journal of Occupational Therapy, 48,* 595–607.

Earle-Grimes, G. (1994). Psychiatric home health care: New horizons for occupational therapy. *Mental Health Special Interest Section Newsletter, 17*(2) 3–4.

Grady, A. P. (1995). Building inclusive community: A challenge for occupational therapy: 1994 Eleanor Clarke Slagle lecture. *American Journal of Occupational Therapy, 49,* 300–310.

Giangreco, M. F. (1995). Related services decision-making: A foundational component of effective education for students with disabilities. *Physical and Occupational Therapy in Pediatrics, 15*(2), 47–68.

Hanft, B. (1988). The changing environment of early intervention services: Implications for practice. *American Journal of Occupational Therapy, 42,* 26–33.

Hasselkus, B. R. (1992). The meaning of activity: Day care for persons with Alzheimer disease. *American Journal of Occupational Therapy, 46,* 199–206.

King, P. M. (1993). Outcome analysis of work-hardening programs. *American Journal of Occupational Therapy, 47,* 595–603.

Leviton, A., Mueller, M., & Kauffman, C. (1992). The family-centered consultation model: Practical applications for professionals. *Infants and Young Children, 4*(3), 1–8.

McCormack, K. F. (1990). Job site analysis. *Occupational Therapy Practice, 1*(2), 35–43.

Niemeyer, L. (1989). Program models for work hardening. In L. Ogden-Niemeyer and K. Jacobs (Eds.), *Work hardening: State of the art* (pp. 13–66). Thorofare, NJ: Slack.

Pizzi, M. (1992). Hospice: The creation of meaning for people with life-threatening illness. *Occupational Therapy Practice, 4*(1), 1–7.

Richert, G. Z. & Merryman, M. B. (1987). The vocational continuum: A model for providing vocational services in a partial hospitalization program. *Occupational Therapy in Mental Health, 7*(3), 6–19.

Wilberding, D. (1991). The quarterway house: More than an alternative of care. *Occupational Therapy in Mental Health, 11*(1), 65–91.

Wyrick, J. M., Niemeyer, L. O., Ellexson, M., Jacobs, K., & Taylor, S. (1991). Occupational therapy work-hardening programs: A demographic study. *American Journal of Occupational Therapy, 45*, 109–112.

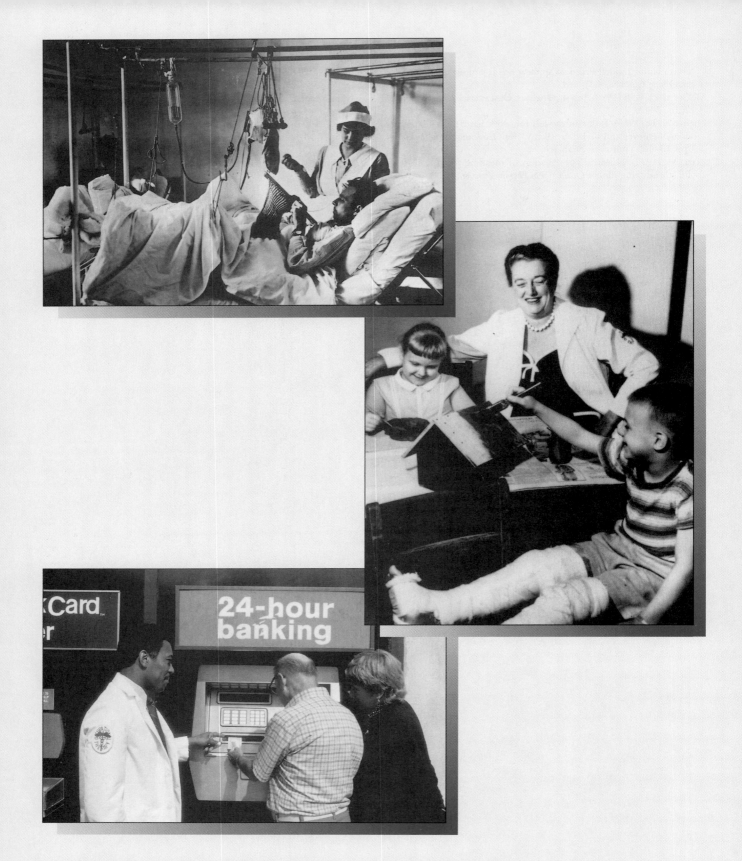

Occupational therapy intervention has evolved in response to the changes in health care and the needs of society. (top) Bedside occupational therapy during World War I: Miss Hitchcock; reconstruction aide; and Cpl. Lane, patient; Base Hospital, Chateauroux, France. (middle) Working with children in the 1950s. (bottom) Learning to use an ATM is part of a community reentry program for a mental health client in the 1990s (Photos courtesy of the Archives of the American Occupational Therapy Association, Inc, Bethesda, MD).

Unit XII

Professional Issues

LEARNING OBJECTIVES

After completing this unit, readers will be able to:

▶ Define ethics, research, and history and explain their importance to occupational therapy practice.

▶ Explain the uses and purposes of a professional code.

▶ Describe the purpose and meaning of each principle in the *Occupational Therapy Code of Ethics*.

▶ Demonstrate a basic understanding of quantitative and qualitative research approaches, and the value of each to the study of occupation and occupational therapy.

▶ Describe the history of occupational therapy relative to the social and political forces that were the catalyst for its creation and continuing development.

▶ Apply knowledge of ethics, research, and history to their professional practice.

▶ Identify crucial professional decisions that will influence occupational therapy's potential contribution to society in the changing environmental context of a new millennium.

Central to the practice of occupational therapy are three interrelated topics: ethics, research, and history. Our professional ethics articulate the core values and beliefs that direct our actions as we provide intervention for the people who seek our services. Our ethics and values also undergird our research priorities and efforts. Consequently, our research is directed toward topics that help us understand how to enable people to lead full, meaningful lives, regardless of their health or disability status. In doing our research, our ethics also direct us to respect the dignity of those we are studying. Finally, our history provides the rich tradition on which our profession was founded. By understanding our history we can discover the common threads that link occupational therapy practitioners from the founders to today. This unit develops these themes and topics and concludes with an essay calling us to embrace the future and its challenges. (*Note*: words in **bold** type are defined in the Glossary.)

Chapter 47

Ethics in Occupational Therapy

Ruth Ann Hansen

Making ethical decisions is part of our daily lives. You may have noticed that *ethics* is a word that is being used more and more frequently by individuals in discussions of their personal lives and of public issues. The public media—television, radio, newspapers, and magazines—have made us all aware of the unethical conduct of public figures.

Struggling with decisions about what is "the right thing to do" can cause both intrapersonal and interpersonal tensions and create stress. We decide what is "right" based on personal, professional, and societal values. Ethical dilemmas occur when we face situations in which the right or correct action is not clear. This may mean there is more than one "right" answer or that you are struggling to select from several less-than-desirable options. Ethical conflicts occur when our values clash with others—friends, relatives, or professional colleagues. These situations cause us to feel uneasy, upset, and perplexed.

What follows is a summary of some of the ethical concepts that are critical when discussing ethical issues within the occupational therapy profession. First we need to understand some basic terminology, which is presented in Box 47–1. Keeping these basic ideas in mind we will then discuss several theoretical perspectives we might use when deliberating ethical issues.

There are associations and relations among many of these terms. In discussions of ethical issues, people will talk about both beneficence and nonmaleficence. Beneficence conveys the idea of doing good or what is best for an individual or group of people, whereas nonmaleficence infers an effort to avoid doing harm either physical, financial, psychological, or social. To examine the difference between these two terms, let us think about a practitioner (occupational therapist or certified occupational therapy assistant) working with someone with severe burns. From one perspective, the treat-ment is beneficent because the ultimate goal is to enable the person to regain as much movement as possible. Treatment, on the other hand, is often quite painful. Some individuals may consider that serious harm (pain and psychological distress) is being inflicted on the person over the short term. Conversely, therapists would be likely to consider that withholding treatment (avoiding pain) would cause long-term harm. The individual would have contractures and serious limitations in range of motion (ROM) and mobility. As you can see, people involved (practitioner, client, family) may describe this treatment in very different ways, depending on their view of the situation.

Autonomy or self-determination, competency, and informed consent are interdependent concepts. In our society, as well as many others, we place a high value on a person's being able to make an independent decision. This right is predicated on the person's ability to make competent decisions, and having the necessary facts on which to make an informed decision. Not everyone is able to make autonomous decisions. Individuals may have a temporary or permanent loss of cognitive or psychological functioning that interferes with their ability to reason and make sound judgments. Those who can not speak are very frequently assumed to be unable to make decisions for themselves. The determination of whether persons are competent to make decisions about their lives is crucial. Making these determinations is not easy. Often, legal judgments are what determine whether individuals are competent, or whether they need a guardian. Those who are competent must have the necessary information available to choose a course of action. As helping professionals, we must remind ourselves that all individuals have the right to make autonomous decisions. Persons who have physical, psychological, or cognitive disabilities, as well as the very young and the very old, have

▼ **BOX 47-1**

Key Terms

Autonomy. The right of an individual to be self-determining. The right to make independent decisions about one's life.

Beneficence. The act or attitude of doing good or causing good to happen for others. The duty to try to do what is best for another person.

Competence. Having the cognitive and psychological ability to make decisions that others judge to be rational. It is also necessary to be able to communicate these decisions to others.

Equity. The belief that all individuals are equal and that being treated equally is a right. This is particularly at issue when scarce resources are being distributed.

Ethics. The values and beliefs that are part of a particular group (social, cultural, professional). These beliefs are a guide for the members of the group when determining right from wrong.

  Metaethics. The branch of philosophy that examines the commonalties in the ways that humans make decisions about what is right or moral.

  Normative ethics. The study of individuals' deliberations about what is right.

Fidelity. The duty to be faithful to another person and to that individual's best interests. Included is the idea of holding information about that person in confidence.

Informed consent. The right to make decisions about health care that occurs after the person has a complete understanding of the options available and the possible consequences of various alternative forms of care.

Justice. Rules for determining how to allocate resources (materials, goods, supplies, money, personnel).

  Compensatory. Provision of resources to a wronged or injured individual.

  Distributive. A method of determining how to dispense or allocate resources (for example, equal shares to all, first-come first-served).

Nonmaleficence. The obligation to avoid doing harm to another or to avoid creating a circumstance in which harm could occur to another.

Paternalism. Acting or making decisions for another. There is usually a presumption that the decision maker is acting in the best interest of the other person and is doing so without that person's consent.

the right (and should be encouraged) to remain as autonomous as possible in their daily lives. We have an obligation in all cases to inform those we serve of the nature of the therapy being provided, the goals of treatment, expected outcomes, and the availability of other treatment options.

Justice is also an important principle. Most people agree that all individuals have the right to fair and equal treatment, but whether that equity extends to equal access to

health, education, and social services is a thorny question. Do all persons have the right to receive all services (resources) that they need or want? Obviously, there are limits to the money, time, personnel, equipment, and other resources that are available. Do the current reimbursement mechanisms assure fair and equal access to treatment? In this era of managed care, third-party payers are making decisions about the types and amount of resources that will be provided. Payment mechanisms determine if persons will receive specific services.

An understanding of this terminology is necessary, but we also must have some knowledge of the basic theoretical foundations in ethics. This next section contains a summary of some of the more fundamental ideas. Familiarity with these ideas will help you understand the different ways that individuals perceive ethical dilemmas and variations in the ways people will make choices about the desirable resolution.

▼ THEORETICAL PERSPECTIVES

Philosophical

Glenn Graber has organized basic philosophical theories used in medical ethics into two groupings: teleological and deontological. Graber (1988) makes three, key comparisons between these two theories of moral obligation. First, when deciding how to determine right from wrong, the teleologist would look at the consequences of the act, whereas the deontologist would weigh the duties that an individual has in the situation. Second, the goal in teleology is to do good and avoid harm. In deontology the emphasis is on being respectful of others' rights. Finally, there is a principle within each theory to help in the resolution of conflict. In the teleological approach producing the greatest good for the greatest number is the guide. From a deontological perspective the way to resolve conflict is to weigh the conflicting duties in the situation and determine which duty is primary.

When reading and talking about ethics, we need to determine the orientation of the author or speaker. Individuals will make very different choices about right action, depending on whether they consider the consequences or the obligation to carry out duties to have the higher priority. Knowing how people set these priorities will aid in understanding why they make certain choices.

Let us go back to the example of the person who has severe burns. The teleologist would examine the consequences of treatment and make a decision about ethical practice by deciding what would cause the greatest good for the greatest number of people involved—the client, the client's family and significant others, and society. The deontologist would decide the right thing to do by balancing the duties that the practitioner has to the various individuals and groups of concern. If you are thinking that this still does not give you the answer, you are correct. What it does is help you understand the thinking process that might be used in coming to a decision.

I hope that this example will help you realize that even though discussions of philosophical theory may seem far removed from everyday decisions, they are not. Conflicts with colleagues about "right" choices may have at their roots a disagreement about how to prioritize duties. In another situation, conflicts may arise because of a disagreement about what is the greatest good or whether that "good" should take priority over a specific duty.

Modern Perspectives

A logical extension of these philosophical foundations is the work of some modern philosophers and educators in the United States. Morrill (1980) organized this information into four categories. I have added the feminist perspective to this list.

1. *Values clarification* helps individuals identify and clarify their personal values and identify those values that are most important. The goal is for persons to be able to establish a personal system of values. This occurs through the active process of choosing and prizing personal beliefs, as well as being able to act on those beliefs (Raths, Harmin, & Simon, 1966).

2. *Values inquiry* provides individuals with the opportunity to examine and try to understand the values that others hold. In this process people become more aware of the general values that motivate human choice and decision making. The goals are a commitment to a reasonably stable set of values and an understanding of that value system within society (McGrath, 1977).

3. *Moral education and moral development* propose that moral reasoning changes and matures in a predictable sequence. Kohlberg proposed six stages of cognitive–moral development that are grounded in concepts of fairness and justice. Each stage is descriptive of a unique pattern of reasoning that the person uses to determine right from wrong. The emphasis from this perspective is on the cognitive structures used to process moral issues rather than on a personal awareness of specific values. The highest or sixth stage of moral reasoning is the Golden Rule: " Do unto others as you would have them do unto you" (Kohlberg, 1984). He maintained that the person first makes moral judgments and then will act on them. The person has a commitment to act on moral judgments (Kohlberg & Candee, 1984).

Numerous individuals have criticized Kohlberg's theory and research. Critics have faulted Kohlberg for interviewing male subjects exclusively when arriving at his original construction of stages. Other critics voice a concern that his theory has a bias toward the Western culture. They maintain that the dominant themes of moral decision making in this culture are the principals of justice,

contract-keeping, and rights. Gilligan (1982) found that women used the ideas of responsibility, caring, and mutuality when deliberating about certain ethical dilemmas (Haste & Baddeley, 1991).

4. *Feminist perspectives* of moral reasoning emerged in the last two decades. In their chapter on moral theory and feminist culture, Haste and Baddeley (1991) discuss their own research and the more current writings of Gilligan. They found a clear association between being female and having a predominant moral orientation of responsibility and caring. They also found that males were more likely to make moral decisions using a "rights and justice" orientation. However, Haste and Baddeley make the important point that each gender can reason from the alternative perspective under appropriate conditions.

While the moral orientations are gender-linked, it is clear that both sexes are aware of each orientation and can use both. . . Such evidence undermines the notion that impermeable boundaries and peculiar experience are the *sine que non* for the development of particular orientations or ways of knowing, but it does not undermine the concept of separate culture per se. (Haste & Baddeley, 1991, pp. 234–235)

"Feminist ethics is best characterized as a special challenge to traditional ethical theory" (Ladd, 1996, p. 30). The more traditional ethical perspectives develop rules to guide and gauge public behavior. Women have, typically, been involved in a domestic role that requires intensely personal relationships with particular, unique individuals (Ladd; Sichel, 1992). Feminist theory shifts the focus to that which is private and personal in peoples' lives. It favors partiality, rather than detachment. As Ladd states, "It is a natural human tendency to favor 'our own.' The question is when, if ever, it is justified to do so. Can partiality be a part of morality?" (p. 30).

5. *Normative and applied ethics* enables individuals to explore and justify the proper right action in a specific and familiar situation. This method is particularly useful to explore issues of professional ethics, professional codes of ethics, and professional responsibility (Morrill, 1980).

I have given you several different ways that experts in the field of ethics discuss and reason about moral issues. Later in this section we will examine the use of various strategies to resolve ethical dilemmas.

▼ OCCUPATIONAL THERAPY ETHICS

Within our profession there are two key AOTA documents that describe aspects of the moral stance of occupational therapy. These documents are the *Core Values and Attitudes of Occupational Therapy Practice* (American Occupational Therapy Association [AOTA], 1993a) (see Appendix A) and the

Occupational Therapy Code of Ethics (AOTA, 1994a) (see Appendix B).

Core Values and Attitudes of Occupational Therapy Practice

The first document is a statement of the values and attitudes that are evident in the official documents of the American Occupational Therapy Association (AOTA). The documents used to write this paper were (1) *Dictionary Definition of Occupational Therapy* (AOTA, 1986), (2) *The Philosophical Base of Occupational Therapy* (AOTA, 1979), (3) *Essentials and Guidelines for an Accredited Educational Program for the Occupational Therapist* (AOTA, 1991a), (4) *Essentials and Guidelines for an Accredited Education Program for the Occupational Therapy Assistant* (AOTA, 1991b), and (5) *Occupational Therapy Code of Ethics* (AOTA, 1988).

These documents directly state or imply the values and beliefs undergirding the occupational therapy profession in the United States. Kanny (1993) identified seven core values and attitudes: altruism, equality, freedom, justice dignity, truth, and prudence (Box 47–2).

▼ **BOX 47-2**

Core Values and Attitudes of Occupational Therapy

Altruism is the unselfish concern for the welfare of others. This concept is reflected in actions and attitudes of commitment, caring, dedication, responsiveness, and understanding.

Dignity emphasizes the importance of valuing the inherent worth and uniqueness of each person. This value is demonstrated by an attitude of empathy and respect for self and others.

Equality requires that all individuals be perceived as having the same fundamental human rights and opportunities. This value is demonstrated by an attitude of fairness and impartiality.

Freedom allows the individual to exercise choice and to demonstrate independence, initiative, and self-direction.

Justice places value on the upholding of such moral and legal principles as fairness, equity, truthfulness, and objectivity.

Truth requires that we be faithful to facts and reality. Truthfulness or veracity is demonstrated by being accountable, honest, forthright, accurate, and authentic in our attitudes and actions.

Prudence is the ability to govern and discipline oneself through the use of reason. To be prudent is to value judiciousness, discretion, vigilance, moderation, care, and circumspection in the management of one's affairs, to temper extremes, make judgments, and respond on the basis of intelligent reflection and rational thought.

(Kanny, pp. 1085–1086).

Occupational Therapy Code of Ethics

The second AOTA document is the *Occupational Therapy Code of Ethics* (AOTA, 1994a). Before examining the contents of this document we need to understand why professions develop codes of ethics. What is the purpose of a professional code of ethics? Members of many professions, particularly health care or service-providing professions, have privileges that are not granted to the nonprofessional. In turn, professions develop principles of conduct or codes of ethics that hold members of that profession to a higher standard of behavior.

For example, as occupational therapy practitioners we have access to personal information about the people we serve. We are also allowed to touch and physically manipulate their bodies to administer therapy. Under most other circumstances this type of access is illegal. Having personal information about another individual is an invasion of privacy, and physical contact can be deemed an assault. Because practitioners have these extraordinary rights, we also have the duty to hold information in confidence, to avoid doing harm, and to respect the client's privacy and integrity.

The *Occupational Therapy Code of Ethics* (AOTA, 1994a) describes correct professional conduct for occupational therapy practitioners (occupational therapists and occupational therapy assistants). The code also provides guidance for occupational therapy students as future practitioners and for all persons, in addition to occupational therapists and occupational therapy assistants, who may be providing occupational therapy services (aides, technicians, or others). The code consists of six principles of conduct. These principles provide general guidance. They are not specific and do not give the solution for a particular ethical dilemma.

Principle 1 states, "Occupational therapy personnel shall demonstrate a concern for the well-being of the recipients of their services (beneficence)" (AOTA, 1994a, p. 1037). This statement reminds us that our services must be provided equitably. We must not exploit the individuals whom we serve in any way. We must take precautions to avoid causing harm to those individuals or to their property. This principle also covers the duty to charge fees that are fair and reasonable.

Principle 2 emphasizes respect for the rights of our clients (autonomy, informed consent, privacy, right to refuse treatment) (AOTA, 1994a). This means that we need to collaborate with our clients in setting treatment goals. Ideally, the client is the one who selects the goals of treatment and the practitioner helps the client find ways of reaching those goals. We must ensure that clients are fully informed about (1) the type of treatment, (2) any risks involved in treatment, and (3) the expected outcomes of therapy. We must respect their right to refuse treatment; and maintain confidentiality about privileged information. The code provides guidance to professionals in a variety of roles: practitioner, educator, researcher, manager. Thus, this principle also covers the rights of research subjects to giving fully informed consent before participation in any study. Subjects must understand the potential risks, as well as the possible outcomes of the study.

Principle 3 describes the duty that we have to remain professionally competent (AOTA, 1994a). We have an obligation to maintain appropriate national and state credentials. First, practitioners must acquire the appropriate entry-level credentials (registered occupational therapist [OTR] or certified occupational therapy assistant [COTA]). Beyond entry level the practitioner must maintain competency. One way to do this is by obtaining recognized advanced credentialing in areas like sensory integration and hand therapy. In addition, the practitioner must seek necessary supervision and training when learning new skills. We must also comply with the AOTA Standards of Practice (AOTA, 1994b, p. 1039), participate in professional development activities, and base our professional activities on accurate and up-to-date information.

Also, we are responsible for the competence of all those we supervise. This means that we must carefully assign tasks to make sure that the person assuming the duties has the qualifications, experience, and training necessary to carry them out safely and responsibly. The supervisor must decide how much and what type of supervision is necessary for the designated individual to carry out the assigned duties. We must always provide adequate supervision in these situations. Finally, if we feel that the services being requested are outside our area of competence, we should refer clients to other providers or consult with those providers.

Principle 4 is a reminder of our duty to comply with all local, state, federal, and institutional laws governing our professional activities (AOTA, 1994a). This includes the responsibility to follow the AOTA policies and guidelines for the profession. Not only must we abide by and comply with these rules, but we must also be sure that our professional colleagues are aware of and follow these regulations including the *Occupational Therapy Code of Ethics*. This principle also covers documentation. All professional documentation must be accurate and complete. This means keeping accurate and complete client records, and billing correctly. It also requires accuracy in our professional resumes, professional presentations, and scholarly writing.

Principle 5 covers the idea of veracity or truthfulness. It states, "Occupational therapy personnel shall provide accurate information about occupational therapy services" (AOTA, 1994a, p. 1038). We must accurately represent our qualifications, education, and level of competence. We must be aware of and report any potential conflict of interest, and we must represent our qualifications, credentials, and capabilities accurately. We must accurately present the scope and limits of our personal expertise and refrain from making exaggerated or unfounded promises or guarantees about the outcomes of the professional services provided.

Principle 6 emphasizes the need for fidelity and veracity. We need to safeguard all confidential information about colleagues and staff, as well as acknowledging the contribu-

tions and findings of colleagues (AOTA, 1994a). Included is the obligation to report the illegal or unethical conduct of professional colleagues to appropriate authorities. *Whistle blowing* is the term used to describe this obligation.

The members of the AOTA write and maintain the *Occupational Therapy Code of Ethics*. The AOTA reviews this document every 5 years to make sure that the content is current and relevant to member concerns. The members of AOTA have designated that the AOTA Commission on Standards and Ethics has the responsibility to maintain, revised and enforce this code. The Representative Assembly must approve all revisions of the code before the document becomes official.

The *Occupational Therapy Code of Ethics* and the *Core Values and Attitudes of Occupational Therapy Practice* are two AOTA documents. They are "key" because they describe the values, attitudes, and moral beliefs that guide occupational therapy practice in the United States. Next we will discuss the agencies that have jurisdiction over the ethical conduct of occupational therapy practitioners.

Ethical Jurisdiction

There are three specific agencies that have jurisdiction and concerns about the ethical conduct of occupational therapy personnel. These three groups are the American Occupational Therapy Association (AOTA), the National Certification Board for Occupational Therapy (NBCOT), and state regulatory boards (SRBs) (licensure, registration, or trademark). This section describes each organization, including the purpose, scope, and regulatory power of each. Following this description are some guidelines for determining which of the three agencies to contact with specific concerns or questions.

AMERICAN OCCUPATIONAL THERAPY ASSOCIATION

The AOTA is a voluntary membership organization that represents and promotes the interests of persons who choose to become members. Because membership is voluntary, AOTA has no direct authority over practitioners (occupational therapists or occupational therapy assistants) who are not members. AOTA has no direct legal mechanism for preventing nonmembers who are incompetent, unethical, or unqualified from practicing. The Commission on Standards and Ethics (SEC) is the volunteer-sector component of AOTA that is responsible for writing, revising and enforcing the *Occupational Therapy Code of Ethics*. SEC is also responsible for informing and educating members about current ethical issues, and for reviewing allegations of unethical conduct by AOTA members.

When the SEC receives a complaint about a member, the chairperson requests that a designated individual conduct a confidential, preliminary investigation. Currently, that individual is the Ethics Program Manager, who is a member of the AOTA National Office Staff. This investigation provides the members of SEC with necessary information to determine if the allegation warrants deliberation by the Commission. If they decide that the allegation is a violation of the Occupational Therapy Code of Ethics, they can impose one of four types of disciplinary action.

1. Reprimand is a formal expression of disapproval of conduct communicated privately by letter from the chairperson of SEC.
2. Censure is a formal expression of disapproval that is public.
3. Suspension requires removal of membership for a specified period of time.
4. Revocation prohibits a person from being a member of AOTA indefinitely. (AOTA, 1996)

NATIONAL BOARD FOR THE CERTIFICATION IN OCCUPATIONAL THERAPY

The NBCOT is currently in the process of reviewing and revising their disciplinary action procedures. NBCOT is the national credentialing agency that certifies qualified persons as registered occupational therapists and certified occupational therapy assistants at the entry level. This is accomplished by successfully passing a written certification examination. This organization, because of it purpose, has jurisdiction over all NBCOT-certified practitioners as well as those currently eligible to "sit" for the next examination.

The three main categories of violations that warrant disciplinary action are incompetence, unethical behavior, and impairment. When NBCOT receives a complaint, they initiate an intensive, confidential review process to determine whether the allegations are warranted. If so, the Disciplinary Action Committee (DAC) may select one of several sanctions, depending on the seriousness of the misconduct. The following is a listing of the available options, starting with the least severe action and progressing to most severe.

1. Reprimand is a formal, written expression of disapproval of conduct communicated privately and retained in the individual's certification file.
2. Censure is a formal expression of disapproval that is publicly proclaimed.
3. Ineligibility to take the certification examination may be determined indefinitely or for a specific time period.
4. Probation requires that the individual fulfill certain conditions, such as education, supervision, or counseling, for a specified time. The individual must meet these conditions to remain certified.
5. Suspension is the loss of certification for a specified time. The DAC uses suspension when they determine that the person must complete specific amounts of public service or participate in a rehabilitation program.
6. Revocation means that the individual loses certification permanently (Hansen, 1992).

STATE REGULATORY BOARDS

SRBs are public bodies created by state legislatures to ensure the health and safety of the citizens of that state. Their specific responsibility is to protect the public from potential harm that incompetent or unqualified practitioners may cause. State regulation may be in the form of licensure, registration, or certification. The legal guidelines of each state usually specify the scope of practice for the profession and the qualifications that professionals must meet to practice. In addition, the board usually provides a description of ethical behavior. In most cases the SRBs have adopted the AOTA Occupational Therapy Code of Ethics for this purpose.

Each SRB has direct jurisdiction over those therapists practicing in that state. By the very nature of this limited jurisdiction, each state can monitor the practitioners in that state more closely than national organizations such as AOTA and NBCOT. They have the authority, by state law, to discipline members of a profession practicing in that state if they have caused harm to citizens of that state. The SRBs can also intervene in situations for which the person has been convicted of an illegal act that directly affects professional practice (for example, the misappropriation of funds through false-billing practices).

The primary concern of each state is to protect the people living in that state. They, therefore, limit their review of complaints to those involving such a threat. When an SRB determines that an individual has violated the law, it can elect several different sanctions as a disciplinary measure. Examples of disciplinary actions are (1) public censure, (2) temporary suspension of practice privileges, and (3) permanent prohibition from practice in that state.

WHERE TO GO FIRST

As you can see the AOTA, NBCOT, and state regulatory boards have specific jurisdictions over occupational therapy. Among the three groups, some areas of concern overlap. Others are separate and distinct. If you need information or want to file a complaint, it is helpful to know which of the three is the most appropriate to contact. To do so you should ask yourself the following three questions:

1. Did the alleged violation take place in a state that regulates occupational therapy practice?
2. Is the individual a member of AOTA?
3. What consequences do I consider appropriate if the complaint is determined to be justified? (Hansen, 1992, pp. 6–7)

Certainly in some instances, you would have a choice of any of the three agencies. For example, all three have concerns if there has been harm or potential harm to a consumer. On the other hand, ethical violations of professional values that have no potential to cause harm would likely be of interest to AOTA, alone. (For example, violation of a verbal contract to provide a continuing education workshop). You should also consider what disciplinary action you would consider appropriate for a particular violation. Do you want to revoke or restrict the person's state licensure? Do you want the organization to either suspend or revoke the individual's certification? Would it be more appropriate in your mind to restrict or prohibit the person's ability to be a member of AOTA? You need to seek advice before filing a complaint to be sure that you have selected the agency with the jurisdiction to achieve the conse-

quences you consider commensurate to the violation. (Hansen, 1994)

Several years ago, AOTA, NBCOT, and the state regulatory boards established a network for communicating and publishing the disciplinary actions of the respective groups. The Disciplinary Action Information Exchange Network (DAIEN) provides a mechanism for notifying the public and other organizations when any disciplinary action is

CASE STUDY

MS. GARCIA

Ms. Garcia is an occupational therapist and an employee of a for-profit, health care agency. In her current position she provides home health services. Mr. Alexander is 68 years old and had a stroke 6 weeks ago. Under the new managed care plan, they will permit six visits. The main goal of therapy is to help Mr. Alexander regain as much self-care independence as possible so that he can remain in his home. Of course, safety is a primary concern, not only because of his physical abilities, but also because his judgment is impaired. His partner is employed full-time. Once the funding runs out for a home health aide, Mr. Alexander will be home alone from 7:30 A.M. to 5:30 P.M. At the end of six visits, Mr. Alexander is able to bath, dress, and groom himself with stand-by verbal cueing and some physical assistance. He must be able to perform these activities with minimal verbal cueing and no physical assistance to stay at home with his partner.

Ms. Garcia has 10 years of experience as an occupational therapist and has primarily worked in home health. Her professional judgment is that with three more visits, Mr. Alexander will be able to reach the goal of safely performing his self-care activities with minimal assistance. The case manager is reluctant to allow more visits and wants Ms. Garcia to discontinue her visits. What should the practitioner do in this situation?

There are several approaches that you could take in this situation. One is to examine the conflict among the therapist's duties to the employer, the third-party payer and Mr. Alexander. You may need more information to develop a solution. Many times a dilemma exists because we do not have all the information that we need to make an educated decision. For now, take this case at face value. What are some of the options that you might consider in bringing this issue to a satisfactory resolution?

The following are some that I have identified:

1. What is the likelihood that the case manager will allow more visits? In the current environment the containment of costs is a primary concern. What sort of "track record" does Ms. Garcia have for obtaining satisfactory outcomes within the specified number of visits? If she has a record of favorable outcomes, the case manager is more likely to allow the extension. There is also the legal concern that the home health agency may be liable if Mr. Alexander is discharged before he can perform his daily living activities safely.
2. What if the case manager refuses? Mr. Alexander does not have resources to have someone in the home at all times, nor do he and his partner have sufficient financial reserves or insurance coverage to pay for an assisted-living facility. Can Ms. Garcia find another way to cover the cost of the three additional visits? What if Ms. Garcia decides to provide the additional visits without cost (otherwise, known as *pro bono*, that is "for the good")?
3. What is the best way to provide the greatest good for the greatest number? To whom does Ms. Garcia have a primary duty? Does she decide what to do by relying on the rules of justice or based on her feelings of partiality for Mr. Alexander and his partner? If she decides to provide free services, does that obligate her to provide similar services for other clients, now and in the future? Can you provide a justification for not providing free occupational therapy services to *all* others, but rather, to only a few.
4. Does the sexual orientation of Mr. Alexander and his partner make a difference in how you decide to resolve this dilemma? Should sexual orientation be an influential factor? Give a rationale for your response.

taken against an occupational therapy practitioner. The NBCOT's newsletter, *The Information Exchange*, and the AOTA's *OT Week* publish the DAIEN list. This is a master list of those individuals who have been subject to disciplinary action since the previous publication of this list. (This usually occurs quarterly.)

Summary

This section is a summary of the various organizations that have ethical jurisdiction over occupational therapy practice. Use this information to guide you when seeking information about ethical issues, and when trying to decide where to file a complaint about an ethical violation.

▼ ETHICAL DILEMMAS FOR DISCUSSION

It is never easy trying to make the transition from abstract ideas to practical solutions. In this section I will try to help you see how you can use the ethical concepts (terms and principles) and translate them into action plans when ethical dilemmas arise. We will use two cases to try out an analysis process that you might find useful. One case describes a practice dilemma, and the other is a management and supervisory predicament.

First, you should read the details of the case and be sure that you understand the situation. Then you will consider a series of questions. By answering these questions you should

---

CASE STUDY

JEREMY

Jeremy is the director of a rehabilitation services department in a large metropolitan hospital. There are now eight occupational therapists, two occupational therapy assistants, and one occupational therapy aide on the rehabilitation team. The corporation that owns the hospital has recently merged with several other health care businesses in the area. They are initiating a plan to "right-size" the organization. They have issued a mandate to all departments to establish cost-saving measures that will reduce cost. Jeremy must also eliminate unnecessary services while providing services of increasingly higher quality. Jeremy has been told to reduce the number of occupational therapists to two and, in their place, to hire more occupational therapy assistants and aides to deliver treatment.

Jeremy believes that some changes in the distribution of levels of occupational therapy personnel are possible. However, his main concern is that the quality of the services provided would be seriously compromised if he initiates such a dramatic change, particularly for those clients who are very seriously and acutely ill. They need very high levels of sophisticated expertise to ensure that they receive safe and competent treatment. An example is the neurology unit where there are currently two occupational therapists and one occupational therapy assistant. The clients on this unit are primarily individuals who have had recent spinal cord injuries and traumatic brain injuries.

What steps should Jeremy take to make sure that there is a proper balance between providing competent treatment and being cost-effective? The fol-

lowing are some questions that he will need to answer. Can you think of others?

1. What are the legal and ethical guidelines that describe the practice of occupational therapists and occupational therapy assistants? What, if any, differences are there between the role of each? What type of supervisor is needed? What credentials must the supervisor have? How much time must the supervisor spend to make sure that the aide or occupational therapy assistant is providing safe and competent services? (The AOTA Roles (1996b) would be a good resource for this discussion.)
2. Would a change in staffing allow the department to maintain all services currently provided, including those in such areas as the neonatal intensive care unit and the neurology unit? If not, how should Jeremy make decisions about what services to discontinue?
3. Are all the occupational therapists now on the staff capable of providing the type of supervision necessary? Are they willing to reduce their direct client contact and take on these supervisory responsibilities? How can Jeremy help them acquire the skills needed to take on new roles? Should he be doing this?
4. Is it realistic to expect that there are occupational therapy assistants and aides available in the community who want to apply for these new positions?
5. If the department is successful in making this transition, does it set a precedent for further shifts in staffing in the future?

be able to come to some a conclusion about what you think should happen. Read the case study on p. 825.

Naturally, you will come up with other questions that you want to take into account. Develop different scenarios and options and discuss them with your colleagues. Try to reach consensus on a plan of action that all, or most of you, can agree on. After doing this, role play the situation of providing this explanation to Mr. Alexander, his partner, the case manager, the employer, and yourself, as Ms Garcia. Read the case study on p. 826.

Obviously, there are not clear answers to the questions in this case study either. Discuss the Jeremy dilemma with your peers. Explore the resources that are available to you that would help you come up with a solution. Try to look at this situation from Jeremy's perspective, the CEO of the health care corporation, the present and future occupational therapy staff, and the clients in the hospital. Again, you can test possible solutions by role playing the explanation of a solution to each of the parties involved in this scenario.

►CONCLUSION

Struggling with right and wrong in given situations is part of everyday life. We find ethical dilemmas throughout our profession—in clinical practice, supervision, management, teaching, research, and consultation. You now have a working knowledge of the terminology, theory, professional code, and analytical process needed to grapple with ethical issues. You are also aware of the three major organizations that have concern for occupational therapy ethics and who have the jurisdiction to impose disciplinary action for infraction of ethical conduct.

The conflicts that are described in the two cases are current versions of common ethical dilemmas. The current health care environment demands cost-effective care and requires major changes in the nature and delivery of services. The conflicts that arise between provision of quality services and cost-effectiveness create serious tensions for all of us—provider and recipient, alike. I hope that these cases will provide a springboard for the discussion and clarification of other ethical dilemmas that you encounter. I urge you to explore the literature on health care and human services ethics more deeply. My hope is that you can remain well versed about the issues involved in the emerging ethical challenges facing us in our professional lives. I also hope that you acquire the understanding and reasoning ability to analyze and confront these challenges.

▼ REFERENCES

American Occupational Therapy Association (AOTA). (1979). The philosophical base of occupational therapy. *American Journal of Occupational Therapy, 33,* 785.

American Occupational Therapy Association. (1986, April). Dictionary definition of occupational therapy. Adopted and approved by the Representative Assembly to fulfill Resolution #596–83.

American Occupational Therapy Association. (1988). Occupational therapy code of ethics. *American Journal of Occupational Therapy, 42,* 795–796.

American Occupational Therapy Association. (1991a). Essentials and guidelines for an accredited educational program for the occupational therapist. *American Journal of Occupational Therapy, 45,* 1077–1084.

American Occupational Therapy Association. (1991b). Essentials and guidelines for an accredited educational program for the occupational therapy assistant. *American Journal of Occupational Therapy, 45,* 1085–1092.

American Occupational Therapy Association. (1993a). Core values and attitudes of occupational therapy practice. *American Journal of Occupational Therapy, 47,* 1085–1086.

American Occupational Therapy Association. (1993b). Occupational therapy roles. *American Journal of Occupational Therapy, 47,* 1087–1099.

American Occupational Therapy Association. (1994a). Occupational therapy code of ethics. *American Journal of Occupational Therapy, 48,* 1037–1038.

American Occupational Therapy Association. (1994b). Standards for practice for occupational therapy. *American Journal of Occupational Therapy, 48,* 1039–1043.

American Occupational Therapy Association. (1996). Enforcement procedure for occupational therapy code of ethics. *American Journal of Occupational Therapy, 50,* 848–852.

Gilligan, C. (1982). *In a different voice: Psychological theory and women's development.* Cambridge, MA: Harvard University Press.

Graber, G. C. (1988). Basic theories in medical ethics. In J. F. Monagle & D. C. Thomasma (Eds.), *Medical ethics: A guide for health professionals* (pp. 462–475). Rockville, MD: Aspen.

Hansen, R. A. (1992). Ethical jurisdiction of occupational therapy: The role of AOTA, AOTCB and state regulatory boards. *OT Week, 6*(3), 6–7.

Hansen, R. A. (1994). Guidelines for responding to questions about ethical dilemmas. Distributed to the members of the Committee of State Presidents, Boston, MA, July 1994.

Haste, H. & Baddeley, J. (1991). Moral theory and culture: The case of gender. In W. M. Kurtines & J. L. Gewirtz (Eds.), *Handbook of moral behavior and development, Volume I: Theory* (pp. 223–249). Hillsdale, NJ: Lawrence Erlbaum Associates.

Kanny, E. (1993). Core values and attitudes of occupational therapy practice. *American Journal of Occupational Therapy, 47,* 1085–1086.

Kohlberg, L. (1984). *Essays on moral development. Volume II. The psychology of moral development. The nature and validity of moral stages.* San Francisco: Harper & Row.

Kohlberg, L. & Candee, D. (1984). The relationship of moral judgment to moral action. In W. Kurtines & J. Gerwitz (Eds.), *Morality, moral behavior and moral development* (pp. 52–73). New York: Wiley Interscience.

Ladd, R. E. (1996). Partiality and the pediatrician. *The Journal of Clinical Ethics, 7,* 29–34.

McGrath, E. (1977). Institutional alternative for an education in values. *Counseling and values, 22,* 5–19.

Morrill, R. (1980). *Teaching values in education.* San Francisco: Josey-Bass.

Raths, L., Harmin, M., & Simon, S. (1966). *Values and teaching.* Columbus, OH: Charles E. Merrill.

Sichel, B. (1992) Ethics of caring and the institutional ethics committee. In H. B. Holmes & L. M. Purdy (Eds.), *Feminist perspectives in medical ethics* (pp. 113–123). Bloomington, IN: Indiana University Press.

Chapter 48

Research: Discovering Knowledge Through Systematic Investigation

Section 1: Introduction to Research

Section 2: Quantitative Research

Section 3: Qualitative Research

Section 4: Qualitative and Quantitative Research: Joint Contributors to the Knowledge Base in Occupational Therapy

Section I

Introduction to Research

Jean C. Deitz

As an occupational therapy practitioner questions are likely to emerge from your daily interaction with the people receiving therapy. You may wonder:

- "Will this splint prevent contractures?"
- "What factors contribute to people wearing the splints that are made for them?"
- "Will more of the residents in the nursing home participate in the walking group if we have a new destination for each walk, as opposed to taking a familiar path each session?"
- "What are the benefits of the walking group from the resident's perspective?"
- "At what age can typically developing children access a computer to play a simple cause and effect game involving switch control?"
- "What are the activity patterns of parents with children who are multiply disabled?"
- "What is the nature of occupational therapy practice in acute care psychiatry?"
- "Does provision of occupational therapy services influ-

ence the quality of life of adults who have impairments as a result of polio during childhood?"

You can answer these practice-related questions through research, which according to Cox and West, is "a systematic approach to the discovery of knowledge" (1982, p. 5). It is a process involving a logical sequence, leading from a question to an answer which, in turn, may result in a new question. Inherent to this process is systematic observation.

Gilfoyle and Christiansen contended that research "is essential to the survival and continued development of occupational therapy" (p. 7). They further maintained that the "challenge that confronts our profession . . . concerns a commitment to inquiry, knowledge development, and responsible (scientifically based) clinical practice" (Gilfoyle & Christiansen, 1987, p. 7). Research is important to occupational therapy for three reasons. First, it develops and extends the knowledge base of the profession; second, it contributes to the development and validation of occupational therapy tests and measurements; and third, it documents the effectiveness of occupational therapy interventions. In the process, research plays an important role in theory testing and building.

There are different types of research, and each is relevant and appropriate for answering different types of questions. Occasionally, however, the same question may be answered by two or more different research approaches. Although research approaches have been classified in a variety of ways, for purposes of this chapter, they are divided into two major types: (1) quantitative research; and (2) qualitative research.

RESEARCH SHOULD DOCUMENT THAT OCCUPATION IS AN EFFECTIVE METHOD OF THERAPEUTIC INTERVENTION

Kenneth J. Ottenbacher

Many important issues face the profession of occupational therapy as it enters the 21st century. The ability to generate a body of knowledge unique to occupational science must remain a high priority. Closely related to this priority is the ability to demonstrate and document that occupation is an effective method of therapeutic intervention. In an editorial written in 1982 describing the need for research in occupational therapy, Christiansen observed that *It is worth noting here that our failure to meet the challenge of research may ultimately lead to our demise as a viable discipline* (Christiansen,

1981, p. 116). Over the past decade occupational therapy has addressed the challenge of research referred to by Christiansen and emerged as a viable and respected health care discipline. Research, however, represents a dynamic challenge that must continue to be a professional priority. The changes in our health care system have generated a new set of research questions and issues. Determining the answers to these questions, and raising new ones, will ensure that occupational therapy remains a viable health care speciality in the 21st century. ■

Christiansen, C. H. (1981). [Editorial] Toward resolution of crisis: Research requisites in occupational therapy. *The Occupational Therapy Journal of Research, 1,* 116–124.

Section 2

Quantitative Research

Jean C. Deitz

Carefully designed and conducted quantitative research enables occupational therapy practitioners to answer questions important for an understanding of occupational science and occupational therapy. Quantitative research of high quality enables practitioners to obtain precise, objective information about one individual or many individuals. The research process always involves a series of logical steps:

1. Identifying a question that merits answering
2. Reviewing existing literature and knowledge related to the question
3. Clarifying the question based on this review
4. Designing a study to answer the question
5. Carrying out the procedures of the study
6. Analyzing the data collected
7. Interpreting the data collected to determine the extent to which the identified question has been answered
8. Identifying new questions that emerge as a result of the research
9. Disseminating research findings

Quantitative research can be subdivided into quantitative group research and quantitative single-system research. The unit of analysis for the former is a group or groups of individuals; whereas the unit of analysis for the latter is the individual. These two types of quantitative research can be further subdivided. Researchers choose the research type and design based on (1) the nature of the research question; (2) the ability to control variables; and (3) the extent of the knowledge base related to the area of concern. Vocabulary related to quantitative research is shown in Box 48–1.

▼ QUANTITATIVE GROUP RESEARCH

Quantitative group research is characterized as being group focused, reductionistic, and carefully controlled. Through this type of research it is possible to obtain extensive information about numerous participants in a parsimonious manner. The designs for this type of research can be categorized into descriptive, correlational, and experimental. To some extent, these designs are sequential. According to Payton (1988), if little or nothing is known about a topic, there is a general sequence of research designs that proceeds from descriptive, to correlational, to experimental. However, in reality, there is some overlap in these designs. For example, the design of a single study may include both descriptive and correlational design elements.

BOX 48-1

Vocabulary Related to Quantitative Research

Operational definition: "a definition based on the observable characteristics of that which is being defined" (Tuckman, 1994; p. 103); method by which you quantify or measure a variable.

Independent variable: treatment variable; a condition that is manipulated by the researcher.

Dependent variable: the outcome or measured variable; the variable used to measure the effect of the independent variable.

Reliability: the consistency or stability of measurement.

Interobserver agreement: the extent to which two or more observers agree in assigning scores or ratings to the performance of a participant or a group of participants.

Procedural agreement: the extent to which the experimental procedures (the independent variables) are applied in accordance to the delineated plan (Billingsley, White, & Munson, 1980).

Validity: the extent to which findings are "accurate or reflect the underlying purpose of the study" (DePoy & Gitlin, 1994; p. 95).

Internal validity: a condition that exists when the observed effect on the dependent variable can be attributed to the independent variable. (A condition that exists when you can attribute the outcome of the study—for the individual or group studied—to the treatment.)

External validity: a condition that exists when generalizations can be made from the sample to the population.

These three basic types of quantitative group research design differ relative to (1) the kind of question asked; (2) the degree to which the researcher manipulates the sample; (3) the statistical tools used to summarize and interpret the data; and (4) the types of statements the researcher makes on the basis of the data collected and analyzed (Payton, 1988).

Before addressing the three types of quantitative group research designs, it is important to discuss populations and samples. A population is a well-defined group of people or objects that meet the criteria set by the researcher. Such groups have some characteristics in common. For example, a population might be adults with multiple sclerosis, or typically developing 4-year-old girls, or individuals treated at the Helpful Hand Clinic in Florida in 1996. In some instances, the participants in a research study may include the entire population. For example, it might be possible to include the population of all individuals treated at the Helpful Hand Clinic in Florida in 1996 in one study. On the other hand, it would be almost impossible to include the 1996 population of all typically developing 4-year-old children in the United States in a study. Instead, the researcher selects a sample (a small subset of the population) designed to be representative of the population. The researcher should

carefully describe the sample selection process and the steps taken to ensure that the sample was representative of the population.

For example, if the researcher desires a sample reflecting the population of 4-year-old girls who are typically developing, the researcher should describe such factors as how it was determined that the girls were typically developing and how he or she ensured that children were included from a variety of ethnic groups and diverse socioeconomic backgrounds. This is desirable because, often when a sample is used, the researcher wants to learn information that is generalizable to the population, in this case, 4-year-old girls who are typically developing. Therefore, it is important to know that the girls in the sample are comparable with those in the population. One of the best ways to ensure this is through random selection. This is exemplified by listing all members of a specified population and using a random numbers table to select the desired number of individuals for the sample.

Descriptive Research

The research question for quantitative descriptive research focuses on the characteristics of a specific group relative to that question. The purpose of such research is to answer a clearly defined question about a specifically identified sample or population. For example, the researcher might ask: "How many people with C5–6 quadriplegia in Michigan, who were initially fitted with wrist-driven splints, continue to wear them 6 months following discharge?" After compiling a list of all facilities in Michigan where individuals with C5–6 quadriplegia are treated, the researcher might randomly select six facilities from the list. Next, the researcher would find the names of all the people in these settings with C5–6 quadriplegia who were discharged between given dates and at the time of discharge were wearing wrist-driven splints. The researcher might then develop a carefully designed questionnaire concerning use of wrist-driven splints and mail it to all of the individuals identified as having such splints at the time of discharge.

Data from this survey might be reported in terms of the number or percentage of individuals answering each of the questions in a given way. Had the research question been phrased in terms of the number of hours persons with C5–6 quadriplegia wear such splints, data would be reported using statistics reflecting the central tendency (mean, median, or mode) and the extent of score spread or dispersion (ie, variance, standard deviation, range) of the responses to a specific item.

Survey and normative studies are examples of quantitative descriptive research. The preceding hypothetical study, as well as a study by Kanny, Anson, and Smith (1991), exemplify the former. The study by Kanny and coworkers had two purposes. The first was to document the status of technological training in entry-level curricula; the second was to "identify the factors that were barriers and those that would facilitate the development of technological training components in entry-level occupational therapy curricula" (Kanny et al., 1991). The population was defined as the 67 schools offering entry-level occupational therapy programs. Therefore, surveys were mailed to these 67 institutions, 59 of which returned their questionnaires. Thus, the response rate was over 88%. The answers to the questions on these surveys were compiled and the final results were reported in a table and a graph. For other examples of survey research relevant to occupational therapy refer to studies by Dewire, White, Kanny, and Glass (1996) on the nature of occupational therapy practice in neonatal intensive care unit (NICU) settings, the training of therapists working in these settings, and the opinions of NICU therapists concerning the necessary education for preparing therapists for this practice arena; by Case-Smith and Cable (1996) on the perceptions of occupational therapists concerning service delivery models in school-based practice; and by DeGangi and Royeen (1994) on current practice among Neurodevelopmental Treatment Association members.

An example of a normative study is that completed by Link, Lukens, and Bush (1995). They collected normative data on spherical grip strength, as measured by the Martin Vigorimeter, and on hand width. The sample consisted of 225 children ranging in age from 3 to 6 years. Means and standard deviations for grip strength and hand width were reported for both right and left hands for each of six age categories (Table 48–1).

Normative information such as this is useful clinically in that it assists in interpreting evaluation results and in setting realistic treatment goals. For additional examples of normative studies refer to test manuals for the *Miller Assessment for Preschoolers* (Miller, 1982); the *Sensory Integration and Praxis Tests* (Ayres, 1989); and the *Manual for Application of the Motor-Free Visual Perception Test to the Adult Population* (Bouska & Kwatny, 1983).

Correlational Research

The purpose of correlational research is to determine the extent to which two or more phenomena tend to occur together. For example, a researcher would use this type of research if he or she wanted to find out the extent to which hyperactivity and scores on a test of sensory integration are related, or to find out the extent to which two tests of hand function measure the same thing. To do this, the researcher uses correlational statistics to examine the degree of relationship between two or more variables. Note, that correlation does not imply causation. For example, relative to the former question, if the researcher determines that hyperactivity and low scores on a test of sensory integration are related, the researcher should not say that poor sensory integration causes hyperactivity or that hyperactivity causes poor sensory integration. Instead, the researcher should only say that hyperactivity and poor sensory integration tend to occur together. Thus, the focus of the conclusions based on

correlational research should be on degree of relationship and not on causation. Such research might lead to questions concerning cause and effect that might then become the focus of future research using experimental research designs.

An investigation by Penny, Mueser, and North (1995) exemplifies a correlational study. This study was designed primarily to examine the relationship between cognitive disability and social skills in adults with psychiatric illness in an acute inpatient setting. For purposes of this study, cognitive disability was operationally defined as scores on the Allen Cognitive Level Test (ACL)-90 (Allen, 1990) and social skills were defined as scores on the Social Interaction Test (SIT) (Trower, Bryant, & Argyle, 1978). The final sample for this study consisted of 55 participants. Scores on the ACL-90 and scores on the SIT were correlated significantly ($r = -0.32, p < 0.01$), thus indicating a tendency for patients with higher cognitive disability to have lower social scores and, conversely, for those with lower cognitive disability to have higher social scores. The correlation is negative because high scores on the ACL-90 reflect higher functioning, whereas, high scores on the SIT are associated with lower social skills. The finding of this significant, though relatively low, correlation is clinically important in that it suggests that patients functioning at different cognitive levels may have corresponding social skills. However, as the authors suggest: "Further research is needed to identify whether deficits in social skills are a result of deficits in cognitive skills, or if both result from a third common factor of mental illness; for example, mental illness may lead to fewer opportunities to learn and to practice the skills required for both cognitive and social functioning" (Trower, Bryant, & Argyle, p. 426). This study exemplifies the type of question answered by correlational research and the way such research can both contribute to clinical practice and suggest directions for future research.

In some studies the primary focus of the research is correlational; in others, such as the study by Case-Smith and Cable (1996), only one component of the study is correlational. Using survey research, Case-Smith and Cable described the perceptions of occupational therapists concerning service delivery models in school-based practice and then, using correlational methods, examined the relationship between a variety of variables and therapists' attitudes toward direct pull-out services and integrative or consultative services. Therefore, the study can be classified as both descriptive and correlational.

For additional examples of correlational research refer to journal articles by Edwards, Baum, and Deuel (1991) on the contributions of constructional apraxia to functional loss in Alzheimer's disease; by Larson (1990) on activity patterns and life changes in people with depression; and by Walker and Burris (1991) on the correlation of scores of normal children on the Sensory Integration and Praxis Tests (Ayres, 1989) and the scores of the same children on the Metropolitan Achievement Tests (Prescott, Balow, Hogan, & Farr, 1978).

Table 48-1. Means and Standard Deviations for Grip Strength and Hand Width

Age Group: Year/Month	N	Left Grip Strength		Right Grip Strength		Right Hand Width		Left Hand Width	
		M	SD	M	SD	M	SD	M	SD
3/0–3/5	16	13.89	4.12	13.64	3.68	2.22	0.15	2.20	0.16
3/6–3/11	38	18.64	6.52	18.21	7.65	2.26	0.19	2.23	0.18
4/0–4/5	53	23.80	6.45	22.23	6.24	2.31	0.15	2.30	0.15
4/6–4/11	47	27.69	6.77	27.15	6.36	2.43	0.15	2.41	0.16
5/0–5/5	50	30.99	7.97	29.70	7.92	2.52	0.19	2.48	0.14
5/6–5/11	20	36.03	8.45	34.35	8.48	2.54	0.13	2.50	0.12

Experimental Research

Experimental research is used when the desire is to establish cause-and-effect relations between variables. With this type of research, the question is generally one of comparison:

- For a particular group, is intervention A better than intervention B relative to a specifically desired outcome?
- For a particular group, is intervention A better than no intervention relative to a specifically desired outcome?

The interpretation of experimental research is in terms of probability. For example, to a research question on whether intervention A or intervention B is more effective relative to a desired outcome, the answer might state that the chances are 5 in 100 of being wrong in saying that intervention B is better than intervention A. In other words, it might be stated that the results were significant at the 0.05 level, a commonly selected minimum standard.

Experimental research designs can be divided into true experimental designs, pre-experimental designs, and quasi-experimental designs (Campbell & Stanley, 1963). All are discussed and evaluated in terms of a series of factors that can jeopardize their internal or external validity. Internal validity (see definition earlier in chapter) is the "basic minimum without which any experiment is uninterpretable" (Campbell & Stanley, p. 5). Consider a study designed to address the foregoing question of whether intervention A is better than intervention B. If that study has good internal validity and the results are significant in favor of intervention A, then the researcher can say that intervention A was better than intervention B for the group studied. If the study does not have good internal validity, the researcher cannot say that intervention A is better than intervention B, even if the results are significant in favor of intervention A.

Internal validity is a prerequisite for good external validity, but it does not ensure external validity (see definitions). To have good external validity the results of the study must be generalizable to other situations. Although good external validity is desirable, within a single study, external validation is usually possible only to a limited extent. This, however, can be improved by replicating the study, provided the results of the two studies are comparable.

A critical concept to the discussion of experimental research is control. Experimental research involves the manipulation of the independent variable (treatment); the control or holding constant of all other variables; and the observation of the effect of the manipulation of the independent variable on the dependent variable (Cox & West, 1982). According to Cox and West, control

... refers to the attempt by the researcher to rule out the effects of any variables, other than the independent variable, on the dependent variable so that statements about the relationship between the independent and dependent variables will be accurate (p. 34).

This relates directly to the validity of the study; it relates to the extent to which the therapist can have confidence in the results of the research. The following are examples of how control can be incorporated into the design of a research study. All examples relate to the internal validity of the described study. Imagine a study having two groups, an experimental group and a control group. An experimental group is the group that experiences the treatment (the independent variable). The control group is a group of participants "whose selection and experiences are identical in every way possible to the treatment or experimental group except that they do not receive the treatment" (Tuckman, 1994, p. 120). In the hypothetical study, the experimental group receives a treatment specifically designed to improve grip strength and a control group receives no treatment. To help rule out the possibility that the participants in one group at the beginning of the study are stronger, the researcher could partially control for this threat to validity by randomly assigning participants to the two groups.

The internal validity of the same study can also be threatened by differences between data collectors. For example, if two data collectors were administering grip strength measures for all participants before the onset of the treatment (pretest) and at the completion of the study (posttest), one data collector might be naturally more encouraging; therefore, the participants tested by this data collector might perform better. This variable can be partially controlled by standardizing the interactions between the data collectors and the participants and checking for procedural agreement. The latter involves checking to see that the data collectors follow the same preset plan for data collection. This variable also can be controlled by counterbalancing, such that each data collector tests 50% of the participants in the control group and 50% of the participants in the experimental group for both the pretest and the posttest.

A shorthand code is used for displaying research designs (Bork, 1993; Campbell & Stanley, 1963). According to this code X designates a treatment; a blank space designates the absence of treatment; O designates an observation (a pretest or a posttest); R indicates random assignment; and a dashed line (---) indicates that intact groups have been used. Bork uses M to indicate matching of participants on a particular characteristic or set of characteristics. The following exemplifies use of this shorthand code.

$$R \quad O \quad X \quad O$$
$$R \quad O \quad \quad O$$

According to the design depicted, participants were randomly divided into two groups. The first group experienced a pretest, a treatment, and a posttest; the second group experienced a pretest and a posttest, but no treatment. An alternative to this design is depicted in the following.

$$O \quad M \quad R \quad X \quad O$$
$$O \quad M \quad R \quad \quad O$$

The only difference between this design and the previous one is that the participants were paired on the basis of a variable believed to be of importance to the study and, then, randomly assigned so that one member of each pair was in the treatment group and one was in the no-treatment group.

TRUE EXPERIMENTAL DESIGNS

With true experimental designs, it is possible to control for threats to internal validity. Two of the most common designs in this category that are appropriate for use in occupational therapy are the pretest–posttest control group design and the posttest-only control group design. The pretest–posttest control group design was previously depicted. According to this design the participants are randomly divided into two groups, a control group receiving no treatment and an experimental group receiving the treatment to be studied. Participants in both groups are pretested before the institution of the treatment and are posttested following the completion of the treatment. This design successfully controls for threats to internal validity, such as history, maturation, and instrumentation.

History refers to events that occur between the first and the second measurement in addition to the experimental variable. In this case, both groups should have similar histories because the participants are randomly assigned. Maturation refers to processes within participants that operate as a function of time, such as becoming tired or hungry, growing older, or changing as a result of a disease process. For example, if the sample for the grip strength study included persons who had had cardiovascular accidents resulting in hemiparesis, their grip strength scores might improve with the passage of time because of the normal course of recovery. If the researcher had only one group, the researcher, when measuring the change in scores, might erroneously attribute that change to the treatment. Instrumentation refers to changes in the observers or scorers or changes in the calibration of the testing instruments. For example, in the grip strength study, the calibration of the dynamometer may change with use, and it may become easier to obtain higher grip strength scores. Because this is true for both groups with a pretest–posttest control group design, it does not lead to the false conclusion that the participants have improved because of the treatment, since the improvement would be observed in both the treatment and the control groups.

The second design, the posttest-only control group design, is depicted as follows:

$$R \quad X \quad O$$
$$R \quad \quad O$$

This design is exemplified by a study entitled "Added-Purpose Versus Rote Exercise in Female Nursing Home Residents" (Yoder, Nelson, & Smith, 1989). Thirty women who were residents in two nursing homes and who met predetermined criteria on the *Parachek Geriatric Rating Scale* were randomly divided into two groups, a rote-exercise group and an added-purpose group. Therefore, 15 women

were in each group. The rote-exercise group participated in an occupation designed to elicit rotary arm exercise; the added-purpose group participated in the same occupation except they had the added purpose of stirring cookie dough. The tested hypothesis was that "the subjects engaged in the added-purpose, occupationally embedded exercise would engage in more exercise repetitions than would the subjects engaged in the rote exercise" (Yoder et al, 1989 p. 584).

This hypothesis was tested using inferential statistics, and the results were significant ($p < 0.05$). The design of this study was strong for threats to internal validity, but was not as strong for external validity because the participants were drawn from only two nursing homes and only two examiners were used. This limits the generalizability of the results. However, when the results of this study are combined with those from other similar studies, the external validity is improved, and together, they provide "support for the traditional occupational therapy idea of embedding exercise within occupation" (Yoder et al, 1989, p. 581).

PRE-EXPERIMENTAL DESIGNS

Pre-experimental designs contain some elements of experimental designs, but they typically do not provide adequate control for threats to internal validity. Two of the more common pre-experimental designs seen in occupational therapy literature are the one-group pretest–posttest design and the intact-group comparison. The one-group pretest–posttest design is depicted as follows.

$$O \quad X \quad O$$

With this design, a group of participants are administered a pretest followed by a treatment, then followed by a posttest. The treatment is considered to be effective if there is a significant difference between pretest and posttest scores. This design is exemplified by a study by Shillam, Beeman, and Loshin (1983) on the effect of occupational therapy intervention on bathing independence of persons with disabilities. The sample consisted of 19 patients who were being treated in an inpatient rehabilitation facility. The pre–post measure was the bathing section of the Klein-Bell Activities of Daily Living Scale. The treatment was specific to the person and involved bathing training including provision and training in the use of adaptive equipment. Results of the study indicated that all participants performed better on the posttest than on the pretest and, as a group, mean scores were significantly higher ($p < 0.01$) on the posttest than on the pretest.

A one-group pretest–posttest design, such as that used in the study by Shillam and colleagues (1983), is subject to threats to internal validity. For example, it is possible that something other than the treatment caused the change in scores from pretest to posttest, such as the participants experiencing spontaneous recovery between the pretest and posttest. This was unlikely in this study because patients with changing pathology were not included and because all patients were reported to have stable medical conditions. Nevertheless, the study design did not rule out the potential effects of other concurrent therapies on the bathing skills of the participants; therefore, caution is indicated in interpreting the results. This design was chosen by the authors because of ethical and practical concerns related to the withholding of treatment from a no-treatment control group.

The second pre-experimental design is the intact-group comparison which is depicted as follows.

$$\begin{array}{c} \underline{X\ \ O} \\ O \end{array}$$

This design includes an experimental group and a comparison group, but participants in the two groups are not selected or assigned randomly. For example, the participants in one group might be all of the patients in one rehabilitation facility, and the participants in the other group might be all of the patients in a second rehabilitation facility. With this design, one group experiences a treatment, after which both groups are tested. The posttest scores of the two groups are compared in an effort to ascertain whether the treatment was effective. This design is subject to threats to validity because steps are not taken to ensure comparability of the two groups. It may be that differences in the outcome are related to inherent differences in the two groups. Also, differences in outcome may be related to differences in the staff in the two facilities, rather than to a specific treatment that is used. Therefore, findings from such studies should be viewed cautiously.

QUASI-EXPERIMENTAL DESIGNS

Quasi-experimental designs are better than pre-experimental designs in that they control for some, but not all, threats to internal validity. Two of the more common are the time-series design and the nonequivalent control group design. The former is depicted as follows.

$$O\ \ O\ \ O\ \ X\ \ O\ \ O\ \ O$$

The time-series design differs from the one-group pretest–posttest design in that a series of pretests are given before the treatment is instituted. The treatment is then followed by a series of posttests. Effectiveness of the treatment is demonstrated if the change between the last test before the treatment and the first test after the treatment is significantly greater than the change between any of the adjacent pretests or posttests.

The nonequivalent control group design is similar to, and an improvement on, the intact-group comparison in that a pretest is added for both groups. This makes it possible to compare the two groups on the dependent variable before implementing the treatment. Ideally, at the time of pretesting, the two groups should be very similar relative to this variable. Then, if posttest differences are revealed, the researcher can have more confidence that the posttest differences were not reflective of initial differences in the dependent variable between the two groups. The nonequivalent control group design is depicted as follows.

$$\begin{array}{c} \underline{O\ \ X\ \ O} \\ O\ \ \ \ \ O \end{array}$$

For additional examples of experimental research, refer to studies by Einarsson-Backes, Deitz, Price, and Hays (1994) on the effect of oral support on the sucking efficiency of preterm infants; by Thomas (1996) on the effects of two approaches to patient education for persons undergoing cardiac surgery; and by Neistadt (1994) on the effects of different treatment activities on functional fine motor coordination in adults with brain injuries.

▼ QUANTITATIVE SINGLE-SYSTEM RESEARCH

Single-system research, sometimes referred to as single-subject research, differs from quantitative group research in that the focus is on a single person or system. The unit of study may be one person or a group considered collectively. With this type of research the participant serves as his or her own control, and there are repeated measurements over time of the same dependent variable or variables. Also, although other factors are held constant, there is the systematic application, withdrawal, or sometimes variation of the treatment (independent variable). Quantitative single-system research methods are suggested for use in occupational therapy for several reasons. First, groups of persons with similar disabilities and characteristics are not required. Therefore, it is applicable in the clinical setting, in which often the therapist has one, or at most a few clients with whom a particular treatment is employed. With group research methods, the effects of the specific treatment on numerous clients from numerous settings would have to be evaluated to address a question on the merits of the treatment. By contrast, with single-system research, the effects of a specific treatment can be evaluated in a systematic way by studying one participant in a single setting. Hence, this method is highly appealing for answering specific questions in the clinical setting related to the effectiveness of treatment, especially for persons with low-incidence diagnoses or disabilities.

The second reason why single-system research is recommended is that this type of experimental research does not require the withholding of treatment from a no-treatment control group. Because each participant serves as his or her own control, the treatment typically is withheld from the participant for one or more periods of time, and then it is instituted or reinstituted. The third reason for recommending this type of research is that the financial and time demands are realistic for the clinical setting because data are maintained on only one or a small number of participants. Also, because of the moderate financial and time demands, this research method is appropriate for pilot studies conducted before beginning more costly group experimental studies involving numerous participants and multiple sites.

Use of Single-System Research to Answer a Clinical Question: Example

An occupational therapist worked in a residential facility with adults with cerebral palsy who were dependent on outside help for eating (Einset, Deitz, Billingsley, & Harris, 1989). In this setting these adults were fed by staff members. Because of cost factors and a desire to increase self-sufficiency, the use of feeding devices to help these adults eat was explored. From her clinical experience with this client group, the therapist identified a specific feeder that she believed would be useful for her clients. She obtained two of these. Before recommending the purchase of more feeders, however, the therapist was interested in determining the extent to which these mechanical feeders were effective relative to three dependent measures: (1) the amount of time needed to eat a meal; (2) the amount of staff time necessary for feeding a client who was physically dependent; and (3) the percentage of food ingested per meal by the client. She also was interested in determining her clients' impressions of the usefulness of the feeder.

Together with others (three faculty members having expertise in the areas of cerebral palsy, measurement, and single-system research), she designed a study to answer her questions. Next, she identified four participants, all of whom (1) had a diagnosis of athetoid cerebral palsy; (2) were being fed by staff; (3) had functional communication skills as determined by a speech pathologist; and (4) were able to remove food from a spoon using lips or teeth. Data were systematically collected for each of the first three dependent measures for each of the participants individually. Each participant experienced a series of days of being fed (baseline phase), followed by training in the use of the mechanical feeder, and a series of days of using the mechanical feeder (treatment phase). Finally, this was followed by a series of days of being fed (return to baseline). Throughout all phases of data collection, efforts were made to hold all factors constant that could potentially have influenced the results of the study. All data collection meals were eaten in the same room and the same therapist provided feeding assistance and collected data.

Data were graphed and examined for each participant individually. For an example of graphed data for one variable (percentage of food intake) for one participant, refer to Figure 48–1. Results for this study indicated that use of the feeder increased the length of the meal for some participants, decreased the amount of staff time needed for feeding for some participants, and decreased the percentage of food eaten by all participants. At the end of the study, only two of the four participants indicated that they would choose to use the feeder regularly. Given these results, the therapist questioned the advisability of using the feeder in her setting on a regular basis, primarily because of the decrease in percentage of food ingested by all participants. This was particularly concerning because each participant, like most people with athetoid cerebral palsy, was thin. However, if this therapist had not systematically collected data in both baseline and treatment conditions she might not have been aware of this difficulty when using the feeder.

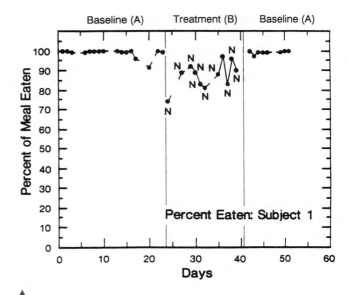

▲

Figure 48-1. Percentage of food intake for participant 1 during three phases (baseline, treatment, and baseline). (Einset, Deitz, Billingsley, & Harris, 1989, p. 46)

Studies such as the one just described assist the therapist in effective decision making and, when shared through professional journals, they assist others in the clinical decision-making process. For additional examples of single-system research studies designed to answer clinical questions in occupational therapy, refer to studies by Dirette and Hinojosa (1994) on the effects of continuous passive motion on the edematous hands of two persons with flaccid hemiplegia; by Casby and Holm (1994) on the effect of music on repetitive disruptive vocalizations of persons with dementia; and by Engel, Rapoff, and Pressman (1994) on the durability of relaxation training in pediatric headache management.

Presentation of Data

Typically, with single-system research, data for each variable for each participant or system are graphed individually, on either equal interval graph paper or the standard behavior chart (sometimes referred to as six-cycle graph paper). The primary benefit of the former is that it is easily understood. Benefits of the standard behavior chart are (1) that behaviors with extremely high or low rates can be recorded on the chart; and (2) the graph progresses in semilog units, thereby facilitating the estimation of linear trends in the data. Carr and Williams (1982) clearly describe the rationale for and use of the standard behavior chart.

Demonstration of Change

With single-system research, effectiveness of treatment is demonstrated by a change in level, trend, or variability between phases when treatment is instituted or withdrawn (Ottenbacher & York, 1984; Wolery & Harris, 1982). For potential patterns of data reflecting change and no change, refer to Figure 48–2.

Common Single-System Designs

A simple notation system is used for single-system designs for which A represents baseline; B represents the intervention or treatment phase; and C and all other letters represent additional treatments or conditions. The design on which all others are built is the A-B design, which can be exemplified by looking at both the first baseline phase (A) and the treatment phase (B) on Figure 48–1 for the electric feeder study. This displays the data for one participant for the percentage of food ingested. The vertical axis of the graph indicates the percentage of the meal eaten, and the horizontal axis indicates the days. During the first baseline phase (A), this participant experienced 16 days of being fed as usual, and data were systematically kept on percentage of food ingested. Note that the participant consistently ingested more than 90% of the food served. On the 17th day of data collection, phase B (intervention) was started. The intervention consisted of use of the feeder and assistance with mealtime tasks as needed. Note that the percentage of the meal eaten dropped substantially during the treatment phase. If the study had stopped after data were collected for only a baseline phase and an intervention phase, this would have been an A-B design.

A common variation of the A-B design is the A-B-C successive intervention design. With this design, a second treatment is introduced in the C phase. For example, the therapist studying the effects of the electric feeder might have chosen to introduce one feeder in the B phase and a totally different feeder in the C phase in an attempt to see if one feeder was more effective for the client than the other. Another variation of the A-B design is the A-B-C changing criterion design (Hartmann & Hall, 1976). With this design, the criterion for success changes with each successive treatment phase. For example, in the B phase, a therapist, working on scissor cutting with a child with fine motor deficits might count how many times the child goes outside 2-inch boundaries when cutting a 10-inch strip of paper. Once the child achieves success with this criterion, the C phase would be entered, and the criterion for success would change to staying within a 1-inch boundary.

With both the A-B and A-B-C designs, no causal statements can be made. In the electric feeder study, if data had been collected only for an initial baseline phase and a treatment phase (see Fig. 48–1), the therapist would not have known if some factor other than the introduction of the electric feeder resulted in the drop in percentage of food ingested. For example, the participant might have become ill on the 17th day of data collection or there might have been a change in cooks in the residential facility in which the participant was eating his or her meals. Therefore, this design is subject to threats to internal validity.

Because of this, the A-B-A or withdrawal design was developed. This design consists of a minimum of three phases: baseline, treatment, and baseline. It is exemplified by the electric feeder study during which the feeder was removed after the treatment phase and data were again collected under baseline conditions (see Fig. 48–1). Because this design involves a return to baseline, it is most appropriate for behaviors that are reversible (likely to return to the original baseline levels when intervention is withdrawn). This is a true experimental design in the sense that causal inferences can be made related to the participant studied. For example, in the electric feeder study, because the percentage of food ingested dropped during the intervention phase and then returned to the original baseline levels during the second baseline phase, it is possible to say that it is likely that the use of the electric feeder by participant 1 resulted in a decrease in the percentage of food ingested.

If the treatment (use of the electric feeder) resulted in a desirable change, the advisability of ending on a baseline

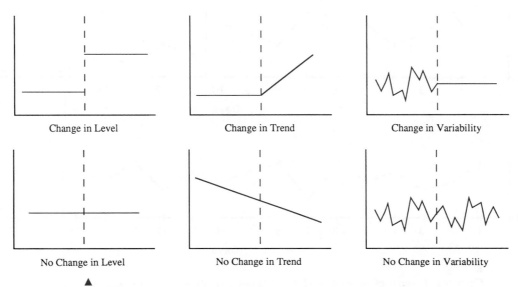

Figure 48-2. Potential patterns of data reflecting change and no change.

phase would be questionable. Thus, the A–B–A–B design was developed for situations in which treatments are expected to be effective. With this design the treatment is reinstated after the second baseline phase.

The next category of designs are the **multiple baseline designs**. These designs require repeated measures of at least three baseline conditions that typically are implemented concurrently, with each successive baseline being longer than the previous one. Multiple baseline designs can be (1) across behaviors; (2) across participants; or (3) across settings.

In a multiple baseline design across behaviors, the same treatment variable is applied sequentially to separate behaviors in a single participant. Consider the hypothetical example of a child in a mental health setting who, when in the presence of other children, frequently displays three aggressive, antisocial behaviors: biting, hitting, and kicking. The therapist is interested in knowing whether or not her intervention (a 5-minute time-out) is successful in reducing or eliminating the frequency of occurrence of these behaviors.

For 5 days, during a 2-hour peer socialization group the researcher collects baseline data on these behaviors in the natural situation making no change in treatment (Fig. 48–3). On the sixth day, the researcher introduces the intervention, thus starting the treatment phase (B) for the first behavior (biting). This involves consequating episodes of

biting with a 5-minute time-out. The researcher makes no change in the intervention program for hitting and kicking. These two behaviors remain in baseline phase (A). After 10 days the researcher initiates the time-out treatment for hitting and, after 15 days, she initiates this same treatment for kicking. Note on the graph that once the intervention is instituted for a behavior it is continued until the end of the study. If the researcher can demonstrate a change in behavior across all three behaviors following the institution of the treatment, this provides support for the effectiveness of time-out in decreasing aggressive, antisocial behaviors in the child studied. This exemplifies a multiple baseline study across behaviors.

With a multiple baseline design across participants, one behavior is treated sequentially across matched participants. For example, if you had three participants with limited wrist extension, you might institute treatment for the first participant on the fourth day, for the second participant on the seventh day, and for the third participant on the tenth day. Figure 48–4 displays hypothetical data for such a study.

The last type of multiple baseline design is that across settings. With this design the same behavior or behaviors are studied in several independent settings. Consider the client with dementia, who is in a nursing home. This client repeatedly interrupts by singing inappropriately. She does this in the dining room during meal times, in the day room during

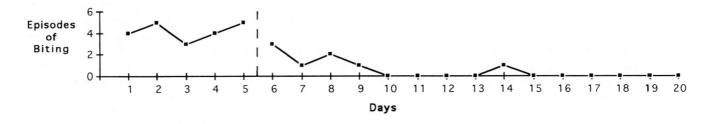

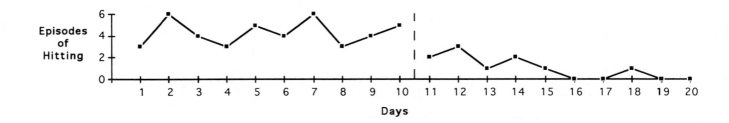

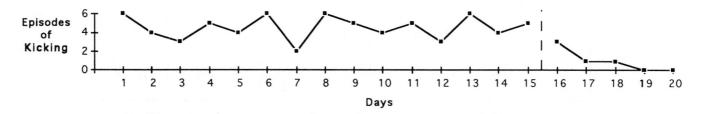

▲

Figure 48-3. Example of graphed data for a study using a multiple baseline design across behaviors.

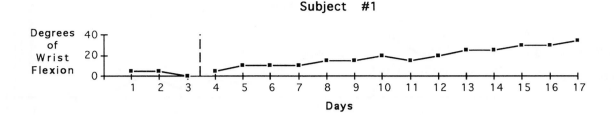

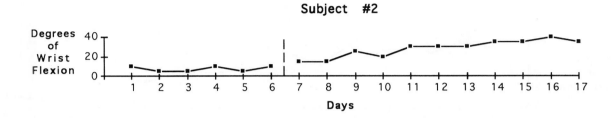

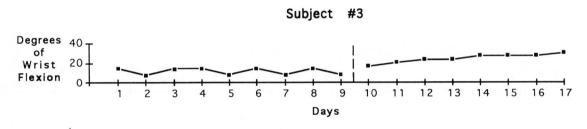

▲
Figure 48-4. Example of graphed data for a study using a multiple baseline design across participants.

movies, and on recreational outings in the van. First, the therapist collects baseline data in all three settings for 4 days. Then, she tries an intervention in the dining room (the first setting), while simultaneously continuing to collect baseline data in the other two settings. After, 3 more days, she introduces the intervention in the second setting (the day room during movies), while continuing to collect baseline data in the third setting. Last, after 2 more days, she introduces the treatment in the third setting (the van during recreational outings). For a graphic display of hypothetical data for such a study, refer to Figure 48–5.

With all of these multiple baseline designs, effectiveness of treatment is demonstrated if a desired change in level, trend, or variability occurs only when treatment is introduced. In addition, the change in performance should be maintained during the treatment phase or there should be a continual improvement as long as treatment is maintained.

Multiple baseline designs have three major strengths. First, they require no reversal or withdrawal of the intervention. This makes them appealing and practical for clinical research for which a second baseline, requiring discontinuation of therapy, often is contraindicated because of the perceived importance of continued therapy to maintain the client's performance at the optimal level.

The second strength of multiple baseline designs is that they are useful when behaviors are not likely to be reversible. Typically, therapists hope that the treatment will cause a difference that will be maintained even when the treatment is withdrawn. For example, once a therapist has taught a client who has had a stroke to eat independently using only his nondominant hand, the therapist expects the client will be able to eat independently, even when therapy is withdrawn. The therapist expects that the effects of therapy will be long lasting. This makes it difficult in some instances to use the withdrawal design discussed earlier, because traditionally, with a withdrawal design, treatment effectiveness is demonstrated by having the behavior return to the original baseline level when treatment is withdrawn.

The third strength of a multiple baseline design is that results of research based on it provide some support for the demonstration of causal relationships because the therapist is showing that change can be effected in multiple situations.

The weakness of multiple baseline designs relates to the requirement of more data collection time because of the staggered starting times for the intervention phases. Also, because of this, some behaviors or participants are required to remain in the baseline phase for longer time periods. Sometimes in clinical settings, these long baseline requirements

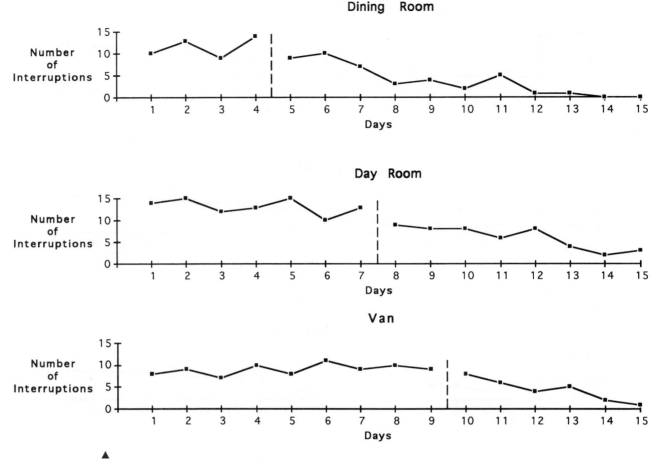

Figure 48-5. Example of graphed data for a study using a multiple baseline design across settings.

can be problematic. For example, in the first hypothetical study involving a child in a mental health setting, the last behavior (kicking) was allowed to continue for 15 days before the institution of treatment. This would be contraindicated for others in the setting because of the potential for injury.

The last type of single-system design is the alternating treatments design (Barlow & Hayes, 1979). This design, or minor variations of it, have also been termed multi-element baseline designs, randomization designs, multiple schedule designs, and simultaneous treatments designs. These designs can be used to compare the effects of treatment and no treatment, or they can be used to compare the effects of two or more distinct treatments. They always involve the fast alternation of two or more different treatments or conditions. They usually have a baseline phase, and they require interventions that will produce immediate and distinct changes in behavior.

Harris and Riffle (1986) used an alternating treatments design when studying the effects of inhibitive ankle-foot orthoses on standing balance in a 4-year-old boy with cerebral palsy who was not walking independently. The researchers wanted to know whether orthoses would improve the child's ability to maintain two-foot standing balance. The independent variable was ankle-foot orthoses, and the dependent variable was duration of two-foot independent standing. See Figure 48–6 for a graph of the data.

During the first phase of the study, baseline data on independent standing were collected for five sessions. The child did not wear ankle-foot orthoses during this phase. Phase 2 began after the child had been wearing a new set of orthoses for 1 week. During this phase, the child's standing balance was measured both with and without orthoses during each session. The order of the two conditions (with and without orthoses) was counterbalanced by random assignment. Therefore, for three of the five sessions in phase 2, duration of standing balance was measured first with orthoses. For the other two sessions, duration of standing balance was measured first without orthoses. As depicted in the graph, the child's ability to maintain independent standing rapidly improved, thereby providing support for the use of orthoses with this child with cerebral palsy. This study exemplifies use of a single-subject alternating treatments design to answer a clinical question.

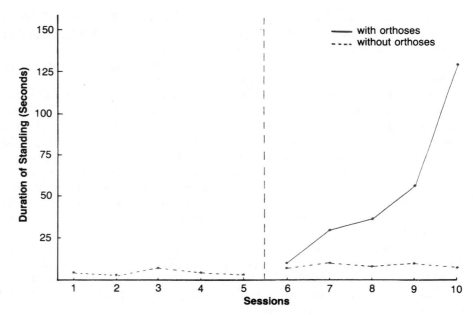

▶ *Figure 48-6.* Example of graphed data for a study using an alternating treatments design: Duration of independent standing with and without orthoses (Harris & Riffle, 1986, p. 665).

The alternating treatments design has three primary strengths. First, it does not require a lengthy withdrawal of the treatment, which may result in a reversal of therapeutic gain. Second, it often requires less time for a comparison to be made because a second baseline is not required. Third, with this design, it is possible to proceed without a formal baseline phase. This is useful in clinical situations for which ethically it is sometimes difficult to justify baseline data collection.

The primary weakness of the alternating treatment design stems from its vulnerability to a validity threat relating to the influence of one treatment on the adjacent treatment. As a partial control for this threat, all variables that could potentially influence the results of the study should be counterbalanced. For example, in the study by Harris and Riffle (1986), the conditions (with orthoses and without orthoses) for measuring duration of two–foot-standing balance were counterbalanced by random assignment. Instead, if the child always had stood first without orthoses and second with orthoses, it is possible that the improved performance might be a function of the practice in the "without orthoses" condition.

▶CONCLUSION

Through well-designed quantitative research it is possible (1) to obtain precise, objective information; and (2) to control for many of the factors that could jeopardize the validity of a study. The latter is facilitated because decisions on the design of quantitative research studies (ie, the operational definitions of variables, the methods by which data will be collected, the ways in which reliability in data collection will be assured) are made a priori. Both

group and single-system quantitative research studies that are well conceived and implemented have contributed and will continue to contribute to the knowledge base in occupational science and occupational therapy.

Section 3

Qualitative Research

Elizabeth Blesedell Crepeau and Jean C. Deitz

Qualitative Research Methods
    Data Collection
    Data Analysis
    Establishing Trustworthiness
Types of Qualitative Research
    Ethnographic Research
    Phenomenological Research
    Grounded Theory
Critiquing Qualitative Research
Conclusion

Qualitative research in occupational therapy is derived from the fields of anthropology, sociology, and philosophy. Currently, there is a lively debate about the belief systems and methods underlying this form of research (Clifford & Marcus, 1986; Denzin & Lincoln, 1994; Rheinharz, 1992; Smith, 1987; Wolf, 1992). Central to this debate is the nature of truth and whether we can actually identify it, the nature of objectivity and whether a researcher can achieve this ideal in any type of research, and the relation of the researcher to the research question and the people being studied. For some qualitative researchers even the terminology used to describe the people being studied is problematic because this terminology is deemed to be a reflection of the power relations inherent in the research process. This raises questions about the role of the people being studied. Are they passive subjects, who simply provide data for the researcher to use to find answers to the research question, or are they research partners who explore with the researcher the questions and the multiple ways of answering them (Rheinharz, 1984; Wolf, 1992)? A full discussion of these issues is beyond the scope of this chapter; however, it is important to be aware that qualitative researchers have not yet developed a consensus on the best ways of conducting this type of research.

Despite these issues, qualitative research represents a valuable addition to the development of knowledge in occupational science and occupational therapy. Its contextual nature and focus on meaning makes it especially compatible with occupational therapy's humanistic values and occupational therapy's focus on occupational performance (Kielhofner, 1982b; Yerxa, 1991). Typically, qualitative research involves studying the social lives of individuals and groups in an effort to understand their experience from their own perspectives (Kielhofner, 1982a). Qualitative research involves observation and interviews of people in their own environments, as well as the use of diaries, letters, memoranda, and other types of documents. As Kielhofner (1982b) maintained:

There is a special harmony between the concerns of occupational therapy and the paradigm and methods of qualitative research. Both focus on the realities of everyday life. Both appreciate the richness of mundane affairs (p. 162).

Because the goal of qualitative research is to explore the meaning and interpretation of experience, much of this research must evolve as the meaning and understanding emerges during the research process. Consequently, one descriptor of qualitative research is that it is "emergent." That is, as the research progresses the questions may change or become more focused as the process continues to unfold (Lincoln & Guba, 1985). For example, the AOTA–AOTF Clinical Reasoning Study began with broad questions about defining competent clinical practice and explicating the clinical reasoning that supports this practice (Cohn, 1991). As the research progressed, more focused questions about the types of clinical reasoning and effective ways to teach clinical reasoning emerged (Fleming, 1991). Further studies beyond the initial AOTA–AOTF Clinical Reasoning Study have continued to explore clinical reasoning from a variety of perspectives (Clark, 1993; Neistadt, 1996; Schell, 1994).

▼ QUALITATIVE RESEARCH METHODS

Data Collection

With qualitative research, the data typically are extensive and are in the form of words rather than numbers. These data are collected through observation; interviews; and review of diaries or letters, official documents (eg, medical records or memos within an organization), audiotapes, and videotapes. Recording data accurately and completely is essential to the process, because the recorded text becomes the source for analysis. Interviews in qualitative research are generally semistructured or unstructured. Open-ended questions enable the researcher to explore the topic from the perspective of the person being interviewed. Follow-up questions evolve as the interview progresses and the researcher gains deeper insights into the topic (Lofland & Lofland, 1984; Mishler, 1986). Although the interview questions are not highly structured, they should be framed to elicit the feelings, thoughts, and interpretations of the interviewee (Lofland & Lofland). The role of the interviewer is a crucial one in this process. Mishler suggested that the interview process itself is an act of knowledge construction between the interviewer and interviewee. As a result, the interviewer needs to be aware of the role he or she plays in this process.

Typically, qualitative researchers write fieldnotes recording their interviews, observations, feelings, and responses. The goal is to obtain an accurate and detailed accounting of everything available to the researcher. Brief notes may be taken at the time of the observation or interview; however, these must be expanded as soon as possible after the event for a complete record (Lofland & Lofland, 1984). This can be an exhausting process because writing the fieldnotes may take at least as long as the observation or interview itself. Careful recording is essential because the research may last many months and important observations may be forgotten over time. Beyond fieldnotes, the researcher also writes memoranda that record insights, musings, questions, and reflections. In this process, data collection merges with interpretation and analysis.

Mechanic (1989) suggested that the researcher write a social biography that enables the reader to identify the perspective from which the researcher approached the research process. This recognizes that it is the researcher who is the "instrument" of measurement. Just as a scale needs to be calibrated to measure accurately, a social biography enables the reader to calibrate the interpretation provided by the researcher (Mechanic, 1989). Drawing from Marcus and Fischer, Hasselkus (1997) eloquently stated, "Each of us as a researcher is 'positioned' in relation to that which we are researching. This 'positioning' is the lens through which every researcher sees her or his research" (p.81).

Data Analysis

Data analysis varies with each type of qualitative research; however, there are several commonalities. Themes, categories, and codes are derived from the data. Typically, these emerge during the analysis, although sometimes preliminary themes from the literature may be identified in advance (McCuaig & Frank, 1991). The researcher strives to remain as close to the data as possible to reflect the interpretations of those being studied. One of the strengths of qualitative research is its capacity to demonstrate that multiple interpretations exist and that a singular view of a complex social world is not likely to be entirely adequate. This includes the interpretations made by both the researcher (Agar, 1986) and those being studied (Gubrium, 1991). Consequently, the goal of the research is to represent these multiple interpretations of a single situation, rather than striving for a singular perspective.

Because meaning is socially constructed, the interpretation of meaning from another culture is accomplished through the values and beliefs of the observer. These values and beliefs reflect the observer's cultural background (Agar, 1986; Mechanic, 1989). Thus, qualitative research of the same group may vary considerably, based on who is conducting the research and his or her interpretive process (Agar; Hasselkus, 1997; Mechanic). The social biography helps with this process by aiding the reader in understanding the perspective of the researcher (Crepeau, 1997; Mechanic). To provide further insight into the interpretive process, Rheinharz (1984) also suggested that the researcher keep a reflexive journal to record feelings, attitudes, and questions that emerge as the research proceeds. Aspects of this journal should be reflected in the final manuscript.

Because fieldnotes can be very extensive, computer programs have been developed to facilitate the mechanics of the coding process (Fielding & Lee, 1991). The writing process is often an extension of the analysis, for it is often through writing that the interpretation and meaning emerge (Richardson, 1994; Wolf, 1992). The final written document may vary in style and voice, dependent on the expected audience and the goals of the author (Van Maanen, 1988).

Establishing Trustworthiness

Rigor in qualitative research is established when the inquiry is perceived to be trustworthy by the reader. Trustworthiness is concerned with the truth value, transferability, dependability, and neutrality of the research (Lincoln & Guba, 1985).

TRUTH VALUE

Truth value relates to the credibility of the research, that is how closely the research reflects the experience of the people being studied. Because qualitative research recognizes that multiple truths exist, credible studies reflect these multiple realities. Five common methods of improving truth value are (1) prolonged engagement, (2) persistent observation, (3) triangulation of sources and methods, (4) peer debriefing, and (5) member checks (Lincoln & Guba, 1985).

Prolonged engagement in the field enables the researcher to become part of the environment so that trust evolves as the people being observed become comfortable with the researcher. This is thought to reduce the influence of the researcher's presence on the behavior of the group (Krefting, 1991). Prolonged engagement carries with it the danger that the researcher becomes enmeshed with the group. Reflexive analysis, as suggested by Rheinharz (1984) may help uncover the conflict between being an outsider or an insider. It is a process by which the researcher examines his or her history, perceptions, and interests in relation to the research (Reinharz, 1984). Rheinharz referred to this as "reclaiming self-awareness" (1984, p. 240). Persistent observation also relates to time spent in the field, but here, it is directed at the researcher learning enough about the field to understand what is important to focus on in relation to the particular research question.

Triangulation refers to the use of different sources or different methods of data collection. For example, Krefting (1989), in her study of individuals with moderate head injuries, used four approaches in an attempt to "experience life" from the perspectives of persons with head injuries (p. 69). The first involved over 80 hours of unstructured interviews with the persons with head injuries, their families, and their friends. Each interview ranged from 1 to 4 hours. The second approach involved participant observations and the recording of the researcher's own actions, the behavior of others, and aspects of the sociocultural situation. To do this, Krefting attended meetings, social events, and treatment sessions, and accompanied the individuals with head injuries with their families on a variety of outings. The third approach was to review documents, such as a diary that had been kept by a person with a head injury, human interest stories from newspapers, and newsletters from organizations concerned with head injury. The last approach involved maintaining a field log in which Krefting noted her thoughts, feelings, ideas, and hypotheses generated by her contact with the persons with head injuries and their families and friends. By triangulating data sources the researcher is assured that a variety of perspectives is represented (Lincoln & Guba, 1985).

Peer debriefing provides a mechanism for the researcher to check observations, impressions, analytic schemes, and conclusions with a knowledgeable, but disinterested, person. It is useful from the beginning of the research process through the end of writing the final report. This mechanism assists with the exploration of aspects of the study that may have been implicit and can be made more explicit through candid and thoughtful conversation with someone knowledgeable about the topic, but not involved directly in the research (Lincoln & Guba, 1985).

Finally, member checking is a way of improving credibility by checking the data itself with the people who have supplied it, as well as reviewing interpretations and analyses with individuals and groups involved in the research to be sure that these interpretations reflect their understandings. For example, Crepeau (1994) in her ethnography of a geropsychiatric team provided transcripts to all people she interviewed. This enabled them to review the transcripts to be sure they were factually accurate and that they reflected their ideas, opinions, and feelings. Through this review, they could correct any factual errors, clarify statements they made, and add to the transcripts if they had additional thoughts or observations to share. Toward the end of her research she reviewed the emerging themes with unit personnel to see if these seemed to accurately reflect aspects of the world of the team and their work together. This enabled her to verify that her interpretations remained true to their experience. Member checking has its dangers in that the group may share common myths that the research may uncover. This may lead to a conflict in interpretations between the researcher and group, and present an ethical dilemma for the researcher in the use of the findings (Lincoln & Guba, 1985). If the disagreement is severe and cannot be resolved, the researcher may feel as if he or she would violate the trust established with the group should the research be submitted for publication.

TRANSFERABILITY

One goal of quantitative research is to be able to generalize the findings of a study to the population at large (Lincoln & Guba, 1985). This ability to apply findings to other groups is limited in qualitative research because settings are likely to be quite different from each other. Consequently, vivid, detailed description must be included in the study to enable the reader to judge the similarity between settings and, therefore, make judgments about the transferability of the findings (Lincoln & Guba).

DEPENDABILITY

Control of variability of data is not the goal of qualitative research; rather, variability is sought to understand the range of experience of research informants (Krefting, 1991). Consistency or dependability of the data is established by assuring that fieldnotes are accurately recorded and logged and that the accounts from these fieldnotes can be traced back to them. An audit trail enables someone not involved in the research to follow the process of data collection and analysis as well as to judge the accuracy of the record, much like an auditor checks the financial records of an organization (Lincoln & Guba, 1985). Lincoln and Guba suggested use of such an audit to assure that the documentation supporting the research is sufficient to have confidence in the findings. Triangulation of data from multiple sources enables evalua-

tion of the data in order to understand where consistency, as well as variation in the data occurs (Krefting).

NEUTRALITY

Finally, neutrality refers to freedom from bias. Because qualitative research represents the particular perspectives of those being studied, the search for researcher objectivity typical of quantitative studies is not appropriate (Lincoln & Guba, 1985). Lincoln and Guba asserted that objectivity of the data should be the focus. This occurs when data are confirmed through the use of an audit, triangulation, entries in a reflexive journal, and peer debriefing (Lincoln & Guba). Keeping a reflexive journal and reporting the researcher's social biography does not remove bias, rather it enables the reader to evaluate the perspective of the researcher in relation to the data and the findings (Mechanic, 1989).

▼ TYPES OF QUALITATIVE RESEARCH

Three major types of qualitative research will be described: ethnographic, phenomenological, and grounded theory. These are well suited to questions related to the development of knowledge in occupational science and occupational therapy. Other forms not covered in this chapter, but of value to the field, are oral histories, case studies, and biographies.

Ethnographic Research

The goal of ethnographic research is to describe the culture being studied from the point of view of the people within the culture (Spradley, 1979). It is concerned with uncovering the stated and unstated forms and meanings in a group and how these are combined to create the culture of the group (Gubrium, 1988). An example of an ethnographic question for a family caregiver would be to ask for a description of the caregiver's day (Hasselkus, 1995). The interpretation of meaning is a central activity in this form of research; consequently, analyzing descriptions of typical days of caregivers enables the ethnographer to understand these experiences from the perspectives of the caregivers, to identify patterns in these experiences, and to identify the meaning of these experiences to the caregivers themselves.

Because the goal of ethnographic research is to develop an understanding of the meanings within a particular group; observation and interviews of members of the group are often a part of the research design. The observations should take place in the natural settings of the group; for example, within the family unit if a family is the focus of the study, in a classroom if understanding the classroom environment is important. Within an organization, internal documents such as memoranda, as well as public documents, such as brochures or press releases, may also be used to gain an understanding of the group (Lofland & Lofland, 1984).

In ethnographic research, as in other forms of qualitative research, the identification of research informants is a critical issue. Because the goal is to develop an understanding of the culture, a variety of perspectives must be identified. The study might begin with key informants such as the leaders of the group, but should include other group members so that all levels of the group are included. For example, in Crepeau's (1994) study of a geropsychiatric team, she began with the director of the unit, a nurse, and the medical director, a psychiatrist. As the study progressed she interviewed all of the direct care day staff including the nurses aide, social worker, nurses, and occupational therapists. In addition to interviews, she observed team meetings; informal conferences; and interactions in the nurses' station, dining room, and other public places on the unit. This provided her with a wide range of views of the work of the team on the unit. Because the primary goal of her research was to study the team and because it would have been too intrusive, she did not observe family meetings nor individual sessions between patients and the professionals on the staff (Crepeau, 1994).

In ethnographic research, data analysis begins at the same time data are being collected. This enables the researcher to focus the data collection as an understanding of the issues emerges. For example, Crepeau (1994) assumed that the concept of team was a clear concept that had a shared meaning for everyone on the geropsychiatric unit. However, as she began to observe and talk to people, a variety of interpretations of this very basic concept emerged. This insight led her to ask more questions about the meaning of team as she conducted her interviews and observed how people used this concept in their day-to-day practices (Crepeau, 1994).

Trustworthiness in ethnographic research can be improved by (1) prolonged engagement in the field, (2) using a variety of data sources and methods to assure a broad view of the group, (3) peer debriefing, and (4) member checks. As in all qualitative research a reflexive journal and clear notes on the feelings of the researcher, as well as delineation of methodological decisions are essential.

AN EXAMPLE OF ETHNOGRAPHIC RESEARCH

McCuaig and Frank (1991) conducted an ethnographic study of Meghan Miller (a pseudonym), a 53-year-old woman with severe athetoid cerebral palsy. Meghan used a power wheelchair for mobility and, because she was unable to speak, she used an augmentative communication system. Although her disability was severe, she did all of her personal care, homemaking, and shopping. McCuaig and Frank's research questions were:

1. What decisive events have contributed to long-term, stable patterns of adaptation in the subject's life?

2. How does the subject accommodate to breakdown, or unusual challenges, within her customary pattern of adaptation? (p. 226)

McCuaig and Frank (1991) used life history methods and participant observation to develop a narrative about Meghan's life and to observe her adaptive capacities in a variety of situations and settings that she encountered on a regular basis. McCauig engaged in 75 hours of contact with Meghan, her sister, doctor, friends, and neighbors. This prolonged engagement enabled her to obtain a full picture of Meghan and her life. McCauig kept fieldnotes that she analyzed by initial categories she derived from independent living and occupational therapy research literature. McCauig and Frank found that Meghan exerted much of her energy in presenting herself as able to those around her. This involved demonstrating to others that she was competent mentally and that she could function independently. For example, she had the practice of taking a letter to the doctor to explain her medical concerns because she knew that this form of communication was more efficient for both of them. This presentation of self required considerable planning and effort on her part, but it was incorporated into her pattern of living so that the strategies Meghan used became "transparent." When unexpected events occurred, such as an unscheduled visit from the wheelchair repairman, her adaptive strategies failed. In this instance Meghan was unable to do the advanced preparation necessary for the interaction and, consequently, was not successful at presenting herself as able.

These findings are credible because they were based on persistent observation and careful documentation, which was clearly explained in the paper itself. McCuaig and Frank (1991) used several extended examples to demonstrate the effectiveness of Meghan's adaptive strategies to present herself to others as able and her failure to do so when she was not able to anticipate events. Through prolonged involvement with Meghan, McCauig was able to identify these strategies and the multiple ways Meghan devised to live successfully in the community. This approach to data collection and analysis enabled McCuaig and Frank to show that these strategies were developed over a lifetime, and that many approaches were derived from Meghan's own creativity and experience, not professional intervention.

Phenomenological Research

Phenomenological research is derived from philosophy and is directed at understanding and explicating the lived experiences of other people. This research strives to uncover meanings and understanding that we may have, but have not expressed, in other words to make the tacit (unstated) explicit (stated). This type of research provides insights that enable a fuller understanding of everyday lived experience (van Manen, 1990). This involves asking the people being studied to reflect on an experience that they had in the past to understand the nature or essence of the experience itself. Hasselkus (1995) explained this relative to a phenomenological study she conducted of caregiving in which she asked caregivers to tell her about one of their caregiving experiences that "was especially satisfying" (Hasselkus, 1995, p. 76). Phenomenological research uses paradigm cases or exemplars, which are "strong cases" drawn from the data. These cases are developed to examine the various meanings of everyday activities of people as accurately as possible (Leonard, 1994). This research is deemed to be trustworthy if the participants comment on the interpretation, "You have put into words what I have always known, but did not have the words to express" (Dreyfus, as cited in Benner, 1994, p. xviii). This means that the researcher has remained true to the experiences of the participant and the meaning the participant ascribes to these experiences, rather than interpreting them from the perspective of the researcher. Leonard (1994) referred to this as "honoring the lived experiences of the research participants" (p. 56).

Phenomenological research is valuable because it provides insights about a particular issue that were not available before (Leonard, 1994). For example, Hasselkus' caregiving research has value to the extent that it illuminates the caregiving experience. Through her research, occupational therapy practitioners can develop a deeper understanding of the meaning of caregiving and use this understanding to interact more effectively with caregivers.

AN EXAMPLE OF PHENOMENOLOGICAL RESEARCH

Hasselkus and Dickie (1994) conducted a phenomenological study examining the "nature of satisfying and dissatisfying experiences in occupational therapy practice" (p. 145). They asked therapists to write a story of a situation from their practice. By a thematic analysis of these stories, Hasselkus and Dickie identified three dimensions of practice: change, community, and craft. Change is exemplified by the therapists sense of making or not making a difference in the lives of their clients. Community is a theme of togetherness and the harmony or disharmony that exists between everyone in the story. Collaboration and teamwork characterize positive narratives of community, whereas lack of community is characterized by discordant beliefs, lack of respect, and not being valued by others. Finally, stories of craft reflect the therapists' role in working with patients, focusing on the skills the therapists used to bring about change and the enjoyment and satisfaction that come from that process. This paper is especially strong because Hasselkus and Dickie clearly explained their research method and the literature that supported the method and the question they pursued. It also provided an additional way to understand the work of occupational therapists that previous research had not examined.

Grounded Theory

Unlike ethnographic and phenomenological research, the goal of grounded theory is theory development. In this approach, theory is derived from systematically collected and analyzed data; hence, the theory is "grounded" in the data (Glaser & Strauss, 1967). With this approach, theory is developed and elaborated to greater levels of abstraction (Glaser & Strauss, 1967). Frequently, multiple studies are used to build the theory (Strauss, Fagerhaugh, Suczek, & Wiener, 1985). For example, Bogdan and Bilken (1992) observed that in staff and parent communication, staff not only communicated with the parents about their children, but used this opportunity to make judgments about the parents on which they based further communication decisions. They explained that they saw parallels in other forms of parent and staff communications. If they studied different settings and found these same processes occurring, they could develop a more generalizable theory about parent and staff communication than they started with in the initial study.

Qualitative data are collected through interviews, observations, diaries, and other documents. Data analysis proceeds with what is called a "constant comparative method." That is, themes and codes are developed from the data and constantly compared back with it. The themes and codes are developed to respond to the researchers' evolving understanding and interpretation of the data. Data collection continues until a saturation point is reached; that is, when the new data for a particular category simply confirm what has already been collected (Glaser & Strauss, 1967). As the data are collected, the theory is modified until it provides the best explanation for the data. Strauss and Corbin (1994) described this as an ongoing conversation between and among the data, the researcher, and the respondents. This openness to change and modification recognizes that theory development is an interpretive process that is bounded by the perspective of the researcher and the particular historical context in which the research occurs (Strauss & Corbin). The use of grounded theory approaches is emerging in our field as we begin to explore the meaning of human occupation and clinical reasoning.

AN EXAMPLE OF GROUNDED THEORY

Clark, Ennevor, and Richardson (1996) articulated a grounded theory of techniques used for occupational storytelling and occupational story making. This theory emerged from Clark's work with Richardson, a stroke survivor. Through analyzing and coding the transcripts of the Clark and Richardson conversations, Clark, Ennevor, and Richardson identified approaches Clark used to facilitate Richardson's recovery. These were building a communal horizon of understanding, occupational storytelling, and occupational story making. Clark and Ennevor, after Richardson's death, further elaborated these themes with more specific techniques of collaboration, empathy building, inclusion of the ordinary, listening, and reflection. This theory applies to the Richardson and Clark relationship; however, it can also be used to sensitize therapists to approaches they can use with their clients. If Clark, Ennevor, or other scholars build on this research with other people, it can also be used as the basis for building a broader theory of occupational storytelling and occupational story making. Through this research theory could evolve to apply to different kinds of situations. For example, the building of empathy between two college professors (Clark & Richardson) is based on the shared experience of being faculty members at the University of Southern California. Would the same kind of storytelling and story making occur when the client is of a different social group? What would be the challenges to the therapist to facilitate this process? Richardson had strong family support and sufficient income to be able to consider season tickets to the opera as a way of expanding her social world (Clark, 1993). What would the effect of poverty or a very limited social network have on the choices of people who survive stroke as they strive to create a new life? How would the theory of occupational story telling and occupational storymaking account for these very different situations? Studies building on this work could address these and related questions. This is an exciting opportunity for research for academicians and clinicians in the field.

▼ CRITIQUING QUALITATIVE RESEARCH

The task of critiquing a qualitative study is challenging, even for the experienced researcher. A critique should focus on whether the researcher "took sufficient steps to validate inferences and conclusions" (Polit & Hungler, 1993, p. 341) and effectively documented the analytic process (Glaser & Strauss, 1967; Lincoln & Guba, 1985). Findings will be more credible to the reader if the researcher has supported them adequately with data and explanations.

►CONCLUSION

Qualitative research is a viable and important method of inquiry in occupational science and occupational therapy. Its value is its ability to articulate meaning and context and how these interrelate in occupational performance, health, and adaptation to illness or disability. Although the tradition of qualitative research in the field is relatively brief, qualitative studies are expanding our understanding of human occupation and occupational therapy.

Section 4

Qualitative and Quantitative Research: Joint Contributors to the Knowledge Base in Occupational Therapy

Jean C. Deitz and Elizabeth Blesedell Crepeau

> Combining Qualitative and Quantitative Research: An Example
> Research Ethics
> Conclusion: Research Skills of Occupational Therapists

Both qualitative research and quantitative research are viable methods of inquiry in occupational science and occupational therapy; studies generated from both methods have contributed to our knowledge base. Both are suited to answering important questions and to expanding knowledge related to occupational performance and the components of function. Sometimes one method is more suited to a particular question than another. When the answer to a question requires precision, quantitative methods are preferred; when the answer to a question involves capturing the complexity in a situation or understanding meaning, qualitative methods are preferred. At other times, the question can potentially be answered using either quantitative or qualitative methods. In such cases, research using one method can be employed to confirm or expand on the findings demonstrated by the other method.

▼ COMBINING QUALITATIVE AND QUANTITATIVE RESEARCH: AN EXAMPLE

Consider a study by Kathy Washington (1996) that was designed (1) to evaluate the effects of one type of adaptive seating device, a contoured foam seat (CFS), on the postural alignment and upper extremity function of young children with neuromotor impairments; and (2) to explore parents' perceptions of the use and effects of the CFS when used at home on a daily basis. The former was addressed through quantitative single-system research, whereas the latter was addressed using qualitative research.

Four children were selected to participate in the study. Each met predetermined criteria, including, but not limited to, being between the ages of 9 and 24 months; receiving

therapy services for neuromotor impairment; having a specified level of head and trunk control; being recommended as
an appropriate candidate for a CFS by the child's treating
therapist; and being able to reach out and grasp a specified
toy. For the quantitative study, the primary dependent variables were (1) percentage of time intervals when the child
maintained postural alignment in midline; and (2) percentage
of time intervals when the child had one or both hands in
contact with a toy with hands and arms free from support. By
using an alternating treatments design to address the first
question, baseline data were collected on both variables while
the child was positioned on the regular highchair seat without the CFS. During the intervention phase, data were systematically collected on both variables under two conditions:
(1) when the child was using the CFS; and (2) when the child
was sitting on the highchair seat with only a very thin layer of
foam on the seat. During the intervention phase of the study,
one probe was conducted with the child positioned on the
regular highchair seat. Results clearly indicated that relative to
postural alignment, the CFS was better for all children than
either the regular highchair seat or the seat covered with a
thin layer of foam. Relative to hand function the results for
one child clearly favored the CFS, whereas no clear effect of
the CFS was observed for the other three children.

Following this standardized data collection, mothers of all
four children were given the contoured foam seats to use for
a minimum of 4 weeks at home. Approximately 1 month
later, the mothers participated in a semistructured interview
during which they were asked open-ended questions. From
this process, two major themes emerged. The first was labeled
"Acceptability: I can't leave home without it." Mothers reported that they used the CFS in their infants' highchairs
consistently and some mothers also used the CFS in alternative ways, such as using it as a floor-sitter. They found it more
convenient to use than previous positioning strategies, such as
placing rolled towels on the sides of the highchair. No negative aspects were reported with use of the insert except one
mother indicated that it stuck to her infant's bottom when
she was trying to remove him from the chair. Thus, she suggested use of Velcro to secure the CFS to the highchair seat.

The second theme was that of greater independence for
both the mothers and their children. For example, mothers
commented on their new ability to perform household and
caregiving responsibilities while their infants were safely
and comfortably positioned. Also, mothers indicated that use
of the CFS improved, not only their children's manipulation
of toys, but also their abilities to interact socially with other
family members, especially at mealtimes.

These findings complemented those from the quantitative component of the study and added depth by providing
insight into what use of the contoured foam seats meant to
the mothers of the children. Had the mothers not valued
the seats, or if they had found them to be difficult to use, it is
likely that they would not have continued to use them at
home. Also, the mothers' clear descriptions of changes in
their lives and those of their children provided information
important for evaluating the use of these devices and directions for determining appropriate dependent variables for
future research. If data collection had focused only on the
operationally defined variables or if a structured interview
had been employed, important information would have
been overlooked. Conversely, if only qualitative methods
had been employed without systematic measurement of two
variables, identified as important from a theoretical perspective, it is possible that these outcomes might have been overlooked. Thus, a more complete picture was obtained by
careful use of both methods, than if either method had been
employed individually.

The issue is not whether one type of research is better
than the other; the issue is how can the two types of research be used to complement one another for the benefit
of knowledge development in occupational science and occupational therapy. These two types of research cannot be
substituted for one another because they facilitate the observation of different aspects of the same reality. This is highlighted by McCracken (1988) who maintained that qualitative research offers the opportunity to glimpse the
complicated character, organization, and logic of culture,
and that the extent to which what is discovered exists in the
rest of the world can best be decided by quantitative meth-

ETHICS NOTE
WHO OWNS INTELLECTUAL PROPERTY?
Penny Kyler and Ruth A. Hansen

Doug is a newly hired instructor in a well-established occupational therapy program. He needs to begin to do research.
He has spent long hours, when he was not on a teaching
contract, working on a grant proposal. He asks his department chairperson to review and evaluate his proposal. The
chair tells him that the proposal needs more work. Six
months later, Doug finds out that, without his knowledge,
the chair submitted Doug's proposal for funding and that, if
funded, the chair will be the project director.

1. Who "owns" the ideas for this grant proposal?
2. Does the department chairperson have the authority and
   the right to submit this grant without Doug's knowledge
   or agreement?
3. What options does Doug have in this situation? What are
   the benefits and risks with each potential course of action? ■

WORKSHEET
Questions to Guide Reading and Critiquing a Quantitative Research Study

Topic:_____

Title:_____

Author(s):_____

Source:_____

Year:_____Volume:_____Pages:_____

1. What was the purpose of the study?

   What questions were asked and were they precisely and clearly stated?

   What hypotheses were stated or implied? Write them in either research or null form.

2. To what extent did the researcher give evidence of having reviewed literature relevant to the study?

   Were any areas of literature that may have been relevant to the study not reviewed?

3. From what population was the sample selected?

   How was the sample selected and how large was it? What was the rationale for how the sample was selected, for sample size, and such?

   Was subject attrition reported? Explain.

   Could the results of the study be generalized to a larger group? Specify.

(Answer 4.a. for descriptive and correlational studies and 4.b. for pre-experimental, experimental, and quasi-experimental studies.)

4.a. What variables were studied and were they consistent with the stated purpose of the study?

   What evidence of instrument reliability and validity was provided?

4.b. What intervention (independent variable) was studied? Was the described intervention consistent with the stated purpose of the study?

   What outcome measures (dependent variables) were used in the study? Were these measures appropriate operational definitions of the variables studied?

   What evidence of instrument reliablity and validity was provided?

5. All aspects of a research project should be controlled except the ones being studied by the researcher. List all factors controlled in the study and how they were controlled.

Controlled Factors	Method of Control
A.	
B.	
C.	
D.	
E.	

   List all factors not controlled in the research study that you believe could have affected the results of the study. Briefly explain how each factor could have influenced the research results.

Uncontrolled Factors	Potential Influence
A.	
B.	
C.	
D.	
E.	

7. How were the data analyzed and what were the results? Were the data analysis procedures appropriate for the design of the study, the sample size, and so on.

8. What were the strengths of the study?

9. Did the researcher(s) describe the limitations of the study? Are there any other limitations to the study that were not described by the researcher(s)?

10. Does the study have implications for practice? What are they?

▲

Figure 48-7. Worksheet: reading and critiquing a quantitative research study.

ods. Therefore, Polit and Hungler (1993) advocated multi-method research involving the judicious combining of qualitative and quantitative methods in a single study to minimize the effects of the limitations of either method used in isolation. In contrast, Bogdan and Bilken (1992) cautioned that multi-method studies are often weak methodologically when one researcher is responsible for understanding and implementing both methods, because the knowledge and mind-set for each is very different. With this caution, it seems advisable in some situations for experts in qualitative research to combine with experts in quantitative research to design and implement multi-method studies capable of providing a more complete view than would be possible if either method was used independently.

▼ RESEARCH ETHICS

Important considerations when designing and conducting both quantitative and qualitative research are ethics as they relate to the researcher and the research process. The researcher has the responsibility to adhere to high scientific

---

WORKSHEET
Questions to Guide Reading and Critiquing a Qualitative Research Study

Topic:_____

Title:_____

Author(s):_____

Source:_____

Year:_____ Volume:_____ Pages:_____

1. What was the purpose of the study?
   Were research questions asked? If so, what were they and were they clearly stated?

2. To what extent did the researcher give evidence of having reviewed literature relevant to the study?
   Were any areas of literature not reviewed that may have been relevant to the study?

3. Who were the participants and what was the rationale behind their selection? Did the researcher provide you with adequate information about the participants and the context of the phenomenon studied?

4. What sources of data were used and what were the methods for data collection and analysis? What were the coding categories and what was the reasoning process for thematic analysis? Did they make sense to you?

5. Was there congruence between the chosen research tradition and the methods for data collection and analysis?

6. What was the role of the researcher in the study? Did the research report provide you with a clear picture of the researcher's role in the research process and his or her biases and characteristics that might have influenced his or her perspective? If not, what additional information would have been helpful?

7. How did the researcher establish the trustworthiness of the data? What is your evaluation of the researcher's process and findings?

8. How did the researcher report his or her involvement in the process and how did the researcher explain the effect of this involvement on the reported results of the study? Do you agree with the researcher's assessment?

9. What were the reported results of the study? Did they make sense to you? Are there other plausible interpretations of the data? Did you find the study to be trustworthy? Why? Why not? Be specific.

10. How do findings from this study link to research findings from other studies? What further research questions did the study inspire?

11. Does the study have implications for clinical practice or for theory refinement or development? Explain.

▲
Figure 48-8. Worksheet: Reading and critiquing a qualitative research study.

standards in designing and conducting research studies, and in analyzing and reporting research findings. Scientific misconduct includes such acts as fabrication, falsification, and plagiarism. In addition, there are ethical implications related to the researcher's decisions and actions concerning the rights of research participants. Researchers need to check with the human subjects' review boards in all of the institutions in which potential participants will be approached. They need to consider whether or not participation in the study could be contraindicated for the potential participant. This consideration should focus not only on physical issues, but also on issues related to such factors as stress and invasion of privacy. Data about a participant must be handled confidentially, and privacy should be respected. Participants or participant advocates must give informed consent before participation in a study, and they must be informed of their right to withdraw from participation at any point, while still maintaining the services to which they are otherwise entitled. For example, consider a hypothetical study designed to examine the effects of 6 weeks of biweekly therapy on functional skills for people 1 year after a cardiovascular accident. Even if a person has agreed to participate for 6 weeks, the person has the right to drop out of the study at any time, without repercussions, even if that decision jeopardizes the validity of the study. Similarly, if a participant in a qualitative study tells about an incident in an interview and then requests that the researcher not use that information, the researcher must abide by the participant's request.

►CONCLUSION: RESEARCH SKILLS OF OCCUPATIONAL THERAPISTS

All occupational therapists have the responsibility to become knowledgeable consumers of research so that they can evaluate and effectively use the research literature relevant to their practice arenas. It is the professional responsibility of therapists to know how to find resources and to be able to read, understand, and critically review the research reported in journal articles, newsletters, and test manuals. To do this, therapists must have a basic understanding of statistics and the different types of research, including their respective strengths and weaknesses. *Research Competencies for Occupational Therapists* (Crepeau & Coster, 1995) delineates and describes five levels of research competence arranged in a developmental hierarchy.

Most professional journals in occupational therapy have a peer review process whereby each manuscript is reviewed and critiqued by a minimum of two or three colleagues with expertise in the area of the research before the manuscript is accepted for publication. Even so, there is great variability in the quality of the articles published. Thus, the last step in the review process is taken by the informed consumer, who critically reads the research literature. To assist in this process, additional readings related to research are included in the bibliography and the reference list. See Figures 48–7 and 48–8 for worksheets containing questions to guide reading and critiquing quantitative and qualitative research studies.

Some therapists extend beyond the role of research consumer to that of researcher. Such therapists may contribute through formulation of research questions, systematic data collection, or the design, implementation, and dissemination of research studies. Often research is the product of many persons (clinicians and academicians) working collaboratively to discover knowledge through the systematic investigation of a problem of mutual interest.

▼ BIBLIOGRAPHY

Babbie, E. R. (1990). *Survey research methods.* Belmont, CA: Wadsworth Publishing.

Bailey, D. M. (1997). *Research for the health professional: A practical guide (2nd ed.).* Philadelphia: F. A. Davis.

Bogdan, R. & Taylor, S. (1984). *Introduction to qualitative research methods.* New York: John Wiley & Sons.

Campbell, P. H. (1988). Using a single-subject research design to evaluate the effectiveness of treatment. *The American Journal of Occupational Therapy, 44,* 732–738.

Dillman, D. A. (1978). *Mail and telephone surveys: The total design method.* New York: John Wiley & Sons.

Elzey, F. F. (1974). *A first reader in statistics.* Belmont, CA: Wadsworth Publishing.

Kazdin, A. E. (1982). *Single-case research designs: Methods for clinical and applied settings.* New York: Oxford University Press.

Ottenbacher, K. (1986). *Evaluating clinical change: Strategies for occupational and physical therapists.* Baltimore: Williams & Wilkins.

Ruyeen, C. B. (1997). *A research primer for occupational and physical therapists.* Bethesda, MD: American Occupational Therapy Association.

▼ REFERENCES

Agar, M. H. (1986). *Speaking of ethnography.* Sage University Paper series on Qualitative Research Methods (Vol. 2). Newbury Park, CA: Sage.

Allen, C. K. (1990). *Allen Cognitive Level Test manual.* Colchester, CT: S & S Worldwide.

Ayres, A. J. (1989). *Sensory Integration and Praxis Tests manual.* Los Angeles: Western Psychological Services.

Barlow, D. H. & Hayes, S. C. (1979). Alternating treatments design: One strategy for comparing the effects of two treatments in a single subject. *Journal of Applied Behavior Analysis, 12,* 199–210.

Benner, P. (1994). Introduction. In P. Benner (Ed.), *Interpretive phenomenology: Embodiment, caring, and ethics in health and illness* (pp. xiii–xxvii). Thousand Oaks, CA: Sage.

Billingsley, F. F., White, O. R., & Munson, R. (1980). Procedural reliability: A rationale and an example. *Behavioral Assessment, 2,* 229–241.

Bogdan, R. C. & Bilken, S. K. (1992). *Qualitative research for education: An introduction to theory and methods* (2nd ed.). Boston: Allyn & Bacon.

Bork, C. E. (1993). *Research in physical therapy.* Philadelphia: J. B. Lippincott.

Bouska, M. J. & Kwatny, E. (1983). *Manual for application of the Motor-Free Visual Perception Test to the adult population.* Philadelphia: P.O. Box 12246.

Campbell, D. & Stanley, J. C. (1963). *Experimental and quasi-experimental designs for research.* Chicago: Rand McNally College Publishing.

Carr, B. S. & Williams, M. (1982). Analysis of therapeutic techniques through use of the standard behavior chart. *Physical Therapy, 52,* 117–183.

Casby, J. A. & Holm, M. (1994). The effect of music on repetitive disruptive vocalizations of persons with dementia. *The American Journal of Occupational Therapy, 48,* 883–889.

Case-Smith, J. & Cable, J. (1996). Perceptions of occupational therapists regarding service delivery models in school-based practice. *The Occupational Therapy Journal of Research, 16,* 23–44.

Clark, F. (1993). Occupation embedded in real life: Interweaving occupational science and occupational therapy, 1993 Eleanor Clark Slagle lecture. *American Journal of Occupational Therapy, 47,* 1067–1078.

Clark, F., Ennevor, B. L., & Richardson, P. L. (1996). A grounded theory of techniques for occupational storytelling and occupational story making. In R. Zemke & F. Clark (Eds.), *Occupational science: The evolving discipline* (pp. 373–392). Philadelphia: F. A. Davis.

Clifford, J. & Marcus, G. E. (Eds.). (1986). *Writing culture: The poetics and politics of ethnography.* Berkeley, CA: University of California Press.

Cohn, E. S. (1991). [Nationally speaking] Clinical reasoning: Explicating complexity. *American Journal of Occupational Therapy, 45,* 969–971.

Cox, R. C. & West, W. L. (1982). *Fundamentals of research for the health professional.* Laurel, MD: RAMSCO Publishing.

Crepeau, E. B. (1991). Achieving intersubjective understanding: Examples from an occupational therapy treatment session. *American Journal of Occupational Therapy, 45,* 1016–1026.

Crepeau, E. B. (1994). Uneasy alliances: Belief and action on a geropsychiatric team. (Doctoral dissertation, University of New Hampshire, 1994). *Dissertation Abstracts International,* 9506410.

Crepeau, E. B. (1997). Social biography and research. *Occupational Therapy Journal of Research, 17,* 105–109.

Crepeau, E. B. & Coster, W. (June, 1995). Resolution for the AOTA Representative Assembly: Research competencies for occupational therapy. Bethesda, MD: American Occupational Therapy Foundation.

DeGangi, G. A. & Royeen, C. B. (1994). Current practice among Neurodevelopmental Treatment Association members. *The American Journal of Occupational Therapy, 48,* 803–809.

Denzin, N. & Lincoln, Y. (Eds.). (1994). *Handbook of qualitative research.* Thousand Oaks, CA: Sage.

DePoy, E. & Gitlin, L. N. (1994). *Introduction to research.* St. Louis: C.V. Mosby.

Dewire, A., White, D., Kanny, E., & Glass, R. (1996). Education and training of occupational therapists for neonatal intensive care units. *The American Journal of Occupational Therapy, 50,* 486–494.

Dirette, D. & Hinojosa, J. (1994). Effects of continuous passive motion on the edematous hands of two persons with flaccid hemiplegia. *The American Journal of Occupational Therapy, 48,* 403–409.

Edwards, D. F., Baum C. M., & Deuel, R. K. (1991). Constructional apraxia in Alzheimer's disease: Contributions to functional loss. *Physical and Occupational Therapy in Geriatrics, 9*(3/4), 53–68.

Einarsson-Backes, L. M., Deitz, J., Price, R., Glass, R., & Hayes, R. (1994). The effect of oral support on sucking efficiency in preterm infants. *The American Journal of Occupational Therapy, 48,* 490–498.

Einset, K., Deitz, J., Billingsley, F., & Harris, S. (1989). The electric feeder: An efficacy study. *The Occupational Therapy Journal of Research, 9,* 38–52.

Engel, J. M., Rapoff, M. A., & Pressman, A. R. (1994). The durability of relaxation training in pediatric headache management. *The Occupational Therapy Journal of Research, 14,* 183–190.

Fielding, N. G. and Lee, R. M. (Eds.). (1991). *Using computers in qualitative research.* Newbury Park, CA: Sage.

Fleming, M. H. (1991). Clinical reasoning in medicine compared with clinical reasoning in occupational therapy. *American Journal of Occupational Therapy, 45,* 988–1006.

Gilfoyle, E. & Christiansen, C. (1987). Research: The quest for truth and the key to excellence. *The American Journal of Occupational Therapy, 41,* 7–8.

Glaser, B. G. & Strauss, A. L. (1967). *The discovery of grounded theory: Strategies for qualitative research.* New York: Aldine de Gruyter.

Gubrium, J. (1988). *Analyzing field reality.* Sage University paper series on qualitative research methods (vol. 8). Beverly Hills, CA: Sage.

Gubrium, J. (1991). *The mosaic of care: Frail elderly and their families in the real world.* New York: Springer.

Harris, S. R. & Riffle K. (1986). Effects of inhibitive ankle-foot orthoses on standing balance in a child with cerebral palsy. *Physical Therapy, 66,* 643–667.

Hartmann, D. P. & Hall, R. V. (1976). The changing criterion design. *Journal of Applied Behavior Analysis, 9,* 527–532.

Hasselkus, B. R. (1995). Beyond ethnography: Expanding our understanding and criteria for qualitative research. *Occupational Therapy Journal of Research, 15,* 75–84.

Hasselkus, B. R. (1997). In the eye of the beholder: The researcher in qualitative research. *Occupational Therapy Journal of Research, 17,* 81–83.

Hasselkus, B. R. & Dickie, V. A. (1994). Doing occupational therapy: Dimensions of satisfaction and dissatisfaction. *American Journal of Occupational Therapy, 48,* 145–154.

Kanny, E., Anson, D., & Smith, R.O. (1991). A survey of technology education in entry-level curricula: Quantity, quality, and barriers. *Occupational Therapy Journal of Research, 11,* 311–319.

Kielhofner, G. (1982a). Qualitative research: Part 1. Paradigmatic grounds and issues of reliability and validity. *Occupational Therapy Journal of Research, 2,* 67–79.

Kielhofner, G. (1982b). Qualitative research: Part 2. Methodological approaches and relevance to occupational therapy. *Occupational Therapy Journal of Research, 2,* 150–164.

Krefting, L. (1989). Reintegration into the community after head injury: The results of an ethnographic study. *Occupational Therapy Journal of Research, 9,* 67–83.

Krefting, L. (1991). Rigor in qualitative research: The assessment of trustworthiness. *The American Journal of Occupational Therapy, 45,* 214–222.

Larson, K. B. (1990). Activity patterns and life changes in people with depression. *The American Journal of Occupational Therapy, 44,* 902–906.

Leonard, V. W. (1994). A Heideggerian phenomenological perspective. In P. Benner (Ed.), *Interpretive phenomenology: Embodiment, caring, and ethics in health and illness* (pp. 43–63). Thousand Oaks, CA: Sage.

Lincoln, Y. S. & Guba, E. G. (1985). *Naturalistic inquiry.* Newbury Park, CA: Sage.

Link, L., Lukens, S., & Bush, M. A. (1995). Spherical grip strength in children 3 to 6 years of age. *American Journal of Occupational Therapy, 49,* 318–326.

Lofland, J. & Lofland, L. H. (1984). *Analyzing social settings: A guide to qualitative observation and analysis* (2nd ed.) Belmont, CA: Wadsworth.

McCracken, G. (1988). *The long interview* (Qualitative Research Methods Series, Vol. 13). Newbury Park, CA: Sage Publications.

McCuaig, M. & Frank, G. (1991). The able self: Adaptive patterns and choices in independent living for a person with cerebral palsy. *American Journal of Occupational Therapy, 45,* 224–234.

Mechanic, D. (1989). Medical sociology: Some tensions among theory, method, and substance. *Journal of Health and Social Behavior, 30,* 147–160.

Miller, L. J. (1982). *Miller assessment for preschoolers.* Littleton, CO: The Foundation for Knowledge in Development.

Mishler, E. G. (1986). *Research interviewing: Context and narrative.* Cambridge, MA: Harvard University Press.

Moritz, C. (Ed.) (1967). *Current biography yearbook.* New York: H. W. Wilson.

Neistadt, M. E. (1994). The effects of different treatment activities on functional fine motor coordination in adults with brain injuries. *The American Journal of Occupational Therapy, 48,* 877–882.

Neistadt, M. E. (1996). Teaching strategies for the development of clinical reasoning. *American Journal of Occupational Therapy, 50,* 676–684.

Ottenbacher, K. & York, J. (1984). Strategies for evaluating clinical change: Implications for practice and research. *The American Journal of Occupational Therapy, 38,* 647–659.

Payton, O. (1988). *Research: The validation of clinical practice*. Philadelphia: F. A. Davis.

Penny, N. H., Mueser, K. T., & North, C. T. (1995). The Allen Cognitive Level Test and social competence in adult psychiatric patients. *The American Journal of Occupational Therapy, 49*, 420–427.

Polit, D. F. & Hungler, B. (1993). *Essentials of nursing research: Methods, appraisal, and utilization*. Philadelphia: J. B. Lippincott.

Prescott, G. A., Balow, I. H., Hogan, T. P., & Farr, R. C. (1978). *Metropolitan Achievement Tests*. New York: The Pyschological Corporation.

Quigley, M. C. (1995). Impact of spinal cord injury on the life roles of women. *The American Journal of Occupational Therapy, 49*, 780–786.

Rheinharz, S. (1984). *On becoming a social scientist: From survey research and participant observation to experiential analysis*. New Brunswick, NJ: Transaction.

Rheinharz, S. (1992). *Feminist methods in social research*. New York: Oxford University Press.

Richardson, L. (1994). Writing: A method of inquiry. In N. K. Denzin & Y. S. Lincoln (Eds.), *Handbook of qualitative research* (pp. 516–529). Thousand Oaks, CA: Sage.

Schell, B. B. (1994). *The effect of practice context on occupational therapist's clinical reasoning* Unpublished doctoral dissertation, University of Georgia.

Shillam, L. L., Beeman, C., & Loshin, P. M. (1983). Effect of occupational therapy intervention on bathing independence of disabled persons. *The American Journal of Occupational Therapy, 37*, 744–748.

Smith, D. E. (1987). *The everyday world as problematic: A feminist sociology*. Boston: Northeastern University Press.

Spradley, J. P. (1979). *The ethnographic interview*. New York; Harcourt, Brace Jovanovich College Publishers.

Strauss, A. & Corbin, J. (1994). Grounded theory methodology: An overview. In N. K. Denzin & Y. S. Lincoln (Eds.), *Handbook of qualitative research* (pp. 273–285). Thousand Oaks, CA: Sage.

Strauss, A., Fagerhaugh, S., Suczek, B., & Wiener, C. (1985). *The social organization of medical work*. Chicago: University of Chicago Press.

Thomas, J. J. (1996). Comparison of patient education methods: Effects on knowledge of cardiac rehabilitation principles. *The Occupational Therapy Journal of Research, 16*, 166–178.

Trower, P., Bryant, B., & Argyle, M. (1978). *Social skills and mental health*. London: Methuen.

Tuckman, B. (1994). *Conducting educational research*. New York: Harcourt Brace Jovanovich.

van Manen, M. (1990). *Researching lived experience: Human science for an action sensitive pedagogy*. London, Ontario, Canada: State University of New York Press.

Van Maanen, J. (1988). *Tales of the field: On writing ethnography*. Chicago: University of Chicago Press.

Walker, K. F. & Burris, B. (1991). Correlation of Sensory Integration and Praxis Test scores with Metropolitan Achievement Test scores in normal children. *Occupational Therapy Journal of Research, 11*, 307–310.

Washington, K. (1996). The effects of an adaptive seating device on postural alignment and upper extremity function in infants with neuromotor impairments. Unpublished doctoral dissertation. University of Washington.

Wolery, M. & Harris, S. (1982). Interpreting results of single-subject research designs. *Physical Therapy, 62*, 445–452.

Wolf, M. (1992). *A thrice told tale: Feminism, postmodernism, and ethnographic responsibility*. Stanford, CA: Stanford University Press.

Yerxa, E. J. (1991). [Nationally speaking] Seeking a relevant, ethical, and realistic way of knowing for occupational therapy. *American Journal of Occupational Therapy, 45*, 199–204.

Yoder, R. M., Nelson, D. L., & Smith, D. A. (1989). Added-purpose versus rote exercise in female nursing home residents. *The American Journal of Occupational Therapy, 43*, 581–586.

Chapter 49

The History of Occupational Therapy

Kathleen Barker Schwartz

The following history describes the development of the profession of occupational therapy in the 20th century. It examines how the ideas of the founders have evolved into our profession today: one that strives to retain both the art and science inherent in the therapeutic process.

▼ THE FOUNDING YEARS

The profession was founded in Clifton Springs, New York on March 15, 1917. The charter members of the National Society for the Promotion of Occupational Therapy (NSPOT; later to be renamed the American Occupational Therapy Association) brought a rich mix of backgrounds, interests, and skills to this first meeting. George Barton, the host of the meeting, was an architect who had tuberculosis; Susan Cox Johnson, a former arts and crafts instructor, was Director of Occupations for the New York City Department of Public Charities; Thomas B. Kidner, a former architect, was the vocational secretary of the Military Hospital Commission of Canada; William Rush Dunton, a psychiatrist, was Assistant Physician at the Shephard and Enoch Pratt Hospital in Towson, Maryland; and Eleanor Clarke Slagle, formerly associated with Hull House, was Director of the Henry B. Favill School of Occupations. The founders' views represented a variety of ideas and movements, some dating back the 1800s, some attaining prominence during the progressive era of 1890 to 1920. They included moral treatment, the arts and crafts movement, scientific medicine ideology, and women's professions and social reform.

Moral Treatment

Bing (1981) suggested that occupational therapy can trace its roots to the moral treatment reforms of the 19th century. Moral treatment originated in Europe when physicians such as Phillipe Pinel and William Tuke, in a departure from the prevalent view that the insane were subhuman, proposed that persons with mental disorders could reason (Bockoven, 1963). The moral treatment regimen was based on the optimistic assumption that a humane approach that used daily routine and occupation would lead to recovery.

The first hospitals to provide moral treatment in the United States included Friend's Asylum built by the Pennsylvania Quakers and McLean Hospital in Massachusetts (Rothman, 1971). Early studies showed the success of small asylums. However, as patient populations grew, the humane familylike atmosphere disappeared (Peloquin, 1989). By necessity, treatment was reduced to custodial care. Thus, what began as a progressive chapter in the treatment of moral illness ended in disappointment (Peloquin).

A half century later Dunton, drawing on the ideas from moral treatment, advocated occupational therapy's role as one that provided a "judicious regimen of activity" (as cited in Bing, 1981 p. 508). This meant treating individuals in a humane and caring way while engaging them in occupation and routine. Adolph Meyer (1922), a psychiatrist who worked with Slagle at Phipps Clinic, asserted that many mental illnesses were "problems of adaptation" that could be addressed through involvement in curative occupations that gave patients the opportunity to "work ... to do, and to plan and create ..."(p. 1).

Arts and Crafts Movement

Founded in England by William Morris, the Arts and Crafts Movement drew on the antimodernist ideas of John Ruskin. Ruskin urged a return to a simpler life in which the body and mind could be engaged in satisfying labor that yielded fine hand-crafted objects (Boris, 1986). This notion attracted those concerned with the negative effects of the rapid social, economic, and industrial changes on the small towns in early 20th century America (Wiebe, 1967). The idea of using arts and crafts as curative occupation was similarly attractive to the founders. Whereas moral treatment provided the idea of using occupations involving labor and manual tasks, such as gardening or carpentry, the arts and crafts movement suggested the potential of crafts for both their curative process and satisfying outcome. According to Johnson (1920)

Handcrafts have a special therapeutic value as they afford occupation that combines the elements of play and recreation with work and accomplishment. They give a concrete return and provide a stimulus to mental activity and muscular exercise at the same time, and afford an opportunity for creation and self-expression. (p. 69)

Johnson also described how crafts could be graded for the desired physical and mental results.

In adapting the arts and crafts ideology to curing the physically and mentally ill, the profession shifted its focus to the medical domain (Schemm, 1994). This created a tension between the humanistic values of the moral treatment and arts and crafts movements and the mechanistic values of scientific medicine ideology.

Scientific Medicine Ideology

In his theory of scientific management, Frederick Taylor (1911) proposed that the engineering values of rationality, efficiency, and systematic observation be applied to all areas of society's ills. Drawing from this ideology, the reformers of the progressive era argued for scientific and efficient medical care. Indeed, the unsanitary, disorganized conditions of the 1800s were giving way to clean, efficient hospitals and more reliable medical treatment based on scientific research.

The desire for a scientific approach to treatment can be seen in the founders' writings. Barton (c. 1920) suggested that Taylor's time and motion studies might provide a model for occupational therapy research. Dunton (1928b) argued that the profession needed individuals capable of systematic inquiry. Slagle (1924) proposed that to validate occupational therapy's efficacy the profession needed research to complement empirical knowledge about occupations.

Beyond advocating scientific inquiry, scientific management ideology promoted a mechanistic view of society. When applied to medicine, the therapist was the factory worker who applied a similar treatment that yielded a predictable result. This perspective failed to take into account individual differences, creating a conflict within occupational therapy practice between a humane and individually focused treatment and an efficient and production-oriented one.

Scientific medicine also promoted a hierarchical model in which the doctor supervised the nurses and therapists. Under this model it was assumed that only doctors had true scientific knowledge and, therefore, should be preeminent. This idea was supported by Dunton (1928a), who wrote ". . . The occupational therapist, therefore, has the same relation to the physician as has the nurse, that is, she is a technical assistant" (p. 10). The notion of a therapist as physician's helper was also in keeping with the commonly accepted idea of the times that "women's" professions were subservient to those of men.

HISTORICAL NOTE
ELEANOR CLARK SLAGLE'S PUSH FOR LEADERSHIP: THE CALL TO LEAD

Suzanne M. Peloquin

Eleanor Clarke Slagle was a leader. Elected vice president at the first meeting of the Society for the Promotion of Occupational Therapy, Slagle eventually held every association office and for longer than anyone else. Men held many positions of authority in those early years. In medical matters, therapists deferred to male physicians; in promotional and organizational efforts, men were most often elected to high positions. Given this context, Slagle's leadership in both ideational and organizational realms is all the more remarkable.

Ora Ruggles, a reconstruction aide during World War I, remembered Slagle's leadership. During the difficult months after the death of her fiance, Ruggles had taken a leave from "occupational work." Slagle asked Ruggles to return, arguing that the occupational therapy movement needed her to "get behind it and push!" (Carlova & Ruggles, 1946, p. 113). Ruggles returned to practice and started occupational therapy programs in many locations across the United States.

Slagle's words teach this worthwhile lesson: A person can move a profession forward from a number of places. One can lead if one agrees to get behind some effort and push!

■

Carlova, J. & Ruggles, O. (1946). The healing heart. New York: Julian Messner.

Women's Professions and Social Reform

Occupational therapy provided a new vocation for the professional women of the progressive era who were seeking to enter the work place (Quiroga, 1995). These women tended to be middle- to upper-class, with some education and a desire to serve (Litterst, 1992). Along with other "women's" professions, such as nursing, settlement work, and teaching, occupational therapy enabled women to extend their sphere of influence and to contribute to society by helping individuals in need. As with nursing, occupational therapy combined the domestic skills and benevolent tendencies ascribed to women with technical expertise acquired through specialized training (Reverby, 1987).

Eleanor Clarke Slagle benefited from such training when she enrolled in a 6-week course in curative occupations given by Julia Lathrop of Hull House, at the Chicago School of Civics and Philanthropy. Hull House at that time was a center for progressive social reform under the leadership of its founders Jane Addams and Ellen Gates Starr (Addams, 1910). It maintained a close association with John Dewey's Laboratory School, which emphasized the belief that learning should involve "active occupation" (Dewey, 1910, p. 224). Several years later, Slagle professed the importance of the course in forming her understanding of the value of "the normalizing effect" of occupations (Loomis, 1992) in returning the patient to "community life and economic usefulness" (Slagle, 1921, p. 43) through "organized occupation" that encouraged self-expression (Slagle, 1924, p. 98).

Summary

The profession of occupational therapy was a product of its time, and the founder's views represented ideas and movements prevalent during the progressive era. Their views reflected a mix of humanitarianism with the mechanistic and scientific perspective of medicine. This combination of two value systems would contribute to the uniqueness of the profession, but would also lead to tensions within the field that continue to the present. Another source of tension was the subservient role of the occupational therapist as the doctor's helper.

The expansive definition of occupational therapy reflects the early idealism of the founders. "The duties of the occupational therapist are broad and far reaching, including as they do something of arts and crafts, social services, trades and industries, and humanity" (American Occupational Therapy Association [AOTA], 1923a). This idealistic definition would prove difficult to achieve (Ambrosi and Schwartz, 1995) and would be challenged by other groups as specialization became prevalent. Thus, the founding years set the stage for the profession's future growth and conflicts.

▼ THE WORLD WARS

World War I: Recognition

The World Wars provided a great impetus for the growth of occupational therapy. Shortly after the profession was founded the United States entered World War I. This prompted a call for volunteers, known as "reconstruction aides," to assist the wounded men at the front (Low, 1992). Unlike nursing, the appointment was a civilian one; therefore, it carried no military status and provided little pay. There were two types of reconstruction aides: physical therapy and occupational therapy. Physical therapy reconstruction aides used exercise and massage; occupational therapy aides gave instruction in crafts. Chosen for their womanly qualities and technical skills, it was assumed that the occupational therapy aides would provide assistance during the initial stages of recovery. Although, at first, they received a cool reception, when their presence increased discipline and improved the mood of the soldiers, they were deemed to be "worth their weight in gold" (Quiroga, 1995, p. 164). By the end of the war nearly 1200 occupational therapy reconstruction aides had contributed their services. The unprecedented call for occupational therapists who could immediately be sent into service prompted the creation of emergency-training programs in Boston, Chicago, New York, and Milwaukee. At the same time, the professional association, NSPOT, served as a clearing house for information on occupational therapy reconstruction aides and attempted to monitor the quality of the educational programs.

World War II: Expansion

World War II resulted in an even greater need for medical services than World War I, partly owing to the recent scientific discoveries of penicillin and sulfur. The war again highlighted the value of occupational therapy for aiding the sick and wounded. Unlike World War I, occupational therapists who served in the war achieved the official recognition of military status (Messick, 1947). Occupational therapy was still viewed as women's work and recruiting material offered commissions to unmarried women younger than the age of 26 with cheerful, outgoing dispositions. However, recruits were warned: "The training course for OTs is stiff, the standards of the profession are high and you'll have to have more than a Florence Nightingale complex to be . . . [a worthy] recruit" (The Gift, 1943, p. 115). As with the first world war, emergency training programs were created to meet the critical need for therapists. By 1945 there were 21 educational programs and 3224 occupational therapists (Arestad & Westmoreland, 1946). To assure minimum educational standards for all programs, in 1935 the American Occupational Therapy Association (AOTA) with the American Medical Association

(AMA) adopted the *Essentials of an Acceptable School of Occupational Therapy* (Essentials, 1935). The first edition of a major textbook, Willard and Spackman's *Principles of Occupational Therapy*, was published in 1947.

The demands of World War II required a change in the therapeutic medium used by occupational therapists. Emphasis on crafts, such as basketry, weaving, and pottery, shifted to more practical job-related skills. Along with the shift from crafts to more functional occupations there was a high demand for therapists to treat those with physical impairments. To care for the war injured, Veterans Administration Hospitals were reorganized, with departments of Physical Medicine and Rehabilitation formed to direct the interdisciplinary team work. This interdisciplinary approach meant that occupational therapy had to negotiate its role among other professions. At this time, the AOTA sought closer ties with the AMA in the hopes of increasing the profession's scientific and medical credibility. The AMA's definition of occupational therapy illustrates this growing alliance: ". . . Occupational therapy is treatment for illness or disability through remedial work actively prescribed by a doctor and directed by trained technicians" (The Gift, 1943, p. 115).

Summary

The World Wars helped increase public awareness of the benefits of occupational therapy and provided an opportunity for therapists to prove their competence and social worth. The wars also more closely aligned occupational therapy with medicine, as did the linkage between the AOTA and the AMA. As the profession negotiated its role with other professionals within the medical system, turf issues arose, such as the differentiation of occupational therapy from physical therapy. To practice within the medical system there was pressure on occupational therapy to narrow its definition of services and relinquish some of the founder's humanistic goals.

▼ FIFTY YEARS AFTER THE FOUNDING

A Time of Change

By 1967, the 50th anniversary of occupational therapy, the country and the profession faced a time of great change. American social, political, and economic structures were challenged by the antiwar and civil rights movements. Advances in science and technology caused knowledge to expand, additionally challenging all aspects of society. Legislation that supported the popular notion that all citizens should have equal opportunity to high-quality health care triggered the growth of the health care industry and accelerated costs of medical care (Starr, 1982).

Mary Reilly (1966) highlighted these uncertainties and opportunities in a paper at the 45th Annual AOTA Conference. Elizabeth Yerxa (1967), in her Slagle lecture, urged the profession to become more autonomous in directing its future, "to move with speed and self-confidence toward true professionalism" (p. 1). She supported the profession's move away from the medical model and argued that the physician's written prescription was no longer seen as "necessary, holy or healthy" (p. 2). The profession should, she proposed, base its practice on treatments that encouraged self-initiated choice and purposeful activity to increase function and promote self-actualization. Wilma West's Slagle lecture (1968) urged the profession to move from an illness model toward one based on wellness and prevention. She said, "We should think more about roles in prevention as well as in treatment and rehabilitation, about socioeconomic and cultural as well as biological causes of disease and dysfunction and about serving health needs of people in many other settings than the hospital" (p. 14). Thus, these leaders called on the profession to respond to the changing health care environment by moving in new directions that encouraged a greater role and increased autonomy for the profession.

There is evidence of new directions in the *American Journal of Occupational Therapy* (AJOT) and the actions of the AOTA. From 1947 to the 1960s, AJOT primarily featured articles written by authors with doctoral degrees (MDs and PhDs) or coauthored with occupational therapists. By the late 1960s, occupational therapists were the main contributors to AJOT. In 1972, the AOTA moved its headquarters from New York to Rockville, Maryland, to enable closer access to the Capitol and other professional organizations (Cromwell, 1972). The newly formed Government Affairs Department with its public relations and lobbying staff followed legislative actions. The Association launched a marketing campaign directed toward physicians, consumers, and third-party payers. AOTA revised its earlier negative view of licensing and began to help state organizations trying to secure licensure. There was substantial activity in education, including the 1965 revision of the *Essentials of an Accredited Occupational Therapy Program*, a curriculum study, and the formulation of national educational objectives for occupational therapy programs (Yerxa, 1967). The first standards for the education of occupational therapy assistants were adopted in 1958 (Crampton, 1958).

Specialization

Occupational therapists were urged to specialize to strengthen treatment techniques, become more credible with physicians, and increase their professional status (Higher Status Near, c. 1960). Legislative, technological, and market changes and pressures within the medical community apparently drove this specialization (Gritzer & Arluke, 1985). However, some practitioners worried that specialization could cause therapists to lose sight of the core of their practice (Diamond, 1956). Reflecting this concern, Gregory Bateson (1956), the well-known anthropologist, spoke at the Annual American Occupational Therapy Conference in San Francisco, of the critical role the occupational therapist played in helping the patient discover inner strengths:

Every act of creation is an act of discovery and the message which [occupational therapy is] trying to communicate is a discovery . . . The modality is somehow to be the carrier for a message to the patient. A message about himself [sic], his relationship to the human universe and the relationship between himself and you (p. 188).

Bateson's words gave eloquent expression to what the founders and succeeding generations of therapists saw as the essence of the therapeutic process. The problem lay in the fact that the therapeutic process Bateson described is not easy to convey. Occupational therapists had to find a way to articulate and practice occupational therapy's art and science within a medical context that primarily rewarded the scientific.

Changes in the delivery of health services required concomitant changes in education, especially related to occupational therapy's role in rehabilitation. In 1956, West and McNary, anticipating these changes, recommended that educational programs needed to place more emphasis on the basic and applied sciences. These included kinesiology and neurology, prosthetics, activities of daily living, adaptive equipment, work simplification, and prevocational evaluation and testing. They further recommended that the teaching of arts and crafts be deemphasized and that occupational therapists be clearer about defining their unique role within the rehabilitation setting.

By 1967 the profession of occupational therapy had two distinct specialty areas: physical disabilities and psychosocial dysfunction, and an emerging one, pediatrics. The growth of physical disability services in occupational therapy resulted from the Rehabilitation Act of 1954 (Public Law [PL] 565) and the Medicare legislation of 1965 (Title 18). Advances in science and new theories, such as neuromuscular education, expanded the treatment possibilities and the opportunities for further specialization into treatment areas such as neurorehabilitation.

While physical disabilities practice coped with its expansion within a medical rehabilitation model, psychosocial dysfunction practice struggled to redefine itself within an environment of changing models of treatment. In tandem with mental health approaches of the 1950s, Gail and Jay Fidler (1954) proposed the use of the psychodynamic approach to occupational therapy intervention. The 1960s brought a shift to ego and behavioral models, reflected in Llorens (1968) early work. This occurred as the deinstitutionalization movement shifted patients from state hospitals to community mental health centers. Community mental health centers adopted milieu treatment. This approach provided the opportunity for occupational therapists to take responsibility for functional evaluation and treatment of patients. Although the movement toward deinstitutionaliza-

tion seemed promising, a retrospective look at its failures shows that the community supports necessary for its success were never fully developed (Mechanic, 1989). By the late 1970s, it became clear that the needs of those with chronic mental illness were not being met in the community, and occupational therapy's value had diminished as psychopharmacological intervention became the treatment of choice.

The third area of practice, pediatrics, emerged in large part because of the passage of the Education of the Handicapped Act (PL 94–142) in 1975. This law provided children with handicaps the needed therapy to ensure participation in the school setting. In addition, pediatric practice was aided by the research and theory development of Jean Ayres (1963), whose work provided a rationale for occupational therapy treatment.

Research in Occupational Science and Occupational Therapy

The founders recognized the need for research to validate occupational therapy practice by forming the Committee on Research and Efficiency (NSPOT, 1917). Unfortunately, no studies of substance were conducted until the 1960s. Several factors contributed to this lag. First, there were few doctorally prepared occupational therapists to conduct this research, nor were other scholars interested in studying the field. Second, there was little pressure within health care to prove efficacy of treatment until the advent of Medicare and third-party payers. In 1965 a group of leaders in occupational therapy established the American Occupational Therapy Foundation (AOTF) to provide the intellectual and financial resources to support research within the field (AOTF, 1975). Today AOTF provides monies for occupational therapy research and supports the *Occupational Therapy Journal of Research*, the primary research journal for the field.

The need for research was highlighted by the call for stronger theoretical underpinnings than the intuitive approach the practice had previously offered. In her Slagle Lecture, Reilly (1962) restated the hypothesis on which the profession was founded. That is, "that man, through the use of his hands as they are energized by mind and will, can influence the state of his own health" (p. 2). To support this hypothesis she said that the field needed a theory that could identify the drive in individuals for occupation; this theory would provide scientific support to an intuitive belief. Reilly articulated this drive as a component of occupational behavior. Her work contributed directly to the development of the Model of Human Occupation and the emergence of the academic discipline of Occupational Science (Clark, 1993). Others during this period shared the concern about lack of theory and were among the early leaders in providing conceptual guidance for practice (Ayres, 1963; Rood, 1958). This period marked the beginning of the research and theory development that continues into the present.

Summary

The late 1960s through the 1980s was a time of rapid change in society and occupational therapy. Occupational therapy practice became specialized and began to expand into areas of health care beyond the hospital. This specialization brought with it more recognition and the opportunity to respond to the increase in technological and medical knowledge. However, specialization threatened the generalist approach to the treatment process that considered all aspects of the patient. The close bond developed with medicine and its reliance on scientific approaches continued to conflict with the art of practice and the humanistic goals of occupational therapy.

►CONCLUSION: THE PRESENT AND THE LESSONS FROM THE PAST

Health care in the 1990s is big business, and occupational therapy has been a beneficiary of this trend. Occupational therapy services are now being delivered in private homes, public schools, nursing homes, hospices, and the work place, as well as hospitals. By 1995, the Accreditation Council for Occupational Therapy Education had accredited 89 professional and 86 technical programs (Listing of Educational Programs, 1995). Demand for occupational therapy services, especially in rehabilitation and long-term care, is expected to continue through the year 2005 (Occupational Outlook Handbook, 1994). This growth is due in part to (1) demographics, in that more elderly people require occupational therapy; (2) legislation, such as PL 94–142, that brought occupational therapy services to school children; and (3) the success of medical insurance, including Medicare, which now covers a substantial portion of the population.

Scientific management ideology, with its focus on efficiency, and fiscal and legislative efforts to control costs, drives health care decisions in the 1990s. All health care professions must show the efficacy of their treatment through outcome measures. The growth of for-profit health care institutions further emphasizes decision making based on financial considerations. Indeed, the idea of managed care is based on the assumption that the treatment of each patient can be rationally managed by having overseers choose the least expensive treatment that will achieve the desired goals. Occupational therapy, similar to all other health care professions, has to respond to the challenges of working in such an environment.

Our history shows us that occupational therapy has benefitted from external forces, such as war and legislation, because the profession's message has been attractive. In its early years occupational therapy offered the promise of arousing "interest, courage and confidence: to exercise mind and body in healthy activity; to overcome disability; and to reestablish capacity for industrial and social usefulness" (AOTA, 1923b). It offers a similar promise today. In the outcome-oriented language of the 1990s, "Occupational therapy is the use of purposeful activity or interventions designed to achieve functional outcomes which promote health, prevent injury or disability and which develop, improve, sustain, or restore the highest possible level of independence . . ." (AOTA, 1994). The profession has struggled to retain its broad purpose, and continues to fight the turf battles that are inevitable with such an expansive mission. Although it has specialized areas of practice, it promises the same result for all who receive its services, despite age or disability. Occupational therapy continues to have as its fundamental concern the individual's capacity to live a satisfying life, to work and play, to meet the needs of family and friends, and to achieve the goals to which he or she aspires.

We face many challenges: (1) the increased use of occupational therapy aides to substitute for fully trained practitioners, (2) financially driven health care and reimbursement policies, (3) a society that places less emphasis on humanistic values and caring, (4) an array of disciplines from psychology to nursing that also claim to address function, and (5) decreased funding for health care services. History provides us a sense of continuity with the past and helps us know that others have addressed similar challenges. We see that the founders and succeeding generations of occupational therapy practitioners have also faced societal and marketplace changes, challenges to their autonomy, turf issues, and indifference toward the individual with disability. That the profession has continued to grow gives testimony to its powerful message, what Reilly (1962) called "one of the great ideas of 20th century medicine" (p. 1).

▼ REFERENCES

Addams, J. (1910). *Twenty years at Hull House.* New York: Macmillan.

Ambrosi, E. & Schwartz, K. B. (1995). The profession's image, 1917–1925, Part II: Occupational therapy as represented by the profession. *American Journal of Occupational Therapy, 49,* 828–832.

American Occupational Therapy Association (AOTA). (1923a). *Bulletin No. 1.* Towson, MD: Sheppard Hospital Press.

American Occupational Therapy Association (AOTA). (1923b). *Bulletin No. 4: Principles of occupational therapy.* Towson MD: Sheppard Hospital Press.

American Occupational Therapy Association. (1994). Definition of occupational therapy practice for state regulation. *American Journal of Occupational Therapy, 48,* 1072–1073.

American Occupational Therapy Foundation (AOTF). (1975). The first decade: 1965–1975. *American Journal of Occupational Therapy, 29,* 636–640.

Arestad, F. H. & Westmoreland, M. G. (1946). Hospital service in the United States. *Journal of the American Medical Association, 130,* 1085.

Ayres, A. J. (1963). Eleanor Clarke Slagle's lecture. The development of perceptual–motor abilities: A theoretical basis for treatment of dysfunction. *American Journal of Occupational Therapy, 17,* 221–225.

Barton, G. E. (c. 1920). *The movies and the microscope.* Manuscript in American Occupational Therapy Archives: Bethesda MD.

Bateson, G. (1956). Communication in occupational therapy. *American Journal of Occupational Therapy, 10*, 188.

Bing, R. K. (1981). Occupational therapy revisited: A paraphasic journey. *American Journal of Occupational Therapy, 35*, 499–518.

Bockoven, J. S. (1963). *Moral treatment in American psychiatry.* New York: Springs Publishing.

Boris, E. (1986). *Art and labor: Ruskin, Morris, and the craftsman ideal in America.* Philadelphia: Temple University.

Clark, F. (1993). Occupation embedded in a real life: Interweaving occupational science and occupational therapy. *American Journal of Occupational Therapy, 47*, 1067–1078.

Crampton, M. W. (1958). Recognition of occupational therapy assistants. *American Journal of Occupational Therapy, 12*, 269–275.

Cromwell, F. (1972). Nationally speaking. *American Journal of Occupational Therapy, 26*, 3–5.

Dewey, J. (1910). *How we think.* Lexington MA: Heath.

Diamond, H. (1956). Some psychiatric problems of the physically disabled. *American Journal of Occupational Therapy, 10*, 113–117.

Dunton, W. R. (1928a). *Prescribing occupational therapy.* Springfield, IL: Charles C. Thomas.

Dunton, W. R. (1928b). The three "r's" of occupational therapy. *Occupational Therapy and Rehabilitation, 7*, 345–348.

Essentials of an acceptable school of occupational therapy. (1935). *Journal of American Medical Association, 104*, 1632–1633.

Fidler, G. S. & Fidler, J. W. (1954). *Introduction to psychiatric occupational therapy.* New York: Macmillian.

Gritzer, G. & Arluke, A. (1985). *The making of rehabilitation.* University of California Press: Berkeley, CA.

Higher status near, doctor tells therapists. (c. 1960). Archives of the Department of Occupational Therapy, San Jose State University, San Jose CA.

Johnson, S. C. (1920). Instruction in handcrafts and design for hospital patients. *The Modern Hospital, 15*(1), 69–72.

Listing of Educational Programs (1995). *American Journal of Occupational Therapy, 49*, 1036–1048.

Litterst, T. A. (1992). Occupational therapy: The role of ideology in the development of a profession for women. *American Journal of Occupational Therapy, 46*, 20–25.

Llorens, L. A. (1968). Changing methods in treatment of psychosocial dysfunction. *American Journal of Occupational Therapy, 22*, 26–29.

Loomis, B. (1992). The Henry B. Favill School of Occupations and Eleanor Clarke. *American Journal of Occupational Therapy, 46*, 34–37.

Low, J. F. (1992). The reconstruction aides. *American Journal of Occupational Therapy, 46*, 38–43.

Mechanic, D. (1989). *Mental health and social policy* (3rd ed.). Englewood Cliffs, NJ: Prentice Hall.

Messick, H. E. (1947). The new women's medical specialist corps. *American Journal of Occupational Therapy, 1*, 298–300.

Meyer, A. (1922). The philosophy of occupation therapy. *Archives of Occupational Therapy, 1*, 1–10.

National Society for the Promotion of Occupational Therapy (NSPOT). (1917). *Constitution of the National Society for the Promotion of Occupational Therapy.* Towson MD: Sheppard Pratt Hospital Press.

Occupational outlook handbook. (1994). Washington, DC: Bureau of Labor Statistics. U.S. Government Printing Office.

Peloquin, S. M. (1989). Moral treatment: Context considered. *American Journal of Occupational Therapy, 43*, 537–544.

Quiroga, V. (1995). *Occupational therapy: The first 30 years, 1990–1930.* Bethesda, MD: American Occupational Therapy Association.

Reilly, M. (1962). Occupational therapy can be one of the great ideas of 20th century medicine. *American Journal of Occupational Therapy, 16*, 1–9.

Reilly, M. (1966). The challenge of the future to an occupational therapist. *American Journal of Occupational Therapy, 20*, 221–225.

Reverby, S. M. (1987). *Ordered to care: The dilemma of American nursing, 1850–1945.* Cambridge: Cambridge University Press.

Rood, M. S. (1958). Every one counts. *American Journal of Occupational Therapy, 12*, 326–329.

Rothman, D. J. (1971). *The discovery of the asylum.* Boston: Little, Brown & Co.

Schemm, R. L. (1994). Bridging conflicting ideologies: The origins of American and British occupational therapy. *American Journal of Occupational Therapy, 48*, 1082–1088.

Slagle, E. C. (1921). To organize an O.T. department. *Hospital Management, 12*, 43–45.

Slagle, E. C. (1924). A year's development of occupational therapy in New York state hospitals. *Modern Hospital, 22*, 98–104.

Starr, P. (1982). *The social transformation of American medicine.* New York: Basic Books.

Taylor, F. (1911). *The principles of scientific management.* New York: Harper.

The gift of healing (1943). *Mademoiselle, 114–115;177–178.* Department scrapbooks, 1943–1954. Archives of the Department of Occupational Therapy. San Jose State University, San Jose, CA.

West, W. L. & McNary, H. (1956). A study of the present and potential role of occupational therapy in rehabilitation. *American Journal of Occupational Therapy, 10*, 150–156.

West, W. L. (1968). 1967 Eleanor Clarke lecture: Professional responsibility in times of change. *American Journal of Occupational Therapy, 22*, 9–15.

Wiebe, R. H. (1967). *The search for order, 1877–1920.* New York: Hill & Wang.

Willard, H. S. and Spackman, C. S. (Eds.). (1947). *Principles of occupational therapy.* Philadelphia: J. B. Lippincott.

Yerxa, E. (1967). 1966 Eleanor Clarke lecture: Authentic occupational therapy. *American Journal of Occupational Therapy, 21*, 1–9.

Dreams, Decisions, and Directions for Occupational Therapy

Elizabeth J. Yerxa

> Context of the Future
> Assumptions
> Crucial Decisions
> Potential Contributions
> Challenges to Students

I shall explore the exciting future of occupational therapy by (1) identifying a probable environmental *context* for the profession; (2) adopting a particular set of *assumptions*; (3) examining crucial *decisions* the profession needs to make; (4) projecting some potential *contributions* of occupational therapy; and (5) raising *challenges* for students.

Context of the Future

The 21st century will certainly usher in an "era of chronicity" (Robinson, 1988). As a result of the triumphs of medicine in preserving life, the population with chronic impairments will increase worldwide. Society will become even more technologically sophisticated, complex, and information driven (Postman, 1992). Organizing our daily life activities, managing time, finding satisfying work (Rifkin, 1995), and achieving valued goals will require even more advanced skills than do today's activities of "surfing the net" or balancing the social roles of worker and mother.

More sophisticated knowledge of the individual human who interacts with specific environments throughout the life span will reveal new resources of adaptation (Montgomery, 1984). For example, we will know more about how humans construct their nervous systems, psyches, and culture through their own purposeful actions in adapting to environmental challenges (Goldfield, 1995). Scientists will increasingly emphasize human individuality, contextual embeddedness, and the human need for mastery (Kagan, 1996). Health, rather than being defined as the absence of pathology, will be viewed as one's capability to achieve vital goals in specific environments through the use of a repertoire of skills (Pörn, 1993). Prevention of disease and injury and promotion of health as a qualitative, positive attribute will be a high priority.

Emphasis will be placed on the significance of the context of action to successful performance, for example, by studying people's activities in the environments in which they actually use their skills in practical en-

deavors (Lave, 1988). Health care systems will provide needed services in the home, work place, and communities in which people live and work.

Assumptions

First, our profession consists of four essential, integrated components that need to nurture one another if it is to go forward. From *practice* arise the questions and puzzles that are worth pursuing because they will generate new knowledge, enabling us to do a better job. Such questions are addressed in the realm of *ideas*. Models, theories or frames of reference that organize and synthesize new knowledge of occupation address the crucial questions from practice and suggest better interventions. These ideas are tested and refined in the crucible of *research*, which enables us to develop confidence in their usefulness to achieve our purposes. New ideas are transmitted back into the profession through *education* as students and practitioners interact with the profession's curriculum and literature. The fruitful interaction among these four components is vital to ensure our ability to progress (Yerxa, 1994).

Second, the crucial goals of occupational therapy are concerned with enduring, significant human needs for survival, challenge, contribution, and mastery. Occupational therapy is committed to improving the life opportunities, health, and capability of all people, including those with chronic impairments, by employing occupation as therapy, contributing new knowledge of occupation to society, and influencing public policy for people with impairments, disabilities, and handicaps.

Third, the profession is founded on values that have energized it for almost 100 years. These include:

- Endorsing the essential humanity of those we serve by seeking higher levels of life satisfaction for patient-agents,* including those with severe impairments;
- Maintaining and enhancing health by discovering and enhancing the healthy aspects of those we serve;
- Fostering self-directedness and responsibility of patient-agents;
- Maintaining a generalist, integrated, nonspecialist

---

*I use the term "patient-agent" for people served by occupational therapy in a medical context. It reminds me of our ethical obligation to help transmute patients into agents of their own intentions.

perspective of the human in interaction with his or her environment

- Utilizing a therapeutic relationship of mutual cooperation and shared authority;
- Viewing those we serve as actors on the environment, rather than passive reactors
- Possessing faith in the patient-agent's potential
- Emphasizing patient-agent productivity and participation in society
- Viewing play and leisure activities along with work and rest as necessary components of a balanced life
- Finally, seeking to understand the subjective experiences or the internal "world" of those we serve (Yerxa, 1983)

These optimistic values need to undergird our profession's goals, science, and future decisions.

Crucial Decisions

Achieving our potential depends on making thoughtful decisions in the present. These need to affirm occupational therapy's importance to society and commit us to a future-oriented perspective, rather than settling for what seems to be present "security" that may be purchased at the high price of reducing our profession to a set of techniques done *to* people, or losing our identity altogether. We might become, for example, hybrid "rehabilitation therapists" (O'Neill, 1993) because executives fail to see how we are different from other professions.

What should be our appropriate *knowledge* base for theory, research, education, and practice? Should it be centered on the natural and physical sciences, as are medicine and physical therapy? Or, should it include relevant medical knowledge, but also emphasize the multileveled, open human system engaged in occupation within multiple environments (occupational science)? Should our knowledge be examined for its consistency with our philosophy and values so that we can better assure its compatibility with practice? For example, focusing unduly on pathology may be incompatible with viewing all people as potentially healthy and resourceful.

What relation should occupational therapy seek with medicine, related professions, and other academic disciplines? Should we practice as members of an interdisciplinary medical hierarchy? Or should we be an autonomous profession and academic discipline that communicates with many professions and disciplines? This decision is significant in enabling occupational

therapists to practice in varied environments, with different groups, according to their needs. Conforming to other professions' often erroneous expectations, instead of defining our own scope of practice will, severely limit our potential to serve humankind (Yerxa, 1995).

Who should be responsible for developing our knowledge and thus defining our practice, occupational therapists or other disciplines? Our profession is beginning to emerge from a long-term "Kuhnian crisis" (Kuhn, 1970) concerning our relevant knowledge and the practice emanating from it. We lacked a consensual paradigm and were frustrated by medicine's failure to address the issue of chronicity. We are beginning to develop, synthesize, and transmit our own ideas. These often create refreshing new models of practice that meet pressing societal needs. For example, instead of delimiting our practice to the use of "physical modalities" in hospitals or clinics, we are helping people with chronic impairments develop independent-living skills, enabling them to manage their lives in satisfying ways in the real world of home and community (Jackson, Rankin, Siefkin, & Clark, 1989). We are learning more about how to develop such skills through creating a "just right" environmental challenge that helps people reclaim their resources (Montgomery, 1984). Developing our own knowledge of occupation, in all of its complexity, will enable us to practice more autonomously and to serve varied populations, such as infants at risk, new mothers, people who are unemployed, troubled adolescents, those with addictions, and other people who want to stay healthy and achieve a decent quality of life.

In an era of increasingly profit-driven, commercialized, "managed" health care, ethical decisions arise almost daily in practice and education. One dilemma is whether we will succumb to environmental pressures to reduce our practice to techniques that are "reimbursable." Or, will we practice according to the needs of patient-agents, advocating for them so that they may obtain what they need, including comprehensive occupational therapy, leading to mastery? The need to practice our profession competently, thoroughly, and thoughtfully is supported by studies showing that occupational therapists overutilize techniques such as exercise and range of motion because they do not "have time," nor do they "receive reimbursement" for developing independent living skills (Pendleton, 1989), talking with patient-agents or family members, or following up to facilitate independence in the human and community. Yet people with chronic impairments living in the community cite major unmet needs for skill development (Burnett & Yerxa, 1980). Will students learn to perceive people as complex, multileveled, whole human beings, who interact with complex environments by employing occupation, or will graduates adopt a specialized perspective, limited to physical or mental pathology, viewing people as "strokes," "bipolar mood disorders" or "traumatic hand injuries?" The latter course not only fragments the people we serve, but it necessarily leads to an overemphasis on sterile, repetitive technique, ignoring significant human needs related to occupation. For example, Robert Murphy (1990), a professor of anthropology, who developed a spinal cord tumor requiring rehabilitation, thought that the exercises he was supposed to do in occupational therapy were "silly." Yet, his vital goals of being able to manage his time, home, and transportation, and continue to work apparently were not addressed by his rehabilitation program.

One of the great strengths of occupational therapy education has been its insistence on preparing students to see people as whole and integrated and to prepare practitioners to deal with any threat to adaptation, be it in the nervous system, the culture, or the physical environment. Occupational therapists engaged in specialized, technical practice could eventually be supplanted by computers or robots (J. Jackson, personal communication, 1995). Yet, as Mary Reilly (1962) observed, the idea of occupational therapy is so vital to society that if the profession ceased to exist tomorrow, a new one soon would arise to take its place.

Potential Contributions

The era of chronicity, in which burgeoning populations of people with impairments try to adapt to the demands of a dizzingly complex world, could be answered by a new millennium of occupation. Through new knowledge of how people become competent and manage their environments, in spite of even severe degrees of impairment and challenge, those with chronic conditions could be helped to reclaim their resources and find their place in the culture. They could learn the skills for self-direction by doing things that are satisfying, worthwhile, and of interest, thereby achieving a goodness of fit with their environments. These occupational goals are not trivial because engagement in occupation, self-responsibility, and autonomy have been associated in several studies with survival, longevity, health, ability to cope effectively with stress, quality of life, and happiness (Langer & Rodin, 1976; Wright, 1983).

Through occupational therapy, which develops competence, people with impairments could be con-

nected with the mainstream of humanity. Consequently, social attitudes would change. Impairment no longer would be perceived as a barrier to full personhood or a "tragedy" that endlessly confers the sick role. Society would gain new appreciation of both the contributions of and satisfaction possible for people with impairments.

Occupational therapy could promote a new concept of health. It would be perceived as possession of a repertoire of skills that enables people to achieve their valued goals in their own environments (Pörn, 1993). People with chronic impairments could be seen as healthy and assured of "equality of capability" (Bickenbach, 1993), to have an environment and receive services that enable them to achieve their desired potential.

Occupational therapy practitioners could learn much more about how to help people develop the adaptive skills, rules, and habits that enable competence through creating a "just right challenge" from the environment to enable an adaptive response. Such "coaching" by occupational therapists could benefit all people who need to develop skills to survive, contribute, and achieve satisfaction in their daily life activities, whether or not they have impairments.

Occupational therapy practitioners could become visible and vocal allies and advocates for people with impairments, disabilities, and handicaps. We could influence social policy to create better life opportunities for such people because our values, optimism, and knowledge demand such action as a reification of our commitment.

Our profession could search vigorously for new knowledge of humans as individuals who are unique, whole, and authors of their lives through their occupations. The significance of engagement in occupation to the health and well-beingness of all humans could be a major area of investigation, as would the influences of varying degrees of environmental challenged on the development of competence and adaptation.

Occupational therapy practitioners who practice in medical environments would be better able to help transmute patients into agents. New knowledge would enable people to achieve higher levels of capability and skills, to achieve their goals, and to manage their own lives. Such new knowledge would support our autonomy in practice.

New models of practice could be developed and tested. Some of these might focus on the prevention of disability and handicap caused by impairment; development of capability across the life span; utilization of the play–work continuum to develop skills, rules, and habits; life organization, including management of one's environment and resources; the development of and nurturance of intrinsic motivation for occupation through the pursuit of one's unique interests; skill development to enable people to make necessary role transitions across the life span; restoration of healthy balances of work, rest, play, and sleep in individual lives; assessment of how to create the just right environmental challenge necessary to enable an adaptive response; and utilizing engagement in occupation to obtain a satisfying and healthy balance of ritual and novelty in one's daily round of activity (Klapp, 1986). The current limited concept of "activities of daily living" could be broadened to include all activities that individuals need and want to do to adapt to their unique environments, obtain personal satisfaction by their own action, and contribute to their cultures.

Challenges to Students

Dyson (1995) observed that many scientists make their most creative contributions when they are new to a field, but deeply immersed in its knowledge. Einstein was only 25 years of age when he published his revolutionary relativity theory, considered the pinnacle of his creativity. Students and other newcomers could contribute revolutionary new ideas to our profession if they are deeply immersed in its concepts and values and are audacious enough to perceive its issues and possibilities with fresh eyes, eschewing oversimplification and "recipes."

Some examples of areas that need to be better understood include environmental "affordances"; resources in the environment that create curiosity, act as attractors, or pose challenges demanding an adaptive response; "just right challenges," neither too difficult nor too easy, that lead to human action, skill development, and confidence in mastery; assessments of individual strengths and identification of personal and environmental resources that could be used, developed, and reclaimed to enable competence in spite of impairments; the significance of people's daily routines to survival, contribution, being in place in one's culture and life satisfaction; patterns of daily living that contribute to health and happiness; the relevance of the play–work continuum to the development of skills, habits, and rules, and its reconstitution in the face of impairment; discovery, development, and nurturance of interests and their relation to intrinsic motivation and capability; cultural differences and similarities in interests, skills, rules, and habits; "coaching" by the occupational therapist to elicit optimal performance and motivation; de-

velopment of competence, autonomy, and self-responsibility among people with impairments, or in danger of becoming social outsiders; and development of new practice environments that provide opportunities for patient-agent choice and self-direction.

Because the occupational therapy profession is founded on complex, vital ideas central to the human condition, it could contribute to society in significant ways. Students will need to become "infected" with the need to know much, much more (M. Reilly, personal communication, 1994), recognizing that understanding occupation and applying it in practice require lifelong study.

Our profession has almost limitless potential to create a significant influence on tomorrow's world. Realizing it will depend on several choices: How well will the profession recognize and nurture its four components of practice, ideas, research, and education? To what extent will today's decisions foster our ethical responsibility to patient-agents, develop our knowledge, further our autonomy and professional self-directedness, and enhance our generalist education and outlook.

To serve humankind well will require that we learn much more about people as agents, in their own environments, engaged in daily occupations. To learn what we need to know requires that we accept the challenge of becoming ardent students of life's daily activities and grapple with the ambiguity and complexity of occupation, the occupational human, and the contexts in which occupation takes place. Only then, will we fulfill our commitment to people with chronic impairments and assure that our humanistic values are reified in the practice of occupational therapy for a new millennium.

References

Bickenbach, J. (1993). *Physical disability and social policy.* Toronto: University of Toronto Press.

Burnett, S. & Yerxa, E. J. (1980). Community-based and college-based needs assessment of physically disabled persons. *American Journal of Occupational Therapy, 34,* 201–207

Dyson, F. (1995). The scientist as rebel. In J. Cornwell (Ed.), *Nature's imagination: The frontiers of scientific vision* (pp. 1–11). Oxford: Oxford University Press.

Goldfield, E. C. (1995). *Emergent forms: Origins and early development of human action and perception.* New York: Oxford University Press

Jackson, J., Rankin, A., Siefkin, S., & Clark, F. (1989). "Options": An occupational therapy transition program for adolescents with developmental disabilities. In J. A. Johnson & D. A. Ethridge (Eds.), *Developmental disabilities: A handbook for occupational therapists* (pp. 197–214). New York: Haworth Press.

Kagan, J. (1996, Jan. 12). Point of view: The misleading

abstractions of social scientists. *The Chronicle of Higher Education, XLII*, A52.

Klapp, O. (1986). *Overload and boredom: Essays on the quality of life in the information society.* New York: Greenwood Press.

Kuhn, T. S. (1970). *The structure of scientific revolutions.* Chicago: University of Chicago Press.

Langer, E. & Rodin, J. (1976). The effects of choice and enhanced personal responsibility for the aged: A field experiment in an institutional setting. *Journal of Personality and Social Psychology, 34*, 191–198

Lave, J. (1988). *Cognition in practice.* New York: Cambridge University Press.

Montgomery, M. (1984). Resources of adaptation for daily living: A classification with therapeutic implications for occupational therapy. *Occupational Therapy in Health Care, 1*, 9–23

Murphy, R. F. (1990). *The body silent.* New York: Norton.

O'Neill, E. H. (1993). *Health professions education for the future: Schools in service to the nation.* San Francisco, CA: PEW Health Professions Commission.

Pendleton, H. (1989). Occupational therapists' current use of independent living skills training for adult inpatients who are physically disabled. *Occupational Therapy in Health Care, 6*, 93–108.

Pörn, I. (1993). Health and adaptedness. *Theoretical Medicine, 14*, 295–303.

Postman, N. (1992). *Technopoly: The surrender of culture to technology.* New York: Alfred A. Knopf.

Reilly, M. (1962). Occupational therapy can be one of the great ideas of 20th century medicine. *American Journal of Occupational Therapy, 16*, 1–9.

Rifkin, J. (1995). *The end of work.* New York: G. P. Putnam's Sons.

Robinson, I. (1988). The rehabilitation of patients with long-term physical impairments: The social context of professional roles. *Clinical Rehabilitation, 2*, 339–347.

Wright, B. (1983). *Physical disability: A psychological approach* (2nd ed.). New York: Harper & Row.

Yerxa, E. J. (1983). Audacious values, the energy sources for occupational therapy practice. In G. Kielhofner (Ed.), *Health through occupation: Theory and practice in occupational therapy* (pp. 149–162). New York: F. A. Davis Co.

Yerxa, E. J. (1994). In search of good ideas for occupational therapy. *Scandinavian Journal of Occupational Therapy, 1*, 7–15.

Yerxa, E. J. (1995). Who is the keeper of occupational therapy's practice and knowledge? *American Journal of Occupational Therapy, 49*, 295–299.

Glossary

Accreditation Council of Occupational Therapy Education of the American Occupational Therapy Association (ACOTE) maintains standards and accredits occupational therapy educational programs

Acquired immune deficiency syndrome (AIDS) a chronic, debilitating disease of the immune system caused by HIV infection that results in health problems such as specific types of cancer, pneumonias, fungal and parasitic infections

Activities of daily living (ADL) self-maintenance tasks considered necessary for meeting the demands of daily living including such activities as bathing, dressing, grooming, oral hygiene, eating, taking medication, and communicating

Acute very severe or sharp, as in pain; disease or symptoms with rapid, severe onset

Americans With Disability Act (ADA) a federal civil rights law in the United States that addresses employment discrimination and reasonable accommodations within the work setting for people with disabilities

Adaptation making the tasks simpler or less physically demanding to promote independent function; changing in response to new demands or expectations

Adapt change task or environment demands to support performance

Adolescent Role Assessment (ARA) a semistructured interview procedure that gathers information in six areas: childhood play, socialization within the family, school functioning, socialization with peers, occupational choice, and anticipated adult work

Adult day care programs run for several hours a day that provide meaningful, structured activities to assist people with physical and/or cognitive disabilities to remain living at home as well as respite for primary care givers

Affect the emotional tone of an individual demonstrated by facial expression and voice inflection

Agnosia inability to recognize familiar objects in spite of intact sensory capacities

Alcoholism a chronic illness characterized by extreme dependence on alcohol and corresponding disturbances in the individual's family, social, and work life

Alter selecting a new context with demands that more closely matches the skills and abilities of a person with a disabling condition such as memory impairment, social withdrawal, apathy, and sleep disturbance

American Occupational Therapy Association (AOTA) the national professional association for occupational therapy with voluntary membership that represents and promotes the interests of persons who choose to become members

American Occupational Therapy Foundation (AOTF) a nonprofit organization dedicated to expanding and refining the knowledge base of occupational therapy. Provides support to research and education through grants and scholarships

Amputation surgical removal of a part of the body, typically all or part of a limb; may also be a congenital defect

Amyotrophic lateral sclerosis (ALS) a degenerative disease that destroys motor neurons in the cortex, brainstem, and spinal cord leading to weakness, muscle atrophy, and death

Anorexia nervosa self-induced starvation, often a chronic condition with medical and psychological components

Aphasia impairment of language. Receptive aphasia—the inability to understand spoken or written language; expressive aphasia—impairment in the use of verbal and written language

Apraxia inability to perform motor activities although sensory motor function is intact and the individual understands the requirements of the task

Arrhythmia irregular beating of the heart

Arterial pressure line (A-line or art line) catheter that is inserted into an artery, most commonly the radial artery in adults, to monitor blood pressure and provide blood gas measurements

Arthritis a common chronic condition of the joints that results in pain, loss of motion, deformity, and associated functional deficits

Arthroplasty surgical intervention to reconstruct or replace a damaged joint

Assessment specific tools or instruments used in the evaluation process

Assessment of Motor and Process Skills (AMPS) assessment used to examine the relationship between motor and process skills and task performance, to establish current level of task competence, and to predict performance in IADL; useful for treatment planning with children, adolescents, and adults with a variety of underlying impairments

Assessment of occupational functioning (AOF) a screening tool using the model of human occupation to assess the function of clients with physical or psychiatric disabilities

Association learning the mental linking between two events or activities so that the occurrence of one triggers initiation of the other

Asymmetrical tonic neck reflex (ATNR) stereotypical reflexive reaction elicited by turning the head, producing extension and abduction of the arm on the face side, with flexion and adduction of the arm on the skull side

Attention the cognitive ability to focus on a task, issue, or object

Attention deficit hyperactivity disorder (ADHD) a disorder characterized by inattention or attention deficit, overactivity, and impulsiveness

Autism a pervasive developmental disorder characterized by deficits in social interaction, communication; people with autism demonstrate restrictive and repetitive behavior

Automatic reactions ability to maintain balance and equilibrium during movement, (including righting and equilibrium reactions) to prevent falling

Automatic thoughts internal speech that involves errors in thinking and distortions

Baltimore Therapeutic Equipment Work Simulator (BTE) equipment to evaluate upper extremity performance by simulating work tasks using devices such as a knob, screwdriver, lever, and so on and measuring the amount of force produced during those simulations

Bilateral integration using both sides of the body in a coordinated manner during activity

Biomechanical frame of reference addresses problems such as diminished strength, endurance, range of motion, and structural stability

Biomedicine human being viewed as an organism made up of organ subsystems and physiological processes

Bipolar disorder also called manic depression; characterized by cycles of mania and depression persisting for at least a week or severe enough for hospitalization

Blood pressure (BP) the force exerted by the circulating blood against the walls of the arteries, veins, and chambers of the heart

Borderline personality disorder a personality disorder characterized by instability of thought, mood, and behavior; difficult relationships with others, poor self-esteem

Bradycardia abnormally slow heart rate, with a pulse less than 60 beats per minute

Bradypnea a slow respiratory rate

Bronchiectasis dilation of a bronchus or bronchi with secretion of large amounts of pus

Bulimia nervosa eating disorder consisting of binge eating followed by self-induced vomiting, or use of laxatives; excessive exercising or fasting to compensate for the binge

Canadian Occupational Performance Measure (COPM) client-centered semistructured interview procedure designed to measure a client's perceptions of his or her occupational performance over time

Cerebral palsy condition caused by damage to the brain, usually occurring before, during, or shortly after birth, with associated impairments that may include visual and auditory deficits, seizures, mental retardation, learning disabilities, and oral–motor and behavioral problems

Cerebrovascular accident (CVA) interruption of blood supply that causes injury to the brain resulting in neurological deficits in a specific area; also called stroke

Certification process of credentialing for practice as an OTR or COTA; National Board for Certification in Occupational Therapy (NBCOT) oversees this process

Certified occupational therapy assistant (COTA) graduate of the 2-year associate degree program in occupational therapy accredited by the ACOTE; individual must also pass the certification examination for occupational therapy assistants administered by NBCOT; works under the supervision of an OTR

Child abuse and neglect occurs when a person responsible for the care of the child injures, sexually abuses, neglects, or mistreats the child

Chronic bronchitis a pulmonary condition characterized by excessive mucous secretion in the bronchial tree, which leads to obstruction of airflow and mucous plugging, with persistent productive cough present for 3 months of 2 consecutive years

Chronic illness illness of long duration, showing little change or with slow progression that can lead to decline in functional ability

Chronic obstructive pulmonary disorder (COPD) a variety of pulmonary disorders including chronic bronchitis, asthma, emphysema, and bronchiectasis; implies irreversible airway damage

Chronic pain pain, often less intense than acute pain, which continues and recurs over a long period of time

Clinical reasoning complex multifaceted thought process used by practitioners to plan, direct, perform, and reflect on client care

Cognition ability to think and reason to solve problems

Cognitive behavior therapy approaches therapeutic change by changing ways of thinking, point of view, and interpretation of events

Cognitive disability frame of reference an approach to intervention that focuses on therapeutic interventions that match the demands of the activities to the person's current level of cognitive function for people with chronic mental disorders resulting in difficulty with reasoning and learning

Community mental health community programs that support people with chronic psychiatric illnesses to prevent decompensation and subsequent inpatient hospitalization

Compensation intervention that changes the task or adapts the objects or performance context to counteract a defect or functional problem

Concept construct or idea

Conduct disorder a repetitive and persistent pattern of behavior in which the basic rights of others or societal norms or rules are violated

Congestive heart failure (CHF) cardiac syndrome in which the heart fails to maintain an adequate blood output, causing decreased blood to the tissues and congestion in the pulmonary or the systemic circulation

Consultation a relationship in which a consultant brings expertise that will assist the consultee in reaching programmatic goals

Context consists of two aspects: temporal and environmental: temporal aspects—chronological, culture, developmental, life cycle, disability status; environmental aspects—physical, social, cultural

Contracture decrease in length of soft tissue that can lead to decreased joint motion

Coordination—fine smooth patterns of movement, typically of the upper extremity, such as those required for buttoning, tying, writing, or typing

Coordination—gross smooth patterns of movement, especially of large muscle groups, such as those required for running, walking, and so on

Correlational research examines the extent to which two or more phenomena tend to occur together

Create interventions that develop improved performance in a person's current context; circumstances that promote more adaptable or complex performance in context

Crepitus a grating sound caused by movement of ends of broken bones or by joint movement when cartilage covering bone ends is rough and pitted

Cumulative trauma disorders injuries to joints, muscles, tendons, or nerves due to activities that are of a repetitive nature, such as carpal tunnel syndrome caused by computer use

Delusions false ideas that may be fragmented and bizarre or organized and systematic

Dementias mental states with symptoms of memory impairment and abstract thinking that are severe enough to impair function in an individual who was previously unimpaired

Depression a mood disorder characterized by extreme sadness, feelings of hopelessness, worthlessness, and dejection that are pervasive and interfere with day-to-day activities; may also be used to describe feelings of sadness and despair of a more transient nature

Developmental delay a deficit in one or more of the following areas of development: cognitive, physical, communication, social or emotional, and adaptive or self-help skills

Developmental disabilities a group of chronic conditions including mental retardation, cerebral palsy, genetic and chromosomal anomalies, autism, learning disabilities, severe orthopedic impairments, visual and hearing impairments, serious emotional disturbances, and traumatic brain injury

Diagnostic and Statistical Manual of Mental Disorders, 4th **Edition (DSM-IV)** guide for the diagnosis of psychiatric conditions, includes diagnostic criteria, symptoms, prevalence, and course

Dignity valuing the inherent worth and uniqueness of each person as demonstrated by an attitude of empathy and respect for self and others

Disability inability to engage in self-care, work, and play or leisure as a result of an impairment (mental or physical)

Disease a disorder with signs and symptoms indicating abnormality of function of the organism

Documentation written reports (evaluations, progress notes, reports to management) recording occupational therapy services and departmental activities to others

Early intervention programs family-focused programs that address the developmental, educational, and social needs of children to the age of 3 who have a disability or developmental delay

Ecological systems analysis a model that presents behavior as the result of interactions between an individual with an inherent biopsychosocial makeup and a given environmental system

Ecology of human performance (EHP) a framework that emphasizes that the ecology, or the interaction between a person and the context, affects human behavior and task performance

Electroconvulsive therapy (ECT) a brief convulsion induced by electrical stimulation; used to treat acute depression

Empathy an attitude exemplified by an understanding of and identification with the feelings and perspective of another person

Emphysema pulmonary disease that causes the destruction of the walls of the bronchioles and alveoli, resulting in abnormally enlarged air spaces and impaired breathing

Endurance the ability to continue an activity over time

Environment physical (geography, buildings, objects) and social (people, culture, surroundings)

Equity the belief that all individuals are equal and that being treated equally is a right

Ergonomics study of work, most especially of the physical demands placed on workers

Establish and restore a therapeutic intervention from the EHP that focuses on improving skills so that individuals can function more effectively within their context

Evaluation a process of gathering information to identify the problems experienced by an individual, at the beginning, during treatment, and at discharge; may involve use of observation, interview, nonstandardized, and standardized assessment instruments.

Executive functions the ability to organize, problem solve, and engage in independent behavior

Explanatory models personal accounts of illness, held by both practitioners and professionals, that describe the nature and origins of the problem and what can be done about it

Family-centered care care enacted through the collaborative efforts of family members and practitioners and typically provided through multidisciplinary and interdisciplinary team structures

Fiduciary a person who stands in a special relation of trust, confidence, or obligation to another

Flow state of deep concentration in which consciousness is well ordered; elements present are a feeling of control, loss of self-consciousness, transformation of time, and concentration on the task at hand

Frame of reference set of interrelated internally consistent concepts, definitions, postulates, and principles that provide a systematic description of and prescription for a practitioner's interaction with clients

Functional capacity evaluation an evaluation designed to identify an individual's current capacity relative to the ability to do work related tasks; includes Physical Capacity Evaluation, ADI, and work simulation activities

Functional Independence Measure (FIM) measures disability associated with physical impairments and provides a mechanism for standardizing data collection nationwide for clients in medical rehabilitation

General adaptation response response to stress that includes three stages: alarm, adaptive, and exhaustion.

Generalization the spontaneous ability to transfer what is learned in one situation to a different situation

General systems theory sees the person and environment as interdependent while they interact in the system of input, throughput, and output

Grading sequentially increasing or decreasing the demands of an activity over time to stimulate improvement in the client's function or respond to diminishing functional capacity

Group dynamics relationships between members of the group, with the leader, and the task of the group

Guillain-Barré syndrome a peripheral nerve disorder characterized by an acute inflammation of multiple nerves, leading to rapid progressive muscular weakness, potential paralysis, and sensory disturbances or loss

Habits automatic behavior that is integrated into more complex patterns that enable people to function on a day-to-day basis; skills that are habituated are typically performed easily and with little effort

Halfway house a program, typically for people with chronic mental illness, which creates a therapeutic milieu to enable people to leave the hospital and reenter the community

Hallucination a false perception having no relation to reality and not accounted for by any exterior stimuli

Handicap inability to perform role-related responsibilities secondary to an impairment or disability and is often the result of inadequate access to health care or inaccessible environments

Health behaviors positive (exercise, regular meals, and so on) and negative (alcohol use, drug abuse, smoking, and so on) behaviors that have been shown to influence health

Health maintenance organizations (HMO) both insurers and providers of care; consumers pay a flat fee to the HMO to cover all services and then must receive those services from HMO providers.

Hemianopsia impaired vision or blindness in half the visual field

Hip spica cast a cast that immobilizes the trunk and hip, used to correct hip deformities and fractures

Human immunodeficiency virus (HIV) the retrovirus that causes AIDS

Holter monitor small recording unit that stores a client's electrocardiogram (ECG) tracings from surface electrodes for a preprogrammed time period

Hospice program that provides care to enhance the quality of life for people who are dying and for their families; provides pain-control strategies, health care services, and increased client autonomy until death

Hypertension (high blood pressure) blood pressure consistently greater than 140/90 mm Hg

Hypertonia high muscle tone that results in slow, difficult movements, requiring excessive effort

Hypertrophic scars connective tissue (formed to fill in a wound) that rises above the skin surface; initially, the areas appear thick, rigid, and congested with blood; scars across joints can limit range of motion (ROM) and function

Hypotension (low blood pressure) blood pressure consistently less than 90/60 mm Hg

Hypotonia low muscle tone that interferes with the balance between stability and mobility required for almost all movement, especially antigravity movement

Illness impairment of an individual's capacity to function on a day-to-day basis secondary to a disease process; also refers to the perspective of the individual versus the perspective of the physician

Illness experience the meaning an individual attaches to an illness, may vary from one person to another with the same diagnosis

Impairment loss or abnormality of physical or psychological structure or functions

Individual education plan (IEP) a plan developed by the school placement team to support the learning of a child with a disability that has an effect on school performance

Instrumental activities of daily living (IADL) activities such as telephone use, shopping, food preparation, housekeeping, medication management, financial management, and getting around one's community

Interdisciplinary team a type of team in which members share responsibility for providing services; team members conduct separate evaluations, but share the results to develop an integrated care plan

Interest checklists self-report measures generally used to determine a client's level of interest in a range of activities

International Classification of Impairments, Disabilities, and Handicaps (ICIDH) classification system that provides a uniform language for documentation of services and assists in tracking outcomes.

Intervention strategies designed to improve the occupational performance of individuals; may involve direct services by occupational therapy practitioners with clients and indirect service as consultation with individuals and groups

Interview a communication process between interviewer and interviewee involving questions and answers; a reciprocal or shared process of discovery

Isometric muscle contraction increase in tension of the muscle fibers without change in length (ie, movement does not occur)

Job description written statement to identify, define, and describe a position; clarifies the role of the position within the organization

Job site analysis examination of the physical demands of the job site including the relationship between equipment and the worker, the steps involved in the tasks of the job, and the physical demands of these tasks

Joint protection techniques designed to minimize stress to joints damaged by arthritis or other musculoskeletal conditions

Kohlman Evaluation of Living Skills (KELS) designed to aid in discharge planning for clients with psychiatric diagnoses by evaluating the ability to live independently and safely in the community

Learned helplessness a belief held by an individual that efforts he or she makes will not be effective in making any change or improvement

Learning disability a chronic condition of neurological origin that interferes with the development, integration, and use of verbal and nonverbal abilities

Leisure activities driven by internal motivation, implies freedom of choice, is not usually done within time constraints

License state regulation that controls the right to practice; many states have licensure laws that regulate occupational therapy practice; all require certification by NBCOT

Life cycle phase refers to the involvement of the person in social roles and life tasks that are common for persons of that age and social status in the culture in which the individual lives

Liminal the period of time between one status and another; typically occurs during rites of passage

Lower motor neuron lesions area of injury within the cell body or axon of nerves that innervate or synapse with the muscle fibers; characterized by a loss of voluntary muscle control and loss of the reflex arc with a consequent decrease in muscle tone

Major depressive disorder severe depression that is present almost all of every day for at least 2 weeks; there is a noticeable change in person's usual mood, evidenced through sadness, and a loss of pleasure in almost everything

Major life events normative (eg, marriage, bereavement, job change) and nonnormative (war, natural disasters) that create stress and may influence health status

Managed care programs that seek to control the patients' use of physicians and other health care providers and services; managed care systems integrate financing and delivery of health care services

Measurement process of assigning numbers to represent quantities of a trait, attribute, or characteristic; or to classify objects that enable therapists to quantify aspects of people, but not people themselves

Medicaid government program in the United States to provide health care for people with limited incomes; states administer the program with matching funds from the federal government

Medicare government program in the United States to provide health care coverage for persons 65 years and older; people on kidney dialysis; and people receiving social security due to disabilities (SSDI)

Memory the ability to register, retain, and recall past experience, knowledge, and sensation

Meningitis inflammation of the membranes of the brain and spinal cord, usually caused by infection

Mental retardation general term used to describe a lifelong developmental disability marked by intellectual and functional skills deficits

Mental status examination formal procedure to examine and diagnose mental functioning, including a general description of a person, notation of emotional expression, identification of perceptual disturbances, and exploration of thought processes and thought content

Metabolic equivalent tables (MET) a measure of oxygen requirements for various activities, one MET is equivalent to an oxygen uptake of 3.5 milliliters per kilogram body weight per minute

Metacognition the ability to think about thinking

Model of human occupation model that incorporates a systems view of the human being, emphasizing that behavior is dynamic and context-dependent, and that occupation is essential to human self-organization

Motor learning acquiring and modifying motor behavior

Motor planning the ability to carry out a skilled, nonhabitual motor activity

Multicultural competence knowledge and attitudes indicating awareness of our own cultural embeddedness and sensitivity to the values of people from other cultures

Multidisciplinary team team approach with members working together in clearly defined roles with specific areas of responsibility; evaluation, planning and therapy take place independently

Multiple sclerosis (MS) progressive disease characterized by a demyelinization or destruction of the myelin sheath that covers the nerve fibers within the central nervous system (brain and spinal cord)

Muscle strength the ability to produce movement or to resist an external force

Muscle tone resistance to stretch or mild contraction of muscle at rest

Myasthenia gravis (MG) progressive, degenerative muscle disease that occurs at the site of the myoneural junction, resulting in muscle weakness from the decrease in the numbers of receptors for neurotransmitters

Myocardial infarction heart attack; damage to the heart muscle from loss of blood supply secondary to atherosclerosis or an embolus

National Board for Certification in Occupational Therapy (NBCOT) independent credentialing agency for occupational therapy practitioners

Neonatal intensive care unit (NICU) a hospital unit designed to care for premature infants

Neoplasm abnormal proliferation of cells, as a tumor or growth

Neural tube defect spinal bifida; spine is cleft or split because the vertebrae do not enclose the spinal cord during the first trimester of pregnancy, resulting in abnormal development of the meninges, nerves, and vertebrae

Neurodevelopmental treatment (NDT) treatment approach used with people with cerebral palsy and cerebrovascular accidents to inhibit abnormal patterns, normalize muscle tone, and foster the normal movement patterns

Occupation the daily activities typical for a culture that form a pattern of activity

Occupational behavior involves interaction with the environment in a range of activities that are consistent with the social roles filled by an individual

Occupational Case Analysis Interview and Rating Scale a semistructured interview based on the model of human occupation for use in short-term adult psychiatric settings

Occupational Performance History Interview a semistructured interview for use with adolescent, adult, and geriatric clients with both physical and psychiatric diagnoses designed to gather information about a client's occupational performance

Occupational Questionnaire a paper-and-pencil measure that gathers data on time use patterns and feelings about time use

Occupational role roles consist of behavioral expectations that fit with an individual's position or status in the social system (eg, student, parent, cub scout)

Occupational science the study of the form, function, and meaning of human occupation

Occupational therapist (OTR) a graduate of an accredited occupational therapy program, who has completed fieldwork, and passed the certification examination administered by NBCOT; also referred to as certified occupational therapist or registered occupational therapist

Occupational Therapy aide an individual assigned by a certified occupational therapist to perform delegated, selected, skilled tasks in specific situations under intense close supervision of occupational therapy practitioners

Occupational Therapy Code of Ethics describes professional conduct for occupational therapy practitioners (OTRs and COTAs)

Occupational therapy practitioners graduates of accredited occupational therapy and occupational therapy assistant programs who meet certification and state licensure requirements; referred to as registered or certified occupational therapist (OTR) and certified occupational therapy assistant (COTA)

Omnibus Budget Reconciliation Acts (OBRA) of 1987 and 1990 federal regulations in the United States that assure the individual rights, autonomy, and quality of life of nursing home residents

Opportunistic infection a disease that generally occurs only in an individual who has lowered immune system resistance, as in someone with HIV, diabetes mellitus, or cancer

Orientation awareness of self in relation to time, place, and identification of others

Orthopedics concerned with the dysfunction of bones, joints, and their related structures: muscles, tendons, ligaments, and nerves

Orthotics the making and fitting of orthopedic appliances

Osteoarthritis degenerative joint disease (DJD), a progressive localized joint disease affecting the joints of the fingers, elbows, hips, knees, and ankles; results in limitation of motion and formation of bony outgrowths at the affected joints

Osteogenesis imperfecta a genetic disease that results in brittle, osteoporotic bones that fracture easily

Oximeter a noninvasive instrument that measures the percentage of hemoglobin saturated with oxygen

Pain discomfort caused by noxious stimulation to the sensory nerve endings; pain is subjective and varies from one individual to another, it is an important diagnostic symptom

Paralysis loss or impairment of motor or sensory function of body part caused by injury to central or peripheral nervous system tissue

Parkinson disease neurological symptom complex characterized by rigidity, tremor, akinesia, and loss of spontaneous and automatic movement

Perception mental process by which intellectual, sensory, and emotional data are organized meaningfully; the process of conscious recognition and interpretation of sensory stimuli

Performance areas activities of daily living, work and productive activity, and play and leisure activities

Performance Assessment of Self-Care Skills (PASS) a criterion-referenced instrument designed to evaluate the independent-living skills of adults

Performance components skills used to engage in daily activities—sensorimotor, cognitive integrative and cognitive, psychosocial skills, and psychological

Performance contexts temporal and environmental factors that influence an individual's engagement in desired or required activities related to activities of daily living, work, and leisure

Perseveration unnecessary and prolonged repetition of a word, phrase, or movement

Phantom limb pain pain (tingling, gripping, clenching, burning, or cramping) that is perceived by the amputee as occurring in the amputated limb

Phenomenology study of consciously reported experiences

Physical Capacity Evaluation (PCE) assesses the physical and biomechanical aspects of the client's level of function, including active range of motion, muscle strength, posture, gait, sensation, and cardiopulmonary status

Physical environment nonhuman aspects of the environment, such as the landscape, buildings, furniture, objects, or tools

PL 94-142 1975 The Education for All Handicapped Children Act mandates free and appropriate education in the least restrictive environment for all children with "handicaps," ages 5 through 21 years in the United States

PL 99-457 amended EHA in 1986 created programs for preschoolers (3 to 5 years) with handicaps, including early intervention for infants and toddlers (birth to 2 years) in the United States

PL 101-476 1990 Individuals with Disabilities Education Act (IDEA) reauthorization of educational services for children with disabilities from 3 to 21 years in the United States; the IEP may include transition and assistive technology services

PL 102-119 The IDEA Amendments reauthorized early intervention; established Federal Interagency Coordinating Council in the United States

Play and leisure activities intrinsically motivating activities that provide pleasure, relaxation, and expression of creativity

Population a group from which a sample is drawn for research or statistical purposes

Posttraumatic amnesia (PTA) a state of confusion or disorientation with no awareness of time or place following a traumatic brain injury; may include severe inattention, restlessness or lethargy and uninhibited behavior

Practice theory theory that provides guidance to practitioners relative to occupational therapy goals and interventions; also called frame of reference

Preferred provider organization (PPO) a form of managed care by a network of providers who compete to provide services to members of an existing group (such as an employed group receiving care from an HMO) for a fixed monthly fee

Press expectation or demands from the physical and social environment

Prevent therapeutic interventions designed to prevent the occurrence or evolution of barriers to performance may address person, context, or task variables

Progressive relaxation a stress management technique involving alternately tensing and relaxing muscle groups

Protective sensation sensory awareness of pain or temperature that alerts individuals to the potential for injury

Psychometrics the process by which psychological and intelligence tests are developed, administered, and interpreted

Pulse the rhythmical dilation of arteries, produced by the blood being pumped into the arteries by the contractions of the heart; indicates heart rate

Range of motion (ROM) the arc through which a joint moves

Rapport conscious, harmonious accord or relationship between people

Reasonable accommodation modifications to a work site, schedule, or job functions to enable a qualified person with a disability to continue to work; these accommodations must not present a financial hardship to the employer

Reflex automatic response of an organism to a specific event in the environment

Reinforcement strengthening a response by using a stimulus immediately after the response (may be positive or negative)

Reliability a characteristic of a test or measurement in which the same results occur with repeated trials; the measure is consistent

Remediation intervention designed to restore clients to previous functional level by addressing performance component deficits (eg, strength, endurance, short-term memory)

Remission abatement or lessening of symptoms of a disease

Representational learning development of an internal image of an event or task so that an action or a series of actions can be repeated without reference to directions

Respiratory rate the number of breaths a person takes per minute, 12–22 breaths per minute is typical for adults

Rheumatoid arthritis (RA) a progressive systemic disease characterized by remissions and exacerbations of destructive inflammation of connective tissue, particularly synovial membranes in synovial joints; results in limitations in range of motion and deformity

Righting reactions reflexes that through various receptors in the labyrinth, eyes, muscles, or skin tend to bring an organism's body into its normal position in space and that resist any force acting to put it into a false position (eg, on its back)

Role Activity Performance Scale a semistructured interview for use with adult psychiatric patients that focuses specifically on role functioning

Roles give people scripts to behave in ways consistent with their social roles, such as student, worker, or parent

Schizophrenia a group of related psychotic disorders that produce disturbed thought processes, leading to difficulties with communication, interpersonal relationships, and reality testing

Scoliosis lateral curvature of the spine

Screening a cursory evaluation to determine if a more intensive evaluation is needed

Self-Assessment of Occupational Functioning (SAOF) a self-report measure designed to gather data on a person's perception of his or her strengths and weaknesses relative to occupational functioning

Self-care activities that individuals engage in on their own behalf to maintain their health and well-being such as eating, bathing, and dressing

Self-report measures Surveys, forms, and checklists that the client completes on his or her own

Sensation the transmission to the brain of nerve impulses caused by stimulation of a sensory receptor site; results in awareness of this stimulation

Sensibility ability to perceive, appreciate, and transmit nerve impulses

Sensory integration the organization of sensation to form perceptions, behaviors, and to learn; a neurological process and a theory of the relationship between the neural organization of sensory processing and behavior

Sensory reeducation a combination of techniques used to teach people with peripheral nerve injuries how to interpret and make functional use of abnormal sensory feedback from regenerated nerves

Service competency the ability to use the identified intervention in a safe and effective manner

Spasticity excessive tone in a muscle, typically caused by an upper motor neuron lesion

Spina bifida a neural tube defect in which the spine is cleft or split because the vertebrae (bones of the spinal column) do not enclose the spinal cord during the first trimester of pregnancy; this results in abnormal development of the meninges, nerves, and vertebrae and leads to paralysis and other developmental problems

Spinal cord injury any traumatic event that causes damage to the spinal cord leading to loss (complete or partial) of function below the level of the injury

Standardized tests instruments that have established and tested norms

Static splint splint with no moving parts; maintains a joint in desired position

Stereognosis perception and identification of the form and nature of an object through the sense of touch

Stress physical, emotional, or intellectual strain or tension disturbing normal equilibrium

Stroke lay terminology for a cerebrovascular accident

Subluxation incomplete or partial dislocation of a joint

Substance abuse impairment secondary to the use of drugs, alcohol, or other substance, that leads to failure in meeting social role obligations or to legal problems

Substance dependence physiological dependence and tolerance to substances that leads to withdrawal symptoms; people with substance dependence also have difficulty meeting social role obligations and may have legal problems

Sundowning increased confusion or disorientation that occurs at the end of the day; typically seen in people with Alzheimer's disease or other dementias

Supervision a dynamic, interactive process in which the supervisor assists in and directs the work and growth of the supervisee

Symptom magnification exaggerated complaints of pain

and functional limitation; may occur with people who have work-related injuries

Synergies combinations or correlated actions of different organs of the body, as of muscles working together

Tachycardia abnormally fast heart rate—a pulse greater than 100 beats per minute

Tactile pertaining to touch

Tactile defensiveness quality of being unable to tolerate touch; resistive to and uncomfortable with certain kinds of touch

Tactile localization ability to determine the location of a cutaneous stimulus

Task-oriented group group whose focus is on reaching a goal, finding a solution to a problem, or making a product

Tenodesis biomechanical effect related to muscles that pass over multiple joints; the position of one joint affects muscle tension over other joints, eg, in the wrist and hand wrist extension accentuates finger flexion

Total hip replacement (THR) surgical removal of the head of the femur and the acetabulum and replacement with metal and plastic components; used for people with severe arthritis or other degenerative hip disease

Tracheostomy surgical formation of an opening into the trachea and suturing of the edges to the skin in the neck for an airway or passage of a tube

Transfer of learning the ability to use something that has been learned in a different situation; also known as generalization

Trauma injury as a result of physical or emotional means or insult

Traumatic brain injury (TBI) damage to the brain as a result of a car accident, fall, gunshot wound or other trauma

Treatment interaction between an occupational therapy practitioner and client directed toward achieving client-centered goals relative to enhanced occupational performance

Tremor alternate contraction and relaxation of opposing groups of muscles resulting in involuntary rhythmic and oscillating movements, such as quivering or trembling

Uniform Terminology a standard terminology developed by AOTA to facilitate use of consistent language for documentation, reimbursement, management, and research

Unilateral inattention also called unilateral neglect, the lack of awareness of stimuli presented to the side opposite the cerebral lesion in individuals who do not have primary sensory or motor impairments

Universal precautions infection control procedures used to prevent transmission of HIV and other infections to others; involves washing hands after each contact with a patient, and the use of protection in the form of gloves, masks, and goggles when contact with body fluids such as blood, urine, or feces, is anticipated

Upper motor neuron lesions area of injury within the central nervous system (cortex and spinal cord) resulting in loss of voluntary muscle control and a loss of inhibition on reflexive movement causing hyperreflexia; results in spasticity or excess muscle tone in the affected muscle

Validity a psychometric property that is concerned with the capacity of the measurement instrument to measure what it is supposed to measure

Values beliefs and commitments that define what is good, right, and important

Vestibular system structures of the inner ear associated with balance and position sense

Visual accommodation ability to focus on an object at varying distances

Visual perception cognitive process of obtaining and interpreting visual information from the environment; includes discrimination, memory, spatial relationships, form constancy, sequential memory, figure-ground, and closure

Vital signs pulse rate, respiration rate, and body temperature

Work and productive activities activities that enable people to contribute to society; to support themselves and others dependent on them through work-related activities, and to manage day-to-day activities such as shopping and cleaning

Work conditioning a program to develop the strength and endurance necessary to return to work, may include strengthening, flexibility, cardiovascular exercises, as well as activities involving lifting, pushing, or pulling

Work hardening therapeutic program that moves the worker from a submaximal level of performance to a level adequate for entry or reentry into the work force

Work simplification performance of a task in an organized, planned, and orderly way, so that body motions, work load, and fatigue are reduced to a minimum

Worker Role Interview (WRI) semistructured interview designed for injured workers regarding psychosocial and environmental factors related to work, such as personal causation, values, interests, roles, and so forth

Workers' compensation federal legislation in the United States that provides temporary income for injured workers and encourages employers to take some responsibility for the safety of their employees

Appendix A

Core Values and Attitudes of Occupational Therapy Practice

INTRODUCTION

In 1985, the American Occupational Therapy Association (AOTA) funded the Professional and Technical Role Analysis Study (PATRA). This study had two purposes: to delineate the entry-level practice of OTRs and COTAs through a role analysis and to conduct a task inventory of what practitioners actually do. Knowledge, skills, and attitude statements were to be developed to provide a basis for the role analysis. The PATRA study completed the knowledge and skills statements. The Executive Board subsequently charged the Standards and Ethics Commission (SEC) to develop a statement that would describe the attitudes and values that undergird the profession of occupational therapy. The SEC wrote this document for use by AOTA members.

The list of terms used in this statement was originally constructed by the American Association of Colleges of Nursing (AACN) (1986). The PATRA committee analyzed the knowledge statements that the committee had written and selected those terms from the AACN list that best identified the values and attitudes of our profession. This list of terms was then forwarded to SEC by the PATRA Committee to use as the basis for the Core Values and Attitudes paper.

The development of this document is predicated on the assumption that the values of occupational therapy are evident in the official documents of the American Occupational Therapy Association. The official documents that were examined are: (a) *Dictionary Definition of Occupational Therapy* (AOTA, 1986), (b) *The Philosophical Base of Occupational Therapy* (AOTA, 1979), (c) *Essentials and Guidelines for an Accredited Educational Program for the Occupational Therapist* (AOTA, 1991a), (d) *Essentials and Guidelines for an Accredited Educational Program for the Occupational Therapy Assistant* (AOTA, 1991b), and (e) *Occupational Therapy Code of Ethics* (AOTA, 1988). It is further assumed that these documents are representative of the values and beliefs reflected in other occupational therapy literature.

A *value* is defined as a belief or an ideal to which an individual is committed. Values are an important part of the base or foundation of a profession. Ideally, these values are embraced by all members of the profession and are reflected in the members' interactions with those persons receiving services, colleagues, and the society at large. Values have a central role in a profession

and are developed and reinforced throughout an individual's life as a student and as a professional.

Actions and attitudes reflect the values of the individual. An attitude is the disposition to respond positively or negatively toward an object, person, concept, or situation. Thus, there is an assumption that all professional actions and interactions are rooted in certain core values and beliefs.

SEVEN CORE CONCEPTS

In this document, the *core values and attitudes* of occupational therapy are organized around seven basic concepts—altruism, equality, freedom, justice, dignity, truth, and prudence. How these core values and attitudes are expressed and implemented by occupational therapy practitioners may vary depending upon the environments and situations in which professional activity occurs.

Altruism is the unselfish concern for the welfare of others. This concept is reflected in actions and attitudes of commitment, caring, dedication, responsiveness, and understanding.

Equality requires that all individuals be perceived as having the same fundamental human rights and opportunities. This value is demonstrated by an attitude of fairness and impartiality. We believe that we should respect all individuals, keeping in mind that they may have values, beliefs, or life-styles that are different from our own. Equality is practiced in the broad professional arena, but is particularly important in day-to-day interactions with those individuals receiving occupational therapy services.

Freedom allows the individual to exercise choice and to demonstrate independence, initiative, and self-direction. There is a need for all individuals to find a balance between autonomy and societal membership that is reflected in the choice of various patterns of interdependence with the human and nonhuman environment. We believe that individuals are internally and externally motivated toward action in a continuous process of adaptation throughout the life span. Purposeful activity plays a major role in developing and exercising self-direction, initiative, interdependence, and relatedness to the world. Activities verify the individual's ability to adapt, and they establish a satisfying balance between autonomy and societal membership. As professionals, we affirm the freedom of choice for each individual to pursue goals that have personal and social meaning.

Justice places value on the upholding of such moral and legal principles as fairness, equity, truthfulness, and objectivity. This means we aspire to provide occupational therapy services for all individuals who are in need of these services and that we will maintain a goal-directed and objective relationship with all those served. Practitioners must be knowledgeable about and have respect for the legal rights of individuals receiving occupational therapy services. In addition, the occupational therapy practitioner must understand and abide by the local, state, and federal laws governing professional practice.

Dignity emphasizes the importance of valuing the inherent worth and uniqueness of each person. This value is demonstrated by an attitude of empathy and respect for self and others. We believe that each individual is a unique combination of biologic endowment, sociocultural heritage, and life experiences. We view human beings holistically, respecting the unique interaction of the mind, body, and physical and social environment. We believe that dignity is nurtured and grows from the sense of competence and self-worth that is integrally linked to the person's ability to perform valued and relevant activities. In occupational therapy we emphasize the importance of dignity by helping the individual build on his or her unique attributes and resources.

Truth requires that we be faithful to facts and reality. Truthfulness or veracity is demonstrated by being accountable, honest, forthright, accurate, and authentic in our attitudes and actions. There is an obligation to be truthful with ourselves, those who receive services, colleagues, and society. One way that this is exhibited is through maintaining and upgrading professional competence. This happens, in part, through an unfaltering commitment to inquiry and learning, to self-understanding, and to the development of an interpersonal competence.

Prudence is the ability to govern and discipline oneself through the use of reason. To be prudent is to value judiciousness, discretion, vigilance, moderation, care, and circumspection in the management of one's affairs, to temper extremes, make judgments, and respond on the basis of intelligent reflection and rational thought.

SUMMARY

Beliefs and values are those intrinsic concepts that underlie the core of the profession and the professional interactions of each practitioner. These values describe the profession's philosophy and provide the basis for defining purpose. The emphasis or priority that is given to each value may change as one's profes-

sional career evolves and as the unique characteristics of a situation unfold. This evolution of values is developmental in nature. Although we have basic values that cannot be violated, the degree to which certain values will take priority at a given time is influenced by the specifics of a situation and the environment in which it occurs. In one instance dignity may be a higher priority than truth; in another prudence may be chosen over freedom. As we process information and make decisions, the weight of the values that we hold may change. The practitioner faces dilemmas because of conflicting values and is required to engage in thoughtful deliberation to determine where the priority lies in a given situation.

The challenge for us all is to know our values, be able to make reasoned choices in situations of conflict, and be able to clearly articulate and defend our choices. At the same time, it is important that all members of the profession be committed to a set of common values. This mutual commitment to a set of beliefs and principles that govern our practice can provide a basis for clarifying expectations between the recipient and the provider of services. Shared values empowers the profession and, in addition, builds trust among ourselves and with others.

REFERENCES

American Association of Colleges of Nursing. (1986). *Essentials of College and University Education for Professional Nursing. Final report.* Washington, DC: Author.

American Occupational Therapy Association. (1986, April). *Dictionary definition of occupational therapy.* Adopted and approved by the Representative Assembly to fulfill Resolution #596-83. (Available from AOTA, 1383 Piccard Drive, PO Box 1725, Rockville, MD 20849–1725.)

American Occupational Therapy Association. (1988). Occupational therapy code of ethics. *American Journal of Occupational Therapy, 42,* 795–796.

American Occupational Therapy Association (1991a). Essentials and guidelines for an accredited educational program for the occupational therapist. *American Journal of Occupational Therapy, 45,* 1077–1084.

American Occupational Therapy Association. (1991b). Essentials and guidelines for an accredited educational program for the occupational therapy assistant. *American Journal of Occupational Therapy, 45,* 1085–1092.

American Occupational Therapy Association. (1979). The philosophical base of occupational therapy. *American Journal of Occupational Therapy, 33,* 785.

Prepared by Elizabeth Kanny, MA, OTR, for the Standards and Ethics Commission (Ruth A. Hansen, PhD, OTR, FAOTA, Chairperson). Approved by the Representative Assembly June 1993.

Occupational Therapy Code of Ethics

T he American Occupational Therapy Association's *Code of Ethics* is a public statement of the values and principles used in promoting and maintaining high standards of behavior in occupational therapy. The American Occupational Therapy Association and its members are committed to furthering people's ability to function within their total environment. To this end, occupational therapy personnel provide services for individuals in any stage of health and illness, to institutions, to other professionals and colleagues, to students, and to the general public.

The *Occupational Therapy Code of Ethics* is a set of principles that applies to occupational therapy personnel at all levels. The roles of practitioner (registered occupational therapist and certified occupational therapy assistant), educator, fieldwork educator, supervisor, administrator, consultant, fieldwork coordinator, faculty program director, researcher–scholar, entrepreneur, student, support staff member, and occupational therapy aide are assumed.

Any action that is in violation of the spirit and purpose of this Code shall be considered unethical. To ensure compliance with the Code, enforcement procedures are established and maintained by the Commission on Standards and Ethics. Acceptance of membership in the American Occupational Therapy Association commits members to adherence to the *Code of Ethics* and its enforcement procedures.

PRINCIPLE 1.
Occupational Therapy Personnel Shall Demonstrate a Concern for the Well-Being of the Recipients of Their Services (Beneficence).

A. Occupational therapy personnel shall provide services in an equitable manner for all individuals.
B. Occupational therapy personnel shall maintain relationships that do not exploit the recipient of services sexually, physically, emotionally, financially, socially or in any other manner. Occupational therapy personnel shall avoid those relationships or activities that interfere with professional judgment and objectivity.
C. Occupational therapy personnel shall take all reasonable precautions to avoid harm to the recipient of services or to his or her property.

From *American Journal of Occupational Therapy, 48,* 1037–1038. Copyright © 1994, American Occupational Therapy Association, Inc. Reprinted with Permission.

D. Occupational therapy personnel shall strive to ensure that fees are fair, reasonable, and commensurate with the service performed and are set with due regard for the service recipient's ability to pay.

PRINCIPLE 2.
Occupational Therapy Personnel Shall Respect the Rights of the Recipients of Their Services (Autonomy, Privacy, Confidentiality).

A. Occupational therapy personnel shall collaborate with service recipients or their surrogate(s) in determining goals and priorities throughout the intervention process.
B. Occupational therapy personnel shall fully inform the service recipients of the nature, risks, and potential outcomes of any interventions.
C. Occupational therapy personnel shall obtain informed consent from subjects involved in research activities indicating they have been fully advised of the potential risks and outcomes.
D. Occupational therapy personnel shall respect the individual's right to refuse professional services or involvement in research or educational activities.
E. Occupational therapy personnel shall protect the confidential nature of information gained from educational, practice, research, and investigational activities.

PRINCIPLE 3.
Occupational Therapy Personnel Shall Achieve and Continually Maintain High Standards of Competence (Duties).

A. Occupational therapy practitioners shall hold the appropriate national and state credentials for providing services.
B. Occupational therapy personnel shall use procedures that conform to the Standards of Practice of the American Occupational Therapy Association.
C. Occupational therapy personnel shall take responsibility for maintaining competence by participating in professional development and educational activities.
D. Occupational therapy personnel shall perform their duties on the basis of accurate and current information.
E. Occupational therapy practitioners shall protect service recipients by ensuring that duties assumed by or assigned to other occupational therapy personnel are commensurate with their qualifications and experience.
F. Occupational therapy practitioners shall provide appropri-

ate supervision to individuals for whom the practitioners have supervisory responsibility.

G. Occupational therapists shall refer recipients to other service providers or consult with other service providers when additional knowledge and expertise are required.

PRINCIPLE 4.
Occupational Therapy Personnel Shall Comply with Laws and Association Policies Guiding the Profession of Occupational Therapy (Justice).

A. Occupational therapy personnel shall understand and abide by applicable Association policies; local, state, and federal laws; and institutional rules.

B. Occupational therapy personnel shall inform employers, employees, and colleagues about those laws and Association policies that apply to the profession of occupational therapy.

C. Occupational therapy practitioners shall require those they supervise in occupational therapy related activities to adhere to the Code of Ethics.

D. Occupational therapy personnel shall accurately record and report all information related to professional activities.

PRINCIPLE 5.
Occupational Therapy Personnel Shall Provide Accurate Information About Occupational Therapy Services (Veracity).

A. Occupational therapy personnel shall accurately represent their qualifications, education, experience, training, and competence.

B. Occupational therapy personnel shall disclose any affiliations that may pose a conflict of interest.

C. Occupational therapy personnel shall refrain from using or participating in the use of any form of communication that contains false, fraudulent, deceptive, or unfair statements or claims.

PRINCIPLE 6.
Occupational Therapy Personnel Shall Treat Colleagues and Other Professionals with Fairness, Discretion, and Integrity (Fidelity, Veracity).

A. Occupational therapy personnel shall safeguard confidential information about colleagues and staff members.

B. Occupational therapy personnel shall accurately represent the qualifications, views, contributions, and findings of colleagues.

C. Occupational therapy personnel shall report any breaches of the Code of Ethics to the appropriate authority.

Prepared by the Commission on Standards and Ethics (SEC) (Ruth Hansen, PhD, OTR, FAOTA, Chairperson).

Approved by the Representative Assembly April 1977.

Revised 1979, 1988, 1994.

Adopted by the Representative Assembly July 1994.

This document replaces the 1988 Occupational Therapy Code of Ethics (*American Journal of Occupational Therapy, 42,* 795–796), which was rescinded by the 1994 Representative Assembly.

Occupational Therapy Roles

This document is a guide to major roles common in the profession of occupational therapy. It is intended to assist the practitioner in identifying career options and developing career paths. *Practitioner* refers to anyone who is certified by the American Occupational Therapy Certification Board (AOTCB) as an occupational therapist (OTR) or an occupational therapy assistant (COTA). Practitioners work in a variety of systems including health care, educational, academic, governmental, social, corporate, and industrial settings. This document can be a resource for planning career ladders, developing job descriptions, and suggesting educational content for formal and continuing education programs.

Roles listed in this document are those frequently held by certified practitioners and are not all inclusive. The nature of the experience as an occupational therapy practitioner prepares individuals for other specialized roles (e.g., activity director, case manager, rehabilitation coordinator, dean). Roles described in this document are valued equally. Although different roles may vary in their scope and in the experience required to perform them, each role fulfills a specific function within the profession and contributes to the profession's growth, development and strength.

An individual's employment setting, method of service delivery, performance competence, and career goals are all interdependent and result in an individualized composite of roles during actual job performance. In this document, roles are not exclusive because jobs performed by practitioners may include aspects of more than one role. For example, an occupational therapist may have a job that includes practitioner and fieldwork educator roles. Another individual may function as a faculty member, researcher, and consultant.

Career progression involves advancement within roles as well as transition to different roles. When transitioning occurs, practitioners need to have demonstrated performance potential and appropriate educational preparation for the new role. Individuals entering into a new role typically require closer supervision and will begin at a relatively lower level of expertise than in their other roles. Preparation for new roles often involves self-reflection, continuing or advanced education, and acquisition of experience and skills required for the new role. The development of a mentoring relationship assists in understanding the context in which role performance will occur. For example, an individual who is an advanced-level administrator in a practice setting may move into an entry-level faculty role in an academic setting. Preparation for this transition may include acquiring appropriate academic degrees; understanding the educational environment; and demonstrating potential for teaching, scholarly activity, and professional service.

ROLE DESCRIPTIONS

Each role in this document consists of the following components: major function, scope of role, performance areas, qualifications, and supervision. These components are described as follows:

Major function: Describes the primary purpose(s) of the role.

Scope of role: Delineates the range of responsibility and complexity that typically occurs within the role.

Key performance areas: Specifies common activities and expectations associated with role function. Performance that occurs within each area is built upon the unique philosophy and perspective of occupational therapy. Practitioners are expected to take personal responsibility for functioning within the ethical code and standards of the profession. Specific knowledge, skills, and attitudes fundamental for performance are beyond the scope of this document.

Individuals develop varying degrees of expertise in role performance. Levels of expertise are those skills that are fundamental to the entry level, those skills that are intermediate, or those skills that require a high degree of proficiency. These three levels describe the professional development process for each role and are described in Table C-1. Progression within a role through the three levels of professional development is based on accumulation of higher level skills through experience, education, guided self-development, and professional socialization. Progression is not simply the amount of time in a role. Each person progresses along this continuum at an individualized pace. Some individuals may remain at one level for the duration of their career and not everyone progresses to the advanced level. An individual may function in more than one role simultaneously. When this occurs, it is possible to function at different levels within each role. For example, a new faculty member may be at an entry level in teaching, though at an advanced level in clinical practice. All roles described in this document build on the performance expectations of the Practitioner–OTR and Practitioner–COTA, as this is the entry point into the profession. Consequently, the entry-level performance areas are considered to be an inherent part of all other roles described in this document.

Supervision: Describes the typical oversight required or recommended for individuals at the various levels of role performance. The amount of supervision required is closely linked to both the role and the level of expertise in a role. The supervision recommended is intended to be a collaborative relation-

Table C-1 Levels of Role Performance

Level	Major Foci	Supervision
Entry	-The development of skills. -Socialization in the expectations related to the organization, peers, and the profession. Acceptance of responsibilities and accountability in role-relevant professional activities is expected.	Close
Intermediate	-Increased independence. -Mastery of basic role functions. -Ability to respond to situations based on previous experience. -Participation in the education of personnel. Specialization is frequently initiated, along with increased responsibility for collaboration with other disciplines and related organizations. Participation in role-relevant professional activities is increased.	Routine or general
Advanced	-Refinement of specialized skills. -Understanding of complex issues affecting role functions. Contribution to the knowledge base and growth of the profession results in being seen as an expert, resource person, or consultant within a role. This expertise is recognized by others within and outside the profession through leadership, mentoring, research, education, and volunteerism.	Minimal

ship that serves to promote quality service and the professional development of the individuals involved. All COTAs will require more than a minimal level of supervision by an OTR when providing services. Formal supervision occurs along a continuum including close, routine, general, and minimal. Refer to Table C-2 for descriptions of these levels.

In addition to formal supervision, individuals may provide or receive functional supervision. Functional supervision implies the provision of information and feedback to coworkers. Individuals who provide functional supervision have specialized knowledge as a result of their own experience and expertise. On the basis of this specialized knowledge or skill, the individual supervises peers relative to this expertise in a particular function. For example, a fieldwork educator may provide functional supervision to coworkers who are supervising students, although he or she is not responsible for evaluating the overall performance of the other therapists.

Qualifications: Lists the critical credentials, education, and work experience necessary as a prerequisite to adequate role performance. Qualifications are listed in a range to reflect changing expectations associated with higher levels of role functioning. As all roles are within the profession, professional certification as a practitioner is a consistent requirement. Additionally, all practitioners are expected to meet state and federal regulatory mandates, adhere to relevant Association policies, and participate in continuing professional development.

PRACTITIONER–OTR

Major Function

Provide quality occupational therapy services, including assessment, intervention, program planning and implementation, discharge planning–related documentation, and communication. Service provision may include direct, monitored, and consultative approaches.

Scope of Role

OTR practitioners advance along a continuum from entry to advanced level based on experience, education, and practice skills. The OTR has the ultimate responsibility for service provision (AOTA, 1990, p. 1093).

Table C-2 Types of Formal Supervision

Type	Description
Close	Daily, direct contact at the site of work.
Routine	Direct contact at least every 2 weeks at the site of work, with interim supervision occurring by other methods such as telephone or written communication.
General	At least monthly direct contact, with supervision available as needed by other methods.
Minimal	Provided only on a need basis, and may be less than monthly.

Key Performance Areas

Entry-level skills

- Responds to requests for service and initiates referrals when appropriate.
- Screens individuals to determine the need for intervention.
- Evaluates individuals to obtain and interpret data necessary for planning intervention and for intervention.
- Interprets evaluation findings to appropriate individuals.
- Develops and coordinates intervention plans, including goals and methods to achieve stated goals.
- Implements the intervention plan directly or in collaboration with others.
- Adapts environment, tools, materials, and activities according to the needs of the individual and his or her social cultural context.
- Monitors the individual's response to intervention and modifies plan as needed.
- Communicates and collaborates with other team members, individuals, family members, or caregivers.
- Follows policies and procedures required in the setting.
- Develops appropriate home and community programming to support performance in natural environment.
- Terminates services when maximum benefit is received and formulates discontinuation and follow-up plans.
- Documents services as required.
- Maintains records required by practice setting, third-party payers, and regulatory agencies.
- Performs continuous quality improvement activities and program evaluation using predetermined criteria.
- Provides inservice education to team members and the community.
- Maintains treatment area, equipment, and supply inventory.
- Identifies and pursues own professional growth and development.
- Schedules and prioritizes own workload.
- Participates in professional and community activities.
- Monitors own performance and identifies supervisory needs.
- Functions according to the AOTA *Code of Ethics* (AOTA, 1988) and *Standards of Practice* (AOTA, 1992) of the profession.

Intermediate skills

- Supervises/teaches occupational therapy practitioners, students, and other staff performing supportive services and/or other aspects of service provision.
- Assists other practitioners in the development of professional skills.
- Participates in committees and activities of larger systems in the development of service operations, policies, and procedures.
- Participates in the fieldwork education process.
- Critically examines own practice and integrates new knowledge.

High-proficiency skills

- Performs advanced, specialized evaluations or interventions.
- Develops protocols and procedures for intervention programs based on current occupational therapy theory and practice.

- Provides expert consultation to practitioners and outside groups about area of expertise.

Qualifications

- Certified by the American Occupational Therapy Certification Board (AOTCB) as an OTR.
- Meets state regulatory requirements.
- Progressive levels of expertise will require one or more of the following: work experience, self-study, continuing education, special certification, or postprofessional education.

Supervision

Practice supervision must be performed by an experienced OTR. Administrative supervision is determined by individual settings and may or may not be performed by an OTR.

- Entry-level Practitioners—OTRs in a particular practice area will require close supervision for service delivery aspects and routine supervision for administrative aspects (AOTA, 1981).
- Intermediate Practitioners—OTRs require routine to general supervision from advanced practitioners.
- Advanced Practitioners—OTRs require minimal supervision within area of expertise and general supervision for administrative aspects.

PRACTITIONER–COTA

Major Function

Provides quality occupational therapy services to assigned individuals under the supervision of an OTR.

Scope of Role

COTA practitioners advance along a continuum from entry to advanced level, based on experience, education, and practice skills. Development along this continuum is dependent on the development of service competency. The OTR has ultimate overall responsibility for service provision (AOTA, 1990, p. 1093).

Key Performance Areas

Entry-level skills

- Responds to request for services in accordance with service agency's policies and procedures.
- Assists with data collection and evaluation under the supervision of an OTR.
- Develops treatment goals under the supervision of an OTR.
- Implements and coordinates intervention plan under the supervision of an OTR.
- Provides direct service that follows a documented routine and accepted procedure under the supervision of an OTR.
- Adapts intervention environment, tools, materials, and activities according to the needs of the individual and his or her sociocultural context under the supervision of an OTR.
- Communicates and interacts with other team members and the individual's family or caregivers in collaboration with an OTR.

- Monitors own performance and identifies supervisory needs.
- Follows policies and procedures required in a setting.
- Performs continuous quality improvement activities or program evaluation in collaboration with an OTR.
- Maintains treatment area, equipment, and supply inventory as required.
- Identifies and pursues own professional growth and development.
- Maintains records and documentation required by work settings under the supervision of an OTR.
- Participates in professional and community activities.
- Functions according to the AOTA Code of Ethics (AOTA, 1988) and Standards of Practice (AOTA, 1992) of the profession.

Intermediate skills
- Schedules and prioritizes own workload.
- Supervises volunteers, COTAs, OTA students, and personnel other than OT practitioners under the direction of an OTR.
- Participates in development of policies and procedures in collaboration with an OTR.
- Participates in the fieldwork education process under the direction of an OTR.
- Selects, adapts, and implements intervention under the supervision of an OTR.
- Administers standardized tests under the supervision of an OTR after service competency has been established.
- Modifies treatment approaches to reflect changing needs under the supervision of an OTR.
- Formulates discontinuation and follow-up plans under the supervision of an OTR.
- Participates in organizational activities and committees.

High-proficiency skills
- Serves as a resource person to the agency in areas of specific expertise.
- Educates others in the area of established service competency under the supervision of an OTR.
- Contributes to program planning and development in collaboration with an OTR.

Qualifications
- Certification by the AOTCB as a COTA.
- Meets state regulatory requirements.
- Progressive levels of expertise will require one or more of the following: work experience, self-study, continuing education, and formal education including advanced degrees.

Supervision

COTAs at all levels require at least general supervision by an OTR. The level of supervision is related to the ability of the COTA to safely and effectively provide those interventions delegated by an OTR. Typically, entry-level COTAs and COTAs new to a particular practice environment will require close supervision, intermediate-level practitioners routine supervision, and advanced-level practitioners general supervision. COTAs will require closer supervision for interventions that are more complex or evaluative in nature and for areas in which service competencies have not been developed. Service competency is the ability to use the identified intervention in a safe and effective manner.

EDUCATOR (CONSUMER, PEER)

Major Function

Develops and provides educational offerings or training related to occupational therapy to consumer, peer, and community individuals or groups.

Scope of Role

Practitioners advance along a continuum of providing informal education to individuals and small groups in the course of service provision, to developing and providing comprehensive educational programs targeted to consumers and peers. At entry level of role, education typically occurs with peers and consumers within the individual's own service system (e.g., patient education, department, or school district inservice). At higher levels of expertise, provision of educational offerings may involve individuals or groups from multiple systems (e.g., provision of injury-prevention programs to industry, caregiver education programs to community, and continuing education seminars).

Key Performance Areas

Entry-level skills
- Implements strategies to assist individual learner to identify own learning needs.
- Develops or collaborates with individual learner in developing learning objectives.
- Implements educational methods designed to support learner's objectives.
- Responds to feedback about the teaching-learning process, and modifies own educational strategies to support learning.
- Supports the evaluation of educational effectiveness.
- Monitors own performance and identifies own development needs.
- Functions according to the AOTA Code of Ethics (AOTA, 1988) and Standards of Practice (AOTA, 1992) of the profession.

Intermediate skills
- Selects or designs strategies to identify individual learner needs.
- Develops program plans and materials for formal program offerings (e.g., conference presentations, workshops, seminars).
- Uses a variety of teaching-learning methods appropriate to the learning objectives and learner needs.

High-proficiency skills
- Evaluates strategies to identify learning needs of individuals and groups.
- Develops program plans and educational methods for extended or multiple program offerings.

- Designs evaluation strategies to assess impact of educational programs.

Qualifications
- Certification by AOTCB as an OTR or a COTA.
- Progressive levels of expertise will require combinations of the following: self-study, continuing education, experience, and post–entry-level formal education.
- Appropriate level of practice or service expertise is necessary as it relates to provision of these education services.

Supervision

Supervision depends on the nature of the project and the skills of the educator. COTAs at all levels usually will require OTR supervision for educational activities that occur related to occupational therapy consumers.

FIELDWORK EDUCATOR (PRACTICE SETTING)

Major Function

Manages Level I or II fieldwork in a practice setting. Provides occupational therapy or occupational therapy assistant students with opportunities to practice and carry out practitioner competencies.

Scope of Role

The fieldwork educator role may range from supervision of an individual student to full responsibility for an entire fieldwork program.

Key Performance Areas

Entry-level skills
- Establishes, mediates, and supports relationships between practice-based and academic personnel.
- Initiates and maintains communication and correspondence between the practice and academic settings.
- Schedules students in collaboration with the academic fieldwork coordinator.
- Provides orientation for student to fieldwork site including policies, procedures, and student responsibilities.
- Facilitates student learning activities to achieve desired student competence.
- Facilitates student's clinical reasoning and reflective practice.
- Evaluates student performance throughout fieldwork.
- Provides the student with both formative and cumulative feedback and supervision.
- Ensures student's integration of professional standards and ethics into practice.
- Ensures students' compliance with agencies' standards, goals, and objectives.
- Attends meetings, programs, or continuing education related to fieldwork education.
- Develops learning objectives for fieldwork in collaboration with academic institution(s) and consistent with current student fieldwork evaluation(s).

- Functions according to the AOTA *Code of Ethics* (AOTA, 1988), and *Standards of Practice* (AOTA, 1992) of the profession.

Intermediate skills
- Provides functional supervision to OTRs and COTAs specific to their roles as student fieldwork supervisors.
- Facilitates assignment of students to appropriate practitioners for supervision.
- Counsels or arbitrates students' concerns.
- Oversees the administrative aspects of the fieldwork program, including the formal agreement with academic programs.
- Conducts ongoing fieldwork program evaluations and monitors changes in program.
- Organizes or participates in appropriate fieldwork education support groups (e.g., local fieldwork councils, Commission on Education).
- Coordinates continuing education and inservice opportunities to develop staff fieldwork education skills.

High-proficiency skills
- Participates at leadership level in appropriate fieldwork groups.
- Facilitates the development of clinical fieldwork programs and related student supervision skills.
- Contributes to student learning by modeling leadership in professional organizations and facilitating student involvement.

Qualifications
- Certified by AOTCB as an OTR or a COTA.
- Meets appropriate state regulatory requirements.
- Continuing education regarding fieldwork education and supervision.
- Entry-level OTRs and COTAs may supervise Level I fieldwork students.
- OTRs with 1 year of practice-based experience may supervise OT and OTA Level II fieldwork students.
- COTAs with 1 year of practice-based experience may supervise OTA Level II fieldwork students.
- Three years of experience are recommended for individuals overseeing programs involving multiple student supervisors and multiple students.

Supervision

Supervision provided by an administrator or specifically designated individual. Level of supervision varies with skills of educator, complexity of setting, and nature of student's learning needs.

SUPERVISOR

Major Function(s)

Manages the overall daily operation of occupational therapy services in a defined practice area(s).

Scope of Role

The supervisor is involved in managing other occupational therapy practitioners, personnel, and volunteers in a defined practice setting or program.

Key Performance Areas

Entry-level skills

- Assists in selection, orientation, and training of staff, students, and volunteers.
- Promotes professional growth through staff development.
- Coordinates scheduling of work assignments.
- Evaluates, monitors, and provides feedback regarding job performance of assigned staff.
- Assists in establishment, implementation, and evaluation of agency goals and objectives.
- Monitors and facilitates staff compliance with established standards and guidelines.
- Provides for acquisition, care, and maintenance of physical facilities, supplies, and equipment.
- Oversees implementation of continuous quality improvement activities.
- Represents personnel, fiscal, professional, and program needs to occupational therapy administrator.
- Functions according to the AOTA *Code of Ethics* (AOTA, 1988) and *Standards of Practice* (AOTA, 1992) of the profession.

Intermediate skills

- Develops, implements, and monitors department policies and procedures in collaboration with occupational therapy administrator.
- Coordinates specific activities for department or service unit.
- Facilitates collaboration among occupational therapy and non–occupational therapy personnel and administrators.

High-proficiency skills

- Serves as liaison to specialty program coordinators and administrators.

Qualifications

- Certified by AOTCB as an OTR or COTA.
- Meets appropriate state regulatory requirements.
- Two to 3 years of practice experience in service area prior to supervising others are recommended.
- One year of experience is recommended prior to supervising a COTA. Experienced COTAs may supervise other COTAs administratively, as long as service protocols and documentation are supervised by an OTR.
- Continuing or postprofessional education relevant to supervisory function.

Supervision

Routine to minimal supervision provided by the occupational therapy administrator. Supervision ranges from routine to minimal, depending on the experience and expertise of the supervisor. Consultation from more advanced practitioners should be available as needed.

ADMINISTRATOR (PRACTICE SETTING)

Major Function

Manages department, program, services, or agency providing occupational therapy services.

Scope of Role

This role encompasses those individuals who organize and manage occupational therapy service units.

Key Performance Areas

Entry-level skills

- Plans, develops, and monitors occupational therapy services to ensure quality service.
- Achieves service unit goals and objectives through allocation of resources.
- Recruits and hires employees.
- Conducts performance evaluation and staff development activities.
- Establishes policies and standard operating procedures.
- Formulates and manages budget.
- Maintains effective information management systems.
- Assures safe work environments, procedures, and methods.
- Develops and monitors reimbursement processes to support services.
- Monitors the acquisition and maintenance of supplies, equipment, and facilities.
- Develops and supervises a continuous quality improvement program.
- Ensures compliance with accreditation, certification, and government standards.
- Advocates for appropriate use of occupational therapy services.
- Oversees fieldwork education process.
- Functions according to the AOTA *Code of Ethics* (AOTA, 1988) and *Standards of Practice* (AOTA, 1992) of the profession.

Intermediate skills

- Establishes a long-range plan for staff recruitment, development, and retention.
- Collaborates with other administrators within the organization to develop and manage organizational systems.
- Collaborates with others outside of the organization regarding pertinent administrative management issues.
- Participates at a leadership level in professional, community organizations.

High-proficiency skills

- Participates in organizational strategic planning and establishes strategic plan for assigned areas.
- Develops and implements marketing strategies for assigned areas.
- Facilitates development of systems supporting clinical research.
- Assumes leadership role within the organization and in interorganizational projects.

Qualifications

- Certification by AOTCB as an OTR.
- Meets appropriate state regulatory requirements.
- Graduate degree or continuing education relevant to management.
- Recommended experience varies with size and scope of department; a minimum of 3 years experience is preferred for small programs and 5 or more years for larger programs.

Supervision

General supervision by administrative personnel within the organization is required. Individuals with fewer than 3 years of experience should have access to an occupational therapy management consultant. Consultation from more advanced practitioners should be available as needed.

CONSULTANT

Major Function

Provides occupational therapy consultation to individuals, groups, or organizations.

Scope of Role

Consultative services may take place within the case, colleague, or systems model. Consultation may relate to practice, education, administration, or research.

Key Performance Areas

Entry-level skills
- Communicates scope of professional expertise.
- Assists consumers in identifying problems to be addressed in the consultative process.
- Collaborates with consumers in developing appropriate consultation outcomes.
- Develops recommendations that are relevant within the cultural context of the consumers' environment.
- Assists consumers in developing and implementing interventions, or identifying alternate resources necessary to obtain consumer objectives.
- Complies with applicable local, state, and federal laws and regulations.
- Functions according to the AOTA *Code of Ethics* (AOTA, 1988) and *Standards of Practice* (AOTA, 1992) of the profession.

Intermediate skills
- Assesses quality of own consultative efforts and identifies own continuing professional development needs.

High-proficiency skills
- Participates at a leadership level in professional, community organizations.

Qualifications
- Certified by AOTCB as an OTR or COTA.
- Meets appropriate state regulatory requirements.
- Intermediate or advanced practice level.
- Recommend minimum of 6 months experience for case consultation, 1 year for colleague consultation, and 3 to 5 years for systems consultation.

Supervision

Practitioners are expected to function as consultants within the scope of practice appropriate to their level of competence. The OTR functioning as a consultant is responsible for obtaining supervision when needed to meet regulatory and professional standards. The COTA functioning as a consultant is expected to seek the appropriate level of OTR supervision to meet regulatory and professional standards.

FIELDWORK COORDINATOR (ACADEMIC SETTING)

Major Function

Manages student fieldwork program within the academic setting.

Scope of Role

The fieldwork coordinator role may be decentralized among the faculty or may be managed entirely by one individual. This encompasses all fieldwork experiences required by a curriculum.

Key Performance Areas

Entry-level skills
- Identifies and secures sites for fieldwork education.
- Reviews the quality and appropriateness of fieldwork sites in collaboration with other academic faculty.
- Develops fieldwork objectives in collaboration with the fieldwork sites.
- Initiates and maintains communication and correspondence between the academic and fieldwork sites.
- Communicates with fieldwork educators regarding the curriculum model, course content, and fieldwork expectations.
- Oversees the administrative aspects of the fieldwork program including agreements with fieldwork sites.
- Assigns students to fieldwork settings.
- Orients students to responsibilities and protocol for fieldwork.
- Maintains communication with fieldwork educators and students during fieldwork.
- Monitors the facilitation of clinical reasoning and reflective practice in Level II fieldwork settings.
- Counsels and arbitrates with students and fieldwork educators on matters of concern.
- Collaborates with the fieldwork educator in assigning the final appraisal (grading) of the student.
- Supports research.
- Functions according to the AOTA *Code of Ethics* (AOTA, 1988) and *Standards of Practice* (AOTA, 1992) of the profession.
- Participates in appropriate fieldwork educational support groups (e.g., local fieldwork councils, Commission on Education).

Intermediate skills
- Provides educational opportunities to prepare and enhance fieldwork educators' knowledge and skills.
- Coordinates continuing education pertaining to fieldwork education processes for clinical fieldwork educators.
- Participates actively in professional, volunteer organizations.
- Supervises support personnel carrying out administrative aspects of fieldwork.

High-proficiency skills
- Participates at leadership level in appropriate fieldwork group.
- Facilitates the development of fieldwork programs and related student supervision skills.

Qualifications
- Certified by AOTCB as an OTR or COTA.
- Three years of practice experience and experience in supervising and advising fieldwork students are recommended.

Supervision

General supervision by academic administrator who is usually the program director. Close to routine supervision for new faculty.

FACULTY

Major Function

Provides formal academic education for occupational therapy or occupational therapy assistant students.

Scope of Role

This role varies among institutions and the subsequent balance expected between teaching, service, and scholarly activities. Progression within this role typically advances from lecturer and instructor to the professorial ranks, including assistant, associate, full, and emeritus professorships. Included in the faculty role may be adjunct, clinical, or academic appointments.

Key Performance Areas

Entry-level skills
- Develops educational course objectives and sequences the content to promote optimal learning.
- Designs and structures effective educational experiences, including methods, media, content areas, and types of student interactions.
- Facilitates students' learning through lectures, discussions, practical and laboratory exercises, or practice-related experiences.
- Evaluates and addresses student learning needs within their social and cultural environmental context.
- Reviews educational media and published resources and selects class readings or supplemental materials.
- Plans and prepares course materials to include course syllabi, lectures, case studies, teaching/learning handouts, and questions for group discussion.
- Prepares evaluation materials and measures student attainment of stated course objectives.
- Develops and maintains proficiency in teaching areas through investigation, formal education, continuing education, or practice.
- Participates in curriculum development.
- Participates in teaching evaluation and uses outcome data to modify teaching.
- Advises students and student groups.

- Serves on department, school, college, or university committees.
- Assists with designated departmental administrative tasks such as student admissions, recruitment, and course scheduling.
- Maintains students' records according to regulations and procedures.
- Functions according to AOTA *Code of Ethics* (AOTA, 1988) and *Standards of Practice* (AOTA, 1992) of the profession.
- Engages in service to the university or community.

Intermediate skills
- Prepares innovative curriculum or instructional methods.
- Evaluates and incorporates emerging research findings and technology into teaching and research.
- Participates in research and scholarly activities.
- Collaborates in the preparation of academic reports and accreditation self-studies.
- Participates actively in professional organizations.

High-proficiency skills
- Provides expert consultation to practitioners, educators, and outside groups about area of expertise.
- Chairs or leads groups or organizations outside the department.
- Mentors students through scholarly investigation process to develop student skills in research.
- Mentors other faculty in the development of their teaching, research, and practice skills.

Qualifications
- Certified by AOTCB as an OTR or COTA.
- For OTR, in professional programs, a doctoral degree is preferred (a master's degree is recommended).
- In technical programs, a master's degree is preferred (a bachelor's degree is recommended).
- Intermediate to advanced skills in primary area of teaching.
- Skills as a classroom instructor and understanding of the educational system.

Supervision

General supervision by academic program director and other appropriate academic administrators. Close to routine supervision by academic program directors for new, adjunct, and part-time faculty.

PROGRAM DIRECTOR (ACADEMIC SETTING)

Major Function

Manages the occupational therapy educational program.

Scope of Role

The program director's role varies depending on the level of the program (e.g., technical, professional, or postprofessional level) and the demands of the academic setting (e.g., technical school, community college, college, university, or health sciences center). The academic program director facilitates the education of competent graduates through faculty development and supervision and effective program management. Dependent on their academic environment, program directors may oversee both academic and practice-related activities, externally funded projects, and continuing education programs.

Key Performance Areas

Entry-level skills

- Oversees student recruitment, selection, evaluation, advisement, retention, and professional development.
- Oversees institutional and professional accreditation activities and reports.
- Manages faculty recruitment, development, evaluation, and retention.
- Assigns and monitors faculty and staff responsibilities.
- Ensures the quality of the program.
- Formulates and implements a fiscal plan.
- Represents the program to university administrators and negotiates for the needs of the program.
- Fosters an academic climate that facilitates faculty, student, and staff learning and professional growth.
- Promotes effective instructional techniques for faculty.
- Oversees student and faculty rights and responsibilities.
- Produces narrative and data-based reports for internal and external communication.
- Facilitates library acquisitions of resources for teaching and research.
- Fosters beneficial relationships among faculty and practitioners.
- Functions according to the AOTA *Code of Ethics* (AOTA, 1988) and *Standards of Practice* (AOTA, 1992) of the profession.

Intermediate skills

- Develops and implements long-range or strategic plans.
- Produces scholarly work.
- Facilitates the development of useful information management systems.
- Participates at the leadership level in professional and community organizations.

High-proficiency skills

- Leads in the acquisition of externally-funded projects.
- Designs and implements marketing for program enhancement.
- Promotes central theme within the occupational therapy programs that contributes to the knowledge base of the profession.

Qualifications

Technical-Level Program Director

- An OTR with a bachelor's degree (a master's degree is preferred) who is certified by AOTCB.
- Recommend 3 years professional practice with experience supervising COTAs.
- Recommend 3 years experience as a faculty member.
- Experience or continuing education in academic management.

Professional-Level Program Director

- An OTR with a master's degree (a doctoral degree is preferred) who is certified by AOTCB.
- Recommend 5 years experience in practice.
- Recommend 5 years experience as a faculty member.
- Experience or continuing education in academic management.

Post-Professional-Level Program Director

- An OTR with a doctoral degree who is certified by AOTCB.
- Recommend 5 years experience in practice.
- Recommend 5 years experience as a faculty member.
- Experience or continuing education in academic management.
- Intermediate to advanced competence as a researcher/scholar.

Supervision

General to minimal administrative supervision from designated administrative officer. Individuals with fewer than 3 years experience shall have access to occupational therapy education and accreditation consultants.

RESEARCHER/SCHOLAR

Major Function

Performs scholarly work of the profession including examining, developing, refining, and evaluating the profession's body of knowledge, theoretical base, and philosophical foundations.

Scope of Role

The role of the researcher ranges from the individual who critically examines and interprets empirical studies to independent investigator. The scholar is an individual who has in-depth knowledge and who engages in examination, development, or refinement of the profession's body of knowledge.

Key Performance Areas

Entry-level skills

- Promotes and engages in research/scholarly activities.
- Reads, interprets, and applies scholarly information relative to occupational therapy.
- Collects research data.
- Assumes responsibility for the ethical concerns in research and complies with institutional bio-ethics committee protocols.
- Functions according to the AOTA *Code of Ethics* (AOTA, 1988) and the *Standards of Practice* (AOTA, 1992) of the profession.

Intermediate skills

- Directs the completion of studies, including data analysis, interpretation, and dissemination of results.
- Collaborates with others to facilitate studies of concern to the profession.

- Monitors resources which facilitate research and scholarly activities.

High-proficiency skills
- Probes methods of science, theoretical information, or research designs to answer questions important to the profession.
- Conceptualizes the body of knowledge in the profession to develop new theories, frames of reference, or models of practice.
- Mentors novice researchers.
- Participates at the leadership level in professional, volunteer organizations.

Qualifications
- Certified by AOTCB as an OTR or COTA.
- Progressive levels of expertise will require combinations of the following: self-study, continuing education, experience, and formal education for independent research or scholarly activities.
- COTAs can contribute to the research process. COTAs need additional academic qualifications to be a principal investigator.

Supervision

Supervision ranges from close to minimal, depending on the nature of the project and the skills of the researcher/scholar.

ENTREPRENEUR

Major Function

Entrepreneurs are partially or fully self-employed individuals who provide occupational therapy services.

Scope of Role

Entrepreneurs may function in a variety of roles, including independent contractor and private practice owner or operator. The form of organization may be sole proprietorship, partnership, corporation, group practice, or joint venture.

Key Performance Areas

Entry-level skills
- Delivers quality occupational therapy services within scope of endeavor.
- Develops and implements business plan designed to ensure viability using financial and legal consultation.
- Establishes a business organization appropriate to nature and scope of activities.
- Negotiates contractual relationships that take into account the setting, services, and reimbursement.
- Uses legal, financial, and practice consultation as needed to support business operations.
- Establishes and collects fees for service, complying with reimbursement requirements.
- Manages business support services.
- Complies with local, state, and federal laws and regulations related to business and practice.

- Complies with standards and guidelines of accrediting or regulating organizations.
- Develops and maintains personnel policies and records.
- Develops and implements marketing strategies, as appropriate.
- Evaluates consumer satisfaction and business operations.
- Develops and implements risk management plan that includes business property, liability, and employee or employer benefits.
- Functions according to the AOTA *Code of Ethics* (AOTA, 1988) and *Standards of Practice* (AOTA, 1992) of the profession, as well as business ethics.

Intermediate skills
- Participates in, supervises, or oversees fieldwork program.
- Participates at a leadership level in professional, community organizations.

Qualifications

- Certified by AOTCB as an OTR or COTA.
- Meets appropriate state regulatory requirements.
- A minimum of 3 years of practice experience.

Supervision

In cases in which a COTA provides direct service, it is the COTA's responsibility to obtain the appropriate level of supervision from an OTR. Expert consultation or mentorship is obtained as needed to support the business, legal, financial, regulatory, and practice aspects of role performance.

REFERENCES

American Occupational Therapy Association. (1981). Guide for supervision of occupational therapy personnel. *American Journal of Occupational Therapy, 35*, 815–816.

American Occupational Therapy Association. (1988). Occupational therapy code of ethics. *American Journal of Occupational Therapy, 42*, 795–796.

American Occupational Therapy Association. (1990). Entry-level role delineation for registered occupational therapists (OTRs) and certified occupational therapy assistants (COTAs). *American Journal of Occupational Therapy, 44*, 1091–1102.

American Occupational Therapy Association. (1992). Standards of practice for occupational therapy. *American Journal of Occupational Therapy, 46*, 1082–1085.

RELATED BACKGROUND MATERIALS

American Occupational Therapy Association. (1991). Essentials and guidelines for an accredited educational program for the occupational therapist. *American Journal of Occupational Therapy, 45*, 1077–1084.

American Occupational Therapy Association. (1991). Essentials and guidelines for an accredited education program for the occupational therapy assistant. *American Journal of Occupational Therapy, 45*, 1085–1092.

American Occupational Therapy Association. (in press). Guide to supervision of occupational therapy personnel. (1988). In *Reference manual of official documents of The American Occupational Therapy Association, Inc.* Rockville, MD: Author. (Original work published 1981, *American Journal of Occupational Therapy, 35*, 815–816.)

Beeler, J. L., Young, P. A., & Dull, S. M. (1990). Professional development framework: Pathway to the future. *Journal of Nursing Staff Development, 6,* 296–301.

Mitchell, M. M. (1985). Professional development: Clinician to academician. *American Journal of Occupational Therapy, 39,* 368–373.

APPENDIX

The need for a broader description of career options for occupational therapy was identified as part of the Entry-Level Study Report (AOTA, 1987) presented to the Representative Assembly (RA). The RA charged the Executive Board to study the recommendation of the Entry-Level Report and develop an action plan. The Executive Board formed a Directions for the Future (DFF) Coordinating Committee and charged that committee to develop an overall action plan. Part of the action plan was the implementation of a DFF Symposium to examine the future needs of practice and education.

Following the symposium, the DFF Coordinating Committee directed the Commission on Education (COE) and Commission on Practice (COP) to form a combined task force of members to develop a document describing a hierarchy of occupational therapy roles. The chairpersons of both commissions selected representatives from a wide variety of arenas in both practice and education. The task force included individuals directly involved in both professional and technical levels of education and practice. Special Interest Section Steering Committee (SISSC) representation was added to the task force to further broaden the scope of the task force. Reference to current professional literature provided a foundation for committee work. The most important references are listed at the end of this section.

Throughout the entire document development process, the document was reviewed by the members of the full COE, COP, COTA Task Force, and SISSC, as well as program directors for professional and technical curricula, thus ensuring both OTR and COTA perspectives. One preliminary review of this document was followed by two formal reviews of drafts. The commission chairpersons recommended that the task force report be sent to the Intercommission Council (ICC) to further ensure that all facets of the Association were represented in the document development process.

As a result of the task force and review processes, an integrated education and practice taxonomy was recommended by the task force rather than a hierarchy. The taxonomy was preferred because it would provide practical information for a variety of uses within the profession. Since this taxonomy is a classification of categories of professional roles, it was decided to entitle the document Occupational Therapy Roles.

An ad hoc task force representing the Commission on Education Steering Committee (COESC), the Commission on Practice (COP), and the Special Interest Sections Steering Committee (SISSC) met in 1991 to 1992 and developed this draft, entitled *Occupational Therapy Roles.* This document is expected to replace and expand on the *Guide to Classification of Occupational Therapy Personnel* (AOTA, 1987).

REFERENCE

American Occupational Therapy Association. (1987). Guide to classification of occupational therapy personnel. In *Reference manual of official documents of The American Occupational Therapy Association, Inc.* Rockville, MD: Author. (Original work published 1985, *American Journal of Occupational Therapy, 39,* 803–810.)

Prepared by the Occupational Therapy Roles Task Force: Patricia A. Crist, PhD, OTR, FAOTA, Chairperson; Julie A. Halom, OTR; Jim Hinojosa, PhD, OTR, FAOTA; Scott McPhee, DrPH, OTR/L, FAOTA; Marlys M. Mitchell, PhD, OTR/L, FAOTA; Barbara A. Boyt Schell, MS, OTR/L, FAOTA; Mary Jane Youngstrom, MS, OTR; Carolyn Harsh, ScD, OTR/L, Staff Liaison; Sarah D. Hertfelder, MEd, MOT, OTR, Staff Liaison; for the Intercommission Council, Catherine Nielson, MPH, OTR/L, Chairperson.

Approved by the Representative Assembly June 1993.

This document replaces the following documents rescinded by the Representative Assembly in June of 1993:

American Occupational Therapy Association (1987). Guide to classification of occupational therapy personnel. In *Reference manual of official documents of The American Occupational Therapy Association, Inc.* Rockville, MD: Author. (Original work published 1985, *American Journal of Occupational Therapy, 39,* 803–810.)

American Occupational Therapy Association. (1990). Supervision guidelines for certified occupational therapy assistants. *American Journal of Occupational Therapy, 44,* 1089–1090.

Guide for Supervision of Occupational Therapy Personnel

The intent of this document is to clarify the supervisory relationships and responsibilities between registered occupational therapists (OTRs), certified occupational therapy assistants (COTAs), and other personnel involved in the provision of occupational therapy services. Supervision is a process in which two or more people participate in a joint effort to promote, establish, maintain, and/or elevate a level of performance and service. Supervision is a mutual undertaking between the supervisor and the supervisee that fosters growth and development; assures appropriate utilization of training and potential; encourages creativity and innovation; and provides guidance, support, encouragement, and respect while working toward a goal. As described here, supervision helps promote quality occupational therapy and fosters professional development of the individuals involved.

The American Occupational Therapy Association (AOTA) holds and maintains the principle that those persons not trained and qualified as occupational therapy practitioners (*occupational therapy practitioners* refers to both registered occupational therapists and certified occupational therapy assistants) are not acceptable to supervise occupational therapy practice. It is recognized that occupational therapy practitioners may be administratively supervised by others, such as principals, facility administrators, or physicians. During the supervision of occupational therapy practice, it is the supervisor who is responsible for setting, encouraging, and evaluating the standard of work performed by the supervisee. The amount of supervision required varies, depending upon the occupational therapy practitioner's clinical experience, responsibilities, and level of expertise. Supervision occurs along a continuum that includes close, routine, general, and minimal.

- *Close supervision* requires daily, direct contact at the site of work.
- *Routine supervision* requires direct contact at least every 2 weeks at the site of work, with interim supervision occurring by other methods, such as telephonic or written communication.
- *General supervision* requires at least monthly direct contact, with supervision available as needed by other methods.

- *Minimal supervision* is provided only on a need basis, and may be less than monthly. (AOTA, 1993a, p. 1088)

The amount, degree, and pattern of supervision a practitioner requires varies depending on the employment setting, method of service provision, the practitioner's competence, and the demands of service (i.e., facility standards, state laws and regulations, diagnoses served, techniques used). The method of supervision is determined by the supervising registered occupational therapist. The method should be the one most suitable to the situation. Methods of supervision should be determined before the individual enters into a supervisor–supervisee relationship and should be reevaluated regularly for effectiveness. In all cases, it is the occupational therapy practitioner's ethical responsibility to ensure that the amount, degree, and pattern of supervision are consistent with the level of role performance. As changes in the practice situation occur, the intensity of required supervision may also change to reflect new demands.

The registered occupational therapist has the ultimate responsibility for service provision. By virtue of their education and training, registered occupational therapists are able to provide services independently. Nevertheless, AOTA recommends that entry-level registered occupational therapists receive close supervision and that intermediate-level registered occupational therapists receive routine or general supervision. Certified occupational therapy assistants at all levels require at least general supervision by a registered occupational therapist. The level of supervision is related to the ability of the certified occupational therapy assistant to safely and effectively provide those interventions delegated by a registered occupational therapist. Typically, entry-level certified occupational therapy assistants and certified occupational therapy assistants new to a particular practice environment will require close supervision, intermediate level practitioners routine supervision, and advanced-level practitioners general supervision. When occupational therapy aides are delegated selected, routine tasks in specific situations, they must work under the close supervision of an occupational therapy practitioner.

These supervision guidelines are to assist occupational therapy practitioners in the provision of occupational therapy services (see Appendix). The guidelines themselves cannot be interpreted to constitute a standard of supervision in any particular locality; rather, they indicate ideal patterns and types of supervision. All practitioners are expected to meet state and federal regulatory mandates, adhere to relevant Association policies regarding supervision standards, and participate in continuing professional development.

From *American Journal of Occupational Therapy, 48,* 1045–1046. Copyright © 1994, American Occupational Therapy Association, Inc. Reprinted with Permission.

Appendix

Occupational Therapy Personnel	Supervision	Supervises:
Entry-level OTR*	Not required. Close supervision by an intermediate-level or an advanced-level OTR recommended.	Occupational therapy aides, technicians, care extenders, all levels of COTAs, volunteers, Level I fieldwork students.
Intermediate-level OTR*	Not required. Routine or general supervision by an advanced-level OTR recommended.	Occupational therapy aides, technicians, care extenders, all levels of COTAs, volunteers, Level I and II fieldwork students, entry-level OTRs.
Advanced-level OTR*	Not required. Minimal supervision by an advanced-level OTR is recommended.	Occupational therapy aides, technicians, care extenders, all levels of COTAs, volunteers, Level I and II fieldwork students, entry-level and intermediate-level OTRs.
Entry-level COTA*	Close supervision by all levels of OTRs, or an intermediate or an advanced-level COTA, who is under the supervision of an OTR.	Occupational therapy aides, technicians, care extenders, volunteers.
Intermediate-level COTA*	Routine or general supervision by all levels of OTRs, or an advanced-level COTA, who is under the supervision of an OTR.	Occupational therapy aides, technicians, care extenders, entry-level COTAs, volunteers, Level I occupational therapy (OT) fieldwork students, Level I and II occupational therapy assistant (OTA) fieldwork students.
Advanced-level COTA*,**	General supervision by all levels of OTRs, or an advanced-level COTA, who is under the supervision of an OTR.	Occupational therapy aides, technicians, care extenders, entry-level and intermediate-level COTAs, volunteers, Level I OT fieldwork students, Level I and II OTA fieldwork students.
Personnel other than occupational therapy practitioners assisting in occupational therapy intervention***	Close supervision by all levels of occupational therapy practitioners.	No supervisory capacity.

*Refer to the Occupational Therapy Roles document for descriptions of entry-level, intermediate-level, and advanced-level OTRs and COTAs (AOTA, 1993a).

**Although specific state regulations may dictate the parameters of certified occupational therapy assistant practice, the American Occupational Therapy Association supports the autonomous practice of the advanced certified occupational therapy assistant practitioner in the independent living setting (AOTA, 1993b, p. 1079).

***Students are not addressed in this category. The study role as a supervisor is addressed in the Essentials and Guidelines of an Accredited Educational Program for the Occupational Therapist and Essentials and Guidelines of an Accredited Program for the Occupational Therapy Assistant (AOTA, 1991a, 1991b).

REFERENCES

American Occupational Therapy Association (1991a). Essentials and guidelines of an accredited educational program for the occupational therapist. *American Journal of Occupational Therapy, 45,* 1077–1084.

American Occupational Therapy Association (1991b). Essentials and guidelines of an accredited educational program for the occupa-tional therapy assistant. *American Journal of Occupational Therapy, 45,* 1085–1092.

American Occupational Therapy Association (1993a). Occupational therapy roles. *American Journal of Occupational Therapy, 47,* 1087–1099.

American Occupational Therapy Association (1993b). Statement: The role of occupational therapy in the independent living movement. *American Journal of Occupational Therapy, 47,* 1079–1080.

Prepared by the Commission on Practice (Jim Hinojosa, PHD, OTR, FAOTA, Chairperson).

Approved by the Representative Assembly March 1981, edited July 1988.

Revised in 1994 and adopted by the Representative Assembly, July 1994.

This replaces the 1981 document "Guide for Supervision of Occupational Therapy Personnel" (*American Journal of Occupational Therapy, 35,* 815–816), which was rescinded by the 1994 Representative Assembly.

Appendix E

Standards of Practice for Occupational Therapy

PREFACE

These standards are intended as recommended guidelines to assist occupational therapy practitioners in the provision of occupational therapy services. These standards serve as a minimum standard for occupational therapy practice and are applicable to all individual populations and the programs in which these individuals are served.

These standards apply to those registered occupational therapists and certified occupational therapy assistants who are in compliance with regulation where it exists. The term *occupational therapy practitioner* refers to the registered occupational therapist and to the certified occupational therapy assistant, both of whom are in compliance with regulation where it exists.

The minimum educational requirements for the registered occupational therapist are described in the current *Essentials and Guidelines of an Accredited Educational Program for the Occupational Therapist* (American Occupational Therapy Association [AOTA], 1991a). The minimum educational requirements for the certified occupational therapy assistant are described in the current *Essentials and Guidelines of an Accredited Educational Program for the Occupational Therapy Assistant* (AOTA, 1991b).

STANDARD I: PROFESSIONAL STANDING

1. An occupational therapy practitioner shall maintain a current license, registration, or certification as required by law.
2. An occupational therapy practitioner shall practice and manage occupational therapy programs in accordance with applicable federal and state laws and regulations.
3. An occupational therapy practitioner shall be familiar with and abide by AOTA's (1994) *Occupational Therapy Code of Ethics.*
4. An occupational therapy practitioner shall maintain and update professional knowledge, skills, and abilities through appropriate continuing education or in-service training or higher education. The nature and minimum amount of continuing education must be consistent with state law and regulation.
5. A certified occupational therapy assistant must receive super-

From *American Journal of Occupational Therapy, 48,* 1039–1043. Copyright © 1994, American Occupational Therapy Association, Inc. Reprinted with Permission.

vision from a registered occupational therapist as defined by official AOTA documents. The nature and amount of supervision must be provided in accordance with state law and regulation.
6. An occupational therapy practitioner shall provide direct and indirect services in accordance with AOTA's standards and policies. The nature and scope of occupational therapy services provided must be in accordance with state law and regulation.
7. An occupational therapy practitioner shall maintain current knowledge of the legislative, political, social, and cultural issues that affect the profession.

STANDARD II: REFERRAL

1. A registered occupational therapist shall accept referrals in accordance with AOTA's *Statement of Occupational Therapy Referral* (AOTA, 1994) and in compliance with appropriate laws.
2. A registered occupational therapist may accept referrals for assessment or assessment with intervention in performance areas, performance components, or performance contexts when individuals have or appear to have dysfunctions or potential for dysfunctions.
3. A registered occupational therapist, responding to requests for service, may accept cases within the parameters of the law.
4. A registered occupational therapist shall assume responsibility for determining the appropriateness of the scope, frequency, and duration of services within the parameters of the law.
5. A registered occupational therapist shall refer individuals to other appropriate resources when the therapist determines that the knowledge and expertise of other professionals is indicated.
6. An occupational therapy practitioner shall educate current and potential referral sources about the process of initiating occupational therapy referrals.

STANDARD III: SCREENING

1. A registered occupational therapist, in accordance with state and federal guidelines, shall conduct screening to determine whether intervention or further assessment is necessary and to identify dysfunctions in performance areas.
2. A registered occupational therapist shall screen indepen-

dently or as a member of an interdisciplinary team. A certified occupational therapy assistant may contribute to the screening process under the supervision of a registered occupational therapist.

3. A registered occupational therapist shall select screening methods that are appropriate to the individual's age and developmental level; gender; education; cultural background; and socioeconomic, medical, and functional status. Screening methods may include, but are not limited to, interviews, structured observations, informal testing, and record reviews.

4. A registered occupational therapist shall communicate screening results and recommendations to appropriate individuals.

STANDARD IV: ASSESSMENT

1. A registered occupational therapist shall assess an individual's performance areas, performance components, and performance contexts. A registered occupational therapist conducts assessments individually or as part of a team of professionals, as appropriate to the practice settings and the purposes of the assessments. A certified occupational therapy assistant may contribute to the assessment process under the supervision of a registered occupational therapist.

2. An occupational therapy practitioner shall educate the individual, or the individual's family or legal guardian, as appropriate, about the purposes and procedures of the occupational therapy assessment.

3. A registered occupational therapist shall select assessments to determine the individual's functional abilities and problems as related to performance areas, performance components, and performance contexts.

4. Occupational therapy assessment methods shall be appropriate to the individual's age and developmental level; gender; education; socioeconomic, cultural, and ethnic background; medical status; and functional abilities. The assessment methods may include some combination of skilled observation, interview, record review, or the use of standardized or criterion-referenced tests. A certified occupational therapy assistant may contribute to the assessment process under the supervision of a registered occupational therapist.

5. An occupational therapy practitioner shall follow accepted protocols when standardized tests are used. Standardized tests are tests whose scores are based on accompanying normative data that may reflect age ranges, gender, ethnic groups, geographic regions, and socioeconomic status. If standardized tests are not available or appropriate, the results shall be expressed in descriptive reports, and standardized scales shall not be used.

6. A registered occupational therapist shall analyze and summarize collected evaluation data to indicate the individual's current functional status.

7. A registered occupational therapist shall document assessment results in the individual's records, noting the specific evaluation methods and tools used.

8. A registered occupational therapist shall complete and document results of occupational therapy assessments within the time frames established by practice settings, government agencies, accreditation programs, and third-party payers.

9. An occupational therapy practitioner shall communicate assessment results, within the boundaries of client confidentiality, to the appropriate persons.

10. A registered occupational therapist shall refer the individual to the appropriate services or request additional consultations if the results of the assessments indicate areas that require intervention by other professionals.

STANDARD V: INTERVENTION PLAN

1. A registered occupational therapist shall develop and document an intervention plan based on analysis of the occupational therapy assessment data and the individual's expected outcome after the intervention. A certified occupational therapy assistant may contribute to the intervention plan under the supervision of a registered occupational therapist.

2. The occupational therapy intervention plan shall be stated in goals that are clear, measurable, behavioral, functional, and appropriate to the individual's needs, personal goals, and expected outcome after intervention.

3. The occupational therapy intervention plan shall reflect the philosophical base of occupational therapy (AOTA, 1979) and be consistent with its established principles and concepts of theory and practice. The intervention planning processes shall include
   (a) formulating a list of strengths and weaknesses
   (b) estimating rehabilitation potential
   (c) identifying measurable short-term and long-term goals
   (d) collaborating with the individual, family members, other caregivers, professionals, and community resources
   (e) selecting the media, methods, environment, and personnel needed to accomplish the intervention goals
   (f) determining the frequency and duration of occupational therapy services
   (g) identifying a plan for reevaluation
   (h) discharge planning.

4. A registered occupational therapist shall prepare and document the intervention plan within the time frames and according to the standards established by the employing practice settings, government agencies, accreditation programs, and third-party payers. The certified occupational therapy assistant may contribute to the formation of the intervention plan under the supervision of the registered occupational therapist.

STANDARD VI: INTERVENTION

1. An occupational therapy practitioner shall implement a program according to the developed intervention plan. The plan shall be appropriate to the individual's age and developmental level, gender, education, cultural and ethnic background, health status, functional ability, interests and personal goals, and service provision setting. The certified occupational therapy assistant shall implement the intervention under the supervision of a registered occupational therapist.

2. An occupational therapy practitioner shall implement the intervention plan through the use of specified purposeful activities or therapeutic methods to enhance occupational performance and achieve stated goals.

3. An occupational therapy practitioner shall be knowledgeable

about relevant research in the practitioner's areas of practice. A registered occupational therapist shall interpret research findings as appropriate for application to the intervention process.

4. An occupational therapy practitioner shall educate the individual, the individual's family or legal guardian, non–certified occupational therapy personnel, and non–occupational therapy staff, as appropriate, in activities that support the established intervention plan. An occupational therapy practitioner shall communicate the risk and benefit of the intervention.

5. An occupational therapy practitioner shall maintain current information on community resources relevant to the practice area of the practitioner.

6. A registered occupational therapist shall periodically reassess and document the individual's levels of functioning and changes in levels of functioning in the performance areas, performance components, and performance contexts. A certified occupational therapy assistant may contribute to the reassessment process under the supervision of a registered occupational therapist.

7. A registered occupational therapist shall formulate and implement program modifications consistent with changes in the individual's response to the intervention. A certified occupational therapy assistant may contribute to program modifications under the supervision of a registered occupational therapist.

8. An occupational therapy practitioner shall document the occupational therapy services provided, including the frequency and duration of the services within the time frames and according to the standards established by the employing facility, government agencies, accreditation programs, and third-party payers.

STANDARD VII: TRANSITION SERVICES

1. The occupational therapy practitioner shall provide community-referenced services, as necessary, to identify occupational performance needs related to transition. Transition involves outcome-oriented actions which are coordinated to prepare or facilitate an individual for change, such as from one functional level to another, from one life stage to another, from one program to another, or from one environment to another.

2. The occupational therapy practitioner shall participate, when appropriate, in preparing a formal individualized transition plan based on the individual's needs and shall assist in the fulfillment of life roles (e.g., independent or community living, self-care, care for others, work, play, and leisure) through activities in such a plan.

3. The occupational therapy practitioner shall facilitate the transition process in cooperation with the individual and the multidisciplinary team or other community support systems (including family members), when appropriate. The registered occupational therapist shall initiate referrals to appropriate community agencies to provide needed services (e.g., direct service, consultation, monitoring).

4. The occupational therapy practitioner shall determine the effectiveness of transition programs and the extent to which individuals have achieved desired transition outcomes (e.g.,

degree to which the individual is integrated and successful in community living and work environments). This is done in conjunction with the individual and other team members, where appropriate.

STANDARD VIII: DISCONTINUATION

1. A registered occupational therapist shall discontinue service when the individual has achieved predetermined goals or has achieved maximum benefit from occupational therapy services.

2. A registered occupational therapist, with input from a certified occupational therapy assistant where applicable, shall prepare and implement a discharge plan that is consistent with occupational therapy goals, individual goals, interdisciplinary team goals, family goals, and expected outcomes. The discharge plan shall address appropriate community resources for referral for psychosocial, cultural, and socioeconomic barriers and limitations that may need modification.

3. A registered occupational therapist shall document the changes between the initial and current states of functional ability and deficit in performance areas, performance components, and performance contexts. A certified occupational therapy assistant may contribute to the process under the supervision of a registered occupational therapist.

4. An occupational therapy practitioner shall allow sufficient time for the coordination and effective implementation of the discharge plan.

5. A registered occupational therapist shall document recommendations for follow-up or reevaluation when applicable.

STANDARD IX: CONTINUOUS QUALITY IMPROVEMENT

1. An occupational therapy practitioner shall monitor and document the continuous quality improvement of practice, which may include outcomes of services, using predetermined practice criteria reflecting professional consensus, recent developments in research, and specific employing facility standards.

2. An occupational therapy practitioner shall monitor all aspects of individual occupational therapy services for effectiveness and timeliness. If actual care does not meet the prescribed standard, it must be justified by peer review or other appropriate means within the practice setting. Occupational therapy services shall be discontinued when no longer necessary.

3. A registered occupational therapist shall systematically assess the review process of patient care to determine the success or appropriateness of interventions. Certified occupational therapy assistants may contribute to the process in collaboration with the registered occupational therapist.

STANDARD X: MANAGEMENT

1. A registered occupational therapist shall provide the management necessary for efficient organization and provision of occupational therapy services.

2. A certified occupational therapy assistant, under the supervi-

sion of a registered occupational therapist, may perform the following management functions:

(a) education of members of other related professions and physicians about occupational therapy

(b) participation in (1) orientation, supervision, training, and evaluation of the performance of volunteers and other non–certified occupational therapy personnel, and (2) developing plans to remediate areas of skill deficit in the performance of job duties by volunteers and other non–certified occupational therapy personnel

(c) design and periodic review of all aspects of the occupational therapy program to determine its effectiveness, efficiency, and future directions

(d) systematic review of the quality of service provided, using criteria established by professional consensus and current research, as well as established standards for state regulation; accreditation; American Occupational Therapy Certification Board (AOTCB) certification; and related laws, policies, guidelines, and regulations

(e) incorporation of a fair and equitable system of admission, discharge, and charges for occupational therapy services

(f) participation in cross-disciplinary activities to ensure that the total needs of the individual are met

(g) provision of support (i.e., space, time, money as feasible)

for clinical research or collaborative research when such projects have the approval of the appropriate governing bodies (e.g., institutional review board), and the results of which are deemed potentially beneficial to individuals of occupational therapy services now or in the future.

REFERENCES

American Occupational Therapy Association. (1979). The philosophical base of occupational therapy. *American Journal of Occupational Therapy, 33,* 785.

American Occupational Therapy Association. (1991a). Essentials and guidelines of an accredited educational program for the occupational therapist. *American Journal of Occupational Therapy, 45,* 1077–1084.

American Occupational Therapy Association. (1991b). Essentials and guidelines of an accredited educational program for the occupational therapy assistant. *American Journal of Occupational Therapy, 45,* 1085–1092.

American Occupational Therapy Association (1994). Occupational therapy code of ethics. *American Journal of Occupational Therapy, 48,* 1037–1038.

American Occupational Therapy Association (1994). Statement of occupational therapy referral. *American Journal of Occupational Therapy, 48,* 1034.

Prepared by the Commission on Practice (Jim Hinojosa, PHD, OTR, FAOTA, Chairperson).

Adopted by the Representative Assembly July 1994.

This document replaces the 1992 Standards of Practice for Occupational Therapy (*American Journal of Occupational Therapy, 46,* 1082–1085) and the 1987 Standards of Practice for Occupational Therapy in Schools (*American Journal of Occupational Therapy, 41,* 804–808), which were rescinded by the 1994 Representative Assembly.

Appendix F

Uniform Terminology for Occupational Therapy—Third Edition

This is an official document of The American Occupational Therapy Association (AOTA). This document is intended to provide a generic outline of the domain of concern of occupational therapy and is designed to create common terminology for the profession and to capture the essence of occupational therapy succinctly for others.

It is recognized that the phenomena that constitute the profession's domain of concern can be categorized, and labeled, in a number of different ways. This document is not meant to limit those in the field, formulating theories or frames of reference, who may wish to combine or refine particular constructs. It is also not meant to limit those who would like to conceptualize the profession's domain of concern in a different manner.

INTRODUCTION

The first edition of Uniform Terminology was approved and published in 1979 (AOTA, 1979). In 1989, *Uniform Terminology for Occupational Therapy—Second Edition* (AOTA, 1989) was approved and published. The second document presented an organized structure for understanding the areas of practice for the profession of occupational therapy. The document outlined two domains. *Performance areas* (activities of daily living [ADL], work and productive activities, and play or leisure) include activities that the occupational therapy practitioner emphasizes when determining functional abilities (*occupational therapy practitioner* refers to both registered occupational therapists and certified occupational therapy assistants). *Performance components* (sensorimotor, cognitive, psychosocial, and psychological aspects) are the elements of performance that occupational therapists assess and, when needed, in which they intervene for improved performance.

This third edition has been further expanded to reflect current practice and to incorporate contextual aspects of performance. *Performance areas, performance components,* and *performance contexts* are the parameters of occupational therapy's domain of concern. *Performance areas* are broad categories of human activity that are typically part of daily life. They are activities of daily living, work and productive activities, and play or leisure activities. *Performance components* are fundamental human abilities that—to varying degrees and in differing combinations—are required for successful engagement in performance areas. These

components are sensorimotor, cognitive, psychosocial, and psychological. *Performance contexts* are situations or factors that influence an individual's engagement in desired and/or required performance areas. Performance contexts consist of *temporal* aspects (chronological age, developmental age, place in the life cycle, and health status) and *environmental* aspects (physical, social, and cultural considerations). There is an interactive relationship among performance areas, performance components, and performance contexts. Function in performance areas is the ultimate concern of occupational therapy, with performance components considered as they relate to participation in performance areas. Performance areas and performance components are always viewed within performance contexts. Performance contexts are taken into consideration when determining function and dysfunction relative to performance areas and performance components, and in planning intervention. For example, the occupational therapist does not evaluate strength (a performance component) in isolation. Strength is considered as it affects necessary or desired tasks (performance areas). If the individual is interested in homemaking, the occupational therapy practitioner would consider the interaction of strength with homemaking tasks. Strengthening could be addressed through kitchen activities, such as cooking and putting groceries away. In some cases, the practitioner would employ an adaptive approach and recommend that the family switch from heavy stoneware to lighter-weight dishes, or use lighter-weight pots on the stove to enable the individual to make dinner safely without becoming fatigued or compromising safety.

Occupational therapy assessment involves examining performance areas, performance components, and performance contexts. Intervention may be directed toward elements of performance areas (e.g., dressing, vocational exploration), performance components (e.g., endurance, problem solving), or the environment aspects of performance contexts. In the latter case, the physical and/or social environment may be altered or augmented to improve and/or maintain function. After identifying the performance areas the individual wishes or needs to address, the occupational therapist assesses the features of the environments in which the tasks will be performed. If an individual's job requires cooking in a restaurant as opposed to leisure cooking at home, the occupational therapy practitioner faces several challenges to enable the individual's success in different environments. Therefore, the third critical aspect of performance is the performance context, the features of the environment that affect the person's ability to engage in functional activities.

This document categorizes specific activities in each of the performance areas (ADL, work and productive activities, play or leisure). This categorization is based on what is considered "typical," and is not meant to imply that a particular individual characterizes personal activities in the same manner as someone else. Occupational therapy practitioners embrace individual differences, and so would document the unique pattern of the individual being served, rather than forcing the "typical" pattern on him or her and family. For example, because of experience or culture, a particular individual might think of home management as an ADL task rather than "work and productive activities" (current listing). Socialization might be considered part of a play or leisure activity instead of its current listing as part of "activities of daily living," because of life experience or cultural heritage.

EXAMPLES OF USE IN PRACTICE

Uniform Terminology—Third Edition defines occupational therapy's domain of concern, which includes performance areas, performance components, and performance contexts. While this document may be used by occupational therapy practitioners in a number of different areas (e.g., practice, documentation, charge systems, education, program development, marketing, research, disability classifications, and regulations), it focuses on the use of uniform terminology in practice. This document is not intended to define specific occupational therapy programs or specific occupational therapy interventions. Examples of how performance areas, performance components, and performance contexts translate into practice are provided below.

- An individual who is injured on the job may have the potential to return to work and productive activities, which is a performance area. In order to achieve the outcome of returning to work and productive activities, the individual may need to address specific performance components, such as strength, endurance, soft tissue integrity, time management, and the physical features of performance contexts, like structures and objects in his or her environment. The occupational therapy practitioner, in collaboration with the individual and other members of the vocational team, uses planned interventions to achieve the desired outcome. These interventions may include activities such as an exercise program, body mechanics instruction, and job site modifications, all of which may be provided in a work-hardening program.
- An elderly individual recovering from a cerebrovascular accident may wish to live in a community setting, which combines the performance areas of ADL with work and productive activities. In order to achieve the outcome of community living, the individual may need to address specific performance components, such as muscle tone, gross motor coordination, postural control, and self-management. It is also necessary to consider the sociocultural and physical features of performance contexts, such as support available from other persons, and adaptations of structures and objects within the environment. The occupational therapy practitioner, in cooperation with the team, utilizes planned interventions to achieve the desired outcome. Interventions may include neuromuscular facilitation, practice of object manipulation, and instruction in the use of adaptive equipment and home safety equipment. The practitioner and in-

dividual also pursue the selection and training of a personal assistant to ensure the completion of ADL tasks. These interventions may be provided in a comprehensive inpatient rehabilitation unit.

- A child with learning disabilities is required to perform educational activities within a public school setting. Engaging in educational activities is considered the performance area of work and productive activities for this child. To achieve the educational outcome of efficient and effective completion of written classroom work, the child may need to address specific performance components. These include sensory processing, perceptual skills, postural control, motor skills, and the physical features of performance contexts, such as objects (e.g., desk, chair) in the environment. In cooperation with the team, occupational therapy interventions may include activities like adapting the student's seating in the classroom to improve postural control and stability, and practicing motor control and coordination. This program could be developed by an occupational therapist and supported by school district personnel.
- The parents of an infant with cerebral palsy may ask to facilitate the child's involvement in the performance areas of activities of daily living and play. Subsequent to assessment, the therapist identifies specific performance components, such as sensory awareness and neuromuscular control. The practitioner also addresses the physical and cultural features of performance contexts. In collaboration with the parents, occupational therapy interventions may include activities such as seating and positioning for play, neuromuscular facilitation techniques to enable eating, facilitating parent skills in caring for and playing with their infant, and modifying the play space for accessibility. These interventions may be provided in a home-based occupational therapy program.
- An adult with schizophrenia may need and want to live independently in the community, which represents the performance areas of activities of daily living, work and productive activities, and leisure activities. The specific performance categories may be medication routine, functional mobility, home management, vocational exploration, play or leisure performance, and social interaction. In order to achieve the outcome of living independently, the individual may need to address specific performance components, such as topographical orientation; memory; categorization; problem solving; interests; social conduct; time management; and sociocultural features of performance contexts, such as social factors (e.g., influence of family and friends) and roles. The occupational therapy practitioner, in cooperation with the team, utilizes planned interventions to achieve the desired outcome. Interventions may include activities such as training in the use of public transportation, instruction in budgeting skills, selection and participation in social activities, instruction in social conduct, and participation in community reintegration activities. These interventions may be provided in a community-based mental health program.
- An individual with a history of substance abuse may need to reestablish family roles and responsibilities, which represent the performance areas of activities of daily living, work and productive activities, and leisure activities. In order to achieve the outcome of family participation, the individual may need to address the performance components of roles;

values; social conduct; self-expression; coping skills; self-control; and the sociocultural features of performance contexts, such as custom, behavior, rules, and rituals. The occupational therapy practitioner, in cooperation with the team, utilizes planned interventions to achieve the desired outcomes. Interventions may include roles and values exercises, instruction in stress management techniques, identification of family roles and activities, and support to develop family leisure routines. These interventions may be provided in an inpatient acute care unit.

PERSON–ACTIVITY–ENVIRONMENT FIT

Person–activity–environment fit refers to the match among the skills and abilities of the individual; the demands of the activity; and the characteristics of the physical, social, and cultural environments. It is the interaction among the performance areas, performance components, and performance contexts that is important and determines the success of the performance. When occupational therapy practitioners provide services, they attend to all of these aspects of performance and the interaction among them. They also attend to each individual's unique personal history. The personal history includes one's skills and abilities (performance components), the past performance of specific life tasks (performance areas), and experience within particular environments (performance contexts). In addition to personal history, anticipated life tasks and role demands influence performance.

When considering the person–activity–environment fit, variables such as novelty, importance, motivation, activity tolerance, and quality are salient. Situations range from those that are completely familiar to those that are novel and have never been experienced. Both the novelty and familiarity within a situation contribute to the overall task performance. In each situation, there is an optimal level of novelty that engages the individual sufficiently and provides enough information to perform the task. When too little novelty is present, the individual may miss cues and opportunities to perform. When too much novelty is present, the individual may become confused and distracted, inhibiting effective task performance.

Humans determine that some stimuli and situations are more meaningful than others. Individuals perform tasks they deem important. It is critical to identify what the individual wants or needs to do when planning interventions.

The level of motivation an individual demonstrates to perform a particular task is determined by both internal and external factors. An individual's biobehavioral state (e.g., amount of rest, arousal, tension) contributes to the potential to be responsive. The features of the social and physical environments (e.g., persons in the room, noise level) provide information that is either adequate or inadequate to produce a motivated state.

Activity tolerance is the individual's ability to sustain a purposeful activity over time. Individuals must not only select, initiate and terminate activities, but they must also attend to a task for the needed length of time to complete the task and accomplish their goals.

The quality of performance is measured by standards generated by both the individual and others in the social and cultural environments in which the performance occurs. Quality is a continuum of expectations set within particular activities and contexts (Fig. 1).

UNIFORM TERMINOLOGY FOR OCCUPATIONAL THERAPY— THIRD EDITION

Occupational therapy is the use of purposeful activity or interventions to promote health and achieve functional outcomes. *Achieving functional outcomes* means to develop, improve, or restore the highest possible level of independence of any individual who is limited by a physical injury or illness, a dysfunctional condition, a cognitive impairment, a psychosocial dysfunction, a mental illness, a developmental or learning disability, or an adverse environmental condition. *Assessment* means the use of skilled observation or evaluation by the administration and interpretation of standardized or nonstandardized tests and measurements to identify areas for occupational therapy services.

Occupational therapy services include, but are not limited to

1. the assessment, treatment, and education of or consultation with the individual, family, or other persons; or
2. interventions directed toward developing, improving, or restoring daily living skills, work readiness or work performance, play skills or leisure capacities, or enhancing educational performance skills; or
3. providing for the development, improvement, or restoration of sensorimotor, oral-motor, perceptual or neuromuscular functioning; or emotional, motivational, cognitive, or psychosocial components of performance.

These services may require assessment of the need for and use of interventions such as the design, development, adaptation, application, or training in the use of assistive technology devices; the design, fabrication, or application of rehabilitative technology such as selected orthotic devices; training in the use of assistive technology, orthotic or prosthetic devices; the application of physical agent modalities as an adjunct to or in preparation for purposeful activity; the use of ergonomic principles; the adaptation of environments and processes to enhance functional performance; or the promotion of health and wellness (AOTA, 1993, p. 1117).

I. Performance Areas
Throughout this document, activities have been described as if individuals performed the tasks themselves. Occupational therapy also recognizes that individuals arrange for tasks to be done through others. The profession views independence as the ability to self-determine activity performance, regardless of who actually performs the activity.

A. *Activities of Daily Living*—Self-maintenance tasks.
  1. *Grooming*—Obtaining and using supplies; removing body hair (use of razors, tweezers, lotions, etc.); applying and removing cosmetics; washing, drying, combing, styling, and brushing hair; caring for nails (hands and feet), caring for skin, ears, and eyes; and applying deodorant.
  2. *Oral Hygiene*—Obtaining and using supplies; cleaning mouth; brushing and flossing teeth; or removing, cleaning, and reinserting dental orthotics and prosthetics.
  3. *Bathing/Showering*—Obtaining and using supplies; soaping, rinsing, and drying body parts; maintaining bathing position; and transferring to and from bathing positions.

I. Performance Areas	II. Performance Components	III. Performance Context

A. Activities of Daily Living
  1. Grooming
  2. Oral Hygiene
  3. Bathing/Showering
  4. Toilet Hygiene
  5. Personal Device Care
  6. Dressing
  7. Feeding and Eating
  8. Medication Routine
  9. Health Maintenance
  10. Socialization
  11. Functional Communication
  12. Functional Mobility
  13. Community Mobility
  14. Emergency Response
  15. Sexual Expression
B. Work and Productive Activities
  1. Home Management
    a. Clothing Care
    b. Cleaning
    c. Meal Preparation Cleanup
    d. Shopping
    e. Money Management
    f. Household Maintenance
    g. Safety Procedures
  2. Care of Others
  3. Educational Activities
  4. Vocational Activities
    a. Vocational Exploration
    b. Job Acquisition
    c. Work or Job Performance
    d. Retirement Planning
    e. Volunteer Participation
C. Play or Leisure Activities
  1. Play or Leisure Exploration
  2. Play or Leisure Performance
	A. Sensorimotor Component
	  1. Sensory
	    a. Sensory Awareness
	    b. Sensory Processing
	      (1) Tactile
	      (2) Proprioceptive
	      (3) Vestibular
	      (4) Visual
	      (5) Auditory
	      (6) Gustatory
	      (12) Olfactory
	    c. Perceptual Processing
	      (1) Stereognosis
	      (2) Kinesthesia
	      (3) Pain Response
	      (4) Body Scheme
	      (5) Right–Left Discrimination
	      (6) Form Constancy
	      (7) Position in Space
	      (8) Visual-Closure
	      (9) Figure Ground
	      (10) Depth Perception
	      (11) Spatial Relations
	      (12) Topographical Orientation
	  2. Neuromusculoskeletal
	    a. Reflex
	    b. Range of Motion
	    c. Muscle Tone
	    d. Strength
	    e. Endurance
	    f. Postural Control
	    g. Postural Alignment
	    h. Soft Tissue Integrity
	  3. Motor
	    a. Gross Coordination
	    b. Crossing the Midline
	    c. Laterality
	    d. Bilateral Integration
	    e. Motor Control
	    f. Praxis
	    g. Fine Coordination/Dexterity
	    h. Visual-Motor Integration
	    i. Oral-Motor Control
	B. Cognititive Integration and Cognitive Components
	  1. Level of Arousal
	  2. Orientation
	  3. Recognition
	  4. Attention Span
	  5. Initiation of Activity
	  6. Termination of Activity
	  7. Memory
	  8. Sequencing
	  9. Categorization
	  10. Concept Formation
	  11. Spatial Operations
	  12. Problem Solving
	  13. Learning
	  14. Generalization
	C. Psychosocial Skills and Psychological Components
	  1. Psychological
	    a. Values
	    b. Interests
	    c. Self-Concept
	  2. Social
	    a. Role Performance
	    b. Social Conduct
	    c. Interpersonal Skills
	    d. Self-Expression
	  3. Self-Management
	    a. Coping Skills
	    b. Time Management
	    c. Self-Control
		A. Temporal Aspects
		  1. Chronological
		  2. Developmental
		  3. Life Cycle
		  4. Disability Status
		B. Environment
		  1. Physical
		  2. Social
		  3. Cultural

▲

Figure 1. Uniform Terminology for Occupational Therapy—Third Edition outline.

4. *Toilet Hygiene*—Obtaining and using supplies; clothing management; maintaining toileting position; transferring to and from toileting position; cleaning body; and caring for menstrual and continence needs (including catheters, colostomies, and suppository management).

5. *Personal Device Care*—Cleaning and maintaining personal care items, such as hearing aids, contact lenses, glasses, orthotics, prosthetics, adaptive equipment, and contraceptive and sexual devices.

6. *Dressing*—Selecting clothing and accessories appropriate to time of day, weather, and occasion; obtaining clothing from storage area; dressing and undressing in a sequential fashion; fastening and adjusting clothing and shoes; and applying and removing personal devices, prostheses, or orthoses.

7. *Feeding and Eating*—Setting up food; selecting and using appropriate utensils and tableware; bringing food or drink to mouth; cleaning face, hands, and clothing; sucking, masticating, coughing, and swallowing; and management of alternative methods of nourishment.

8. *Medication Routine*—Obtaining medication, opening and closing containers, following prescribed schedules, taking correct quantities, reporting problems and adverse effects, and administering correct quantities by using prescribed methods.

9. *Health Maintenance*—Developing and maintaining routines for illness prevention and wellness promotion, such as physical fitness, nutrition, and decreasing health risk behaviors.

10. *Socialization*—Accessing opportunities and interacting with other people in appropriate contextual and cultural ways to meet emotional and physical needs.

11. *Functional Communication*—Using equipment or systems to send and receive information, such as writing equipment, telephones, typewriters, computers, communication boards, call lights, emergency systems, Braille writers, telecommunication devices for the deaf, and augmentative communication systems.

12. *Functional Mobility*—Moving from one position or place to another, such as in-bed mobility, wheelchair mobility, transfers (wheelchair, bed, car, tub, toilet, tub/shower, chair, floor). Performing functional ambulation and transporting objects.

13. *Community Mobility*—Moving self in the community and using public or private transportation, such as driving, or accessing buses, taxi cabs, or other public transportation systems.

14. *Emergency Response*—Recognizing sudden, unexpected hazardous situations, and initiating action to reduce the threat to health and safety.

15. *Sexual Expression*—Engaging in desired sexual and intimate activities.

B. *Work and Productive Activities*—Purposeful activities for self-development, social contribution, and livelihood.
1. *Home Management*—Obtaining and maintaining personal and household possessions and environment.
   a. *Clothing Care*—Obtaining and using supplies; sorting; laundering (hand, machine, and dry clean); folding; ironing; storing; and mending.
   b. *Cleaning*—Obtaining and using supplies; picking up; putting away; vacuuming; sweeping and mopping floors; dusting; polishing; scrubbing; washing windows; cleaning mirrors; making beds; and removing trash and recyclables.
   c. *Meal Preparation and Cleanup*—Planning nutritious meals; preparing and serving food; opening and closing containers, cabinets, and drawers; using kitchen utensils and appliances; cleaning up and storing food safely.
   d. *Shopping*—Preparing shopping lists (grocery and other); selecting and purchasing items; selecting method of payment; and completing money transactions.
   e. *Money Management*—Budgeting, paying bills, and using bank systems.
   f. *Household Maintenance*—Maintaining home, yard, garden, appliances, vehicles, and household items.
   g. *Safety Procedures*—Knowing and performing preventive and emergency procedures to maintain a safe environment and to prevent injuries.

2. *Care of Others*—Providing for children, spouse, parents, pets, or others, such as giving physical care, nurturing, communicating, and using age-appropriate activities.

3. *Educational Activities*—Participating in a learning environment through school, community, or work-sponsored activities, such as exploring educational interests, attending to instruction, managing assignments, and contributing to group experiences.

4. *Vocational Activities*—Participating in work-related activities.
   a. *Vocational Exploration*—Determining aptitudes; developing interests and skills, and selecting appropriate vocational pursuits.
   b. *Job Acquisition*—Identifying and selecting work opportunities, and completing application and interview processes.
   c. *Work or Job Performance*—Performing job tasks in a timely and effective manner; incorporating necessary work behaviors.
   d. *Retirement Planning*—Determining aptitudes; developing interests and skills; and selecting appropriate avocational pursuits.
   e. *Volunteer Participation*—Performing unpaid activities for the benefit of selected individuals, groups, or causes.

C. *Play or Leisure Activities*—Intrinsically motivating activities for amusement, relaxation, spontaneous enjoyment, or self-expression.
1. *Play or Leisure Exploration*—Identifying interests, skills, opportunities, and appropriate play or leisure activities.
2. *Play or Leisure Performance*—Planning and participating in play or leisure activities. Maintaining a balance of play or leisure activities with work and productive activities, and activities of daily living. Obtaining, utilizing, and maintaining equipment and supplies.

II. Performance Components

A. *Sensorimotor Component*—The ability to receive input, process information, and produce output.
1. *Sensory*
   a. *Sensory Awareness*—Receiving and differentiating sensory stimuli.
   b. *Sensory Processing*—Interpreting sensory stimuli:

(1) *Tactile*—Interpreting light touch, pressure, temperature, pain, and vibration through skin contact/receptors.

(2) *Proprioceptive*—Interpreting stimuli originating in muscles, joints, and other internal tissues that give information about the position of one body part in relation to another.

(3) *Vestibular*—Interpreting stimuli from the inner ear receptors regarding head position and movement.

(4) *Visual*—Interpreting stimuli through the eyes, including peripheral vision and acuity, and awareness of color and pattern.

(5) *Auditory*—Interpreting and localizing sounds, and discriminating background sounds.

(6) *Gustatory*—Interpreting tastes.

(7) *Olfactory*—Interpreting odors.

c. *Perceptual Processing*—Organizing sensory input into meaningful patterns.

(1) *Stereognosis*—Identifying objects through proprioception, cognition, and the sense of touch.

(2) *Kinesthesia*—Identifying the excursion and direction of joint movement.

(3) *Pain Response*—Interpreting noxious stimuli.

(4) *Body Scheme*—Acquiring an internal awareness of the body and the relationship of body parts to each other.

(5) *Right–Left Discrimination*—Differentiating one side from the other

(6) *Form Constancy*—Recognizing forms and objects as the same in various environments, positions, and sizes.

(7) *Position in Space*—Determining the spatial relationship of figures and objects to self or other forms and objects.

(8) *Visual-Closure*—Identifying forms or objects from incomplete presentations.

(9) *Figure Ground*—Differentiating between foreground and background forms and objects.

(10) *Depth Perception*—Determining the relative distance between objects, figures, or landmarks and the observer, and changes in planes of surfaces.

(11) *Spatial Relations*—Determining the position of objects relative to each other.

(12) *Topographical Orientation*—Determining the location of objects and settings and the route to the location.

2. *Neuromusculoskeletal*

a. *Reflex*—Eliciting an involuntary muscle response by sensory input.

b. *Range of Motion*—Moving body parts through an arc.

c. *Muscle Tone*—Demonstrating a degree of tension or resistance in a muscle at rest and in response to stretch.

d. *Strength*—Demonstrating a degree of muscle power when movement is resisted, as with objects or gravity.

e. *Endurance*—Sustaining cardiac, pulmonary, and musculoskeletal exertion over time.

f. *Postural Control*—Using righting and equilibrium adjustments to maintain balance during functional movements.

g. *Postural Alignment*—Maintaining biomechanical integrity among body parts.

h. *Soft Tissue Integrity*—Maintaining anatomical and physiological condition of interstitial tissue and skin.

3. *Motor*

a. *Gross Coordination*—Using large muscle groups for controlled, goal-directed movements.

b. *Crossing the Midline*—Moving limbs and eyes across the midsagittal plane of the body.

c. *Laterality*—Using a preferred unilateral body part for activities requiring a high level of skill.

d. *Bilateral Integration*—Coordinating both body sides during activity.

e. *Motor Control*—Using the body in functional and versatile movement patterns.

f. *Praxis*—Conceiving and planning a new motor act in response to an environmental demand.

g. *Fine Coordination/Dexterity*—Using small muscle groups for controlled movements, particularly in object manipulation.

h. *Visual-Motor Integration*—Coordinating the interaction of information from the eyes with body movement during activity.

i. *Oral-Motor Control*—Coordinating oropharyngeal musculature for controlled movements.

B. *Cognitive Integration and Cognitive Components*—The ability to use higher brain functions.

1. *Level of Arousal*—Demonstrating alertness and responsiveness to environmental stimuli.

2. *Orientation*—Identifying person, place, time, and situation.

3. *Recognition*—Identifying familiar faces, objects, and other previously presented materials.

4. *Attention Span*—Focusing on a task over time.

5. *Initiation of Activity*—Starting a physical or mental activity.

6. *Termination of Activity*—Stopping an activity at an appropriate time.

7. *Memory*—Recalling information after brief or long periods of time.

8. *Sequencing*—Placing information, concepts, and actions in order.

9. *Categorization*—Identifying similarities of and differences among pieces of environmental information.

10. *Concept Formation*—Organizing a variety of information to form thoughts and ideas.

11. *Spatial Operations*—Mentally manipulating the position of objects in various relationships.

12. *Problem Solving*—Recognizing a problem, defining a problem, identifying alternative plans, selecting a plan, organizing steps in a plan, implementing a plan, and evaluating the outcome.

13. *Learning*—Acquiring new concepts and behaviors.

14. *Generalization*—Applying previously learned concepts and behaviors to a variety of new situations.

C. *Psychosocial Skills and Psychological Components*—The ability to interact in society and to process emotions.

1. *Psychological*

a. *Values*—Identifying ideas or beliefs that are important to self and others.

b. *Interests*—Identifying mental or physical activities that create pleasure and maintain attention.

c. *Self-Concept*—Developing the value of the physical, emotional, and sexual self.

2. *Social*
   a. *Role Performance*—Identifying, maintaining, and balancing functions one assumes or acquires in society (e.g., worker, student, parent, friend, religious participant).
   b. *Social Conduct*—Interacting by using manners, personal space, eye contact, gestures, active listening, and self-expression appropriate to one's environment.
   c. *Interpersonal Skills*—Using verbal and nonverbal communication to interact in a variety of settings.
   d. *Self-Expression*—Using a variety of styles and skills to express thoughts, feelings, and needs.

3. *Self-Management*
   a. *Coping Skills*—Identifying and managing stress and related factors.
   b. *Time Management*—Planning and participating in a balance of self-care, work, leisure, and rest activities to promote satisfaction and health.
   c. *Self-Control*—Modifying one's own behavior in response to environmental needs, demands, constraints, personal aspirations, and feedback from others.

III. Performance Contexts

Assessment of function in performance areas is greatly influenced by the contexts in which the individual must perform. Occupational therapy practitioners consider performance contexts when determining feasibility and appropriateness of interventions. Occupational therapy practitioners may choose interventions based on an understanding of contexts, or may choose interventions directly aimed at altering the contexts to improve performance.

A. *Temporal Aspects*
   1. *Chronological*—Individual's age.
   2. *Developmental*—Stage or phase of maturation.
   3. *Life cycle*—Place in important life phases, such as career cycle, parenting cycle, or educational process.
   4. *Disability status*—Place in continuum of disability, such as acuteness of injury, chronicity of disability, or terminal nature of illness.

B. *Environment*
   1. *Physical*—Nonhuman aspects of contexts. Includes the accessibility to and performance within environments having natural terrain, plants, animals, building, furniture, objects, tools, or devices.
   2. *Social*—Availability and expectations of significant individuals, such as spouse, friends, and caregivers. Also includes larger social groups which are influential in establishing norms, role expectations, and social routines.
   3. *Cultural*—Customs, beliefs, activity patterns, behavior standards, and expectations accepted by the society of which the individual is a member. Includes political aspects, such as laws that affect access to resources and affirm personal rights. Also includes opportunities for education, employment, and economic support.

REFERENCES

American Occupational Therapy Association. (1979). *Occupational therapy product output reporting system and uniform terminology for reporting occupational therapy services.* Rockville, MD: Author.

American Occupational Therapy Association. (1989). Uniform terminology for occupational therapy—Second edition. *American Journal of Occupational Therapy, 43,* 808–815.

American Occupational Therapy Association. (1993). Association policies—Definition of occupational therapy practice for state regulation (Policy 5.3.1). *American Journal of Occupational Therapy, 47,* 1117–1121.

Prepared by The Terminology Task Force: Winifred Dunn, PhD, OTR, FAOTA, Chairperson; Mary Foto, OTR, FAOTA; Jim Hinojosa, PhD, OTR, FAOTA; Barbara Schell, PhD, OTR/L, FAOTA; Linda Kohlman Thomson, MOT, OTR, FAOTA; Sarah D. Hertfelder, MEd, MOT, OTR/L.—Staff Liaison, for The Commission on Practice (Jim Hinojosa, PhD, OTR, FAOTA, Chairperson).

Adopted by the Representative Assembly July 1994.

This document replaces the following documents, all of which were rescinded by the 1994 Representative Assembly: *Occupational Therapy Product Output Reporting System* (1979), *Uniform Terminology for Reporting Occupational Therapy Services—First Edition* (1979), "Uniform Occupational Therapy Evaluation Checklist" (1981, *American Journal of Occupational Therapy, 35,* 817–818), and "Uniform Terminology for Occupational Therapy—Second Edition" (1989, *American Journal of Occupational Therapy, 43,* 808–815).

Elements of Clinical Documentation (Revision)

These elements are provided to assist occupational therapy practitioners to document occupational therapy services. Occupational therapy practitioners determine the appropriate type of documentation and document the services provided within the time frames established by facilities, government agencies, and accreditation organizations. These elements do not address the specific content of documentation which is unique to occupational therapy intervention for particular ages and types of impairments.

The purpose of documentation is to:

1. Provide a chronological record of the consumer's condition which details the complete course of therapeutic intervention.
2. Facilitate communication among professionals who contribute to the consumer's care.
3. Provide an objective basis to determine the appropriateness, effectiveness, and necessity of therapeutic intervention.
4. Reflect the practitioner's reasoning.

TYPES OF DOCUMENTATION

I. Evaluation Report
   A. Identification and Background Information
   B. Assessment Results
   C. Intervention or Treatment Plan
II. Contact, Treatment, or Visit Note
III. Progress Report
IV. Re-evaluation Report
V. Discharge or Discontinuation Report

I. Evaluation Report

Used to document the initial contact with the consumer, the data collected, the interpretation of the data, and the intervention plan. When an abbreviated evaluation process is used, such as screening, it is documented using only limited content areas applicable to the consumer and situation.

A. Identification and Background Information (see Table G-1)
B. Assessment Results (see Table G-2)
C. Intervention or Treatment Plan (see Table G-3)

Table G-1 Identification and Background Information

Content	Clarification
1. Name, age, sex, date of admission, treatment diagnosis, and date of onset of current diagnosis	Name may be omitted, depending on facility and department policies and procedures.
2. Referral source, services requested, and date of referral to occupational therapy	Who requested occupational therapy services, what specific services were requested, and date services were requested.
3. Medical history and secondary problems or preexisting conditions, prior therapy	Additional problems or conditions that may affect consumer function or outcomes.
4. Precautions and contraindications	May be identified by referral source or occupational therapy practitioners.
5. Pertinent history that indicates prior levels of function and support systems	Applicable developmental, educational, vocational, cultural, and socioeconomic history.
6. Present levels of function in performance areas determined by examination[a]	Brief description of the consumer's level of performance in activities of daily living, work and productive activities, and play or leisure activities.
7. Performance contexts determined by examination[a]	Description of those temporal aspects (chronological, developmental, life cycle, health status) and environmental (physical, social, cultural) features that affect the consumer's function in performance areas.
8. Consumer and family expectations	Brief description of expected outcome of occupational therapy intervention.

[a]Refer to *Uniform Terminology for Occupational Therapy, Third Edition* (AOTA, 1994a), for specific performance areas, performance components, and performance contexts.

Table G-2 Assessment Results

Content	Clarification
1. Tests and assessments administered and the results	Name and type of assessment or test and the results; may include comparison with previous testing. State if standardized procedure not followed.
2. References to other pertinent reports and information	Any additional sources of data or assessments results used.
3. Summary and analysis of evaluation findings	State the type and severity of impairments identified and the functional limitations caused by the impairments in objective, functional, and measurable terms. Include the functional diagnosis.
4. Projected functional outcome(s)	Prognosis and anticipated level of performance (activities of daily living [ADL], work or productive activities, and play or leisure activities) the consumer will be able to achieve as a result of therapeutic intervention. May include a statement indicating the consumer does not have the potential to improve beyond current status.

Table G-3 Intervention or Treatment Plan

Content	Clarification
1. Long-term functional goals	Functional limitations that must change in order to achieve the projected functional outcome.
	Degree the functional limitations will be decreased.
	Rationale for decreasing functional limitations.
	Functional change to occur by end of intervention.
	Consumer and/or family agreement with goals.
2. Short-term goals	Directly relate to long-term functional goals.
	Impairment that must change in order to achieve the projected functional outcome.
	Degree the impairment will be decreased.
	Functional ability that will result from a decrease in level of impairment.
	Change to occur in a brief period of time (e.g., 7, 14, or 30 days).
	Consumer and/or family agreement with goals.
3. Intervention or treatment procedures	Activities, techniques, and modalities selected to be used and how they relate to goals. May include family training and home programs.
	Identify assistive/adaptive equipment, orthotics, and/or prosthetics to meet consumer's environmental adaptation needs.
4. Type, amount, frequency, and duration of intervention or treatment	State skill and performance areas to be addressed and estimate the number, duration, and frequency of sessions to accomplish goals.
5. Recommendations	Need for OT services and necessary referrals to other professionals.

Table G-4 Contact, Treatment, or Visit Note

Content	Clarification
1. Attendance and participation	Therapy occurrence or reason for therapy not occurring as scheduled. May be indicated by checklist or brief statement.
2. Activities, techniques, and modalities used	
3. Assistive/adaptive equipment, prosthetics, and orthotics if issued or fabricated, and specific instructions for the application and/or use of the item	State the device; note whether it was fabricated, sold, rented, or loaned; and state the effectiveness of the device.
4. Consumer's response to therapy	Level of performance and anything unusual or significant that was a result of occupational therapy intervention.

Table G-5 Progress Report

Content	Clarification
1. Activities, techniques, and modalities used	Brief statement of intervention process.
2. Consumer's response to therapy, and the progress toward short- and long-term goal attainment and comparison with previous functional status	State the consumer's physical and behavioral response to therapy, whether the goals are being achieved, if change has occurred, and how much change has occurred.
3. Goal continuance	Explanation for no or slow progress, reason for not meeting short-term goal(s), or need to continue current goal(s).
4. Goal modification when indicated by the response to therapy or by the establishment of new consumer needs	State new goals and rationale for changes or additions.
5. Change in anticipated time to achieve goals	If, for any reason, the therapy time frame is altered, include the reason for the change and the new anticipated time frame.
6. Assistive/adaptive equipment, prosthetics, and orthotics, if issued or fabricated, and specific instructions for the application and/or use of the item	State the device; note whether it was fabricated, sold, rented, or loaned; and state the effectiveness of the device.
7. Consumer-related conferences and communication	If occupational therapy practitioners participated in a conference or made a pertinent contact with a family member, agency, or health care professional, state this information with a brief summary of the conference or communication.
8. Home programs	Include a copy of the home program as established with the consumer. Include a statement regarding the consumer's ability to follow the program.
9. Consumer/caretaker instruction	What instruction was provided and in what format (i.e., verbal or written).
10. Plan	Specific procedures, communication, or consultations to be done in the future to address the goals.

II. Contact, Treatment, or Visit Note

Used to document individual occupational therapy session or care coordination. May be very brief, such as in the use of a checklist, flow chart, or short narrative-type notation (see Table G-4).

III. Progress Report

Used periodically to document care coordination, interventions, progress toward functional goals, and to update goals and intervention or treatment plan (see Table G-5).

IV. Re-evaluation Report

Used to document sessions in which portions of the evaluation process are repeated or readministered. Usually occurs monthly or quarterly, depending on the setting (see Table G-6).

V. Discharge or Discontinuation Report

Used to document a summary of the course of therapy and any recommendations (see Table G-7).

Table G-6 Re-evaluation Report

Content	Clarification
1. Tests and assessments readministered and the results	Name and type of test readministered. State if standardized procedure is not followed.
2. Comparative summary and analysis of previous evaluation findings	Results analyzed and compared with previous testing.
3. Reestablishment of projected functional outcome(s)	Anticipated level of performance (ADL, work or productive activities, and play or leisure activities) the consumer will be able to achieve as a result of therapeutic intervention. May include a statement of changes in previously established functional outcome(s) based on revised potential or goals or consumer.
4. Update of intervention or treatment plan	Revised or continued long-term functional goals; short-term goals; treatment procedures; and type, amount, and frequency of therapy.

Table G-7 Discharge or Discontinuation Report

Content	Clarification
1. Therapy process	Summary of interventions used, consumer's responses, and number of sessions.
2. Goal attainment	Degree to which short- and long-term functional goals were achieved.
3. Functional outcome	Comparison of functional status prior to therapy and at discharge.
4. Home programs	Include the actual written home program that is to be followed after discharge.
5. Follow-up plans	State the schedule and specific plans.
6. Recommendations	State any recommendations pertaining to the consumer's future needs.
7. Referral(s) to other health care providers and community agencies	Indicate referral(s) or recommendations for referral(s) when additional or new services are needed.

FUNDAMENTAL ELEMENTS OF DOCUMENTATION

Each consumer of occupational therapy services must have a case record maintained as a permanent file. The record should be organized, legible, concise, clear, accurate, complete, current, and objective. Correct grammar and spelling should be used.

The following 10 elements should be present:

1. Consumer's full name and case number on each page of documentation.
2. Date stated as month, day, and year for each entry; time of intervention; and length of session.
3. Identification of type of documentation and department name.
4. Practitioner's signature with a minimum of first name or initial, last name, and professional designation.
5. Signature of the recorder directly at the end of the note without space left between the body of the note and the signature.
6. Countersignature by a registered occupational therapist (OTR) on documentation written by students and certified occupational therapy assistants (COTA) when required by law or the facility.
7. Compliance with confidentiality standards.
8. Acceptable terminology as defined by the facility.
9. Facility-approved abbreviations.
10. Errors corrected by drawing a single line through an error, and the correction initialed (liquid correction fluid and erasures are not acceptable), or facility requirements followed.

Prepared by Linda Kohlman Thomson, OT, OTR, OT(C), Mary Foto, OTR, FAOTA, for The Commission on Practice (Jim Hinojosa, PhD, OTR, FAOTA, Chairperson).

Approved by the Representative Assembly April 1986.

Revised 1994 and sent to the Representative Assembly FYI.

This document replaces the 1986 Guidelines for Occupational Therapy Documentation. (*American Journal of Occupational Therapy, 40,* 830–832).

Note. If a document is revised, the previous version is superseded and, according to Parliamentary procedure, is automatically rescinded.

REFERENCES

American Occupational Therapy Association. (1994a). Uniform terminology for occupational therapy—Third edition. *American Journal of Occupational Therapy, 48,* 1047–1054.

American Occupational Therapy Association. (1994b). Uniform terminology—Third edition: Application to practice. *American Journal of Occupational Therapy, 48,* 1055–1059.

BIBLIOGRAPHY

Allen, C. K., Earhart, C. A., & Blue, T. (1992). *Occupational therapy treatment goals for the physically and cognitively disabled.* Bethesda, MD: American Occupational Therapy Association.

Allen, C., Foto, M., Moon-Sperling, T., & Wilson, D. (Eds.). (December 1989). A medical review approach to medicare outpatient documentation. *American Journal of Occupational Therapy, 43,* 793–800.

American Occupational Therapy Association. (1989). Reports that work. *AOTA self study series: Assessing function* (Chapter 9). Bethesda, MD: Author.

American Occupational Therapy Association. (1992). *Effective documentation for occupational therapy.* Bethesda, MD: Author.

American Occupational Therapy Association. (1994). Standards of practice for occupational therapy. *American Journal of Occupational Therapy, 48,* 1039–1043.

Hopkins, H. L., & Smith, H. D. (1993). *Willard and Spackman's occupational therapy* (8th ed.). Philadelphia: Lippincott.

Stewart, D. L., & Abeln, S. H. (Eds.). (1993). *Documenting functional outcomes in physical therapy.* St. Louis: Mosby.

Sample Print Resources
for Person–Task–Environment
Transaction Enhancement

Michele Ciofalo

PRINT RESOURCES AVAILABLE FROM:

American Association of Retired Persons (AARP)
601 E. Street, N.W.
Washington, DC 20049
(The Do Able Renewable Home: Making Your Home Fit Your
    Needs (DI2470)

Association for Retarded Citizens (ARC)
500 E. Border Street, Suite 300
Arlington, TX 76010

Barrier-Free Design Centre
2075 Bayview Ave.
Toronto, Ontario M4N 3M5
Canada

Clearinghouse on Disability Information
Office of Special Education and Rehabilitative Services
U.S. Department of Education
Room 3132, Switzer Bldg.
Washington, DC 20202-2524

Council for Exceptional Children
1920 Association Drive
Reston, VA 22091

In Door Sports Club, Inc.
1145 Highland Street
Napoleon, OH 43545

Mental Health Law Project
2021 L Street N.W., Suite 800
Washington, DC 20036

National Information Center for Children and Youth with
    Disabilities
PO Box 1492
Washington, DC 20013

National Organization on Disability
910 16th Street N.W., Suite 600
Washington, DC 20006

The Association of Persons with Severe Handicaps (TASH)
29 West Susquehanna Ave.
Baltimore, MD 21204

The Research and Training Center for Accessible Housing
North Carolina State University School of Design
Box 8613
Raleigh, ND 27695-8613

Appendix I

Sample Toll-Free and Telephone Resources for Person–Task–Environment Transaction Enhancement

Ronald G. Stone and Michele Ciofalo

SAMPLE RESOURCE ORGANIZATIONS

(800) 555-1212	Toll-Free Directory number (for updates or numbers not listed)
(800) 344-2666	Al-Anon Family Group Headquarters, Inc.
(800) 621-0379	Alzheimer's Disease Association
(800) 749-2257	American Association of Kidney Patients
(800) 424-3410	American Association of Retired Persons
(800) 548-2876	American Burn Association
(800) 424-8666	American Council of the Blind
(800) 232-3472	American Diabetes Association, Inc.
(800) 223-0179	The American Liver Foundation
(800) 729-2682	American Occupational Therapy Association
(800) 223-2732	American Parkinson Disease Association
(800) 556-7890	American Trauma Society
(800) 782-4747	Amyotrophic Lateral Sclerosis Association
(800) 727-8462	Asthma and Allergy Foundation of America
(800) 233-1222	AT&T National Special Needs Center
(800) 833-3232	(TDD)
(800) 669-7079	Blinded Veterans Association
(800) 955-0906	BRS Information Technologies
(800) 237-6213	Captioned Films/Video for the Deaf Program
(800) 726-9119	Center for Rehabilitation Technology
(800) 242-4453	Children's Hospice International
(800) 753-2357	Cornelia deLange Syndrome Foundation
(800) 344-4823	Cystic Fibrosis Foundation
(800) 535-3323	Deafness Research Foundation
(800) 222-3277	Dial A Hearing Screening Test
(800) 332-1000	Epilepsy Foundation of America
(800) 548-4337	Guide Dog Foundation for the Blind, Inc.
(800) 245-2691	HUD User
(800) 526-7234	Job Accommodation Network
(800) 558-0121	Lupus Foundation of America, Inc.
(800) 541-5454	Myasthenia Gravis Foundation
(800) 342-2437	National AIDS Hotline
(800) 344-7432	National AIDS Hotline (Spanish language)
(800) 458-5231	National AIDS Information Clearinghouse
(800) 243-0701	(TDD)
(800) 424-8666	National Alliance of Blind Students
(800) 331-5362	National Association for the Dually Diagnosed
(800) 221-4602	National Down Syndrome Society
(800) 662-4357	National Drug Treatment Referral & Information Hotline
(800) 221-6827	National Easter Seal Society
(800) 222-3937	National Foundation of the American Academy of Ophthalmology Public Service Programs
(800) 843-2256	National Headache Foundation
(800) 658-8898	National Hospice Organization
(800) 541-3259	National Lymphedema Network
(800) 969-6642	National Mental Health Association
(800) 323-7938	National Neurofibromatosis Foundation
(800) 999-6673	National Organization for Rare Disorders
(800) 346-2742	National Rehabilitation Information Center
(800) 221-3004	National Society to Prevent Blindness
(800) 962-9629	National Spinal Cord Injury Association
(800) 369-7433	North American Riding for the Handicapped Association
(800) 422-6237	Office of Cancer Communications
(800) 457-6676	Parkinson's Disease Foundation, Inc.
(800) 888-2876	Phoenix Society for Burn Survivors, Inc.
(800) 221-4792	Recording for the Blind and Dyslexic
(800) 421-8453	Sickle Cell Disease Association of America
(800) 772-1213	Social Security Administration
(800) 325-0778	(TDD)
(800) 872-5827	United Cerebral Palsy Associations, Inc.
(800) 728-5483	United Leukodystrophy Foundation
(800) 426-2547	Visiting Nurse Association of America

Note: Updated lists can be obtained from Jamal Mazrui, National Council on Disability, Email: 74444.1076@compuserve.com.

SAMPLE NATIONAL CIVIL GROUPS

(317) 875-8755	Kiwanis International (focus on children)
(708) 571-5466	Lions International (focus on blind or visually-impaired)
(215) 988-1917	Masons/Shriners Lodge (may fund assistive devices)
(708) 859-2000	Moose Club (may fund initiatives for individuals with disabilities)

(816) 333-8300   Sertoma International (focus on speech/hearing impairments)

(816) 756-3390   Veterans of Foreign Wars (focus on veterans)

SAMPLE LISTINGS OF THE TOLL-FREE DIRECTORY OF DISABILITY SERVICES AND SUPPLIES

(800) 858-5116   Ability Access (Escondido, CA)

(800) 344-9301   Accessible Work Systems (Bellevue, OH)

(800) 748-3695   Adaptive Automotive (Denver, CO)

(800) 225-2610   Alimed (Dedham, MA)

(800) 325-6233   Alternative Unlimited Inc (Whitinsville, MA)

(800) 961-3273   EASE2000 Environmental Assessment and Prescription Software (New Brighton, MN)

(800) 323-6598   E-Z-On Product Inc (Jupiter, FL)

(800) 548-7905   Electric Mobility (Sewell, NJ)

(800) 841-8923   Environmental Health Science Inc (Princeton, NJ)

(800) 952-2248   Ford Mobility Motoring Program (Ruston, LA)

(800) 833-0312   (TDD)

(800) 548-4337   Guide Dog Foundation For The Blind (Smithtown, NY)

(800) 536-9383   Handicapped - Getaway Cruises (Saddle River, NJ)

(800) 622-0623   Independent Mobility Systems (Farmington, NM)

(800) 829-0500   Lighthouse Low Vision Products (Long Island City, NY)

(800) 443-4926   Maddak Inc (Wayne, NJ)

(800) 421-1221   National Accessible Apartment Clearinghouse (Washington, DC)

(800) 253-4391   Office Systems For Visually/Physically Impaired (Chicago, IL)

(800) 262-1984   Prentke Romich (Wooster, OH)

(800) 548-8531   Right Start Catalog (Westlake Village, CA)

(800) 448-8434   Salem Coach & Equip (Salem, VA)

(800) 323-5547   Sammons - Preston (Burr Ridge, IL)

(800) 422-7382   Wheelchair Getaway and See Go Van (Las Vegas, NV)

(800) 452-2085   Special Mobility Services (Portland, OR)

(800) 832-8697   Toys For Special Children (Hastings On Hudson, NY)

(800) 327-1911   Tub-Master (Orlando, FL)

(800) 531-1678   Visions Technology (Vero Beach, FL)

(800) 221-6501   Wheelchair Getaways (Lancaster, PA)

Appendix J

Sample Internet/Software Resources for Person–Task–Environment Transaction Enhancement

Ronald G. Stone and Michele Ciofalo

SAMPLE RESOURCE WEB SITES

http://trace.wisc.edu/tcel/abledata/index.html
ABLEDATA on the Internet

http://abe.www.ecn.purdue.edu/ABE/Extension/BNG/Index.html
Breaking New Ground
Adaptive technologies for farmers with disabilities

http://otpt.ups.edu/Rehabilitation/AdapTec.html
Adaptive Technology Links (OTPT Pages - University of Puget Sound)

http://janweb.icdi.wvu.edu/kinder
Americans with Disabilities Act Document Center

http://www2.apple.com/disability/welcome.html
Apple Computer's Disability Connection

http://bilbo.isu.edu/ota/ota/html
Archives of the Office of Technology Assessment
The Office of Technology Assessment closed in 1995, however, its archives are housed at Idaho State University.

http://www.asel.udel.edu/at-online/assistive.html
Assistive Technology On-Line

http://www.resna.org/resna/webres.htm
Assistive Technology Web Pages from RESNA

http://cosmos.ot.buffalo.edu/aztech.html
AZtech (A to Z Technology) www page

http://nz.com/webnz/ability/
Canterbury Community Internet Access Project (CCIA)

http://www.gsa.gov/coca/
CITA (Center for Information Technology Accommodation)

http://www.closingthegap.com/
Closing the Gap
Microcomputer technology for persons with special needs

http://www.eskimo.com/~jlubin/disabled/cmpyinfo.htm
Disability-related product information

http://codi.buffalo.edu/
Cornucopia of Disability Information (CODI)

http://weber.u.washington.edu/~doit/Brochures/internet_resources.html
DO-IT (Disabilities, Opportunities, Internetworking, and Technology).
Program for persons with disabilities to explore careers in science, engineering, and mathematics.

EASE2000 is a comprehensive software package for guiding home assessments that includes local and national database resources for prescribing environmental adaptations—individualized for each client. Information can be obtained from:
Lifease, Inc., Suite D, 2451 15th Street N.W., New Brighton, MN 55112

http://www.isc.rit.edu/~easi/
EASI Project (Equal Access to Software & Information)

gopher://sjuvm.stjohns.edu/II/disabled/
Electronic Rehabilitation Resources (St. John's University)

http://disability.com/
Evan Kemp Associates, Inc.
Comprehensive resource for disability and assistive technology information

http://www.ndepot.com/idi/
Independence Dogs, Inc. Service dogs for the mobility-impaired

http://www.eskimo.com/~jlubin/disabled.html
Jim Lubin's Disability Resource List
A comprehensive compendium of disability-related links

OT FACT uses dynamic question sets, generated from a computer software program, to compile and organize large quantities of patient evaluation data so that they can be meaningfully interpreted.

Smith R. O. (1992). *OT FACT software and operating manual.* Bethesda, MD: American Occupational Therapy Association.

http://otpt.ups.edu/
OTPT Pages - University of Puget Sound

http://www.resna.org/resna/reshome.htm
RESNA (rehabilitation engineering and assistive technology society of north america) RESNA is an interdisciplinary association for the advancement of rehabilitation and assistive technologies

http://www.psych.org
The American Psychiatric Association's site for information on public policy, resources, news, and links to other mental health web sites

http://www.databahn.net/connection/technability/index.htm
TechnAbility

http://www.trace.wisc.edu/
Trace Research and Development Center (University of WI, Madison)

http://www.yahoo.com/yahoo/Society_and_Culture/Disabilities/
Yahoo online index of disability web sites

http://www.tc.umn.edu/nlhome/g258/vitlink/heathl.html
Vast Spaces and Stone Walls: Overcoming Barriers to Postsecondary Education for Rural Students with Disabilities

Note: For an up-to-date version of this listing, go to:
http://otpt.ups.edu/Rehabilitation/Resources.html

INDEX